# THE HUMAN FRONTAL LOBES

# THE HUMAN FRONTAL LOBES

## Functions and Disorders

### SECOND EDITION

*Edited by*

## BRUCE L. MILLER
## JEFFREY L. CUMMINGS

*Series Editor's Note by Robert A. Bornstein*

**THE GUILFORD PRESS**
New York       London

© 2007 The Guilford Press
A Division of Guilford Publications, Inc.
72 Spring Street, New York, NY 10012
www.guilford.com

Printed in the United States of America

This book is printed on acid-free paper.

Last digit is print number:   9   8   7   6   5   4   3   2   1

**Library of Congress Cataloging-in-Publication Data**

The human frontal lobes : functions and disorders / edited by Bruce L. Miller, Jeffrey L. Cummings.—2nd ed.
    p. cm.—(The science and practice of neuropsychology)
    Includes bibliographical references and index.
    ISBN-10: 1-59385-329-7   ISBN-13: 978-1-59385-329-7 (hardcover)
    1. Frontal lobes—Physiology.   2. Frontal lobes—Pathophysiology.
3. Frontal lobes—Physiology.   4. Frontal lobes—Pathophysiology.
I. Miller, Bruce L., 1949–   .  II. Cummings, Jeffrey L., 1948–   .
III. Series.
    [DNLM: 1. Frontal Lobe—physiology.  2. Brain Diseases.  3. Mental
Disorders.    WL 307 H918 2007]
    QP382.F7H85 2007
    612.8′25—dc22
                                 2006002478

# About the Editors

**Bruce L. Miller, MD,** is Professor of Neurology at the University of California at San Francisco (UCSF), where he holds the A.W. & Mary Margaret Clausen Distinguished Chair. He is also the clinical director of the aging and dementia program at UCSF, where he heads the State of California Research and Clinical Center and a new National Alzheimer's Disease Research Center. For nearly two decades, Dr. Miller has been the scientific director of the John Douglas French Foundation for Alzheimer's Disease, for which he has organized conferences, scientific consortiums, and grant programs. He has been listed in *The Best Doctors in America* since 1996. Dr. Miller directs a National Institutes of Health–funded program on frontotemporal dementia (FTD) called "FTD: Genes, Images, and Emotions." He has published more than 250 articles.

**Jeffrey L. Cummings, MD,** is Director of the Alzheimer's Disease Research Center and the Deane F. Johnson Center for Neurotherapeutics at the University of California at Los Angeles (UCLA). He is the Augustus S. Rose Professor of Neurology and Professor of Psychiatry and Biobehavioral Sciences in the David Geffen School of Medicine at UCLA. Dr. Cummings is past president of the American Neuropsychiatric Society and the Behavioral Neurology Society. He is the recipient of several prestigious awards, including the Henderson Lectureship of the American Neurological Society. Dr. Cummings has lectured, pursued research, and produced a body of research-related publications on the topics of neuropsychiatry, behavioral neurology, neurotherapeutics, and drug development. He has contributed to the understanding of the role of the frontal–subcortical circuits in the behavior of normal individuals and of persons with brain disorders and is the author of the Neuropsychiatric Inventory, a tool used to assess behavioral changes in patients with neurological diseases.

# Contributors

**Judith Aharon-Peretz, MD**, Cognitive Neurology Unit, Rambam Health Care Campus, Haifa, Israel

**Serena Amici, MD**, Memory and Aging Center, Department of Neurology, University of California, San Francisco, California

**Michel Benoit, MD, PhD**, Centre Mémoire de Ressources et de Recherche, Centre Hospitalier Universitaire de Nice, Nice, France

**Antonello Bonci, MD, PhD**, Memory and Aging Center, Department of Neurology, University of California, San Francisco, California

**Adam L. Boxer, MD, PhD**, Memory and Aging Center, Department of Neurology, University of California, San Francisco, California

**Arne Brun, MD, PhD**, Department of Pathology, Lund University Hospital, Lund, Sweden

**Hervé Caci, MD, PhD**, Pédopsychiatre, Centre Hospitalier Universitaire de Nice, Nice, France

**Nigel J. Cairns, PhD**, Department of Neurology, Washington University in St. Louis, St. Louis, Missouri

**Danielle Andrea Carlin, BA**, Memory and Aging Center, Department of Neurology, University of California, San Francisco, California

**Tiffany W. Chow, MD**, Departments of Medicine (Neurology Division) and Psychiatry (Geriatric Psychiatry Division), University of Toronto, and Rotman Research Institute, Baycrest, Toronto, Ontario, Canada

**Helena Chui, MD**, Department of Neurology, Keck School of Medicine, University of Southern California, Los Angeles, California

**Julia A. Chung, MD**, Department of Psychiatry and Biobehavioral Science, Harbor–UCLA Medical Center, Torrance, California

**Jeffrey L. Cummings, MD**, Department of Neurology and Alzheimer's Disease Research Center, University of California, Los Angeles, California

**David Dean, BA**, Memory and Aging Center, Department of Neurology, University of California, San Francisco, California

**Mary G. DeMay, MD,** Memory and Aging Center, Department of Neurology, University of California, San Francisco, California

**Mark D'Esposito, MD,** Department of Psychology, University of California, Berkeley, California

**Bruno Dubois, MD,** Fédération de Neurologie, Hôpital de la Salpêtrière, Paris, France

**Laura B. Dunn, MD,** Department of Psychiatry, University of California, San Diego, La Jolla, California

**Denys Fontaine, MD,** Neurochirurgie, Centre Hospitalier Universitaire de Nice, Nice, France

**Adam Gazzaley, MD, PhD,** Departments of Neurology and Physiology, University of California, San Francisco, California, and Department of Neuroscience, University of California, Berkeley, California

**Daniel H. Geschwind, MD, PhD,** Departments of Neurology and Psychiatry and Biobehavioral Sciences, University of California, Los Angeles, California

**Michael D. Geschwind, MD, PhD,** Memory and Aging Center, Department of Neurology, University of California, San Francisco, California

**Jill Goldman, MA, MPhil,** Memory and Aging Center, Department of Neurology, University of California, San Francisco, California

**Maria Luisa Gorno-Tempini, MD, PhD,** Memory and Aging Center, Department of Neurology, University of California, San Francisco, California

**Cheryl L. Grady, PhD,** Department of Psychiatry, University of Toronto, and Rotman Research Institute, Baycrest, Toronto, Ontario, Canada

**Jordan Grafman, PhD,** Cognitive Neuroscience Section, National Institute of Neurological Disorders and Stroke, National Institutes of Health, Bethesda, Maryland

**Murray Grossman, MD,** Department of Neurology, University of Pennsylvania, Philadelphia, Pennsylvania

**Elizabeth Head, PhD,** Department of Neurology, University of California, Irvine, California

**Argye E. Hillis, MD,** Department of Neurology, Johns Hopkins School of Medicine, Baltimore, Maryland

**Marco Iacoboni, MD, PhD,** Departments of Neurology, Psychiatry and Biobehavioral Sciences, and Psychology, University of California, Los Angeles, California

**Harry J. Jerison, PhD,** Department of Psychiatry and Biobehavioral Sciences, University of California, Los Angeles, California

**Julene K. Johnson, PhD,** Memory and Aging Center, Department of Neurology, University of California, San Francisco, California

**Susan Jones, PhD,** Department of Physiology, Development and Neuroscience, University of Cambridge, Cambridge, United Kingdom

**Jason H. T. Karlawish, MD,** Division of Geriatric Medicine, Department of Medicine, University of Pennsylvania, Philadelphia, Pennsylvania

**Daniel I. Kaufer, MD,** Department of Neurology, University of North Carolina School of Medicine, Chapel Hill, North Carolina

**Joel H. Kramer, PsyD,** Memory and Aging Center, Department of Neurology, University of California, San Francisco, California

**Ae Young Lee, MD,** Department of Neurology, Chungnam National University School of Medicine, Taejon, Korea

**Virginia M.-Y. Lee, PhD,** Department of Pathology and Laboratory Medicine, University of Pennsylvania School of Medicine, Philadelphia, Pennsylvania

**Ira M. Lesser, MD,** Department of Psychiatry and Biobehavioral Science, Harbor-UCLA Medical Center, Torrance, California

**Brian Levine, PhD,** Department of Psychology, University of Toronto, and Rotman Research Institute, Baycrest, Toronto, Ontario, Canada

**Irene Litvan, MD,** Department of Neurology, University of Louisville School of Medicine, Louisville, Kentucky

**Vianney Mattei, MD,** Psychiatrie, Centre Hospitalier Universitaire de Nice, Nice, France

**Ian G. McKeith, MD,** School of Neurology, Neurobiology, and Psychiatry, University of Newcastle upon Tyne, and Wolfson Research Centre, Newcastle General Hospital, Newcastle upon Tyne, United Kingdom

**Margaret C. McKinnon, PhD,** Department of Psychology, University of Toronto, and Rotman Research Institute, Baycrest, Toronto, Ontario, Canada

**Bruce L. Miller, MD,** Memory and Aging Center, Department of Neurology, University of California, San Francisco, California

**Jennifer Ogar, MS,** Center for Aphasia and Related Disorders, VA Northern California Health Care System, Martinez, California

**Barton W. Palmer, PhD,** Department of Psychiatry, University of California, San Diego, La Jolla, California

**Danijela Pavlic, BS,** Memory and Aging Center, Department of Neurology, University of California, San Francisco, California

**William Perry, PhD,** Department of Psychiatry, University of California, San Diego, La Jolla, California

**Bernard Pillon, PhD,** Centre de Neuropsychologie, Fédération de Neurologie, Hôpital de la Salpêtrière, Paris, France

**Bruce H. Price, MD,** Department of Neurology, McLean Hospital, Harvard Medical School, Belmont, Massachusetts

**Lovingly Quitania, BA,** Memory and Aging Center, Department of Neurology, University of California, San Francisco, California

**Katherine P. Rankin, PhD,** Memory and Aging Center, Department of Neurology, University of California, San Francisco, California

**Scott L. Rauch, MD,** Department of Psychiatry, Massachusetts General Hospital, Harvard Medical School, Charlestown, Massachusetts

**Philippe H. Robert, MD,** Centre Mémoire de Ressources et de Recherche, Centre Hospitalier Universitaire de Nice, Nice, France

**Susan A. Legendre Ropacki, PhD,** Department of Psychology, Loma Linda University, Loma Linda, California

**Howard Rosen, MD,** Memory and Aging Center, Department of Neurology, University of California, San Francisco, California

**Carole Samango-Sprouse, EdD,** Department of Pediatrics, George Washington University, Washington, DC

**Douglas W. Scharre, MD,** Department of Neurology, Ohio State University, Columbus, Ohio

**William W. Seeley, MD,** Memory and Aging Center, Department of Neurology, University of California, San Francisco, California

**W. Dale Stevens, MSc,** Department of Psychology, Harvard University, Cambridge, Massachusetts

**Virginia E. Sturm, MD,** Department of Psychology, University of California, Berkeley, California

**Donald T. Stuss, PhD,** Departments of Medicine and Psychology, University of Toronto, and Rotman Research Institute, Baycrest, Toronto, Ontario, Canada

**Eva Svoboda, PhD,** Department of Psychology, University of Toronto, and Rotman Research Institute, Baycrest, Toronto, Ontario, Canada

**Rachel Tomer, PhD,** Department of Psychology, University of Haifa, Haifa, Israel

**John Q. Trojanowski, PhD,** Department of Pathology and Laboratory Medicine, University of Pennsylvania School of Medicine, Philadelphia, Pennsylvania

**Irene van Balkan, MD,** Department of Neurology, University of Louisville School of Medicine, Louisville, Kentucky

**Pei-Ning Wang, MD,** Neurological Institute, Taipei Veterans General Hospital, and Department of Neurology, National Yang-Ming University School of Medicine, Taipei, Taiwan

**Anthony P. Weiss, MD,** Department of Psychiatry, Massachusetts General Hospital, Harvard Medical School, Charlestown, Massachusetts

**Grace Yoon, MD,** Memory and Aging Center, Department of Neurology, University of California, San Francisco, California

# Series Editor's Note

The second edition of *The Human Frontal Lobes* represents a window into the rapid growth of our knowledge on the functions of the frontal lobe. In the few years since the first edition was released, the sophistication of our understanding, and the technologies and techniques that have been developed, continue to expand the horizons of our appreciation of frontal lobe functions and their centrality in human behavior.

This edition reflects the vast increase in knowledge that has been accrued over the past 8 years. Drs. Miller and Cummings have assembled an all-star team of basic and clinical scientists who provide a comprehensive review of the frontal lobes, including cytoarchitectonics, neurotransmitter systems, and neuroimaging. In keeping with the rapid growth in knowledge and evolving technologies, the section on imaging techniques has been significantly expanded. Similarly, the sections on neurological and psychiatric diseases reflect the increasing awareness of the frontal lobes in a broad range of disorders, as well as our enhanced understanding of the pathophysiological mechanisms underlying these diseases.

The first edition of this book was the inaugural volume of the Guilford series The Science and Practice of Neuropsychology. The goal of this series is to integrate the scientific foundations and clinical applications of knowledge of brain–behavior relationships. The study of the frontal lobes is in many regards at the leading edge of the neuroscience knowledge explosion that has fundamentally revised many traditional concepts and constructs. This second edition demonstrates how rapidly the field is advancing.

ROBERT A. BORNSTEIN, PhD

# Preface

Since the publication of the first edition of *The Human Frontal Lobes* in 1999, scientific understanding of the frontal lobes has greatly advanced, with the fields of neuropsychology, neuroimaging, and neuroscience all contributing to a rapidly changing perspective on the role of the frontal lobes in behavior and cognition. Not only are these advances important for understanding the neuroanatomy, neurophysiology, and neurochemistry of frontal lobe function, but they have also altered clinical approaches to the evaluation of patients with frontal lobe disorders. This changing landscape is reflected in this book's new edition. This second edition of *The Human Frontal Lobes* brings an international perspective to the organization, function, and role in disease of the frontal lobes, and the chapter authors come from a wide variety of specialties.

The neuroanatomical section of this book is reorganized and expanded to reflect the evolving understanding of frontal lobe divisions. Increasingly, frontal lobe divisions are influenced by a better understanding of the circuits and connections associated with specific frontal areas. Harry J. Jerison contributes a fascinating chapter on evolution that challenges existing paradigms regarding selective growth of prefrontal regions. Daniel H. Geschwind and Marco Iacoboni, leaders in our understanding of brain asymmetries, further pursue novel aspects of prefrontal anatomy by describing differences in left versus right prefrontal structure, changes that reflect these unique aspects of human anatomy. Other chapters in this section explore the anatomy of prefrontal cortex from the histological to the gross morphological level. These contributions are lively and accessible to a broad audience ranging from clinicians to basic scientists. Similarly, the neurochemistry section of this book reflects new concepts regarding the roles of serotonin, acetylcholine, and dopamine in the cognitive and emotional functions of the frontal lobe. The role of dopamine in reward and learning is emphasized in a new chapter from Antonello Bonci and Susan Jones.

Over the past 7 years the field of functional imaging has expanded, leading to a comprehensive picture of the circuitry that contributes to the cognitive and emotional underpinnings of frontal lobe function. The sections on functional and structural imaging and on neuropsychological functions reflect this evolving story. Howard Rosen and David Dean offer a new chapter on structural imaging and Adam L. Boxer describes the role that the frontal lobes play in the planning of movement. A new chapter from Margaret McKinnon and colleagues discusses the key role of frontal cortex in autobiographical memory, and Adam Gazzaley and Mark D'Esposito outline the anatomy and testing of working memory.

The neuropsychology section has chapters that range from practical to theoretical. Joel H. Kramer and Lovingly Quitania offer a practical approach to bedside neuropsychological testing, while Donald T. Stuss explores more experimental approaches to frontal testing. The critical roles of the frontal lobes in personality and emotion are described in a new chapter from Katherine P. Rankin.

The clinical chapters reflect an explosion of new findings regarding the critical functions of the frontal lobes in the major degenerative disorders. A new series of chapters explore the clinical (Pei-Ning Wang and Bruce L. Miller), imaging (Murray Grossman), and neuropathological (Nigel J. Cairns and colleagues) features of frontotemporal dementia and related disorders. Finally, the wide range of neurological and psychiatric syndromes that are driven by loss of function in prefrontal cortex are described.

*The Human Frontal Lobes* is recommended for readers who enjoyed the first edition of this book and for new readers interested in the rapidly evolving story regarding the role of the prefrontal cortex in human disease.

# Dedication and Acknowledgments

We dedicate this book to Milton Miller (Bruce L. Miller's father), who succumbed to a brain tumor in 2005 during the preparation phase of this book. As a physician and psychiatrist, Milton was enormously influential, modeling interactions with patients that would affect generations of students. As a chair of psychiatry at Harbor–UCLA Medical Center in Los Angeles, he was a leader in the psychiatric community and improved the care of thousands of indigent patients with mental illnesses. As a thinker and philosopher, he was able to see his way through complex ideas and develop a vision that others could follow. As a father, he was remarkable and his wonderful wit and wisdom will live on in his sons.

We both were highly influenced by D. Frank Benson, MD. Frank was a leader in behavioral neurology in Boston before becoming the Augustus S. Rose Professor of Neurology at UCLA. Dr. Cummings worked with Dr. Benson as a resident and fellow in Boston and as a colleague throughout the time Frank lived in Los Angeles. Dr. Miller was one of the first fellows to be trained in Los Angeles after Frank's move to UCLA. As an insightful clinician and enthusiastic teacher, he inspired all who had the privilege of studying with him. He was particularly fascinated by the frontal lobe disorders, and our interest in the clinical phenomenology of frontal lobe dysfunction can be traced largely to his influence.

We have the good fortune of being in departments that have outstanding leaders who promote and encourage our investigation into the clinical neurobiology of human behavior. We gratefully acknowledge the support of Dr. Stephen Hauser at UCSF and Dr. John Mazziotta at UCLA.

Our work on the frontal lobes and particularly the frontotemporal dementias has been greatly facilitated by center and program project grants from the National Institute on Aging. Neil Buckholtz, Tony Phelps, and Elizabeth Koss were instrumental in facilitating these studies.

Academic productivity and scholarship can exist only where there is support from one's family and loved ones. I (B. L. M.) have the great joy of Debbie's unstinting love and encouragement. And I (J. L. C.) found new light in life with Kate (Xue) Zhong.

# Contents

# PART III. NEUROCHEMISTRY

# PART IV. FUNCTIONAL AND STRUCTURAL IMAGING APPROACHES

# PART V. NEUROPSYCHOLOGICAL FUNCTIONS

## PART VI. NEUROLOGICAL DISEASES

### A. Frontotemporal Dementia and Related Disorders

### B. Other Neurological Disorders

# PART I

## OVERVIEW OF THE FRONTAL LOBES

# CHAPTER 1

# The Human Frontal Lobes

## AN INTRODUCTION

*Bruce L. Miller*

Recent research into the functions of the frontal lobes is transforming our understanding of this important brain region. This chapter offers an overview of the frontal lobes and introduces the major topics discussed in greater detail throughout this book. A historical review emphasizes the key developments in frontal lobe research generated over the past two centuries. Also, it describes the important new imaging techniques that play an increasingly central role in the study of the frontal lobes; new cognitive, social, and pharmacological approaches to frontal lobe functions; and human neurological and psychiatric diseases in which frontal lobes or frontal–subcortical connections to the frontal lobes are particularly vulnerable. Frontotemporal dementia, traumatic brain injury, anterior cerebral artery stroke, schizophrenia, and depression are introduced as model systems for understanding frontal function. Links between subcortical and frontal structures are noted, and future approaches to frontal lobe research are outlined.

## HISTORICAL OVERVIEW OF CLINICAL ADVANCES

During the 19th century, Dr. John Harlow's description of the social changes in Phineas Gage following traumatic injury to the orbitofrontal cortex (Macmillan, 2001) and Broca's delineation of the language functions of dominant

frontal cortex (Berker, Berker, & Smith, 1986) forever changed the way that brain–behavior relationships would be perceived. With the emergence of new histological and anatomical techniques by von Economo and Broadmann, and the growth of experimental psychology, Tilney suggested in 1928 that the 20th century would become "the century of the frontal lobes." Yet for the first 60 years of the 20th century, biologically oriented studies of frontal cortex were exceedingly uncommon, and opportunities to understand the sequelae of frontal lesions associated with stroke, tumor, trauma, seizures, infections, and neurodegenerative or psychiatric disorders were routinely ignored. Even when procedures such as the frontal leukotomy emerged as a routine practice for patients with disabling psychiatric conditions, there was never a systematic attempt to understand the effects of this procedure on cognition or behavior.

In retrospect, this lack of scientific progress had many causes. Undoubtedly, the formal separation of the fields of psychiatry and neurology at the end of the 19th century had a negative influence, leaving higher cortical functions neglected by both fields. For nearly a century, the dominant focus of psychiatry was no longer brain–behavior relationships, whereas neurology became the study of motor and sensory, but not higher cortical functions. Also, the frontal lobes did not prove easily tractable to clinicians; the cognitive and behavioral deficits associated with frontal injury were not readily apparent or easily characterized. The concepts of executive control and behavioral disorders due to frontal lobe pathology were foreign to the field. Similarly, imaging and the technologies needed to measure frontal lobe function or structures were lacking. By midcentury, Tilney's predictions appeared premature.

However, by the 1960s, a few investigators began seriously to tackle questions regarding the function of the frontal lobes. In the area of motor systems, Penfield's intraoperative stimulation work facilitated understanding of the functional organization of motor and premotor cortex. Penfield's work helped to elucidate the concept that the frontal lobes has three major anatomical divisions: the motor strip involved with fine coordination of movement; the premotor area, a region involved with the overall organization of movement; and the prefrontal region. Stimulation of the motor strip resulted in simple movements of the affected muscles and muscle groups, whereas with premotor stimulation, complex organized movements were seen (Penfield, 1954). Yet Penfield seemed to run into a brick wall when he electrically stimulated prefrontal cortex. These prefrontal areas were "silent," and Penfield was unable to explain the functions of these regions based upon these stimulation studies.

Paul Yakovlev's anatomical studies of the frontal lobes and their connections strongly influenced neurologists and pathologists, including Norman Geschwind, D. Frank Benson, and Arne Brun, who went on to do important research into frontal lobe function. Yakovlev focused these emerging investigators on the phylogenetic and developmental origins of frontal cortex and the subcortical–limbic connections to the frontal regions (Yakovlev, 1968). This work eventually led to important new studies that explored the clinical syndromes associated with frontal injury from stroke, trauma, tumor, and neurodegeneration. In the second half of the 20th century, Alexander Luria and D. Frank Benson began to focus their research on the vast space of the frontal lobes. Luria (1970), the innovative Russian psychologist, developed novel and, even by today's standards, remarkably modern theories about frontal lobe functions. His theories about frontal lobe organization were highly theoretical, but many components of Luria's ideas were shaped and sharpened by his clinical

experiences with patients who had focal lesions.

The advent of behavioral neurology under the leadership of Norman Geschwind and D. Frank Benson stimulated a whole generation of neurologists and psychologists to explore the anatomical basis for cognition and behavior. Benson, a student and colleague of Geschwind, was particularly intrigued by functions of the frontal lobes and even traveled to Russia to observe Luria's patient-based approach to frontal lobe function (Benson, 1996). Benson liked to tell how Luria's patients and their families approached him with profound formality, respecting his place in Russia's rigid hierarchy. Patients with frontal lobe injury were different, often greeting Luria like an old friend, entering inappropriately into his personal space.

Benson realized that the frontal lobes had a strong connection to social cognition, and he was one of the first investigators to include the study of behavior in the evaluation of frontal lobe function. The importance of his studies and their influence on his students cannot be underemphasized. Benson stressed the importance of bedside observation. He believed that capturing phenomenology was the first step, with theories coming later. Theories were greatly bolstered if they were based upon careful clinical observations. Among the behavioral neurologists of his generation, Benson was most willing to explore the interface between neurology and psychiatry, and he realized that the frontal lobes played an important role in the genesis of behaviors that were considered psychiatric in origin.

Some of his most original work came from his study of the role of the frontal cortex in disorders that were considered psychiatric in origin: syndromes such as reduplicative paramnesia and confabulation associated with amnesia. Benson hypothesized that one possible mechanism for delusions was the patient's altered monitoring of distorted or incomplete information (Mercer, Wapner, Gardner, & Benson, 1977). In the case of reduplicative paramnesia, the combination of distorted visual information from a posterior nondominant temporal–parietal lesion and abnormal monitoring due to a frontal lesion led to delusions about the identity of a place (Benson et al., 1976). With confabulation associated with amnesia, frontal injury led a patient to fill in the amnesia with false information, whereas without the frontal injury, the confabulation would not occur (Benson et al., 1996; Stuss & Benson, 1986).

Benson and his colleague and friend Don Stuss evaluated the effects of leukotomy on frontal lobe function (Stuss et al., 1981). This work required finding patients in whom leukotomy has had been performed. In many instances, Stuss and Benson found patients in whom the procedure had been performed years or even decades earlier. It represented the beginning of a new era, and Stuss and Benson eventually modified Luria's classification by suggesting that the prefrontal cortex has three major anatomical divisions: orbitofrontal, cingulate, and dorsolateral. Whereas the orbitofrontal cortex modulated social control and the cingulate cortex was responsible for the generation of goal-directed behavior, the neuropsychological functions of the frontal cortex were localized within dorsolateral prefrontal regions (Stuss & Benson, 1986). These concepts have proven remarkably durable across many approaches, whether lesion-based or studied in healthy controls with functional magnetic resonance imaging (fMRI).

Others continue to evaluate the frontal lobes from distinctive perspectives. The concept of working memory pioneered by Alan Baddeley (2003) began the parcellation of specific frontal lobe neuropsychological functions localized to different regions in the frontal cortex. Patricia Goldman-Rakic and colleagues (e.g., Chafee & Goldman-Rakic, 1998) emphasized the role of a frontoparietal system in visual attention/working memory tasks and showed the role and anatomy of the dopaminergic components of this circuit. Mark D'Esposito and colleagues (e.g., Ranganath & D'Esposito, 2005), Cheryl Grady (2002), and others have successfully used functional imaging techniques such as fMRI to evaluate this working memory system *in vivo*. Marsel Mesulam's (1998) histological and phylogenetic approaches to cortical organization have emphasized the functional organization of cortex based on connections to primary sensory or motor areas. With his single-cell recording in rodents, Edmund Rolls's (2004) pioneering research has demonstrated the important function of orbitofrontal cortex in reward and eating-related behaviors. Finally, Antonio Damasio's (2003) "somatic marker" theory suggests that the orbitofrontal cortex is involved with the interpretation of autonomic information in decision making.

## IMAGING

Neuroimaging research continues as the pre-eminent technique for evaluation of the frontal lobes. Computed tomography (CT) became widely available in the late 1970s; prior to that, clinicians had few ways to visualize the structure or function of frontal cortex. Older tools, pneumoencephalography and angiography, were highly invasive, painful, and sometimes dangerous, and offered only crude outlines of frontal anatomy. With CT, suddenly clinical–anatomical correlations could be made *in vivo*, and the presence and extent of structural lesions associated with stroke, demyelination, tumor, or trauma became visible prior to death. CT allowed researchers to explore the relationship between volume of frontal injury and clinical status with trauma, tumor, stroke, and neurodegeneration. Measurement of atrophy became a way to differentiate between normal aging and dementia, and to separate the distinctive dementia syndromes from each other. Yet CT had constraints related to the frontal lobes. In particular, artifacts generated from adjacent bone diminished visualization of orbitofrontal and anterior frontal structures. Also, resolution between gray and white matter was limited.

Development of MRI in the early 1980s circumvented some of the problems associated with CT. Better resolution of gray and white matter, and disappearance of artifacts associated with bone made MRI the technique of choice for the evaluation of the frontal lobes. MRI allowed quantitative measurement of frontal volumes, facilitating studies on the role of frontal cortex, or subfrontal white matter lesions in the pathogenesis of a wide variety of cognitive and behavioral syndromes.

Volumetric region-of-interest (ROI) measures of normal or pathological tissue, correlated with specific cognitive or behavioral parameters, remain a widely used approach to the study the sequelae from frontal injury. Hand-drawn measures (ROIs) in different frontal regions have facilitated the study of neurological and psychiatric disorders. However, because this approach is slow and interrater reliability is a methodological concern, automatic ROI methods are being developed for measuring the frontal lobes in their entirety and for selective regional analyses.

Other MRI-based techniques have facilitated study of brain–behavior relationships related to the frontal lobes, including voxel-based-morphometry (VBM) and deformation–tensor morphometry (DTM). With these techniques, the brains from two groups can be compared with regards to overall patterns of atrophy. Often a disease cohort is compared to age-matched controls, and VBM and DTM also allow comparisons between an individual patient and a control group (Ashburner & Friston, 2001; Studholme et al., 2004). Or, a patient's results can be compared with use of images obtained at different times. Unlike ROI approaches, VBM and DTM require no a priori hypotheses and allow comparisons of the whole brain (or specific frontal regions) between patient cohorts and controls. These techniques have proven particularly powerful for delineating the most vulnerable brain regions in different conditions that cause dementia.

Structural MRI still holds great promise for facilitating a better understanding of the frontal lobes. VBM and ROI approaches are still relatively new, and studies combining these techniques with newer cognitive approaches should offer many new insights into structural and functional relationships related to the frontal lobes. Movement from 0.5 to 1.5 T (tesla) magnets has improved resolution of frontal regions and has facilitated better separation of gray matter from white matter. Furthermore, more powerful magnets (3, 4, and 7 T magnets) will offer even greater advantages for structural resolution of the frontal lobes in the coming decade.

Functional methods using radionuclides such as single-photon emission computed tomography (SPECT) and positron emission tomography (PET) have contributed to a better understanding of the frontal lobes. SPECT and PET have helped to show the frontal component of a wide variety of disease states, including depression (Mayberg, 2002), obsessive–compulsive disorder (Saxena et al., 2004), schizophrenia (Hill et al., 2004), attention deficit disorder (Schweitzer et al., 2003), Alzheimer's disease (Craig et al., 1996), and frontotemporal dementia (Miller et al., 1991). Similarly, frontal contributions to working memory, generation, executive function, apathy, and disinhibition continue to be explored with these functional techniques. Both SPECT and PET still have great potential for imaging the brain receptor systems described in Chapters 12–17, this volume.

Increasingly, MRI is being explored as a way to supplement, or even replace, SPECT and PET techniques for measuring brain metabolism. Perfusion MRI (Callen, Black, Caldwell, & Grady, 2004) offers better resolution and is less invasive than either SPECT or PET, but systematic comparisons between perfusion MRI, SPECT, and PET are still lacking. A newly funded National Institutes of Health (NIH) initiative on imaging in dementia will compare the relative value of perfusion MRI and PET, facilitating more scientific selection of imaging techniques in the future.

fMRI is a new and powerful tool that has dramatically changed research into the frontal lobes by allowing noninvasive evaluation *in vivo*. Relying upon changes in the MRI signal that occur when the brain undergoes metabolic activity (the BOLD signal), fMRI allows study of brain activity associated with specific cognitive tasks (Frackowiak, 2000–2001). Frontal brain regions that are active during working memory, self-reflection, word generation, temporal sequencing, set shifting, and many other cognitive paradigms are being evaluated by psychologists, psychiatrists, and neurologists with this technique (Baron-Cohen, 2004). Another exciting development with fMRI has been the mapping of networks activated with cognitive tasks or during rest (Greicius, Krasnow, Reiss, & Menon, 2003). This elucidates an understanding of what brain systems work together during specific activities. No technique has ever generated quite so much new data regarding the functional organization of the frontal lobes, and it will be many years before this data can be fully understood.

Magnetoencephalography, transcranial magnetic stimulation, and nuclear magnetic resonance spectroscopy represent other imaging approaches that have been applied to the study of frontal lobe function in healthy or disease states. Whatever the technique, it is clear that neuroimaging will continue to influence of our understanding of the frontal lobes.

## NEUROANATOMICAL/FUNCTIONAL ORGANIZATION

The frontal lobes are no longer considered a single functional entity. Rather, there are a variety of ways to anatomically subdivide this brain region, all based upon distinctive constructs. Most researchers accept that the frontal lobes have three major divisions: motor, premotor, and prefrontal regions. Motor and premotor areas are considered distinctive functional units, whereas prefrontal cortex is more complex, requiring further subdivision. One system to subdivide the frontal cortex relies on the distinctive functions of different prefrontal regions. Another approach considers regional connections to and from specific subcortical regions. Additionally, the left and right frontal lobes are increasingly differentiated: The left frontal lobes are more specialized for language-related functions, and the right frontal region is dominant in social cognition and emotion. Analyzing regional histology represents another way to subdivide the frontal lobes.

A functional approach suggested by Stuss and Benson (1986) divides prefrontal cortex into orbital, dorsolateral, and cingulate regions. Increasingly, these gross divisions are being further parcellated into smaller functional units. Baddeley (2003) and others have shown a dorsal prefrontal (Brodmann's area [BA] 46) parietal system involved with working memory (left verbal working memory and right visual working memory). A more ventral frontal–parietal system is involved with mirror movements, (Rizzolatti, Fogassi, & Gallese, 2002), speech initiation (Dronkers, 1996), and affect matching (Rosen et al., 2004). Orbitofrontal cortex has important medial–lateral and right–left divisions. Medial orbitofrontal cortex is strongly connected with hypothalamic nuclei, whereas lateral orbital cortex is more strongly connected with anterior temporal and insular regions. In certain behavioral paradigms orbitofrontal regions show antagonistic functions. For example, the medial area activates when an individual is hungry, whereas the lateral region activates when the same individual is sated (Small, Zatorre, Dagher, Evans, & Jones-Gotman, 2001).

"Executive control," a broad term used to describe the neuropsychological functions of the frontal lobes, incorporates many distinctive cognitive processes. Neuropsychologists are now attempting to subdivide neuropsychological functions into their anatomically driven subcomponents. Working memory is a core constituent of executive function, and when there are deficits in working memory, nearly all other tests of executive control are vulnerable. Other components of executive control include generation, inhibition, set shifting, concept for-

mation, temporal sequencing, insight, interpersonal perspective taking (theory of mind), and social and real-world executive performance. Distinctive tasks that capture these different aspects of executive control are in development. Similarly, the anatomical components of these tasks are under investigation. This topic is explored by Kramer and Quitania in Chapter 18, this volume. Left versus right frontal lobe functions are now under careful scrutiny. Linguistic functions of Broca's area in prefrontal cortex has been understood for nearly 150 years, but only recently have investigators begun to formally address the preeminence of the right prefrontal cortex for social and emotional behavior. For example, in a recent imaging study of a large cohort of patients with dementia, Rosen and colleagues (2004) found that repetitive compulsive behaviors were strongly associated with right supplementary motor area atrophy, disinhibition with atrophy in the right orbitofrontal cortex, and apathy with atrophy in the right cingulate cortex. Right insular atrophy correlated with abnormalities in eating. fMRI approaches to behavior suggest that self-reflection, reading the emotional expressions of others, and many other aspects of social cognition activate more right compared to left frontal regions. The specifics of behavioral specialization of right frontal cortex still remain poorly understood, but the combination of fMRI and lesion studies should elucidate many of these details in the coming decades.

Earlier, Yakovlev (1968), but more recently Flaherty and Graybiel (1995), Tekin and Cummings (2002), and others, have emphasized the intimate connections between subcortical and frontal structures, and this connectivity has helped to organize the frontal lobes into distinctive units. The presence of these anatomical circuits suggests one way to classify the organization of the frontal lobes. Tekin and Cummings suggest that there are five distinctive frontal subcortical systems: (1) supplementary motor area, (2) frontal eye fields, (3) dorsolateral prefrontal, (4) orbitofrontal, and (5) anterior cingulate cortex. With each circuit, specific neurochemical systems transmit their functional activity. Lesions in these different frontal or subcortical circuits lead to distinctive clinical syndromes. With supplementary motor dysfunction, deficits in controlled movement and repetitive motor behaviors emerge (Gorno-Tempini, Murray, Rankin, Weiner, & Miller,

2004); with eye movement injury, control of gaze is diminished (Chou & Lisberger, 2004); with dorsolateral dysfunction, there is loss of executive control and neuropsychological deficits in the area of working memory, and alternation and planning deficits emerge (Boone et al., 1999); orbitofrontal dysfunction causes social deficits, including disinhibition with sparing of cognition (Damasio, 2003); and cingulate lesions lead to "amotivational" states (Tekin & Cummings, 2002). Psychiatric syndromes are strongly linked to these frontal–subcortical circuits, in particular, depression, mania, and obsessive–compulsive disorders. The relationship of these psychiatric syndromes to frontal lobe dysfunction is discussed extensively in this book. Finally, movement disorders are particularly prominent when the basal ganglia component of frontal–subcortical circuits is affected.

Mesulam (1998) considers anatomical connectivity and histology in his approach to cortical organization of the frontal regions. His system emphasizes limbic, paralimbic, and cortical divisions. Cortical regions are divided into four subtypes—primary, unimodal, heteromodal, and supramodal cortex—based on the nature of these regions' other cortical connections. With this system, the first-order regions include primary motor (BA 4), sensory (BA 3), visual (BA 17), auditory (BA 42), and gustatory cortex (BA 43). These regions are theoretically bound together by the fact that they are the first cortical regions that connect with subcortical areas that translate information from or to the external milieu. Unimodal regions have efferent connections from the primary areas and process only one type of sensory stimuli (visual, auditory, or gustatory). Heteromodal regions are areas that connect with unimodal areas and are involved with multiple types of sensory processing. In the final, supramodal division, many prefrontal regions are considered supramodal because they are remote from sensory processing, and involved with higher order processing.

Finally, in recent years, the role of a histologically unique neuron, the spindle cell, is being explored in relation to the distinctive functions of the frontal lobes in humans. Originally described by von Economo, these large, spindle-shaped cells found in layer 5b of the ventral frontal anterior cingulate and anterior insular regions are more strongly localized to the right frontal area. These cells first appeared in great apes but are only abundant in humans. They first appeared in orangutans but are far more abundant in gorillas. Spindle cells show still greater abundance in bonobo chimpanzees and have 1,000-fold greater concentration in humans than in chimps. Spindle cells are absent in gibbons, New World monkeys, Old World monkeys, and all other mammals studied (Allmann, Hakeem, & Watson, 2002; Nimchinsky et al., 1999). The role of these cells in social cognitive paradigms will be extensively studied in the coming decade.

## NEUROLOGICAL DISORDERS OF THE FRONTAL LOBES

One important approach to understanding frontal function is to examine neurological disorders that selectively attack the frontal regions. Neuroimaging has facilitated this approach by allowing investigators to outline brain areas affected by distinctive pathological processes. Many neurological disorders involve the frontal lobes either directly or through frontal–subcortical connections. Alzheimer's disease (AD) is an example of a disease in which frontal cortex is not the primary site of injury but is usually affected at some time in the course of the illness (Johnson, Vogt, Kim, Cotman, & Head, 2004). With AD, the combination of imaging, behavioral, and cognitive approaches has helped to clarify the role of the cingulate cortex in a variety of psychological processes, including apathy and compulsions. There are also a few conditions in which frontal cortex is the primary site of disease. Frontotemporal lobar degeneration (FTLD) is one such example, and this disorder has become a powerful model for the investigation of frontal function. Three subtypes of FTLD exist, all defined by distinctive clinical syndromes (Rosen et al., 2002). The core features of the major subtype, frontotemporal dementia (FTD), include loss of social and personal conduct, loss of insight, and emotional blunting. The most profound atrophy with FTD is in the anterior cingulate, insular, and orbitofrontal cortex. The right hemisphere is more severely affected than the left. In the second subtype, progressive nonfluent aphasia, the atrophy involves these same frontal regions but is more severe on the left than on the right side. With semantic dementia, the third FTLD subtype, the insula and orbitofrontal cortex, amygdala, and anterior temporal lobes are bilaterally atrophic. These distinctive anatomies facilitate exploration of the functions of the right versus left frontal cortex and different frontal regions. Each patient with FTLD shows slightly distinctive involvement of dorsolateral, orbital, cingulate, or insular regions. This allows comparison of individuals, or groups of patients, with unique anatomical patterns, with the goal of parceling out the specific functions of these frontal regions.

There are other neurological disease models for the evaluation of frontal lobe function. Beginning with Harlow's descriptions of Phineas Gage, trauma has helped to delineate the functional anatomical divisions in the frontal lobes. Often, trauma selectively injures orbitofrontal cortex while sparing dorsolateral regions (Alexander & Stuss, 2000). In patients with these selective injuries, profound deficits in social behavior and intelligence, with sparing of the cognitive components of frontal lobe function, led to the recognition that orbitofrontal and dorsolateral components of the frontal lobes are distinctive. Similarly, from the clinical study of patients with selective injury to the cingulate cortex associated with anterior cerebral artery stroke or psychosurgery (Brower & Price, 2001), researchers now suspect that this area is particularly important for initiation of behavior.

## PSYCHIATRIC DISORDERS AND THE FRONTAL LOBE

An important paradigm shift in psychiatry has been the recognition of dysfunction in the prefrontal cortex or within frontal–subcortical circuitry in many psychiatric disturbances. This conceptual shift has been driven by converging evidence generated through a wide variety of approaches: cognitive, behavioral, neuroimaging, and neuropathological. Schizophrenia represents one such disorder in which all of these distinctive parameters suggest frontal dysfunction.

Neuropsychological testing of many patients with schizophrenia shows deficits in frontal/executive skills compared to controls (Kremen, Seidman, Faraone, Toomey, & Tsuang, 2004). Similarly, the behavioral features of patients with schizophrenia have many parallels to patients with frontal injury. The negative symp-

tom complex found in many patients with schizophrenia is similar to the apathetic syndromes caused by frontal injury (Boone, Miller, Swartz, Lu, & Lee, 2003). Furthermore, patients with schizophrenia who have the most severe negative symptoms, such as apathy, tend to have the smallest frontal brain volumes, further linking specific symptoms in schizophrenia to the frontal lobes (Roth, Flashman, Saykin, McAllister, & Vidaver, 2004). Also, a wide-variety of PET and fMRI studies show metabolic abnormalities at rest and during activation in prefrontal cortex (Davidson & Heinrichs, 2003). Finally, autopsies of many patients with schizophrenia reveal neuropathological abnormalities. Most of these changes are found in the hippocampus, but recent work suggests that abnormalities in the frontal regions (Webster, O'Grady, Kleinman, & Weickert, 2005).

Schizophrenia represents just one of the many psychiatric illnesses in which behavioral disturbance is linked to the frontal lobes. Major depression is associated with hypometabolism in the dorsal and orbitofrontal cortex (Mayberg, 2002). Metabolic changes have also been noted in the anterior cingulate and insular regions. Similarly, disproportionate atrophy in the orbitofrontal cortex is seen in elderly patients with depression or bipolar disorder. Also, injury to frontal cortex is often followed by depressive syndromes, and right orbitofrontal injury can trigger secondary manic syndromes. Frontal–subcortical circuits have also been hypothesized to participate in obsessive–compulsive disorder, and this hypothesis is supported by both structural and functional imaging. Finally, attention deficit disorder is clearly associated with dysfunction in the prefrontal cortical, attentional, and executive systems.

## SUMMARY

The frontal lobes are a large brain region representing 30% of the cortical surface. The coming decade will see a more definitive exploration of the structural, functional, neurochemical, and histological underpinnings of the frontal lobes. Understanding the frontal lobes will lead to advances against a wide variety of neurological and psychiatric conditions. These new developments are outlined throughout this book.

## REFERENCES

Alexander, M. P., & Stuss, D. T. (2000). Disorders of frontal lobe functioning. *Seminars in Neurology, 20,* 427–437.

Allman, J., Hakeem, A., & Watson, K. (2002). Two phylogenetic specializations in the human brain. *Neuroscientist, 8,* 335–346.

Ashburner, J., & Friston, K. J. (2001). Why voxel-based morphometry should be used. *NeuroImage, 14,* 1238–1243.

Baddeley, A. (2003). Working memory: Looking back and looking forward. *Nature Reviews: Neuroscience, 4,* 829–839.

Baron-Cohen, S. (2004). The cognitive neuroscience of autism. *Journal of Neurology, Neurosurgery, and Psychiatry, 75,* 945–948.

Benson, D. F. (1996). My day with Luria. *Journal of Geriatric Psychiatry and Neurology, 9,* 120–122.

Benson, D. F., Gardner, H., & Meadows, J. C. (1976). Reduplicative paramnesia. *Neurology, 26,* 147–151.

Benson, D. F., Djenderedjian, A., Miller, B. L., Pachana, N. A., Chang, L., Itti, L., et al. (1996). The neural basis of confabulation. *Neurology, 46,* 1239–1243.

Berker, E. A., Berker, A. H., & Smith, A. (1986). Translation of Broca's 1865 report: Localization of speech in the third left frontal convolution. *Archives of Neurology, 43,* 1065–1072.

Boone, K. B., Miller, B. L., Lee, A., Berman, N., Sherman, D., & Stuss, D. (1999). Neuropsychological patterns in right versus left frontotemporal dementia. *Journal of the International Neuropsychological Society, 5,* 616–622.

Boone, K. B., Miller, B. L., Swartz, R., Lu, P., & Lee, A. (2003). Relationship between positive and negative symptoms and neuropsychological scores in frontotemporal dementia and Alzheimer's disease. *Journal of the International Neuropsychological Society, 9,* 698–709.

Brower, M. C., & Price, B. H. (2001). Neuropsychiatry of frontal lobe dysfunction in violent and criminal behaviour: A critical review. *Journal of Neurology, Neurosurgery, and Psychiatry, 71,* 720–726.

Callen, D. J., Black, S. E., Caldwell, C. B., & Grady, C. L. (2004). The influence of sex on limbic volume and perfusion in AD. *Neurobiology and Aging, 25,* 761–770.

Chafee, M. V., & Goldman-Rakic, P. S. (1998). Matching patterns of activity in primate prefrontal area 8a and parietal area 7ip neurons during a spatial working memory task. *Journal of Neurophysiology, 79,* 2919–2940.

Chou, I. H., & Lisberger, S. G. (2004). The role of the frontal pursuit area in learning in smooth pursuit eye movements. *Journal of Neuroscience, 24,* 4124–4133.

Craig, A., Cummings, J. L., Fairbanks, L., Itti, L., Miller, B. L., & Mena, I. (1996). Cerebral blood flow correlates of apathy in Alzheimer's disease. *Archives of Neurology, 53,* 1116–1120.

Damasio, A. (2003). Feelings of emotion and the self. *Annals of the New York Academy of Sciences, 1001,* 253–261.

Davidson, L. L., & Heinrichs, R. W. (2003). Quantification of frontal and temporal lobe brain-imaging findings in schizophrenia: A meta-analysis. *Psychiatry Research, 122,* 69–87.

Dronkers, N. F. (1996). A new brain region for coordinating speech articulation. *Nature, 14,* 159–161.

Flaherty, A. W., & Graybiel, A. M. (1995). Motor and somatosensory corticostriatal projection magnifications in the squirrel monkey. *Journal of Neurophysiology, 74,* 2638–2648.

Frackowiak, R. S. (2000–2001). Forthergillian Lecture: Imaging human brain function. *Transactions of the Medical Society of London, 117,* 53–63.

Gorno-Tempini, M. L., Murray, R., Rankin, K., Weiner, M. W., & Miller, B. L. (2004). Clinical, cognitive and anatomical evolution from nonfluent progressive aphasia to corticobasal syndrome: A case report. *Neurocase, 10,* 426–436.

Grady, C. L. (2002). Introduction to the special section on aging, cognition, and neuroimaging. *Psychology and Aging, 17,* 3–6.

Greicius, M. D., Krasnow, B., Reiss, A. L., & Menon, V. (2003). Functional connectivity in the resting brain: A network analysis of the default mode hypothesis. *Proceedings of the National Academy of Sciences, 100,* 253–258.

Hill, K., Mann, L., Laws, K. R., Stephenson, C. M., Nimmo-Smith, I., & McKenna, P. J. (2004). Hypofrontality in schizophrenia: A meta-analysis of functional imaging studies. *Acta Psychiatrica Scandinavica, 110,* 243–256.

Johnson, J. K., Vogt, B. A., Kim, R., Cotman, C. W., & Head, E. (2004). Isolated executive impairment and associated frontal neuropathology. *Dementia and Geriatric Cognitive Disorders, 17,* 360–367.

Kremen, W. S., Seidman, L. J., Faraone, S. V., Toomey, R., & Tsuang, M. T. (2004) Heterogeneity of schizophrenia: A study of individual neuropsychological profiles. *Schizophrenia Research, 71,* 307–321.

Luria, A. R. (1970). The functional organization of the brain. *Scientific American, 222,* 66–72.

Macmillan, M. (2001). John Martyn Harlow: "Obscure country physician"? *Journal of the History of the Neurosciences, 10*(2), 149–162.

Mayberg, H. (2002). Images in Neuroscience Depression: II: Localization of pathophysiology. *American Journal of Psychiatry, 159,* 1979.

Mercer, B., Wapner, W., Gardner, H., & Benson, D. F. (1977). A study of confabulation. *Archives of Neurology, 34,* 429–433.

Mesulam, M. M. (1998). From sensation to cognition. *Brain, 121,* 1013–1052.

Miller, B. L., Cummings, J. L., Villanueva-Meyer, J., Boone, K., Mehringer, C. M., Lesser, I. M., et al. (1991). Frontal lobe degeneration: Clinical, neuropsychological and SPECT characteristics. *Neurology, 41,* 1374–1382.

Nimchinsky, E. A., Gilissen, E., Allman, J. M., Perl, D. P., Erwin, J. M., & Hof, P. R. (1999). A neuronal morphologic type unique to humans and great apes. *Proceedings of the National Academy of Sciences*, 96, 5268–5273.

Penfield, W. (1954). Mechanisms of voluntary movement. *Brain*, 77, 1–17.

Ranganath, C., & D'Esposito, M. (2005). Directing the mind's eye: Prefrontal, inferior and medial temporal mechanisms for visual working memory. *Current Opinion in Neurobiology*, 15, 175–182.

Rizzolatti, G., Fogassi, L., & Gallese, V. (2002). Motor and cognitive functions of the ventral premotor cortex. *Current Opinion in Neurobiology*, 12, 149–154.

Rolls, E. T. (2004). Convergence of sensory systems in the orbitofrontal cortex in primates and brain design for emotion. *Anatomical Record*, 281, 1212–1225.

Rosen, H. J., Gorno-Tempini, M. L., Goldman, W. P., Perry, R. J., Schuff, N., Weiner, M., et al. (2002). Common and differing patterns of brain atrophy in frontotemporal dementia and semantic dementia. *Neurology*, 58, 198–208.

Rosen, H. J., Pace-Savitsky, C., Perry, R. J., Kramer, J. H., Miller, B. L., & Levenson, R. W. (2004). Recognition of emotion in the frontal and temporal variants of FTD. *Dementia and Geriatric Cognitive Disorders*, 17, 277–281.

Roth, R. M., Flashman, L. A., Saykin, A. J., McAllister, T. W., & Vidaver, R. (2004). Apathy in schizophrenia: Reduced frontal lobe volume and neuropsychological deficits. *American Journal of Psychiatry*, 161, 157–159.

Saxena, S., Brody, A. L., Maidment, K. M., Smith, E. C., Zohrabi, N., Katz, E., et al. (2004). Cerebral glucose metabolism in obsessive–compulsive hoarding. *American Journal of Psychiatry*, 161, 1038–1048.

Schweitzer, J. B., Lee, D. O., Hanford, R. B., Tagamets, M. A., Hoffman, J. M., Grafton, S. T., et al. (2003). A positron emission tomography study of methylphenidate in adults with ADHD: Alterations in resting blood flow and predicting treatment response. *Neuropsychopharmacology*, 28, 967–973.

Small, D. M., Zatorre, R. J., Dagher, A., Evans, A. C., & Jones-Gotman, M. (2001). Changes in brain activity related to eating chocolate: From pleasure to aversion. *Brain*, 124, 1720–1733.

Studholme, C., Cardenas, V., Blumenfeld, R., Schuff, N., Rosen, H. J., Miller, B. L., et al. (2004). Deformation tensor morphometry of semantic dementia with quantitative validation. *NeuroImage*, 21, 1387–1398.

Stuss, D., & Benson, D. F. (1986). *The frontal lobes*. New York: Raven.

Stuss, D. T., Kaplan, E. F., Benson, D. F., Weir, W. S., Naeser, M. A., & Levine, H. L. (1981). Long-term effects of prefrontal leukotomy—an overview of neuropsychologic residuals. *Journal of Clinical Neuropsychology*, 3, 13–32.

Tekin, S., & Cummings, J. L. (2002). Frontal–subcortical neuronal circuits and clinical neuropsychiatry: An update. *Journal of Psychosomatic Research*, 53, 647–654.

Webster, M. J., O'Grady, J., Kleinman, J. E., & Weickert C. S. (2005). Glial fibrillary acidic protein mRNA levels in the cingulate cortex of individuals with depression, bipolar disorder and schizophrenia. *Neuroscience*, 133, 453–461.

Yakovlev, P. I. (1968). Telencephalon "impar," "semipar" and "totopar" (morphogenetic, tectogenetic and architectonic definitions). *International Journal of Neurology*, 6, 245–265.

# CHAPTER 2

# Conceptual and Clinical Aspects
# of the Frontal Lobes

*Jeffrey L. Cummings*
*Bruce L. Miller*

The human frontal lobes mediate the behaviors that most distinguish man from animals. Even higher nonhuman primates lack the empathy, regret, sarcasm, social awareness, planning, and judgment characteristic of human behavior. These frontally mediated behaviors define the highest level of human culture and achievement. Frontal executive functions are also among the most vulnerable of all human capabilities and are compromised by a variety of neurological illnesses, including stroke, demyelinating disorders, neurodegenerative diseases, traumatic brain injury, and neoplasms. Developmental disorders frequently find their most severe expressions in frontal executive dysfunction.

Disorders of frontal lobe function and executive abilities are commonly encountered in clinical circumstances. The assessment and interpretation of frontal executive skills are complex and require substantial clinical expertise. Neuropsychological measures have evolved that capture aspects of frontal executive behavior, and advances are being made in developing bedside tests that provide insight into frontal executive abnormalities. In this brief chapter, an overview of frontal executive dysfunction is provided, methods of assessment are described, and disorders commonly affecting these functions are discussed. The anatomical underpinnings of distinct aspects of frontal executive functions are correlated with clinical and functional descriptions.

## FRONTAL LOBE FUNCTIONS

Several major categories of function are mediated by the frontal lobes. Elemental neurological functions, speech and language abilities, volitional eye movements, motivational behaviors, social competency, and executive abilities are mediated by discrete regions within the frontal lobe.

### Elemental Neurological Functions

Basic neurological functions mediated by the frontal lobes include pyramidal motor functions, control of continence, and olfaction. Olfaction depends on the integrity of the olfactory bulb, olfactory nerve, and olfactory tract. The olfactory bulbs and nerves lie on the inferior surface of the orbitofrontal cortex, where they are vulnerable to damage by orbitofrontal injury. Traumatic contusions and subfrontal neoplasms (e.g., meningiomas) are not infrequent causes of acquired olfactory dysfunction. The medial olfactory track projects into the septal region of the basal forebrain within the inferior medial frontal lobe.

The pyramidal motor tract begins in the motor strip and projects through the internal capsule and peduncle to the basis pontis and the medullary decussations before descending to the anterior horn cells. Pyramidal lesions cause a characteristic posture featuring extension of the lower limb and flexion of the upper limb. This posture is the typical hanging posture of the nonhuman primate and reflects the evolutionary history of the nonpyramidal motor system. There is concomitant spasticity of the involved limbs, with a gradual crescendo of tone, culminating in sudden cessation of resistance as Golgi tendon organs release the spastic resistance. The pyramidal motor system mediates fine finger and lip movements, as well as upper limb reach into the environment. This upper limb reach, and hand and lip dexterity allow for fine motor control of writing and speech, which contribute importantly to human enterprise and culture.

## Ocular Motor Functions

Volitional eye movements are mediated by the frontal eye fields anterior to the motor strip. Saccadic eye movements depend on the integrity of this system. Supranuclear eye movement abnormalities reflecting an involvement of the frontal eye fields or disconnection of the fields from the ocular nuclei occur in progressive supranuclear palsy, Huntington's disease, and a variety of other neurological disorders. Seizures produce ocular deviation away from the affected frontal eye field, and ocular eye deviation toward the affected side is characteristic of a postictal state or a focal lesion.

## Frontal Release Signs

Frontal release signs, more properly called "primitive reflexes," represent evolutionarily derived motor programs that facilitate the existence of the infant but are normally lost as frontal cortex matures and frontal function suppresses these more primitive motor programs. The suck reflex represents the innate sucking response necessary for infant survival. It reappears in advanced neurological disorders or diseases specifically affecting the frontal lobes. Similarly, the grasp reflex enhances the chance of survival in tree-dwelling primates, whose survival from infancy depends on unlearned reflexes to hang from parents or branches. The grasp reflex reappears in patients with diffuse neurological dysfunction or frontal lobe disorders. The extensor plantar represents a portion of the triple flexion withdrawal reflex, a protective response to distal limb stimulation.

The palmomental reflex can occur in normal individuals but may occur asymmetrically or be elicitable after multiple stimulations in individuals with frontal dysfunction. It has been hypothesized that the palmomental reflex represents a primitive growl response associated with upper limb simulation.

## Sphincter Control

The urethral and anal sphincters are represented anatomically in the medial inferior frontal cortex, inferior to the leg area of the medial primary motor cortex. Involvement of this region through anterior cerebral artery stroke or degeneration results in loss of sphincter control and urinary or fecal incontinence.

## Speech and Language Functions

Speech and language functions are mediated by frontal lobe structures. A frontal dysarthria has been described with lesions anterior to the mouth area of the primary frontal cortex. Aphemia is a syndrome that begins with mutism and evolves into a "foreign accent syndrome." It is associated with small lesions confined to Broca's area of the left hemisphere. Larger Broca's area lesions produce the syndrome of Broca's aphasia, with nonfluent verbal output, largely intact comprehension, and compromised repetition. Medial left frontal lesions produce a transcortical motor aphasia characterized by nonfluent output, preserved comprehension, and preserved repetition. An executive aprosodia with impaired speech occurs with lesions of the right hemisphere in the location equivalent to Broca's area on the left. More anterior lesions of the right hemisphere contribute to a language output syndrome of verbal dysdecorum, featuring lewd remarks, sarcasm, or inappropriate humor (Alexander, Benson, & Stuss, 1989). Thus, frontal lobe lesions may produce a variety of speech and language disorders. The syndromes tend to be specific for left or right hemisphere.

## Prefrontally Mediated Skills and Syndromes

The prefrontal cortex is parcellated into orbitofrontal, dorsolateral prefrontal, and medial frontal/anterior cingulate regions. Each of these mediates a separate set of skills and produces a distinct clinical syndrome when rendered dysfunctional (described below). Disorders affecting the medial frontal cortex produce an apathetic amotivational syndrome; disorders of the orbitofrontal cortex produce a disinhibited, impulse control disorder; and lesions of the dorsolateral prefrontal cortex result in executive dysfunction (Cummings, 1998; Sarazin et al., 1998).

## FRONTAL–SUBCORTICAL CIRCUITS

Frontal–cortical regions are connected to a complex circuitry of subcortical structures (Figure 2.1). Frontal motor cortex and frontal eye fields connect to subcortical motor and ocular control nuclei through descending pathways involving the basal ganglia and thalamus. The behaviorally relevant cortical regions of medial frontal cortex, orbitofrontal cortex, and dorsolateral prefrontal cortex each project to distinct areas of the striatum. These striatal regions in turn project to subdivisions of the substantia nigra and globus pallidus. Nigral and pallidal structures project to discrete nuclei of the dorsomedial thalamic nuclei. The final limb of the circuit projects back to frontal cortex, as well as more widely to parietal and temporal regions (Cummings, 1998). Each frontal–subcortical circuit has both a direct and an indirect pathway. The indirect pathway projects from globus pallidus externa to the subthalamic nucleus and back to globus pallidus

interna before connecting to thalamic nuclei. The direct circuit projects from globus pallidus interna to medial thalamic regions. The dynamic balance between direct and indirect circuitry provides the basis for some types of motoric and behavioral disturbances emanating from disorders of one of the component pathways (Litvan, Paulsen, Mega, & Cummings, 1998).

Each of the frontal–subcortical circuits is relatively discrete, with communication between circuits occurring primarily at the level of the frontal cortex. This anatomical arrangement emphasizes the unique function of the frontal cortex as an integrator across functional complexes.

The principal pathways outlined here share common transmitters, as well as an overall common anatomical structure (while remaining largely discrete within those structures). Glutamate is the principal cortical transmitter, both from cortex to striatum, and from thalamus to cortex. The main excitatory transmitter within the circuits is also primarily glutamate, whereas the common inhibitory transmitter is $\gamma$-aminobutyric acid (GABA). These pathways receive modulating input from serotonergic and dopaminergic nuclei. In addition, cholinergic interneurons comprise a population within the striatal structures. Differential expression of receptor subtypes distinguishes among the frontal–subcortical circuits.

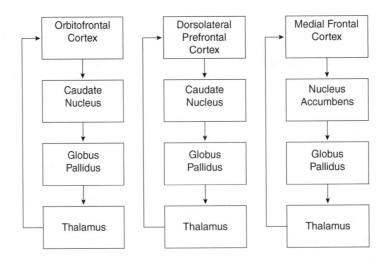

FIGURE 2.1.  Principal anatomic structures of frontal–subcortical circuits.

## MEDIAL FRONTAL CORTEX

The medial frontal cortex comprises the supplementary motor area and the anterior cingulate cortex. The anterior cingulate is intimately involved in motivated behavior, and the principal behavioral product of anterior cingulate dysfunction is an amotivational apathetic state. Apathy has several dimensions (Table 2.1). *Motoric apathy* is manifested by diminished motor activity, reduced gesturing, and diminished verbal output. *Cognitive apathy* is manifested by decreased curiosity and altered interest in learning, deducing, and drawing logical conclusions. *Affective apathy* includes diminished vocal inflection and reduced facial expression of internal emotional states. *Emotional apathy* is evidenced by reduced social interest, diminished affection, and compromised enthusiasm. *Motivational apathy* includes reduced initiation and poor maintenance of implemented activities. The independence and anatomical and neurobiological correlates of these different forms of apathy have not been determined.

Apathy occurs with degenerative, ischemic, neoplastic, and infectious conditions affecting the anterior cingulate cortex, nucleus accumbens, globus pallidus, thalamus, or connecting white matter tracts. Apathy is particularly striking in some patients with frontotemporal dementia, individuals with thalamic stroke, and persons with human immunodeficiency virus (HIV) encephalopathy.

## ORBITOFRONTAL CORTEX

The orbitofrontal cortex, particularly the right-hemispheric orbitofrontal regions, mediates the rules of social convention. Patients with orbitofrontal lesions are socially disabled, manifesting interpersonal disinhibition, poor social judgment, impulsive decision making, lack of consideration for the impact of their behavior, absence of an appreciation for the effect of their behavior or comments on others, and lack of empathy for others. This orbitofrontal syndrome has been labeled a "pseudopsychopathic" disorder, linking it to the sociopathic or psychopathic behavior exhibited by individuals with character disorders who manifest a disregard for accepted social conventions. Like individuals with sociopathy, patients with orbitofrontal syndromes may commit minor crimes, such as shoplifting, and may come to clinical attention through manifestations of criminal behavior (Miller, Darby, Benson, Cummings, & Miller, 1997). Other behaviors that frequently co-occur with the orbitofrontal disinhibition syndrome include apathy, restlessness, stereotypes, indifference, euphoria, disinterestedness, cheerfulness, diminished attention, dependence or hyperdependence on stimuli in the physical environment, planning disorders, and impairment of emotional control (Sarazin et al., 1998). When orbitofrontal injury is sustained in childhood, a similar behavioral complex emerges but, in addition, the patients exhibit defective social and moral reasoning (Anderson, Bechara, Damasio, Tranel, & Damasio, 1999). "Theory of mind" tests reveal that the ability to infer the mental state of others depends explicitly on right orbitofrontal function (Stuss, Gallupp, & Alexander, 2001). Orbitofrontal dysfunction is frequently apparent in individuals exhibiting the environmental dependence syndrome manifested by imitation and utilization behavior (Lhermitte, 1986; Lhermitte, Pillon, & Serdaru, 1986).

## DORSOLATERAL PREFRONTAL CORTEX AND EXECUTIVE FUNCTION

The dorsolateral prefrontal cortex is responsible for organizing a volitional response to environmental contingencies, recalling past events and planning current actions in a temporally informed manner, programming motor acts to follow volitional command, implementing programs to achieve the intended goal, monitoring the results of the action to determine the success of the intervention, and adjusting or stopping the action depending on the outcome of the assessment (Royall et al., 2002) (Figure 2.2). Each of these component processes is an

**TABLE 2.1. Components of the Apathetic Syndrome**

| |
|---|
| Motoric |
| Cognitive |
| Affective |
| Emotional |
| Motivational |

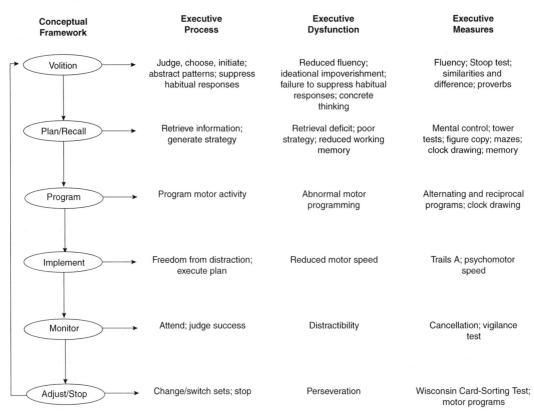

| Conceptual Framework | Executive Process | Executive Dysfunction | Executive Measures |
|---|---|---|---|
| Volition | Judge, choose, initiate; abstract patterns; suppress habitual responses | Reduced fluency; ideational impoverishment; failure to suppress habitual responses; concrete thinking | Fluency; Stoop test; similarities and difference; proverbs |
| Plan/Recall | Retrieve information; generate strategy | Retrieval deficit; poor strategy; reduced working memory | Mental control; tower tests; figure copy; mazes; clock drawing; memory |
| Program | Program motor activity | Abnormal motor programming | Alternating and reciprocal programs; clock drawing |
| Implement | Freedom from distraction; execute plan | Reduced motor speed | Trails A; psychomotor speed |
| Monitor | Attend; judge success | Distractibility | Cancellation; vigilance test |
| Adjust/Stop | Change/switch sets; stop | Perseveration | Wisconsin Card-Sorting Test; motor programs |

FIGURE 2.2. Components of frontal executive function abnormalities and relevant assessments.

executive process, and each may be impaired independently of the others. Thus, patients with executive dysfunction disorders may manifest any of a diverse array of clinical phenomena reflecting the complex organizational framework mediating executive function. Not all patients with frontal lobe or frontal–subcortical circuit disorders exhibit abnormalities in all executive function domains. Prefrontal functions are conceptualized as a nested series of hierarchical functions, with the first, lowest level involved in selecting motor actions and motor programs, the second providing contextual control and involved in selecting premotor representations contingent on external circumstances, and a third, episodic control level placing the volitional act in a temporally relevant and situationally informed context (Koechlin, Ody, & Kouneiher, 2003).

Executive function depends on the integrity of instrumental functions, such as language, memory, praxis, and visuospatial skills. One cannot abstract proverbs, a function that depends on assigning two meanings to language, in the presence of a primary language deficit. Likewise, the typical memory syndromes associated with prefrontal dysfunction, such as a retrieval deficit disorder, cannot be exhibited in the presence of a frank amnesia associated with temporal lobe dysfunction. Strategies associated with resolution of complex visuospatial challenges cannot be developed and applied in the absence of elementary visual perceptual and visuospatial functions. In the course of assessment, relative functional capacity of instrumental functions must be ensured before conclusions can be derived about the integrity of executive functions.

Many executive function tasks assess multiple types of executive processes. For example, the Wisconsin Card Sorting Test assesses both abstraction and preservation. The clock drawing task tests both visual strategy and freedom from distraction. Failure of a specific executive function task rarely implicates a single, unique executive process. Rules that apply to assessing frontal disorders are summarized in Table 2.2.

## TABLE 2.2. Observations Guiding the Assessment of Frontal Lobe Functions

- Executive function has many dimensions, including choosing, planning, programming, implementing, monitoring, and adjusting or ending a volitional act.
- Individual component processes of executive functions can be affected independently.
- Not all component processes are affected in patients with frontal lobe disorders simultaneously.
- Assessment of multiple component processes should be included in the evaluation of patients with a suspected frontal lobe dysfunction.
- Executive function depends on intact instrumental functions such as language, memory, praxis, perception, and visuospatial processing.
- Many tests of frontal lobe function simultaneously assess more than one component process.
- Executive function is synthetic, creative, and generative; the constrained and structured circumstances of many testing situations minimize the effects of frontal dysfunction.
- Executive functions, motivation, and social behavior depend on frontal–subcortial circuitry in addition to integrity of frontal cortex.
- "Frontal" disorders may occur with subcortical lesions (basal ganglia, thalamus) linked to frontal cortex through fontal–subcortical circuits.
- Three relatively distinct frontal lobe syndromes are recognized: An amotivational syndrome reflects dysfunction of the anterior cingulate and medial frontal cortex; disinhibition is associated with disturbances of the inferior frontal cortex; and executive dysfunction is associated with dysfunction of the dorsolateral prefrontal cortex.

## Component Procedures of Executive Function

### Volition

There are few pure tests of volition. Assessment of this domain is best accomplished by investigating the patient's insight and determining his or her understanding of the illness, disability, and likelihood of regaining employment status. Verbal fluency testing contains a generative intellectual component relevant to the assessment of volition. Patients must volitionally search their lexicon to identify members of a specific category, such as animals or words beginning with the letter "a."

Volitional activity demands the ability to suppress habitual responses in favor of novel activity, an ability tested by the Stroop Color–Word Test. This ability is critical to implementing programs in response to environmental contingencies (Peterson et al., 1999). Volition also requires abstraction of a pattern from the background. Abstraction is assessed by the Wisconsin Card Sorting Test and tests of similarities, differences, and proverb interpretation (Goldstein, Obrzut, John, Ledakis, & Armstrong, 2004; Rezai et al., 1993).

### Planning and Recalling

This component of executive function mediates development of a plan and puts it into a temporal context of previously accomplished activities. Assessments relevant to this executive function level include mental control tasks and the ability to hold the task in mind, such as reciting the months of the year in reverse order or spelling the word "world" backwards, tower tests that require extensive planning, complex figure copy tasks that require a sophisticated strategy to best accomplish the copy, maze tasks that require the patient to anticipate and plan maze moves, and a clock-drawing task that requires the patient to exhibit spatial planning (Royall, Cordes, & Polk, 1998). Memory functions rendered abnormal by prefrontal cortex dysfunction include problems retrieving information from semantic stores, impairments of temporal ordering, decrements of source memory (where or when something was learned), increased susceptibility to interference in the course of memory testing, compromised strategies for encoding and retrieval, impaired metamemory or insight into memory function, and increased rates of confabulatory and false memory responses (Wheeler, Stuss, & Tulving, 1995). Patients have difficulty retrieving remote memories, just as they do retrieving recent memories, and there is less of a recent–remote dissociation in frontally based retrieval deficit syndromes compared to temporally based amnestic disorders (Mangels, Gershberg, Shimamura, & Knight, 1996). Procedural or motor learning is impaired in patients with prefrontal lesions (Gomez Beldarrain, Grafman, Pascual-Leone, & Garcia-Monco, 1999).

### Motor Programs

Appropriate programming involves both selecting and implementing a program and resisting or inhibiting alternative responses. Commonly used motor program tests include alternating programs, reciprocal programs, and the go/no-go test.

### Implementation of Volitional Activity

The actual implementation phase of volitional activity is mediated by frontal motor cortex or, in the case of eye movements, by frontal eye fields. Relevant measures of motor activity include the Trail Making A test, the grooved pegboard test, and the finger-tapping test.

### Monitoring the Effects of Volitional Activity

A variety of vigilance and abstraction tasks are required to monitor the impact of a volitional effect. Cancellation tasks assess vigilance, as do digit span and continuous performance tasks.

### Adjusting and Stopping Volitional Activity

Adjusting and stopping volitional activity is as critical as implementing it. Perseveration is a commonly observed clinical phenomenon that represents an inability to stop an action appropriately. This is tested clinically with multiple loops or motor programming tasks, such as alternating programs. The Wisconsin Card Sorting Test and the Trail Making B Test also elicit perseverative behavior.

## BEDSIDE ASSESSMENT
## OF FRONTAL LOBE FUNCTION

Orbitofrontal, medial frontal, and some aspects of dorsolateral prefrontal dysfunction are best assessed by careful observation during the course of an interview. Is the patient disinhibited, impulsive, and tactless? Is the patient apathetic, agestural, and without motivation? Does the patient have poor judgment, failing to grasp the implications of his or her illness or disability?

Bedsides mental status testing can assess a substantial number of component executive processes. Lexical search strategies are assessed by verbal fluency; information and recall search is assessed through tests of recent and remote recall; strategy generation can be determined through complex figure copy tasks; mental control is assessed by asking the patient to repeat the months of the year in reverse order, to spell the word "world" backward, or to execute serial subtractions. Abstraction is assessed through interpretation of proverbs or derivation of the meaning of differences or similarities. Motor tasks include motor programming tasks such as go/no-go tasks and serial hand sequences. Freedom from distraction can be assessed by asking the patient to draw the face of a clock and set it for the time of 11:10. Vigilance and concentration are examined with a continuous performance test, and the ability to shift sets can be determined by asking the patient to perform oral trails (alternating between counting and reciting the alphabet).

In addition to these individual components of a bedside assessment of frontal lobe functions, several relevant rating scales and questionnaires have been developed and may assist in identifying and characterizing frontal lobe disorder. The EXIT-25, which provides a brief assessment of several component frontal executive functions, may be used in conjunction with the CLOX, a method of scoring clock drawing that emphasizes executive function (Royall et al., 1998). The Frontal Assessment Battery (FAB; Dubois, Slachevsky, Litvan, & Pillon, 2000) also assesses several processes relevant to frontal lobe function and has been shown to identify patients with frontal lobe syndromes. The Montreal Cognitive Assessment (MoCA; Nasreddine et al., 2005) is a 30-item cognitive assessment with an emphasis on evaluation of executive function.

Assessment of neuropsychiatric symptoms may assist in identifying patients with frontal lobe dysfunction. The Neuropsychiatric Inventory (NPI; Cummings et al., 1994) had been used to assess patients with frontotemporal degeneration, where it reveals a characteristic profile of disinhibition and euphoria (Levy, Miller, Cummings, Fairbanks, & Craig, 1996). The Frontal Systems Behavior Scale (Stout, Ready, Grace, Malloy, & Paulsen, 2003) includes ratings of apathy and disinhibition and measures of executive dysfunction, and is useful in assessment of patients with frontal lobe disorders.

## FUNCTIONAL IMAGING AND THE EXPLORATION OF FRONTALLY MEDIATED ABILITIES

Functional magnetic resonance imaging (fMRI) has emerged as a tool uniquely suited to explore aspects of frontal lobe function. In these assessments, an individual is challenged with a unique situation or test. Activation of a specific region of the frontal lobes in response to the challenge implies participation of that region in generating the response. This methodology has been successfully applied to the exploration of higher-order human cognitive functions. For example, regret has been shown to depend on the integrity of orbitofrontal cortex (Camille et al., 2004). Conflict monitoring has been ascribed by fMRI to the anterior cingulate, a concept consistent with the idea that absence of conflict monitoring would result in an apathetic syndrome (Kerns et al., 2004). Activation of the presupplementary motor area, as well as right dorsolateral prefrontal region was observed when patients paid attention to their volitional activity (Lau, Rogers, Haggard, & Passingham, 2004). Participation of the anterior cingulate cortex has been demonstrated in monitoring situations in which errors are likely to occur (Carter et al., 1998), and the orbitofrontal cortex was found to participate in reward-dependent activity in nonhuman primates (Roesch & Olson, 2004). This approach has been unusually valuable in linking regions of frontal cortex to specific behaviors.

## DIFFERENTIAL DIAGNOSIS OF CONDITIONS PREDOMINANTLY AFFECTING FRONTAL CORTICAL FUNCTION

A variety of neurological disorders can have disproportionate impact on frontal function (Table 2.3). Among vascular disorders, occlusion of the anterior cerebral artery produces an anterior cingulate syndrome, whereas occlusion of the superior branch of the middle cerebral artery affects dorsolateral prefrontal cortex. Rupture of anterior communicating artery aneurysms may produce orbitofrontal injury and a disinhibition syndrome. Frontal cortical degenerations likewise produce a prominent frontal disorder (Miller, Boone, Cummings, Read, & Mishkin, 2000).

**TABLE 2.3. Conditions Producing a Disproportionate Impact on Frontal and Frontal–Subcortical Function**

Vascular disorders
  Anterior cerebral artery occlusion
  Middle cerebral artery occlusion
  Anterior communicating artery aneurysm rupture
  Cerebrovascular disease affecting small vessels
Degenerative disorders
  Frontotemporal dementia
  Primary progressive aphasia
  Frontal variant of Alzheimer's disease
  Progressive supranuclear palsy
  Corticobasal degeneration
  Parkinson's disease
Multiple sclerosis
Infections
  Syphilis
  HIV infection
Traumatic brain injury
Brain neoplasms
  Butterfly gliomas
  Subfrontal meningiomas
Hydrocephalus

Frontotemporal dementia affecting primarily right anterior temporal or frontal structures produces a disinhibition syndrome, whereas asymmetric involvement of the left frontal cortex produces primary progressive aphasia. A frontal variant of Alzheimer's disease has been recognized, in which prominent frontal features co-occur with a typical amnestic type of memory disorder (Johnson, Head, Kim, Starr, & Cotman, 1999). Disorders of frontal–subcortical circuits, such as progressive supranuclear palsy and corticobasal degeneration, also produce a frontal-type syndrome. Demyelinating disorders, particularly multiple sclerosis, affecting frontal lobe white matter tracks can produce a prominent frontal-type syndrome. Traumatic brain injury not infrequently has disproportionate effects on the orbitofrontal cortex, resulting in an orbitofrontal disinhibition syndrome in the posttraumatic state. Syphilis and HIV are two examples of infectious disorders that can have disproportionate effects on frontal function. Patients with brain tumors, particularly butterfly gliomas involving the frontal lobes bilaterally, or subfrontal meningiomas that compress the orbitofrontal cortex from below, may present with prominent frontal lobe dysfunction. Obstructive hydrocephalus may produce a frontal-type syndrome.

## TREATMENT

Most disorders of the frontal lobe await discovery of disease-modifying treatments to ameliorate their impact on frontal function. Disease-specific therapies may be useful in ameliorating progression of stroke or multiple sclerosis affecting frontal lobe functions. Symptomatic treatments may sometimes provide useful relief of symptoms. Cholinesterase inhibitors have modest effects on executive dysfunction in Parkinson's disease dementia (Emre et al., 2004), and selective serotonin reuptake inhibitors may improve behavior in frontal degenerations (Swartz, Miller, Lesser, & Darby, 1997).

## REFERENCES

Alexander, M. P., Benson, D. F., & Stuss, D. T. (1989). Frontal lobes and language. *Brain and Language, 37,* 656–691.

Anderson, S. W., Bechara, A., Damasio, H., Tranel, D., & Damasio, A. R. (1999). Impairment of social and moral behavior related to early damage in human prefrontal cortex. *Nature Neuroscience, 2,* 1032–1037.

Camille, N., Coricelli, G., Sallet, J., Pradat-Diehl, P., Duhamel, J. R., & Sirigu, A. (2004). The involvement of the orbitofrontal cortex in the experience of regret. *Science, 304,* 1167–1170.

Carter, C. S., Braver, T. S., Barch, D. M., Botvinick, M. M., Noll, D., & Cohen, J. D. (1998). Anterior cingulate cortex, error detection, and the online monitoring of performance. *Science, 280,* 747–749.

Cummings, J. L. (1998). Frontal–subcortical circuits and human behavior. *Journal of Psychosomatic Research, 44,* 627–628.

Cummings, J. L., Mega, M., Gray, K., Rosenberg-Thompson, S., Carusi, D. A., & Gornbein, J. (1994). The Neuropsychiatric Inventory: Comprehensive assessment of psychopathology in dementia. *Neurology, 44,* 2308–2314.

Dubois, B., Slachevsky, A., Litvan, I., & Pillon, B. (2000). The FAB: A Frontal Assessment Battery at bedside. *Neurology, 55*(11), 1621–1626.

Emre, M., Aarsland, D., Albanese, A., Byrne, E. J., Deuschl, G., De Deyn, P. P., et al. (2004). Rivastigmine for dementia associated with Parkinson's disease. *New England Journal of Medicine, 351*(24), 2509–2518.

Goldstein, B., Obrzut, J. E., John, C., Ledakis, G., & Armstrong, C. L. (2004). The impact of frontal and non-frontal brain tumor lesions on Wisconsin Card Sorting Test performance. *Brain and Cognition, 54,* 110–116.

Gomez Beldarrain, M., Grafman, J., Pascual-Leone, A., & Garcia-Monco, J. C. (1999). Procedural learning is impaired in patients with prefrontal lesions. *Neurology, 52,* 1853–1860.

Johnson, J. K., Head, E., Kim, R., Starr, A., & Cotman, C. W. (1999). Clinical and pathological evidence for a frontal variant of Alzheimer's disease. *Archives of Neurology, 56,* 1233–1239.

Kerns, J. G., Cohen, J. D., MacDonald, A. W., III, Cho, R. Y., Stenger, V. A., & Carter, C. S. (2004). Anterior cingulate conflict monitoring and adjustments in control. *Science, 303,* 1023–1026.

Koechlin, E., Ody, C., & Kouneiher, F. (2003). The architecture of cognitive control in the human prefrontal cortex. *Science, 302,* 1181–1185.

Lau, H. C., Rogers, R. D., Haggard, P., & Passingham, R. E. (2004). Attention to intention. *Science, 303,* 1208–1210.

Levy, M. L., Miller, B. L., Cummings, J. L., Fairbanks, L. A., & Craig, A. (1996). Alzheimer disease and frontotemporal dementias: Behavioral distinctions. *Archives of Neurology, 53,* 687–690.

Lhermitte, F. (1986). Human autonomy and the frontal lobes: Part II. Patient behavior in complex and social situations: The "environmental dependency syndrome." *Annals of Neurology, 19,* 335–343.

Lhermitte, F., Pillon, B., & Serdaru, M. (1986). Human autonomy and the frontal lobes: Part I. Imitation and utilization behavior: A neuropsychological study of 75 patients. *Annals of Neurology, 19,* 326–334.

Litvan, I., Paulsen, J. S., Mega, M. S., & Cummings, L. (1998). Neuropsychiatric assessment of patients with hyperkinetic and hypokinetic movement disorders. *Archives of Neurology, 55,* 1313–1319.

Mangels, J. A., Gershberg, F. B., Shimamura, A. P., & Knight, R. T. (1996). Impaired retrieval from remote memory in patients with frontal lobe damage. *Neuropsychology, 10,* 32–41.

Miller, B. L., Boone, K., Cummings, J. L., Read, S. L., & Mishkin, F. (2000). Functional correlates of musical and visual ability in frontotemporal dementia. *British Journal of Psychiatry, 176,* 458–463.

Miller, B. L., Darby, A., Benson, D. F., Cummings, J. L., & Miller, M. H. (1997). Agressive, socially, disruptive and antisocial behavior associated with frontotemporal dementia. *British Journal of Psychiatry, 170,* 150–155.

Nasreddine, Z. S., Phillips, N. A., Bedirian, V., Charbonneau, S., Whitehead, V., Collin, I., et al. (2005). The Montreal Cognitive Assessment, MoCA: A brief screening tool for mild cognitive impairment. *Journal of the American Geriatric Society, 53,* 695–699.

Peterson, B. S., Skudlarski, P., Gatenby, J. C., Zhang, H., Anderson, A. W., & Gore, J. C. (1999). An fMRI study of Stroop word–color interference: Evidence for cingulate subregions subserving multiple distributed attentional systems. *Biological Psychiatry, 45,* 1237–1258.

Rezai, K., Andreasen, N. C., Alliger, R., Cohen, G.,

Swayze, V., II, & O'Leary, D. S. (1993). The neuropsychology of the prefrontal cortex. *Archives of Neurology, 50,* 636–642.

Roesch, M. R., & Olson, C. R. (2004). Neuronal activity related to reward value and motivation in primate frontal cortex. *Science, 304,* 307–310.

Royall, D. R., Cordes, J. A., & Polk, M. (1998). CLOX: An executive clock drawing task. *Journal of Neurology, Neurosurgery, and Psychiatry, 64,* 588–594.

Royall, D. R., Lauterbach, E. C., Cummings, J. L., Reeve, A., Rummans, T. A., Kaufer, D. I., et al. (2002). Executive control function: A review of its promise and challenges for clinical research [Report from the Committee on Research of the American Neuropsychiatric Association]. *Journal of Neuropsychiatry and Clinical Neurosciences, 14,* 377–405.

Sarazin, M., Pillon, B., Giannakopoulos, P., Rancurel, G., Samson, Y., & Dubois, B. (1998). Clinico-metabolic dissociation of cognitive functions and social behavior in frontal lobe lesions. *Neurology, 51,* 142–148.

Stout, J. C., Ready, R. E., Grace, J., Malloy, P. F., & Paulsen, J. S. (2003). Factor analysis of the Frontal Systems Behavior Scale (FrSBe). *Assessment, 10,* 79–85.

Stuss, D. T., Gallup, G. G., Jr., & Alexander, M. P. (2001). The frontal lobes are necessary for "theory of mind." *Brain, 124,* 279–286.

Swartz, J. R., Miller, B. L., Lesser, I. M., & Darby, A. L. (1997). Frontotemporal dementia: treatment response to serotonin selective reuptake inhibitors. *Journal of Clinical Psychiatry, 58,* 212–216.

Wheeler, M. A., Stuss, D. T., & Tulving, E. (1995). Frontal lobe damage produces episodic memory impairment. *Journal of the International Neuropsychological Society, 1,* 525–536.

# PART II

## ANATOMY

# CHAPTER 3

# Frontal–Subcortical Circuits

*Tiffany W. Chow*
*Jeffrey L. Cummings*

Frontal–subcortical circuits (FSCs) incorporate complex input from the central nervous system to modulate the expression of cognition and emotion through behavior and movement. Alexander, DeLong, and Strick (1986) used the concept of the motor thalamocortical circuit as an architectural template to build the concept of other FSCs. Their description of five cortically anchored circuits provided a basis for subsequent elucidation of how those circuits influence behavior and movement. This chapter presents the clinical neuropsychiatric syndromes associated with disturbances of these circuits. These FSCs include those behaviorally relevant circuits originating in dorsolateral prefrontal, superior medial frontal, and orbitofrontal cortices. In addition, there are important roles for inferotemporal and posterior parietal cortical regions via open connections to these circuits.

This chapter begins with an orientation to features shared by all FSCs. We describe the balanced inhibitory and excitatory influences that modulate cortical activation within each circuit. Each circuit has a direct pathway that generally enhances cortical activity; there is also a mechanism for inhibition within each circuit via an indirect pathway. The manifestations of direct or indirect pathway dominance allow a wide repertoire of adaptive responses to shifting internal priorities or external environmental stimuli. The manifestation of a particular neuropsychiatric symptom can reflect a loss of the balancing mechanism within one

or more FSCs. After introducing the generic neuroanatomy and connectivity of the circuits, this chapter presents cognitive and behavioral functions of the FSCs. The following section describes the impact of clinical neuropsychiatric syndromes on the cognitive, behavioral, and motor FSCs. Subsequent chapters of this book detail further the assessment of FSC function.

## THE FSC PROTOTYPE

### Shared Anatomy and Neurochemistry of the FSCs

As illustrated in Figure 3.1, FSCs share a common template of topography and physiology. Each circuit enjoins the same member structures, but the circuits are arranged in parallel, largely segregated from each other. The relative

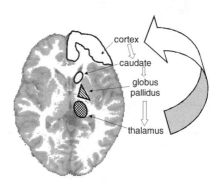

FIGURE 3.1. Basic structural template for the FSCs.

25

**TABLE 3.1. Neurotransmitters and Neuropeptides of the FSCs**

| | |
|---|---|
| Glutamate | Enkephalin |
| GABA | Neurotensin |
| Dopamine | Substance P |
| Acetylcholine | Dynorphin |
| Serotonin | Adenosine |
| Norepinephrine | Neuropeptide Y |

anatomical positions of the circuits are preserved as they pass through striatum (caudate and putamen), globus pallidus, substantia nigra, and thalamus (Mega & Cummings, 1994). In addition to sharing anatomical components, each circuit makes use of the same neurotransmitters and neuropeptides, although the distribution of neuroreceptor subtypes might mediate different activations for each circuit (see Table 3.1). Figures 3.2 to 3.5 show the cortical areas involved in FSCs; although these figures illustrate one cerebral hemisphere, the FSCs are present bilaterally.

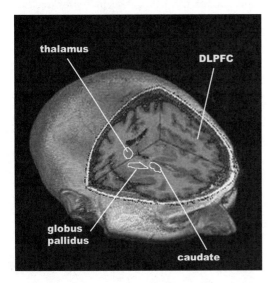

FIGURE 3.2. Dorsolateral prefrontal–subcortical circuit. Brodmann's areas 9 and 46 from DLPFC serve as the origins. Each of these BAs has a dorsal and ventral stream by which it relays to the dorsal aspect of the head of the caudate. These four subcircuits continue to specific regions within GPi and/or the substantia nigra (not shown). From those destinations, the circuit proceeds to ventroanterior, ventrolateral, or dorsomedial thalamic nuclei before returning to the cortical origins (Middleton & Strick, 2000).

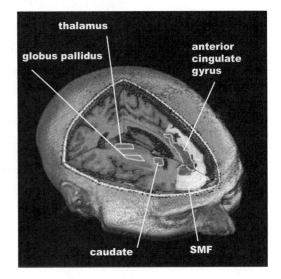

FIGURE 3.3. The superior medial FSC. Input travels from neurons of the anterior cingulate and other superior medial frontal (SMF) regions to the ventral striatum, which includes the ventromedial caudate, ventral putamen, nucleus accumbens, and the olfactory tubercle (Middleton & Strick, 2000; Selemon & Goldman-Rakic, 1985). Projections then innervate areas of the globus pallidus and substantia nigra (not shown). This FSC continues to the ventroanterior and dorsomedial nuclei of the thalamus and closes with projections back to cortex (Middleton & Strick, 2000).

Each FSC has a direct pathway that results in sustained activation of the cortical component. Cortical projections release glutamate (GLU) to the corresponding regions of the striatum, which usually includes the caudate nucleus; some FSCs involve the putamen or ventral striatum, which consists mainly of the nucleus accumbens. Binding of GLU at N-methyl-D-aspartate receptors in the striatum triggers release of γ-aminobutyric acid (GABA) at the internal segment of the globus pallidus interna (GPi) and substantia nigra. This diminishes GABA release from the GPi to the thalamic component of the circuit. The disinhibited thalamus then enhances glutamatergic excitation of cortical regions.

There is also an indirect pathway for each circuit to balance the direct pathway. The indirect pathway diverges from the direct pathway when striatal efferents project to the globus pallidus externa (GPe). GABA-ergic pallidal fi-

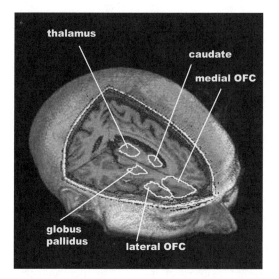

FIGURE 3.4. Lateral and medial orbitofrontal–sub-cortical circuits. The lateral OFC (lateral and or-bital aspects of Brodmann's area 12) connects as two subcircuits with ventromedial caudate, then medial GPi and substantia nigra (not shown), then dorsomedial and ventroanterior thalamic nuclei, before returning to lateral OFC. The medial OFC begins from Brodmann's area 13 and insular transitional cortex, projecting to the ven-tromedial caudate, similar to the lateral orbito-frontal circuit, but also with projections to the ventral striatum similar to the superior medial FSC. The next destination of the medial OFC subcircuits is ventral pallidum and substantia nigra (not shown). Thalamic nuclei for this circuit include ventroanterior, dorsomedial, and ventro-lateral.

bers extend to the subthalamic nucleus, which then stimulates the GPi of the direct pathway with GLU. This glutamatergic influence on the GPi counterbalances the direct pathway's GABA-ergic input at the GPi, which would otherwise lead to inhibition of cortical activa-tion via the thalamus.

The direct pathway of the circuit disinhibits the thalamus, whereas the indirect pathway in-hibits it. The relative influences of the direct and indirect pathways determine the control of the thalamocortical connections and the motor, cognitive, or behavioral output of the circuit. Both pathways begin with excitatory, gluta-matergic projections from the frontal cortex to specific areas within the striatum. Striatal out-put neurons then project to either GPi or Gpe

to the direct or the indirect pathway, respec-tively.

The direct and indirect pathways diverge in neuroanatomical connectivity at the cytoarchi-tectural level. The division of striatal neurons into striosomes and matrix allows for the bifur-cation of circuits to direct and indirect path-ways. Both striosomes and matrix produce GABA, but striosomes project onward to GPi (the direct pathway), and the matrix efferents take the other route (indirect pathway), pro-jecting to GPe. The pathways also differ in neuroreceptors expressed: The striosomal di-rect pathway features dopamine type 1 recep-tors, whereas the matrix indirect pathway has dopamine type 2 receptors.

Several neurotransmitters and neuropeptides have impacts on the cortex, striatum, and glo-bus pallidus within the FSCs. Neurotransmit-ters and neuropeptides with effects on the FSCs are listed in Table 3.1. Neurotransmitter influ-ences on the circuits are complex. No single neurotransmitter has one simple role in activat-ing or inhibiting a given circuit. The heteroge-neity of receptors for each neurotransmitter (e.g., at least five dopamine receptor families have been described) and different localization of these receptors on components of the circuit

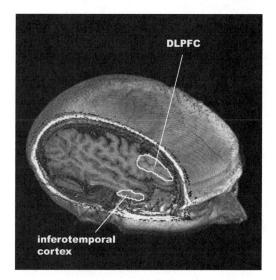

FIGURE 3.5. Lateral view of cortical contributions to DLPFC and inferotemporal subcortical circuit. The inferotemporal circuit echoes the FSC's corti-cal connectivity to basal ganglia with reflection back to via thalamus for modulation of cortical visuomotor processing (see Table 3.2).

make it difficult to predict the outcome of activating a single neurotransmitter receptor. Circuit physiology also enjoys a reputation for plasticity that reflects shifts in pre- and postsynaptic neuroreceptor activation. Neurotransmitters also affect one another; for example, cholinergic agonism can enhance dopamine release in the striatum. Pharmacological manipulations of the FSCs are therefore challenging, because benefits in one axis of behavior, cognition, or motor function may bear undesirable effects in another. A classic example is the production of extrapyramidal rigidity when dopamine receptor blockade is used to treat psychosis.

## FSC Connections

Each FSC has three orders of connectivity: (1) connections within each circuit's direct and indirect pathways, (2) corticocortical connections with the other circuits, and (3) open connections to areas outside the FSCs (see Figure 3.6). Open elements of the circuits relate systematically to brain regions that mediate related functions and have similar phylogenetic origins to the FSC. Neuroanatomical structures with which the circuits share open connections are more easily understood in the context of the clinical syndromes specific to each circuit and are discussed below.

## BEHAVIORALLY RELEVANT FSCs

Lesion studies and functional neuroimaging reveal the roles of the FSCs in cognition, motivation, affect, and motor control. Classically, three FSCs were linked to executive dysfunction, akinetic mutism, and disinhibition; more recent neuropsychological and neuroimaging studies have confirmed major roles for the dorsolateral prefrontal (DLPFC), superior medial frontal (formerly known as anterior cingulate), and medial orbitofrontal–subcortical (OFC) circuits, as well as a contribut-

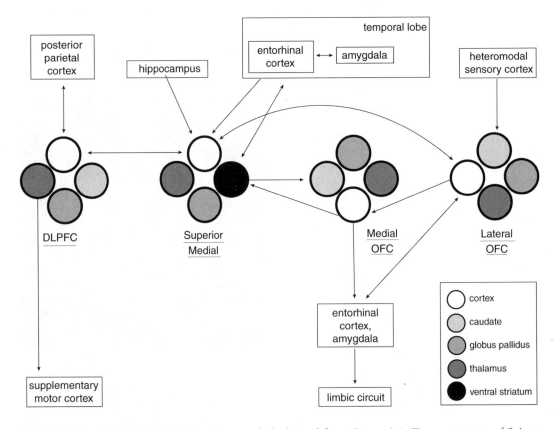

FIGURE 3.6. Connectivity of the FSCs, using symbols derived from Figure 3.1. Figure courtesy of Sajung Yun.

## Executive Functions

Examples of executive activities include the ability to organize a behavioral response to solve a complex problem (e.g., learning new information, copying complicated figures), systematically searching memory, activation of remote memories, appropriate prioritization of external stimuli, attention, generation of motor programs, and use of verbal skills to guide behavior. As described in more detail by Stuss (Chapter 19, this volume), basic working processes for these activities include (1) task setting, (2) initiation of the task, (3) detecting error, and (4) behavioral self-regulating functions.

These processes are modulated by more than one FSC. Superior medial cortex includes the anterior cingulate gyri. Task setting correlates with activity in the left DLPFC, whereas error detection correlates with right DLPFC activation (Stuss, Binns, Murphy, & Alexander, 2002). The laterality of DLPFC FSC contributions to cognition highlights the presence of FSC connectivity in both hemispheres, with the potential for differentiation between hemispheres. Initiation of a new task involves both left and right superior medial frontal FSCs (Stuss, Floden, Alexander, Levine, & Katz, 2001). Behavioral self-regulation can be defective after disruption of the medial OFC circuit. Impulsivity can cause difficulty with executive function by enhancing distractibility and impairing prioritization of external stimuli.

The separation of executive function into basic processes helps to explain how lesions in different frontal areas can cause a patient to do poorly on tests of executive function, such as the Wisconsin Card Sorting Test (WCST), while performing adequately on other tests. Errors may be made to different degrees and for different reasons, based on the type and number of FSCs disrupted. For example, an individual may show impairment on the WCST because of slowed response time after resection of a butterfly glioma that intruded upon superior medial frontal cortex. Another individual with a lesion to the left DLPFC may have no difficulty initiating a response but will make multiple errors due to faulty task setting whenever

the examiner shifts the rules for matching the cards (e.g., matching by color instead of shape). A third individual who has suffered a hemorrhagic infarct in the left head of the caudate nucleus, disrupting both the superior medial frontal and DLPFC FSCs, would show marked impairment on the WCST in slow processing time and perseverative errors.

Four of the FSCs and their open connections therefore contribute to executive function. Brain lesions outside of the FSC proper may cause FSC dysfunction if they affect open connections. Posterior parietal Brodmann's area (BA) 7a is richly interconnected to prefrontal BA 46 of the DLPFC (Yeterian & Pandya, 1993). BA 7a participates in visual processing, attending to significant visual stimuli, visually guided reaching, and planning visuospatial strategies. This is distinct from the inferotemporal subcortical circuit, which contributes input to the motor FSC (see Table 3.2).

The number of FSCs disrupted will change behavior. The exact location of a lesion along the FSC may also determine the type of cognitive impairment that results. Lesions of the dorsolateral cortex and caudate nucleus result in poor recall, with relative preservation of recognition abilities (Butters, Wolfe, Granholm, & Martone, 1986), whereas further along the circuit, thalamic lesions produce impairment of both recall and recognition (Stuss, Guberman, Nelson, & Larochelle, 1988). Lesions in the thalamus usually combine the amnesia of medial limbic dysfunction and executive impairment (Deymeer, Smith, DeGirolami, & Drachman, 1989; Eslinger, Warner, Grattan, & Easton, 1991; Stuss et al., 1988), because the thalamus is poised at the intersection of the FSCs, with the limbic circuit comprised of the hippocampus, fornix, and hypothalamus.

We present the functional neuroimaging findings that support these linkages in the context of circuit-related neuropsychiatric syndromes later in this chapter.

## Motivational Function

Akinetic mutism occurs with bilateral lesions of the anterior cingulate cortex (Barris & Schuman, 1953; Fesenmeier, Kuzniecky, & Garcia, 1990; Nielsen & Jacobs, 1951). With bilateral lesions, patients are profoundly apathetic or abulic; rarely moving, they are incontinent, eat and drink only when fed, and may have speech limited to monosyllabic responses

**TABLE 3.2. Symptoms of Neuropsychiatric Syndromes That Relate to FSCs**

| | DLPFC | Superior medial FSC | Lateral OFC | Medial OFC | Inferotemporal subcortical circuit |
|---|---|---|---|---|---|
| Dementia | Impaired task setting and monitoring, depression | Apathy, amotivational syndrome, depression | Irritability, obsessive–compulsive features | Loss of empathy and social skills | Impaired visual discrimination, visual hallucinations |
| Primary psychiatric disorders | Impaired task setting and monitoring, depression, mania (psychosis?) | Apathy, amotivational syndrome, depression, mania, agitation | Depression, obsessive–compulsive disorder, Klüver–Bucy syndrome | Loss of empathy and social skills, mood instability | Psychosis, visual hallucinations |
| Movement disorders | Impaired task setting and monitoring, depression | Apathy, amotivational syndrome, depression | Irritability, obsessive–compulsive features | Visual hallucinations (usually iatrogenic) | |
| Vasculitis, encephalitis | Impaired task setting and monitoring, depression | Apathy, amotivational syndrome, depression | Irritability, obsessive–compulsive features | Loss of empathy and social skills, mood instability | Impaired visual discrimination, visual hallucinations |

to others' questions. Displaying no response to pain or emotions, patients show complete indifference to their circumstances. Unilateral lesions produce less dramatic apathetic syndromes, including transient akinetic mutism (Damasio & Damasio, 1989). Patients also experience a diminished ability to conceive new thoughts or participate in creative thought processes. Lesions outside the anterior cingulate gyrus but within other areas of the superior medial frontal cortex (e.g., the supplementary motor area) and its subcortical circuit can also cause difficulty in task initiation or motivation to continue the task to completion (Bechara & Van der Kooy, 1989). The superior medial FSC has open connections with the limbic and hippocampal systems: It receives afferents from the entorhinal cortex, the perirhinal area, and the hippocampus (see Figure 3.6). The amygdala also contributes to the superior medial FSC as a minor open afferent. Whereas the superior medial FSC is the externally directed arm of the limbic system, enabling the intentional selection of environmental stimuli based on the internal relevance of those stimuli for the organism, the OFC is phylogenetically older and involved with the internal state of the organism. For its part, the medial OFC circuit

relays its prioritization of internal drives (aversive, appetitive) to the superior medial FSC (Mega & Cummings, 1994). As shown in Figure 3.6, the superior medial FSC has an afferent connection from the medial OFC circuit to the ventral striatum. There also are opportunities for mutual influences between these FSCs in their connections to amygdala and entorhinal cortex. These convergences may relate to the anhedonia, apathy, and psychomotor retardation seen in depressive states.

Akinetic mutism has occurred in the context of midline pathology due to craniopharyngiomas and neoplasms of the third ventricle, resulting in obstructive hydrocephalus. Apathy occurs as a component of many neuropsychiatric syndromes (listed later in this chapter).

### Dysregulation of Affect and Social Behavior

In general, the two OFCs (medial and lateral) mediate empathic, civil, and socially appropriate behavior. An individual's patterned set of social behaviors defines his or her personality to others, and personality change is the hallmark of orbitofrontal dysfunction (Damasio, Grabowski, Frank, Galaburda, & Damasio, 1994). (See also Rankin, Chapter 23, this volume.) Patients with lesions of the OFC, often from traumatic brain injury, may develop irritability, lability, tactlessness, and fatuous euphoria (Bogousslavsky & Regli, 1990; Hunter, Blackwood, & Bull, 1968; Logue, Durward, Pratt, Piercy, & Nixon, 1968). Patients do not respond appropriately to social cues, show undue familiarity, and cannot empathize with the feelings of others. Enslavement to environmental cues, exemplified by utilization behavior (inappropriate automatic use of tools and utensils in the patient's environment), and automatic imitation of the gestures and actions of others may occur with large lesions (Cummings, 1993; Lhermitte, Pillon, & Serdaru, 1986). Patients with primarily orbitofrontal dysfunction may perform card-sorting tasks normally (Laiacona et al., 1989; Stuss et al., 2000). As described earlier in the section on executive functions, this would reflect intact DLPFC and superior medial FSCs. Behavioral changes similar to those of patients with OFC lesions are evident in patients with dysfunction of the subcortical structures of the orbitofrontal–subcortical circuit, including patients with Huntington's disease (caudate abnormalities) and manganese intoxication (globus pallidus lesions) (Folstein, 1989; Mena et al., 1967).

The medial and lateral OFC circuits play distinct but complementary roles in affect and social behavior. Both the medial and lateral OFC circuits mediate the individual's affect, impulse control, and recognition of reinforcing stimuli. Lesions in either OFC can result in emotional incontinence and disinhibition, but individuals with these lesions manifest impairments differently. A patient with an impaired medial OFC shows abnormal autonomic responses to socially meaningful stimuli and has difficulty extinguishing unreinforced behavior. These characteristics correlate with antisocial behavior.

The medial OFC includes structures of the prototypical FSC, along with the ventral striatum. The medial OFC has open connections with limbic and paralimbic regions (see Figure 3.6). Paralimbic input merges with the medial OFC at the ventral striatum (Nauta, 1979; Zald & Kim, 1996a). The ventral striatum itself receives projections from the basolateral nucleus of the amygdala, entorhinal cortex, perirhinal cortex, and temporal lobe (Zald & Kim, 1996a) (see Figure 3.6). The ventral striatum is also a major recipient of efferents from the superior medial FSC, po-

tentially explaining the co-occurrence of amotivational syndromes with symptoms of medial OFC disruption.

The medial OFC constitutes the only major efferent prefrontal projection to entorhinal cortex (Van Hoesen, Pandya, & Butters, 1975), which may influence memory. The clinical characteristics of patients with medial OFC lesions imply failure to assign emotional valence to an event, which would otherwise facilitate episodic memory or learning. The superior medial FSC also has connections with entorhinal cortex and the amygdala (see Figure 3.6).

In addition to its singular relationship with entorhinal cortex, the medial OFC possesses the strongest reciprocal association with the amygdala of the FSCs (Zald & Kim, 1996a). Because the amygdala is also the major source of efferents to the brainstem and hypothalamus, emotional processing by the medial OFC impacts a spectrum of endocrine, autonomic, and involuntary behavioral responses (Amaral, Price, Pitkaenen, & Carmichael, 1992). An example of this type of response is abnormally diffident skin galvanometry in patients with medial OFC lesions when they view affective stimuli (Critchley, Elliott, Mathias, & Dolan, 2000). The medial OFC sends unreciprocated efferents to other limbic structures, which further amplify its role in regulating visceral responses to stimuli via the olfactory-centered paralimbic belt (Mesulam, 1985; Nauta, 1971, 1973).

In contrast to patients with a medial OFC circuit dysfunction, a patient with a lateral OFC lesion is more likely to show irritability, mood disorders, utilization behaviors, undue familiarity with strangers, imitation behavior, and acquired obsessive–compulsive disorder (OCD) (Berthier, Kulisevsky, Gironell, & Heras, 1996). The lateral OFC has a corticocortical connection with the medial OFC and open connections with the superior temporal gyrus and the inferotemporal gyrus (see Figure 3.6). The inferotemporal subcortical circuit is important to the integration of visual discrimination with visuomotor associations. This may bear upon the utilization and imitative behaviors that arise after a lesion to the lateral OFC.

Other important lateral OFC open connections involve projections to its caudate component from heteromodal sensory cortex (Zald & Kim, 1996a). Here, information from every sensory modality (olfactory, gustatory, visual, auditory, somatosensory), preprocessed by heteromodal areas of the temporal pole and insula, can be integrated with lateral OFC efferents (Chavis & Pandya, 1976; Jones & Powell, 1970; Mesulam & Mufson, 1982a, 1982b). Whereas the medial OFC has an efferent role for visceral function via the autonomic system, the lateral OFC receives afferents monitoring visceral stimuli.

Disruption of each of the four behaviorally relevant FSCs leads to recognizable clinical signs and syndromes described earlier. A disease process may affect more than one FSC to produce a complex neuropsychiatric syndrome (see Table 3.2). The following section describes how neuropsychiatric syndromes manifest as combinations of deficits in executive function, motivation, affect and social behavior, and motor control.

## CLINICAL SYNDROMES

### Neuropsychiatric Syndromes Affecting Executive Function

Executive dysfunction is a hallmark feature of neurodegenerative dementias that affect the basal ganglia. Neurodegenerative disorders with tauopathy seem especially prone to manifest with signs of FSC disruption (Cummings, 2003). Examples of tauopathies include progressive supranuclear palsy, frontotemporal degeneration, and Alzheimer's disease (AD). Progressive supranuclear palsy is described below with other hypokinetic movement disorders.

Frontotemporal degeneration (FTD) is an early-onset (mean age at onset is approximately 55) dementia characterized by regional atrophy in frontal and/or temporal lobes. Consensus criteria highlight loss of empathy, social awareness, concern for personal hygiene, and frontal executive function (Neary et al., 1998); patients also develop new preference for sweets and obsessive–compulsive behaviors (Wang & Miller, Chapter 24, this volume). FTD studies report lateralized neuropsychiatric sequelae. Right-sided atrophy in FTD patients most commonly presents first with disinhibition. Aprosodia, mania, bizarre affect, and OCD are other features. In contrast, left-dominant FTD manifests predominantly with aphasia (at least anomia). In addition, patients with right-sided behavioral presentation of FTD demonstrate more impaired task monitoring on the WCST, whereas the patients with more degenerative changes on the left have more difficulty with

Stroop word reading and color naming (task setting) (Boone et al., 1999). FTD has served as a revealing model of the consequences of asymmetric disruption to FSCs.

AD is the most common dementia among persons over the age of 65 years. Although patients most frequently complain of short-term memory loss and anomia, retrieval memory deficits and frontal dysexecutive syndrome may also be apparent as early features on formal neuropsychological testing. Despite the more posterior cerebral involvement of AD at presentation, global cognitive decline proceeds. Cortical atrophy involves frontal regions paralleling the cognitive decline. Cortical regions outside of the frontal lobe that contribute to open connections also impact the function of these FSCs.

Several movement disorders affect both neurobehavioral and motor FSCs, specifically through debilitation of the basal ganglia and the substantia nigra. Patients with Parkinson's disease (PD) with dementia characteristically manifest long response latency, apathy or depressed mood, retrieval-type memory deficits, and motor abnormalities, typically including dysarthria and gait disturbance (Albert, Feldman, & Willis, 1974; Cummings, 1990). Loss of dopaminergic neurons from the substantia nigra has long been associated with the pathogenesis of PD. The substantia nigra contributes to the direct pathway for all FSCs, which could explain the constellation of impairments that involve not only the motor FSC but also neurobehavioral FSCs.

Functional magnetic resonance imaging (fMRI) studies for PD have examined both dopamine function and cortical metabolic activity. Imaging techniques that specifically focus on markers of dopaminergic function indicate that the DLPFC is impaired at the level of the caudate nucleus (Carbon et al., 2004). In addition, fluoro-deoxyglucose positron emission tomography (FDG-PET) studies on patients with PD reveal a correlation between dysexecutive function and hypometabolism in the left DLPFC (Lozza et al., 2004; Nagano-Saito et al., 2004).

Surgical treatment of PD with pallidotomy (lesioning of the GPi) can result in lateralized executive dysfunction: A more rostral left pallidotomy could impair verbal memory and verbal fluency (Green & Barnhart, 2000; Lombardi et al., 2000; Masterman et al., 1998; Stebbins, Gabrieli, Shannon, Penn, & Goetz,

2000; Trepanier, Saint-Cyr, Lozano, & Lang, 1998), whereas a right pallidotomy could disrupt visuospatial function (Trepanier et al., 1998).

Other hypokinetic movement disorders affecting cognitive and motor function through the FSCs include corticobasal degeneration (CBD) and progressive supranuclear palsy (PSP). CBD shares many features with FTD, such as frontal executive impairment, anomia, obsessive–compulsive behaviors and disinhibition (Boeve, Lang, & Litvan, 2003). In addition, though, there is impairment of visuospatial skills and cortical sensation that correlates with degenerative changes in the parietal region ipsilateral to the subcortical lesions. Patients with CBD are not as perseverative as those with PSP (Boeve et al., 2003).

Hyperkinetic movement disorders also can cause executive dysfunction. Huntington's disease and Tourette's syndrome are hyperkinetic movement disorders caused by basal ganglia pathology. Patients with these movement disorders frequently have impaired executive function. Huntington's disease and Tourette's syndrome are detailed in a later section in this chapter on affect and social behavior.

Some psychiatric disorders are accompanied by executive dysfunction. Psychosis is a circuit-related behavior. Neuropsychological testing of patients with schizophrenia reveals impairment of stimulus prioritization to the same degree as that in patients who have lesions along the DLPFC (Braff & Beyer, 1990; Grebb, Weinberger, & Wyatt, 1992; Swerdlow & Koob, 1990). PET studies using fluoro-L-dopa as a tracer demonstrate transient increased binding in the striatum of patients with schizophrenia or with psychosis secondary to temporal lobe epilepsy. Reith and colleagues (1994) hypothesize that this indicates dopamine receptor upregulation in response to frontal cortical insufficiency. It is not yet clear whether this explains the dysexecutive syndrome seen in schizophrenia.

Depression in different contexts has variable neuroanatomical correlates. Structural neuroimaging of patients with major depressive disorder can reveal atrophy in frontal and temporal lobes relative to nondepressed control subjects, but functional imaging with FDG-PET indicates more specific localization of structures that correlate with active symptoms of depression. FDG-PET studies of primary depression reveal decreased metabolism in the dorsolateral prefrontal cortex and the caudate nucleus (Baxter et al., 1989). In addition, positive antidepressant response to the selective serotonergic reuptake inhibitor, fluoxetine, has been accompanied by decreases in FDG-PET signal in the subgenual cingulate gyrus, anterior and posterior cingulate, and the DLPFC (Mayberg et al., 2000). Depression is also closely linked with lesions of the temporal lobes; thus, the disorder is not circuit-specific (Cummings, 1993; Irle, Peper, Wowra, & Kunze, 1994; Mayberg, 1994).

Secondary depression has been linked to lesions in two structures of the FSCs: the frontal cortex and the caudate nucleus. Stroke in the dorsolateral prefrontal area can manifest with depression and anxiety (Folstein, 1989; Robinson & Starkstein, 1990; Starkstein, Cohen, et al., 1990). Lesion analysis shows that caudate dysfunction from stroke and basal ganglia disorders can also result in depression.

Core clinical features for the diagnosis of attention deficit disorder include inattentiveness and impulsivity. Additional hyperactivity may be present. Patients with attention-deficit/hyperactivity disorder (ADHD) have difficulty maintaining concentration and staying on task. Structural MRI findings in ADHD have been contradictory in terms of right versus left laterality, but most studies report atrophy in at least one caudate nucleus (Hale, Hariri, & McCracken, 2000).

Symptoms of ADHD may be relieved with psychostimulants. Structural MRI in this population has more consistently predicted therapeutic response than it has clarified pathophysiology: Those patients with smaller and more symmetrical caudate nuclei and left frontal cortex atrophy are more likely to respond to psychostimulants (Rilipek et al., 1997). The separation by imaging of responders and nonresponders indicates that heterogeneous brain changes can lead to similar clinical presentations. fMRI, on the other hand, has yielded more information about relative inactivity of FSCs in ADHD that would indicate pathological dominance of the indirect pathway. FDG-PET reveals diffuse hypometabolism across DLPFC, superior medial, and posterior frontal regions in untreated hyperactive adults (Zametkin et al., 1990). It is not yet clear whether the pathogenesis begins at the cortical or subcortical level in ADHD, but responders to methylphenidate show related posttreatment increases in both frontal and striatal activation on fMRI (Vaidya et al., 1998).

Disruption of the FSCs is not necessarily the etiology of autism, but patients with autism show impairment in executive function and attention (Courchesne et al., 1994; Ozonoff, Strayer, McMahon, & Filloux, 1994). These findings, along with structural imaging studies, indicate at least an association between frontal system dysfunction and autism (Minshew, 1997).

## Neuropsychiatric Syndromes Affecting Motivation

Neurodegenerative dementias and the movement disorders listed earlier also cause apathy. Severe apathy in AD correlates with cortical cerebral blood flow deficits in DLPFC, OFC, and anterior temporal regions (Craig et al., 1996). Apathy in AD also correlates with the degree of neurofibrillary tangle pathology in the left anterior cingulate region (Tekin et al., 2001). Apathy is not specific to AD; in the form of loss of empathy, it is one of the consensus criteria for the clinical diagnosis of FTD (Neary et al., 1998). Volumetric MRI analyses reveal atrophy in anterior cingulate and orbitofrontal areas in groups of patients with FTD, the majority of whom endorsed apathy symptoms (Chow et al., 2006; Liu et al., 2004; Rosen et al., 2002, 2005; Williams, Nestor, & Hodges, 2005). None of these studies has found a significant correlation between the apathetic behavior and atrophy specific to a brain region. The type of apathy common to FTD, arguably more of an affective deficit than one of behavioral motivation, may be linked to the insular atrophy reported by Rosen and others (e.g., Rosen et al., 2002). The insular cortex shares open loop connectivity with the lateral OFC and therefore may add additional weight to SMFSC lesions to produce symptoms of apathy.

PD, Huntington's disease, globus pallidus lesions, and thalamic lesions, which affect the subcortical links of the superior medial FSC, commonly manifest apathy (Burns, Folstein, Brandt, & Folstein, 1990; Helgason, Wilbur, & Weiss, 1988; Starkstein, Fedoroff, Price, Leiguarda, & Robinson, 1993; Starkstein et al., 1992; Stuss et al., 1988). In addition to dysfunctional basal ganglia structures involved in the superior medial FSC, fMRI techniques have identified superior medial frontal cortical deficits in patients with severe apathy due to PD (Nagano-Saito et al., 2004) and PSP (Aarsland,

Litvan, & Larsen, 2001; Juh, Kim, Moon, Choe, & Suh, 2004).

Behavioral disturbances may occur after pallidotomy for PD, ranging from apathy in some patients to disinhibition and mania in others (Trepanier et al., 1998). The adverse events could be transient or permanent, with a worse prognosis for bilateral pallidotomy (Saint-Cyr, Boronstein, & Cummings, 2002). Not all neuropsychological outcomes of the unilateral procedure were negative: Most caudal pallidotomies improved attention scores in PD (Lombardi et al., 2000).

## Neuropsychiatric Syndromes Resulting in Affective or Behavioral Control Disorders

### Secondary Depression

Depressive symptoms may arise after several types of insult to FSCs. Patients with subcortical ischemic vascular dementia characteristically manifest apathy, as well as long response latency, retrieval-type memory deficits, and depressed mood (Albert et al., 1974; Cummings, 1990). Left-hemisphere lesions due to traumatic brain injury and stroke tend to produce negative expressions of mood (crying or depression) (Mendez, Adams, & Lewandowski, 1989; Starkstein, Preziosi, Bolduc, & Robinson, 1990; Starkstein, Robinson, & Price, 1987), whereas those on the right tend to produce mood-incongruent or inappropriate laughter (Bogousslavsky et al., 1988; Cummings & Mendez, 1984; Jorge et al., 1993; Starkstein, Pearlson, Boston, & Robinson, 1987).

Subacute or chronic changes to the frontal lobes due to neurodegenerative diseases may also result in depression. Hypometabolism in left anterior cingulate and bilateral superior frontal regions on FDG-PET correlates with depressive symptoms in AD, which implicates the superior medial FSC (Hirono et al., 1998). Patients with PD tend to develop depression. Depression has been reported in up to 40% of patients with PD and may be the initial manifestation of the disease, as well as a component of its later stages. Deep brain stimulation (DBS) as a surgical intervention for refractory PD targets a variety of subcortical components of the FSC. Occasionally, adverse effects of these surgeries confirm the role of FSCs in depression. Stimulation of the subthalamic nucleus or the left substantia nigra has resulted in depressive symptoms that are novel to the individual and reversible (Bejjani et al., 1999; Piasecki & Jefferson, 2004). Studies of depression associated with PD, Huntington's disease, or complex partial seizures demonstrate reduced metabolic activity in the OFC and caudate nucleus (Goldman-Rakic, 1994; Mayberg et al., 1990, 1992).

## Bipolar Affective Disorder

Bipolar affective disorder (BAD) is another circuit-related but not circuit-specific behavior. Imaging studies are sometimes complicated by the potential confound of chronic use of antidepressants or mood stabilizers (e.g., lithium). Structural imaging reports atrophy in the DLPFC and superior medial FSC and, inconsistently, significant enlargement of the thalamus (Haldane & Frangou, 2004). fMRI shows reduced DLPFC activity during phases of depression; meanwhile, manic states are associated with reduced superior medial frontal and OFC activity. Both these states normalize when the patient's mood stabilizes (Haldane & Frangou, 2004). As in the case of ADHD, a relative hypoactivity in cortex can lead to an externally hyperactive state. Haldane and Frangou (2004) speculate that the efferent open connection from the hypoactive medial OFC inadequately inhibits the amygdala in BAD.

## Secondary Mania

Findings in acquired mania echo those during the manic phase of patients with primary BAD. Secondary mania occurs with lesions or degenerative disorders affecting the OFC, caudate nucleus, and perithalamic areas (Bogousslavsky et al., 1988; Cummings & Mendez, 1984; Kulisevsky, Berthier, & Pujol, 1993; Starkstein, Pearlson, et al., 1987; Trautner, Cummings, Read, & Benson, 1988). Lesions of the inferior temporal lobe regions and amygdala also produce mania, which follows from their open connections with the OFC (see Figure 3.6) (Berthier, Starkstein, Robinson, & Leiguarda, 1990; Lykestos et al., 1993; Starkstein, Pearlson, et al., 1987). Subcortical lesions affecting the caudate nucleus and thalamus tend to produce a bipolar type of mood disorder, with alternating periods of mania and depression, whereas lesions of the cortex that produce mania are not typically followed by a cyclic mood disorder (Starkstein, Fedoroff, Berthier,

& Robinson, 1991). Nearly all focal lesions producing secondary mania have involved the right hemisphere (Cummings, 1995).

## Secondary Psychosis

Psychosis may result from many disease entities that affect FSCs and the inferotemporal subcortical circuit either structurally or neurochemically. Systemic lupus erythematosus and vascular dementia may cause psychosis due to infarction at the cortical or subcortical level. HIV dementia or AIDS dementia complex, metachromatic leukodystrophy, and neoplasms that manifest with psychosis may disrupt white matter tracts that constitute the subcortical component of the circuits (Hyde, Ziegler, & Wieinberger, 1992). Late-life psychosis has been associated with infarctions of frontal lobe white matter, normal pressure hydrocephalus (Miller, Benson, Cummings, & Neshkes, 1986), and basal ganglia calcification (Cummings, Gosenfeld, Houlihan, & McCaffrey, 1983). Psychosis may be iatrogenic: Dopaminergic pharmacotherapy can alleviate symptoms of PD, but visual hallucinations can arise as an adverse effect, potentially by overstimulating the inferotemporal subcortical circuit (Middleton & Strick, 1996).

As in the case of depression, there are many links between psychosis and temporal lobe dysfunction. Caudate dysfunction in Huntington's disease is associated with psychosis (Cummings et al., 1983; Folstein, 1989), but most lesions producing delusional syndromes involve the temporal lobe, particularly medial temporal–limbic structures (Gorman & Cummings, 1990). Studies of patients with temporal lobe epilepsy and psychosis describe onset of postictal psychosis after resection of either temporal lobe (Leinonen, Tuunainen, & Lepola, 1994). FDG-PET scans of patients with AD and psychosis show hypometabolism in temporal and frontal lobes relative to those with AD but without psychosis (Sultzer et al., 1995).

## Impulsivity

The spectrum of impulse control disorders spans OCD, Tourette's syndrome, attention deficit disorders, suicidality, eating disorders, and criminal behaviors. fMRI has indicated roles for FSCs in some of these disorders. Structural neuroimaging has localized lesions in FSCs associated with the acquired syndromes.

Both primary and acquired OCD are highly related to the lateral OFC. Primary OCD is a disorder characterized by the presence of intrusive and contextually inappropriate ideas, thoughts, urges, and images (obsessions), as well as repetitive cognitive and physical activities performed in a ritualistic way (compulsions) (American Psychiatric Association, 1994). Obsessive–compulsive spectrum disorders include pathological gambling, kleptomania, risk-seeking behavior, and body dysmorphic disorder. The balance between direct and indirect pathways of the lateral OFC has provided the basis for several biological models of OCD. Patients with idiopathic and acquired OCD display similar behavioral disturbances and neuropsychological dysfunction. Aberrant motor behaviors, which approximate acquired obsessive–compulsive behaviors, in patients with AD are associated with neurofibrillary tangle density in the left OFC (Tekin et al., 2001). The same behaviors in patients with FTD have been associated with loss of gray matter volume in the SMFSC (Williams et al., 2005). Other etiologies for acquired OCD include pericallosal neoplasms compressing the posterior cingulate gyrus or unilateral temporal lobe anomalies, left anterior temporal or bitemporal arachnoid cysts, subcortical lesions (particularly involving the caudate nucleus), infarction of the right posterior putamen, posttraumatic orbitofrontal contusions (Berthier et al., 1996), and autoimmune disorders. Immune responses to the group A β-hemolytic streptococcal infection may be the pathogenic basis for OCD seen in pediatric autoimmune neuropsychiatric disorders associated with streptococcal infections (PANDAS). Other clinical diagnostic criteria for PANDAS include presence of tic disorder and motoric hyperactivity. The antibodies cross-react with basal ganglia, and the clinical manifestations indicate involvement of OFC and motor subcortical circuits (Kim et al., 2004).

These observations provide clinicopathological evidence of the significance of FSCs in OCD, both at the cortical and at the subcortical level.

On the basis of the neurochemical properties of the basal ganglia loops, several authors have hypothesized that the core pathology of OCD arises from excessive thalamic disinhibition promoting the direct pathway (Baxter, 1990; Modell, Mountz, Curtis, & Greden, 1989; Rapoport & Wise, 1988). Positive feedback loops would cause the OFC FSC to process information in a perseverative manner (Zald & Kim, 1996b).

Functional imaging supports this hyperactivity model. Pre- and posttreatment PET studies show that responders to behavioral therapy for primary OCD decrease abnormal hypermetabolism in the caudate nucleus bilaterally. Other investigators note cortical hypermetabolic activity in right-sided orbital gyri to accompany similar hyperactivity in the ipsilateral caudate nucleus and thalamus (Schwartz, Stoessel, Baxter, Martin, & Phelps, 1996). Unlike ADHD, in which a dominant indirect pathway results in hyperactive behavior, the direct pathway drives the overactivated mental and physical state of OCD.

Surgical interventions for OCD also support an FSC-based etiology. In cases of severe OCD that is refractory to pharmacotherapy, DBS has been effective. The electrodes seem to work regardless of placement in ventral caudate (Aouizerate et al., 2004), subthalamic nucleus (STN) (Fontaine et al., 2004), the zona incerta (near the STN) (Mallet et al., 2002), the anterior limb of the internal capsule (Anderson & Ahmed, 2003; Cosyns, Gabriels, & Nuttin, 2003; Gabriels, Cosyns, Nuttin, Demeulemeester, & Gybels, 2003; Nuttin, Cosyns, Demeulemeester, Gybels, & Meyerson, 1999; Nuttin et al., 2003), or ventral striatum (Sturm et al., 2003). In the context of disinhibited hyperactivity causing the obsessions and compulsions, DBS applied to the STN would increase the influence of the indirect pathway. The other DBS contact points could decrease output along the OFC FSC direct pathway or increase activity of the indirect pathway.

Impulsivity is frequently seen in Huntington's disease, but the nature of the psychiatric manifestation cannot be generalized across all patients: Behaviors may be obsessive–compulsive, explosive, psychotic, or suicidal (Anderson, Louis, Stern, & Marder, 2001; Cummings & Cunningham, 1992; Paulsen, Ready, Hamilton, Mega, & Cummings, 2001). Caudate atrophy is a hallmark finding on structural neuroimaging and is usually followed by signs of frontal lobe atrophy.

Tourette's syndrome is a neuropsychiatric and movement disorder accompanied frequently by obsessions and compulsions, impulsivity, coprolalia, self-injurious behavior, echolalia, depression, and measures of attentional and visuospatial dysfunction. As in the case of OCD, functional neuroimaging with FDG-PET reveals a hyperactive abnormality. Areas identified as hypermetabolic in association with active behavioral and cognitive symptoms include the OFC and putamen (Braun et al., 1995). Patients with either Huntington's disease or Tourette's syndrome express agitation, irritability, anxiety, and euphoria, but those with Tourette's syndrome may have the more exaggerated presentation. Kulisevsky and colleagues (2001) attribute these symptoms to superior medial FSC and OFC disruption.

Lack of autonomic response to an emotionally disturbing stimulus can indicate lesions of the medial OFC. Although it is tempting to draw a causal relationship between medial OFC circuit dysfunction and criminally violent behaviors, not all patients with OFC lesions show such severe changes in behavior. In fact, forensic neuroimaging has failed to reveal a consistent functional imaging pattern to correlate with homicidal and sadistic tendencies, aberrant sexual drive, violent impulsivity, and psychopathic and sociopathic personality traits (Mayberg, 1996). Part VI of this book discusses the lateral OFC in the contexts of OCD and criminality in more detail.

## Neuropsychiatric Syndromes Impairing Motor Control

As described earlier, both hypokinetic and hyperkinetic movement disorders bear aspects of cognitive and behavioral impairment. Of hypokinetic movement disorders, PD has been the most well characterized. The cardinal signs of PD are bradykinesia, rigidity, resting tremor, and postural instability. Classic PD responds to treatment with dopaminergic agonists. Motor dyskinesias in PD may arise from similar disinhibition of thalamic output during dopaminergic pharmacotherapy, which affects the motor FSC (Albin, Young, & Penney, 1989; DeLong, 1990). FDG-PET reveals that DBS at the STN increases metabolic activity in both globus pallidus regions, premotor areas, and anterior cingulate cortices. This effect is accompanied by decreased activity in the left limbic lobe and both inferior frontal cortical regions (Zhao, Sun, Li, & Wang, 2004).

A related hypokinetic movement disorder, CBD, is an asymmetrical, progressive parkinsonian syndrome that precedes the onset of cognitive deficits, and the asymmetry may manifest as alien limb syndrome. Functional

imaging with PET reveals asymmetrical hypometabolism in the striatum, thalamus, and peri-Rolandic cortex (Coulier, de Vries, & Leenders, 2003).

PSP causes executive dysfunction, apathy, and behavioral changes consistent with disruption of the FSCs. Patients with PSP can be difficult to distinguish from FTD, CBD, PD, diffuse Lewy body disease, and multiple-system atrophy (MSA). The constellation of supranuclear vertical gaze palsy, moderate or severe postural instability, symmetrical bradykinesia, absence of tremor-dominant disease, absence of alien limb syndrome, lack of a response to L-dopa, and the absence of delusions can distinguish PSP from the other syndromes (Litvan et al., 1997).

Clinical diagnostic criteria for MSA include non- or poorly L-dopa responsive parkinsonism, severe symptomatic autonomic failure (e.g., orthostatic hypotension), urinary dysfunction, and/or cerebellar or pyramidal signs (e.g., gait ataxia) (Litvan et al., 1997). Patients with PD have lower metabolic activity over the lateral prefrontal cortex on FDG-PET but do not show the same subcortical hypometabolism as those with PSP or MSA (Juh et al., 2004). The MSA group shows additional significant hypometabolism in the putamen.

The motor FSC shows damage in many neurological disorders associated with aging. Neurodegenerative tauopathies (FTD, AD) may manifest parkinsonism late in the course of illness. Patients with subcortical ischemic vascular dementia characteristically exhibit dysarthria and gait disturbance (Albert et al., 1974; Cummings, 1990).

Hyperkinetic movement disorders include Huntington's disease, Tourette's syndrome, and ADHD. Huntington's disease is characterized by a triad of hyperkinetic movements (chorea and athetosis), psychiatric disturbance, and dementia. The clinical presentation indicates motor, oculomotor, DLPFC, and superior medial FSC and OFC involvement. Impaired facial recognition and discrimination may occur early in the illness due to disruption of the inferotemporal subcortical circuit at the level of the caudate tail (Jacobs, Shuren, & Heilman, 1995; Vonsattel et al., 1985).

Tourette's syndrome is characterized by repetitive vocal and/or motor tics. Although patients can suppress these vocalizations and movements, inhibiting them leads to feelings of restlessness and anxiety that are more difficult to tolerate than consequences of expressing the tic. Midbrain, ventral striatum, parahippocampal gyrus, supplementary motor area, lateral premotor, and Rolandic cortices appear hypermetabolic in patients with Tourette's syndrome compared to controls and support pathology in both the superior medial frontal and motor FSCs as causes of the tics (Braun et al., 1993).

The hyperactivity that may accompany attention deficit disorder is less circumscribed as the choreoathetotic movements of Huntington's disease or the tics of Tourette's syndrome. The restlessness of ADHD resembles the iatrogenic hyperkinesia of PD patients on dopaminergic therapy and appears concurrently with impulsive behaviors and impatience.

## CONCLUSIONS

The frontal lobe evolved to manage the pyramidal pathway and to implement cognitive decisions in adaptation to a dynamic environment. Cognitive and emotional processes temper the body's actions. The body's actions constitute behaviors in patterns characteristic of the individual or in response to changing environmental stimuli. To manage these actions requires a flexible system that can incorporate a wealth of sensory input, use higher cognitive functions to prioritize that input, and choose the most effective response to serve shifting needs of the individual, initiate the action, and monitor its execution. The individual must function not only against the elements but also within a society.

The FSCs provide an architectural template from which the frontal lobe manages the pyramidal pathway. The same general flow of control from frontal cortex to striatum to globus pallidus to thalamus back to cortex supports motor, cognitive, and emotional output. This chapter has focused on FSCs that manage executive function, motivation, and social interactions. In addition to creating integral connectivity between dedicated frontal cortex and the basal ganglia, the FSCs afford intercommunication for related cognitive functions and social behaviors. Open connections allow for a full complement of sensory afferents to the FSCs, as well as efferents from the FSCs to limbic systems, to reinforce the emotional state of the individual.

The manifestation of a particular neuropsychiatric symptom reflects an imbalance of the direct and indirect pathways within a frontal–subcortical circuit. Events that can destabilize the normal state of equilibrium between these two pathways include cortical or subcortical structural lesions along the circuit, input from the limbic system or other open connections, and neurotransmitter effects on the striatal striosome matrix. Similarly, current therapeutic interventions seeking to restore the equilibrium would either suppress the relatively dominant pathway or bolster the relatively dormant one.

## ACKNOWLEDGMENTS

We appreciate the assistance of Joanna Szewczyk and Christina Pataky in formatting and referencing this manuscript. Anda Pacurar assisted with development of Figures 3.2–3.5.

## REFERENCES

Aarsland, D., Litvan, I., & Larsen, J. P. (2001). Neuropsychiatric symptoms of patients with progressive supranuclear palsy and Parkinson's disease. *Journal of Neuropsychiatry and Clinical Neurosciences*, *13*(1), 42–49.

Albert, M. L., Feldman, R. G., & Willis, A. L. (1974). The "subcortical dementia" of progressive supranuclear palsy. *Journal of Neurology, Neurosurgery and Psychiatry*, *37*, 121–130.

Albin, R. L., Young, A. B., & Penney, J. B. (1989). The functional anatomy of basal ganglia disorders. *Trends in Neuroscience*, *12*, 355–375.

Alexander, G. E., DeLong, M. R., & Strick, P. L. (1986). Parallel organization of functionally segregated circuits linking basal ganglia and cortex. *Annual Review of Neuroscience*, *9*, 357–381.

Amaral, D. G., Price, J. L., Pitkaenen, A., & Carmichael, S. T. (1992). Anatomical organization of the primate amygdaloid complex. In J. P. Aggleton (Ed.), *The amygdala: Neurobiological aspects of emotion, memory, and mental dysfunction* (pp. 1–66). New York: Wiley.

American Psychiatric Association. (1994). *Diagnostic and statistical manual of mental disorders* (4th ed.). Washington, DC: Author.

Anderson, D., & Ahmed, A. (2003). Treatment of patients with intractable obsessive–compulsive disorder with anterior capsular stimulation. *Journal of Neurosurgery*, *98*(5), 1104–1108.

Anderson, K. E., Louis, E. D., Stern, Y., & Marder, K. S. (2001). Cognitive correlates of obsessive and compulsive symptoms in Huntington's disease. *American Journal of Psychiatry*, *158*, 799–801.

Aouizerate, B., Cuny, E., Martin-Guehl, C., Guehl, D., Amieva, H., Benazzouz, A., et al. (2004). Deep brain stimulation of the ventral caudate nucleus in the treatment of obsessive–compulsive disorder and major depression. *Journal of Neurosurgery, 101*(4), 682–686.

Barris, R. W., & Schuman, H. R. (1953). Bilateral anterior cingulate gyrus lesions: Syndrome of the anterior cingulate gyri. *Neurology, 3,* 44–52.

Baxter, L. R. (1990). Brain imaging as a tool in establishing a theory of brain pathology in obsessive–compulsive disorder. *Journal of Clinical Psychiatry, 51*(Suppl.), 22–26.

Baxter, L. R., Schwartz, J. M., Phelps, M. E., Mazziotta, J. C., Guze, B. H., Selin, C. E., et al. (1989). Reduction of prefrontal cortex glucose metabolism common to three types of depression. *Archives of General Psychiatry, 43*(3), 243–250.

Bechara, A., & Van der Kooy, D. (1989). The tegmental pedunculopontine nucleus: A brainstem output of the limbic system critical for the conditioned place references produced by morphine and amphetamine. *Journal of Neuroscience, 9,* 3440–3449.

Bejjani, B.-P., Damier, P., Arnulf, I., Thivard, L., Bonnet, A.-M., Dormont, D., et al. (1999). Transient acute depression induced by high-frequency deep-brain stimulation. *New England Journal of Medicine, 340*(19), 1476–1480.

Berthier, M. L., Kulisevsky, J., Gironell, A., & Heras, J. A. (1996). Obsessive–compulsive disorder associated with brain lesions: Clinical phenomenology, cognitive function, and anatomic correlates. *Neurology, 47*(2), 353–361.

Berthier, M. L., Starkstein, S. E., Robinson, R. G., & Leiguarda, R. (1990). Limbic lesions in a patient with recurrent mania [Letter]. *Journal of Neuropsychiatry and Clinical Neurosciences, 2*(2), 235–236.

Boeve, B. F., Lang, A. E., & Litvan, I. (2003). Corticobasal degeneration and its relationship to progressive supranuclear palsy and frontotemporal dementia. *Annals of Neurology, 54*(Suppl. 5), S15–S19.

Bogousslavsky, J., Ferrazzini, M., Regli, F., Assal, G., Tanabe, H., & Delaloye-Bischof, A. (1988). Manic delirium and frontal-like syndrome with paramedian infarction of the right thalamus. *Journal of Neurology, Neurosurgery and Psychiatry, 51*(1), 116–119.

Bogousslavsky, J., & Regli, F. (1990). Anterior cerebral artery territory infarction in the Lausanne stroke registry. *Archives of Neurology, 47*(2), 144–150.

Boone, K. B., Miller, B. L., Lee, A., Berman, N., Sherman, D., & Stuss, D. T. (1999). Neuropsychological patterns in right versus left frontotemporal dementia. *Journal of the International Neuropsychological Society, 5,* 616–622.

Braff, D. L., & Beyer, M. A. (1990). Sensorimotor gating and schizophrenia: Human and animal studies. *Archives of General Psychiatry, 47,* 181–188.

Braun, A. R., Randolph, C., Stoetter, B., Mohr, E., Cox, C., Vladar, K., et al. (1995). The functional neuroanatomy of Tourette's syndrome: An FDG-PET Study: II. Relationships between regional cerebral metabolism and associated behavioral and cognitive features of the illness. *Neuropsychopharmacology, 13*(2), 151–168.

Braun, A. R., Stoetter, B., Randolph, C., Hsiao, J. K., Vladar, K., Gernet, J., et al. (1993). The functional neuroanatomy of Tourette syndrome: An FDG-PET study: I. Regional changes in cerebral glucose metabolism differentiating patients and controls. *Neuropsychopharmacology, 9,* 277–291.

Burns, A., Folstein, S., Brandt, J., & Folstein, M. (1990). Clinical assessment of irritability, aggression, and apathy in Huntington and Alzheimer disease. *Journal of Nervous and Mental Disease, 178*(1), 20–26.

Butters, N., Wolfe, J., Granholm, E., & Martone, M. (1986). An assessment of verbal recall, recognition and fluency abilities in patients with Huntington's disease. *Cortex, 22*(1), 11–32.

Carbon, M., Ma, Y., Barnes, A., Dhawan, V., Chaly, T., Ghilardi, M., et al. (2004). Caudate nucleus: Influence of dopaminergic input on sequence learning and brain activation in Parkinsonism. *NeuroImage, 21*(4), 1497–1507.

Chavis, D. A., & Pandya, D. N. (1976). Further observations on corticofrontal connections in the rhesus monkey. *Brain Research, 117*(3), 369–386.

Chow, T. W., Binns, M. A., Freedman, M., Stuss, D., Ramirez, J., & Black, S. E. (2006). The diagnostic utility of regional atrophy in frontotemporal degeneration. *Archives of Neurology.* Manuscript submitted for publication.

Cosyns, P., Gabriels, L., & Nuttin, B. (2003). Deep brain stimulation in treatment refractory obsessive compulsive disorder. *Verhandelingen–Koninklijke Academie voor Geneeskunde van Belgie, 65*(6), 385–399.

Coulier, I. M., de Vries, J. J., & Leenders, K.L. (2003). Is FDG-PET a useful tool in clinical practice for diagnosing corticobasal ganglionic degeneration? *Movement Disorders, 18*(10), 1175–1178.

Courchesne, E., Townsend, J. P., Akshoomoff, J. P., Yeung-Courchesne, R., Press, G. A., Murakami, J. W., et al. (1994). A new finding: Impairment in shifting attention in autistic and cerebellar patients. In S. H. Broman & J. Grafman (Eds.), *Atypical cognitive deficits in developmental disorder: Implications for brain function* (pp. 101–137). Hillsdale, NJ: Erlbaum.

Craig, A. H., Cummings, J. L., Fairbanks, L., Itti, L., Miller, B. L., Li, J., & Mena, I. (1996). Cerebral blood flow correlates of apathy in Alzheimer disease. *Archives of Neurology, 53*(11), 1116–1120.

Critchley, H. D., Elliott, R., Mathias, C. J., & Dolan, R. J. (2000). Neural activity relating to generation and representation of galvanic skin conductance responses: A functional magnetic resonance imaging study. *Neuroscience, 20*(8), 3033–3040.

Cummings, J. L. (1990). Introduction. In J. L. Cummings (Ed.), *Subcortical dementia* (pp. 3–16). New York: Oxford University Press.

Cummings, J. L. (1993). The neuroanatomy of depression. *Journal of Clinical Psychiatry, 54*(Suppl.), 14–20.

Cummings, J. L. (1995). Anatomic and behavioral aspects of frontal–subcortical circuits. In J. Grafman, K. J. Holyoak, & F. Boller (Eds.), *Structure and functions of the human prefrontal cortex* (Vol. 769, pp. 1–13). New York: New York Academy of Sciences.

Cummings, J. L. (2003). Toward a molecular neuropsychiatry of neurodegenerative diseases. *Annals of Neurology, 54*(2), 147–154.

Cummings, J. L., & Cunningham, K. (1992). Obsessive–compulsive disorder in Huntington's disease. *Biological Psychiatry, 31*, 263–270.

Cummings, J. L., Gosenfeld, L. F., Houlihan, J. P., & McCaffrey, T. (1983). Neuropsychiatric disturbances associated with idiopathic calcification of the basal ganglia. *Biological Psychiatry, 18*(5), 591–601.

Cummings, J. L., & Mendez, M. F. (1984). Secondary mania with focal cerebrovascular lesions. *American Journal of Psychiatry, 141*(9), 1084–1087.

Damasio, H., & Damasio, A. R. (1989). *Lesion analysis in neuropsychology.* New York: Oxford University Press.

Damasio, H., Grabowski, T., Frank, R., Galaburda, A. M., & Damasio, A. R. (1994). The return of Phineas Gage: Clues about the brain from the skull of a famous patient. *Science, 264*, 1102–1105.

DeLong, M. R. (1990). Primate models of movement disorders of basal ganglia origin. *Trends in Neuroscience, 13*, 281–285.

Deymeer, R., Smith, T. W., DeGirolami, U., & Drachman, D. A. (1989). Thalamic dementia and motor neuron disease. *Neurology, 60*, 102–107.

Eslinger, P. J., Warner, G. C., Grattan, L. M., & Easton, J. D. (1991). "Frontal lobe" utilization behavior associated with paramedian thalamic infarction. *Neurology, 41*(3), 450–452.

Fesenmeier, J. T., Kuzniecky, R., & Garcia, J. H. (1990). Akinetic mutism caused by bilateral anterior cerebral tuberculous obliterative arteritis. *Neurology, 40*(6), 1005–1006.

Folstein, S. E. (1989). *Huntington's disease: A disorder of families.* Baltimore: Johns Hopkins University Press.

Fontaine, D., Mattei, V., Borg, M., von Langsdorff, D., Magnie, M. N., Chanalet, S., et al. (2004). Effect of subthalamic nucleus stimulation on obsessive–compulsive disorder in a patient with Parkinson disease. *Journal of Neurosurgery, 100*(6), 1084–1086.

Gabriels, L., Cosyns, P., Nuttin, B., Demeulemeester, H., & Gybels, J. (2003). Deep brain stimulation for treatment-refractory obsessive–compulsive disorder: Psychopathological and neuropsychological outcome in three cases. *Acta Psychiatrica Scandinavica, 107*(4), 275–282.

Goldman-Rakic, P. S. (1994). Working memory dysfunction in schizophrenia. *Journal of Neuropsychiatry and Clinical Neurosciences, 6*(4), 348–357.

Gorman, D. G., & Cummings. (1990). Organic delusional syndrome. *Seminars in Neurology, 10*(3), 229–238.

Grebb, J. A., Weinberger, D. R., & Wyatt, R. J. (1992). Schizophrenia. In A. K. Asbury, G. M. McKhann, & W. I. McDonald (Eds.), *Diseases of the nervous system: Clinical neurobiology* (2nd ed., Vol. 1, pp. 839–848). Philadelphia: Saunders.

Green, J., & Barnhart, H. (2000). The impact of lesion laterality on neuropsychological change following posterior pallidotomy: A review of current findings. *Brain and Cognition, 42*, 379–398.

Haldane, M., & Frangou, S. (2004). New insights help define the pathophysiology of bipolar affective disorder: Neuroimaging and neuropathology findings. *Progress in Neuropsychopharmacology and Biological Psychiatry, 28*(6), 943–960.

Hale, T. S., Hariri, A. R., & McCracken, J. T. (2000). Attention-deficit/hyperactivity disorder: Perspectives from neuroimaging. *Mental Retardation and Developmental Disabilities Research Reviews, 6*, 214–219.

Helgason, C., Wilbur, A., & Weiss, A. (1988). Acute pseudobulbar mutism due to discrete bilateral capsular infarction in the territory of the anterior choroidal artery. *Brain and Cognition, 111*, 507–519.

Hirono, N., Mori, E., Ishii, K., Ikejiri, Y., Imamura, T., Shimomura, T., et al. (1998). Frontal lobe hypometabolism and depression in Alzheimer's disease. *Neurology, 50*(2), 380–383.

Hunter, R., Blackwood, W., & Bull, J. (1968). Three cases of frontal meningiomas presenting psychiatrically. *British Medical Journal, 3*(609), 9–16.

Hyde, T. M., Ziegler, J. C., & Wieinberger, D. R. (1992). Psychiatric disturbances in metachromatic leukodystropy: Insights into the neurobiology of psychosis. *Archives of Neurology, 49*(4), 401–406.

Irle, E., Peper, M., Wowra, B., & Kunze, S. (1994). Mood changes after surgery for tumors of the cerebral cortex. *Archives of Neurology, 51*(2), 164–174.

Jacobs, D. H., Shuren, J., & Heilman, K. M. (1995). Impaired perception of facial identity and facial affect in Huntington's disease. *Neurology, 45*(6), 1217–1218.

Jones, E. G., & Powell, T. P. (1970). An anatomical study of converging sensory pathways within the cerebral cortex of the monkey. *Brain, 93*, 793–820.

Jorge, R. E., Robinson, R. G., Starkstein, S. E., Arndt, S. V., Forrester, A. W., & Geisler, F. H. (1993). Secondary mania following traumatic brain injury. *American Journal of Psychiatry, 137*, 1275–1276.

Juh, R., Kim, J., Moon, D., Choe, B., & Suh, T. (2004). Different metabolic patterns analysis of Parkinsonism on the $^{18}$F-FDG PET. *European Journal of Radiology, 51*(3), 223–233.

Kim, S. W., Grant, J. E., Kim, S. I., Swanson, T. A., Bernstein, G. A., Jaszcz, W. B., et al. (2004). A possible association of recurrent streptococcal infections and acute onset of obsessive–compulsive disorder. *Journal of Neuropsychiatry and Clinical Neurosciences, 16*(3), 252–258.

Kulisevsky, J., Berthier, M. L., & Pujol, J. (1993). Hemiballismus and secondary mania following right thalamic infarction. *Neurology, 43*(7), 1422–1424.

Kulisevsky, J., Litvan, I., Berthier, M. L., Pascual-

Sedano, B., Paulsen, J. S., & Cummings, J. L. (2001). Neuropsychiatric assessment of Gilles de la Tourette patients: Comparative study with other hyperkinetic and hypokinetic movement disorders. *Movement Disorders, 16*(6), 1098–1104.

Laiacona, M., De Santis, A., Barbarotto, R., Basso, A., Spagnoli, D., & Capitani, E. (1989). Neuropsychological follow-up of patients operated for aneurysms of anterior communicating artery. *Cortex, 25*(2), 261–273.

Leinonen, E., Tuunainen, A., & Lepola, U. (1994). Postoperative psychoses in epileptic patients after temporal lobectomy. *Acta Neurologica Scandinavica, 90*(6), 394–399.

Lhermitte, F., Pillon, B., & Serdaru, M. (1986). Human autonomy and the frontal lobes. I: Imitation and utilization behavior, a neuropsychological study of 75 patients. *Annals of Neurology, 19*(4), 326–334.

Litvan, I., Campbell, G., Mangone, C. A., Verny, M., McKee, A., Chaudhuri, K. R., et al. (1997). Which clinical features differentiate progressive supranuclear palsy (Steele–Richardson–Olszewski syndrome) from related disorders?: A clinicopathological study. *Brain, 120*(1), 65–74.

Liu, W., Miller, B. L., Kramer, J. H., Rankin, K., Wyss-Coray, C., Gearhart, R., et al. (2004). Behavioral disorders in the frontal and temporal variants of frontotemporal dementia. *Neurology, 62*(5), 742–748.

Logue, V., Durward, M., Pratt, R. T., Piercy, M., & Nixon, W. L. (1968). The quality of survival after an anterior cerebral aneurysm. *British Journal of Psychiatry, 114*, 137–160.

Lombardi, W. J., Gross, R. E., Trepanier, L. L., Lang, A. E., Lozano, A. M., & Saint-Cyr, J. A. (2000). Relationship of lesion location to cognitive outcome following microelectrode-guided pallidotomy for Parkinson's disease: Support for the existence of cognitive circuits in the human pallidum. *Brain, 123*, 746–758.

Lozza, C., Baron, J. C., Eidelberg, D., Mentis, M. J., Carbon, M., & Marie, R. M. (2004). Executive processes in Parkinson's disease: FDG-PET and network analysis. *Human Brain Mapping, 22*(3), 236–245.

Lykestos, C., Stoline, A. M., Longstreet, P., Ranen, N. G., Lesser, R., Fisher, R., et al. (1993). Mania in temporal lobe epilepsy. *Neuropsychiatry, Neuropsychology, and Behavioral Neurology, 6*, 19–25.

Mallet, L., Mesnage, V., Houeto, J.-L., Pelissolo, A., Yelnik, J., Behar, C., et al. (2002). Compulsions, Parkinson's disease, and stimulation. *Lancet, 360*, 1302–1304.

Masterman, D., DeSalles, A., Baloh, R. W., Frysinger, R., Foti, D., Behnke, E., et al. (1998). Motor, cognitive, and behavioral performance following unilateral ventroposterior pallidotomy for Parkinson's disease. *Archives of Neurology, 55*, 1201–1208.

Mayberg, H. (1994). Frontal lobe dysfunction in secondary depression. *Journal of Neuropsychiatry and Clinical Neurosciences, 6*(4), 428–442.

Mayberg, H. (1996). Medical–legal inferences from functional neuroimaging evidence. *Seminars in Clinical Neuropsychiatry, 1*(3), 195–201.

Mayberg, H., Starkstein, S. E., Peyser, C. E., Brandt, J., Dannals, R. F., & Folstein, S. E. (1992). Paralimbic frontal lobe hypometabolism in depression associated with Huntington's disease. *Neurology, 42*(9), 1791–1797.

Mayberg, H., Starkstein, S. E., Sadzot, B., Preziosi, T., Andrezejewski, P. L., Dannals, R. F., et al. (1990). Selective hypometabolism in inferior frontal lobe in depressed patients with Parkinson's disease. *Annals of Neurology, 28*(1), 57–64.

Mayberg, H. S., Brannan, S. K., Tekell, J. L., Silva, J. A., Mahurin, R. K., McGinnis, S., et al. (2000). Regional metabolic effects of fluoxetine in major depression: Serial changes and relationship to clinical response. *Biological Psychiatry, 48*(8), 830–843.

Mega, M. S., & Cummings, J. L. (1994). Frontal–subcortical circuits and neuropsychiatric disorders. *Journal of Neuropsychiatry and Clinical Neurosciences, 6*(4), 358–370.

Mena, I., Marin, O., Fuenzalida, S., Horiuchi, K., Burke, K., & Cotzias, G. C. (1967). Chronic manganese poisoning. *Neurology, 17*(2), 128–136.

Mendez, M. F., Adams, N. L., & Lewandowski, K. S. (1989). Neurobehavioral changes associated with caudate lesions. *Neurology, 39*, 349–354.

Mesulam, M. M. (1985). Patterns in behavioral neuroanatomy: Association areas, the limbic system, and hemispheric specialization. In *Behavioral neurology* (pp. 1–70). Philadelphia: Davis.

Mesulam, M. M., & Mufson, E. J. (1982a). Insula of the Old World Monkey: II. Afferent cortical output and comments on the claustrum. *Journal of Comparative Neurology, 212*(1), 23–37.

Mesulam, M. M., & Mufson, E. J. (1982b). Insula of the Old World Monkey: III. Efferent cortical output and comments on function. *Journal of Comparative Neurology, 212*(1), 38–52.

Middleton, F. A., & Strick, P. L. (1996). The temporal lobe is a target of output from the basal ganglia. *Proceedings of the National Academy of Sciences of the United States of America, 93*(16), 8683–8687.

Middleton, F. A., & Strick, P. L. (2000). Basal ganglia output and cognition: Evidence from anatomical, behavioural and clinical studies. *Brain and Cognition, 42*, 183–200.

Miller, B. L., Benson, D. F., Cummings, J. L., & Neshkes, R. (1986). Late-life paraphrenia: An organic delusional syndrome. *Journal of Clinical Psychiatry, 47*(4), 204–207.

Minshew, N. J. (1997). Pervasive developmental disorders: Autism and similar disorders. In T. E. Feinberg & M. J. Farrah (Eds.), *Behavioral neurology and neuropsychology* (pp. 817–826). New York: McGraw-Hill.

Modell, J. G., Mountz, J. M., Curtis, G. C., & Greden, J. F. (1989). Neurophysiologic dysfunction in basal ganglia/limbic striatal and thalamocortical circuits as a pathogenetic mechanism of obsessive–compulsive disorder. *Journal of Neuropsychiatry and Clinical Neurosciences, 1*(1), 27–36.

Nagano-Saito, A., Kato, T., Arahata, Y., Washimi, Y., Nakamura, A., Abe, Y., et al. (2004). Cognitive- and motor-related regions in Parkinson's disease: FDOPA and FDG PET studies. *NeuroImage, 22*(2), 553–556.

Nauta, W. J. H. (1971). The problem of the frontal lobe: A reinterpretation. *Journal of Psychiatric Research, 8*(3), 167–187.

Nauta, W. J. H. (1973). Connections of the frontal lobe with the limbic system. In L. V. Laitinen & K. E. Livingston (Eds.), *Surgical approaches in psychiatry* (pp. 303–314). Baltimore: University Park Press.

Nauta, W. J. H. (1979). A proposed conceptual reorganization of the basal ganglia and telencephalon. *Neuroscience, 4*(12), 1875–1881.

Neary, D., Snowden, J. S., Gustafson, L., Passant, U., Stuss, D., Black, S., et al. (1998). Frontotemporal lobar degeneration: A consensus on clinical diagnostic criteria. *Neurology, 51*(6), 1546–1554.

Nielsen, J. M., & Jacobs, L. L. (1951). Bilateral lesions of the anterior cingulate gyri. *Bulletin of the Los Angeles Neurological Society, 16*, 231–234.

Nuttin, B. J., Gabriëls, L. A., Cosyns, P. R., Meyerson, B. A., Andréewitch, S., Sunaert, S. G., et al. (2003). Long-term electrical capsular stimulation in patients with obsessive–compulsive disorder. *Neurosurgery, 52*(6), 1263–1274.

Nuttin, B. J., Gabriëls, L. A., van Kuyck, K., & Cosyns, P. (2003). Electrical stimulation of the anterior limbs of the internal capsules in patients with severe obsessive–compulsive disorder: Anecdotal reports. *Neurosurgery Clinics of North America, 14*(2), 267–274.

Ozonoff, S., Strayer, D. L., McMahon, W. M., & Filloux, F. (1994). Executive function abilities in autism: An information processing approach. *Journal of Child Psychology and Psychiatry, 35*, 659–685.

Paulsen, J. S., Ready, R. E., Hamilton, J. M., Mega, M. S., & Cummings, J. L. (2001). Neuropsychiatric aspects of Huntington's disease. *Journal of Neurology, Neurosurgery, and Psychiatry, 71*, 310–314.

Piasecki, S. D., & Jefferson, J. W. (2004). Psychiatric complications of deep brain stimulation for Parkinson's disease. *Journal of Clinical Psychiatry, 65*(6), 845–859.

Rapoport, J. L., & Wise, S. P. (1988). Obsessive–compulsive disorder: Evidence for basal ganglia dysfunction. *Psychopharmacology Bulletin, 24*(3), 380–384.

Reith, J., Benkelfat, C., Sherwin, A., Yasuhara, Y., Kuwabara, H., Andermann, F., et al. (1994). Elevated dopa decarboxylase activity in living brain of patients with psychosis. *Proceedings of the National Academy of Sciences of the United States of America, 91*(24), 11651–11654.

Rilipek, P. A., Semrud-Clikemann, M., Steingard, R. J., Renshaw, P. F., Kennedy, D. N., & Biederman, J. (1997). Volumetric MRI analysis comparing subjects having attention-deficit hyperactivity disorder with normal controls. *Neurology, 48*, 589–601.

Robinson, R. G., & Starkstein, S. E. (1990). Current research in affective disorders following stroke. *Journal of Neuropsychiatry and Clinical Neurosciences, 2*(1), 1–14.

Rosen, H. J., Allison, S. C., Schauer, G. F., Gorno-Tempini, M. L., Weiner, M. W., & Miller, B. L. (2005). Neuroanatomical correlates of behavioural disorders in dementia. *Brain, 128*(11), 2612–2625.

Rosen, H. J., Gorno-Tempini, M. L., Goldman, W. P., Perry, R. J., Schuff, N., Weiner, M., et al. (2002). Patterns of brain atrophy in frontotemporal dementia and semantic dementia. *Neurology, 58*(2), 198–208.

Saint-Cyr, J. A., Boronstein, Y. L., & Cummings, J. L. (2002). Neurobehavioral consequences of neurosurgical treatments and focal lesions of frontal-subcortical circuits. In D. T. Stuss & R. T. Knight (Eds.), *Principles of frontal lobe function* (pp. 408–427). New York: Oxford University Press.

Schwartz, J. M., Stoessel, P. W., Baxter, L. R., Jr., Martin, K. M., & Phelps, M. E. (1996). Systematic changes in cerebral glucose metabolic rate after successful behavior modification treatment of obsessive–compulsive disorder. *Archives of General Psychiatry, 53*(2), 109–113.

Selemon, L. D., & Goldman-Rakic, P. S. (1985). Longitudinal topography and interdigitation of corticostriatal projections in the rhesus monkey. *Journal of Neuroscience, 5*(3), 776–794.

Starkstein, S. E., Cohen, B. S., Fedoroff, P., Parikh, R. M., Price, T. R., & Robinson, R. G. (1990). Relationship between anxiety disorders and depressive disorders in patients with cerebrovascular injury. *Archives of General Psychiatry, 47*(3), 246–251.

Starkstein, S. E., Fedoroff, J. P., Berthier, M. L., & Robinson, R. G. (1991). Manic–depressive and pure manic states after brain lesions. *Biological Psychiatry, 29*(2), 149–158.

Starkstein, S. E., Fedoroff, J. P., Price, T. R., Leiguarda, R., & Robinson, R. G. (1993). Apathy following cerebrovascular lesions. *Stroke, 24*, 1625–1630.

Starkstein, S. E., Mayberg, H. S., Preziosi, T. J., Andrezejewski, P., Leiguarda, R., & Robinson, R. G. (1992). Reliability, validity, and clinical correlates of apathy in Parkinson's disease. *Journal of Neuropsychiatry and Clinical Neurosciences, 4*(2), 134–139.

Starkstein, S. E., Pearlson, G. D., Boston, J., & Robinson, R. G. (1987). Mania after brain injury: A controlled study of causative factors. *Archives of Neurology, 44*(10), 1069–1073.

Starkstein, S. E., Preziosi, T. H., Bolduc, P. L., & Robinson, R. G. (1990). Depression in Parkinson's disease. *Journal of Nervous and Mental Disease, 178*, 27–31.

Starkstein, S. E., Robinson, R. G., & Price, T. R. (1987). Comparison of cortical and subcortical lesions in the production of post-stroke mood disorders. *Brain, 110*, 1045–1059.

Stebbins, G. T., Gabrieli, J. D. E., Shannon, K. M., Penn, R. D., & Goetz, C. G. (2000). Impaired frontostriatal cognitive functioning following posteroventral pallidotomy in advanced Parkinson's disease. *Brain and Cognition, 42*, 348–363.

Sturm, V., Lenartz, D., Koulousakis, A., Treuer, H., Herholz, K., Klein, J., et al. (2003). The nucleus accumbens: A target for deep brain stimulation in obsessive–compulsive and anxiety disorders. *Journal of Chemical Neuroanatomy, 26*(4), 293–299.

Stuss, D. T., Binns, M. A., Murphy, K. J., & Alexander, M. P. (2002). Dissociations within the anterior attentional system: Effects of task complexity and irrelevant information on reaction time speed and accuracy. *Neuropsychologia, 16*, 500–513.

Stuss, D. T., Floden, D., Alexander, M. P., Levine, B., & Katz, D. (2001). Stroop performance in focal lesion patients: Dissociation of processes and frontal lobe lesion location. *Neuropsychologia, 39*, 771–786.

Stuss, D. T., Guberman, A., Nelson, R., & Larochelle, S. (1988). The neuropsychology of paramedian thalamic infarction. *Brain and Cognition, 8*(3), 348–378.

Stuss, D. T., Levine, B., Alexander, M. P., Hong, J., Palumbo, C., Hamer, L., et al. (2000). Wisconsin Card Sorting Test performance in patients with focal frontal and posterior brain damage: Effects of lesion location and test structure on separable cognitive processes. *Neuropsychologia, 30*, 388–402.

Sultzer, D. L., Mahler, M. E., Mandelkern, M. A., Cummings, J. L., van Gorp, W. G., Hinkin, C. H., et al. (1995). The relationship between psychiatric symptoms and regional cortical metabolism in Alzheimer's disease. *Journal of Neuropsychiatry and Clinical Neurosciences, 7*(4), 476–484.

Swerdlow, N. R., & Koob, G. F. (1990). Toward a unified hypothesis of cortico–striato–pallido–thalamus function. *Behavioral and Brain Sciences, 13*, 168–177.

Tekin, S., Mega, M. S., Masterman, D. M., Chow, T., Garakian, J., Vinters, H. V., et al. (2001). Orbitofrontal and anterior cingulate cortex neurofibrillary tangle burden is associated with agitation in Alzheimer's disease. *Annals of Neurology, 49*, 355–361.

Trautner, R. J., Cummings, J. L., Read, S. L., & Benson, D. F. (1988). Idiopathic basal ganglia calcification and organic mood disorder. *American Journal of Psychiatry, 145*(3), 350–353.

Trepanier, L. L., Saint-Cyr, J. A., Lozano, A. M., & Lang, A. E. (1998). Neuropsychological consequences of posteroventral pallidotomy for the treatment of Parkinson's disease. *Neurology, 51*, 207–215.

Vaidya, C. J., Austin, G., Kirkorian, G., Ridlehuber, H. W., Desmond, J. E., Glover, G. H., et al. (1998). Selective effects of methylphenidate in attention deficit hyperactivity disorder: A functional magnetic resonance study. *Proceedings of the National Academy of Sciences of the United States of America, 95*(25), 14494–14499.

Van Hoesen, G. W., Pandya, D. N., & Butters, N. (1975). Some connections of the entorhinal (area 28) and perirhinal (area 35) cortices of the rhesus monkey: II. Frontal lobe afferents. *Brain Research, 95*, 25–38.

Vonsattel, J. P., Myers, R. H., Stevens, T. J., Ferrante, R. J., Bird, E. D., & Richardson, E. P. (1985). Neuropathological classification of Huntington's disease. *Journal of Neuropathology and Experimental Neurology, 44*(6), 559–577.

Williams, G. B., Nestor, P. J., & Hodges, J. R. (2005). Neural correlates of semantic and behavioural deficits in frontotemporal dementia. *NeuroImage, 24*(4), 1042–1051.

Yeterian, E. H., & Pandya, D. N. (1993). Striatal connections of the parietal association cortices in rhesus monkeys. *Journal of Comparative Neurology, 332*(2), 175–197.

Zald, D. H., & Kim, S. W. (1996a). Anatomy and function of the orbital frontal cortex: I. Anatomy, neurocircuitry, and obsessive–compulsive disorder. *Journal of Neuropsychiatry and Clinical Neurosciences, 8*(2), 125–138.

Zald, D. H., & Kim, S. W. (1996b). Anatomy and function of the orbital frontal cortex: II. Function and relevance to obsessive–compulsive disorder. *Journal of Neuropsychiatry and Clinical Neurosciences, 8*(3), 249–261.

Zametkin, A. J., Nordahl, T. E., Gross, M., Semple, W. E., Rumsey, J., Hamburger, S., et al. (1990). Cerebral glucose metabolism in adults with hyperactivity of childhood onset. *New England Journal of Medicine, 323*(20), 1361–1366.

Zhao, Y. B., Sun, B. M., Li, D. Y., & Wang, Q. S. (2004). Effects of bilateral subthalamic nucleus stimulation on resting-state cerebral glucose metabolism in advanced Parkinson's disease. *Chinese Medical Journal, 117*(9), 1304–1308.

# CHAPTER 4

# The Dorsolateral and Cingulate Cortex

*Daniel I. Kaufer*

The dorsolateral prefrontal cortex (DLPFC) and the anterior cingulate cortex (ACC) have contrasting anatomical positions but jointly execute important transactions within the frontal lobe. Whereas the DLPFC lies superficially on the lateral aspect of the cerebral hemisphere, the ACC resides in the medial portion of the interhemispheric fissure. The microscopic cellular architectures of the DLPFC and the ACC are also notably different, reflecting neocortical association and paralimbic cortices, respectively. However, from a functional perspective, neural circuits spanning these two regions subserve and integrate attention, working memory, and other executive cognitive functions. This chapter reviews basic principles of functional anatomy and cortical connectivity regarding the prefrontal cortex, with a particular focus on the DLPFC and the ACC.

The classification of frontal lobe regions, as with other areas of cerebral cortex, is based on morphological features of varying resolution, ranging from gross surface landmarks to the microscopic analysis of constituent neurons. At the microscopic level, cytoarchitectonic maps of human, nonhuman primate, and mammalian cerebral cortex have been constructed over the last century, whereby regions are parcellated based on the laminar distribution and packing density of neurons (e.g., Brodmann, 1909/1994; Sanides, 1972; Walker, 1940; reviewed in Zilles, 1990; see also Geschwind & Iacoboni, Chapter 6, this volume). Among human cytoarchitectonic maps, that of Brodmann, published in 1909 (English translation, 1994), has been most widely adopted as a ref-

erence standard (Damasio & Damasio, 1989; Mesulam, 1985; Talairach & Tournoux, 1988). Despite methodological differences, intersubject variation, and the absence of uniform morphological criteria, there has been general agreement among different human architectonic maps. However, compared to nonhuman primates, a striking feature of the human brain is the increased relative size of the frontal lobe, including a greater degree of hemispheric asymmetry and differentiation of nonmotor regions (see Ogar & Gorno-Tempini, Chapter 5, and Carlin, Chapter 7, this volume). Some of the cross-species discrepancies between human and monkey brain architectonic maps arising from earlier work (Brodmann, 1909/1994; Walker, 1940) have been reconciled, allowing for greater cross-talk between animal and human research (Petrides, 2005; Petrides & Pandya, 1994). The structural and functional similarities of prefrontal cortex across human and nonhuman primates allow for extrapolating data from animal studies in shaping current hypotheses of the neural circuitry underlying human frontal lobe functions (Goldman-Rakic, 1987; Petrides, 2005; Vogt, Vogt, Farber, & Bush, 2005; see also Amici & Boxer, Chapter 10, this volume).

## FRONTAL LOBE ANATOMY

### Functional Regions

The surface boundaries of the frontal lobes are demarcated by the central sulcus caudally and the lateral sulcus in each hemisphere (Figure

4.1). Within these gross borders, three primary functional regions on the lateral surface of the frontal lobes are recognized: motor, premotor, and prefrontal, essentially forming a caudal to rostral continuum (Nieuwenhuys, Voogd, & van Huijzen, 1988; Zilles, 1990). A fourth functional region, paralimbic or limbic, is located deep in the medial portion of the frontal lobes (Damasio, 1991; Damasio & Damasio, 1989; Mesulam, 1985). More detailed anatomical features of these frontal lobe regions are presented in Table 4.1.

## Cortical Types

Following the nomenclature of Mesulam (1985, 1997), cerebral cortical areas are classified into three types: *idiotypic* (koniocortex), *homotypic* (isocortex), and *paralimbic* (proisocortex and periallocortex) (Barbas & Pandya, 1989; Sanides, 1972). In general, idiotypic and homotypic cortices (neocortex) have six distinct cellular layers at some stage of development, whereas paralimbic regions may have fewer recognizable lamina, reflecting a transi-

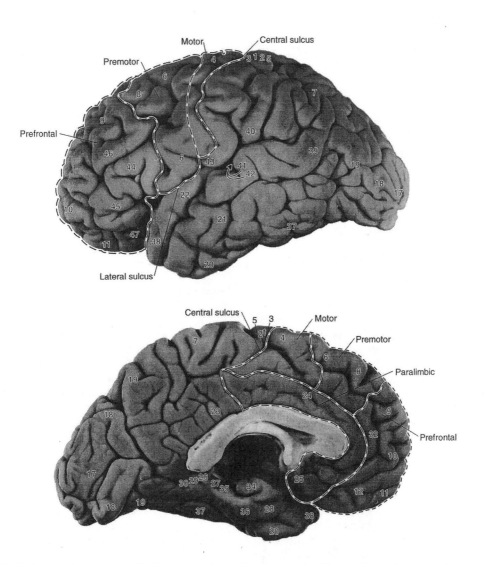

FIGURE 4.1. Lateral (top) and medial (bottom) views of the left cerebral hemisphere of a human brain, indicating the subdivisions of the frontal lobe. Numbers indicate the approximate location of Brodmann's areas.

**TABLE 4.1. Frontal Lobe Anatomy**

| Brodmann's area | Anatomical description | Cortical type | Functional region |
|---|---|---|---|
| 4 | Primary motor cortex | Primary motor | Motor |
| 6 | Premotor/supplementary motor area | Primary motor (caudal) Unimodal motor (rostral) | Premotor |
| 44[a,b] | Pars opercularis | Unimodal motor | |
| 8[c] | Motor association cortex | Unimodal motor (caudal) Heteromodal (rostral) | |
| 46 | Dorsolateral prefrontal cortex | Heteromodal | Prefrontal |
| 9 | Superior prefrontal cortex | Heteromodal | (dorsolateral) |
| 10 | Inferior prefrontal cortex | Heteromodal | |
| 45[a,b] | Pars triangularis | Heteromodal | Prefrontal |
| 47[a] | Pars orbitalis | Heteromodal | (ventrolateral) |
| 11[d] | Lateral orbitofrontal cortex | Heteromodal | Prefrontal |
| 12[d] | Medial orbitofrontal cortex | Heteromodal (rostral) Paralimbic (caudal) | (orbitofrontal) |
| 32 | Medial frontal cortex | Heteromodal (rostral) Paralimbic (caudal) | Paralimbic (medial frontal) |
| 24 | Anterior cingulate | Paralimbic | |
| 25 | Paraolfactory region (subcallosal area) | Paralimbic | |

*Note.* After Mesulam (1985) and Damasio and Damasio (1989).
[a] Frontal operculum.
[b] Broca's area (left hemisphere).
[c] Frontal eye fields.
[d] Region numbers are reversed in nonhuman primates (Walker, 1940).

tional spectrum with more primitive limbic-associated cortical and nuclear regions. General trends in architectonic features spanning the range from paralimbic to idiotypic cortex include a progressively more distinct laminar organization, an increase in myelin content, an emergent granular layer (layer IV), increased pyramidal cell size, and increased cellular density, particularly in the supragranular layers (Barbas & Pandya, 1989; Mesulam, 1985; Zilles, 1990).

Primary motor cortex (area 4) is the only idiotypic cortex in the frontal lobe. Giant pyramidal neurons (Betz cells) in layer V, which project to the spinal cord, are a prominent feature. A well-developed inner granular layer (IV) characteristic of primary sensory idiotypic (koniocortical) areas is absent in BA 4, leading to its designation as agranular cortex.

The most abundant cortical type in the frontal lobe is homotypic cortex, which carries the functional connotation of association cortex. There are two types of homotypical cortex, unimodal association or modality-specific, and heteromodal association, representing multimodal or higher-order cortical regions. Functional properties, as opposed to cytoarchitectonic differences, are the primary basis for distinguishing unimodal and heteromodal association cortices. For example, an individual neuron in a given unimodal association area is typically responsive only to a single sensory (auditory, visual, somatosensory) or motor input; neurons in heteromodal association cortices, by contrast, respond to or influence the activity of neurons in multiple sensory modalities or are involved in integrated sensory and motor processing. Within the frontal lobes, area 6 and part of area 8 are unimodal motor association areas, whereas areas 9–11, 45–47, and portions of areas 8, 12, and 32 are integrative heteromodal association regions. Cognitive associative functions putatively mediated by rostral prefrontal areas have been referred to as a "supramodal" association region (Benson, 1993).

Paralimbic cortex is structurally heterogenous and exhibits gradations of features between more highly differentiated isocortex (idiotypic and homotypic) and less differentiated allocortex (hippocampus and olfactory cortex). A continuous belt of paralimbic cortex including portions of the frontal and temporal lobes (Broca's "limbic lobe") circumscribes the corpus callosum along the medial and basal hemispheric surface. Phylogenetically, paralimbic regions are composed of two intersecting allocortical lines. One is the hippocampal trend, which includes the hippocampus, parahippocampal, and cingulate regions, forming the caudal and superior portions of the "paralimbic belt"; the other is the olfactory-based line, emanating from olfactory piriform cortex, and extending into orbitofrontal, insular, and anterior temporal polar regions (Barbas & Pandya, 1989, 1991; Mesulam, 1985, 1997; Sanides, 1972).

## Structure–Function Relationships

The laminar pattern and distribution of cortical projection systems have important implications for functional connectivity (Barbas & Pandya, 1989; Selemon & Goldman-Rakic, 1988; Zilles, 1990). First, limbic regions with less well-delineated lamina typically have numerous local and long-distance connections, whereas primary sensory and motor areas generally have relatively few connections. The DLPFC, representing heteromodal association cortex, has an intermediate number of connections and is strongly interconnected with the ACC. The latter, reflecting paralimbic cortex, has relatively few connections with highly organized primary sensory or motor cortex. Within prefrontal cortices, connections from a given area generally project in both directions to more highly and less differentiated regions (Barbas, 1992).

Short corticocortical association fibers most commonly arise from neurons in cortical layers II and superficial III; long corticocortical association tracts and commissural (interhemispheric) fibers are primarily associated with lamina III and, to a lesser extent, infragranular layers V and VI. In contrast, cortical–subcortical (i.e., striatum, thalamus, brainstem) pathways traverse infragranular cortical lamina. A similar pattern of laminar distribution has also been suggested to occur among cortical areas based on their degree of differentiation (Barbas, 1986; Barbas & Pandya, 1989). Frontally directed cortical projections

from less differentiated areas tend to have their cells of origin in infragranular layers V and VI, whereas projections from more differentiated cortical areas generally arise from supragranular layers. Within prefrontal areas, interconnections originating from a more highly developed laminar pattern to a less developed region generally terminate into a column that spans all six cortical layers. By contrast, interconnections starting from a less differentiated prefrontal region and terminating in a more highly differentiated prefrontal region (e.g., paralimbic to association cortex) are typically concentrated in layer I.

As initially described in the visual and auditory systems, functionality based on the direction of information flow is linked to the laminar distribution of neural pathways (Galaburda & Pandya, 1983; Nieuwenhuys et al., 1988; Pandya & Yeterian, 1985; Rockland & Pandya, 1979; van Essen & Mausell, 1983). Feed-forward pathways, transferring information from primary sensory areas to secondary association areas, arise in supragranular areas and principally terminate in layer IV. Feedback projections in the reverse direction originate from both supra- and infragranular layers of association cortices and terminate outside of layer IV. These two types of projections underscore the fact that most interconnections between cortical association areas are reciprocal (Felleman & van Essen, 1991).

## Dorsolateral Prefrontal Cortex

The classic human cerebral cortical map of Brodmann (1909/1994) depicts areas 46 and 9 as occupying the middle and lateral portions of the prefrontal cortical surface. Area 46 is contained within the middle frontal gyrus, whereas area 9 occupies portions of the superior and middle frontal gyri caudal to area 46. This depiction of area 9 as an intermediate zone between areas 46 and 8 in the human is at odds with Walker's map of the macaque monkey brain (1940), which shows areas 46 and 8 to be contiguous and area 9 to be confined to the superior frontal gyrus (Petrides, 2005). To reconcile these differences, the classic work of Petrides and Pandya (1994) identified homologous features of a poorly developed layer IV and the presence of large pyramidal cells in the deeper part of layer III that were common to area 9 of the monkey (Walker, 1940) and the portion of area 9 confined to the superior frontal gyrus. By contrast, area 46 is distinguished from area 9 by two features: a well-developed layer IV and small- to medium-size pyramidal neurons in the deeper part of layer III. The portion of area 9 lying on the middle frontal gyrus and contained within Walker's area 46 has a well-developed layer IV but contains large pyramidal neurons deep in layer III. The mixed cytoarchitectonic features of this region led Petrides and Pandya to rename this area 46/9 to reflect its transitional properties between Walker's monkey and Brodmann's human cortical maps (Petrides, 2005). These authors further divided the DLPFC into dorsal and ventral components (46/9v and 46/9d), using the principal sulcus in the monkey brain as a boundary (Figure 4.2).

Area 10 lies rostral in the frontopolar region and is similar in the human and monkey brain (Petrides & Pandya, 1994). It is bordered laterally by areas 9, 46, and 47, inferiorly by areas 11 and 14, and medially by areas 9, 32, and 14.

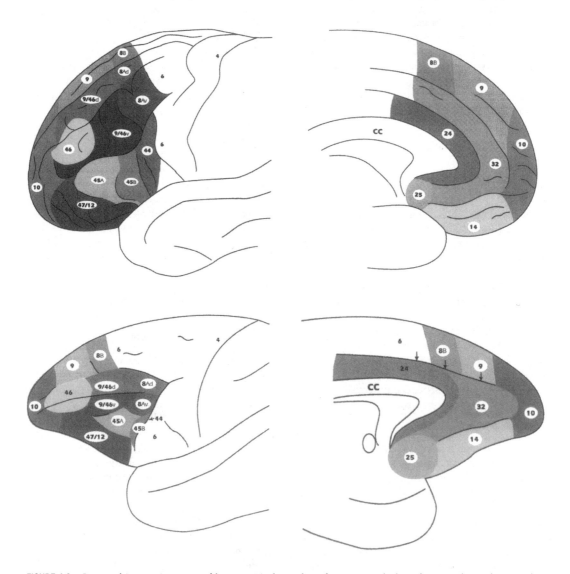

FIGURE 4.2. Cytoarchitectonic maps of human (A, lateral surface; B, medial surface) and monkey (C, lateral surface; D, medial surface) prefrontal cortical regions. Downward arrows refer to lateral extension of areas 32 and 24. From Petrides and Pandys (1994). Copyright 1994 by Elsevier. Adapted by permission.

The cellular structure and connectivity of area 10 is similar to that of dorsal area 46, although area 10 has lower cell density, particularly in layer III.

The functional organization of the DLPFC has been suggested to lie along a dorsal–ventral axis (Petrides, 2005; Petrides & Pandya, 1994). The dorsal DLPFC is viewed to be primarily active in monitoring information in working memory, whereas the ventral DLPFC is thought to regulate the active encoding and retrieval of information stored in posterior cortical association regions based on selective judgments. Both of these higher-order control processes involve the integration of sensory, motor, and cognitive information, and reflect widespread interconnections with other cortical and subcortical regions. Based on its interconnections with other DLPFC and medial temporal regions, area 10 has been hypothesized to play a superordinate role in working memory (hypermonitoring) (Petrides, 2005).

## Anterior Cingulate Cortex

The ACC lies on the medial surface of the cingulate gyrus, wrapping around the anterior portion of the corpus callosum (Barbas, 1992; Vogt et al., 2005). Area 24 occupies the cingulate gyrus and extends caudally to area 6 (premotor region) and rostrally around the genu and rostrum of the corpus callosum, where it is contiguous with area 25. The most salient cellular characteristics of area 24 are an absent layer IV and a prominent layer V composed of medium to large pyramidal neurons. Subdivisions of area 24 (a, b, and c) extend from area 25 in the subcallosal gyrus superiorly to area 9 and reflect minor variations in cellular architecture area. Area 25 occupies the subcallosal gyrus and is similar to area 24, in that both are proisocortex by virtue of well-developed infragranular layers and the absence of layer IV. Together, areas 25 and 24a are referred to as subgenual cortex (Vogt et al., 2005). The main cellular difference between areas 25 and 24 is that the former also has a prominent layer VI. Area 32 surrounds area 24, lying more superficially in the paralimbic gyrus, and is distinguished from it by a denser layer III that contains small- to medium-size pyramidal cells and a less well-developed layer VI. A thin intervening layer IV in area 32 underlies its description as dysgranular cortex.

Other borders of area 32 include area 10 rostrally, paramedian areas 8 and 9 dorsally, and area 14 (Brodmann's areas 11 and 12) ventrally.

The functional organization of the ACC reflects its central role as an integrative center for cognitive-behavioral (e.g., attention–motivation) and emotional–autonomic–motor neural networks (Bush, Luu, & Posner, 2000; Vogt, Finch, & Olson, 1992). The diverse functional affiliations of the ACC reflect its widespread connections to the DLPFC and other cortical and subcortical regions. A detailed cytoachitectonic map of monkey ACC describes four primary functional regions of cingulate cortex that are homologous to the human ACC (Vogt et al., 2005). Rostral and ventral portions of the ACC are more strongly affiliated with emotional processing and depression, whereas dorsal portions of the ACC have been implicated to participate in cognitive processing and skeletomotor activity.

## CORTICAL CONNECTIVITY

Prefrontal regions are reciprocally connected with temporal, parietal, and occipital cortices, where they receive higher-level visual, auditory, and somatosensory information. In addition, prefrontal regions have strong connections with limbic structures such as the hippocampus and amygdala, which mediate processes such as learning and memory, emotional and affective tone, autonomic regulation, drive, and motivation. Prefrontal association and paralimbic cortices play a major role integrating information about the external world and internal states that guides executive behavior. A schematic summary of major interconnections of the DLPFC and ACC is presented in Figure 4.3.

## Visual System

Two functionally and topographically segregated visual systems are recognized: a dorsal system, composed of visual association cortices in parietal–occipital areas (caudal area 7 and dorsal portions 18 and 19), and a ventral system, composed of regions extending rostrally from the temporal–occipital border along the inferior and middle temporal gyri (ventral areas 18 and 19, and areas 37, 20, and 21) (Mishkin, Ungerleider, & Macko, 1983; van

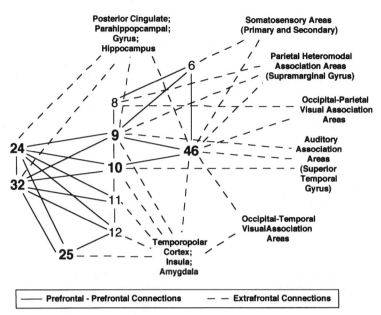

FIGURE 4.3. Schematic diagram of interconnections between the DLPFC and ACC regions (Brodmann's areas in boldface type) and their principal corticocortical connections. This diagram is intended primarily as a heuristic graphical summary.

Essen & Maunsell, 1983). Functionally, the dorsal system is primarily involved in processing motion and spatial dimensions of visual information ("where"); the ventral system is mainly associated with discriminative visual feature processing ("what"). Spatial information from peripheral visual fields is principally carried by projections from dorsal occipital and caudal parietal regions that travel rostrally within the intrahemispheric white matter to terminate in area 8, and the dorsal and caudal regions of areas 46 and 9. Object-related information originates in striate cortex mediating central vision and travels via ventral occipital and caudal temporal–visual projections to inferotemporal cortices. From there projections via the uncinate fasciculus extend to lateral orbitofrontal regions and the ventral part of area 46 (Barbas, 1992; Cavada & Goldman-Rakic, 1989; Petrides & Pandya, 1984; Selemon & Goldman-Rakic, 1988). Single neuron recordings in monkeys have demonstrated that the parallel, segregated visuospatial and object-processing streams associated with working memory remain functionally and anatomically distinct in these respective DLPFC regions (Wilson, Scalaidhe, & Goldman-Rakic, 1993).

## Auditory System

Functionally segregated processing streams akin to the "what" (ventral) and "where" (dorsal) visual systems have not been described for cortical auditory pathways. Linguistic and nonlinguistic auditory processing represents the principal basis of functional segregation in cortical auditory pathways that are topographically distributed between the left and right hemispheres. Projections from auditory association cortex (area 22) in the superior temporal gyrus to dorsal area 8, lateral prefrontal areas 10 and 46, and medial frontal areas 32 and 25 are the main frontal–auditory cortical connections (Barbas, 1992; Barbas & Pandya, 1991). Topographically, the latter projections and those to medial frontal paralimbic areas originate from anterior superior temporal regions; lateral frontal auditory pathways emanate from more posterior superior temporal areas. Wernicke's area includes a portion of auditory association cortex in the posterior one-third of the superior temporal gyrus and adjacent heteromodal regions in the left (dominant) hemisphere. Connections from Wernicke's to Broca's area in the frontal operculum (areas 44 and 45) accompany auditory association projections to ventral premotor areas (Nieuwenhuys et al., 1988).

## Somatosensory System

Projections from postcentral somatosensory areas extend to the rostral inferior parietal lobule (supramarginal gyrus), which, together with fibers from the parietal operculum, traverse the ventral portion of the superior longitudinal fasciculus and terminate in the ventral portion of area 9/46, premotor area 6, and the frontal opercular region (Petrides & Pandya, 1984). Reciprocal pathways from ventral prefrontal cortex provide feedback to the rostral inferior parietal lobule and parietal operculum, forming a putative loop for monitoring oral, facial, and limb movements underlying gestural communication. Lesions in the rostral inferior parietal region and adjacent white matter are associated with ideomotor apraxia.

## Medial Temporal Limbic System

Prefrontal cortices are richly connected to paralimbic and allocortical areas (Amaral & Price, 1984; Carmichael & Price, 1995; Rosene & Van Hoesen, 1987). A general rostrocaudal gradient of limbic innervation has been described, whereby medial frontal and ventral orbital areas have the highest proportion of limbic inputs, followed by lateral prefrontal (DLPFC) regions, with premotor areas having the least (Barbas, 1992; Barbas & Mesulam, 1981). Limbic input to the ACC arises primarily from the amygdala and entorhinal cortex, in addition to a small projection from the subiculum. DLPFC regions are indirectly linked to limbic regions of the parahippocampal gyrus through connections with the ACC and posterior cingulate (area 23) and retrosplenial cortex (area 30), which forms the ventral bank of the posterior cingulate and lies dorsal to the corpus callosum (Barbas, 1992; Vogt et al., 2005). In addition, sparse connections between the DLPFC and entorhinal, presubicular, and caudal parahippocampal regions (caudomedial lobule) have been described (Goldman-Rakic, Selemon, & Schwartz, 1984). Although the functional significance of these indirect and direct connections are not well-defined, they represent parallel pathways between the DLPFC and hippocampal formation that have been implicated to play a role in maintaining contextual infor-

mation on a moment-by-moment basis (i.e., working memory) (Goldman-Rakic, 1987).

## Interhemispheric Connectivity

It is estimated that 2–3% of all cortical neurons send projections to the contralateral hemisphere, most of which cross in the corpus callosum (Lamantia & Rakic, 1990). In general, patterns of interhemispheric cortical connectivity parallel intrahemispheric associational relationships (Innocenti, 1986; Pandya & Seltzer, 1986). Homotopic connections interconnect similar cortical areas in both hemispheres; heterotopic commissural fibers typically project to contralateral areas that correspond to the intrahemispheric distribution of fibers from that region but are usually less abundant than ipsilateral connections. Higher-order association areas tend to have the greatest density of commissural projections, whereas fewer interhemispheric connections are present between primary sensory and motor cortices.

The general pattern of callosal connectivity between prefrontal regions, as with other cerebral cortices, broadly reflects cortical topography along the anterior–posterior hemispheric axis (Figure 4.4) (Barbas, 1992; Barbas & Pandya, 1984; Pandya & Seltzer, 1986). Commissural fibers from the DLPFC generally cross in the genu of the corpus callosum, rostral to premotor and motor axons. Interhemispheric axons from dorsal regions of the DLPFC typically occupy more caudal regions of the genu relative to those from ventral DLPFC regions. The most rostral areas of the corpus callosum (lower genu and rostrum) contain commissural axons from rostromedial frontal (areas 25 and rostral area 32) and orbitofrontal areas. Commissural projections from the ACC are distributed throughout the rostral half of the corpus callosum, intermingling with fibers from premotor and motor areas in the superior portion of the callosum.

## MODULAR ORGANIZATION OF CORTICOCORTICAL CONNECTIONS

The preceding discussion has reviewed general aspects of frontal lobe anatomy and cortical connectivity, focusing on architectonic features and topographically distributed functional circuitry. At a superordinate level of organization, contemporary models of brain function are

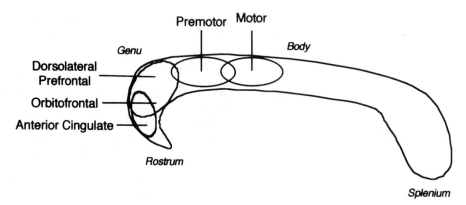

FIGURE 4.4. Prefrontal commisural fiber trajectories within the corpus callosum. ACC fibers also project throughout rostral half of the corpus callosum. After Pandya and Seltzer (1986) and Barbas (1992).

based on multifocal patterns of synchronous activity in distributed networks consisting of neural nodes or modules (Damasio & Damasio, 1989; Mesulam, 1990). Although the physiological determinants of temporal coactivation within network circuitry remain speculative, insight into the anatomical substrates of spatially distributed network activity derives from axon terminal labeling experiments in rhesus monkeys (Selemon & Goldman-Rakic, 1988). In this work, axon terminals from labeled neurons in lateral prefrontal (areas 9 and 10) and posterior parietal (area 7) heteromodal regions were observed to converge in 15 different cortical regions. Among these common areas of intersection, two general, but not all-inclusive, patterns of laminar terminal organization were identified (Figure 4.5). The first pattern is characterized by the interdigitation of convergent prefrontal and posterior parietal inputs. As schematically illustrated (Figure 4.5, left), prefrontal and parietal fiber terminations were observed to span all cortical layers (being slightly more prominent in layer I), and typically formed adjacent, horizontally oriented columns. This pattern of fiber terminal segregation was observed throughout paralimbic cingulate regions. A different pattern of labeling was observed in heteromodal superior temporal cortex, as well as the frontoparietal operculum (Figure 4.5, right). In these regions, alternating columns exhibited a vertically oriented pattern of laminar segregation; prefrontal terminals typically occupied layers I, III, and V, with alternating or "complementary" terminal labeling of layers

IV and VI by fibers of parietal origin. In addition, convergent prefrontal and parietal fiber terminals were observed in the contralateral superior temporal cortex, which may account for the unlabeled intervening columnar spaces in the ipsilateral superior temporal cortex. In previous work, the same investigators (Schwartz & Goldman-Rakic, 1984) also observed columnar organization of contiguous, alternating ipsilateral parietal and contralateral prefrontal inputs to prefrontal cortex in rhesus monkeys. More recently, a similar type of cortical modular organization has been demonstrated for both intrinsic (i.e., local circuit) and long-distance associational connections within monkey prefrontal cortex (Pucak, Levitt, Lund, & Lewis, 1996). Together, these findings suggest that corticocortical connections exhibit a modular functional architecture responsible for channeling patterns of activation in multifocal intra- and interhemispheric networks.

## FRONTAL CORTICAL CONNECTIVITY IN HUMAN DISEASE

### Callosal Morphometry and Degenerative Dementias

Selective cortical neuronal loss in degenerative dementias such as Alzheimer's disease (AD) and frontotemporal dementia (FTD) involve differential pathological topographies (see Grossman, Chapter 26, this volume). In AD, medial temporal limbic and temporoparietal association cortices are the sites of primary involvement, with relative sparing of primary

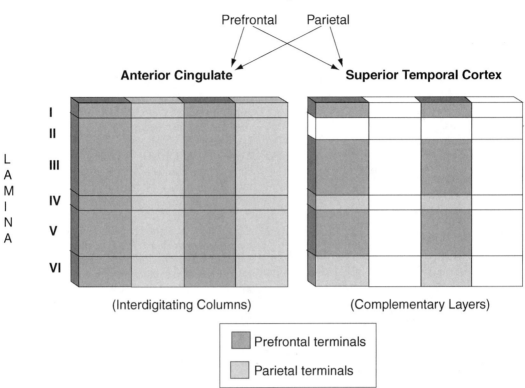

FIGURE 4.5. Schematic illustration of two general patterns of terminations observed for convergent prefrontal and posterior parietal labeled fibers in representative cortical areas of the rhesus monkey. See text for details. From Selemon and Goldman-Rakic (1988). Copyright 1988 by the Society for Neurosience. Adapted by permission.

sensory and motor areas (Arnold, Hyman, Flory, Damasio, & Van Hoesen, 1991). In contrast, pathological alterations in FTD predominantly affect frontal and anterior temporal lobe regions, typically being most concentrated in the DLPFC and the ACC (Lund and Manchester Groups, 1994). Relative differences in the anterior–posterior topographic distribution of pathological involvement may largely account for the distinctive, yet overlapping, clinical features of AD and FTD.

Although much is known about functional cerebral laterality, the fundamental mechanisms and clinical implications of impaired interhemispheric transmission between homotopic and heterotopic regions are poorly understood. Investigating regional callosal morphometry in degenerative and other neurological disorders may facilitate investigations of these interactions and provide insight into their functional significance. Kaufer and colleagues

(1997) examined regional cross-sectional area of the corpus callosum in patients with AD and FTD, and observed marked focal atrophy of anterior (rostrum and genu) callosal areas in subjects with FTD (Figure 4.6). In contrast, subjects with AD exhibited more diffuse atrophy in the genu and body of the corpus callosum compared to the others, consistent with previous findings (Biegon et al., 1994; Janowsky, Kaye, & Carper, 1996). Regional measures of the pericallosal cerebrospinal fluid (CSF) space showed that enlargement of the anterior portions, reflecting local atrophy of the adjacent ACC, was a more robust discriminant of FTD subjects. The overall degree of dementia severity showed no correlation with any callosal area measures in FTD, but was directly correlated to the size of the anterior portion of the callosum in AD, presumably reflecting the loss of commissural projections between prefrontal association and paralimbic areas. The

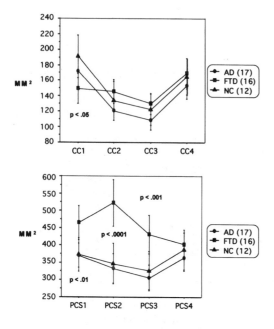

FIGURE 4.6. Comparison of regional areas of the corpus callosum (CC) and pericallosal space (PCS) from midsagittal MRI in subjects with Alzheimer's disease (AD), frontotemporal dementia (FTD), and normal control subjects (NC). Regions 1–4 indicate rostral to caudal location.

observed relationship between dementia severity and anterior callosal area in AD is consistent with other reports (Janowsky et al., 1996), including findings that the strongest correlate of cognitive impairment in AD identified to date is reduced synaptic density or loss of synaptic markers in prefrontal (medial) lobe regions (DeKosky & Scheff, 1990; Terry, Masliah, & Salmon, 1991).

## Intrinsic Prefrontal Circuitry and Schizophrenia

Multiple lines of evidence implicate dysfunction of the DLPFC in the pathophysiology of schizophrenia (see Ropacki & Perry, Chapter 36, this volume). Deficits in spatial working memory are associated with DLPFC lesions (Goldman-Rakic, 1987) and these types of cognitive disturbances are a common feature of schizophrenia (Weinberger, Berman, & Illowsky, 1988). Developmental considerations suggest another link between the DLPFC and schizophrenia; schizophrenia typically has its onset in the postpubertal period, and perfor-

mance on DLPFC-dependent tasks tends to reach adult levels around the time of puberty (Levin, Culhane, Hartmann, Evankovich, & Mattson, 1991). Within the DLPFC, excitatory pyramidal cells in layers II and III send intrinsic axon collaterals horizontally through the supragranular layers, and the terminal fields of these axons are organized as a series of stripes separated by similar size gaps (Levitt, Lewis, Yoshioka, & Lund, 1993). The projections between interconnected stripes are reciprocal, and the majority of these axon terminals synapse on dendritic spines of other pyramidal cells (Lewis, 1997; Pucak et al., 1996) (Figure 4.7). Thus, the reciprocal monosynaptic connections between stripes may provide the anatomical substrate for reverberating excitatory circuits that maintain the activity of functionally related populations of DLPFC cells, a critical feature of working memory (Lewis & Anderson, 1995). During adolescence, the number of these pyramidal cell interconnections typically decreases, suggesting that the pruning of the intrinsic connections of layer III pyramidal neurons in the DLPFC may confer a selective vulnerability related to the clinical onset of schizophrenic symptoms after maturity (Lewis & Levitt, 2002). Consistent with this interpretation, layer III pyramidal cells have been reported to be decreased in size (Rajkowska, Selemon, & Goldman-Rakic, 1994), and to have fewer dendritic spines (Glantz & Lewis, 1995) in subjects with schizophrenia. In addition, the activity of layer III pyramidal cells is modulated by inputs from certain inhibitory γ-aminobutyric acid–containing local circuit neurons, as well as by dopamine afferent fibers. These components of DLPFC circuitry also undergo substantial refinements during adolescence, and have been reported to be altered in schizophrenia (Lewis, Volk, & Hashimoto, 2004).

## SUMMARY AND EMERGING PERSPECTIVES

This survey of the DLPFC and ACC has emphasized general features of architectonic differentiation, functional topographic relationships, and associated patterns of connectivity. The complex functional circuitry of prefrontal association and paralimbic areas reflects the widespread connectivity of these areas to both cortical and subcortical areas, particularly

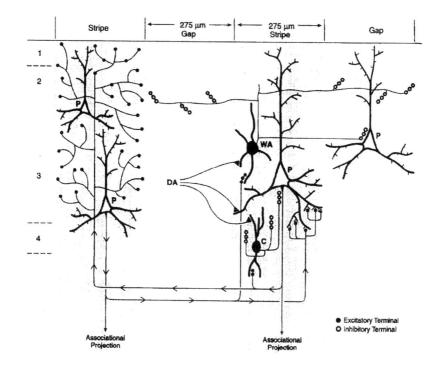

FIGURE 4.7. Schematic summary of intrinsic connectivity in monkey DLPFC. Layer 3 pyramidal neurons (P) furnish horizontal axon collaterals (lower part of figure) which terminate in stripe-like arrays approximately 275 microns wide in the superficial cortical layers. Many of these excitatory axon terminals target dendritic spines of pyramidal neurons that provide reciprocal connections between stripes. A smaller proportion of these excitatory axon terminals also project to chandelier (C) and wide arbor (WA) neurons, which may respectively form inhibitory synapses within the same stripe and in adjacent gaps. Dopamine (DA) afferents project to the dendritic spines and shafts of excitatory pyramidal cells, as well as to local circuit inhibitory neurons. Courtesy of Dr. David Lewis.

limbic-related cortices and nuclei (Barbas, 1992; Barbas & Pandya, 1989, 1991; Mesulam, 1985). Two examples of altered frontal cortical connectivity in human disease, differential patterns of corpus callosum atrophy in AD and FTD, and aberrant DLPFC local circuit interactions in schizophrenia, illustrate contrasting dimensions of frontal circuitry in terms of the level of analysis (gross vs. microscopic), the proximity of interaction (interhemispheric vs. local circuit), and age-related pathophysiological alterations (degenerative vs. developmental).

Although structure–function relationships have primarily been discussed from a frame of reference provided by Brodmann-defined areas, structural and functional heterogeneity within such regions suggest a modular functional organization of prefrontal association

cortices (Goldman-Rakic, 1987; Pucak et al., 1996). Consistent with descriptions of posterior visual cortices in terms of functional modules (van Essen & Maunsell, 1983), detailed architectonic mapping of orbital and medial prefrontal regions have identified at least 22 different areas that may constitute discrete functional zones or modules (Carmichael & Price, 1994, 1995). Concepts of modular cerebral cortical organization and functionally segregated, topographically distributed parallel pathways that have emerged from anatomical and electrophysiological studies in nonhuman primates have important implications for the study of functional connectivity in humans. Newer structural magnetic resonance imaging techniques, such as diffusion tensor imaging, offer the prospect of mapping neural pathways *in vivo* and complementing functional brain-mapping techniques. In addition, neural network models based on the computational theory of parallel-distributed processing have been described, involving both large-scale, distributed functional networks (Mesulam, 1990) and individual neuronal interactions within local (prefrontal) circuits (Cohen & Servan-Schreiber, 1992). Together, these tools may offer complementary avenues for generating and testing hypotheses related to normal and pathological functioning of the human frontal lobes.

## REFERENCES

Amaral, D. G., & Price, J. L. (1984). Amygdalo-cortical projections in the monkey (*Macaca fascicularis*). *Journal of Comparative Neurology, 230,* 465–496.

Arnold, S. E., Hyman, B. T., Flory, J., Damasio, A. R., & Van Hoesen, G. W. (1991). The topographical and neuroanatomical distribution of neurofibrillary tangles and neuritic plaques in the cerebral cortex of patients with Alzheimer's disease. *Cerebral Cortex, 1,* 103–116.

Barbas, H. (1986). Pattern in the laminar origin of corticocortical connections. *Journal of Comparative Neurology, 252,* 415–422.

Barbas, H. (1992). Architecture and cortical connections of the prefrontal cortex in the rhesus monkey. In P. Chauvel & H. V. Delgado-Escueta (Eds.), *Advances in neurology* (Vol. 57, pp. 91–115). New York: Raven.

Barbas, H., & Mesulam, M.-M. (1981). Organization of afferent input to subdivisions of area 8 in the rhesus monkey. *Journal of Comparative Neurology, 200,* 407–431.

Barbas, H., & Pandya, D. N. (1984). Topography of commissural fibers of the prefrontal cortex in the rhesus monkey. *Experimental Brain Research, 55,* 187–191.

Barbas, H., & Pandya, D. N. (1989). Architecture and intrinsic connections of the prefrontal cortex in rhesus monkeys. *Journal of Comparative Neurology, 286,* 353–375.

Barbas, H., & Pandya, D. N. (1991). Patterns of connections of the prefrontal cortex in the rhesus monkey associated with cortical architecture. In H. S. Levin, H. M. Eisenberg, & A. L. Benton (Eds.), *Frontal lobe function and dysfunction* (pp. 35–58). New York: Oxford University Press.

Benson, D. F. (1993). Progressive frontal dysfunction. *Dementia, 4,* 149–153.

Biegon, A., Eberling, J. L., Richardson, B. E., Roos, M. S., Wong, T. S., Reed, B. R., et al. (1994). Human corpus callosum in aging and Alzheimer's disease: A magnetic resonance imaging study. *Neurobiology of Aging, 15,* 393–397.

Brodmann, K. (1994). *Localization in the cerebral cortex.* London: Smith-Gordon. (Original work published 1909)

Bush, G., Luu, P., & Posner, M. I. (2000). Cognitive and emotional influences in anterior cingulate cortex. *Trends in Cognitive Sciences, 4,* 215–222.

Carmichael, S. T., & Price, J. L. (1994). Architectonic subdivision of the orbital and medial prefrontal cortex in the macaque monkey. *Journal of Comparative Neurology, 346,* 366–402.

Carmichael, S. T., & Price, J. L. (1995). Limbic connections of the orbital and medial prefrontal cortex in macaque monkeys. *Journal of Comparative Neurology, 363,* 615–641.

Cavada, C., & Goldman-Rakic, P. S. (1989). Posterior parietal cortex in rhesus monkeys: II. Evidence for segregated corticocortical networks linking sensory and limbic areas with the frontal lobes. *Journal of Comparative Neurology, 287,* 422–445.

Cohen, J. D., & Servan-Schreiber, D. (1992). Context, cortex, and dopamine: A connectionist approach to behavior and biology in schizophrenia. *Psychology Review, 99,* 45–77.

Damasio, H. C. (1991). Neuroanatomy of frontal lobe *in vivo*: A comment on methodology. In H. S. Levin, H. M. Eisenberg, & A. L. Benton (Eds.), *Frontal lobe function and dysfunction* (pp. 92–124). New York: Oxford University Press.

Damasio, H., & Damasio, A. R. (1989). *Lesion analysis in neuropsychology.* New York: Oxford University Press.

DeKosky, S. T., & Scheff, S. W. (1990). Synapse loss in frontal cortex biopsies in Alzheimer's disease: Correlation with cognitive severity. *Annals of Neurology, 27,* 457–464.

Felleman, D. J., & van Essen, D. C. (1991). Distributed hierarchical processing in the primate cerebral cortex. *Cerebral Cortex, 1,* 1–47.

Galaburda, A. M., & Pandya, D. N. (1983). The intrinsic architectonic and connectional organization of the superior temporal region of the rhesus monkey. *Journal of Comparative Neurology, 221,* 169–184.

Glantz, L. A., & Lewis, D. A. (1995). Assessment of spine density on layer III pyramidal cells in the prefrontal cortex of schizophrenic subjects. *Society of Neuroscience Abstracts, 21,* 239.

Goldman-Rakic, P. S. (1987). Circuitry of primate prefrontal cortex and regulation of behavior by representational memory. In F. Plum (Ed.), *Handbook of physiology: The nervous system* (Vol. 5, pp. 373–417). Bethesda, MD: American Physiological Society.

Goldman-Rakic, P. S., Selemon, L. D., & Schwartz, M. S. (1984). Dual pathways connecting the dorsolateral prefrontal cortex with the hippocampal formation and parahippocampal cortex in the rhesus monkey. *Journal of Neuroscience, 12,* 719–743.

Innocenti, G. M. (1986). General organization of callosal connections in the cerebral cortex. In E. G. Jones & A. Peters (Eds.), *Cerebral cortex* (Vol. 5, pp. 291–353). New York: Plenum Press.

Janowsky, J. S., Kaye, J. A., & Carper, R. A. (1996). Atrophy of the corpus callosum in Alzheimer's disease versus healthy aging. *Journal of the American Geriatric Society, 44,* 798–803.

Kaufer, D. I., Miller, B. L., Itti, L., Fairbanks, L., Li, J., Fishman, J., et al. (1997). Midline cerebral morphometry distinguishes frontotemporal dementia and Alzheimer's disease. *Neurology, 48,* 978–985.

Konishi, M. (1995). Neural mechanisms of auditory image formation. In M. S. Gazzaniga (Ed.), *The cognitive neurosciences* (pp. 269–278). Cambridge, MA: MIT Press.

Lamantia, A. S., & Rakic, P. (1990). Cytological and quantitative characteristics of four cerebral commissures in the rhesus monkey. *Journal of Comparative Neurology, 291,* 520–537.

Levin, H. S., Culhane, K. A., Hartmann, J., Evankovich, K., & Mattson, A. J. (1991). Developmental changes in performance on tests of purported frontal lobe functioning. *Developmental Neuropsychology, 7,* 377–395.

Levitt, J. B., Lewis, D. A., Yoshioka, T., & Lund, J. S. (1993). Topography of pyramidal neuron connections in macaque monkey prefrontal cortex (areas 9 and 46). *Journal of Comparative Neurology, 338,* 360–376.

Lewis, D. A. (1997). Development of the prefrontal cortex during adolescence: Insights into vulnerable schizophrenic circuits in schizophrenia. *Neuropsychopharmacology, 16,* 385–398.

Lewis, D. A., & Anderson, S. A. (1995). The functional architecture of the prefrontal cortex and schizophrenia. *Psychological Medicine, 25,* 887–894.

Lewis, D. A., Hayes, T. L., Lund, J. S, & Oeth, K. M. (1992). Dopamine and the neural circuitry of primate prefrontal cortex: Implications for schizophrenia research. *Neuropsychopharmacology, 6,* 127–134.

Lewis, D. A., & Levitt, P. (2002). Schizophrenia as a disorder of neurodevelopment. *Annual Review of Neuroscience, 25,* 409–432.

Lewis, D. A., Volk, D. W., & Hashimoto, T. (2004). Selective alterations in prefrontal cortical GABA neurotransmission in schizophrenia: A novel target for the treatment of working memory dysfunction. *Psychopharmacology (Berlin), 174,* 143–50.

The Lund and Manchester Groups. (1994). Clinical and neuropathological criteria for frontotemporal dementia: The Lund and Manchester Groups. *Journal of Neurology, Neurosurgery, and Psychiatry, 57,* 416–418.

Mesulam, M. (1997). Anatomic principles in behavioral neurology and neuropsychology. In T. E. Feinberg & M. J. Farah (Eds.), *Behavioral neurology and neuropsychology* (pp. 55–68). New York: McGraw-Hill.

Mesulam, M.-M. (1985). Patterns in behavioral neuroanatomy: Association areas, the limbic system, and hemispheric specialization. In *Principles of behavioral neurology* (pp. 1–70). Philadelphia: Davis.

Mesulam, M.-M. (1990). Large scale neurocognitve net-works and distributed processing for attention, language, and memory. *Annals of Neurology, 28,* 597–613.

Mishkin, M., Ungerleider, L. G., & Macko, K. A. (1983). Object vision and spatial vision: Two cortical pathways. *Trends in Neuroscience, 6,* 414–417.

Nieuwenhuys, R., Voogd, J., & van Huijzen, C. (1988). *The human central nervous system: A synopsis and atlas* (3rd rev. ed.). Berlin: Springer-Verlag.

Pandya, D. N., & Seltzer, B. (1986). The topography of commissural fibers. In F. Lepore, M. Ptito, & H. H. Jasper (Eds.), *Two hemispheres—one brain* (pp. 47–73). New York: Liss.

Pandya, D. N., & Yeterian, E. H. (1985). Architecture and connections of cortical association areas. In A. Peters & E. Jones (Eds.), *Cerebral cortex: Vol. 4. Association and auditory cortices* (pp. 3–61). New York: Plenum Press.

Petrides, M. (2005). Lateral and prefrontal cortex: architectonic and functional organization. *Philosophical Transactions of the Royal Society, 360,* 781–795.

Petrides, M., & Pandya, D. N. (1984). Projections to the frontal lobes from the posterior-parietal region in the rhesus monkey. *Journal of Comparative Neurology, 228,* 105–116.

Petrides, M., & Pandya, D. N. (1994). Comparative architectonic analysis of the human and macaque frontal cortex. In F. Boller & J. Grafman (Eds.), *Handbook of neuropsychology* (Vol. 9, pp. 17–58). Amsterdam: Elsevier.

Pucak, M. L., Levitt, J. B., Lund, J. S., & Lewis, D. A. (1996). Patterns of intrinsic and associational excitatory circuitry in monkey prefrontal cortex. *Journal of Comparative Neurology, 376,* 614–630.

Rajkowska, G., Selemon, L. D., & Goldman-Rakic, P. (1994). Reduction in neuronal sizes in prefrontal cortex of schizophrenics and Huntington patients. *Society of Neuroscience Abstracts, 20,* 620.

Rockland, K. S., & Pandya, D. S. (1979). Laminar origins and terminations of cortical connections of the occipital lobe in the rhesus monkey. *Brain Research, 179,* 3–20.

Rosene, D. L., & Van Hoesen, G. W. (1987). The hippocampal formation of the primate brain. In E. G. Jones & A. G. Peters (Eds.), *Cerebral cortex* (pp. 345–456). New York: Plenum Press.

Sanides, F. (1972). Representation in the cerebral cortex and its areal lamination pattern. In G. H. Bourne (Ed.), *The structure and function of nervous tissue* (Vol. 5, pp. 329–453). New York: Academic Press.

Schwartz, M. S., & Goldman-Rakic, P. S. (1984). Callosal and intrahemispheric connectivity of the prefrontal association cortex in rhesus monkey: Relation between intraparietal and principal sulcal cortex. *Journal of Comparative Neurology, 226,* 403–420.

Selemon, L. D., & Goldman-Rakic, P. S. (1988). Common cortical and subcortical targets of the dorsolateral prefrontal and parietal cortices in the rhesus monkey: Evidence for a distributed neural network subserving spatially guided behavior. *Journal of Neuroscience, 8*, 4049–4068.

Talaraich, J., & Tournox, P. (1988). Co-planar stereotaxic atlas of the human brain. New York: Thieme.

Terry, R. D., Masliah, E., & Salmon, D. P. (1991). Physical basis of cognitive alterations in Alzheimer's disease: Synapse loss is the major correlate of cognitive impairment. *Annals of Neurology, 30,* 572–580.

van Essen, D. C., & Maunsell, J. H. R. (1983). Hierarchical organization and functional streams in the visual cortex. *Trends in Neuroscience, 6,* 370–375.

Vogt, B. A., Finch, D. M., & Olson, C. R. (1992). Functional heterogeneity in cingulate cortex: The anterior executive and posterior evaluative regions. *Cerebral Cortex, 2,* 435–443.

Vogt, B. A., Vogt, L., Farber, N. B., & Bush, G. (2005). Architecture and neurocytology of the monkey cingulate gyrus. *Journal of Comparative Neurology, 485,* 218–239.

Walker, A. E. (1940). A cytoarchitectural study of the prefrontal area of the macaque monkey. *Journal of Comparative Neurology, 73,* 59–86.

Weinberger, D. R., Berman, K. F., & Illowsky, B. P. (1988). Physiological dysfunction of dorsolateral prefrontal cortex in schizophrenia: III. A new cohort and evidence for a monoaminergic mechanism. *Archives of General Psychiatry, 45,* 609–615.

Wilson, F. A. W., Scalaidhe, S. P. O., & Goldman-Rakic, P. S. (1993). Dissociation of object and spatial processing domains in primate prefrontal cortex. *Science, 260,* 1955–1958.

Zilles, K. (1990). Cortex. In G. Paxinos (Ed.), *The human nervous system* (pp. 757–802). San Diego, CA: Academic Press.

# CHAPTER 5

# The Orbitofrontal Cortex and the Insula

*Jennifer Ogar*
*Maria Luisa Gorno-Tempini*

The cerebral cortex can be partitioned in two ways: structurally or functionally. Cytoarchitechtonic maps, of which Brodmann's (1909) is probably the most widely used, have provided one way to divide structurally related areas of cortex. Functionally, five subtypes of cortex have been proposed: (1) primary sensory–motor; (2) unimodal association; (3) heteromodal association; (4) paralimbic; and (5) limbic (Mesulam, 1985a). The paralimbic subtype is further separated into a temporal–insular–orbitofrontal region and a hippocampocentric subdivision (Mesulam, 1998). Together, these components of the paralimbic system work to appropriately direct emotional and motivational components of behavior (Mesulam, 1998). The temporal–insular–orbitofrontal region is largely devoted to olfaction and acts as a transition zone between olfactory allocortex and homotypical cortex (Mesulam, 1998). This chapter focuses on the anatomy of the orbitofrontal cortex (OFC) and the insula; two major components of the paralimbic belt.

## THE OFC

The OFC plays a critical role in human emotion, and damage to this brain region has been linked to altered personality, behavior, social conduct, and emotion (Hornak et al., 2003; Rolls & Baylis, 1994). Also, the OFC is recognized as an area important for learning the re-ward and punishment value of stimuli given its rich reciprocal connections with primary sensory, somatosensory, and visceral brain regions. Imaging studies have shown that OFC regions are activated by pleasant and painful touch, taste, and smell stimuli, as well as abstract reinforcements such as winning and losing money (Rolls, 2004). The OFC contains secondary taste cortex, as well as secondary and tertiary olfactory areas. As an end-stage site for projections from sensory cortex, the OFC has a role in determining the reward value of taste, as well as the identity and reward value of odor (Rolls, 2004).

## Boundaries and Cytoarchitecture

The OFC is part of the prefrontal cortex (PFC), which is divided into three zones: medial frontal, orbitofrontal, and dorsolateral. The OFC comprises the most ventral portion of the PFC and is composed of five gyri: (1) the *gyrus rectus*, which forms the boundary between the ventral and medial surface of the PFC; (2) the *medial orbital gyrus*; (3) the *middle orbital gyrus*; (4) the *lateral orbital gyrus*; and (5) the *orbital portion of the inferior frontal gyrus* (see Figure 5.1). It should be noted that the middle orbital gyrus has also been divided into anterior and posterior orbital gyri. Two sulci divide the OFC. The *olfactory sulcus* separates the gyrus rectus and the medial orbital gyrus. The olfactory bulb lies within the olfactory sulcus. An H-shaped, second OFC *sulcus*, also known as the

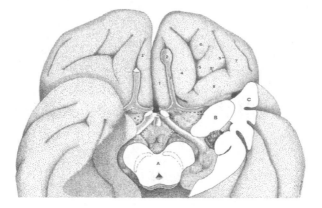

FIGURE 5.1. The OFC. The brainstem (A), uncus (B), and temporal pole (C), have been removed. 1, gyrus rectus; 2, olfactory bulk; 2', medial orbital sulcus (olfactory sulcus); 3, olfactory tract; 4, medial orbital gyrus; 5, H-shaped sulcus; 5', arcuate orbital sulcus; 6, anterior orbital gyrus; 7, lateral orbital gyrus; 8, posterior orbital gyrus. From Duvernoy (1999). Copyright 1999 by Springer-Verlag/Wien. Reprinted by permission.

*arcuate* or *transverse orbital sulcus*, separates the middle orbital gyrus into anterior and posterior zones (Zald & Kim, 2001).

Anatomical variations within the human OFC have led to some confusion regarding the labeling of specific and gyri and sulci. For this reason, some anatomists label all OFC regions between the olfactory sulci and the inferior frontal gyrus "orbital gyri" and "orbital sulci" (Ono, Kubuk, & Abernathy, 1990).

Brodmann's first cytoarchitectonic map detailed only three OFC areas in the human brain: 10, 11, and 47 (Brodmann, 1909). Further analysis with classical histological techniques revealed less homogeneity in the OFC, and researchers have subsequently expanded upon Brodmann's initial maps. Studying the macaque monkey, Walker (1940) noted five separate areas: 10, 11, 12, 13, and 14. Area 12 and 13 occupy the lateral and medial orbital zones; area 14 denotes the region near the gyrus rectus; area 10 comprises the frontal pole, and area 11 refers to the anterior OFC. Walker's map is thought to correspond well to the human OFC, with some further delineations noted by other researchers (Carmichael, Clugnet, & Price, 1994; Hof, Mufson, & Morrison, 1995; Petrides & Pandya, 1994). Of note, Petrides and Pandya attempted to resolve discrepancies between the human and monkey OFC maps by proposing to label lateral parts of the orbitofrontal gyri "47/12," a common notation in the OFC literature. (For more comprehensive reviews of OFC cytoarchitecture,

see Barbas, 1995a; Carmichael et al., 1994; Ongur & Price, 2000; Pandya & Yeterian, 1996; Petrides & Pandya, 1994.)

Kringelbach notes that the OFC and the medial PFC should be regarded as a singular orbitomedial prefrontal cortex (OMPFC) given the region's cytoarchitectural and functional similarities (Kringelbach & Rolls, 2004; Ongur & Price, 2000). Within this proposal, the OMPFC would also include parts of the anterior cingulate cortex. The orbital pathway receives extensive afferents from all sensory systems and visceral areas as well, whereas the medial pathway provides many visceromotor efferents. Together, via these pathways, the OMPFC would function as an important region for regulating eating behavior (Kringelbach & Rolls, 2004).

### Connectivity

The OFC receives input from all sensory modalities: olfactory, gustatory, auditory, visual, and somatosensory, and from visceral systems as well (Rolls, 2004). Given that the OFC receives input from the ventral temporal lobe visual stream, Rolls has proposed that this region has a unique role in processing the "what" of stimuli (as opposed to the "where"). Links to primary sensory cortex also underlie the OFC's role in multimodal stimulus–reinforcement association learning (Rolls, Critchley, Browning, Hernadi, & Lenard, 1999; Rolls, Yaxley, & Sienkiewicz, 1990). Damage to the OFC, therefore, has been found to impair learning and the ability to differentiate between rewarding and nonrewarding situations or appropriate behavior alteration when reinforcements change (Rolls, 2004). For example, macaques with OFC lesions may continue to respond to stimuli that are no longer rewarded or vice versa (Rolls, 2004). Irresponsibility, lack of affect, and apathy (common behavioral changes seen in patients with OFC damage) may be related to this inability to alter responses (Damasio, Grabowski, Frank, Galaburda, & Damasio, 1994; Rolls, 2004).

Unimodal olfactory and taste neurons, as well as single neurons that respond to both gustatory and olfactory stimuli, are found in the OFC (Baylis, Rolls, & Baylis, 1995; Rolls, 2004). This convergence of taste- and smell-related neurons may give rise to the representation of flavor in the OFC (Baylis et al., 1995; Rolls, 2004). The OFC's extensive links have also led some researchers to propose that it is one of the most polymodal regions in the cortex, along with anterior regions of the temporal lobe (Barbas, 1988; see Figure 5.2).

## Inputs

As noted earlier, the OFC receives input from all sensory systems and indirectly from the viscera (primarily via the thalamus). A portion of the lateral OFC has been recognized as secondary taste cortex (Rolls et al., 1990), which receives inputs from primary taste regions in the anterior insula and adjacent frontal operculum via the ventral posteromedial nucleus of the thalamus (Baylis et al., 1995; Kringelbach & Rolls, 2004; Rolls et al., 1990).

Olfactory and auditory information also reach the OFC. Secondary olfactory areas (Iam, Iamp, and 13) and tertiary olfactory areas (area 11) have been identified within medial OFC (Carmichael et al., 1994; Critchley & Rolls, 1996; Rolls, 1996; Rolls & Baylis, 1994). These OFC olfactory areas receive input from primary olfactory cortex and pyriform cortex via posterior OFC cortex (area 13a) (Barbas, 1993; Carmichael et al., 1994; Morecraft, Geula, & Mesulam, 1992; Price, 1991; Rolls, 2004). Auditory projections arrive in the OFC (areas 11 and 47/12) from superior temporal cortex (Barbas, 1988, 1993; Morecraft et al., 1992; Romanski, Bates, & Goldman-Rakic, 1999).

Lateral OFC (area 47/12) receives visual projections, particularly those related to object processing, from inferior temporal cortex, superior temporal sulcus regions, and the temporal pole (Barbas, 1988, 1993, 1995a, 1995b; Barbas & Blatt, 1995; Barbas & Pandya, 1989; Carmichael et al., 1994). Face-processing areas in the temporal lobe and superior temporal sulcus regions also reach the OFC (Hasselmo, Rolls, & Baylis, 1989; Hasselmo, Rolls, Baylis, & Nalwa, 1989). See Figure 5.2. Damage to the OFC, therefore, may impair one's ability to interpret facial and vocal expression (Hornak, Rolls, & Wade, 1996).

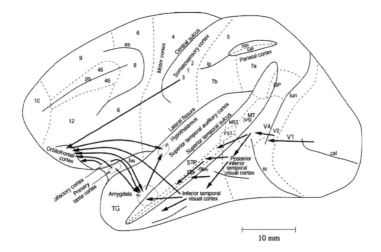

FIGURE 5.2. Connections of the OFC. From Rolls (2004). Copyright 2004 by Elsevier. Reprinted by permission.

The OFC receives projections from somato-sensory regions, the amygdala, and the cingulate gyrus as well. Inputs from the insula and somatosensory areas 1, 2, and S II in the frontal and pericentral operculum project to the OFC (area 47/12) (Barbas, 1988; Carmichael et al., 1994). Visceral input arrives at the caudal OFC from the ventrolateral posteromedial thalamic nucleus (Barbas & Pandya, 1989; Carmichael et al., 1994; Cavada, Company, Tejedor, Cruz-Rizzolo, & Reinoso-Suarez, 2000; Morecraft et al., 1992; Ongur & Price, 2000). Cavada and colleagues (2000) note direct ipsilateral projections from the hippocampus to predominantly medial OFC areas.

The OFC differentiates itself from other PFC areas, in that it receives inputs from the magnocellular, medial nucleus of the mediodorsal thalamus (Fuster, 1979). Other PFC regions receive projections from different parts of the mediodorsal thalamus: The dorsolateral PFC receives input from the lateral, parvocellular part of the mediodorsal thalamic nucleus and the frontal eye fields via projections from the paralamellar part of the mediodorsal nucleus of the thalamus (Kringelbach & Rolls, 2004).

Neurons of the OFC are innervated by cholinergic and aminergic subcortical fibers (Morecraft et al., 1992). The OFC also sends outputs to the nucleus basalis and may therefore control cholinergic input the entire cerebral cortex (Mesulam, Mufson, Levey, & Wainer, 1984).

## Outputs

The majority of OFC connections we have detailed are reciprocal, meaning that the OFC sends outputs back to the amygdala, inferior temporal lobe, entorhinal cortex, hippocampus (Kringelbach & Rolls, 2004; Rolls, 2004; Rolls et al., 1999), and cingulate cortex (Insausti, Amaral, & Cowan, 1987a, 1987b). OFC outputs also project to the lateral hypothalamus, the ventral tegmentum, and preoptic regions (Johnson, Rosvold, & Mishkin, 1968; Nauta, 1964; Rolls et al., 1999), as well as the head of the caudate nucleus (Kemp & Powell, 1970). The OFC also shares reciprocal connections with the hypothalamus and the periaqueductal gray (Rempel-Clower & Barbas, 1998). Rolls has hypothesized that the OFC–periaqueductal gray pathway could underlie the OFC's role in goal-directed behavior (Rolls et al., 1999).

## THE INSULA

### Anatomy

The connectivity and functions of the human insula have remained somewhat more elusive than those of the brain's other lobes. This is largely due to the insula's remote location, buried beneath the frontal, temporal, and parietal lobes. In the last few decades, connections between the insula and adjacent cortical and subcortical areas have been studied extensively in the monkey (Augustine, 1985, 1996; Mesulam & Mufson, 1982a, 1982b). In humans, some insight into the fundamental functions of the insula have been described through the use of classical cortical electrophysiological stimulation (Penfield & Faulk, 1955) and, more recently, with techniques such as functional magnetic resonance imaging (fMRI) (disgust, taste) and positron emission tomography (PET). Findings related to insular functions also arise from studies of patients, because the insula is a common site for focal epileptic discharges, strokes, and tumors (Mesulam & Mufson, 1982a). Today, the insula's role in visceral sensory, motor, vestibular, and somatosensory processes has been widely accepted (Augustine, 1985, 1996). Specifically, an area within the anterior insula (area G) is now recognized as primary gustatory cortex. The insula's precise role in emotion processing and speech praxis is still a matter of some debate.

### Boundaries

Within Brodmann's classic cortical map, the insula, or "the island of Reil," is considered to be the fifth and smallest lobe of the brain, comprising Brodmann's areas 13–16 (Brodmann, 1909). It lies beneath the convergence of the frontal, temporal, and parietal lobes, and can be seen only when these lobes are retracted. In the human insula, three short gyri appear anteriorly and two longer gyri define the posterior insula (Carpenter, 1985; Clark, 1896). It is somewhat triangular in shape, with the anterior and posterior regions separated by a central insular sulcus that is aligned with the central sulcus of the cerebral hemisphere (Clark, 1896; Cunningham, 1891a). The main branch of the middle cerebral artery lies within this sulcus (Clark, 1896). The brain's basal nuclei lie medial to the insula, whereas the insula's topmost portion is defined by the opercula of the inferior frontal gyrus, inferior parietal lobe, and the superior temporal gyrus. The entrance into the insula at the junction of these regions is referred to as the limen insula, or the falciform fold (Cunningham, 1891a; see Figure 5.3).

Insular sulci are fully formed by 32nd week of development and closely correspond with their respective sulci on the lateral hemispheres (Cunningham, 1891a, 1891b). The left insula grows for a longer period of time and is subsequently larger than the right insula (Clark, 1896; Clark & Russel, 1939; Cunningham, 1891a, 1891b). This size difference has led some researchers to speculate that the left insula may play some role in the human-specific ability that is language (Flynn, Benson, & Ardila, 1999).

## Cytoarchitecture

The human insula, though much larger than that of the rhesus monkey, is nearly identical in cellular organization (Mesulam & Mufson, 1982a, 1982b). It shares the cytoarchitecture of the adjacent lateral orbital cortex and temporal pole, so that together these structures comprise part of the paralimbic belt (Mesulam, 1985b; Mesulam & Mufson, 1982a).

Cytoarchitectonically, the insula can be divided into three distinct zones: anterior agran-

ular (Ia), dysgranular (Id), and granular (Ig), moving rostrocaudally (Augustine, 1996; Flynn et al., 1999; Mesulam & Mufson, 1982a, 1982b). Myelin concentration is higher in anterior regions, whereas acetylcholinesterase levels are higher posteriorly (Mesulam & Mufson, 1982a). The anterior insula (Ia) is agranular–allocortical and consists of three cellular layers: the outer contains small pyramidal cells that are contiguous with the pyramidal cell layer of the prepiriform cortex. The intermediate layer (Id) consists of larger, hyperchromic pyramidal cells that are contiguous with layer V of the dysgranular cortex located more dorsally. The innermost layer (Ig) contains polymorphic cells that connect with the deep layer of the prepiriform cortex and the underlying claustrum (Flynn et al., 1999; Mesulam & Mufson, 1982a).

A dysgranular zone lies between the anterior and posterior insular regions. Granulation within this area can be difficult to differentiate. In the area adjoining agranular cortex, layer II contains some granule cells, and laminar organization is absent in layer III rostroventrally. Columnar arrangement can be visualized in dorsal–caudal regions. Layer V is more readily visualized rostrally, and layer VI is difficult to separate from layer V and underlying white

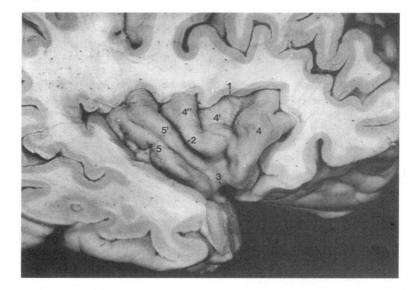

FIGURE 5.3. Lateral aspect of the right insula after ablation of frontal, parietal, and temporal opercila (×1.4). 1, circular insular sulcus; 2, central insular sulcus; 3, falciform fold; 4,4',4", short insular gyri; 5,5', long insular gyri. From Duvernoy (1999). Copyright 1999 by Springer-Verlag/Wien. Reprinted by permission.

matter (Flynn et al., 1999; Mesulam & Mufson, 1982a).

The posterior insula is a granular–isocortical area with greater cortical differentiation than dysgranular regions (Flynn et al., 1999). Layers II and IV are notably granular, and there is an easily visible division between layers V and VI (Flynn et al., 1999). Flynn and colleagues note that sublamination occurs in layer III, and infragranular layers are not clearly defined.

## Cortical Connections

The insula in humans and primates connects primarily with five cortical and subcortical regions, including (1) the cerebral cortex (frontal, temporal, and parietal lobes), (2) cingulate cortex, (3) the basal ganglia, (4) amygdala, (5) other limbic areas (including entorhinal and perirhinal cortex), and (6) the dorsal thalamus (Augustine, 1996; Flynn et al., 1999; Mesulam & Mufson, 1982a, 1982b).

The Ia shares connections primarily with other allocortical orbitofrontal and frontal opercular areas (Augustine, 1996; Mesulam & Mufson, 1982a, 1982b). Specifically, efferent and afferent connections have been visualized between the anterior insula and the prepiriform olfactory area, the frontal operculum, OFC, the dorsal and ventral temporal pole, rhinal fissure, supratemporal plane, the anterior and middle cingulate gyrus, and the somatosensory and opercular areas of the parietal lobe (Flynn et al., 1999; Mesulam & Mufson, 1982a, 1982b).

The Ia is thought to play a role in autonomic and visceral activities, particularly to integrate visceral senses with emotional events (Saper, 1982). Taste, speech praxis, and emotion processing have been associated with the Ia, and cardiovascular and gastrointestinal changes have been documented with IA stimulation. PET has been used to demonstrate increased cerebral blood flow in the Ia during emotion-generating tasks (happiness, sadness, and disgust), compared to emotionally neutral tasks (Reiman, 1996).

Within the Id region, which lies between the Ia and Ig insula, projections move in an anterior–posterior direction (Flynn et al., 1999; Mesulam & Mufson, 1982b). This is thought to underlie Ig's role in integrating information from all five senses. While the Ia connects primarily with frontal lobe areas, the Ig primarily shares connections with regions within the parietal lobe, although some frontal lobe connections also exist (Flynn et al., 1999; Mesulam & Mufson, 1982a, 1982b). In particular, the Ig shares connections with the supplementary motor area, the primary and secondary somatosensory cortex, the primary and secondary auditory cortex, the parietal lobe, and the retroinsular area (Flynn et al., 1999; Mesulam & Mufson, 1982a, 1982b).

The Ig is associated primarily with somatosensory functions and serves as a link between primary somatosensory regions and limbic structures below. For this reason, Ig is thought to be related to functions such as pain perception, tactile recognition, and as a secondary sensory area for the entire body (Mesulam & Mufson, 1982a, 1982b). Odor and taste aversion has been associated with caudal and central insular regions (Bermudez-Rattoni, Introini-Collison, Coleman-Mesches, & McGaugh, 1997; Lasiter, 1985; Lasiter, Deems, & Glanzman, 1985; Naor & Dudai, 1996).

## Subcortical Connections

Subcortically, the anterior insula shares connections primarily with limbic structures (the anterior hippocampus), the amygdala, and brainstem areas. Efferent projections from posterior insular regions terminate in the basal ganglia, specifically within the lentiform nucleus (Showers & Lauer, 1961), caudal–ventral putamen and the tail of the caudate (Forbes & Moskowitz, 1974; Turner, Mishkin, & Knapp, 1980). There are vast connections between the claustrum and the Ig; specifically, many efferents from the Ig terminate in the claustrum terminate (Mesulam & Mufson, 1982a, 1982b; Turner et al., 1980).

Thalamic afferent projections (from sensory and motor areas) terminate in Ig and Id regions (Augustine, 1985; Burton & Jones, 1976; Clark & Russel, 1939; Roberts & Akert, 1963). Projections from the ventral posterior medial and mediodorsal thalamic nuclei terminate primarily in the Ia (Guldin & Markowitsch, 1984). Researchers have delineated vast efferent connections from posterior and midinsular regions to the thalamus, ending in sensory areas of the thalamus, including the ventral posterior lateral nucleus, ventroposterior inferior, centromedian, and parafascicular nuclei (Mesulam et al., 1984; Wirth, 1973).

## Amygdala, Limbic, and Brainstem Connections

Connections between the amygdala and the insula are greatest within the Ia–Id regions (Mufson, Mesulam, & Pandya, 1981). Ia connections to basolateral areas and corticomedial areas within the amygdala have been described (Aggleton, Burton, & Passingham, 1980; Mufson et al., 1981; Turner et al., 1980). Many limbic connections, particularly to the anterior hippocampus, entorhinal cortex, periamygdala regions, and olfactory bulb have been demonstrated (Chikama, McFarland, Amaral, & Haber, 1997; Kaada, 1951; Pribram & Lennox, 1950; Pribram & MacLean, 1953; Saper, 1982; Wright & Groenewegen, 1996). Other researchers have demonstrated connections from the insula to brainstem autonomic and reticular nuclei (Ruggiero, Mraovitch, Granata, Anwar, & Reis, 1987).

## REFERENCES

Aggleton, J. P., Burton, M. J., & Passingham, R. E. (1980). Cortical and subcortical afferents to the amygdala of the rhesus monkey (*Macaca mulatta*). *Brain Research*, 190(2), 347–368.

Augustine, J. R. (1985). The insular lobe in primates including humans. *Neurological Research*, 7(1), 2–10.

Augustine, J. R. (1996). Circuitry and functional aspects of the insular lobe in primates including humans. *Brain Research: Brain Research Reviews*, 22(3), 229–244.

Barbas, H. (1988). Anatomic organization of basoventral and mediodorsal visual recipient prefrontal regions in the rhesus monkey. *Journal of Comparative Neurology*, 276(3), 313–342.

Barbas, H. (1993). Organization of cortical afferent input to orbitofrontal areas in the rhesus monkey. *Neuroscience*, 56(4), 841–864.

Barbas, H. (1995a). Anatomic basis of cognitive-emotional interactions in the primate prefrontal cortex. *Neuroscience and Biobehavioral Reviews*, 19(3), 499–510.

Barbas, H. (1995b). Pattern in the cortical distribution of prefrontally directed neurons with divergent axons in the rhesus monkey. *Cerebral Cortex*, 5(2), 158–165.

Barbas, H., & Blatt, G. J. (1995). Topographically specific hippocampal projections target functionally distinct prefrontal areas in the rhesus monkey. *Hippocampus*, 5(6), 511–533.

Barbas, H., & Pandya, D. N. (1989). Architecture and intrinsic connections of the prefrontal cortex in the rhesus monkey. *Journal of Comparative Neurology*, 286(3), 353–375.

Baylis, L. L., Rolls, E. T., & Baylis, G. C. (1995). Afferent connections of the caudolateral orbitofrontal cortex taste area of the primate. *Neuroscience*, 64(3), 801–812.

Bermudez-Rattoni, F., Introini-Collison, I., Coleman-Mesches, K., & McGaugh, J. L. (1997). Insular cortex and amygdala lesions induced after aversive training impair retention: Effects of degree of training. *Neurobiology of Learning and Memory*, 67(1), 57–63.

Brodmann, K. (1909). *Vergleichende Lokalisationslehre der Grosshinrinde in ihren Prinzipien dargestellt auf Grund des Zellenbaues* [Comparative localization studies in the brain cortex, its fundamentals represented on the basis of its cellular architecture]. Leipzig: Barth.

Burton, H., & Jones, E. G. (1976). The posterior thalamic region and its cortical projection in New World and Old World monkeys. *Journal of Comparative Neurology*, 168(2), 249–301.

Carmichael, S. T., Clugnet, M. C., & Price, J. L. (1994). Central olfactory connections in the macaque monkey. *Journal of Comparative Neurology*, 346(3), 403–434.

Carpenter, M. (1985). *Core text of neuroanatomy*. Baltimore: Williams & Wilkins.

Cavada, C., Company, T., Tejedor, J., Cruz-Rizzolo, R. J., & Reinoso-Suarez, F. (2000). The anatomical connections of the macaque monkey orbitofrontal cortex: A review. *Cerebral Cortex*, 10(3), 220–242.

Chikama, M., McFarland, N. R., Amaral, D. G., & Haber, S. N. (1997). Insular cortical projections to functional regions of the striatum correlate with cortical cytoarchitectonic organization in the primate. *Journal of Neuroscience*, 17(24), 9686–9705.

Clark, T. E. (1896). The comparative anatomy of the insula. *Journal of Comparative Neurology*, 6, 59–100.

Clark, W. E. L., & Russel, W. R. (1939). Observations on the efferent connections of the centre median nucleus. *Journal of Anatomy*, 73, 255–262.

Critchley, H. D., & Rolls, E. T. (1996). Olfactory neuronal responses in the primate orbitofrontal cortex: Analysis in an olfactory discrimination task. *Journal of Neurophysiology*, 75(4), 1659–1672.

Cunningham, D. J. (1891a). The development of the gyri and sulci on the surface of the island of Reil of the human brain. *Journal of Anatomical Physiology*, 25, 338–348.

Cunningham, D. J. (1891b). The Sylvian fissure and the island of Reil in the primate brain. *Journal of Anatomical Physiology*, 25, 286–291.

Damasio, H., Grabowski, T., Frank, R., Galaburda, A. M., & Damasio, A. R. (1994). The return of Phineas Gage: Clues about the brain from the skull of a famous patient. *Science*, 264, 1102–1105.

Duvernoy, H. M. (1999). *The human brain: Surface, blood supply, and three-dimensional sectional anatomy*. New York: Springer.

Flynn, F. G., Benson, D. F., & Ardila, A. (1999). Anatomy of the insula—functional and clinical correlates. *Aphasiology*, 13(1), 55–78.

Forbes, B. F., & Moskowitz, N. (1974). Projections of auditory responsive cortex in the squirrel monkey. *Brain Research, 67*(2), 239–254.

Fuster, J. M. (1979). *The prefrontal cortex.* New York: Raven.

Guldin, W. O., & Markowitsch, H. J. (1984). Cortical and thalamic afferent connections of the insular and adjacent cortex of the cat. *Journal of Comparative Neurology, 229*(3), 393–418.

Hasselmo, M. E., Rolls, E. T., & Baylis, G. C. (1989). The role of expression and identity in the face-selective responses of neurons in the temporal visual cortex of the monkey. *Behavioral Brain Research, 32*(3), 203–218.

Hasselmo, M. E., Rolls, E. T., Baylis, G. C., & Nalwa, V. (1989). Object-centered encoding by face-selective neurons in the cortex in the superior temporal sulcus of the monkey. *Experimental Brain Research, 75*(2), 417–429.

Hof, P. R., Mufson, E. J., & Morrison, J. H. (1995). Human orbitofrontal cortex: Cytoarchitecture and quantitative immunohistochemical parcellation. *Journal of Comparative Neurology, 359*(1), 48–68.

Hornak, J., Bramham, J., Rolls, E. T., Morris, R. G., O'Doherty, J., Bullock, P. R., et al. (2003). Changes in emotion after circumscribed surgical lesions of the orbitofrontal and cingulate cortices. *Brain, 126*(7), 1691–1712.

Hornak, J., Rolls, E. T., & Wade, D. (1996). Face and voice expression identification in patients with emotional and behavioural changes following ventral frontal lobe damage. *Neuropsychologia, 34*(4), 247–261.

Insausti, R., Amaral, D. G., & Cowan, W. M. (1987a). The entorhinal cortex of the monkey: II. Cortical afferents. *Journal of Comparative Neurology, 264*(3), 356–395.

Insausti, R., Amaral, D. G., & Cowan, W. M. (1987b). The entorhinal cortex of the monkey: III. Subcortical afferents. *Journal of Comparative Neurology, 264*(3), 396–408.

Johnson, T. N., Rosvold, H. E., & Mishkin, M. (1968). Projections from behaviorally-defined sectors of the prefrontal cortex to the basal ganglia, septum, and diencephalon of the monkey. *Experimental Neurology, 21*(1), 20–34.

Kaada, B. R. (1951). Somato-motor, autonomic and electrocorticographic responses to electrical stimulation of rhinencephalic and other structures in primates, cat, and dog: A study of responses from the limbic, subcallosal, orbito-insular, piriform and temporal cortex, hippocampus–fornix and amygdala. *Acta Physiolica Scandinavica Supplement, 24*, 1–262.

Kemp, J. M., & Powell, T. P. (1970). The cortico-striate projection in the monkey. *Brain, 93*(3), 525–546.

Kringelbach, M. L., & Rolls, E. T. (2004). The functional neuroanatomy of the human orbitofrontal cortex: Evidence from neuroimaging and neuropsychology. *Progress in Neurobiology, 72*(5), 341–372.

Lasiter, P. S. (1985). Thalamocortical relations in taste aversion learning: II. Involvement of the medial ventrobasal thalamic complex in taste aversion learning. *Behavioral Neuroscience, 99*(3), 477–495.

Lasiter, P. S., Deems, D. A., & Glanzman, D. L. (1985). Thalamocortical relations in taste aversion learning: I. Involvement of gustatory thalamocortical projections in taste aversion learning. *Behavioral Neuroscience, 99*(3), 454–476.

Mesulam, M. M. (1985a). Patterns in behavioral neuroanatomy: Association areas, the limbic system, and hemispheric specialization. In *Principles of behavioral neurology.* Philadelphia: Davis.

Mesulam, M. M. (1985b). *Principles of behavioral and cognitive neurology.* Oxford, UK: Oxford University Press.

Mesulam, M. M. (1998). From sensation to cognition. *Brain, 121*(6), 1013–1052.

Mesulam, M. M., & Mufson, E. J. (1982a). Insula of the Old World monkey: I. Architectonics in the insulo-orbito-temporal component of the paralimbic brain. *Journal of Comparative Neurology, 212*(1), 1–22.

Mesulam, M. M., & Mufson, E. J. (1982b). Insula of the Old World monkey: III. Efferent cortical output and comments on function. *Journal of Comparative Neurology, 212*(1), 38–52.

Mesulam, M. M., Mufson, E. J., Levey, A. I., & Wainer, B. H. (1984). Atlas of cholinergic neurons in the forebrain and upper brainstem of the macaque based on monoclonal choline acetyltransferase immunohistochemistry and acetylcholinesterase histochemistry. *Neuroscience, 12*(3), 669–686.

Morecraft, R. J., Geula, C., & Mesulam, M. M. (1992). Cytoarchitecture and neural afferents of orbitofrontal cortex in the brain of the monkey. *Journal of Comparative Neurology, 323*(3), 341–358.

Mufson, E. J., Mesulam, M. M., & Pandya, D. N. (1981). Insular interconnections with the amygdala in the rhesus monkey. *Neuroscience, 6*(7), 1231–1248.

Naor, C., & Dudai, Y. (1996). Transient impairment of cholinergic function in the rat insular cortex disrupts the encoding of taste in conditioned taste aversion. *Behavioral Brain Research, 79*(1–2), 61–67.

Nauta, W. J. H. (1964). Some efferent connections of the prefrontal cortex in the monkey. In J. M. Warren & K. Akert (Eds.), *The frontal granular cortex and behavior* (pp. 397–409). New York: McGraw-Hill.

Ongur, D., & Price, J. L. (2000). The organization of networks within the orbital and medial prefrontal cortex of rats, monkeys and humans. *Cerebral Cortex, 10*(3), 206–219.

Ono, M., Kubuk, S., & Abernathy, C. D. (1990). *Atlas of the cerebral sulci.* New York: Thieme.

Pandya, D. N., & Yeterian, E. H. (1996). Comparison of prefrontal architecture and connections. *Philosophical Transactions of the Royal Society of London: Series B, Biological Sciences, 351*, 1423–1432.

Penfield, W., & Faulk, M. E., Jr. (1955). The insula: Further observations on its function. *Brain, 78*(4), 445–470.

Petrides, M., & Pandya, D. N. (1994). Comparative architectonic analyses of the human and the macaque frontal cortex. In F. Boller et al. (Eds.), *Handbook of neuropsychology* (pp. 17–58). Amsterdam: Elsevier.

Pribram, K. H., & Lennox, M. A. (1950). Some connections of the oribitofrontotemporal, limbic and hippocampal areas of *Macaca mulatta. Journal of Neurophysiology, 13,* 127–135.

Pribram, K. H., & MacLean, P. D. (1953). Neuronographic analysis of medial and basal cerebral cortex: II. Monkey. *Journal of Neurophysiology, 16,* 324–340.

Price, J. L. (1991). The central olfactory and accessory olfactory systems. In T. E. Finger & W. L. Silver (Eds.), *Neurobiology of taste and smell* (pp. 179–203). Malabar, FL: Krieger.

Reiman, E. M. (1996). *PET studies of anxiety, emotion and their disorders.* Annual meeting of the World Congress of Psychiatry, Madrid, Spain.

Rempel-Clower, N. L., & Barbas, H. (1998). Topographic organization of connections between the hypothalamus and prefrontal cortex in the rhesus monkey. *Journal of Comparative Neurology, 398*(3), 393–419.

Roberts, T. S., & Akert, K. (1963). Insular and opercular cortex and its thalamic projection in *Macaca mulatta. Sweitzer Archive fur Neurologie, Neurochirurgie und Psychiatrie, 92,* 1–43.

Rolls, E. T. (1996). The orbitofrontal cortex. *Philosophical Transactions of the Royal Society of London: Series B, Biological Sciences, 351,* 1433–1443; discussion, 1443–1444.

Rolls, E. T. (2004). The functions of the orbitofrontal cortex. *Brain and Cognition, 55*(1), 11–29.

Rolls, E. T., & Baylis, L. L. (1994). Gustatory, olfactory, and visual convergence within the primate orbitofrontal cortex. *Journal of Neuroscience, 14*(9), 5437–5452.

Rolls, E. T., Critchley, H. D., Browning, A. S., Hernadi, I., & Lenard, L. (1999). Responses to the sensory properties of fat of neurons in the primate orbitofrontal cortex. *Journal of Neuroscience, 19*(4), 1532–1540.

Rolls, E. T., Yaxley, S., & Sienkiewicz, Z. J. (1990). Gustatory responses of single neurons in the caudolateral orbitofrontal cortex of the macaque monkey. *Journal of Neurophysiology, 64*(4), 1055–1066.

Romanski, L. M., Bates, J. F., & Goldman-Rakic, P. S. (1999). Auditory belt and parabelt projections to the prefrontal cortex in the rhesus monkey. *Journal of Comparative Neurology, 403*(2), 141–157.

Ruggiero, D. A., Mraovitch, S., Granata, A. R., Anwar, M., & Reis, D. J. (1987). A role of insular cortex in cardiovascular function. *Journal of Comparative Neurology, 257*(2), 189–207.

Saper, C. B. (1982). Convergence of autonomic and limbic connections in the insular cortex of the rat. *Journal of Comparative Neurology, 210*(2), 163–173.

Showers, M. J., & Lauer, E. W. (1961). Somatovisceral motor patterns in the insula. *Journal of Comparative Neurology, 117,* 107–115.

Turner, B. H., Mishkin, M., & Knapp, M. (1980). Organization of the amygdalopetal projections from modality-specific cortical association areas in the monkey. *Journal of Comparative Neurology, 191*(4), 515–543.

Walker, A. E. (1940). A cyroarchitechural study of the prefrontal area of the macaque monkey. *Journal of Comparative Neurology, 73,* 59–86.

Wirth, F. P. (1973). Insular–diencephalic connections in the macaque. *Journal of Comparative Neurology, 150*(4), 361–392.

Wright, C. I., & Groenewegen, H. J. (1996). Patterns of overlap and segregation between insular cortical, intermediodorsal thalamic and basal amygdaloid afferents in the nucleus accumbens of the rat. *Neuroscience, 73*(2), 359–373.

Zald, D. H., & Kim, S. W. (2001). The orbitofrontal cortex. In S. P. Salloway, P. F. Malloy, & J. D. Duffy (Eds.), *The frontal lobes and neuropsychiatric illness* (pp. 33–69). Washington, DC: American Psychiatric Press.

# CHAPTER 6

# Structural and Functional Asymmetries of the Human Frontal Lobes

*Daniel H. Geschwind*
*Marco Iacoboni*

One of the most fundamental divisions of the human brain is that of the left and right cerebral hemispheres. Numerous studies have revealed the consistent presence of both behavioral and anatomical asymmetries that reflect the specialized capacities of each hemisphere (Annett, 1985; Bogen, 1993; Galaburda, 1991; Gazzaniga, 1970; Geschwind & Galaburda, 1985). The significance of several of these asymmetries is controversial in many cases, and surprisingly little is known about asymmetries in the frontal lobe, arguably the area that contributes most to human cognitive and behavioral attributes. This chapter is not meant to solve all of the mysteries of lateralized functions of the frontal lobes, but merely to highlight anatomical and functional asymmetries as they relate to language, complex motor behaviors, and sensorimotor integration—areas in which the most is currently known with regard to lateralized frontal lobe functions. Additionally, we briefly discuss the lateralization of prosody and emotion. The focus of our review is on patients with focal brain lesions, and on structural and functional brain imaging in healthy volunteers. Chronic progressive conditions such as progressive aphasia (Snowden, Neary, Mann, Goulding, & Testa, 1992) and the right frontal lobe variant of frontal–temporal dementia (Miller, Chang, Mena, Boone, & Lesser, 1993) present intriguing examples of lateralized behaviors, but do not lend

themselves as well to localization and are therefore not included in this brief review. Clinical lesion data are presented first, when applicable, followed by functional imaging and morphological data relevant to each section.

It is often assumed that anatomical asymmetries invariably reflect functional asymmetries. However, physiological asymmetries, asymmetries in gene expression, or subtle differences in neuronal cytoskeletal architecture may play a more significant role in hemispheric specialization than gross anatomical or cytoarchitectonic asymmetries. The identification of morphological asymmetries associated with language is important because of a wealth of evidence that these asymmetries are functionally relevant (Galaburda, LeMay, Kemper, & Geschwind, 1978; Geschwind & Galaburda, 1985; Geschwind & Levitsky, 1968; Witelson, 1977, 1992). Furthermore, a number of studies support the general notion that the amount of cerebral cortex dedicated to a particular function may reflect the brain capabilities in that area (Eccles, 1977; Garraghty & Kaas, 1992; Jerison, 1977).

However, the size of a brain region is not always positively correlated with its capabilities. Often, a larger cerebral hemisphere can be observed due to neuronal migration abnormalities or other cortical malformations. In the domain of language more specifically, the brains of individuals with dyslexia appear to be more symmetrical, with a larger than usual planum temporale on the right, rather than a smaller planum temporale on the left (Galaburda, 1993; Kushch et al., 1993). Thus, anatomical asymmetries, whether gross or fine, cannot be viewed in isolation and must eventually be considered in the context of the physiology of the neuronal systems to which they contribute.

## ASYMMETRIES IN LANGUAGE

Functional and anatomical asymmetries related to language functions have been the most widely studied asymmetries of the frontal lobes. In the last two decades, functional imaging has provided a revealing view of areas involved in healthy and neurologically impaired subjects (Binder et al., 1995; Klein, Milner, Zatorre, Meyer, & Evans, 1995; Petersen, Fox, Posner, Mintun, & Raichle, 1988; Roland, 1984; Warburton et al., 1996). However, the study of hundreds of patients with aphasia over the last century has provided the bulk of the fundamental observations related to language localization. Most observant clinicians have remarked on the variability and overlap of aphasic syndromes, especially in the immediate period following brain injury, as well as the individual differences in symptoms between patients with apparently similar lesions (Benson, 1986; Galaburda, Rosen, & Sherman, 1990). Individual variability in the gross morphology (see Figure 6.1) and detailed cytoarchitecture in humans (Adrianov, 1979; Rajkowska & Goldman-Rakic, 1995) and nonhuman primates (Lashley & Clarke, 1946) has been well demonstrated and is likely to underlie the variability in clinical syndromes in humans. In light of this variability, the left-hemisphere superiority and proficiency for the majority of vocal, motor, and language functions is striking (Benson, 1986; Geschwind, 1970). The correspondence between this functional asymmetry for language and the anatomical asymmetries described later in this chapter provides the most compelling example of a structure–function relationship underlying cerebral hemispheric specializations. Even so, the extent to which these anatomical asymmetries contribute to functional asymmetry has not been totally clarified. The lateralization of any function including language is unlikely to be an all-or-none phenomenon, because language consists of many components. Thus,

some language capacity exists in most right hemispheres (Iacoboni & Zaidel, 1996). Especially relevant to the discussion of the frontal lobes is the predominance of the right frontal lobe in the production of the melodic components that contribute to prosody, as well as the expression of the emotional content of language, which we discuss later.

Because spoken and written language are human specializations, detailed animal models of the role of different frontal subregions serving language are not available. This is in contrast to frontal lobe participation in other cognitive functions, such as working memory and sensorimotor integration, in which studies in primates have vastly accelerated our knowledge of regional subspecializations and provided models that can be tested in humans (Funahashi, Bruce, & Goldman-Rakic, 1989; Fuster, 1995; Goldman-Rakic, 1987; Petrides, 1994; Wilson, Scalaidhe, & Goldman-Rakic, 1993). Thus, our discussion of structure–function relationships in frontal lobe language is relatively crude compared with the latter topics. Although the hope is that functional imaging studies will remedy this deficiency, the complexity of language tasks presents unique challenges in experimental design.

### Clinical Lesion Studies in Aphasia

Broca's original belief that lesions confined to the posterior portion of the third left frontal gyrus (Figure 6.1) caused loss of articulatory language function (*aphemie*) occurred on the background of the conviction, shared by his contemporaries, that the left and right frontal lobes were identical in size and anatomy (Berker, Berker, & Smith, 1986; Broca, 1865; Flourens, 1824). The recovery of language function occurred through the compensatory efforts of homologous, essentially equipotential regions in the right frontal lobe. Broca (1865) stated that the specialization of articulatory language and other functions occurred due to the earlier development of the left hemisphere (hence the preponderance of right-handers as well) and did not imply an underlying functional difference between the two hemispheres. Broca's conclusions were based on extensive lesions that encompassed regions beyond the pars triangularis and opercularis to include the primary motor cortex (see Figure 6.2). However, his fundamental observation of a cerebral asymmetry related to language pro-

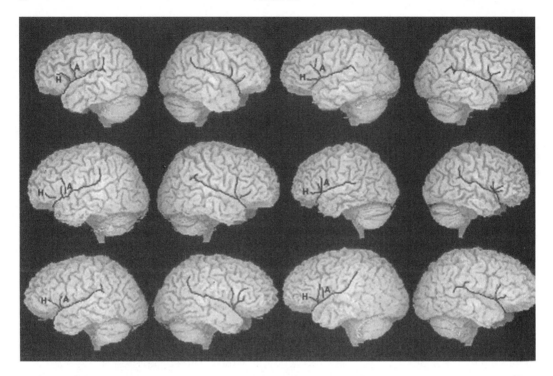

FIGURE 6.1. Variability in frontal cortex surface anatomy. Three-dimensional reconstructions of left and right MRIs from six different Caucasian volunteers demonstrate the variability in surface morphology and emphasize the difficulty in defining Broca's region using surface landmarks alone. The sylvian fissure and the horizontal (H) and ascending (A) rami, which define the anterior and posterior boundary of the pars triangularis (Brodmann's area 45) are traced and labeled in the left side view of each pair. The pars opercularis (Brodmann's area 44) is directly posterior to the ascending ramus and extends posteriorly to border on the precentral gyrus in most individuals. The morphology of these fissures differs considerably between individuals and, in some cases, the landmarks that define Broca's area are difficult to identify. Given these ambiguities, cytoarchitectonic measurement of these areas may be necessary for a meaningful demonstration of morphological hemispheric asymmetries.

vided the foundation for modern brain laterality research.

Following Broca, numerous cases supported the left-hemispheric localization of language in right-handers, while expanding the cerebral territory responsible for language functions (Broca, 1888; Jackson, 1880, 1915; Wernicke, 1874). Jackson (1868) presented the first case of a left-handed man with aphasia and a right-sided lesion, further supporting a connection between hand dominance and language lateralization. More recent lesion studies have confirmed the functional localization of language to the left hemisphere in 99% of right-handers (Annett, 1985; Benson, 1986; Hécaen, De Agostini, & Monzon-Montes, 1981). This relationship is less certain in left-handers, with most demonstrating either left-hemisphere or

bilateral language, and less frequently, right-hemisphere language (Geschwind, 1970; Geschwind & Galaburda, 1985; Hécaen et al., 1981).

However, the precise nature of the lesion necessary to produce nonfluent aphasia remains controversial (Hécaen & Consoli, 1973; Marie, 1906; Mohr et al., 1978; Moutier, 1908; Nielsen, 1946; Zangwill, 1975). The majority of the frontal lobe anterior to Broca's area, the first frontal opercular gyrus, and all of the right hemisphere can be removed in patients with intractable epilepsy without producing lasting aphasia. In contrast, the removal of the first two to three gyri of the left frontal operculum pars opercularis (area 44) and triangularis (area 45) anterior to Brodmann's area 4 on the left in epilepsy surgery resulted in

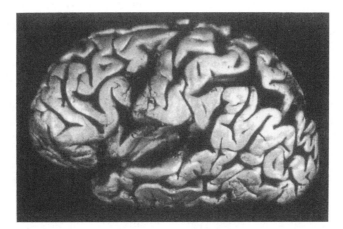

FIGURE 6.2. Lateral left view of Broca's second case, which illustrates the gross extent of this patient's lesion. The area of damaged cortex extends beyond pars triangularis anteriorly and pars opercularis posteriorly, thus encompassing a region slightly larger than the posterior portion of the inferior frontal gyrus anterior to the motor strip (Brodmann's areas 44 and 45). The extent of surface damage supports the argument that lesions encompassing more than areas 44 and 45 are necessary to produce the full syndrome of nonfluent aphasia. Furthermore, this brain was not sectioned or examined histologically to determine the extent of subcortical injury. From *Origins of Neuroscience: A History of Explorations into Brain Function* by Stanley Finger, Copyright 1994 by Oxford University Press, Inc. Used by permission of Oxford University Press, Inc.

nonfluent aphasia in every case except one (Penfield & Roberts, 1959). Cortical stimulation studies by these same investigators demonstrated speech arrest from stimulation of the first two opercular gyri on the left, but never on the right. Stimulation of the left supplementary motor area (SMA), and not right, produced speech arrest (Penfield & Roberts, 1959). Lesions of the left SMA can produce transcortical motor aphasia, whereas similar lesions on the right do not, consistent with the proposed role of the SMA in speech initiation (Freedman, Alexander, & Naeser, 1984; Masdeau, 1980). Further evidence from neuroimaging studies seems to support the contribution of the left SMA to language (see "Functional Imaging" section), but no morphological asymmetries of the SMA have been documented.

Lesion studies support the presence of an anterior frontal lobe language area that encompasses Broca's area and additional perisylvian areas more posteriorly. In a series of patients with left-sided lesions of the posterior part of the inferior frontal gyrus, 17 out of 19 patients had difficulties in language fluency (Hécaen & Consoli, 1973). The two patients without language difficulties suffered from congenital lesions, and it is likely that these anomalies displaced Broca's region. Patients with lesions largely confined to the cortical surface corresponding to Broca's region did not have significant agrammatism, or writing difficulties, whereas those with deeper lesions tended to have more profound language impairment. None of 15 patients with a homologous right-sided lesion demonstrated any language or articulatory deficits, confirming the relative specialization of the left inferior frontal gyrus for language output.

Numerous case studies have underscored the relationship between the extension of lesion into cortical regions adjacent to the third frontal gyrus and the severity of the Broca's aphasia (Tonkonogy & Goodglass, 1981). Articulatory disturbances (dysarthria and dysprosody) are typically associated with lesions that extend into the opercular precentral gyrus (Alexander, Naeser, & Palumbo, 1990). A combination of word-finding difficulties, paraphasias, and slowness in speech is observed with lesions of the pars triangularis and pars opercularis. Involvement of both regions typically leads to a more severe and lasting nonfluent aphasia. Mohr and coworkers (1978) have also demonstrated that lesions localized to Broca's area lead to nonfluent aphasia or nonmotor articulatory disturbance, as well as persistent apraxia and dysprosodia, but not frank agrammatism, as is paradigmatic in many current formulations of nonfluent (Broca's) aphasia. Those with typical Broca's aphasia have larger lesions that encompassed deeper white matter structures, the anterior insula, and adjacent perisylvian regions (Alexander et al., 1990; Mohr et al., 1978). So, although the minimally sufficient lesion necessary to cause nonfluent aphasia in right-handers remains controversial, it is clear that even larger acute lesions on the right only rarely cause a similar disturbance in language function (Benson, 1986; Geschwind, 1970; Geschwind & Galaburda, 1985; Jackson, 1915; Moutier, 1908).

## Functional Imaging

Many functional imaging studies within the last decade employing positron emission tomography (PET) and functional magnetic resonance imaging (fMRI) have supported the functional specialization of the left frontal cortex in language and language-related tasks (Binder et al., 1995; Frith, Friston, Liddle, & Frackowiak, 1991; Just, Carpenter, Keller, Eddy, & Thulborn, 1996; Klein et al., 1995; McCarthy, Blamire, Rothman, Gruetter, & Shulman, 1993). Indeed, widespread areas of lateral frontal hypometabolism are even seen in patients with aphasia and lesions in parietal and temporal cortex, further implicating the lateral left frontal cortex in language function and recovery (Metter, 1991). These imaging studies have also confirmed that even simple language tasks, although highly lateralized, activate a network of widely distributed left-hemisphere cortical areas (Binder et al., 1995; Just et al., 1996; Petersen et al., 1988). The left-hemisphere activations are highly variable and extend beyond Broca's region, including the SMA and cingulate medially, and the dorsolateral prefrontal cortex and the premotor area laterally. Additionally, in most careful PET or fMRI studies of language, homologous regions are often activated on the right side, although typically at far lower levels than those on the left (Habib, Demonet, & Frackowiak, 1996; Just et al., 1996; Warburton et al., 1996).

One of the factors confounding the interpretation of PET language data is the variability in activated areas across different studies. The overall variability in language PET studies is due to a variety of factors, including (1) intersubject differences in cortical representation of language functions, (2) differences in activation tasks, and (3) differences in PET methodologies. However, in spite of this variability, left perisylvian regions in general, and Broca's area in particular, show consistent activation in language tasks. So, although language is a highly complex function that requires the activation of different cortical areas, the PET data support the wide body of data in patients with brain injury, demonstrating that Broca's area is a critical cortical structure for language. However, the precise role of this famous section of frontal cortex in language remains controversial.

Indeed, it is unlikely that Broca's region should be considered an area dedicated solely to language output. It is probable that since Broca's region comprises cytoarchitectonically and physiologically diverse areas, it may serve several language-related functions (Poppel, 1996). For instance, lesion studies, intraoperative electrical stimulation, and PET imaging studies confirm its role in phonological processing (Demonet, Price, Wise, & Frackowiak, 1994; Denny-Brown, 1975; Lecours & Lhermitte, 1970; Ojemann & Mateer, 1979; Zatorre, Meyer, Gjedde, & Evans, 1996). The phonemic paraphasias seen more typically with Broca's than with Wernicke's aphasia are consistent with these observations. PET data indicate that Broca's region is activated in a wide variety of non-output-related language tasks, including listening tasks (Roland, 1984). Phonological discrimination tasks often engage verbal working memory functions, which are typically associated with left frontal lobe predominance as well (Milner & Petrides, 1984; Paulesu, Frith, & Frackowiak, 1993; Petrides, Alivisatos, Meyer, & Evans, 1993). Thus, it is conceivable that Broca's region comprises contiguous areas serving separate functions that can be simultaneously engaged in the same task. Later, in the section "Asymmetries in Sensorimotor Integration," we review some data pertaining to the activation of Broca's area in lip reading and grasping that are particularly relevant and raise important evolutionary considerations. Remarkable in this regard are the observations of Denny-Brown (1965, 1975), initiated over 30 years ago, on the importance of visual input in language acquisition and visual influences on aphasia caused by lesions of Broca's area. Disruption of the integration of these visual inputs with other processing streams is likely a component of the literal alexia that can sometimes be observed in patients with Broca's area lesions (Benson, 1977; Boccardi, Bruzzone, & Vignolo, 1984).

## Morphological Asymmetries

The recognition of the functional asymmetry for language observed over a century ago prompted investigators to search for morphological asymmetries underlying this left frontal lobe specialization. Due to methodological constraints prior to the latter half of this century, investigators were limited to studying gross measures of asymmetry. Comparison of the weights of both hemispheres yielded variable and inconclusive results (Aresu, 1914; Broca, 1875; Thurnam, 1866; von Bonin, 1962). Most morphometric studies demonstrated a larger right frontal lobe and total right-hemisphere size overall. However, these studies did not consider the surface area accounted for by the vast amount of cortex contained in the folds of sulci. In this vein, the specific gravity of the left hemisphere is greater than the right, suggesting more cortical surface area overall on the left (von Bonin, 1962).

Most gross morphological asymmetries of the frontal lobes described in humans are the result of indirect measurements taken of indentations in the skull, called petalias, that reflect outgrowth of the adjacent cerebral hemisphere. Although one of the most consistent findings is the presence of marked left occipital petalia, the nature of frontal lobe asymmetries has been less obvious (Hadziselmovic & Cus, 1966; Tilney, 1927). However, most careful quantitative studies in adequate numbers of cases show a predominance of the right frontal petalia (Geschwind & Galaburda, 1985; Hadziselmovic & Cus, 1966).

LeMay and Kido (1978) made direct measurements of the frontal lobes and demonstrated that the width of the right frontal region was greater in 58% of right-handed patients and extended further forward in 31%, as opposed to only 14% that extended further forward on the left. A trend toward symmetry was observed in left-handers. This gross structural asymmetry has been consistently observed in more recent studies (Bear, Schiff, Saver, Greenberg, & Freeman, 1986; Geschwind & Galaburda, 1985; Glicksohn & Myslobodsky, 1993). However, the meaning of

these observations is unclear. The petalias and even direct gross morphometry are imprecise measurements that do not reflect the total extent of cortical surface area in a given region, because much surface area is contained in the sulcal folds. This explanation is likely to hold for the studies of Wada, Clarke, and Hamm (1975) that demonstrated a right-side size advantage when only the lateral cortical surface of areas 44 and 45 were measured. Nonhuman primates, including orangutans, chimpanzees, gorillas, New World and Old World monkeys also show a right frontal petalia, suggesting that these asymmetries are not related to strictly human cognitive abilities, such as language (Falk et al., 1990; Galaburda et al., 1978; Geschwind & Galaburda, 1985; Holloway, De La Coste-Lareymondie, 1982).

One of the first detailed measurements based on cytoarchitechtonic divisions of the frontal lobes were carried out by Kononova (1936; cited in Adrianov, 1979). This work on five right-handed subjects not only showed that the total area of the left frontal lobe was larger than the right by 16%, but also that Brodmann's areas 45 and 47 were larger on the left by a margin of 30% and 45%, respectively. Intriguingly, the results were reversed in the one left-handed patient studied. Kononova also observed a large amount of individual variation in these and other regions of the frontal lobe, highlighting the difficulty in drawing firm conclusions from this study of only six cases. Galaburda's (1980) detailed study of the magnocellular region of the pars opercularis, which largely coincides with area 44, demonstrated the left side to be larger than the right in the majority of 10 cases.

More recent investigations have demonstrated a population of magnopyramidal neurons that are 15% larger in left Brodmann's area 45 than on the right (Hayes & Lewis, 1993). No difference was seen between similar large pyramidal neurons in area 4 (Hayes & Lewis, 1995). However, in area 46 of the dorsolateral prefrontal cortex, the magnopyramidal neurons were about 10% smaller on the left. These differences are not large, and how these asymmetries relate to lateralization of frontal cortical functions is unknown. An additional problem in interpreting these findings is the small sample sizes studied, especially in light of current knowledge that highlights the striking individual variability in morphology (Figure 6.1) and cytoarchitechtonics of the human frontal lobes (Adrianov, 1979; Rajkowska & Goldman-Rakic, 1995).

Other investigators have demonstrated consistent morphological asymmetries in more extensive regions of the third or inferior frontal gyrus using autopsy material and MRI in living patients (Albanese, Merlo, Albanese, & Gomez, 1989; Falzi, Perrone, & Vignolo, 1982; Foundas, Leonard, Gilmore, Fennell, & Heilman, 1996; Foundas, Leonard, & Heilman, 1995). Foundas and colleagues (1996) demonstrated a striking correlation between the direction of pars triangularis (area 45) asymmetry and hemispheric language lateralization, providing the most convincing evidence to date of the correspondence between language and anatomical asymmetries in the frontal lobe. Nine of 10 patients with Wada test–proven lateralization of language to the left hemisphere displayed asymmetry in favor of the left pars triangularis. This is a striking finding, especially given the well-described individual differences in the surface landmarks that define this region and other frontal lobe areas (e.g., Figure 6.2).

Although it is most likely that an increased neuron number underlies the larger areas 44 and 45 of the left hemisphere (Galaburda, 1993), an increase in neuropil size could also account for the left-hemispheric predominance. Both pars triangularis and pars opercularis have been shown to have increased complexity of higher-order dendritic branching on the left relative to the primary motor cortex in both hemispheres, and pars triangularis and pars opercularis on the right (Scheibel et al., 1985; Simonds & Scheibel, 1989). However, these dendritic specializations may develop independently of gross anatomical asymmetry, and their significance is uncertain. Since the majority of synapses occur on dendritic spines, it is possible that the shape and complexity of these dendritic arbors reflect the influence of experience on synapse elimination during the critical period of language acquisition.

## ASYMMETRIES OF PROSODY AND EMOTION

Speech involves not only the communication of vocabulary and grammatical content but also social and emotional content. The rhythmic, melodic intonation in speech that contributes these additional elements of meaning to language is termed "prosody." Several studies show that patients with right-hemisphere lesions can demonstrate deficiency in interpreting and expressing the emotional content of speech (Ross & Mesulam, 1979). The lesions described in loss of expressive prosody mostly involve large portions of the frontal lobe and often extend into the parietal lobe, hindering precise anatomical localization (Dordain, Degos, & Dordain, 1971; Ross & Mesulam, 1979). To what extent these lesions disrupt prosody by damaging frontal–subcortical circuits is an important, unresolved issue given the involvement of the basal ganglia in prosody, as demonstrated by lesion studies (Cancelliere & Kertesz, 1990; Starkstein, Federoff, Price, Leiguarda, & Robinson, 1994).

It is proposed that the prosodic deficit in cases of frontal lobe damage corresponds to the right-hemisphere homologue of Broca's region (Ross, 1981). The critical role of the right hemisphere in the melodic and musical aspects of speech and language output is also supported by the observation of preservation of simple singing ability in many patients with nonfluent aphasia (Yamadori, Osumi, Masuhara, & Okubo, 1977). In addition, a PET study supports the role of the right lateral prefrontal cortex in simple pitch discrimination, analogous to the role of Broca's area in phoneme perception (Zatorre, Evans, & Meyer, 1994). A PET study of emotional prosody comprehension also suggests that right prefrontal cortex is preferentially active in tasks requiring perception and interpretation of emotional prosody, and is not simply dedicated to prosodic expression (George et al., 1996).

The deficit in prosody observed after right frontal lesions is not entirely limited to the expression of emotional and melodic content, however, and can extend into nonemotional semantic aspects, such as syllable stress (Weintraub, Mesulam, & Kramer, 1981). In addition, prosodic elements of speech comprehension and expression can also be impaired in anterior left-hemisphere lesions resulting in a Broca's aphasia (Benson, 1986; Danly & Shapiro, 1982). In the foreign accent syndrome, which can result from left frontal lesions involving Broca's area, and neighboring cortical and subcortical regions, inappropriate syllable stress, phoneme misproduction, rhythm, and pauses occur, changing a patient's accent, often without chronically altering other aspects of language (Monrad-Krohn, 1947).

However, other nonlinguistic elements of prosody, such as the ability to sing and to produce melodic speech, are preserved, consistent with a right-hemisphere role in these functions. Exaggerated prosody, sometimes observed in nonfluent aphasia, reflects the speaker's attempts to communicate using retained right frontal abilities in the face of minimal linguistic capabilities. Thus, although the evidence is not overwhelming, the left and right frontal lobes appear to have different relative contributions when it comes to prosody, with the right frontal lobe specializing in melody and emotional valence, while the left typically specializes in the linguistic elements.

The role of the orbital frontal lobes in the regulation of emotion and mood has been well established in studies of patients with brain injury (Benson & Stuss, 1986). Asymmetries in frontal cortex in the mediation of emotional behavior have also been described in several studies of patients with unilateral brain damage. Left frontal damage, especially damage to the anterior frontal lobes, is far more likely to cause depression than similar lesions on the right (Gainotti, 1972; Robinson, Kubos, Starr, Rao, & Price, 1984; Sackeim et al., 1982; Starkstein et al., 1991). Lesions on the right more frequently lead to mania (Jorge et al., 1993), especially regions of the orbitofrontal cortex (Starkstein et al., 1989; Starkstein, Pearlson, Boston, & Robinson, 1987). In healthy subjects, left prefrontal cortex cerebral blood flow increases when patients induce a state of dysphoria by thinking sad thoughts (George et al., 1995; Pardo, Pardo, & Raichle, 1993). More recently, transcranial magnetic stimulation (causing transient hypofunctioning) of the left, but not right prefrontal cortex, resulted in decreased self-report of happiness and a significant increase in sadness ratings (Pascual-Leone et al., 1996).

Davidson (1992) has developed a compelling model of human emotion, in which frontal lobe asymmetries reflect affective reactivity and, hence, the potential for mania or depression given the appropriate stimulus. Electrophysiological evidence suggests that the left frontal lobe is more specialized for positive emotions related to approach and exploratory mechanisms and the right for negative, avoidance-related reactions (Davidson, 1992; Davidson & Sutton, 1995). Similar frontal lobe asymmetries in electrical activity can predict a child's likelihood to engage in separation from his or her parents to explore novel elements in the environment, consistent with this model (Davidson, 1992). Because withdrawal and exploration are within the behavioral domain of nonhuman primates and lower animals, if this model were correct, similar asymmetries should exist in these lower species as well. Perhaps, more precise physioanatomical models of lateralized frontal lobe contributions to emotional states and behavior can be developed in nonhuman primates in the future.

## ASYMMETRIES IN SENSORIMOTOR INTEGRATION

The frontal lobe is undeniably one of the most critical cerebral structures involved in sensorimotor integration. Different regions of the frontal lobe receive segregated cortical inputs from a variety of cortical areas of sensory significance. In addition, the frontal lobe controls voluntary action through planning of movements in prefrontal areas, preparation of movements in premotor areas, and execution of movements in primary motor areas (Fuster, 1995). In this section, we review evidence from neurological patients and from functional neuroimaging studies that support the existence of functional asymmetries in the sensorimotor integration processes subserved by frontal lobe areas. Evidence concerning asymmetries in sensorimotor integration, first in the lateral wall, and then in the medial wall of the frontal lobe, is reviewed. Unfortunately, little relevant data on structural asymmetries relate to functional asymmetries in any of these processes.

The reader should be advised that we use sensorimotor integration in its broadest sense. Hence, in this section we discuss known asymmetries in a number of cognitive functions that are necessary components of sensorimotor integration but that, in principle, are distinct cognitive functions (e.g., visuospatial working memory, complex motor functions, conditional motor learning and attention).

### Lateral Wall (Prefrontal, Premotor, and Primary Motor Cortex)

The lateral wall of the frontal lobe can be subdivided in three main sectors along the anterior–posterior axis: prefrontal, premotor, and primary motor. Each of these sectors can further be subdivided in subsectors that are anatomically and functionally differentiated

(Cavada & Goldman-Rakic, 1989; Fogassi et al., 1996; Fujii, Mushiake, & Tanji, 1996; Geyer et al., 1996; Matelli, Luppino, & Rizzolatti, 1985; Petrides, 1994; Rizzolatti, Fadiga, Gallese, & Fogassi, 1996; Stepniewska, Preuss, & Kaas, 1993). We review evidence for asymmetries in sensorimotor processes lateralized to the different sectors of the lateral wall of the frontal lobe, starting from the prefrontal cortex, moving then to the premotor cortex, and finally concluding with the primary motor cortex.

### Prefrontal Cortex: A Role in Working Memory

The prefrontal cortex in the lateral wall of the two cerebral hemispheres is known to be primarily involved in working memory processes (Goldman-Rakic, 1987). Neurophysiological studies in nonhuman primates and functional neuroimaging studies in humans have provided detailed models of the functional anatomy of the lateral prefrontal cortex and are reviewed later in this section. Lesion studies in neurological patients have not provided the same type of detailed information; thus, they are only briefly discussed here. However, these lesion studies in humans provided the foundations of laterality investigations in the prefrontal cortex, leading to models that were subsequently refined by neurophysiological and neuroimaging investigations.

### LESION STUDIES

In patients with brain injury, left frontal lobe damage typically leads to more profound verbal recall deficits than right-sided damage, whereas right frontal damage causes deficits primarily in categorization (Incisa della Rocchetta, 1986; Incisa della Rocchetta & Milner, 1993; Milner & Petrides, 1984). Although deficits in verbal fluency occur with either left or right frontal lesions, performance is worse with left frontal damage (Benson & Stuss, 1986). Deficits in the retrieval of verbal material in patients with left frontal damage may be specific to certain lexical categories, in that injury to the left, but not the right, premotor areas produced a specific deficit in verb, but not noun, retreival (Damasio & Tranel, 1993).

Consistent with the left-language, right-visuospatial specialization, patients with right frontal lesions are more likely to demonstrate poor use and representation of visuospatial data in a variety of tasks that require working memory, and those with left frontal lesions are more likely to have disordered memory for episodic information (Kolb & Whishaw, 1985; Milner, 1995). Of patients with unilateral frontal damage, those with right frontal damage show the poorest performance in design fluency tasks (Benson & Stuss, 1986).

However, left-hemisphere deficits in short-term or working memory are not limited to the sphere of language and suggest the importance of the left prefrontal cortex in programming strategies, control of executive functions, and motor responses (Milner & Petrides, 1984). Left frontal lesions, but not those on the right, are more likely to cause impaired recall of words, especially when the task is based on an internal search strategy generated through the mental effort of the subject (Incisa della Rocchetta & Milner, 1993). In this regard, cueing, or providing the patient with connected discourse, ameliorates the retrieval difficulties patients with left frontal damage experience, emphasizing the importance of the dorsolateral left frontal lobe when a search strategy is not externally provided. Patients with frontal lesions that spare the dorsolateral prefrontal cortex do not exhibit these deficits (Goldman-Rakic, 1987). So, whereas the known specialization of the left hemisphere for language and the right for visuospatial information is well supported in lesion studies of the frontal lobes, the use of internally and externally generated problem-solving strategies may be functionally lateralized as well.

### FUNCTIONAL IMAGING STUDIES

A specific framework of the neural substrates of human planning and executive functions comprising working memory suggests that the dorsolateral prefrontal cortex serves mechanisms of active manipulation and monitoring of sensorimotor information within working memory. In this model, the ventrolateral prefrontal cortex serves only working memory mechanisms that support simple retrieval of information for sensory-guided sequential behavior (Petrides, 1994). The anatomical and physiological evidence presented here support the functional distinction between these two systems.

The lateral prefrontal cortex receives strong input from extrastriate cortical areas of visual significance (Milner & Goodale, 1995). Hence, it is not surprising that some aspects of lateral prefrontal cortex organization replicate the pattern described in occipitofugal corticocortical pathways. The occipitofugal corticocortical pathways consist of a dorsal occipitoparietal stream and a ventral occipitotemporal stream. Initially the dorsal stream was conceived as concerned with the processing of spatial relationships, and the ventral stream as mainly concerned with the processing of object identity (Ungerleider & Mishkin, 1982). This view has been refined, in that the dorsal stream is thought to be primarily related to pragmatic aspects of spatial behavior, whereas the ventral stream is primarily related to semantic aspects of spatial behavior (Goodale & Milner, 1992; Jeannerod, Arbib, Rizzolatti, & Sakata, 1995).

Single-cell recordings in nonhuman primates have supported the differential role of dorsal and ventral aspects of the lateral prefrontal cortex in working memory. Working memory for spatial locations is served by the dorsolateral prefrontal cortex, whereas working memory for object identity is served by the ventrolateral prefrontal cortex (Funahashi, Chatee, & Goldman-Rakic, 1993; Wilson et al., 1993). In the nonhuman primate, however, a lateralization of working memory functions has not been convincingly demonstrated. Again, mirroring the organizational principles of the posterior occipitofugal streams, these two prefrontal areas can be regarded as the neural substrates of the pragmatic aspects of working memory mechanisms (the dorsolateral prefrontal cortex) and of semantic aspects of working memory mechanisms (the ventrolateral prefrontal cortex). Both dorsolateral and ventrolateral prefrontal cortex appear lateralized in the type of information they process.

Indeed, PET studies have shown that listening to digits activates the left dorsolateral prefrontal cortex in normal subjects when active monitoring and manipulation of external information held in memory are required only to make judgements about the same stimuli, and no active manipulation is required (Petrides et al., 1993). Similarly, visuospatial information activates the right dorsolateral prefrontal cortex in normal subjects when active manipulation and monitoring of information is required. The same visuospatial information activates only the right ventrolateral prefrontal cortex

when only "reproduction" of information without active manipulation and monitoring is demanded by the task (Owen, Evans, & Petrides, 1996). Other PET studies on working memory, where the differentiation between active monitoring and passive reproduction of information was not specifically addressed, have confirmed the general pattern of lateralization of verbal working memory functions to the left frontal lobe and of visuospatial working memory functions to the right frontal lobe (Smith, Jonides, & Koeppe, 1996), consistent with the clinical lesion data.

The dorsolateral prefrontal cortex seems to be a critical structure in a number of delayed-response and conditional sensorimotor learning tasks in nonhuman primates (Goldman-Rakic, 1987). One functional aspect of the dorsolateral prefrontal cortex that makes this cerebral structure critical to delayed-response tasks and to conditional sensorimotor learning seems to be related to the learning of association rules between stimuli and responses (Fuster, 1995). In conditional motor learning to visuospatial stimuli in normal volunteers, learning-related changes in regional cerebral blood flow (rCBF) in the dorsolateral prefrontal cortex of the left hemisphere have been observed (see Figure 6.3; Iacoboni, Woods, & Mazziotta, 1996b), consistent with neurophysiological evidence showing that the neuronal discharge in dorsolateral prefrontal neurons of monkeys performing conditional sensorimotor tasks is dependent upon the learning component of the task (Fuster, 1995). Learning-related rCBF increases seem to be lateralized to the left dorsolateral prefrontal cortex even when learning effects in conditional motor tasks are largely parallel in both hands (Iacoboni et al., 1996b). This suggests that transfer of learning might occur through the anterior regions of the corpus callosum, interconnecting the prefrontal cortex of the two cerebral hemispheres (Iacoboni & Zaidel, 1995). In keeping with this, callosal lesions in primates interfere with transfer of visuomotor conditional learning (Eacott & Gaffan, 1990). The lateralization of conditional sensorimotor learning to the left prefrontal cortex may not be specific to the human brain. Indeed, a lateralized left prefrontal learning-dependent activity during sensorimotor learning has been reported in a nonhuman primate (Gemba, Miki, & Sasaki, 1995).

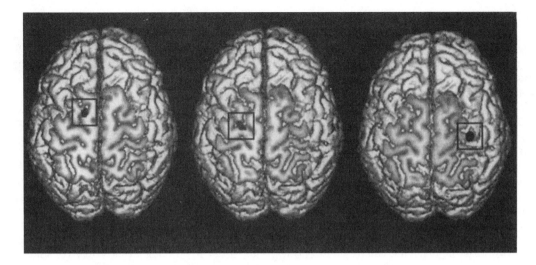

FIGURE 6.3. Functional asymmetries in sensorimotor integration in the human frontal lobe. Left: Rostral dorsal premotor activation in the left frontal lobe, subserving explicit stimulus–response associations. Center: Caudal dorsal premotor activation in the left frontal lobe, subserving implicit sensorimotor learning. Right: primary motor activation in the right frontal lobe, subserving the merging of extrapersonal and personal space.

## Premotor Cortex

There are four different cortical premotor fields in the lateral wall of the frontal lobe in the macaque brain. A variety of different nomenclatures have been used for these cortical fields. We follow here a nomenclature that seems the most intuitive. Independent anatomical and physiological evidence in nonhuman primates (Fogassi et al., 1996; Fuji et al., 1996; Matelli et al., 1985; Rizzolatti, Fadiga, Gallese, et al., 1996), and PET data in humans (Iacoboni et al., 1996a; Rizzolatti, Fadiga, Matelli, et al., 1996) support the division of premotor cortex into four fields: a rostral (PMdr) and a caudal (PMdc) field in the dorsal premotor cortex, and a rostral (PMvr) and a caudal (PMvc) field in the ventral premotor cortex. Neurophysiological evidence from studies of nonhuman primates suggests that PMdr is associated with saccade-, arm- and eye-, eye position–, and stimulus-related activity, whereas PMdc is associated with arm motor preparation– and arm movement–related activity (Fuji et al., 1996). The ventral premotor cortex seems to be associated with grasp representations and action recognition in PMvr (Rizzolatti, Fadiga, Gallese, et al., 1996), and with peripersonal space coding of somatosensory and visual stimuli in PMvc (Fogassi et al., 1996).

### LESION STUDIES

The dorsal premotor cortex is traditionally associated with neglect in extrapersonal space, with the selection and preparation of movements guided by external sensory stimuli, and with the retrieval of responses associated with specific sensory stimuli (Halsband & Freund, 1990; Passingham, 1993). The ventral premotor cortex is associated with neglect in peripersonal space (Rizzolatti, Matelli, & Pavesi, 1983). There are no convincing data from studies of humans with focal premotor cortical damage that address the issue of functional or anatomical lateralization of premotor cortex.

### FUNCTIONAL IMAGING STUDIES

PET evidence seems to suggest a left-hemisphere lateralization in the human PMvr (inferior frontal gyrus, Brodmann's area 45) for the observation/execution matching system of grasping actions (Grafton, Arbib, Fadiga, & Rizzolatti, 1996; Rizzolatti, Fadiga, Matelli, et al., 1996). This functional lateralization seems consistent with the hypothesis that primate communicative gestures could be the precursors of human language and that the "grammar" of communicative gestures could be represented in nonhuman primate PMvr, considered as the anatomical homologue of human Broca's area (Rizzolatti, Fadiga, Gallese, et al., 1996). One of the interpretational limitations of these PET studies is that subjects were required to grasp objects or to imagine grasping objects, or to observe others grasping objects, only with the dominant right hand. Thus, a left-hemisphere lateralization of brain activity might simply be caused by an asymmetry in the activation task. More convincingly, it has been shown with PET that the left PMvr (Brodmann's area 45) is activated in normal subjects while observing others making silent monosyllable mouth movements ("lip reading"), whereas no acoustic or language receptive areas were activated (Grafton, Fadiga, Arbib, & Rizzolatti, 1996). This would be consistent with the hypothesis that visual information feeds forward directly to Broca's area in the left hemisphere, as emphasized by Denny-Brown (1975).

With regard to PET studies of dorsal premotor cortex in humans, there seems to be a left PMdr superiority in establishing explicit stimulus–response associations, and a left PMdc superiority in implicit sensorimotor learning (see Figure 6.3; Iacoboni et al., 1996a). This would suggest a functional rostrocaudal fractionation of human dorsal premotor cortex similar to the one observed in nonhuman primates. The lateralization to the left dorsal premotor cortex also supports the notion, suggested by chronometric investigations, that the human left hemisphere is superior in tasks in which stimulus–response associations and response selection are required (Anzola, Bertoloni, Buchtel, & Rizzolatti, 1977). Finally, as in the dorsolateral prefrontal cortex, sensorimotor learning seems to be associated only with blood flow increases in PMdc. This suggests that, in contrast with other types of learning that may be associated with blood flow decreases (Raichle et al., 1994), frontal lobe mechanisms of sensorimotor learning are generally associated with blood flow increases that correspond to an increase in neural activity.

### Primary Motor Cortex

One of the most striking lateralized behaviors in humans is hand preference, which is typically, although not invariably, associated with manual skill (Annett, 1985). Fine manual coordination is lateralized to the left motor cortex in most right-handed individuals (Annett,

1985; Goldberg, 1985; Liepmann & Mass, 1907). Recent fMRI studies in humans demonstrate asymmetric activation of primary motor cortex during volitional fine movements of the hand (Kawashima et al., 1993; Kim, Ashe, Hendrich, & Ellerman, 1993). However, these activations involve a variety of prefrontal motor areas and are not restricted to primary motor cortex.

Some anatomical evidence suggests that the primary motor cortex in human and nonhuman primates is divided into a rostral sector and a caudal sector (Geyer et al., 1996; Stepniewska et al., 1993). It has been proposed that this anatomical differentiation corresponds to a functional differentiation (Geyer et al., 1996). However, the functional asymmetries of the primary motor cortex that we discuss here, do not differentiate between rostral and caudal sectors.

### LESION AND PHYSIOLOGICAL STUDIES

Hemispatial neglect is typically associated with right temporal–parietal lesions, but it is observed with right frontal lobe lesions as well (Heilman & Valenstein, 1972; Heilman, Watson, & Valenstein, 1993). Patients with right pre-Rolandic lesions, often encompassing primary motor areas, tend not to move the hand ipsilateral to the lesion in the contralateral hemispace (Bisiach, Geminiani, Berti, & Rusconi, 1990) and exhibit motor impersistence as well, which is thought to reflect an attentional deficit (Benson & Stuss, 1986). Under free vision, these patients typically fail to mark short lines lying on the left side of a paper sheet. Under mirror-reversed vision, in which only left–right mirror image is possible, patients have to mark the lines on the *left* side of the paper sheet to mark the lines that they see on the *right*. Paradoxically, these patients tend to neglect lines *seen* on the *left* under free vision, and lines *seen* on the *right* under mirror-reversed vision (Bisiach et al., 1995). Furthermore, a double dissociation in patients with unilateral neglect is often seen: Some patients have unilateral neglect only for near space; others have unilateral neglect only for far space (Halligan & Marshall, 1991). This double dissociation suggests that the representations of extrapersonal and personal space are differentiated and segregated in the human brain.

In the nonhuman primate, there is evidence for two parietal–frontal circuits subserving extrapersonal and personal space. A dorsal parietal–frontal circuit comprises area 7a, lateral intraparietal area (LIP), and dorsal premotor cortex, and codes extrapersonal space. A ventral parietal–frontal circuit comprises area 7b, anterior intraparietal area, and ventral premotor cortex, and codes personal space. These two circuits are anatomically largely independent, but both input to primary motor cortex (Passingham, 1993). PET data, reviewed in the next section, seem to suggest that the right motor cortex is involved in merging the information from these two parietal–frontal circuits.

FUNCTIONAL IMAGING STUDIES

A PET observation has suggested that the right motor cortex is a critical structure in mapping extrapersonal onto personal space (Iacoboni, Woods, Lenzi, & Mazziotta, 1997). To test whether the merging of the two spaces occurred in primary motor cortex, rCBF was measured in normal volunteers performing a task that required the coding of external stimuli in extrapersonal space and of motor responses in personal space. The critical manipulation was to ask subjects to respond half of the times with uncrossed arms (each arm in its homonymous hemispace) and half of the times with crossed arms (each hand in its heteronymous hemispace (i.e., left hand in right hemispace and right hand in left hemispace). The crossed arms response position produced slower reaction times and increased rCBF in primary motor cortex in the right hemisphere (Figure 6.3). These increases in blood flow correlated with the lengthening of reaction times.

A number of fMRI studies have suggested a major role for the primary motor cortex in motor learning (for a brief review, see Grafton, 1995). Most of these studies have also resulted in lateralized activation of the left primary motor cortex. However, these studies are inconclusive with regard to issues of functional asymmetries in motor learning, given that subjects were generally asked to use only the dominant right hand. The only fMRI studies of which we are aware that have used an unbiased learning paradigm in which left- and right-hand motor activity was completely counterbalanced (Iacoboni et al., 1996a, 1996b; Iacoboni, Woods, Lenzi, & Mazziotta, 1997) have resulted in blood flow increases consistently lateralized to the left frontal lobe. These blood flow increases occurred mainly in dorsal premotor cortex (Figure 6.3) and in dorsolateral prefrontal cortex, and only sporadically in primary motor cortex (Iacoboni et al., 1996b).

## Medial Wall (SMA and Anterior Cingulate Cortex)

Two main regions of the medial wall of the frontal lobe have a critical role in sensorimotor integration mechanisms, the SMA, and the anterior cingulate cortex. We review evidence from neurological literature and from neuroimaging techniques suggesting anatomical and functional parcellation, and anatomical and functional asymmetries in these two areas.

### Supplementary Motor Area

According to anatomical and physiological evidence, two distinct areas can be differentiated in this region: a rostral area called pre-SMA and a caudal area called SMA-proper. In macaques, the pre-SMA is located mainly anterior to the genu of the arcuate sulcus, whereas SMA-proper is located posterior to the genu of the arcuate sulcus. In the human brain, the pre-SMA is located rostral to the level of the anterior commissure, and the SMA-proper is located caudal to the level of the anterior commissure. Anatomical and neurophysiological evidence suggests that the pre-SMA is related to selection and preparation of movements, whereas the SMA-proper is more related to aspects of motor execution (Picard & Strick, 1996).

LESION STUDIES

Evidence for asymmetrical functions of the SMA in general, without a precise distinction between pre-SMA and SMA-proper, comes from observations in neurological patients. Patients with long-term unilateral medial frontal lobe lesions in the left hemisphere benefit from preparatory information regarding a motor response and can inhibit inappropriate responses. In contrast, patients with similar long-term lesions in the right hemisphere cannot benefit from preparatory information regarding a motor response and cannot inhibit an inappropriate motor response (Verfaellie & Heilman, 1987). In other words, it seem there is a differential effect of contextual cues on motor performance in the left and right SMA. We present evidence from PET studies of healthy subjects that is compatible with this hypothesis later in this section.

Another functional asymmetry that is observed in right-handed neurological patients with unilateral SMA lesions is related to the temporal control of movement sequences, a function generally subserved by the SMA (Tanji & Shima, 1994). Patients with left SMA lesions are much more impaired in reproducing rhythm patterns using the left hand, the right hand, or both hands in an alternating manner, than patients with right SMA lesions (Halsband, Ito, Tanji, & Freund, 1993). Furthermore, patients with left SMA lesions are more disturbed in the chronology of memory-guided saccade sequences than patients with right SMA lesions (Gaymad, Rivaud, & Pierrot-Deseilligny, 1993).

The evidence for a differential role of the left and right SMA in sequential control of movements, at least in right-handers, might also explain why strategically placed callosal lesions producing motor disconnection tend to be associated with alien hand syndrome in the nondominant hand, but not in the dominant hand in right-handers (Geschwind et al., 1995). If the motor areas of the right hemisphere that control the left hand do not receive inputs on sequential control of movements from the right SMA because of a callosal disconnection, then motor control disturbances in the left hand are likely to appear. We propose that this pathophysiological mechanism might be a unitary mechanism of praxis disturbances following callosal lesions (for a brief review, see Gonzalez-Rothi, Raade, & Heilman, 1994).

FUNCTIONAL IMAGING STUDIES

A robust phenomenon in sensorimotor learning that may be associated with functional asymmetries in the medial wall of the frontal lobe in both the SMA and cingulate cortex is the contextual interference effect. When subjects perform sensorimotor tasks, practice in blocked fashion (where each task pattern is practiced separately from the others) produces a faster learning slope than practice in random fashion (where each practiced task pattern is mixed with the others; Stelmach, 1996).

In a PET experiment on sensorimotor conditional learning, we have observed that contextual interference affects learning in the right hand more than in the left hand. This was associated with blood flow increases in the left

SMA-proper (Iacoboni, 2000). In other words, the left SMA-proper seems to be more sensitive to contextual interference than the right SMA-proper, which might suggest that the differential contextual effect observed in patients with left and right SMA lesions occurs more specifically at the level of the SMA-proper. An additional area of the medial wall of the frontal lobe that showed blood flow changes related to contextual interference effect is in the cingulate cortex, which is discussed in the following section.

### Anterior Cingulate Cortex

In the macaque, three areas, buried in the cingulate sulcus, seem to have significance in sensorimotor processes: the rostral cingulate motor area (CMAr), located anterior to the genu of the arcuate sulcus, and the dorsal (CMAd) and the ventral (CMAv) cingulate motor areas, located caudal to the genu of the arcuate sulcus (Picard & Strick, 1996). A review of PET findings in humans has suggested at least two cortical fields in the human anterior cingulate cortex: a large rostral one, anterior to the anterior commissure, associated with complex sensorimotor tasks and with a somatotopic arrangement; and a small caudal one, posterior to the anterior commissure, associated with simple tasks and not showing a clear somatotopy (Picard & Strick, 1996).

FUNCTIONAL IMAGING STUDIES

The anterior cingulate has been associated with attentional functions (Bench et al., 1993; Posner & Dehaene 1994). However, asymmetries in the anterior cingulate in attentional mechanisms have not been systematically described (Pardo et al., 1991). Furthermore, widespread areas of right dorsolateral prefrontal cortex are preferentially activated during a variety of attentional tasks (Bench et al., 1993; Lewin et al., 1996; Vendrell et al., 1995). In terms of functional asymmetries, lateralized fMRI findings should be interpreted with caution in midline structures, such as the cingulate region, given the spatial proximity of left and right cingulate cortex. If in fMRI studies the behavioral performance can be monitored online, then lateralized findings in the anterior cingulate are more likely to be reliable. For instance, in the contextual interference experiment cited in the previous section, we observed a slower learning in the right hand in subjects practicing in a random fashion, associated with blood flow increases in the left SMA-proper and in the left rostral anterior cingulate area, in a region overlapping with the arm representation in the human anterior cingulate cortex, according to Picard and Strick (1996). Taken together, behavioral data and rCBF findings suggest a greater sensitivity of the left rostral cingulate region to contextual cues. This is in line with a general role of the cingulate cortex in context-specific learning in other mammals (Freeman, Cuppernell, Flannery, & Gabriel, 1996).

## ANATOMICAL ASYMMETRIES

The most striking asymmetry in the anterior cingulate region is at morphological level. In the left hemisphere, there are often two cerebral sulci in the cingulate region, the cingulate sulcus and the paracingulate sulcus, whereas in the right hemisphere, there is generally only one sulcus, the cingulate sulcus. It has been speculated that this asymmetry might be related to certain aspects of effortful versus automatic vocalization (Paus et al., 1996). Indeed, in a PET study that compared reversed speech (effortful) with overpracticed speech, foci of activation were largely observed overlapping with the paracingulate sulcus in the left hemisphere (Paus, Petrides, Evans, & Meyer, 1993). Whether this asymmetry is related to the motor or linguistic components of speech remains to be clarified.

## THE MIRROR SYSTEM: VENTRAL PREMOTOR AND PARIETAL CORTEX

A special class of neurons was discovered in the inferior frontal cortex of the macaque brain. These neurons were found in area F5, the rostral sector of the ventral premotor cortex (Matelli et al., 1985). These premotor neurons fire not only when the monkey performs goal-directed actions, such as grasping objects, but also when holding, tearing, manipulating, and so forth. Surprisingly, these neurons also fire when the monkey is simply watching somebody else performing goal-directed actions (di Pellegrino, Fadiga, Fogassi, Gallese, & Rizzolatti, 1992; Gallese, Fadiga, Fogassi, & Rizzolatti, 1996). Because of these properties, these neurons were dubbed "mirror" neurons

(Gallese et al., 1996). There is generally a good congruence—often a very strict one—between the action coded motorically and the action coded visually by mirror neurons; that is, if a mirror neuron fires during the monkey's execution of a precision grip, it will also likely fire when the monkey sees a precision grip rather than a whole-hand prehension.

Later studies provided further insights into the properties of mirror neurons. For instance, mirror neurons fire even when the sight of the hand grasping the object is occluded, as long as the monkey can see the initial movement of the hand toward the object (Umilta et al., 2001). Moreover, they fire also when the monkey—in complete darkness—hears the sound associated with an action, for instance, breaking a peanut (Kohler et al., 2002). Moreover, mirror neurons also code for mouth actions, some of which are communicative actions for monkeys, such as lipsmacking (Ferrari, Gallese, Rizzolatti, & Fogassi, 2003). These findings suggest that mirror neurons may implement very abstract representations of actions, and that they can map actions of others onto actions of the self, a fundamental functional step for understanding other people.

In terms of their laterality, as usual, the single-unit data do not offer striking asymmetries. In one of the original reports (Gallese et al., 1996), however, some interesting laterality patterns were observed. About 40% of mirror neurons tested demonstrated a discharge influenced by the laterality of the observed hand. The majority of these neurons responded more strongly when the observed hand was ipsilateral to the recorded hemisphere (i.e., a left-hand action triggered stronger discharge in mirror neurons in the left ventral premotor cortex, compared to a right-hand action). Another interesting finding was related to the direction of the observed reach-and-grasp action. About two-thirds of mirror neurons tested demonstrated directional preference. The great majority (more than 80%) of these neurons preferred the direction toward the recorded side, that is, from right to left for mirror neurons in the left hemisphere (Gallese et al., 1996).

Area F5 is connected with the rostral part of the inferior parietal lobule (area PF). Mirror neurons have also been observed in area PF (Fogassi et al., 2005). Thus, the mirror neuron system in macaques is composed of two major centers—one in the posterior inferior frontal cortex and the other in the rostral inferior parietal cortex—that are strongly interconnected.

Several brain-imaging studies have addressed the properties of the human homologue of the macaque mirror neuron system. In good accordance with the monkey data, areas with mirror properties have been described in the posterior inferior frontal and rostral inferior parietal cortex in humans (Buccino et al., 2004; Iacoboni et al., 1999, 2005). With regard to the laterality of the human mirror neuron system, robust lateralized responses have been observed in some cases.

In one of the original reports (Iacoboni et al., 1999), a human left inferior frontal area was described as responding to action observation, action execution, and even more so during action imitation. In light of the evolutionary hypothesis of a link between mirror neurons and language (Rizzolatti & Arbib, 1998), the left lateralization reported in this study has been often taken as suggesting that the whole mirror neuron system in humans is left-lateralized (Corballis, 2003). This lateralization, however, should be interpreted as a specific asymmetry related to a specific form of imitation. In that study, right-hand actions imitated left-hand observed actions. As we have seen, even the monkey data would have predicted a left-lateralized pattern in this case (Iacoboni et al., 1999). In fact, a reanalysis of seven fMRI studies of imitation adopting various forms of hand imitation has shown a fairly bilateral activation pattern in the posterior inferior frontal cortex (Molnar-Szakacs, Iacoboni, Koski, & Mazziotta, 2005).

A robust left-hemisphere mirror neuron response has been observed in a recent transcranial magnetic stimulation (TMS) study probing corticospinal excitability. A highly reproducible effect that is likely due to the mirror neuron system is the increase in excitability of the motor corticospinal system during action observation. When a TMS pulse is applied over the primary motor hand area, a motor response is evoked in the contralateral hand. If subjects are also watching somebody else's actions, this motor evoked response is much stronger when compared to watching some visual control stimuli (Aziz-Zadeh, Maeda, Zaidel, Mazziotta, & Iacoboni, 2002; Fadiga, Craighero, & Oliver, 2005; Fadiga, Fogassi, Pavesi, & Rizzolatti, 1995). This effect is likely due to the activation of mirror neurons in premotor cortex that feed directly onto primary motor regions (Cerri, Shimazu, Maier, & Lemon, 2003;

Shimazu, Maier, Cerri, Kirkwood, & Lemon, 2004). A similar effect has been observed for action sounds. When subjects are listening to action sounds, their corticospinal excitability is facilitated (Aziz-Zadeh, Iacoboni, Zaidel, Wilson, & Mazziotta, 2004). This effect, likely mediated by mirror neurons that respond to the sound of an action (Kohler et al., 2002), is completely lateralized to the left hemisphere in humans (Aziz-Zadeh et al., 2004). This strong left-hemisphere lateralization suggests that a fundamental step in the hypothesized evolutionary progression from action recognition to language may be the multimodal representation of action that only the left hemisphere appears to have in humans.

Two robust right-lateralized responses in the human mirror neuron system have recently been reported. In the first case, right-hemisphere lateralization was observed during imitation and observation of facial emotional expressions (Carr, Iacoboni, Dubeau, Mazziotta, & Lenzi, 2003). This pattern fits well the general pattern of right-hemisphere competence for emotional processing. In the second case, a strongly lateralized response in a mirror neuron area was observed in an action observation task in which the context of the actions provided the observers information to predict the intention of the actor, in other words, to predict the following (unseen) action (Iacoboni et al., 2005). Here, too, the lateralization pattern seems to fit well evidence from other research that suggests a link between the right hemisphere and the capacity to "read the mind" of other people (Happe, Brownell, & Winner, 1999; Winner, Brownell, Happe, Blum, & Pincus, 1998).

Taken together, the laterality findings in the human mirror neuron system suggest that this system is not lateralized to the left or right hemisphere, but that asymmetries may emerge in the system on the basis of the function tapped by specific tasks. These asymmetries seem to follow general patterns of lateralization seen in other domains.

## THE LAST FRONTIER: MOLECULAR ASYMMETRY

The molecular basis of the structural and functional asymmetries evident in the human brain is an important area, with great relevance to both disease and the evolution of cognition, which has received little experimental attention. We have embarked on a program to begin to study the ontogeny of gene expression asymmetries during human fetal brain development, based on the notion that such transcriptional asymmetries underlie the structural asymmetries that are most evident at later stages (Geschwind & Miller, 2001). Recent studies in twins clearly support a genetic basis (Geschwind, Miller, De Carli, & Carmelli, 2002). The driving goal of this work is to connect gene expression patterns to the brain (neural systems), and to behavior and cognition.

We originally tested genes known to be involved in visceral asymmetry in vertebrates and were not able to identify any that were asymmetrically expressed during brain development in humans (Geschwind & Miller 2001; Sun et al., 2005). Subsequently, we have taken a number of genetic screening approaches in our own laboratory, including microarray studies and subtraction studies. Most recently, serial analysis of gene expression was performed in Chris Walsh's laboratory at Boston Children's Hospital and, in collaboration, we were able to show clear asymmetric gene expression in the human brain for the first time (Sun et al., 2005). The asymmetry was variable between individuals and quite regional, being most marked in perisylvian regions for the genes studied in most detail. Strikingly, the pattern of asymmetry in mouse was random for the case of one gene, *LMO4*, whereas it was clearly enriched in right perisylvian cortex in the majority of humans. We have yet to identify any genes with a predominantly frontal asymmetry, although several genes we identified using microarrays in our other screens have frontal lobe enrichment. Such genes are candidates for patterning of frontal lobe structures and can be used to probe the evolutionary conservation of frontal lobe regions across primate species and lower mammals (e.g., Preuss, Caceres, Oldham, & Geschwind, 2004).

This raises one very important issue that is often avoided in neuroscience research—the relevance of animal models to human development and function. It is often assumed that what happens in the mouse is relevant to humans, but over and over again, many human diseases have proven hard to model in the mouse. Similarly, with a few exceptions (e.g., Abu-Khalil, Fu, Grove, Zecevic, & Geschwind, 2003), there are few human studies of important patterning molecules or signaling centers involved in mouse brain patterning. Thus, it will be important to determine experimentally the similarities and differences between the basic patterning of the cerebral cortex in mouse and man, because the mouse is being used as a model for so many key developmental and functional issues.

## CONCLUDING REMARKS

In conclusion, we ask, Is a comprehensive model of frontal lobe lateralization realistic? One model of frontal specialization proposes a dichotomy in which the right frontal lobe is specialized for novelty and the left frontal lobe, for the routine (Goldberg & Podell, 1995). That the right frontal lobe is predominant in novelty processing fits with its role in attentional mechanisms (Heilman, Watson, & Valenstein, 1993). PET studies in healthy volunteers demonstrate strikingly increased blood flow and metabolic activity in the right prefrontal cortex, including Brodmann's areas 8, 9, 44, and 46 during selective attention tasks in different sensory modalities (Bench et al., 1993; Lewin et al., 1996; Pardo et al., 1991; Roland, 1984). The lateralized role of the primary motor area in the merging of personal and extrapersonal space was discussed earlier. However, the role of the right hemisphere in attention or novelty processing does not necessarily relegate the left hemisphere to the routine.

The dichotomization and polarization of the functions of the two cerebral hemispheres are recurrent themes in models of cerebral lateralization. In contrast, we believe that the specialization of one hemisphere for a given function does not require that the contralateral hemisphere not be involved in that function, or that it serve the polar opposite function. Recent PET and fMRI data demonstrate frequent bilateral (although still asymmetrical) activations in homologous regions in tasks previously considered completely lateralized. Furthermore, we have seen in this chapter that the frontal lobes comprise numerous functionally distinct areas on cytoarchitectonic and physiological grounds, and that these functionally distinct frontal areas demonstrate different laterality patterns. Furthermore, the first molecular asymmetries observed early in development are not "whole hemispheric"; rather, they are quite variable and regional. Thus, any attempt to unify lateralized frontal lobe functions under one model is simplistic and likely to be flawed.

In spite of the large number of frontal lobe functions that appear lateralized, the only functional asymmetry for which a corresponding structural asymmetry has been supported by a body of converging evidence is that of language and Broca's area. We anticipate that as physiological and anatomical studies in primates, and functional imaging studies in humans, continue to aid in the segregation of functional units within the frontal lobe, the morphological, physiological, and molecular asymmetries that contribute to these functional asymmetries will be elucidated. Now, with the identification of a first set of asymmetry genes, we have ability to study carefully their conservation in nonhuman primates and understand the evolution of asymmetry.

It is becoming clear that many of the functional asymmetries discussed in this chapter are in functions for which nonhuman primates are well adapted. Thus, a detailed study of the degree of lateralization in these nonlanguage functions and their anatomical correlates in primates should provide important insights into the evolutionary origins of frontal lobe asymmetries: Our emerging notions of the mirror neuron system provides one salient example of how such work can be accomplished. In the same vein, how functional asymmetries in sensorimotor integration in humans correspond to language lateralization in individual subjects should be of great interest.

## ACKNOWLEDGMENTS

We gratefully acknowledge support from the McDonnell-Pew Foundation in Cognitive Neuroscience (to D.H.G.), the International Human Frontier Science Program (to M.I.), and the National Institutes of Health (Grant Nos. NS01849, R01 MH60233, and R56 MH60233 to D.H.G. and Nos. NS20187 and MH00179 to M.I.).

## REFERENCES

Abu-Khalil, A., Fu, L., Grove, E. A., Zecevic, N., & Geschwind, D. H. (2004). Wnt genes define distinct boundaries in the developing human brain: Implications for human forebrain patterning. *Journal of Comparative Neurology, 474,* 276–288.

Adrianov, O. S. (1979). Structural basis for functional interhemispheric brain asymmetry. *Human Physiology, 5,* 359–363.

Albanese, E., Merlo, A., Albanese, A., & Gomez, E. (1989). Anterior speech region: Asymmetry and weight-surface correlation. *Archives of Neurology, 46,* 307–310.

Alexander, M. P., Naeser, M. A., & Palumbo, C. (1990). Broca's area aphasias: Aphasia after lesions including the frontal operculum. *Neurology, 40,* 353–362.

Annett, M. (1985). *Left, right, hand and brain: The right shift theory.* London: Erlbaum.

Anzola, G. P., Bertoloni, G., Buchtel, H. A., & Rizzolatti, G. (1977). Spatial compatibility and anatomical factors in simple and choice reaction time. *Neuropsychologia, 15,* 295–302.

Aresu, M. (1914). La superficie cerebrale nell uomo. *Archivio italiano di anatomia e di embriologia* [Italian Journal of Anatomy and Embriology], *12,* 380–433.

Aziz-Zadeh, L., Iacoboni, M., Zaidel, E., Wilson, S., & Mazziotta, J. (2004). Left hemisphere motor facilitation in response to manual action sounds. *European Journal of Neuroscience, 19*(9), 2609–2612.

Aziz-Zadeh, L., Maeda, F., Zaidel, E., Mazziotta, J., & Iacoboni, M. (2002). Lateralization in motor facilitation during action observation: A TMS study. *Exerimental Brain Research, 144*(1), 127–131.

Bear, D., Schiff, D., Saver, J., Greenberg, M., & Freeman, R. (1986). Quantitative analysis of cerebral asymmetries: Fronto-occipital correlation, sexual dimorphism and association with handedness. *Archives of Neurology, 43,* 598–603.

Bench, C. J., Frith, C. D., Grasby, P. M., Friston, K. J., Paulesu, E., Frackowiak, R. S., et al. (1993). Investigations of the functional anatomy of attention using the Stroop test. *Neuropsychologia, 31,* 907–922.

Benson, D. F. (1977). The third alexia. *Archives of Neurology, 34,* 327–331.

Benson, D. F. (1986). Aphasia and the lateralization of language. *Cortex, 22,* 71–86.

Benson, D. F., & Stuss, D. T. (1986). *The frontal lobes.* New York: Raven.

Berker, E. A., Berker, A. H., & Smith, A. (1986). Translation of Broca's 1865 report: Localization of speech in the third left frontal convolution. *Archives of Neurology, 43,* 1065–1072.

Binder, J. R., Rao, S. M., Hammeke, T. A., Frost, J. A., Bandettini, P. A., Jesmanowicz, A., et al. (1995). Lateralized human brain language systems demonstrated by task subtraction functional magnetic resonance imaging. *Archives of Neurology, 52,* 593–601.

Bisiach, E., Geminiani, G., Berti, A., & Rusconi, M. L. (1990). Perceptual and premotor factors of unilateral neglect. *Neurology, 40,* 1278–1281.

Bisiach, E., Tegner, R., Ladavas, E., Rusconi, M. L., Mijovic, D., & Hjaltason, H. (1995). Dissociation of ophthalmokinetic and melokinetic attention in unilateral neglect. *Cerebral Cortex, 5,* 439–447.

Boccardi, E., Bruzzone, M. G., & Vignolo, L. A. (1984). Alexia in recent and late Broca's aphasia. *Neuropsychologia, 22,* 745–754.

Bogen, J. E. (1993). The callosal syndromes. In K. M.

Heilman & E. Valenstein (Eds.), *Clinical neuropsy-chology* (pp. 337–407). New York: Oxford University Press.

Broca, P. (1865). Sur la faculté du language articulé [On spoken language function]. *Bulletin de la Societé Anatomique de Paris*, 6, 493–494.

Broca, P. (1875). Instructions craniologiques et craniometriques de la Societé d'Anthropologie. *Bulletin de la Societé d'Anthropologie (Paris)*, 6, 534–536.

Broca, P. (1888). *Memoires sur le Cerveau de l'homme*. Paris: Reinwald.

Buccino, G., Vogt, S., Ritzl, A., Fink, G. R., Zilles, K., Freund, H. J., et al. (2004). Neural circuits underlying imitation learning of hand actions: An event-related fMRI study. *Neuron*, 42(2), 323–334.

Cancelliere, A. E., & Kertesz, A. (1990). Lesion localization in acquired deficits of emotional expression and comprehension. *Brain and Cognition*, 13(2), 133–147.

Carr, L., Iacoboni, M., Dubeau, M. C., Mazziotta, J. C., & Lenzi, G. L. (2003). Neural mechanisms of empathy in humans: A relay from neural systems for imitation to limbic areas. *Proceedings of the National Academy of Sciences of the United States of America*, 100(9), 5497–5502.

Cavada, C., & Goldman-Rakic, P. S. (1989). Posterior parietal cortex in rhesus monkey: II. Evidence for segregated corticocortical networks linking sensory and limbic areas with the frontal lobe. *Journal of Comparative Neurology*, 287, 422–445.

Cerri, G., Shimazu, H., Maier, M. A., & Lemon, R. N. (2003). Facilitation from ventral premotor cortex of primary motor cortex outputs to macaque hand muscles. *Journal of Neurophysiology*, 90(2), 832–842.

Corballis, M. C. (2003). From mouth to hand: Gesture, speech, and the evolution of right-handedness. *Behavioral Brain Sciences*, 26(2), 199–208.

Damasio, A. R., & Tranel, D. (1993). Nouns and verbs are retrieved with differently distributed neural systems. *Proceedings of the National Academy of Sciences of the United States of America*, 90, 4957–4960.

Danly, M., & Shapiro, B. (1982). Speech prosody in Broca's aphasia. *Brain and Language*, 16(2), 171–290.

Davidson, R. J. (1992). Anterior cerebral asymmetry and the nature of emotion. *Brain and Cognition*, 20, 125–151.

Davidson, R. J., & Sutton, S. K. (1995) .Affective neuroscience: The emergence of a discipline. *Current Opinion in Neurobiology*, 5, 217–224.

Demonet, J. F., Price, C., Wise, R., & Frackowiak, R. S. (1994). A PET study of cognitive strategies in normal subjects during language tasks: Influence of phonetic ambiguity and sequence processing on phoneme monitoring. *Brain*, 117(4), 671–682.

Denny-Brown, D. (1965). Physiologic aspects of disturbances of speech. *Australian Journal of Experimental Biology and Medical Science*, 43, 455–474.

Denny-Brown, D. (1975). Cerebral dominance. In K. J.

Zulch, O. Creutzfeldt, & G. C. Galbraith (Eds.), *Cerebral localization* (pp. 306–307). New York: Springer-Verlag.

di Pellegrino, G., Fadiga, L., Fogassi, L., Gallese, V., & Rizzolatti, G. (1992). Understanding motor events: A neurophysiological study. *Exerimental Brain Research*, 9, 176–180.

Dordain, M., Degos, J. D., & Dordain, G. (1971). [Voice disorders in left hemiplegia]. *Revue de Laryngologie Otologie Rhinologie*, 92(3), 178–188.

Eacott, M. J., & Gaffan, D. (1990). Interhemispheric transfer of visuomotor conditional learning via the anterior corpus callosum of monkeys. *Behavioral Brain Research*, 38, 109–116.

Eccles, J.C. (1977). Evolution of the brain in relation to the development of the self-conscious mind. *Annals of the New York Academy of Sciences*, 299, 161–178.

Fadiga, L., Craighero, L., & Olivier, E. (2005). Human motor cortex excitability during the perception of others' action. *Current Opinion in Neurobiology*, 15(2), 213–218.

Fadiga, L., Fogassi, L., Pavesi, G., & Rizzolatti, G. (1995). Motor facilitation during action observation: A magnetic stimulation study. *Journal of Neurophysiology*, 73, 2608–2611.

Falk, D., Hildebolt, C., Cheverud, J., Vannier, M., Helmkamp, R. C., & Konigsberg, L. (1990). Cortical asymmetries in frontal lobes of rhesus monkeys (*Macaca mulatta*). *Brain Research*, 512(1), 40–45.

Falzi, G., Perrone, P., & Vignolo, L. A. (1982). Right–left asymmetry in anterior speech region. *Archives of Neurology*, 39, 239–240.

Ferrari, P. F., Gallese, V., Rizzolatti, G., & Fogassi, L. (2003). Mirror neurons responding to the observation of ingestive and communicative mouth actions in the monkey ventral premotor cortex. *European Journal of Neuroscience*, 17(8), 1703–1714.

Finger, S. (1994). *Origins of neuroscience: A history of explorations into brain function*. New York: Oxford University Press.

Flourens, P. (1824). *Recherches experimentales sur les propriétés et les fonctions du système nerveux dans les animaux vertébrés*. Paris: Crevot.

Fogassi, L., Ferrari, P. F., Gesierich, B., Rozzi, S., Chersi, F., & Rizzolatti, G. (2005). Parietal lobe: From action organization to intention understanding. *Science*, 308(5722), 662–667.

Fogassi, L., Gallese, V., Fadiga, L., Luppino, G., Matelli, M., & Rizzolatti, G. (1996). Coding of peripersonal space in inferior premotor cortex. *Journal of Neurophysiology*, 76, 140–157.

Foundas, A. L., Leonard, C. M., Gilmore, R. L., Fennell, E. B., & Heilman, K. M. (1996). Pars triangularis asymmetry and language dominance. *Proceedings of the National Academy of Sciences of the United States of America*, 93, 719–722.

Foundas, A. L., Leonard, C. M., & Heilman, K. M. (1995). Morphologic cerebral asymmetries and handedness: The pars triangularis and planum temporale. *Archives of Neurology, 52*, 501–508.

Freedman, M., Alexander, M. P., & Naeser, M. A. (1984). Anatomic basis of transcortical motor aphasia. *Neurology, 34*(4), 409–417.

Freeman, J. H., Jr., Cuppernell, C., Flannery, K., & Gabriel, M. (1996). Context-specific multi-site cingulate cortical, limbic thalamic, and hippocampal neuronal activity during concurrent discriminative approach and avoidance training in rabbits. *Journal of Neuroscience, 16*, 1538–1549.

Frith, C. D., Friston, K. J., Liddle, P. F., & Frackowiak, R. S. (1991). A PET study of word finding. *Neuropsychologia, 29*, 1137–1148.

Fujii, N., Mushiake, H., & Tanji, J. (1996). Rostrocaudal differentiation of dorsal premotor cortex with physiological criteria [Abstract]. *Society for Neuroscience, 22*, 2024.

Funahashi, S., Bruce, C. J., & Goldman-Rakic, P. S. (1989). Mnemonic coding of visual space in the monkey's dorsolateral prefrontal cortex. *Journal of Neurophysiology, 61*, 331–349.

Funahashi, S., Chafee, M. V., & Goldman-Rakic, P. S. (19930. Prefrontal neuronal activity in rhesus monkeys performing a delayed anti-saccade task. *Nature, 365*, 753–756.

Fuster, J. M. (1995). *Memory in the cerebral cortex.* Cambridge, MA: MIT Press.

Gainotti, G. (1972). Emotional behavior and hemispheric side of the lesion. *Cortex, 8*, 41–55.

Galaburda, A. M. (1980). [Broca's region: Anatomic remarks made a century after the death of its discoverer]. *Revue Neurologique (Paris), 136*, 609–616.

Galaburda, A. M. (1991). Asymmetries of cerebral neuroanatomy. In J. Marsh & M. J. Bock (Eds.), *Biological asymmetry and handedness* (pp. 219–226). New York: Wiley.

Galaburda, A. M. (1993). Neurology of developmental dyslexia. *Optometry and Vision Science, 70*, 343–347.

Galaburda, A. M., LeMay, M., Kemper, T. L., & Geschwind, N. (1978). Right–left asymmetries in the brain. *Science, 199*, 852–856.

Galaburda, A. M., Rosen, G. D., & Sherman, G. F. (1990). Individual variability in cortical organization: Its relationship to brain laterality and implications to function. *Neuropsychologia, 28*, 529–546.

Gallese, V., Fadiga, L., Fogassi, L., & Rizzolatti, G. (1996). Action recognition in the premotor cortex. *Brain, 119*, 593–609.

Garraghty, P. E., & Kaas, J. H. (1992). Dynamic features of sensory and motor maps. *Current Opinion in Neurobiology, 2*, 522–527.

Gaymard, B., Rivaud, S., & Pierrot-Deseilligny, C. (1993). Role of the left and right supplementary motor areas in memory-guided saccade sequences. *Annals of Neurology, 34*, 404–406.

Gazzaniga, M. S. (1970). *The bissected brain.* New York: Appleton-Century-Crofts.

Gemba, H., Miki, N., & Sasaki, K. (1995). Field potential change in the prefrontal cortex of the left hemisphere during learning processes of reaction time hand movement with complex tone in the monkey. *Neuroscience Letters, 190*, 93–96.

George, M. S., Ketter, T. A., Parekh, P. I., Horwitz, B., Herscovitch, P., & Post, R. M. (1995). Brain activity during transient sadness and happiness in healthy women. *American Journal of Psychiatry, 152*, 341–351.

George, M. S., Parekh, P. I., Rosinsky, N. Ketter, T. A., Kimbrell, T. A., Heilman, K. M., et al. (1996). Understanding emotional prosody activates right hemisphere regions. *Archives of Neurology, 53*, 665–670.

Geschwind, D. H., Iacoboni, M., Mega, M. S., Zaidel, D. W., Cloughesy, T., & Zaidel, E. (1995). The alien hand syndrome: Interhemispheric motor disconnection due to a lesion in the midbody of the corpus callosum. *Neurology, 45*, 802–808.

Geschwind, D. H., & Miller, B. L. (2001). Molecular approaches to cerebral laterality: Development and neurodegeneration. *American Journal of Medical Genetics, 101*, 370–381.

Geschwind, D. H., Miller, B. L., DeCarli, C., & Carmelli, D. (2002). Heritability of lobar brain volumes in twins supports genetic models of cerebral laterality and handedness. *Proceedings of the National Academy of Sciences of the United States of America, 99*(5), 3176–3181.

Geschwind, N. (1970). The organization of language and the brain. *Science, 170*, 940–944.

Geschwind, N., & Galaburda, A. (1985). Cerebral lateralization: Biological mechanisms, associations, and pathology. *Archives of Neurology, 42*, 428–458, 521–552.

Geschwind, N., & Levitsky, W. (1968). Human brain: Left–right asymmetries in temporal speech region. *Science, 161*, 186–187.

Geyer, S., Ledberg, A., Schleicher, A., Kinomura, S., Schorman, T., Burgelu, A., et al. (1996). Two different areas within the primary motor cortex of man. *Nature, 382*, 805–807.

Glicksohn, J., & Myslobodsky, M. S. (1993). The representation of patterns of structural brain asymmetry in normal individuals. *Neuropsychologia, 31*, 145–159.

Goldberg, E., & Podell, K. (1995). Lateralization in the frontal lobes. In H. H. Jasper, S. Riggio, & P. Goldman-Rakic (Eds.), *Epilepsy and the functional anatomy of the frontal lobe* (pp. 85–96). New York: Raven.

Goldberg, G. (1985). Supplementary motor area structure and function: Review and hypotheses. *Behavioral and Brain Sciences, 8*, 567–616.

Goldman-Rakic, P. S. (1987). Circuitry of primate prefrontal cortex and regulation of behavior by representational memory. In V. B. Mountcastle (Ed.), *Handbook of physiology—the nervous system* (pp. 373–417). Bethesda, MD: American Physiological Society.

Gonzalez-Rothi, L. G., Raade, A. S., & Heilman, K. M.

(1994). Localization of lesions in limb and bucco-facial apraxia. In A. Kertesz (Ed.), *Localization and neuroimaging in neuropsychology* (pp. 407–428). San Diego, CA: Academic Press.

Goodale, M. A., & Milner, A. D. (1992). Separate visual pathways for perception and action. *Trends in Neurosciences, 15,* 20–25.

Grafton, S. T. (1995). Mapping memory systems in the human brain. *Seminars in Neuroscience, 7,* 157–163.

Grafton, S. T., Arbib, M. A., Fadiga, L., & Rizzolatti, G. (1996). Localization of grasp representations in humans by positron emission tomography: Observation compared with imagination. *Experimental Brain Research, 112,* 103–111.

Grafton, S. T., Fadiga, L., Arbib, M. A., & Rizzolatti, G. (1996). Activation of frontal motor areas during silent lip reading [Abstract]. *Society of Neuroscience, 22,* 1109.

Habib, M., Demonet, J. F., & Frackowiak, R. (1996). [Cognitive neuroanatomy of language: Contribution of functional cerebral imaging]. *Revue Neurologique (Paris), 152,* 249–260.

Hadziselmovic, H., & Cus, M. (1966). The appearance of internal structures of the brain in relation to configuration of the human skull. *Acta Anatomica, 63,* 289–299.

Halligan, P., & Marshall, J. (1991). Left neglect near but not for far space in man. *Nature, 350,* 498–500.

Halsband, U., & Freund, H. J. (1990). Premotor cortex and conditional motor learning in man. *Brain, 113,* 207–222.

Halsband, U., Ito, N., Tanji, J., & Freund, H. J. (1993). The role of premotor cortex and the supplementary motor area in the temporal control of movement in man. *Brain, 116,* 243–266.

Happe, F., Brownell, H., & Winner, E. (1999). Acquired "theory of mind" impairments following stroke. *Cognition, 70*(3), 211–240.

Hayes, T. L., & Lewis, D. A. (1993). Hemispheric differences in layer III pyramidal neurons of the anterior language area. *Archives of Neurology, 50,* 501–505.

Hayes T. L., & Lewis, D. A. (1995). Anatomical specialization of the anterior motor speech area: Hemispheric differences in magnopyramidal neurons. *Brain and Language, 49,* 289–308.

Hécaen, H., & Consoli, S. (1973). Analyse des troubles de langage au cours des lesions de l'aire de Broca [Analysis of language disorders in lesions of Broca's area]. *Neuropsychologia, 11,* 377–388.

Hécaen, H., De Agostini, A. M., & Monzon-Montes, M. A. (1981). Cerebral organization in left-handers. *Brain and Language, 12,* 261–284.

Heilman, K. M., & Valenstein, E. (1972). Frontal lobe neglect in man. *Neurology, 22,* 660–664.

Heilman, K. M., Watson, R. T., & Valenstein, E. (1993). Neglect and related disorders. In K. M. Heilman & E. Valenstein (Eds.), *Clinical neuropsychology* (pp. 279–336). New York: Oxford University Press.

Holloway, R. L., & De La Coste-Lareymondie, M. (1982). Brain endocast asymmetry in pongids and hominids: Some preliminary findings on the paleontology of cerebral dominance. *American Journal of Physical Anthropology, 58,* 101–110.

Iacoboni, M. (2000). Attention and sensorimotor integration: Mapping the embodied mind. In A. Toga & J. C. Mazziotta (Eds.), *Brain mapping: Systems* (pp. 463–490). San Diego, CA: Academic Press.

Iacoboni, M., Molnar-Szakacs, I., Gallese, V., Buccino, G., Mazziotta, J. C., & Rizzolatti, G. (2005). Grasping the intentions of others with one's own mirror neuron system. *PLoS Biology, 3*(3), e79.

Iacoboni, M., Woods, R. P., Brass, M., Bekkering, H., Mazziotta, J. C., & Rizzolatti, G. (1999). Cortical mechanisms of human imitation. *Science, 286,* 2526–2528.

Iacoboni, M., Woods, R. P., Lenzi G. L., & Mazziotta, J. C. (1997). Space coding by right motor cortex in the human brain. *NeuroImage, 3,* S368.

Iacoboni, M., Woods, R. P., Lenzi G. L., & Mazziotta, J. C. (1997). Merging of oculomotor and somatomotor space coding in the human right precentral gyrus. *Brain, 120,* 1635–1645.

Iacoboni, M., Woods, R. P., & Mazziotta, J. C. (1996a). Blood flow increases in left dorsal premotor cortex during sensorimotor integration learning. *Society for Neuroscience Abstracts, 22,* 720.

Iacoboni, M., Woods, R. P., & Mazziotta, J. C. (1996b). Brain–behavior relationships: Evidence from practice effects in spatial stimulus–response compatibility. *Journal of Neurophysiology, 76,* 321–331.

Iacoboni, M., & Zaidel, E. (1995). Channels of the corpus callosum: Evidence from simple reaction times to lateralized flashes in the normal and the split brain. *Brain, 118,* 779–788.

Iacoboni, M., & Zaidel, E. (1996). Hemispheric independence in word recognition: Evidence from unilateral and bilateral presentations. *Brain and Language, 53,* 121–140.

Incisa della Rocchetta, A., & Milner, B. (1993). Strategic search and retrieval inhibition: The role of the frontal lobes. *Neuropsychologia, 31,* 503–524.

Incisa della Rocchetta, A. I. (1986). Classification and recall of pictures after unilateral frontal or temporal lobectomy. *Cortex, 22,* 189–211.

Jackson, J. H. (1868). Deficit of intellectual expression (aphasia) with left hemiplegia. *Lancet, 1,* 457.

Jackson, J. H. (1880). On aphasia, with left hemiplegia. *Lancet, 1,* 637–638.

Jackson, J. H. (1915). Hughlings Jackson on aphasia and kindred affections of speech, together with a complete bibliography of his publications on speech and a reprint of some of the more important papers. *Brain, 38,* 1–190.

Jeannerod, M., Arbib, M. A., Rizzolatti, G., & Sakata, H. (1995). Grasping objects: The cortical mechanisms of visuomotor transformation. *Trends in Neurosciences, 18,* 314–320.

Jerison, H. J. (1977). The theory of encephalization. *Annals of the New York Academy of Sciences, 299,* 146–160.

Jorge, R. E., Robinson, R. G., Starkstein, S. E., Arndt, S. V., Forrester, A. W., & Geisler, F. H. (1993). Secondary mania following traumatic brain injury. *American Journal of Psychiatry, 150*(6), 916–921.

Just, M. A., Carpenter, P. A., Keller, T. A., Eddy, W. F., & Thulborn, K. R. (1996). Brain activation modulated by sentence comprehension. *Science, 274,* 114–116.

Kawashima, R., Yamada, K., Kinomura, S., Yamaguchi, T., Matsui, H., Yoshioka, S., et al. (1993). Regional cerebral blood flow changes of cortical motor areas and prefrontal areas in humans related to ipsilateral and contralateral hand movement. *Brain Research, 623*(1), 33–40.

Kim, S. G., Ashe, J., Hendrich, K., & Ellerman, J. M. (1993). Functional magnetic imaging of motor cortex: Hemispheric asymmetry and handedness. *Science, 261,* 615–616.

Klein, D., Milner, B., Zatorre, R. J., Meyer, E., & Evans, A. C. (1995). The neural substrates underlying word generation: A bilingual functional-imaging study. *Archives of Neurology, 92,* 2899–2903.

Kohler, E., Keysers, C., Umilta, M. A., Fogassi, L., Gallese, V., & Rizzolatti, G. (2002). Hearing sounds, understanding actions: Action representation in mirror neurons. *Science, 297,* 846–848.

Kolb, B., & Whishaw, I. Q. (1985). *Fundamentals of human neuropsychology* (2nd ed.). San Francisco: Freeman.

Kushch, A., Gross, G. K., Jallad, B., Lubs, H., Rabin, M., & Feldman, E. (1993). Temporal lobe surface area measurements on MRI in normal and dyslexic readers. *Neuropsychologia, 31,* 811–821.

Lashley, K. S., & Clark, D. (1946). The cytoarchitecture of the cerebral cortex of *Ateles:* A critical examination of architectonic studies. *Journal of Comparative Neurology, 85,* 223–305.

Lecours, A. R., & Lhermitte, F. (1970). *L'Aphasie.* Paris: Flammarion.

Le May, M., & Kido, D. K. (1978). Asymmetries of the cerebral hemispheres on computed tomograms. *Journal of Computer Assisted Tomography, 2,* 471–476.

Leipmann, H., & Mass, O. (1907). Fall von linksseitiger agraphie und apraxie bei techtsseitiger lahmung. *Journal für Psychologie und Neurologie, 10,* 214–227.

Lewin, J., Friedman, L., Wu, D., Miller, D. A., Thompson, L. A., Klein, S. K., et al. (1996). Cortical localization of human sustained attention: Detection with functional MR using a visual vigilance paradigm. *Journal of Computer Assisted Tomography, 20,* 695–701.

Marie, P. (1906). La troisieme circumvolution frontale gauche ne joue aucun role special dans la fonction du langage. *Semaine Médicale, 26,* 241–247.

Masdeu, J. C., Schoene, W. C., & Funkenstein, H. (1978). Aphasia following infarction of the left supplementary motor area: A clinicopathologic study. *Neurology, 28,* 1220–1223.

Matelli, M., Luppino, G., & Rizzolatti, G. (1985). Patterns of cytochrome oxidase activity in the frontal agranular cortex of the macaque monkey. *Behavioural Brain Research, 18,* 125–136.

McCarthy, G., Blamire, A. M., Rothman, D. L., Gruetter, R., & Shulman, R. G. (1993). Echo-planar magnetic resonance imaging studies of frontal cortex activation during word generation in humans. *Proceedings of the National Academy of Sciences of the United States of America, 90,* 4952–4956.

Metter, E. J. (1991). Brain–behavior relationships in aphasia studied by positron emission tomography. *Annals of the New York Academy of Science, 620,* 153–164.

Miller, B. L., Chang, L., Mena, I., Boone, K., & Lesser, I. M. (1993). Progressive right frontotemporal degeneration: Clinical, neuropsychological and SPECT characteristics. *Dementia, 4,* 204–213.

Milner, A. D., & Goodale, M. A. (1995). *The visual brain in action.* New York: Oxford University Press.

Milner, B. (1995). Aspects of human frontal lobe function. *Advances in Neurology, 66,* 67–81.

Milner, B., & Petrides, M. (1984). Behavioral effects of frontal-lobe lesions in man. *Journal of Neuroscience, 7,* 403–407.

Mohr, J. P., Pessin, M. S., Finkelstein, S., Funkenstein, H. H., Duncan, G. W., & Davis, K. R. (1978). Broca aphasia: Pathologic and clinical. *Neurology, 28,* 311–324.

Molnar-Szakacs, I., Iacoboni, M., Koski, L., & Mazziotta, J. C. (2005). Functional segregation within pars opercularis of the inferior frontal gyrus: Evidence from fMRI studies of imitation and action observation. *Cerebral Cortex, 1,* 986–994.

Monrad-Krohn, G. H. (1947). Dysprosody or alteration in "melody of language." *Brain, 70,* 405–415.

Moutier, F. (1908). *L'Aphasie de Broca* [Broca's aphasia]. Paris: Steinheil.

Nielsen, J. M. (1946). *Agnosia, apraxia, aphasia: Their value in cerebral localization.* New York: Hoeber.

Ojemann, G., & Mateer, C. (1979). Human language cortex: Localization of memory, syntax, and sequential motor–phoneme identification systems. *Science, 205,* 1401–1403.

Owen, A. M., Evans, A. C., & Petrides, M. (1996). Evidence for a two-stage model of spatial working memory processing within the lateral frontal cortex: A positron emission tomography study. *Cerebral Cortex, 6,* 31–38.

Pardo, J. V., Fox, P. T., & Raichle, M. E. (1991). Localization of a human system for sustained attention by positron emission tomography. *Nature, 34*(9), 61–64.

Pardo, J. V., Pardo, P. T., & Raichle, M. E. (1993). Neural correlates of self-induced dysphoria. *American Journal of Psychiatry, 150*(5), 713–719.

Pascual-Leone, A., Catala, M. D., & Pascual-Leone, P. A. (1996). Lateralized effect of rapid-rate transcranial magnetic stimulation of the prefrontal cortex on mood. *Neurology, 46,* 499–502.

Paulesu, E., Frith, C. D., & Frackowiak, R. S. (1993).

The neural correlates of the verbal component of working memory. *Nature, 362,* 342–345.

Passingham, R. E. (1993). *The frontal lobes and voluntary action.* New York: Oxford University Press.

Paus, T., Petrides, M., Evans, A., & Meyer, E. (1993). Role of the human anterior cingulate cortex in the control of oculomotor, manual, and speech responses: A positron emission tomography study. *Neurophysiology, 70,* 453–469.

Paus, T., Tomaiuolo, F., Otaki, N., MacDonald, D., Petrides, M., Atlas, J., et al. (1996). Human cingulate and paracingulate sulci: Pattern, variability, asymmetry, and probabilistic map. *Cerebral Cortex, 6*(2), 207–214.

Penfield, W., & Roberts, L. (1959). *Speech and brain mechanisms.* Princeton, NJ: Princeton University Press.

Petersen, S. E., Fox, P. T., Posner, M. I., Mintun, M., & Raichle, M. E. (1988). Positron emission tomographic studies of the cortical anatomy of single-word processing. *Nature, 331,* 585–589.

Petrides, M. (1994). Frontal lobes and working memory: Evidence from investigations of the effects of cortical excisions in nonhuman primates. In F. Boller & J. Grafman (Eds.), *Handbook of neuropsychology* (Vol. 9, pp. 59–82). Amsterdam: Elsevier.

Petrides, M., Alivisatos, B., Meyer, E., & Evans, A. C. (1993). Functional activation of the human frontal cortex during the performance of verbal working memory tasks. *Proceedings of the National Academy of Sciences of the United States of America, 90,* 878–882.

Picard, N., & Strick, P. L. (1996). Motor areas of the medial wall: A review of their location and functional activation. *Cerebral Cortex, 6,* 342–353.

Poppel, D. (1996). Some remaining questions about studying phonological processing with PET: Response to Demonet, Fiez, Paulesu, Petersen, and Zatorre. *Brain and Language, 55,* 380–385.

Posner, M. I., & Dehaene, S. (1994). Attentional networks. *Trends in Neurosciences, 2,* 75–79.

Preuss, T. M., Caceres, M., Oldham, M. C., & Geschwind, D. H. (2004). Human brain evolution: Insights from microarrays. *Nature Reviews: Genetics, 5,* 850–860.

Raichle, M. E., Fiez, J. A., Videen, T. O., MacLeod, A. M., Pardo, J. V., Fox, P. T., et al. (1994). Practice-related changes in human brain functional anatomy during nonmotor learning. *Cerebral Cortex, 4,* 8–26.

Rajkowska, G., & Goldman-Rakic, P. (1995). Cytoarchitectonic definition of prefrontal areas in the normal human cortex: II. Variability in locations of areas 9 and 46 and relationship to the Talaraich coordinate system. *Cerebral Cortex, 5,* 323–337.

Rizzolatti, G., & Arbib, M. (1998). Language within our grasp. *Trends in Neurosciences, 2,* 188–194.

Rizzolatti, G., Fadiga, L., Matelli, M., Bettinardi, V., Paulesu, E., Perani, D., et al. (1996a). Localization of grasp representations in humans by PET: 1. Observa-tion versus execution. *Experimental Brain Research, 111,* 246–252.

Rizzolatti, G., Fadiga, L., Gallese, V., & Fogassi, L. (1996b). Premotor cortex and the recognition of motor actions. *Cognitive Brain Research, 3,* 131–141.

Rizzolatti, G., Matelli, M., & Pavesi, G. (1983). Deficits in attention and movement following the removal of postarcuate (area 6) and preacruate (area 8) cortex in macaque monkeys. *Brain, 106,* 655–673.

Robinson, R. G., Kubos, K. L., Starr, L. B., Rao, K., & Price, T. R. (1984). Mood disorders in stroke patients: Importance of location of lesion. *Brain, 107*(1), 81–93.

Roland, P. E. (1984). Metabolic measurements of the working frontal cortex in man. *Trends in Neurosciences, 7*(11), 430–435.

Ross, E. D. (1981). The aprosodias: Functional–anatomic organization of the affective components of language in the right hemisphere. *Archives of Neurology, 38,* 561–569.

Ross, E. D., & Mesulam, M.-M. (1979). Dominant language functions of the right hemisphere?: Prosody and emotional gesturing. *Archives of Neurology, 36,* 144–148.

Sackeim, H. A., Greenberg, M. S., Weiman, A. L., Gur, R. C., Hungerbuhler, J. P., & Geschwind, N. (1982). Hemispheric asymmetry in the expression of positive and negative emotions. Neurologic evidence. *Archives of Neurology, 39,* 210–218.

Scheibel, A. B., Paul, L. A., Fried, I., Forsythe, A. B., Tomiyasu, U., Wechsler, A., et al. (1985). Dendritic organization of the anterior speech area. *Experimental Neurology, 87,* 109–117.

Shimazu, H., Maier, M. A., Cerri, G., Kirkwood, P. A., & Lemon, R. N. (2004). Macaque ventral premotor cortex exerts powerful facilitation of motor cortex outputs to upper limb motoneurons. *Journal of Neuroscience, 24*(5), 1200–1211.

Simonds, R. J., & Scheibel, A. B. (1989). The postnatal development of the motor speech area: A preliminary study. *Brain and Language, 37,* 42–58.

Smith, E. E., Jonides, J., & Koeppe, R. A. (1996). Dissociating verbal and spatial working memory using PET. *Cerebral Cortex, 6,* 11–20.

Snowden, J. S., Neary, D., Mann, D. M., Goulding, P. J., & Testa, H. J. (1992). Progressive language disorder due to lobar atrophy. *Annals of Neurology, 31,* 174–183.

Starkstein, S. E., Bryer, J. B., Berthier, M. L., Cohen, B., Price, T. R., & Robinson, R. G. (1991). Depression after stroke: The importance of cerebral hemisphere asymmetries. *Journal of Neuropsychiatry and Clinical Neurosciences, 3*(3), 276–285.

Starkstein, S. E., Federoff, J. P., Price, T. R., Leiguarda, R. C., & Robinson, R. G. (1994). Neuropsychological and neuroradiologic correlates of emotional prosody comprehension. *Neurology, 44*(3, Pt. 1), 515–522.

Starkstein, S. E., Pearlson, G. D., Boston, J., & Robinson, R. G. (1987). Mania after brain injury: A controlled study of causative factors. *Archives of Neurology, 44*(10), 1069–1073.

Starkstein, S. E., Robinson, R. G., Honig, M. A., Parikh, R. M., Joselyn, J., & Price, T. R. (1989). Mood changes after right-hemisphere lesions. *British Journal of Psychiatry, 155,* 79–85.

Stelmach, G. E. (1996). Motor learning: Toward understanding acquired representations. In J. R. Bloedel, T. J. Ebner, & S. P. Wise (Eds.), *The acquisition of motor behavior in vertebrates* (pp. 391–408). Cambridge, MA: MIT Press.

Stepniewska, I., Preuss, T. M., & Kaas, J. H. (1993). Architectonics, somatotopic organization, and ipsilateral cortical connections of the primary motor area (M1) of owl monkey. *Journal of Comparative Neurology, 330,* 238–271.

Sun, T., Patoine, C., Abu-Khalil, A., Visvader, J., Sum, E., Cherry, T. J., et al. (2005). Early asymmetry of gene transcription in embryonic human left and right cerebral cortex. *Science, 308,* 1794–1798.

Tanji, J., & Shima, K. (1994). Role for supplementary motor area cells in planning several movements ahead. *Nature, 371,* 413–416.

Thurnam, J. (1866, April). On the weight of the brain and the circumstances affecting it. *Journal of Mental Science.*

Tilney, F. (1927). The brain of prehistoric man. *Archives of Neurology and Psychiatry, 17,* 723–769.

Tonkonogy, J., & Goodglass, H. (1981). Language function, foot of the third frontal gyrus, and Rolandic operculum. *Archives of Neurology, 38,* 486–490.

Umilta, M. A., Kohler, E., Gallese, V., Fogassi, L., Fadiga, L., Keysers, C., et al. (2001). "I know what you are doing": A neurophysiological study. *Neuron, 31,* 155–165.

Ungerleider, L. G., & Mishkin, M. (1982). Two cortical visual systems. In D. J. Ingle, M. A. Goodale, & R. J. W. Mansfield (Eds.), *Analysis of visual behavior* (pp. 549–586). Cambridge, MA: MIT Press.

Vendrell, P., Junque, C., Pujol, J., Jurado, M. A., Molet, J., & Grafman, J. (1995). The role of prefrontal regions in the Stroop task. *Neuropsychologia, 33,* 341–352.

Verfaellie, M., & Heilman, K. M. (1987). Response preparation and response inhibition after lesions of the medial frontal lobe. *Archives of Neurology, 44,* 1265–1271.

von Bonin, G. (1962). Anatomical asymmetries of the cerebral hemispheres. In V. B. Mountcastle (Ed.), *Interhemispheric relations and cerebral dominance* (pp. 1–6). Baltimore: Johns Hopkins University Press.

Wada, J. A., Clarke, R., & Hamm, A. (1975). Cerebral hemispheric asymmetry in humans. *Archives of Neurology, 32,* 239–246.

Warburton, E., Wise, R. J., Price, C. J., Weiller, C., Hadar, U., Ramsay, S., et al. (1996). Noun and verb retrieval by normal subjects: Studies with PET. *Brain, 119,* 159–179.

Weintraub, S., Mesulam, M.-M., & Kramer, L. (1981). Disturbances in prosody: A right-hemisphere contribution to language. *Archives of Neurology, 38*(12), 742–744.

Wernicke, C. (1874). *Der aphasische symtomenkomplex* [Symptoms of aphasia]. Breslau: Max Cohn & Weigert.

Wilson, F. A., Scalaidhe, S. P., & Goldman-Rakic, P. S. (1993). Dissociation of object and spatial processing domains in primate prefrontal cortex. *Science, 260,* 1955–1958.

Winner, E., Brownell, H., Happe, F., Blum, A., & Pincus, D. (1998). Distinguishing lies from jokes: Theory of mind deficits and discourse interpretation in right hemisphere brain-damaged patients. *Brain and Language, 62*(1), 89–106.

Witelson, S. F. (1977). Anatomic asymmetry in the temporal lobes: Its documentation, phylogenesis and relationship to functional asymmetry. *Annals of the New York Academy of Sciences, 299,* 328–354.

Witelson, S. F. (1992). Cognitive neuroanatomy: A new era [Editorial comment]. *Neurology, 42,* 709–713.

Yamadori, A., Osumi, Y., Masuhara, S., & Okubo, M. (1977). Preservation of singing in Broca's aphasia. *Journal of Neurology, Neurosurgery, and Psychiatry, 40*(3), 221–224.

Zangwill, O. (1975). Excision of Broca's area without persistent aphasia. In K. J. Zulch, O. Creutzfeldt, & G. C. Galbraith (Eds.), *Cerebral localization* (pp. 258–263). New York: Springer-Verlag.

Zatorre, R. J., Evans, A. C., & Meyer, E. (1994). Neural mechanisms underlying melodic perception and memory for pitch. *Journal of Neuroscience, 14,* 1908–1919.

Zatorre, R. J., Meyer, E., Gjedde, A., & Evans, A. C. (1996). PET studies of phonetic processing of speech: Review, replication, and reanalysis. *Cerebral Cortex, 6*(1), 21–30.

# CHAPTER 7

# Gross Morphology and Architectonics

*Danielle Andrea Carlin*

The study of cortical architecture has enjoyed a rich history throughout the 19th and 20th centuries. Although the notion of skull structure connoting function has now been replaced by more modern theories, Franz Gall's work in the late 18th and early 19th century can be considered the start of what has become two centuries of effort aimed at organizing and delineating the cellular and molecular architecture of the brain. Since Gall's time, more sophisticated means of characterizing cortical structure and function have evolved, with modalities such as cytoarchitectonics, functional brain mapping, and computational, molecular, and chemical architectonics. Most of these means of organization have arisen both in conjunction with and as a result of technological innovation. And like maps of the world created by various sensory modalities, we may now lay these separate cortical maps atop one another, with hope of providing for ourselves an even more complex and multifaceted understanding of the cortex, and in particular, the frontal lobes. In this chapter, I address how these maps can be used to elucidate frontal lobe structure and morphology. Beginning with a brief overview of frontal lobe morphology, I then move forward to development, cytoarchitecture, and molecular and neuroarchitectonics of the frontal lobes.

## GROSS MORPHOLOGY

It is surprisingly difficult to subdivide the frontal lobes by gross anatomical landmarks. The frontal lobes comprise the anterior (Joseph, 1996) half of the cerebral cortex and are separated from the parietal cortex by the central sulcus, and from the temporal lobes by the lateral sulcus. The precentral sulcus lies anterior to the central sulcus, dividing motor cortex in the precentral gyrus from prefrontal cortex. Anterior to the precentral sulcus run three horizontal gyri, superior, middle and inferior, which grossly divide the prefrontal cortex. The inferior frontal gyrus extends anteriorly and inferiorly and is divided by both the anterior and ascending limbs of the lateral sulcus into three sections: the pars opercularis posteriorly, the pars orbitalis anteriorly, and the pars triangularis between the two (Duvernoy & Bourgouin, 1999; Nolte & Sundsten, 2002; Stuss & Benson, 1986). These three regions are known collectively as the frontal operculum.

As viewed from a medial perspective, the frontal lobes are bordered inferiorly by the lateral fissure and posteriorly by the central sulcus (or rather, by picturing an imaginary line dropped downward from the central sulcus to the corpus callosum) (Duvernoy & Bourgouin, 1999; Stuss & Benson, 1986). The most conspicuous landmark on the medial frontal surface is the anterior cingulate gyrus, which arises from the lateral recess of the callosal sulcus and circles around the corpus callosum in a C-shaped configuration (Figure 7.1). Rostral to the posterior cingulate sulcus rests the paracentral lobule, and anterior to the paracentral lobule, the medial surface of the superior frontal gyrus (Duvernoy & Bourgouin, 1999). It should be mentioned here, however,

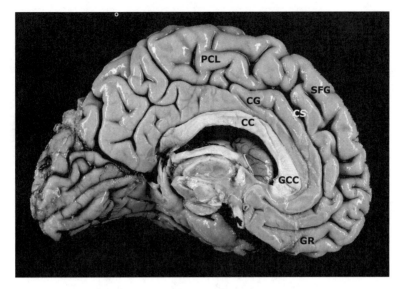

FIGURE 7.1. Frontal lobe from a medial perspective. Note the conspicuous cingulate gyrus. CC, corpus callosum; CG, cingulate gyrus; CS, cingulate sulcus; GCC, genu of the corpus callosum; GR, gyrus rectus; PCL, paracentral lobule.

that sulcal patterns on the medial surface of the frontal lobes, in particular, show notable individual variation (Vogt, Nimchinsky, Vogt, & Hof, 1995).

Finally, when viewed inferiorly, removal of the temporal poles reveals the insula at the posterior border of the frontal lobes. The olfactory bulbs are evident within the olfactory sulcus, and medial to the olfactory sulcus is the gyrus rectus (Duvernoy & Bourgouin, 1999).

## DEVELOPMENT

The cerebral cortex originates from the most rostral segment of the developing brain, the telencephalon. The specific part of the early telencephalon that will grow into the cerebral cortex is the suprastriatal telencephalic vesicle (Parent & Carpenter, 1996). Three concentric zones make up the early suprastriatal telencephalon, with formation of the third and final zone occurring by approximately 16–18 weeks of gestation (Chan, Lorke, Tiu, & Yew, 2002). These zones include the germinal matrix, which surrounds the lateral ventricle and is the site of primitive neuroblast generation, the intermediate zone (destined to become white matter), and the cortical plate, fated to be future neocortex.

Formation of the cortical plate of the telencephalon is a complex process, dependent upon the generation of cells within the germinal zone (GZ; also referred to as the ventricular zone [VZ]) and their subsequent migration outward along radial glia to form the eventual lamina of the cortical plate. This migration occurs between 8 and 18 weeks of gestation (Chan et al., 2002; Levitt, 2003).

The first step in laminar formation of the cerebral cortex is the formation of the preplate, through the early migration of postmitotic cells toward the pial surface (Figure 7.2) (Honda, Tabata, & Nakajima, 2003; Meyer, De Rouvroit, Goffinet, & Wahle, 2003). Radial migration occurs in one of at least two ways. The earliest developing neurons of the VZ, forming the preplate, intermediate zone, and deepest layers of the cortex, use somal translocation as a means of migration (Nadarajah, Brunstrom, Grutzendler, Wong, & Pearlman, 2001; Super, Martinez, Del Rio, & Soriano, 1998). Later developing neuroblasts, originating in the VZ and ventral telencephalon, locomote along radial glia (although some future interneurons appear to use a form of tangential migration, which is addressed below) (Marin & Rubenstein, 2003; Nadarajah et al., 2001; Super et al., 1998). Some have questioned, however, whether radial glia are appro-

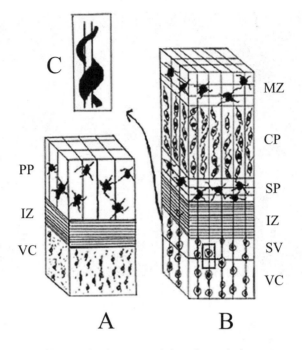

FIGURE 7.2. Cortical lamination during development of the telencephalon. (A) Pioneer neurons form the early PP. These early neurons reach their destination from the VZ, independent of radial glial cells, and instead using somal translocation. (B) Neuroblasts migrate along radial glia, forming a CP and splitting the PP into two regions, the SP and the MZ. The CP lies between the two. The MZ of the neocortex will become layer I, and the CP layers II–VI of the cortex. The SP becomes layer VIb, which will disappear in the adults of most species. (C) Example of a neuron locomoting along a radial glia process. CP, cortical plate; IZ, intermediate zone; MZ, marginal zone; PP, preplate; SP, subplate; SV, subventricular zone; VC, ventricular zone.

priately named, as they may in fact be neuronal precursors themselves (Parnavelas & Nadarajah, 2001). Creation of the cortical plate by these neuroblasts splits the original preplate into two layers, the marginal zone and the subplate. The marginal zone of the neocortex will eventually develop into layer I of the cortex, and the cortical plate into layers II–VI. The subplate will become layer VIb, which disappears in the adults of most species (Reep, 2000; Super et al., 1998; Super & Uylings, 2001). Molecular signaling cascades and inhibitory proteins direct this process (Honda et al., 2003). Site and order of neuroblast generation, rather than location of migration, is predictive of the future fate of neural differentiation. Neuroblasts destined to become pyramidal neurons are generated in the GZ of the dorsal telencephalon. In contrast, most, if not all, neuroblasts destined to become interneurons are generated within the ventral telencephalon (Kriegstein & Noctor, 2004). Laminar formation within the cortical plate

(layers II–VI) occurs as an inside-out process, with the oldest cells forming the deepest layers of cortex first, and the newest cells forming progressively more superficial layers (Marin & Rubenstein, 2003; Super & Uylings, 2001).

In addition to the two modes of radial migration that establish the general cytoarchitectural structure of the forebrain, a significant number of cortical γ-aminobutyric acid (GABA) interneurons are generated through tangential migration of neuroblasts from the ganglionic eminences to the cerebral cortex (Marin & Rubenstein, 2003). These neurons use a wide variety of movements to reach their destinations, which include following developing axons, and in fact sometimes responding to the same molecular signals that guide growing axons (Marin & Rubenstein, 2003; Tessier-Lavigne & Goodman, 1996; Wonders & Anderson, 2005). Some of these tangentially migrating interneurons switch to radial migration upon reaching the cortex (Marin & Rubenstein, 2003). Unlike some of the radical laminar changes seen with disruption to the normal process of radial migration (see lissencephaly, below), more subtle alterations in cortical activity and physiology may occur when there is a disruption to tangential migration (Marin & Rubenstein, 2003; Powell et al., 2003; Powell, Mars, & Levitt, 2001). Researchers have documented these multiple means of early neural migration using elegant genetic models in both rodents and humans, which add to our knowledge of the tremendous diversity of neuronal subpopulations (Letinic & Rakic, 2001; Powell et al., 2001, 2003).

After migrating to their destination site, neuroblasts differentiate into specific classes of neurons, dependent upon the order in which they were generated, rather than by their final position within the cortex (Marin & Ruben-

stein, 2003). Unlike the more subtle morphological changes that may occur with disruption of tangential migration, disturbance of the radial migratory process can have consequences that are seen on the gross anatomical level. An example is lissencephaly (LIS), in which only four of the six neocortical layers form (Ferrer, Alcantara, & Marti, 1993; Miller, 1999). In the X-linked form (XLIS) of this disorder, these laminar derangements are most severe in the frontal lobes and result in an effacement of the normal sulcal and gyral pattern, producing instead a smooth, agyric, cortical surface (Figure 7.3) (Golden, 2001).

The developing zones of the telencephalon remain grossly smooth until approximately the 10th to 12th weeks of gestation, after which sulci and gyri begin to form (Chi, Dooling, & Gilles, 1977). Sulci develop in a phylogeneti-

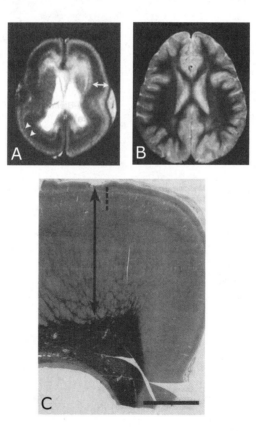

FIGURE 7.3. (A) MRI showing grade 1, X-linked lissencephaly, with a smooth (lacking the normal gyral pattern) and thickened cortex (double arrow). (B) For comparison, MRI of normal cortex, with a normal gyral pattern and cortical width. (C) A coronal section through the frontal cortex of the patient with XLIS depicted in (A). The double arrow demarcates the cortical mantle, which is abnormally thickened. As a comparison, the dashed line indicates the normal thickness of cortex. From Ross et al. (1997). Copyright 1997 by Oxford University Press. Adapted by permission.

cally congruent pattern. The lateral sulcus and callosal sulcus form in the 14th week, the cingulate sulcus in the 18th week, and the central sulcus in the 20th week of gestation (Chi et al., 1977). The frontal lobes continue to form, with emergence of the precentral sulcus at gestational week 24, and the superior and inferior frontal sulci by weeks 25 and 28, respectively, of gestation (Chi et al., 1977).

Neuroimaging and morphometric studies of the frontal lobes indicate that the prefrontal regions, in particular, myelinate late compared to other brain regions, with myelination beginning postnatally and continuing through adolescence (Fuster, 2002; Pfefferbaum et al., 1994; Sowell et al., 2002). Structural imaging of myelination within the cerebral hemisphere shows frontal lobe myelination beginning at 8–12 months of age (Levitt, 2003; Paus et al., 2001), with progressive increases in white matter volume until early (Fuster, 2002; Klingberg, Vaidya, Gabrieli, Moseley, & Hedehus, 1999) and, perhaps in some cases, middle adulthood (Bartzokis et al., 2001). This progressive myelination through adulthood is strongly tied to multiple cognitive, behavioral, and motor developmental milestones acquired by developing children and young adults (Casey, Giedd, & Thomas, 2000; Nagy, Westerberg, & Klingberg, 2004).

In addition to white matter changes, volume of prefrontal gray matter increases dramatically after birth, reaching a maximum between approximately 4 and 12 years of age (Fuster, 2002; Giedd, 2004; Gogtay et al., 2004). Using a series of magnetic resonance images in developing children, Gogtay and colleagues (2004) showed that prepubertal cortical gray matter density increases in a phylogenetically consistent, posterior to anterior progression (i.e. primary sensorimotor regions mature earlier than phylogenetically newer association areas). This pattern can be seen in the frontal lobes, with maturation of the primary motor cortex occurring earliest, with subsequent spread (anteriorly) to the prefrontal cortex. This back to front pattern of maturation in the frontal lobes occurs with the exception of the frontal pole, which matures at approximately the same age as the primary motor cortex (Gogtay et al., 2004).

Although density of cortical gray matter increases in postnatal, prepubertal development, and adult neurogenesis in the hippocampus and olfactory bulb has been confirmed in numerous studies (Kornack & Rakic, 2001;

Taupin, 2005), the question of adult neurogenesis in the cerebral cortex is ardently debated (Altman, 1962; Alvarez-Buylla, Garcia-Verdugo, & Tramontin, 2001; Gould, Vail, Wagers, & Gross, 2001; Koketsu, Mikami, Miyamoto, & Hisatsune, 2003; Kornack & Rakic, 2001; Rakic, 2002; Taupin, 2005). The traditional view of adult neocortical neurogenesis is one of primary stability, with neurogenesis and synapse formation concluded by the end of neocortical development (Bourgeois, Goldman-Rakic, & Rakic, 1994; Brand & Rakic, 1984; Koketsu et al., 2003). Recent studies have challenged this view with evidence that neurons are generated throughout life in primate prefrontal, inferior temporal, and posterior parietal cortex (Figure 7.4) (Gould, Reeves, Graziano, & Gross, 1999; Gould et al., 2001). Animal studies also suggest that neocortical neurogenesis in adulthood remains a possibility (Takemura, 2005), and use of endogenous neural precursors has induced neurogenesis in the neocortex (Arlotta, Magavi, & Macklis, 2003). The role that adult neurogenesis (either innate or induced) will play in the future of neuroscience and the possible treatment of neurological disease processes remains to be seen.

## CYTOARCHITECTURE

The absence of straightforward anatomical and functional margins of the cerebral cortex has paved the way for multiple approaches to its subdivision. Mesulam (2000) organized these approaches into two general groups, one based on structural (architectonic) features of the cortex and the other on functional features. The second type of approach is described in other chapters throughout this book. The structural approach can be split into two spheres, one based on describing the pattern of neuronal organization (cytoarchitecture), and the other on the pattern of molecular expression (molecular neuroarchitecture).

Neurons found within the frontal lobes can be classified into pyramidal, granular, and fusiform types. A fourth identified type, present only in great apes and humans, have been called "spindle cells," or, to reduce confusion with other cells by the same name, "Von Economo neurons" (VENs) (Allman, Watson, Tetreault, & Hakeem, 2005), as tribute to the author who most extensively described them (von Economo & Koskinas, 1925). *Pyramidal*

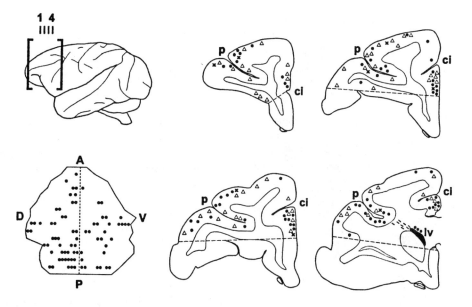

FIGURE 7.4. Bromodeoxyuridine (BrdU) labeling of proliferating cells in the PFC of adult macaques. Immunohistochemistry markers for mature neurons (NeuN, neuronal nuclei) and astrocytes (GFAP, glial fibrillary acidic protein) were used to differentiate proliferating neurons. (A) A lateral view of the anterior cingulate sulcus and principal sulcus. The highlighted area shows sections 1–4 of the coronal slices shown in (B). (B) Coronal sections through the region highlighted in (A). Triangles represent BrdU-labeled neurons staining for NeuN. "X's" represent BrdU-labeled neurons staining for GFAP. Dots represent BrdU-labeled neurons not staining for either NeuN or GFAP. (C) A map of a coronal section from the principal sulcus region, lain flat. Dots represent BrdU-labeled neurons. A, anterior; V, ventral; D, dorsal; P, posterior; p, principal sulcus; ci, cingulate sulcus; lv, lateral ventricle. From Gould, Reeves, Graziano, and Gross (1999b). Copyright 1999 by the American Association for the Advancement of Science. Adapted by permission.

neurons have an apical dendrite, multiple basal dendrites, and an axon emerging from the base of the cells. *Granular* neurons, interneurons with dark-staining nuclei, often act as inhibitors of pyramidal cells. They in turn can be classified into subtypes based on their pattern of dendritic branching (e.g., bitufted neurons) and their density of dendrites (e.g., smooth vs. spinous). Bitufted neurons themselves include two subgroups: chandelier cells, which connect with pyramidal neuron axons, and double bouquet cells, which connect with pyramidal cell dendrites (Miller, 1999; Parent & Carpenter, 1996). *Fusiform* neurons exist mainly in the deepest layer of cortex and have dendrites extending outwards from each pole of the cell. Lower dendrites extend out within the same layer, whereas upper dendrites reach toward more superficial laminae (Parent & Carpenter, 1996). VENs are elongated, bipolar, and spindle-shaped, and can be distinguished from pyramidal cells by their single basal dendrite (Figure 7.5). They are found specifically in

layer Vb of the frontoinsular and anterior cingulate regions of the cortex (von Economo & Koskinas, 1925). This histology is the basis for distinguishing between the six layers of cerebral cortex (Figure 7.6).

The history of 20th-century frontal lobe cytoarchitectonics is almost as interesting, if not more interesting, than the complex conclusions the field has reached during the 21st century. In 1884, Meynert recognized that the cortex was heterogeneous, and suggested that neocortex could be distinguished histologically from underlying mesencephalon (Ffytche & Catani, 2005). In 1905, Campbell, a 19th-century pathologist and clinician, created detailed descriptions of cortical structure and potential functional subdivisions that are now eerily similar to 21st-century conceptions of functional and structural subdivisions (Ffytche & Catani, 2005).

Campbell's work was followed closely by that of his laboratory mate Brodmann (1909), whose cytoarchitectural maps of both human

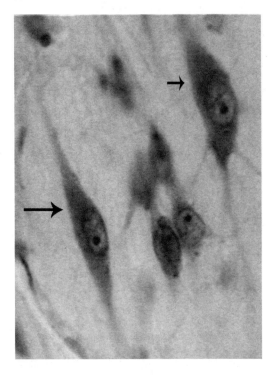

FIGURE 7.5. Nissl stain of a VEN (large arrow) on the left and comparable pyramidal neuron on the right (small arrow; as taken from layer Vb in area 24b of the ACC). Note the elongated, spindle shape of the VEN and presence of a single basal dendrite.

(Brodmann, 1905, 1909; Walker, 1940). Walker attempted to reconcile some of these differences in the monkey literature by using a numbering system in the macaque more closely related to Brodmann's original human map. Walker did not, however, directly compare monkey and human PFC, leading again to inconsistencies (Petrides & Pandya, 1994, 1999). Petrides and Pandya (1994, 1999, 2002) attempted to resolve some of these differences by redefining area 47/12, and likewise, area 9/46 (in addition to area 9 and area 46), both of which correspond to equivalent areas in monkey and human cortex.

In their study detailing orbital and medial prefrontal cortex (OMPFC), Ongur, Ferry, and Price (2003) also compared the OMPFC of macaques and humans, distinguishing 23 separate architectonic areas within human OMPFC that paralleled the OMPFC of the macaque, and which could be used to compare experimental

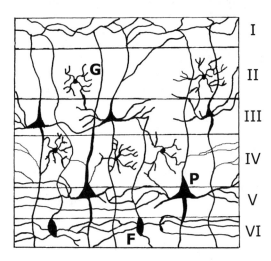

FIGURE 7.6. (I) Molecular or plexiform layer containing dendrites extending from deeper layers of the cortex, and axons traveling to or from connections within the layer. (II) External granular layer, consisting of closely packed granular cells and a few small pyramidal cells. (III) External pyramidal layer, consisting of two sublayers of pyramidal neurons. A few granule cells are found in this layer. (IV) Internal granular layer, consisting mainly of closely packed granular cells and a few pyramidal cells. (V) Internal pyramidal layer containing a mix of medium and large pyramidal cells, in addition to a few granule cells. (VI) Polymorphic or fusiform layer with a range of cells types, but most prominently, fusiform cells. P, pyramidal cell; G, granular cell; F, fusiform cell.

and macaque cortex are highly referenced today (Ffytche & Catani, 2005). Brodmann's work was critiqued frequently by subsequent cartographers, who argued that many of Brodmann's areas did not correspond between monkey and human (Amunts & Zilles, 2001). Brodmann himself, in his original 1909 text, mentioned with forthrightness that his use of labels across species had not been consistent, and that he felt this to be particularly true within the prefrontal cortex (PFC) (Petrides & Pandya, 2002).

There have been numerous efforts throughout the 20th century to reconcile these discrepancies. Walker (1940) investigated the architectonic organization of PFC in macaque monkeys, and found that though some of Brodmann's areas corresponded between monkey and human (e.g., area 10), other areas did not correspond (e.g., area 12 in Walker's map of the macaque corresponded to area 47 in Brodmann's human brain, and areas 45 and 46 were missing from Brodmann's monkey map) data from monkey and human PFC. Interestingly, they noted that the granular cortex at the frontal pole, corresponding to Brodmann's areas 10 and 11, had undergone the most significant expansion between human and macaque.

Nevertheless, perhaps more because they are accessible, organized, and easier to understand than many of the subsequent maps that have been developed, Brodmann's designations have remained widely applied in neuroscience. According to Brodmann's scheme, the frontal lobe includes areas 4, 6, 8–11, and 43–47 along the lateral surface, areas 6, 8–12, 24, 25, 32, and 33 along the medial surface, and areas 10, 11–13, 25, and 47 along the inferior surface (Brodmann, 1909; Stuss & Benson, 1986).

Brodmann's organization of the cortex was followed by von Economo and Koskinas (1925), who divided the cortex into five basic histological types, with each type defined by the relative percentages of the six histological layers within it. von Economo described three of these five types in the frontal lobes, including agranular motor, frontal granular and transitional cortex. Motor and premotor regions of the frontal lobes (BA 4 and 6) are made up of heterotypical frontal agranular cortex, distinguished by a relative paucity of granular layers

II and IV. In contrast, the more anterior PFC is largely made up of granular homotypical cortex, distinguished by a prominence of granular layers II and IV, and correspondingly less prominent pyramidal cell layers (von Economo & Koskinas, 1925; Stuss & Benson, 1986). In von Economo's maps, transitional cortex lies between the agranular motor and frontal granular regions, with a corresponding gradient of increasing granularization and decreasing pyramidalization (Figure 7.7) (von Economo & Koskinas, 1925; Stuss & Benson, 1986).

Various modifications to these maps of human and macaque monkey cortex followed Brodmann and von Economo, including but not limited to von Bonin and Bailey (1947), Beck (1949), and Sarkissov, Filimonoff, Konowa, Preobrascherskaja, and Kekvew (1955) (Figure 7.8). Additional modifications have been made in an attempt to match equivalent structural areas of the frontal cortex in the macaque monkey and human brain, with further differentiation of areas 47/12 and 32 (Ongur et al., 2003), as well as to characterize previous discrepancies between cartographers in assignment of human frontal lobe demarcations (Rajkowska & Goldman-Rakic, 1995).

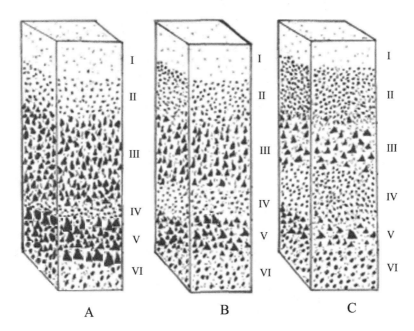

FIGURE 7.7. (A) Agranular, (B) transitional, and (C) granular cortex. Note the increasing granularization and decreasing pyramidalization (layers II/IV and layers III/V, respectively) as one moves from agranular to granular-type cortex.

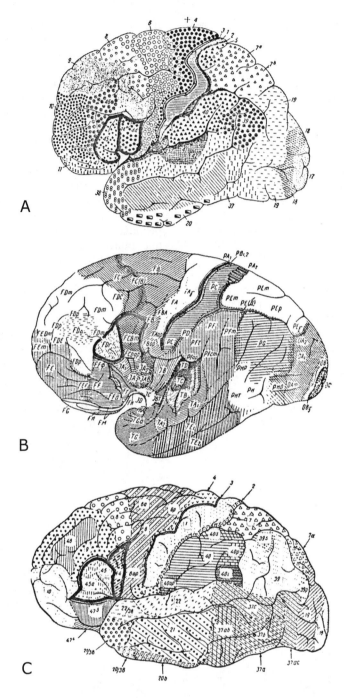

FIGURE 7.8. Twentieth-century cytoarchitectural maps of the human brain, as viewed from a lateral perspective. (A) Brodmann's (1909) areas. (B) Lettered parcellations by von Economo and Koskinas (1925). (C) Sarkissov et al. (1955). Brodmann's areas 44 and 45 are highlighted in all three maps. From Amunts et al. (1999). Copyright 1999 by Williams & Wilkins. Adapted by permission.

A more topographical means of characterizing frontal lobe architecture that uses a combination of cytoarchitectonic, functional, and anatomical approaches, is the subdivision of neocortex into paralimbic, homotypical, and idiotypical subtypes (Filimonoff, 1947; Mesulam, 2000). The transition from paralimbic to homotypical to idiotypical cortex is one of increasing phylogenetic complexity, and is characterized by an increasingly prominent granular layer, more differentiated layers of cortex, and an increasing pattern of myelination (Barbas & Pandya, 1989; Kaufer & Lewis, 1999). The *paralimbic* cortices within the frontal lobes include the orbitofrontal cortex (posterior parts of Brodmann's areas 11–12 and 13), the agranular insula, and the anterior cingulate complex. These areas generally have less well-differentiated layers II and IV and limited differentiation between layer IV and V (Mesulam, 2000). Anterior cingulate cortex (ACC) is agranular and for the most part, has a prominent layer Va. Within the ACC, area 24a has definable layers II and III, and a thinner but still prominent layer Va (Vogt et al., 1995). Area 24b contains the thickest layer Va of the ACC, has a population of large pyramidal neurons, and, like Area 24a, contains VENs. Area 24c also has an obvious layer Va and prominent clumps of pyramidal neurons in layer Vb. Finally, Brodmann's areas 33 and 25 of the ACC show poor differentiation between cortical layers (Vogt et al., 1995).

Primary motor cortex (BA 4) is the only *idiotypical* cortex within the frontal lobes, and because it lacks a well-developed layer IV, is referred to as agranular idiotypical cortex. *Homotypical* cortex makes up the remaining regions of the frontal lobes and can be separated functionally into unimodal (motor) and heteromodal regions (Mesulam, 2000).

## MOLECULAR NEUROARCHITECTONICS

A third means of understanding the structural organization of the frontal lobes is by profiling the molecular expression patterns of distinctive cortical areas. Various neural antigens in cortical and subcortical regions of interest are used to generate monoclonal antibodies (MAb's) (Hinton, Henderson, Blanks, Rudnicka, & Miller, 1988; Reichardt, 1984), which can then be utilized to characterize the neurochemical distribution patterns of particular subpopu-

lations of neurons, including enzymes involved in neuropeptide synthesis, membrane receptors, cytoskeletal proteins, and proteins unique to synaptic endings. Several successful examples of this approach include characterizing specific calcium-binding proteins expressed by separate subclasses of pyramidal neurons, linking of specific proteoglycans to subpopulations of neurons within the frontal lobes, and defining cytoskeletal proteins localized to distinct neuronal subpopulations (Hinton et al., 1988; Reichardt, 1984; Valentino, Winter, & Reichardt, 1985). Normal molecular distribution patterns in the frontal cortex can then be compared with the molecular architecture of diseased frontal cortex, in effort to isolate molecular correlates of neurological disease states.

The OMPFC of the frontal lobe has been mapped in detail using MAb techniques. SMI-32, a monoclonal antibody directed toward a nonphosphorylated neurofilament epitope (cytoskeletal protein), shows immunoreactivity throughout the OMPFC, and most particularly in layers III and V. In the macaque monkey, motor areas of the cingulate are distinguished by a population of layer III/V pyramidal neurons, which stain heavily for SMI-32 (Nimchinsky, Hof, Young, & Morrison, 1996). Ongur and colleagues (2003) noted that this same pattern of SMI-32 activity is seen in a particular region of human area 32 (which they characterized as area 32ac), and hypothesized a correspondence of this area to the cingulate motor areas. Parvalbumin, a calcium-binding protein, is found most prominently in layers V and VI of the OMPFC, and stains a particular type of multipolar neuron that may represent basket cells (Hof, Mufson, & Morrison, 1995; Ongur et al., 2003). Another group of parvalbumin-reactive bipolar neurons is found in layers II and III of the OMPFC, which, in contrast, may represent chandelier-type cells (Kisvarday et al., 1990; Ongur et al., 2003). Acetylcholine (ACh-positive) fibers are found most prominently in the posterior OMPFC but can be seen throughout the remainder of the OMPFC, particularly in cortical layers I and II. ACh-positive neurons are seen most noticeably in layers III and V of the rostral OMPFC (Ongur et al., 2003).

Findings related to MAb and neurotransmitter distribution have also included the characterization of glycine receptors in the apical dendrites of pyramidal neurons in layers II and V of frontal cortex, as well as the distribution pattern of pyramidal and interneuron glutamate receptors within the frontal cortex (Miller, 1999; Naas et al., 1991).

MAb's allow us to examine differences in molecular architecture between normal and diseased cortex. For example, specific proteoglycan Mab's have been implicated in the pathogenesis of Alzheimer's disease (AD) (DeWitt, Silver, Canning, & Perry, 1993; Diaz-Nido, Wandosell, & Avila, 2002; Small et al., 1996; Snow et al., 1988). Proteoglycans are of two main types, chondroitin sulfate (CSPG) and heparin sulfate (HSPG), and play a significant role in patterning neural migration and controlling axon growth during development (Carulli, Laabs, Geller, & Fawcett, 2005). In adult brains, CSPGs are inhibitory both to axon regeneration after neural injury and to plasticity in the central nervous system (Carulli et al., 2005). CSPGs and HSPGs are found in β-amyloid plaques and neurofibrillary tangles of AD, and have been implicated in neurodegenerative process, including the pathogenesis of β-amyloid polymerization in AD (DeWitt et al., 1993; Diaz-Nido et al., 2002; Small et al., 1996; Snow et al., 1988). Recently it has been shown that ADAMTS-1, a chromosome 21–derived metalloproteinase and disintegrin, whose substrates include the proteoglycans aggrecan, versican, and brevican, is overexpressed in the brain tissue of various neurodegenerative disease states, including AD, Pick's disease (PD), and Down's syndrome (DS) (Miguel, Pollak, & Lubec, 2005). This includes a fivefold overexpression of ADAMTS-1 in frontal autopsy specimens of patients with DS, a more than sevenfold overexpression in frontal autopsy specimens of patients with AD, and a more than 10-fold overexpression in frontal autopsy specimens of patients with PD compared to controls. Because proteoglycans are the substrate of ADAMTS-1, overexpression of ADAMTS-1 has been suggested as a mechanism to counteract excess β-amyloid polymerization in the neurodegenerative disease process (Miguel et al., 2005).

MAb studies of calcium-binding proteins in the frontal cortex suggest that neurons expressing calretinin and parvalbumin are resistant to the neurodegeneration of AD (Hof et al., 1991; Hof, Nimchinsky, Celio, Bouras, & Morrison, 1993). Calretinin is immunoreactive to interneurons in all layers of neocortex, but particularly within layers II and III (Hof et al., 1999). A group of pyramidal neurons restricted to the superficial portion of layer V of the ACC (areas 24 and 25 in apes, and 24, 25, and 32 in humans) are also characterized by their expression of calretinin, and are found exclusively in great apes and humans (Hof, Nimchinsky, Perl, & Erwin, 2001). In contrast, calretinin is not expressed by VENs, which are thought to be selectively vulnerable in AD and possibly other neurodegenerative disorders as well (Allman et al., 2005; Hof et al., 2001; Nimchinsky, Vogt, Morrison, & Hof, 1995). Another calcium-binding protein, calbindin, has shown extensive immunoreactivity in the ACC, as well as in a subset of interneurons in PFC layers II, III, V, and VI, and a group of pyramidal neurons in mid/deep layer III (Hof & Morrison, 1991; Nimchinsky, Vogt, Morrison, & Hof, 1997). Interestingly, calbindin-associated interneurons in the superficial layer II are unaffected in AD cases, whereas calbindin-associated pyramidal neurons in layer III and calbindin-associated interneurons in layers V and VI are significantly affected in AD, in direct proportion to the degree of density of neurofibrillary tangle burden (Hof & Morrison, 1991).

The hypothesis that neurodegenerative disease process affects specific neuronal subsets with particular molecular and anatomic characterizations is supported by evidence that AD has a broad impact on calcium-binding protein expression throughout the human cortex (Ichimiya, Emson, Mountjoy, Lawson, & Heizmann, 1988). Recent studies from a transgenic mouse model of AD show a prominent reduction in calbindin expression in the hippocampus (Palop et al., 2003). In addition, there is a strong correlation between the reduction in calbindin expression, defects in the expression of immediate early gene c-fos, and learning/memory deficits. Neuronal depletion of calcium-dependent proteins in the dentate gyrus is tightly linked to AD-related cognitive deficits (Palop et al., 2003).

Populations of frontal cortex neurons that show immunoreactivity to SMI-32 have also been extensively studied in the pathology of AD (Gottron, Turetsky, & Choi, 1995). In the human PFC, SMI-32 reactivity is shown most predominantly in large pyramidal neurons of layers III and V. In the brains of patients with AD compared to controls, there is a dramatic loss of SMI-32 immunoreactive cells. This has been suggested as evidence that decreased or incorrect phosphorylation of these cytoskeletal proteins may occur in the progression of AD

(Hof, Cox, & Morrison, 1990). And like the calbindin studies described earlier, loss of SMI-32-reactive neurons in the brains of patients with AD is highly correlated with increasing neurofibrillary tangle count (Hof et al., 1990).

## CONCLUSIONS

Our conception of frontal lobe architecture has grown remarkably throughout the 19th and 20th centuries with the creation of multiple morphological, cytoarchitectural, molecular, and chemical mapping techniques. When laid atop one another, these maps provide a window into the striking complexity of frontal lobe architecture and offer clues to architectural correlates of neurological disease states. Knowledge of this intricate architecture will only continue to grow, with techniques of microarray profiling within discrete neuronal populations, advanced neuroimaging to detect specific structural correlates of function, neurotransmitter profiling, and assessment of connectivity patterns between adjacent areas of brain. A solid framework of frontal lobe structural anatomy will be crucial in guiding these future directions of frontal lobe research and theory.

## ACKNOWLEDGMENTS

I wish to thank Dr. Eric Huang and Dr. Brandy Matthews for their thoughtful manuscript review and editing, and Dr. William Seeley for discussion of anatomical issues, manuscript review, and providing templates of Figures 7.2 and 7.6.

## REFERENCES

Allman, J. M., Watson, K. K., Tetreault, N. A., & Hakeem, A. Y. (2005). Intuition and autism: A possible role for von Economo neurons. *Trends in Cognitive Science, 9*(8), 367–373.

Altman, J. (1962). Are new neurons formed in the brains of adult mammals? *Science, 135,* 1127–1128.

Alvarez-Buylla, A., Garcia-Verdugo, J. M., & Tramontin, A. D. (2001). A unified hypothesis on the lineage of neural stem cells. *Nature Reviews: Neuroscience, 2*(4), 287–293.

Amunts, K., Schleicher, A., Burgel, U., Mohlberg, H., Uylings, H. B., & Zilles, K. (1999). Broca's region revisited: Cytoarchitecture and intersubject variability. *Journal of Comparative Neurology, 412*(2), 319–341.

Amunts, K., & Zilles, K. (2001). Advances in cyto-

architectonic mapping of the human cerebral cortex. *Neuroimaging Clinics of North America, 11*(2), 151–169, vii.

Arlotta, P., Magavi, S. S., & Macklis, J. D. (2003). Induction of adult neurogenesis: Molecular manipulation of neural precursors in situ. *Annals of the New York Academy of Sciences, 991,* 229–236.

Barbas, H., & Pandya, D. N. (1989). Architecture and intrinsic connections of the prefrontal cortex in the rhesus monkey. *Journal of Comparative Neurology, 286*(3), 353–375.

Bartzokis, G., Beckson, M., Lu, P. H., Nuechterlein, K. H., Edwards, N., & Mintz, J. (2001). Age-related changes in frontal and temporal lobe volumes in men: A magnetic resonance imaging study. *Archives of General Psychiatry, 58*(5), 461–465.

Beck, E. A. (1949). A cytoarchitectural investigation into the boundaries of cortical areas 13 and 14 in the human brain. *Journal of Anatomy, 3,* 147–157.

Bourgeois, J. P., Goldman-Rakic, P. S., & Rakic, P. (1994). Synaptogenesis in the prefrontal cortex of rhesus monkeys. *Cerebral Cortex, 4*(1), 78–96.

Brand, S., & Rakic, P. (1984). Cytodifferentiation and synaptogenesis in the neostriatum of fetal and neonatal rhesus monkeys. *Anatomy and Embryology (Berlin), 169*(1), 21–34.

Brodmann, K. (1905). Beitraege zur histologischen Lokalisation der Grosshirnrinde: III. Mitteilung: Die RIndenfelder der niederen Affen. *Journal of Psychology and Neurology, 4,* 177–206.

Brodmann, K. (1909). *Vergleichende Lokalisationslehre der Grosshirnrinde in ihren Prinzipien dargestallt auf Grun des Zellenbaues.* Leipzig: Barth.

Carulli, D., Laabs, T., Geller, H. M., & Fawcett, J. W. (2005). Chondroitin sulfate proteoglycans in neural development and regeneration. *Current Opinion in Neurobiology, 15*(1), 116–120.

Casey, B. J., Giedd, J. N., & Thomas, K. M. (2000). Structural and functional brain development and its relation to cognitive development. *Biological Psychology, 54*(1–3), 241–257.

Chan, W. Y., Lorke, D. E., Tiu, S. C., & Yew, D. T. (2002). Proliferation and apoptosis in the developing human neocortex. *Anatomical Record, 267*(4), 261–276.

Chi, J. G., Dooling, E. C., & Gilles, F. H. (1977). Gyral development of the human brain. *Annals of Neurology, 1*(1), 86–93.

DeWitt, D. A., Silver, J., Canning, D. R., & Perry, G. (1993). Chondroitin sulfate proteoglycans are associated with the lesions of Alzheimer's disease. *Experimental Neurology, 121*(2), 149–152.

Diaz-Nido, J., Wandosell, F., & Avila, J. (2002). Glycosaminoglycans and beta-amyloid, prion and tau peptides in neurodegenerative diseases. *Peptides, 23*(7), 1323–1332.

Duvernoy, H. M., & Bourgouin, P. (1999). *The human brain: Surface, three-dimensional sectional anatomy with MRI, and blood supply.* Wien: Springer-Verlag.

Ferrer, I., Alcantara, S., & Marti, E. (1993). A four-layered "lissencephalic" cortex induced by prenatal X-irradiation in the rat. *Neuropathology and Applied Neurobiology, 19*(1), 74–81.

Ffytche, D. H., & Catani, M. (2005). Beyond localization: From hodology to function. *Philosophical Transactions of the Royal Society of London, Series B: Biological Sciences, 360,* 767–779.

Filimonoff, I. (1947). A rational subdivision of the cerebral cortex. *Archives of Neurological Psychiatry, 58,* 296–311.

Fuster, J. M. (2002). Frontal lobe and cognitive development. *Journal of Neurocytology, 31*(3–5), 373–385.

Giedd, J. N. (2004). Structural magnetic resonance imaging of the adolescent brain. *Annals of the New York Academy of Sciences, 1021,* 77–85.

Gogtay, N., Giedd, J. N., Lusk, L., Hayashi, K. M., Greenstein, D., Vaituzis, A. C., et al. (2004). Dynamic mapping of human cortical development during childhood through early adulthood. *Proceedings of the National Academy of Sciences of the United States of America, 101*(21), 8174–8179.

Golden, J. A. (2001). Cell migration and cerebral cortical development. *Neuropathology and Applied Neurobiology, 27*(1), 22–28.

Gottron, F., Turetsky, D., & Choi, D. (1995). SMI-32 antibody against non-phosphorylated neurofilaments identifies a subpopulation of cultured cortical neurons hypersensitive to kainate toxicity. *Neuroscience Letters, 194*(1–2), 1–4.

Gould, E., Reeves, A. J., Graziano, M. S., & Gross, C. G. (1999). Neurogenesis in the neocortex of adult primates. *Science, 286,* 548–552.

Gould, E., Vail, N., Wagers, M., & Gross, C. G. (2001). Adult-generated hippocampal and neocortical neurons in macaques have a transient existence. *Proceedings of the National Academy of Sciences of the United States of America, 98*(19), 10910–10917.

Hinton, D. R., Henderson, V. W., Blanks, J. C., Rudnicka, M., & Miller, C. A. (1988). Monoclonal antibodies react with neuronal subpopulations in the human nervous system. *Journal of Comparative Neurology, 267*(3), 398–408.

Hof, P. R., Cox, K., & Morrison, J. H. (1990). Quantitative analysis of a vulnerable subset of pyramidal neurons in Alzheimer's disease: I. Superior frontal and inferior temporal cortex. *Journal of Comparative Neurology, 301*(1), 44–54.

Hof, P. R., Cox, K., Young, W. G., Celio, M. R., Rogers, J., & Morrison, J. H. (1991). Parvalbumin-immunoreactive neurons in the neocortex are resistant to degeneration in Alzheimer's disease. *Journal of Neuropathology and Experimental Neurology, 50*(4), 451–462.

Hof, P. R., Glezer, I. I., Conde, F., Flagg, R. A., Rubin, M. B., Nimchinsky, E. A., et al. (1999). Cellular distribution of the calcium-binding proteins parvalbumin, calbindin, and calretinin in the neocortex of mammals: Phylogenetic and developmental patterns. *Journal of Chemical Neuroanatomy, 16*(2), 77–116.

Hof, P. R., & Morrison, J. H. (1991). Neocortical neuronal subpopulations labeled by a monoclonal antibody to calbindin exhibit differential vulnerability in Alzheimer's disease. *Experimental Neurology, 111*(3), 293–301.

Hof, P. R., Mufson, E. J., & Morrison, J. H. (1995). Human orbitofrontal cortex: Cytoarchitecture and quantitative immunohistochemical parcellation. *Journal of Comparative Neurology, 359*(1), 48–68.

Hof, P. R., Nimchinsky, E. A., Celio, M. R., Bouras, C., & Morrison, J. H. (1993). Calretinin-immunoreactive neocortical interneurons are unaffected in Alzheimer's disease. *Neuroscience Letters, 152*(1–2), 145–148.

Hof, P. R., Nimchinsky, E. A., Perl, D. P., & Erwin, J. M. (2001). An unusual population of pyramidal neurons in the anterior cingulate cortex of hominids contains the calcium-binding protein calretinin. *Neuroscience Letters, 307*(3), 139–142.

Honda, T., Tabata, H., & Nakajima, K. (2003). Cellular and molecular mechanisms of neuronal migration in neocortical development. *Seminars in Cell and Developmental Biology, 14*(3), 169–174.

Ichimiya, Y., Emson, P. C., Mountjoy, C. Q., Lawson, D. E., & Heizmann, C. W. (1988). Loss of calbindin-28K immunoreactive neurons from the cortex in Alzheimer-type dementia. *Brain Research, 475*(1), 156–159.

Joseph, R. (1996). *Neuropsychiatry, neuropsychology, and clinical neuroscience: Emotion, evolution, cognition, language, memory, brain damage, and abnormal behavior.* Baltimore: Williams & Wilkins.

Kaufer, D., & Lewis, D. (1999). Frontal lobe anatomy and cortical Connectivity. In B. Miller & J. Cummings (Eds.), *The human frontal lobes: Functions and disorders* (pp. 27–44). New York, London: Guilford Press.

Kisvarday, Z. F., Gulyas, A., Beroukas, D., North, J. B., Chubb, I. W., & Somogyi, P. (1990). Synapses, axonal and dendritic patterns of GABA-immunoreactive neurons in human cerebral cortex. *Brain, 113*(3), 793–812.

Klingberg, T., Vaidya, C. J., Gabrieli, J. D., Moseley, M. E., & Hedehus, M. (1999). Myelination and organization of the frontal white matter in children: A diffusion tensor MRI study. *NeuroReport, 10*(13), 2817–2821.

Koketsu, D., Mikami, A., Miyamoto, Y., & Hisatsune, T. (2003). Nonrenewal of neurons in the cerebral neocortex of adult macaque monkeys. *Journal of Neuroscience, 23*(3), 937–942.

Kornack, D. R., & Rakic, P. (2001). Cell proliferation without neurogenesis in adult primate neocortex. *Science, 294,* 2127–2130.

Kriegstein, A. R., & Noctor, S. C. (2004). Patterns of neuronal migration in the embryonic cortex. *Trends in Neuroscience, 27*(7), 392–399.

Letinic, K., & Rakic, P. (2001). Telencephalic origin of human thalamic GABAergic neurons. *Nature Neuroscience, 4*(9), 931–936.

Levitt, P. (2003). Structural and functional maturation of the developing primate brain. *Journal of Pediatrics, 143*(Suppl. 4), S35–S45.

Marin, O., & Rubenstein, J. L. (2003). Cell migration in the forebrain. *Annual Review of Neuroscience, 26*, 441–483.

Mesulam, M. M. (2000). *Principles of behavioral and cognitive neurology.* New York: Oxford University Press.

Meyer, G., De Rouvroit, C. L., Goffinet, A. M., & Wahle, P. (2003). Disabled-1 mRNA and protein expression in developing human cortex. *European Journal of Neuroscience, 17*(3), 517–525.

Miguel, R. F., Pollak, A., & Lubec, G. (2005). Metalloproteinase ADAMTS-1 but not ADAMTS-5 is manifold overexpressed in neurodegenerative disorders as Down syndrome, Alzheimer's and Pick's disease. *Brain Research: Molecular Brain Research, 133*(1), 1–5.

Miller, C. A. (1999). Gross morphology and architectonics of the frontal lobes. In B. L. Miller & J. L. Cummings (Eds.), *The human frontal lobes: Functions and disorders* (pp. 71–82). New York: Guilford Press.

Naas, E., Zilles, K., Gnahn, H., Betz, H., Becker, C. M., & Schroder, H. (1991). Glycine receptor immunoreactivity in rat and human cerebral cortex. *Brain Research, 561*(1), 139–146.

Nadarajah, B., Brunstrom, J. E., Grutzendler, J., Wong, R. O., & Pearlman, A. L. (2001). Two modes of radial migration in early development of the cerebral cortex. *Nature Neuroscience, 4*(2), 143–150.

Nagy, Z., Westerberg, H., & Klingberg, T. (2004). Maturation of white matter is associated with the development of cognitive functions during childhood. *Journal of Cognitive Neuroscience, 16*(7), 1227–1233.

Nimchinsky, E. A., Hof, P. R., Young, W. G., & Morrison, J. H. (1996). Neurochemical, morphologic, and laminar characterization of cortical projection neurons in the cingulate motor areas of the macaque monkey. *Journal of Comparative Neurology, 374*(1), 136–160.

Nimchinsky, E. A., Vogt, B. A., Morrison, J. H., & Hof, P. R. (1995). Spindle neurons of the human anterior cingulate cortex. *Journal of Comparative Neurology, 355*(1), 27–37.

Nimchinsky, E. A., Vogt, B. A., Morrison, J. H., & Hof, P. R. (1997). Neurofilament and calcium-binding proteins in the human cingulate cortex. *Journal of Comparative Neurology, 384*(4), 597–620.

Nolte, J., & Sundsten, J. W. (2002). *The human brain: An introduction to its functional anatomy.* St. Louis, MO: Mosby.

Ongur, D., Ferry, A. T., & Price, J. L. (2003). Architectonic subdivision of the human orbital and medial prefrontal cortex. *Journal of Comparative Neurology, 460*(3), 425–449.

Palop, J. J., Jones, B., Kekonius, L., Chin, J., Yu, G. O., Raber, J., et al. (2003). Neuronal depletion of calcium-dependent proteins in the dentate gyrus is tightly linked to Alzheimer's disease-related cognitive deficits. *Proceedings of the National Academy of Sciences of the United States of America, 100*(16), 9572–9577.

Parent, A., & Carpenter, M. B. (1996). *Carpenter's human neuroanatomy.* Baltimore: Williams & Wilkins.

Parnavelas, J. G., & Nadarajah, B. (2001). Radial glial cells: Are they really glia? *Neuron, 31*(6), 881–884.

Paus, T., Collins, D. L., Evans, A. C., Leonard, G., Pike, B., & Zijdenbos, A. (2001). Maturation of white matter in the human brain: A review of magnetic resonance studies. *Brain Research Bulletin, 54*(3), 255–266.

Petrides, M., & Pandya, D. N. (1999). Dorsolateral prefrontal cortex: Comparative cytoarchitectonic analysis in the human and the macaque brain and corticocortical connection patterns. *European Journal of Neuroscience, 11*(3), 1011–1036.

Petrides, M., & Pandya, D. N. (2002). Comparative cytoarchitectonic analysis of the human and the macaque ventrolateral prefrontal cortex and corticocortical connection patterns in the monkey. *European Journal of Neuroscience, 16*(2), 291–310.

Petrides, M. P., & Pandya, D. N. (1994). Comparative cytoarchitectonic analysis of the human and macaque frontal cortex. In J. G. F. Boller (Ed.), *Handbook of neuropsychology* (Vol. 9, pp. 17–58). Amsterdam: Elsevier Science.

Pfefferbaum, A., Mathalon, D. H., Sullivan, E. V., Rawles, J. M., Zipursky, R. B., & Lim, K. O. (1994). A quantitative magnetic resonance imaging study of changes in brain morphology from infancy to late adulthood. *Archives of Neurology, 51*(9), 874–887.

Powell, E. M., Campbell, D. B., Stanewood, G. D., Davis, C., Noebels, J. L., & Levitt, P. (2003). Genetic disruption of cortical interneuron development causes region- and GABA cell type-specific deficits, epilepsy, and behavioral dysfunction. *Journal of Neuroscience, 23*(2), 622–631.

Powell, E. M., Mars, W. M., & Levitt, P. (2001). Hepatocyte growth factor/scatter factor is a motogen for interneurons migrating from the ventral to dorsal telencephalon. *Neuron, 30*(1), 79–89.

Rajkowska, G., & Goldman-Rakic, P. S. (1995). Cytoarchitectonic definition of prefrontal areas in the normal human cortex: I. Remapping of areas 9 and 46 using quantitative criteria. *Cerebral Cortex, 5*(4), 307–322.

Rakic, P. (2002). Neurogenesis in adult primate neocortex: An evaluation of the evidence. *Nature Reviews: Neuroscience, 3*(1), 65–71.

Reep, R. L. (2000). Cortical layer VII and persistent subplate cells in mammalian brains. *Brain Behavior and Evolution, 56*(4), 212–234.

Reichardt, L. F. (1984). Immunological approaches to the nervous system. *Science, 225*, 1294–1299.

Ross, M. E., Allen, K. M., Srivastava, A. K., Featherstone, T., Gleeson, J. G., Hirsch, B., et al.

(1997). Linkage and physical mapping of X-linked lissencephaly/SBH (XLIS): A gene causing neuronal migration defects in human brain. *Human Molecular Genetics, 6*(4), 555–562.

Sarkissov, S. A., Filimonoff, I. W., Konowa, F. P., Preobrascherskaja, I. S., & Kekvew, L. D. (1955). *Atlas of the cytoarchitectonics of the human cerebral cortex.* Moscow: Medgiz.

Small, D. H., Williamson, T., Reed, G., Clarris, H., Beyreuther, K., Masters, C. L., et al. (1996). The role of heparan sulfate proteoglycans in the pathogenesis of Alzheimer's disease. *Annals of the New York Academy Sciences, 777,* 316–321.

Snow, A. D., Mar, H., Nochlin, D., Kimata, K., Kato, M., Suzuki, S., et al. (1988). The presence of heparan sulfate proteoglycans in the neuritic plaques and congophilic angiopathy in Alzheimer's disease. *American Journal of Pathology, 133*(3), 456–463.

Sowell, E. R., Thompson, P. M., Rex, D., Kornsand, D., Tessner, T. D., Jernigan, T. L., et al. (2002). Mapping sulcal pattern asymmetry and local cortical surface gray matter distribution *in vivo*: Maturation in perisylvian cortices. *Cerebral Cortex, 12*(1), 17–26.

Stuss, D. T., & Benson, D. F. (1986). *The frontal lobes.* New York: Raven.

Super, H., Martinez, A., Del Rio, J. A., & Soriano, E. (1998). Involvement of distinct pioneer neurons in the formation of layer-specific connections in the hippocampus. *Journal of Neuroscience, 18*(12), 4616–4626.

Super, H., & Uylings, H. B. (2001). The early differenti-ation of the neocortex: A hypothesis on neocortical evolution. *Cerebral Cortex, 11*(12), 1101–1109.

Takemura, N. U. (2005). Evidence for neurogenesis within the white matter beneath the temporal neocortex of the adult rat brain. *Neuroscience, 134*(1), 121–132.

Taupin, P. (2005). Adult neurogenesis in the mammalian central nervous system: Functionality and potential clinical interest. *Medical Science Monitor, 11*(7), RA247–RA252.

Tessier-Lavigne, M., & Goodman, C. S. (1996). The molecular biology of axon guidance. *Science, 274,* 1123–1133.

Valentino, K. L., Winter, J., & Reichardt, L. F. (1985). Applications of monoclonal antibodies to neuroscience research. *Annual Review of Neuroscience, 8,* 199–232.

Vogt, B. A., Nimchinsky, E. A., Vogt, L. J., & Hof, P. R. (1995). Human cingulate cortex: Surface features, flat maps, and cytoarchitecture. *Journal of Comparative Neurology, 359*(3), 490–506.

von Bonin, G., & Bailey, P. (1947). *The neocortex of Macaca mulatta.* Urbana: University of Illinois Press.

von Economo, C., & Koskinas, G. N. (1925). *Die Cytoarchitektonik der Hirnrinde Des Erwachsenen Menschen.* Wien: Springer-Verlag.

Walker, E. (1940). A cytoarchitectural study of the prefrontal area of the macaque monkey. *Journal of Comparative Neurology, 73,* 59–86.

Wonders, C., & Anderson, S. A. (2005). Cortical interneurons and their origins. *Neuroscientist, 11*(3), 199–205.

# CHAPTER 8

# Evolution of the Frontal Lobes

*Harry J. Jerison*

There is a fossil record of the evolution of the brain that provides insight into the evolution of human frontal neocortex. The evidence is from brain-like endocasts, molded by the cranial cavities of fossil animals. One can use this evidence to understand the evolution of the brain by comparing these endocasts to brains in living species and relating the external morphology of the brain revealed in endocasts to its internal anatomy and functions.

In mammals and birds, endocasts are superficially like freshly prepared brains. They are in a real sense "fossil brains" (Edinger, 1929). The endocast of the Neandertal[1] on the left in Figure 8.1 is a plaster cast prepared from a cleaned skull. On the right, the Taung australopithecine skull shows some of an endocast made by natural processes after death (see also Figure 8.5, p. 112), when sand and other debris replaced soft tissue and became packed tightly in the cranial cavity, and the skull and its contents hardened and fossilized. Mammalian endocasts, whether natural or cast from a cleaned skull, can be treated as if they were brains with dura intact. Direct information from an endocast is on the size and shape of the brain, but by analogy to living brains, the fossils can also tell us about the capacity of brains to process information. In this chapter I review what we know about the evolution of the frontal lobes, emphasizing fossil endocasts and interpreting them as if they were living fresh brains of similar size and shape.

The frontal lobes form an elaborate information-processing system anterior to the cerebral central sulcus. Within the frontal lobes

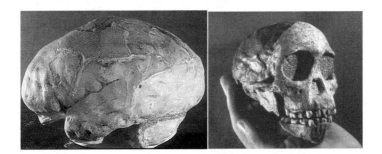

FIGURE 8.1. Left: Endocast of the 40,000-year-old La Chapelle-aux-Saints *Homo neanderthalensis;* length = 18 cm, volume = 1,620 ml (Boule & Anthony, 1911). Right: Skull and natural endocast of the 2.6 million-year-old Taung child, *Australopithecus africanus.* The hand holding the skull is that of Professor Phillip Tobias of the University of Witwatersrand, South Africa, to suggest scale; endocast volume is about 410 ml.

are localized projections for motor control of body, limbs, and eye movements; executive functions in the prefrontal cortex; autonomic and emotion-control in the orbital area; and a lateralized Broca's area for language functions, usually in the left hemisphere. An important limitation on the evolutionary analysis of neural structure and function is that localization in the frontal lobes and elsewhere in the brain is not purely genetic. Frontal lobes in human adults, like much of the rest of the brain, are "programmed" by epigenetic factors, that is, by the way a brain develops in its prenatal, as well as postnatal, environment. This may be most obvious in the human species for the neural control of language, which is determined to a significant extent by learning and socialization. A second language, for example, may be localized differently in the brain from the language learned in infancy. It should, therefore, be appreciated that although the evolution of the complex systems localized in the frontal lobes involved genetic control, it also involved the environments in which the growth and development of the brain takes place. The nature–nurture issue as it affects our knowledge of the brain is reviewed insightfully by Krubitzer and Kahn (2003).

The evolutionary picture presented here emphasizes the brain's *nature* as determined from fossil endocasts. *Nurture* is represented only by scenarios of selection pressures that may have made some neural adaptations more appropriate than others for changing environments. Important developments in evolutionary analyses, such as the reconstruction of phylogenies ("cladistics") and molecular approaches, are considered only in passing.

Evolutionary change in the frontal lobes may be recorded in endocasts such as those shown in Figure 8.1, and in the other endocasts described in this chapter. Their quantitative analysis depends on inferences from the comparative neuroanatomy of living brains. Although primate endocasts typically show a few cortical fissures, such as the rhinal fissure that separates neocortex from paleocortex, they rarely show a central sulcus. It has been possible to prove that the neocortex as a whole evolved to relatively larger size in mammals in which the rhinal fissure is visible in the endocast (Jerison, 1990), but without an objective way to locate the central sulcus, one cannot measure the size of the frontal lobes with sufficient precision for a quantitative analysis. With the help of com-

parative neuroanatomy, however, fossils can be used for inferences about the evolution of similarities and differences among living species and how these developed over time.

## QUANTITATIVE COMPARATIVE NEUROANATOMY

We have had quantitative data on the frontal lobes of living primates beginning with Brodmann's (1913) work, now significantly extended with modern methods (Falk & Gibson, 2001; Fuster, 1997; Semendeferi, Damasio, Frank, & Van Hoesen, 1997; Semendeferi, Lu, Schenker, & Damasio, 2002). On the basis of thalamic projections from the *nucleus medialis dorsalis*, Uylings and Van Eden (1990) have been able to measure the size of prefrontal cortex in rats, as well as in primates, enabling one to think of the evolution of the frontal lobes as a feature of the evolution of the mammalian brain. Of the fossils, Edinger (1975) has catalogued most of the specimens, and I (Jerison, 1973, 1990) have analyzed many of them quantitatively. Falk (1992), Holloway, Broadfield, and Yuan (2004), Martin (1990), Radinsky (1970, 1974), and Tobias (1971) have published more specialized reviews that feature primate fossil endocasts. Although dated in some ways, Gerhardt von Bonin's (1963) essay is very much worth examining for his insights into the problems of quantification and his conclusions about the evidence.

How should we treat the available quantitative evidence? Size matters. That is the first point. The gross size of the brain provides important information about the brain's function. The reason is that brain size estimates information-processing capacity in mammals, which may be inferred from Figure 8.2.

The graph in Figure 8.2 shows how cortical surface area is related to brain size in living mammals. To two significant figures the correlation is perfect, suggesting an almost deterministic connection. The relationship to processing capacity reflects the efficient packing of neurons in the brain. For example, Powell's group at the University of Cambridge reported that the number of neurons under a given surface area of cortex is very similar in several diverse mammal species (Rockel, Hiorns, & Powell, 1980; cf. Haug, 1987). The number of cortical neurons is thus estimated by the total area of the cortex. [The numbers are quite large, about 10 million neurons per square cen-

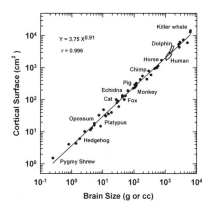

FIGURE 8.2. Cortical surface area as a function of brain size in 50 species of living mammals. Correlation: $r = .996$; regression: $Y = 3.75\ X^{0.91}$. A few of the species are labeled to suggest the diversity of the sample. Human and dolphin data are presented as minimum convex polygons based on 23 points for humans and 13 points for dolphins, and suggest within-species diversity for this measure. Data from Brodmann (1913), Elias and Schwartz (1971), Ridgway (1981), and Ridgway and Brownson (1984). Data from Jerison (1991).

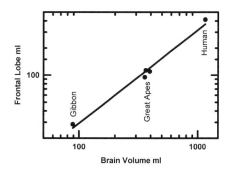

FIGURE 8.3. Frontal lobe volume as a function of the size of the brain in selected hominids. Correlation: $r = .986$; regression: $Y = .26X^{1.03}$. Data from Semendeferi, Damasio, Frank, and Van Hoesen (1997) brain volume.

timeter of neocortical surface. These lead to the order of $2 \times 10^{10}$ for humans and about $10^7$ for a mouse (Braitenberg & Schüz, 1998; Packenberg & Gundersen, 1997).] Since neurons are basic information-processing units in the brain, and brain size estimates their number, brain size also estimates overall information-processing capacity by the cerebral cortex.

Extending this inference to our view of the frontal lobes is straightforward. First, a multivariate analysis of the sizes of major brain structures such as basal ganglia, cerebellum, and neocortex in a large number of mammal species reveals that a general "size factor" accounts for much of the variance in the sizes of the parts of the brain (Jerison, 1997; cf. Stephan, Frahm, & Baron, 1981). In a bivariate analysis, Semendeferi and colleagues (1997) showed that this is specifically true for the volume of the frontal lobes in hominids (humans and apes, including gibbons). The relationship is of special interest for this chapter, and is graphed in Figure 8.3.

That the exponent in Figure 8.3 is slightly greater than 1.0 implies an interesting rule for the size of the frontal lobes in these primates. According to that rule, as hominid brains become larger, the frontal lobes become disproportionately enlarged. One can determine that the gibbon's frontal lobes make up 32% of its brain, whereas in humans it is 37%. Had the great apes not contributed data to Figure 8.3, which enabled one to calculate the regression equation, one might have guessed that the very large human frontal lobes represented a uniquely human advance. The orderliness of the regression in Figure 8.3 makes it easier to think of a genetic instruction based on brain size that is common at least to hominids. The rule is that a brain programmed to reach a particular size will have frontal lobes of the size required by the equation. The rule should be interpreted as showing that there is no uniquely human program for an enlarged frontal lobe. There is, incidentally, no special problem in imagining a genetic program to control an equation; it is conceptually equivalent to a computer program doing the same thing. Other genetic instructions presumably tell the developing nervous systems to "grow" a brain to a particular adult size, and these instructions are probably unique, determining the encephalization of each species.

An independent set of data by Uylings and Van Eden (1990) indicated that a similar rule works for prefrontal cortex as a mammalian feature (Figure 8.4). As I mentioned earlier, they defined prefrontal cortex conventionally as cortex receiving projections from the dorsomedial nucleus of the thalamus and measured its volume in a rat, as well as in primates (for more on this identification, see Jerison, 1997; Preuss, 1995). In other reports on the size of

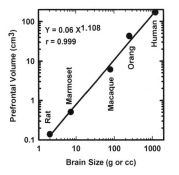

FIGURE 8.4. Prefrontal cortex volume as a function of brain size. Correlation: $r = .999$; regression: $Y = 0.06 X^{1.08}$. Data from Uylings and Van Eden (1990) and Jerison (1997).

the prefrontal area, Semendeferi and her colleagues (2002) verified the Uylings and Van Eden (1990) results for primates, basing their identification on cytoarchitectonic criteria.

As evolutionary evidence, the functional relationships in Figures 8.3 and 8.4 can be treated as representing a trait shared by the species on the graphs. For a cladistic phylogenetic analysis, this implies that the trait was present in their common ancestor. According to present evidence, which I review again in a later section of this chapter, the common ancestor for the hominid species in Figure 8.3 lived at least 30 million years ago, during the Oligocene Epoch. If the analysis in Figure 8.4 is correct, showing that a similar rule works for rats, this would associate prefrontal specialization with the evolution of neocortex. Neocortical localization of motor functions comparable to those localized in the primate frontal lobes is, of course, a trait in all living mammals (Johnson, 1990; cf. Benjamin & Golden, 1985; Kolb & Tees, 1990). At least some of the functions of the frontal lobes, therefore, must have arisen in the common ancestor of all living mammals.

Neocortex was definitely present in mammals 70 million years ago, in late Cretaceous times. A rhinal fissure is visible in endocasts of mammals living then, and from data on living brains, we know that brain dorsal to this fissure is neocortex. The traits that generate the functions of Figures 8.3 and 8.4 were therefore present at least 70 million years ago.

To complete this review of the "age" of the brain, let us recognize that neocortex as a brain structure is present only in mammals, and in no

other living vertebrates. It may, therefore, have appeared in the earliest mammals during the Triassic Period, over 200 million years ago (Jerison, 1990). Regardless of how we date neocortex and the frontal lobes, the brain trait governing the functions in Figures 8.3 and 8.4 is an ancient adaptation. According to this evolutionary evidence, any living mammal can serve as an animal model for studying frontal lobes structure and function.

In a discussion of the evolution of prefrontal neocortex a few years ago, I pointed out that its acknowledged executive functions have to involve connections with much of the rest of the brain (Jerison, 1997). We should, therefore, expect the size of prefrontal neocortex to be related to the size of the parts of the brain that it controls, which add up to pretty much the whole brain. The results graphed in Figure 8.4 should not surprise us. The results in Figure 8.3 are also expected, given the way the brain hangs together. Major structures within the brain tend to be correlated with one another in size as reflected in multivariate analyses that identify a "general size" factor. With respect to the utility of animal models, one may also remember that cognitive control in the prefrontal lobes was first discovered and clearly established by research on baboons (Jacobsen, 1931).

The quantitative neuroanatomical functions presented in Figures 8.2–8.4 are those most useful for interpreting fossil endocasts. Because endocasts do not record the precise position of the central sulcus, it is impossible to analyze of the evolution of the frontal lobes quantitatively with the evidence of fossil endocasts alone. Instead, the fossil evidence reviewed here in Figure 8.1 and Figures 8.5–8.7 provide a gallery of specimens that document all of the past 55 million years of brain evolution in primates, in effect, a qualitative analysis of the available information. All of these primate endocasts display temporal lobes as in living primates and suggest the position of a sylvian fissure. Frontal lobe was almost certainly differentiated in all primates.

In passing, a morphological observation well known to those who have dissected a variety of primate brains: The "orbital" surface of the frontal lobe in primates is the ventral anterior projection of the frontal lobes that covers the orbits of the eyes. It is surprising that some illustrations that present human and other primate brain–skull relations miss this relationship and typically place the whole brain, even including the olfactory bulbs, posterior to the orbits. The shape of the primate brain in the region of the frontal lobes is related to the way the brain grows to its adult shape, molded by pressures related to its fitting into the space available for it. Primate brains are more globular than brains of other mammals, because of the space into which they grow. They squeeze into this space, and the anterior portion of the brain squeezes in above the eyeballs.

## THE FOSSILS

In approaching fossil evidence, including that on the evolution of the frontal lobes as a part of the brain, we rely on the time-honored uniformitarian "hypothesis" developed by geologists in Darwin's time. This is a parsimony principle, which asserts that present structure–function relationships have been true in the past. It continues to be universally accepted (Simpson, 1970).

The first question we ask of fossils is their dating. Because frontal lobes are a feature of the brain of all living primates, and we assume that the relationships in Figures 8.3 and 8.4 are present for all anthropoid primates, the history of anthropoid frontal lobes as brain structures begins no later than the late Eocene, about 40 million years ago, when a common ancestor was alive. The history is at least 15 million years older, dating to the early Eocene, about 55 million years ago, the dating of the oldest known primate endocast sketched below in Figure 8.6. A still older history should be assumed, because the earliest mammals in which there is presently firm evidence of neocortex lived during the Cretaceous Period, and neocortex in all living mammals includes localized motor cortex homologous to primate motor cortex in the frontal lobes. The history of frontal lobes should thus be dated to at least 70 million years ago according to present evidence.

An earlier Cretaceous mammal, *Repenomamus robustus*, which lived about 130 million years ago, has just been discovered (Hu, Meng, Want, & Li, 2005), and an unpublished computed tomography (CT) scan of this animal has been prepared to show the dorsal surface. It appears to show a rhinal fissure, and if this is verified, it would push back the known history of neocortex to that time. As more fossils are analyzed, there is no reason to reject the idea that neocortex appeared with the earliest mammals, more than 200 million years ago.

## HOMININ FOSSILS

There is only speculation that can be added to the obvious information in Figures 8.1 and 8.5 about the appearance of the frontal lobes in the more direct human (hominin) lineage. The Neandertal endocast shown in Figure 8.1, with a volume of 1,600 ml signifies a 1.5 kg brain. (Living human brains fill about 95% of the cranial cavity.) The Neandertal brain was large but well within the range of living brains (Pakkenberg & Voigt, 1960; cf. Allen, Damasio, & Grabowski, 2002). In any event, it is unlikely that this large brain did not have frontal lobes as large as living humans. Perhaps we need a reminder that although brain size gives us useful information, it is not the same as intelligence, and the fossil evidence tells us little about the intelligence of our cousins among the hominins. To the extent that brain size is relevant, however, it tells us that this brain was comparable in size to ours. It is enough to note that frontal lobes are almost certainly not larger on average in living humans than they were in our cousins, the Neandertals.

The 40,000-year-old La Chapelle-aux-Saints Neandertal in Figure 8.1 is unusual among hominid endocasts in a more interesting way, because lateral frontal gyri are visible. There is a fairly clear impression of part of the third frontal convolution of the left hemisphere, which would be in Broca's speech area in a living brain. Figure 8.1 shows that these convolutions had appeared at least 40,000 years ago. One does not know whether the area functioned as a speech area, as in living humans, of course, nor do we know that it did not. From other remains, such as the appearance of the base of the skull, phoneticians have been able to argue about the kinds of sounds that Chapelle-aux-Saints could generate and the vowel structure of those sounds. These may have been more limited than those of living humans, but we know that linguistic communication is possible for us, even with limited capacities for vocalization. From the size of their brains, one would assume that Neandertals could handle the same amount of information as living humans, though we have no way of specifying the information. There is enough evidence not to rule out the evolution of the ca-

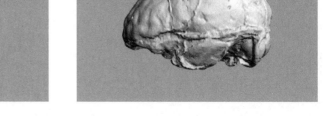

FIGURE 8.5. Endocasts of two australopithecines; the Taung child found in 1923 (right hemisphere) is on the left, and Sts60 (left hemisphere) is on the right. These fossils are presently dated at between 2 and 3 million years ago. Endocast volumes are about 410 ml.

pacity for language at least 40,000 years ago, and it would presumably have been present in the earliest Neandertals, perhaps 200,000 years ago.

The issue has been discussed in more detail by Tattersall (1995; cf. Stringer & McKie, 1996). A similar argument has been presented for the evidence from convolutions in the Taung australopithecine (Falk, 1992; Holloway et al., 2004), which would push the neural history of the speech and language areas back more than 2 million years. Figure 8.5 presents some of the bones of contention, additional views of australopithecine endocasts.

An interesting argument might be developed from the possibility of structural lateralization in the brain. It has been possible to show that in living brains, there is some morphological lateralization, a measurable difference between the left and right hemisphere, mainly in details in the pattern of convolutions. The clearest lateralized difference of superficial features is in the appearance of the sylvian fissure in living humans (Sowell, Thompson, & Toga, 2004). This difference is related to the only well-established functional morphological difference between the right and left hemisphere in the living human brain, that is, in the size and shape of the planum temporale hidden on the temporal lobes within the sylvian fissure and not visible on endocasts. The extent of the planum in the left hemisphere has been related to the adaptation for speech and language. It is usually somewhat expanded in the left hemisphere, and it affects the length and shape of the sylvian fissure, but the sylvian fissure does not leave clear enough impressions on human

endocasts to enable one to measure the possible lateralization in fossils. One would wish it were otherwise—that endocasts might provide clearer clues about the history of this uniquely human trait. Despite the recognized asymmetries in living brains, their utility for functional analysis remains unclear (Walker, 2003). Fossil skulls are not well-enough preserved to be able to argue based on asymmetries.

At this time, on the basis of molecular dating of the evidence of mitochondrial DNA and verified by newly discovered fossils, the human lineage appears to have become differentiated from that of apes about 6 million years ago. We nevertheless share about 99% of our genes with our cousins, the apes (Deacon, 1997), although the remaining 1% is undoubtedly the significant fraction for us, because it presumably includes regulator genes governing the growth of the brain to human size and perhaps the evolution of specialized circuitry related to the language sense (Pinker, 1994).

In the two endocasts of *Australopithecus africanus* shown in Figure 8.5, there is no clear demarcation of the sylvian fissure, but in both there appears to be the impression of the middle cerebral artery. This is typical of the impression of the hominin brain as revealed in an endocast (von Bonin, 1963) and appears on the endocasts of most of them. Other features have been discussed, most curiously the impression of the *Affenspalte* (the human lunate sulcus), which is the anterior border of primary visual cortex. It has been debated that it may be evidence of the first appearance of a language area homologous to Wernicke's area (Falk, 1992). At this time, the issues in that debate remain unresolved, although if a language system can be identified, the origins of language would be pushed back in time even further, to the earliest evidence of australopithecines about 5 million years ago.

## A GALLERY OF FOSSIL PRIMATE ENDOCASTS

Qualitative evidence on the evolution of the frontal lobe can be viewed in fossil endocasts. We have already seen some of it, beginning with Figure 8.1, in which we saw a Neandertal endocast and a partially hidden australopithecine endocast not completely removed from the fossil skull. The latter is of the first australopithecine discovery in 1923, at Taung in South Africa. It is important for our knowledge of brain evolution, because it proved that the brain became enlarged later in human evolution than did other traits defining hominins (Tobias, 1971). The famous and infamous Piltdown fraud of 1913, which married a human cranium to an orangutan jaw, was designed to support evolutionary speculations of a century ago that the "missing link" in human evolution implied a coupling human intelligence, as mirrored in the large brain with an ape's body. The discovery at Taung destroyed that simpleminded paradigm by uncovering a skull with features closer to those of humans than to apes, but with an ape-size brain. It was also obviously much older than the Neandertal or the pithecanthropine (*Homo erectus*) fossils known at the time, and it demonstrated that brain enlargement followed the evolution of other traits within the human lineage. A more complete picture of the Taung endocast and a second australopithecine endocasts were added to the gallery as Figure 8.5.

The fossil record of the primate brain begins much earlier. Fifty-five million years ago, early in the Eocene Epoch, the remains of *Tetonius homunculus*, a prosimian related to living tarsiers, were left to fossilize in what is now the Bighorn Basin in Wyoming. From a sketch of its endocast in Figure 8.6, it is evident that *Tetonius* had visibly identifiable cortical structures that were almost certainly frontal lobes. Figure 8.6 sketches the endocasts of a number of living and fossil prosimian primates, which are discussed more fully in Jerison (1973). Like their living relatives, all of these prosimians had similarly shaped brains, with enough of a suggestion of temporal lobes and a sylvian fis-

sure to identify frontal lobes fairly as having evolved by that time. Two later tarsier-related specimens, *Notharctus* and *Rooneyia*, are also illustrated. The adapids, another lineage of prosimian primates related to living lemurs, are known from middle and late Eocene strata, about 40 or 50 million years ago. The endocasts of two of them, *Smilodectes* from North America and *Adapis* from France, are sketched in Figure 8.6, and also indicate the presence of frontal lobes.

Figure 8.7 completes the gallery with additional lemuroid evidence, the endocast of the fossil *Adapis parisiensis* compared to the brain of the living bushbaby, *Galago senegalensis*. Figure 8.7 shows how good an endocast can be as a representation of the brain. It is, incidentally, also evidence of the evolutionary trend in some mammalian groups, in which brains became more encephalized. The bushbaby is a fairly small primate, weighing about 250 g. Its Eocene relative, the lemuroid, *Adapis parisiensis*, probably weighed about 1,600 g, yet its brain was about the same size as the bushbaby's. This is an example of encephalization within the primate lineage, which was analyzed graphically in Jerison (1973, Figure 16.6). According to that analysis, galagos are somewhat more encephalized than average living mammals, and Eocene lemuroids were less encephalized. As a group, the living prosimians are average among the mammals in encephalization. Living monkeys and apes are about twice as encephalized as the average, and living humans are about five times as encephalized. The specimens in Figure 8.6 are representative of a prosimian assemblage, the adapids on the low end, about half as encephalized as average living mammals, and the tarsier-like fossils very near average for living mammals. On the frontal lobes, lacking data comparable to Figure 8.3 for these animals, one is limited to the qualitative judgment that can be made from the sketches. The basic judgment should be that the frontal lobes expand as the brain as a whole expands. During the 50 million years of evolution represented by the species in Figure 8.6, we expect the frontal lobes to follow the same trend as the brain as a whole. The particular species, the adapids of the Eocene and the living galagos, have very different environmental niches, of course, and brains tend to be appropriate to the niches. Other data, however, support the view that, across a wide range of niches, there was increased encephalization

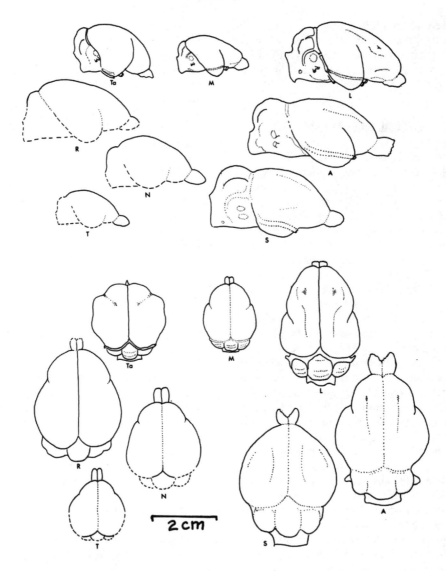

FIGURE 8.6. Three living and five fossil prosimian endocasts in lateral and dorsal view. Ta, *Tarsier spectrum* (living); M, *Microcebus murinus* (mouse lemur, the smallest living primate); L, *Lepilemur ruficaudatus* (living); R, *Rooneyia viejaensis* (Oligocene); A, *Adapis parisiensis* (late Eocene); T, *Tetonius homunculus* (early Eocene); N, *Necrolemur antiquus* (middle Eocene); S, *Smilodectes gracilis* (middle Eocene). From Jerison (1973, Figure 16.3 and Table 16.1).

across the 50-million-year interval. It is likely that the frontal lobes were part of this trend.

The evidence in Figures 8.6 and 8.7 is on prosimian brain evolution. The fossil evidence on anthropoid (monkey, ape, and human) origins available at this writing goes back to the late Eocene, about 40 million years ago, but it begins mainly with postcranial skeleton and teeth, and not the brain. At least one late Eocene or early Oligocene species, however, *Aegyptopithecus xeusis*, is now classified with the anthropoid primates, and its endocast has been described by Radinsky (1967, 1974). Although the animal was probably about the same size as living gibbons, its brain was evidently only half as large. It is not sketched here, because it is little different from the prosimian endocasts sketched in Figure 8.6. Further en-

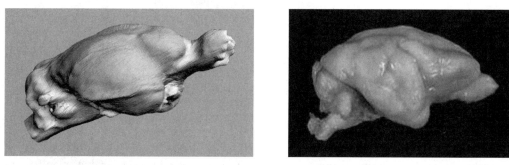

FIGURE 8.7. Endocast of the late Eocene prosimian *Adapis parisiensis* and the brain of the living bushbaby, *Galago crassidens*. Endocast from the Field Museum of Natural History in Chicago (FM 59259); brain from the University of Wisconsin (62–172): brainmuseum.org/.

cephalization in the anthropoid lineage occurred later, probably during the Miocene Epoch, about 15 or 20 million years ago.

The olfactory bulbs and tract in living anthropoid primates, including humans, are reduced in size compared to all other living land mammals. This feature has misled biologists into thinking of reduced olfactory bulbs as evidence of an evolutionary advance. It is a primate trait, shared with cetaceans. Prosimians are intermediate between most mammals and the anthropoids in the reduction of olfactory bulbs, and in this respect, *Aegyptopithecus* was more like prosimians than like anthropoids. The reduction evidently occurred within the anthropoid lineage and appeared later in their evolution. It was completed during the Miocene Epoch, perhaps 15 million years ago. Fossils of that time are similar to living monkeys and apes in the reduction in the olfactory system.

I have speculated on this as related to the evolution of language in primates, specifically in humans, a fairly convoluted just-so story, which may even be correct. I will not repeat the speculations here (see Jerison, 1991, 2001), but one conclusion was that chimpanzee "language" is fundamentally different neurologically from human language. Specifically, I guessed that appropriate brain scans such as positron emission tomography (PET) would reveal different patterns of activation in humans and language-trained chimpanzees. That guess appears to be correct, although the appropriate experiments are, of course, difficult to perform. The results of PET scans on a chimpazee while it worked on a language-like task (pressing one

of an array of response keys representing various linguistic cues) have been reported in a preliminary way (Rilling et al., 1999). Activation in the chimpanzee brain during such work was not lateralized and did not involve regions of the brain homologous to language areas in humans. PET scans in people working on the same task showed unilateral activation in Wernicke's area as expected, whereas both human and chimpanzee scans showed activation in motor cortex and frontal eye fields, as expected for performance involved in gazing at and operating the response keys on the response boxes.

## CONCLUSIONS

The greatest disappointment in preparing this chapter is that, at this writing, there is not enough evidence to permit a quantitative analysis of the evolution of the frontal lobes based on the fossil record. However, from a qualitative perspective, there is no question that frontal lobes as primate brain structures were present in the earliest records of primate brains. Furthermore, from the evidence on living anthropoid brains, in particular, the evidence in Figures 8.3 and 8.4, substantial frontal and prefrontal neocortex were present. The uniformitarian hypothesis leads to the view that frontal lobes were functioning as they do in living primates. Most human functions that have also been studied with appropriate animal models (Fuster, 1997; Rumbaugh & Washburn, 2003) would be present in our ancestors within our lineage. Whether there was specialization for a language sense is impossible to determine.

What are the lessons for neurology from the evolutionary perspective? First, size matters. Brain size is an important variable for evolutionary analysis, and it is worth a closer look in other contexts. The importance of body size in different species has been recognized for some time as a determinant of the success of species in different ecological niches. Brain size, on the other hand, has had a sorrier fate. Its use a century ago in racist and sexist arguments was followed by critical analysis of the errors and bias (Gould, 1981). The evidence, nevertheless, is that size matters in biological systems (Schmidt Nielsen, 1984), including the brain and the frontal lobes. In this chapter, some of the story was told in the graphs showing the interdependence of measures, and how brain size as an independent variable estimates total information-processing capacity. One should be encouraged to take and report these simple measurements routinely, even when they are not required for a particular research protocol. When any animal model is used, it is appropriate routinely to include gross measures on the specimen, such as brain and body weight, sex, and age, and if the study uses modern imaging techniques such as CT or MRI, there are usually computer programs available that can provide measurements from the scans, such as surface area and volumes (cf. Semendeferi et al., 2002).

Second, and perhaps most important for research in neurology, is the suggestion about constraints on the use of animal models. Some human frontal lobe motor functions can be studied in other mammal species, whereas other functions, such as language, may be uniquely human. The organization of motor systems is likely to be similar in many different species, whereas an animal model for language is chancy, even in our nearest relatives, such as chimpanzee or bonobo.

A nuts and bolts conclusion: Given the imprint of cerebral circulation in some endocasts, it would be helpful to be able to correlate that vasculature with localized regions of the brain. Gerhardt von Bonin (1963) discussed such relationships four decades ago, and although the methods of gross anatomy may seem old-fashioned, here is a case in which discoveries remain to be made. It might enable one to do a quantitative analysis on the evolution of the frontal lobes by correlating the location of the central sulcus in living brains with the position of the vasculature, such as the middle cerebral artery in living and fossil species.

A final lesson is recognition of the limits of genetic relationships and the importance of development in a normal environment as determining the structure and function of the adult nervous system. That constraint was not emphasized in this chapter, except by citation of the important review by Krubitzer and Kahn (2003).

## ACKNOWLEDGMENTS

The photograph of the La Chapelle-aux-Saints Neandertal endocast was provided by Dominique Grimaud-Herve (Département de Préhistoire; Muséum national d'Histoire naturelle, Paris). I also thank Jin Meng and Susan K. Bell (American Museum of Natural History, New York), and R. D. Martin and William Turnbull (Field Museum of Natural History, Chicago) for discussion of the fossil materials, and I thank Almut Schüz (Max Planck Institute for Cybernetics in Tuebingen, Germany) and Katerina Semendeferi (University of California at San Diego) for discussion of anatomical issues.

## NOTE ON ORTHOGRAPHY

1. It is conventional in taxonomy to spell genus with an initial capital and species in lowercase, both in italics. The spelling of "Neandertal" adopted here follows modernized German as adopted in 1908, but capitalized, as are German nouns. Taxonomic convention dictates maintaining original spellings, and the spelling of the species *neanderthalensis* is retained, because it was named prior to 1908 with the old spelling.

## REFERENCES

Allen, J. S., Damasio, H., & Grabowski, T. J. (2002). Normal neuroanatomical variation in the human brain. *American Journal of Physical Anthropology, 118*, 341–358.

Benjamin, R. M., & Golden, G. T. (1985). Extent and organization of opossum prefrontal cortex defined by anterograde and retrograde transport methods. *Journal of Comparative Neurology, 238*, 77–91.

Boule, M., & Anthony, R. (1911). L'encéphale de l'homme fossile de La Chapelle-aux-Saints [The brain of the Chapelle-aux-Saints fossil man.]. *L'Anthropologie, 22*, 129–196.

Braitenberg, V., & Schüz, A. (1998). *Anatomy of the*

*cortex: Statistics and geometry* (2nd ed.). New York: Springer-Verlag.

Brodmann, K. (1913). *Neue Forschungsergebnisse der Grosshirnrindenanatomie mit besonderer Beruck-sichtung anthropologischer Fragen* [New contributions on cortical anatomy with separate considerations of anthropological questions]. Transactions of the 85th Assembly of German Naturalists and Physicians in Vienna, pp. 200–240.

Deacon, T. W. (1997). *The symbolic species: The co-evolution of language and the brain.* New York: Norton.

Edinger, T. (1929). *Die fossilen Gehirne* [Fossil brains]. *Advances in Anatomy and Developmental Biology, 28,* 1–249.

Edinger, T. (1975). Paleoneurology 1804–1966: An annotated bibliography. *Advances in Anatomy, Embryology and Cell Biology, 49,* 12–258.

Elias, H., & Schwartz, D. (1971). Cerebro cortical surface areas, volumes, lengths of gyri and their interdependence in mammals, including man. *Zeitschrift für Saugetierkunde, 36,* 147–163.

Falk, D. (1992). *Braindance.* New York: Holt.

Falk, D., & Gibson, K. R. (Eds.). (2001). *Evolutionary anatomy of the primate cerebral cortex.* Cambridge, UK: Cambridge University Press.

Fuster, J. M. (1997). *The prefrontal cortex: Anatomy, physiology, and neuropsychology of the frontal lobe* (3rd ed.). Philadelphia: Lippincott-Raven.

Gould, S. J. (1981). *The mismeasure of man.* New York: Norton.

Haug, H. (1987). Brain sizes, surfaces, and neuronal sizes of the cortex cerebri: A stereological investigation of man and his variability and a comparison with some mammals (primates, whales, marsupials, insectivores, and one elephant). *American Journal of Anatomy, 180,* 126–142.

Holloway, R. L., Broadfield, D. C., & Yuan, M. S. (2004). *The human fossil record: Vol. 3. Brain endocasts, the paleoneurological evidence.* Hoboken, NJ: Wiley.

Hu, Y., Meng, J., Want, Y., & Li, C. (2005). Large Mesozoic mammals fed on young dinosaurs. *Nature (London), 433,* 149–152.

Jacobsen, C. F. (1931). A study of cerebral function in learning: The frontal lobes. *Journal of Comparative Neurology, 52,* 271–340.

Jerison, H. J. (1973). *Evolution of the brain and intelligence.* New York: Academic Press.

Jerison, H. J. (1990). Fossil evidence on the evolution of the neocortex. In E. G. Jones & A. Peters (Eds.), *Cerebral cortex: Vol. 8A. Comparative structure and evolution of cerebral cortex, Part I* (pp. 285 309). New York: Plenum Press.

Jerison, H. J. (1991). *Brain size and the evolution of mind* (59th James Arthur Lecture on the Evolution of the Human Brain). New York: American Museum of Natural History.

Jerison, H. J. (1997). Evolution of prefrontal cortex. In N. A. Krasnegor, R. Lyon, & P. S. Goldman-Rakic (Eds.), *Development of the prefrontal cortex: Evolution, neurobiology, and behavior* (pp. 9–26). Baltimore: Brookes.

Jerison, H. J. (2001). Adaptation and preadaptation in hominid evolution. In P. V. Tobias, M. A. Raath, J. Moggi-Cecchi, & G. A. Doyle (Eds.), *Humanity from African Naissance to coming millennia* (pp. 373–378). Florence, Italy: Firenze University Press; and Johannesburg, South Africa: Witwatersrand University Press.

Johnson, J. I. (1990). Comparative development of somatic sensory cortex. In E. G. Jones & A. Peters (Eds.), *Cerebral cortex: Vol. 8B. Comparative structure and evolution of cerebral cortex, Part II* (pp. 335–449). New York: Plenum Press.

Kolb, B., & Tees, R. C. (Eds.). (1990). *The cerebral cortex of the rat.* Cambridge, MA: MIT Press.

Krubitzer, L., & Kahn, D. M. (2003). Nature versus nurture revisited: An old idea with a new twist. *Progress in Neurobiology, 70,* 33–52.

Martin, R. D. (1990). *Primate origins and evolution: A phylogenetic reconstruction.* London: Chapman & Hall.

Pakkenberg, B., & Gundersen, H. J. G. (1997). Neocortical neuron number in humans: Effect of sex and age. *Journal of Comparative Neurology, 385,* 312–320.

Pakkenberg, H., & Voigt, J. (1964). Brain weights of Danes. *Acta Anatomica, 56,* 297–307.

Pinker, S. (1994). *The language instinct: How the mind creates language.* New York: Morrow.

Radinsky, L. (1974). The fossil evidence of anthropoid brain evolution. *American Journal of Physical Anthropology, 41,* 15–28.

Radinsky, L. B. (1967). The oldest primate endocast. *American Journal of Physical Anthropology, 27,* 385–388.

Radinsky, L. B. (1970). The fossil evidence of prosimian brain evolution. In C. R. Noback & W. Montagna (Eds.), *The primate brain* (pp. 209–224). New York: Appleton.

Ridgway, S. H. (1981). Some brain morphometrics of the bowhead whale. In T. T. Albert (Ed.), *Tissues, structural studies, and other investigations on the biology of endangered whales in the Beaufort Sea* [Final Report to the Bureau of Land Management, U.S. Department of the Interior] (Vol. 2, pp. 837–844). College Park: University of Maryland.

Ridgway, S. H., & Brownson, R. H. (1984). Relative brain sizes and cortical surfaces of odontocetes. *Acta Zoologica Fennica, 172,* 149–152.

Rilling, J. K., Kilts, C., Williams, S., Kelley, J., Beran, M., Giroux, M., et al. (1999). Functional neuroimaging of linguistic processing in chimpanzees. *Society for Neuroscience Abstracts, 25*(2), p. 2170.

Rockel, A. J., Hiorns, R. W., & Powell, T. P. S. (1980). The basic uniformity in structure of the neocortex. *Brain, 103,* 221–244.

Rumbaugh, D. M., & Washburn, D. A. (2003). *Intelligence of apes and other rational beings*. New Haven, CT: Yale University Press

Schmidt Nielsen, K. (1984). *Scaling: Why is animal size so important?* Cambridge, UK: Cambridge University Press.

Semendeferi, K., Damasio, H., Frank, R., & Van Hoesen, G. W. (1997). The evolution of the frontal lobes: A volumetric analysis based on three-dimensional reconstructions of magnetic resonance scans of human and ape brains. *Journal of Human Evolution, 32*, 375–388.

Semendeferi, K., Lu, A., Schenker, N., & Damasio, H. (2002). Humans and great apes share a large frontal cortex. *Nature Neuroscience, 5*, 272–276.

Simpson, G. G. (1970). Uniformitarianism: An inquiry into principle, theory, and method in geohistory and biohistory. In M. K. Hecht & W. C. Steere (Eds.), *Essays in evolution and genetics in honor of Theodosius Dobzhansky* (pp. 43–96). Amsterdam: North Holland.

Sowell, E. R., Thompson, P. M., & Toga, A. W. (2004). Mapping changes in the human cortex throughout the span of life. *Neuroscientist, 10*, 372–392.

Stephan, H., Frahm, H., & Baron, G. (1981). New and revised data on volumes of brain structures in insectivores and primates. *Folia Primatologica, 35*, 1–29.

Stringer, C., & McKie, R. (1996). *African exodus: The origins of modern humanity*. New York: Henry Holt.

Tattersall, I. (1995). *The last Neanderthal*. New York: Macmillan.

Tobias, P. V. ( 1971). *The brain in hominid evolution*. New York: Columbia University Press.

Uylings, H. B., & Van Eden, C. G. (1990). Qualitative and quantitative comparison of the prefrontal cortex in rat and in primates, including humans. *Progress in Brain Research, 85*, 31–62.

von Bonin, G. (1963). *The evolution of the human brain*. Chicago: University of Chicago Press.

Walker, S. F. (2003). Misleading asymmetries of brain structure. *Behavioral and Brain Sciences, 26*, 240–241.

# PART III

## NEUROCHEMISTRY

# CHAPTER 9

# Serotonin and the Frontal Lobes

*Philippe H. Robert*
*Michel Benoit*
*Hervé Caci*

Serotonin, or 5-hydroxytryptamine (5-HT), initially identified in peripheral tissues, was first detected in the mammalian central nervous system 40 years ago. Very rapidly its heterogeneous distribution suggested that this amine could be a cerebral neurotransmitter. It is now clearly established that neurons that synthesize and release 5-HT participate in the control of many central functions, and that alterations of 5-HT-ergic transmission are associated with various neuropsychiatric conditions such as depression, anxiety, impulsivity, and behavioral disorders in dementias. In addition, relations between 5-HT and the dopaminergic system imply that 5-HT is involved in schizophrenic disorders and in complex cognitive-behavioral interactions. It should be noted that frontal dysfunctions have been described in most of these disorders.

This chapter is thus divided into three main sections. The first is devoted to the description of central 5-HT receptors. The second describes relationships between alterations of the serotoninergic system and the neuropsychiatric manifestations usually associated with frontal dysfunction. Finally, the third section deals with potential therapeutic uses of 5-HT receptor ligands.

## SEROTONIN RECEPTOR SUBTYPES

In evolutionary terms, 5-HT is one of the oldest neurotransmitters. 5-HT neurons arise from midbrain nuclei. 5-HT cell bodies are systematically organized in the median and dorsal raphe nuclei. Ascending fibers from the dorsal raphe project preferentially to the cortex and striatal regions, whereas the median raphe projects to the limbic regions (Jacobs & Azmitia, 1992). Cowen (1991) reported that each projecting 5-HT neuron sends over 500,000 terminals to the cerebral cortex. Indeed, the average density of 5-HT innervations in the cortex is greater than that of dopamine (DA) or noradrenaline. Most of the different 5-HT receptor subtypes are located on the postsynaptic targets of 5-HT-ergic neurons. Furthermore, some receptors are located on the soma and dendrites ($5\text{-HT}_{1A}$ somatodendritic autoreceptors) or on the terminals ($5\text{-HT}_{1B}/5\text{-HT}_{1D}$ presynaptic autoreceptors) of 5-HT-ergic neurons (Hamon & Gozlan, 1993). 5-HT receptors with at least 14 members represent one of the most complex families of neurotransmitter receptors.

The general definition of a receptor is now relatively consensual. The three most important criteria are the operational aspect (drug-related characteristics; agonists, antagonists, and ligand-binding affinities), the transductional aspect (receptor–effect coupling events), and the structural aspect (gene and receptor structural sequence). The information provided here is based on the current classification of the International Union of Pharmacology Committee on Receptor Nomenclature and Classification (NC-IUPHAR) (Hoyer et al., 1994) that has been progressively adapted to accommo-

date new information and favors an alignment of nomenclature with the human genome to avoid species differences (Hartig, Hoyer, Humphrey, & Martin, 1996; Hoyer & Martin, 1997). Table 9.1, derived from the nomenclature proposed by the NC-IUPHAR subcommittee on 5-HT receptors (Hoyer, Hannon, & Martin, 2002), summarizes the operational characteristics and main locations of each receptor subtype. It should be noted that, with

**TABLE 9.1. Operational Characteristics and Locations of 5-HT Receptor Subtypes**

| Receptor | Radioligands | Selective agonists | Selective antagonists | Localization |
|---|---|---|---|---|
| 5-HT$_{1A}$ | [$^3$H]8-OH-DPAT<br>[$^3$H]WAY 100635 | 8-OH-DPAT | [$^3$H]WAY 100635 | Limbic system<br>Raphe<br>Prefrontal cortex |
| 5-HT$_{1B}$ | [$^{125}$I]GTI<br>[$^3$H]Sumatriptan | Sumatriptan<br>L694247 | SB 224289<br>SB 236057 | Striatum<br>Frontal cortex |
| 5-HT$_{1D}$ | [$^{125}$I]GTI<br>[$^3$H]Sumatriptan | Sumatriptan | BRL 15572 | Frontal cortex<br>Hippocampus<br>Substantia nigra |
| 5-HT$_{1E}$ | [$^3$H]5-HT | | | Frontal cortex |
| 5-HT$_{1F}$ | [$^3$H]LI 334370<br>[$^{125}$I]LSD | LI 334370 | | Dorsal raphe<br>Striatum<br>Hippocampus |
| 5-HT$_{2A}$ | [$^3$H]Ketanserine<br>[$^{125}$I]DOI | DOI | Ketanserin<br>MDL 100907 | Frontal cortex<br>Claustrum<br>Limbic system |
| 5-HT$_{2B}$ | [$^3$H]5-HT | Methyl-5-HT<br>SB 204 741 | Mesulergine | Mainly peripheral |
| 5-HT$_{2C}$ | [$^3$H]Mesulergine<br>[$^{125}$I]LSD | RO 600175 | Mesulergine | Basal ganglia<br>Limbic system<br>Choroid plexus |
| 5-HT$_3$ | [$^3$H]Zacopride<br>[$^3$H]Tropisetron | SR 57227 | Tropisetron<br>Odansetron | Limbic system |
| 5-HT$_4$ | [$^3$H]GR 113808 | RS 67506<br>GR 113808 | SB204070<br>GR 11 3808 | Frontal cortex |
| 5-HT$_5$ orphan receptor | [$^{125}$I]LSD<br>[$^3$H]5-HT | | | |
| 5-HT$_6$ | [$^{125}$I]LSD<br>[$^3$H]5-HT | | RO 630563<br>SB 271046 | Hippocampus<br>Striatum<br>Nucleus accumbens |
| 5-HT$_7$ | [$^3$H]5-CT<br>[$^3$H]5-HT | | SB 258719<br>SB 269970 | Limbic system |

the exception of the 5-$HT_3$ subtype, all 5-HT receptors are coupled to G proteins (i.e., G-protein-coupled receptors [GPCRs]).

## 5-$HT_1$ Receptors

These were first identified in the course of radioligand-binding studies on brain homogenates with [$^3$H]5-HT (Peroutka & Snyder, 1979), through their high affinity for 5-HT. 5-$HT_{1A}$ receptors were located not only in limbic structures, such as the hippocampus, septum, and amygdala, but also in the frontal cortex (Biegon, Kargman, Snyder, & McEwen, 1986; Dillon, Gross-Isseroff, Israeli, & Biegon, 1991; Radja et al., 1991), striatum, and raphe nuclei. A recent study of human brain areas obtained from autopsied samples (Marazziti et al., 1994) showed that the highest density of 5-$HT_{1A}$ receptors in the human brain, labeled with the selective ligand [$^3$H]8-OH-DPAT, was found in the hippocampus, followed by the prefrontal cortex and striatum. The human 5-$HT_{1A}$ receptor is located on chromosome 5q11.2-q13. Activation of 5-$HT_{1A}$ receptors causes neuronal depolarization. The proposed role of 5-$HT_{1A}$ receptors in modulating anxiety-related behaviors is supported by studies using 5-$HT_{1A}$ receptor knockout mice demonstrating increased anxiety (Heisler et al., 1998; Parks, Robinson, Sibille, Shenk, & Toth, 1998). 5-$HT_{1A}$ receptor agonists, such as buspirone or gepirone, are being developed for the treatment of anxiety and depression (Den Boer, Bosker, & Slaap, 2000). In addition the 5-$HT_{1A}$ receptor antagonist blocker, pindolol, was reported to enhance the therapeutic efficacy of selective serotonin reuptake inhibitors (SSRIs) when coadministered in depressed patients.

The strongest concentration of 5-$HT_{1B}$ receptor-binding sites was found in the basal ganglia, striatum, and frontal cortex. The human 5-$HT_{1B}$ receptor is located on chromosome 6q13. 5-$HT_{1B}$ receptors serve as terminal autoreceptors and may also act as a terminal heteroreceptor controlling the release of other neurotransmitters, such as acetylcholine, glutamate, DA, noradrenaline, and $\gamma$-aminobutyric acid (GABA) (Pauwels, 1997). 5-$HT_{1B}$ receptor agonists have been developed, taking into account the antimigraine properties of sumatripan, a nonselective 5-$HT_{1B/D}$ receptor agonist (Leysen et al., 1996). Finally, little is known about 5-$HT_{1E}$ and 5-$HT_{1F}$ receptors.

## 5-$HT_2$ Receptors

It is now clear that at least three 5-$HT_2$ receptor subtypes exist. 5-$HT_{2A}$ receptors are present in different regions of the cortex (Cook et al., 1994; Hoyer, Pazos, Probst, & Palacios, 1986; Pazos, Cortes, & Palacios, 1985) and the limbic system. They are situated on postsynaptic targets of 5-HT-ergic neurons. The human 5-$HT_{2A}$ receptor is located on chromosome 13q14.2-q21. In an *in vivo* study based on positron-emission tomography (PET) with the ligand F18N-methylspiperone, Wang and colleagues (1995) showed a gradual decay of these receptors with age that was more marked in the frontal cortex than in the occipital cortex. 5-$HT_{2A}$ receptor activation stimulates hormone secretion (Van de Kar et al., 2001). 5-$HT_{2A}$ receptor antagonists such as risperidone, ritanserin, Seroquel, and olanzapine have been indicated for the treatment of schizophrenia and psychotic symptoms.

Human 5-$HT_{2C}$ receptor has been mapped to chromosome Xq24. 5-$HT_{2C}$ receptor activation has been shown to exert a tonic, inhibitory influence on frontocortical DA-ergic and adrenergic transmission (Jorgensen, Knigge, Kjaer, & Warberg, 1999; Millan, Dekeyne, & Gobert, 1998).

## 5-$HT_3$ Receptors

Contrary to the receptors just described, which are all coupled to G proteins, 5-$HT_3$ is an "ion-channel receptor" whose stimulation opens a sodium–potassium channel (Yakel, Shao, & Jackson, 1990). In the central nervous system, it is most abundant in the amygdala, the CA1 pyramidal cell layer in the hippocampus, and entorhinal cortex (Laporte, Kidd, Verge, Gozlan, & Hamon, 1992). Since 5-$HT_3$ receptor activation in the brain leads to DA release and 5-$HT_{2C}$ receptor antagonists produce central effect comparable to those of antipsychotics and anxiolytics, schizophrenia and anxiety were considered as potential indication. However at this time there are no clinical data.

## 5-$HT_{4,6,7}$ Receptors

These receptors are positively coupled to adenylate cyclase. 5-$HT_4$ receptors appear to be present in the frontal cortex (Monferini et al., 1993). The human 5-$HT_4$ receptor is located on chromosome 5q31-33. 5-$HT_4$ receptors appear to modulate neurotransmitter release and enhance synaptic transmission, and they may play a role in memory enhancement. To date, there are no clinical data.

Rat and human 5-HT$_6$ receptors are located in the striatum, amygdala, nucleus accumbens, hippocampus, and cortex. The human 5-HT$_6$ receptor is located on chromosome 1p35-p36. Several studies indicate a potential role for 5-.he HT$_6$ receptor in the control of central cholinergic function (Woolley, Bentley, Sleight, Marsden, & Fone, 2001). Furthermore, several antipsychotic agents (clozapine, Seroquel, olanzapine) and antidepressant (clomipramine, amitryptyline) have high affinity and act as antagonists at 5-HT$_6$ receptors.

5-HT$_7$ receptor is located in the limbic system and thalamocortical regions. The human 5-HT$_7$ receptor is located on chromosome 10q23.3-q24.4. On a clinical point of view atypical antipsychotics such as clozapine and risperidone have high affinity for the 5-HT$_7$ receptor (Roth et al., 1994), and a downregulation of 5-HT$_7$ receptors occurs after chronic antidepressant treatment (Mullins, Gianutsos, & Eison, 1999).

### Serotonin–Dopamine Interactions

There is growing evidence for 5-HT-ergic influences on DA transmission. The majority of studies demonstrated that 5-HT transmission plays an inhibitory role on DA-ergic activity (Kapur & Remington, 1996; Korsgaard, Gerlach, & Christensson, 1985; Sasaki-Adams & Kelley, 2001), but some studies also suggested the opposite view (De Deurwaerdere, Bonhomme, Lucas, Le Moal, & Spampinato, 1996; Hallbus, Magnusson, & Magnusson, 1997; Yoshimoto et al., 1996). These divergences could be partially explained by the variety of subtypes and actions of 5-HT receptors. For example, 5-HT$_{2C}$ agonists inhibit DA-ergic effects (Walsh & Cunningham, 1997), whereas 5-HT$_{1B}$ and 5-HT$_3$ agonists enhance DA release (De Deurwaerdere, Stinus, & Spampinato, 1998).

These interactions are important for frontal lobe function. One of the major DA-ergic pathways is mesocortical, with numerous terminations in prefrontal cortex. Their synapses are regulated by frontal 5-HT$_2$ heteroreceptors activated by 5-HT-ergic neurons projecting from the medial raphe (Ugedo, Grenhoff, & Svensson, 1989). Serotoninergic projections inhibit

also DA-ergic activity in the striatum. The repartition and interaction of DA-ergic and 5-HT-ergic neurons supports the hypothesis of a 5-HT–DA balance, which plays a major role in the regulation of transmission between prefrontal cortex and subcortical structures (Kapur, Zipursky, & Remington, 1999). In fact, it seems possible to enhance DA-ergic activity in prefrontal cortex with 5-HT$_{2A}$ and 5-HT$_{2C}$ inhibitors. The combination of DA D$_2$ and 5-HT$_{2A}$ receptor antagonism may explain the antipsychotic activity of atypical antipsychotics and, in this way, these interactions may have major therapeutic consequences.

## NEUROPSYCHIATRIC MANIFESTATIONS

Many studies have shown a relationship between frontal region dysfunction and clinical behavioral disorders (Mega & Cummings, 1994). At the same time, the role of 5-HT was demonstrated in a wide variety of human and animal disorders (Table 9.2).

Several paradigms have been developed to study *in vivo* the 5-HT function in depression and anxiety, either static (e.g., cerebrospinal fluid [CSF] 5-hydroxyindoleacetic acid [5-HIAA], blood platelet binding) or dynamic. The so-called neuroendocrine challenges consist of measuring the change in a function thought to be under 5-HT-ergic control after administration of some 5-HT agonist. There is compelling evidence that 5-HT neurons regulate the hypothalamus–pituitary–adrenal axis. Thus, the outcome can affect hormonal response adrenocorticotropin hormone ([ACTH], cortisol, prolactin), body temperature, and behavior. There are two types of 5-HT probes: those that increase the 5-HT function (e.g., *d,l*-fenfluramine, tryptophan) and those that act directly on the 5-HT receptors (e.g., metachlorophenylpiperazine (mCPP), 5-HT$_{1A}$ agonists).

### Serotonin Depression and Anxiety

The cerebral 5-HT represents less than 5% of the total 5-HT. Thus, it is not surprising that peripheral measures have been proposed, with the underlying assumption that these measures reflect the central 5-HT-ergic function. For example, specific high-affinity binding sites for [$^3$H]imipramine or [$^3$H]paroxetine have been found in brain and platelet membranes (Paul,

**TABLE 9.2. Behavioral and Affective Disturbances Related to Frontal Lobe and to Serotoninergic System Abnormalities**

| Domains | Symptoms | 5-HT system disturbances[a] |
|---|---|---|
| Emotional disturbances | Depressive mood | + |
| | Anxiety disorders | + |
| Loss of control | Perseveration | + |
| | Compulsion | + |
| | Emotional lability | + |
| | Disinhibition | + |
| | Impulsivity | + |
| Motivational disturbances | Apathy | |
| | Lack of initiative | |
| | Lack of interest | |
| Other disturbances | Aggressiveness | + |
| | Agitation | + |
| | Sleep disorders | + |
| | Eating disorders | + |
| | Pathological gambling | + |

*Note.* Disturbances are divided in three main domains (emotional disturbances, loss of control, and motivational disturbances). An additional category is included (other) for disturbances that are clearly explained by different mechanisms (e.g., pathological gambling could be explained by motivational and control disturbances).
[a]Even if the relation between 5-HT dysfunction and the behavioral disturbances is strong, there is no evidence indicating that the relation is exclusive.

Rehavi, Skolnick, & Goodwin, 1980), and a decreased binding has been reported in patients with depression (Raisman, Sechter, Briley, Zarifian, & Langer, 1981). Patients with panic disorder do not show such a decrease, suggesting a different pathogenesis. Platelets have been also used as a peripheral marker of presynaptic 5-HT function in the brain, and patients with depression have shown a diminished platelet 5-HT uptake (Meltzer, Perline, Tricou, Lowy, & Robertson, 1984). Finally, the platelet membrane has $5\text{-HT}_{2A}$ binding sites. A high density of these $5\text{-HT}_{2A}$ binding sites may be a trait marker for panic disorder (Butler, O'Halloran, & Leonard, 1992).

Asberg, Traskman, and Thoren (1976) were the first to study links between behavioral and biological disturbances. These authors demonstrated the existence of two subgroups of depressed subjects, one with low levels of 5-HIAA in the CSF and the other with normal levels. This bimodal distribution has been confirmed (Brown & Linnolia, 1990; Van Praag, 1982), but clinical characterization of these "low-serotonin" patients with depression has remained unconvincing (Goodwin, Post, Dunner, & Gordon, 1973). The strongest cor-

relation was with a history of attempted suicide (Asberg, Schalling, Taskman-Bendz, & Wagner, 1987), and it is now admitted that low 5-HIAA characterizes a subtype of depression in which violent suicide or aggression is present. One study reported the similarity of the CSF 5-HIAA between patients with panic disorder and age- and sex-matched controls (Eriksson, Westberg, Alling, Thuresson, & Modigh, 1991), tentatively suggesting a different pathogenesis from that of depression. The relative few number of studies on CSF 5-HIAA can be explained by methodological problems that may cast doubt on the reliability of the results. Obviously, CSF 5-HIAA is most related to impulsivity and aggression rather than to any diagnosis based on Axis I *Diagnostic and Statistical Manual of Mental Disorders* (DSM) criteria.

Studies on endocrine responses to agents increasing central serotoninergic activity have the potential advantage of examining the physiological operation of the 5-HT-ergic system. Through their hypothalamic connections, central monoaminergic systems act on the endocrine hypothalamus–pituitary axis. Intravenous tryptophan and oral fenfluramine

(Cowen & Charig, 1986) both increase plasma prolactin levels and have been used to explore the serotoninergic system. Cocaro, Siever, Owen, and Davis (1990) demonstrated a fall in the prolactin response to fenfluramine in 33% of depressed subjects with a history of suicide attempts compared to only 6% of other depressed subjects.

Extending the fenfluramine methodology, Mann and colleagues (1996a) used the PET [$^{18}$F] fluoro-2-deoxyglucose ($^{18}$FDG) method to examine the fenfluramine-induced changes in regional cerebral glucose metabolic rate (rCMR$_{glu}$) as an indicator of changes in regional neuronal activity and therefore in 5-HT responsivity. These authors demonstrated in healthy subjects an increase of rCMR$_{glu}$ in the anterior cingulate and the lateral prefrontal cortex. In contrast, using the same fenfluramine challenge test, patients with depression (Mann et al., 1996b) had no areas of increase in frontal rCMR$_{glu}$. This result provides the first direct *in vivo* evidence of a blunted regional brain response to 5-HT release in patients with depression.

Fenfluramine challenge tends to also support the hypothesis of an increased 5-HT receptor function in panic disorder (Apostolopoulos, Judd, Burrows, & Norman, 1993). The studies using mCPP also favor this hypothesis, although the lack of specificity of this agent is problematic (Kahn, Van Praag, Weltzer, Asnis, & Barr, 1988). The diminution of the mCPP-induced increases in anxiety and prolactin in normal controls by a pretreatment with ritanserin suggests that these responses are mediated through 5-HT$_{2C}$ receptors (Seibyl et al., 1991).

In obsessive–compulsive disorder (OCD), results are inconsistent regarding the behavioral effects of oral versus intravenous administration of mCPP (Charney et al., 1988; Hollander et al., 1992; Pigott et al., 1993). Finally, some results indicate a supersensivity of postsynaptic 5-HT receptors in patients with social phobia (Sheehan, Raj, Trehan, & Knapp, 1993). But the main issue is the effectiveness of serotonin-omimetics such as buspirone, a 5-HT$_{1A}$ agonist, and ondansetron, a 5-HT$_3$ antagonist, on social phobia symptoms.

### Transnosological Approach

As stated earlier with regard to CSF 5-HIAA, it is possible to isolate a cluster of symptoms that cuts across the boundaries of different DSM Axis I and Axis II diagnostic criteria. This is the so-called "transnosological," or dimensional approach, which can be more relevant than the categorical approach to resolve the discrepancies between clinical classifications and biological features. From this point of view, it has been made clear that 5-HT is involved in various behavioral disturbances (Benkelfat, 1993) and one of the most important of these is represented by impulsivity and aggressivity, which are also common in frontal lobe dysfunction.

Impulsivity, taken in the broad sense of a lack of control, is present in all age groups, with a classical intensification in adolescence. For example, impulsive behavior is found in children with attention-deficit/hyperactivity disorder, and in adolescents and adults with personality disorders or affective disorders (Moeller, Barratt, Dougherty, Schmitz, & Swann, 2001). The measurement of impulsivity by means of a questionnaire (Caci, Nadalet, Bayle, Robert, & Boyer, 2003) is well established, although lacking clear transcultural validity (Caci, 2004). Recently, it has been shown that neurobehavioral disinhibition, a construct that encompasses executive cognitive capacity, affect modulation, and behavior control, measured in 16 year-old boys predicts suicide propensity between ages 16 and 19 (Tarter, Kirisci, Reynolds, & Mezzich, 2004). Indeed, suicide attempts are best predicted by both hopelessness and impulsivity in a sample of depressed subjects.

Recently, New and colleagues (2004) replicated previous studies in a much larger sample and found a blunted prolactin response to *d,l*-fenfluramine of male, but not female, patients with personality disorders in relation to impulsive aggression and to suicide attempts. This gender effect has been often reported and is specific to impulsivity and aggression, and independent of the diagnosis of borderline personality disorder (Soloff, Kelly, Strotmeyer, Malone, & Mann, 2003). Furthermore, New and colleagues (2002) reported on a lack of activation in the left anteriomedial orbital cortex in response to mCPP in patients with impulsive aggression, but not in their age- and sex-matched controls. Therefore, the difficulty in modulating aggressive impulsive behavior may be a consequence of the decreased activation of inhibitory regions in response to a 5-HT-ergic stimulus.

Researchers in the field of suicide prevention admit that 5-HT is involved through its inhibitory function on other neuronal systems (Golden, Gilmore, & Carson, 1991), but it remains unclear whether this is a trait or a state feature of suicide attempters (Abbar, Amadeo, & Malafosse, 1992). In a preliminary short-term, longitudinal study of depressed subjects who attempted suicide compared to age- and sex-matched normal controls, we showed that impulsivity acted as a trait marker and hopelessness (i.e., a pervasive pessimism about future), as a state marker that decreased 4 months after the suicide attempt (Caci, Vallier, Robert, & Dossios, 2004).

Postmortem studies of brain 5-HT neurochemistry face strong methodological issues that may explain the discrepancies found in the literature (Aubin-Brunet, Beau, Asso, Robert, & Darcourt, 1996; Mann et al., 1992). Horton (1992) reported on the lack of evidence regarding the altered 5-HIAA levels in cortical areas and the lowered imipramine binding in the cortex in suicide victims. Mann, McBride, and Stanley (1986) described an increase of brain $5HT_2$ receptors in suicides, but the subsequent findings have been contradictory: whether the suicides used violent means or not (Arora & Meltzer, 1989; Lowther, De Paermentier, Crompton, Katona, & Horton, 1994) or whether the act was related to the diagnosis of major depression itself.

Many studies (for a review, see Virkkunen, Roy, & Linnolia, 1990) that have also explored CSF 5-HIAA levels in aggressive patients have indicated a decrease in 5-HIAA in the CSF of impulsively violent criminals, mothers who kill their children and then attempt to commit suicide, impulsive arsonists, compulsive gamblers, and people with antisocial or borderline personality disorders. 5-HT is also involved in the inability to delay actions and to tolerate frustration.

It is interesting to note that the frontal lobe plays an important role in controlling both impulsive behavior (Miller, 1992) and central 5-HT turnover (Linnolia, Virkkunen, & Higley, 1993). Finally, it must be stressed that the 5-HT-ergic system is also involved in pain (Basbaum & Fields, 1984), sleep (Hartmann & Greewald, 1984), alcoholism (Ballanger, Goodwin, & Major, 1979), and eating disorders (Fernstrom, 1985) such as carbohydrate "bingeing" and nocturnal bulimia (Brewerton, Brandt, Lessem, Murphy, & Jimerson, 1990). Taking into account that the serotoninergic system is involved in phenomena as varied as de-

pression and anxiety, behavioral disorders occurring in various disorders, and physiological functions, the Aubin and Jouvent Rating Scale (AJRS) was designed to identify and measure the preceding manifestations, with a particular emphasis on potential relationships between these clinical dimensions and serotoninergic dysfunctions. The AJRS counts 10 items scored from 0 to 6, and has been validated in a sample of subjects over 60 years of age. In her first study, Aubin-Brunet (1993) found four components accounting for 78% of the total variance in a sample of 155 elderly patients with various disorders. The secondary loadings of each item were low, indicating somewhat unidimensional components, namely, loss of control, anxiety and insomnia, and depression and physiological disturbances.

## Cognition and Behavior

Recent functional brain imaging studies have shown the involvement of orbitofrontal cortex and the ventral striatum in the prediction and perception of reward (Berns, McClure, Pagnoni, & Montague, 2001; Breiter, Aharon, Kahneman, Dale, & Shizgal, 2001; O'Doherty, Dayan, Friston, Critchley, & Dolan, 2003). In parallel, neural circuitry in ventral prefrontal cortex has been implicated in cognitive domains such as decision making and reversal learning, which are closely related to complex behavior (Clark, Cools, & Robbins, 2004). Interestingly, there are also psychopharmacological studies in this field. Decision making requires the evaluation of multiple response options, followed by the selection of the optimal response. The Iowa Gambling Task, a test to investigate decision making in human subject, demonstrated activations in orbitofrontal, anterior cingulate, and dorsolateral prefrontal cortex (Ernst et al., 2002). From a pharmacological viewpoint, administration of fenfluramine to patients with conduct disorders reduced impulsive responding to another test, the delayed reward paradigm (Cherek & Lane, 2000). This is in line with animal studies reporting increases in impulsive responding at the same task after animals have been given selective lesions of the ascending 5-HT projection (Mobini, Chiang, Ho, Bradshaw, & Szabadi, 2000).

The reversal learning paradigm, requiring the adaptation of behavior according to changes in stimulus–reward contingencies, is relevant to social and emotional behavior (Rolls, 1999). In the pathologically impaired, reversal learning has been attributed to the loss of inhibitory control of affective responding (Dias, Robbins, & Roberts, 1996). Consistent with animal studies indicating that reversal learning is modulated by 5-HT manipulations (Millan et al., 1998), two studies in healthy human volunteers showed that 5-HT suppression by acute tryptophan depletion impairs reversal learning (Park et al., 1994; Rogers et al., 1999). However, this effect generalized to the other learning step of the protocol.

The role of the 5-HT-ergic system in the reward process seems therefore different from the role of the DA-ergic system. In this field, Tanaka and colleagues (2004) demonstrated that when human subjects learned actions on the basis of immediate rewards, significant activity was seen in the lateral orbitofrontal cortex and the striatum, whereas when subjects learned to act in order to obtain large future rewards while incurring small immediate losses, the dorsolateral prefrontal cortex, inferior parietal cortex, dorsal raphe nucleus, and cerebellum were also activated. The authors suggest that different subloops of the corticobasal ganglia network are specialized for reward prediction at different time scales, and that they are activated differently by the ascending 5-HT-ergic system. This hypothesis is in line with studies emphasizing that the low activity of the central 5-HT-ergic system is associated with impulsive behavior in humans (Rogers et al., 1999), and that animals with lesions in the ascending 5-HT-ergic pathway tend to choose small immediate rewards over large future reward (Evenden & Ryan, 1996).

## THERAPEUTIC IMPLICATIONS

At the exclusion of a very limited case report describing the direct and full effect of a serotoninergic drug on very specific symptoms, such as impulsivity, it seems difficult to find a single explanatory relation between a specific behavioral disturbances and a specific neurotransmitter dysfunction.

Knowledge of the relationships between 5-HT and the frontal lobe has already found therapeutic applications. The best known is the treatment of depression and anxiety disorders. Indeed, SSRIs increase the extracellular concentration of 5-HT, leading to the stimulation of the various classes of specific receptors by endogenous neurotransmitters. However, some of these receptors are autoreceptors whose activation inhibits central 5-HT-ergic transmission (i.e., the opposite phenomenon to the aim of treatment). This explains the potential value of $5\text{-HT}_{1A/B/D}$ autoreceptor antagonists. Finally, it should be remembered that $5\text{-HT}_{1A}$ receptors are directly involved in the control of mood and emotions, and that agonists of these receptors (buspirone, ipsapirone) have proven clinical efficacy, notably in anxiety disorders.

Another implication arises in the treatment of schizophrenia. Since stimulating $5\text{-HT}_1$ receptors may alleviate catalepsy symptoms, it was early hypothesized that negative symptoms of the disease (emotional blunting, social withdrawal, anhedonia, and lack of motivation) could be improved when reinforcing 5-HT transmission in prefrontal and limbic areas (Invernizzi, Cervo, & Samani, 1998). However, the use of SSRIs in this indication did not yield significant positive results, and the actual focus is on antipsychotics using the DA–5-HT interaction. Until the end of the 1980s, classic neuroleptics blocking DA receptors were widely used. The reduction of $D_2$ transmission in the striatum and limbic DA pathways has for a long time been associated with not only their therapeutic effect on positive symptoms but also adverse effects such as dystonia, parkinsonism, or elevation of prolactin.

Atypical antipsychotics such as clozapine, risperidone, or olanzapine have relatively little affinity for $D_2$ receptors, and are to a larger extent $5\text{-HT}_{2A/C}$ receptor antagonists (Kapur et al., 1999). It is suggested after many clinical trials that a compound with a $5\text{-HT}_2$–$D_2$ affinity ratio greater than 1 may have the best therapeutic/tolerability balance (Meltzer, 1992). Large amounts of clinical data suggest that the blockade of $5\text{-HT}_2$ receptors, enhancing DA release in prefrontal cortex, is a therapeutic support for the treatment of negative symptoms and cognitive deficit in schizophrenia. These affinities do not explain the atypical nature of antipsychotics in all cases. Some compounds that do not have a significant 5-HT affinity are efficient in the treatment of negative symptomatology of schizophrenia. This is the case for amisulpride, a $D_{2/3}$ antagonist, and a newer partial $D_2$ agonist, aripiprazole (Kane et al., 2002). More than the balance of DA activity through 5-HT regulation, a profile of low $D_2$ affinity and fast dissociation from receptors may be more relevant for a therapeutic effect with fewer motor adverse effects (Kapur & Seeman, 2001).

A third therapeutic implication is in the treatment of behavioral disorders in patients with dementias. In Alzheimer's disease, for example, clinical trials have demonstrated the efficacy of serotoninergic agents (Nyth & Gottfries, 1990). In addition, the preservation of postsynaptic $5-HT_{1A}$ receptors in these patients (Chen, Adler, & Bowen, 1996) suggests that subjects with depressive symptoms could benefit from SSRI or even $5-HT_{1A}$ agonists. Similarly, the selective preservation of $5-HT_{2A}$ receptors in the orbitofrontal and temporal neocortex of anxious patients with Alzheimer's disease patients (Chen et al., 1994) suggests that products acting on $5-HT_{2A}$ receptors would be of value (Esiri, 1996).

Behavioral disorders are a major problem in frontotemporal dementia (FTD). Some symptoms observed in FTD such as bulimia, impulsivity, or personality changes, are comparable to those related to 5-HT-ergic dysfunction. In parallel several studies indicating that 5-HT-ergic changes are frequent in FTD (Anderson, Scott, & Harborne, 1996; Procter, Qurne, & Francis, 1999; Sparks & Markesbery, 1991) suggested the benefits of SSRIs in FTD (Chow, 2003; Moretti, Torre, Antonello, Cazzato, & Bava, 2003; Swartz, Miller, Lesser, & Darby, 1997). This is also the case for trazodone (Lebert, Pasquier, & Petit, 1994), which is an atypical 5-HT-ergic agent (moderate 5-HT reuptake inhibition and a 5-HT-ergic antagonist effect). Recently Lebert, Stekke, Hasenbroekx, and Pasquier (2004) conducted a randomized, double-blind, placebo-controlled crossover trial with trazodone in 31 patients with FTD. Participants were randomly assigned to one of the two-treatment sequences (placebo–trazodone or trazodone–placebo). Assessment with the Neuropsychiatric Inventory (NPI) was performed on the last day of each 6-week period. Results indicated a clearly significant decrease in the NPI total score after trazodone treatment compared with placebo. This overall reduction was associated with improvement observed specifically in eating disorders, agitation, irritability, and depression.

## Case Study

The following case report demonstrates the utility and the limitation of serotoninergic treatment in a patient with FTD.

Mrs. A, a right-handed, 60-year-old woman with higher education and no psychiatric history, presented in late November 1994, accompanied by her daughter. For about 6 months, she had been sad, impatient, and sometimes irritable. This was out of character, and her daughter persuaded her to consult a physician when she started having morbid ideas. Mrs. A continued to play bridge regularly and to visit her grandchildren, but she seemed to have lost interest. A neuropsychological examination was done in December 1994 (Mini-Mental State Examination: 28/30, Signoret Amnesic Efficiency Battery: 61.5, a score normal for age and education; Wisconsin Card Sorting Test: 3/6 categories completed, and increased number of perseverations). Cerebral scintigraphy with the [$^{99m}$Tc] hexamethyl propylenemaine oxime (HMPAO) tracer showed discrete orbitofrontal hypoperfusion. During a subsequent visit in January 1995, Mrs. A's daughter reported inappropriate behavior. She had caught her mother stealing a packet of sweets in a shop. On another occasion she left a café without paying. Antidepressive treatment with paroxetine (10 mg for 7 days, then 20 mg) considerably improved her emotional disorders and inappropriate behavior: "She seems to be more present when she's with us, is interested in more things and, especially, no longer has morbid ideas, and no longer does silly things."

In July 1995, during another visit, Mrs. A's children reported that she had stopped taking her treatment for 3 weeks. She had started to become withdrawn, lying on her bed and reading, watching TV games, and chatting to the portrait of her husband, who had died 19 years previously. The interview showed that Mrs. A was again having morbid ideas and pessimistic thoughts, although she broached these subjects without sadness. On the contrary, she was very lively, and even socially disinhibited (she lay on a table in the waiting room and greeted the doctor with a kiss). In addition, her daughter reported the following events:

"She only shoplifted once, in a department store, but what is new is that she has become very careful with her money. Sometimes she even goes to the kitchen in a restaurant to discuss the price of a meal. . . . She is also more and more interested in games. She wants to go on playing bridge, but I think she's finding it difficult to get someone to play with her. According to what she has told me, she has been to the casino several times. . . . What's more, she tries to pick up men and is quite successful! Finally, she has put on weight, but it's true that she does eat a lot. I am amazed by the size of the meals she eats. Meals seem to have become very important. At home, she can't bear waiting once the meal is on the table!"

Mrs. A agreed with what her daughter said, then asked when the interview would end, because it was "time to be getting home." Renewed treatment with paroxetine led to a disappearance of depressive ideas, a reduction in her appetite, and less interest in games. In September 1996, a new neuropsychological examination was undertaken (Mini-Mental State Examination: 15/30, altered immediate recall and inability to complete memory tests). Her daughter said that Mrs. A had again stopped taking her treatment during the summer. Her behavior had changed. She would spend long hours lying in bed, was no longer interested in games, and went out for only two reasons: the church and the supermarket. She had recently become very religious and often attended services; she would ask the priest questions on irrelevant subjects during the services. Her eating behavior had also changed. She said she only liked minced steak, bought a great deal of it, and ate two helpings at each meal. Furthermore, she no longer tolerated the cold; her favorite drink was a mint cordial with warm water. This time, paroxetine only partially improved Mrs. A's apathy and had no effect on the other disorders.

Dementias illustrate the value of 5-HT-ergic agents in the treatment of behavioral disorders observed during the course of various neuropsychiatric conditions. Controlled clinical trials are now required to determine the effect of different 5-HT-ergic agents on behavioral disorders that are clearly defined from a clinical standpoint.

## REFERENCES

Abbar, M., Amadeo, S., & Malafosse, A. (1992). An association study between suicidal behavior and tryptophan hydroxylase markers. *Clinical Psychopharmacolgy, 15*(Suppl. 1), 299–290.

Anderson, I. M., Scott, K., & Harborne, G. (1996). Serotonin and depression in frontal lobe dementia (Letter). *American Journal of Psychiatry, 152,* 645–640.

Apostolopoulos, M., Judd, F. K., Burrows, G. D., & Norman, T. R. (1993). Prolactin response to *d,l*-fenfluramine in panic disorder. *Psychoneuroendocrinology, 18,* 337–342.

Arora, R. C., & Meltzer, H. Y. (1989). Serotonergic measures in the brains of suicide victims: 5-HT2 binding sites in the frontal cortex of suicide victims and control subjects. *American Journal of Psychiatry, 146,* 730–736.

Asberg, M., Schalling, D., Taskman-Bendz, L., & Wagner, A. (1987). Psychobiology of suicide, impulsivity, and related phenomena. In H. Y. Meltzer (Ed.), *Psychopharmacology: Third generation of progress* (pp. 665–668). New York: Raven Press.

Asberg, M., Traskman, L., & Thoren, P. (1976). 5-HIAA in the cerebrospinal fluid: A biochemical suicide predictor? *Archives of General Psychiatry, 33,* 1193–1197.

Aubin-Brunet, V. (1993). Echelle d'évaluation clinique du déficit sérotoninergique chez les personnes âgées. *L'Encéphale, 19,* 413–416.

Aubin-Brunet, V., Beau, C. H., Asso, G., Robert, P. H., & Darcourt, G. (1996). Serotoninergic symptomatology in dementia. In E. Giacobini, R. Becker, & P. H. Robert (Eds.), *Alzheimer disease: Therapeutic strategies* (pp. 520–525). Boston: Birkhauser.

Ballanger, J. C., Goodwin, F. K., & Major, L. F. (1979). Alcohol and central serotonin metabolism in man. *Archives of General Psychiatry, 36,* 224–229.

Basbaum, A. I., & Fields, H. L. (1984). Endogenous pain controls systems: Brainstem spinal pathways and endorphin circuits. *Annual Review of Neuroscience, 7,* 309–338.

Benkelfat, C. (1993). Serotonergic mechanisms in psychiatric disorders: New research tools, new ideas. *International Clinical Psychopharmacology, 8* (Suppl. 2), 53–62.

Berns, G. S., McClure, S. M., Pagnoni, G., & Montague, P. R. (2001). Predictability modulates human brain response to reward. *Journal of Neuroscience, 21,* 2793–2798.

Biegon, A., Kargman, S., Snyder, L., & McEwen, B. (1986). Characterization and localization of serotonin receptors in human brain postmortem. *Brain Research, 363,* 91–98.

Breiter, H. C., Aharon, I., Kahneman, D., Dale, A., & Shizgal, P. (2001). Functional imaging of neural responses to expectancy and experience of monetary gains and losses. *Neuron, 30,* 619–639.

Brewerton, T. D., Brandt, H. A., Lessem, M. D., Murphy, D. L., & Jimerson, D. C. (1990). Serotonin and eating disorders: Serotonin in major psychiatric disorders. In E. F. Coccaro & D. L. Murphy (Eds.), *Progress in psychiatry* (pp. 153–184). Washington, DC: American Psychiatric Press.

Brown, G. L., & Linnolia, M. (1990). Serotonin metabolite (5-HIAA) studies in depression, impulsivity, and violence. *Journal of Clinical Psychiatry, 51*(Suppl. 4), 31–41.

Butler, J., O'Halloran, A., & Leonard, B. E. (1992). The Galway Study of Panic Disorder: II. Changes in some peripheral markers of noradrenergic and serotonergic function in DSM-III-R panic disorder. *Journal of Affective Disorders, 26*, 89–99.

Caci, B., Vallier, E., Robert, P. H., & Dossios, C. (2004). Impulsivity and affect in suicide attempter: A short-term longitudinal study. *International Journal of Neuropsychopharmacology, 7*, 455.

Caci, H. (2004). The cross cultural assessment of impulsivity. *Journal of Neuropsychopharmacology, 7*, 132.

Caci, H., Nadalet, L., Bayle, F. J., Robert, P., & Boyer, P. (2003). Functional and dysfunctional impulsivity: Contribution to the construct validity. *Acta Psychiatrica Scandinavica, 107*, 34–40.

Charney, D. S., Goodman, W. K., Price, L. H., Woods, S. W., Rasmussen, S. A., & Heninger, G. R. (1988). Serotonin function in obsessive–compulsive disorder: A comparison of the effects of tryptophan and m-chlorophenylpiperazine in patients and healthy subjects. *Archives of General Psychiatry, 45*, 177–185.

Chen, C. P., Adler, J. T., & Bowen, D. M. (1996). Presynaptic serotonergic markers in community-acquired cases of Alzheimer's disease: Correlations with depression and medication. *Journal of Neurochemistry, 66*, 1592–1598.

Chen, C. P., Hope, R. A., Adler, J. T., Keene, J., McDonald, B., Francis, P. T., et al. (1994). Loss of 5-HT$_{2A}$ receptors in Alzheimer's disease neocortex is associated with disease severity while preservation of 5-HT$_{2A}$ receptors is associated with anxiety. *Annals of Neurology, 36*, 308–309.

Cherek, D. R., & Lane, S. D. (2000). Fenfluramine effects on impulsivity in a sample of adults with and without history of conduct disorder. *Psychopharmacology (Berlin), 152*, 149–156.

Chow, T. W. (2003). Frontotemporal dementias: Clinical features and management. *Seminars in Clinical Neuropsychiatry, 8*, 58–70.

Clark, L., Cools, R., & Robbins, T. W. (2004). The neuropsychology of ventral prefrontal cortex: Decision-making and reversal learning. *Brain and Cognition, 55*, 41–53.

Coccaro, E. F., Siever, L. J., Owen, K., & Davis, K. L. (1990). Serotonin in mood and personality disorders. In E. F. Coccaro & D. L. Murphy (Eds.), *Serotonin in major psychiatric disorders* (pp. 69–98). Washington, DC: American Psychiatric Press.

Cook, E. H., Fletcher, K. E., Wainwright, M., Marks, N., Yan, S., & Leventhal, B. L. (1994). Primary structure of the human platelet serotonin 5-HT$_{2A}$ receptor: Identity with frontal cortex serotonin 5-HT$_{2A}$ receptor. *Journal of Neurochemistry, 63*, 465–469.

Cowen, P. J. (1991). Serotonin receptor subtypes: Implications for psychopharmacology. *British Journal of Psychiatry, 159*(Suppl. 12), 7–14.

Cowen, P. J., & Charig, E. M. (1986). 5-HT in neuroendocrinology: Recent advances: The biology of depression. *Royal College of Psychiatrists*, 71–89.

De Deurwaerdere, P., Bonhomme, N., Lucas, G., Le Moal, M., & Spampinato, U. (1996). Serotonin enhances striatal dopamine outflow *in vivo* through dopamine uptake sites. *Journal of Neurochemistry, 66*, 210–215.

De Deurwaerdere, P., Stinus, L., & Spampinato, U. (1998). Opposite change of *in vivo* dopamine release in the rat nucleus accumbens and striatum that follows electrical stimulation of dorsal raphe nucleus: Role of 5-HT$_3$ receptors. *Journal of Neuroscience, 18*, 6528–6538.

Den Boer, J. A., Bosker, F. J., & Slaap, B. R. (2000). Serotonergic drugs in the treatment of depressive and anxiety disorders. *Human Psychopharmacology, 15*, 315–336.

Dias, R., Robbins, T. W., & Roberts, A. C. (1996). Dissociation in prefrontal cortex of affective and attentional shifts. *Nature, 380*, 69–72.

Dillon, K. A., Gross-Isseroff, R., Israeli, M., & Biegon, A. (1991). Autoradiographic analysis of serotonin 1A receptor binding in the human brain postmortem: Effects of age and alcohol. *Brain Research, 554*, 56–64.

Eriksson, E., Westberg, P., Alling, C., Thuresson, K., & Modigh, K. (1991). Cerebrospinal fluid levels of monoamine metabolites in panic disorder. *Psychiatry Research, 36*, 243–251.

Ernst, M., Bolla, K., Mouratidis, M., Contoreggi, C., Matochik, J. A., Kurian, V., et al. (2002). Decision-making in a risk-taking task: A PET study. *Neuropsychopharmacology, 26*, 682–691.

Esiri, M. M. (1996). The basis for behavioural disturbances in dementia [Editorial]. *Journal of Neurology, Neurosurgery, and Psychiatry, 61*, 127–130.

Evenden, J. L., & Ryan, C. N. (1996). The pharmacology of impulsive behaviour in rats: The effects of drugs on response choice with varying delays of reinforcement. *Psychopharmacology (Berlin), 128*, 161–170.

Fernstrom, J. D. (1985). Dietary effects on brain serotonin synthesis: Relationship to appetite regulation. *American Journal of Clinical Nutrition, 42*, 1072–1082.

Golden, N. R., Gilmore, J. H., & Carson, S. W. (1991). Serotonin, suicide, and aggression: Clinical studies. *Journal of Clinical Psychiatry, 52*(Suppl. 12), 61–69.

Goodwin, F. K., Post, R. M., Dunner, D. L., & Gordon, E. K. (1973). Cerebrospinal fluid amine metabolites in affective illness: The probenecid technique. *American Journal of Psychiatry, 130*, 73–79.

Hallbus, M., Magnusson, T., & Magnusson, O. (1997). Influence of 5-HT$_{1B/1D}$ receptors on dopamine release in the guinea pig nucleus accumbens: A microdialysis study. *Neuroscience Letters, 225*, 57–60.

Hamon, M., & Gozlan, H. (1993). Les récepteurs centraux de la sérotonine. *Médecine/Sciences, 9*, 21–30.

Hartig, P. R., Hoyer, D., Humphrey, P. P., & Martin, G. R. (1996). Alignment of receptor nomenclature with the human genome: Classification of 5-HT$_{1B}$ and 5-HT$_{1D}$ receptor subtypes. *Trends in Pharmacological Science, 17*, 103–105.

Hartmann, E., & Greewald, D. (1984). Tryptophan and

human sleep: An analysis of 43 studies. In H. G. Schlossberger, W. Kochen, & B. Linzen (Eds.), *Tryptophan and serotonin research* (pp. 297–304). Berlin: de Gruyter.

Heisler, L. K., Chu, H. M., Brennan, T. J., Danao, A., Bajwa, P., Parsons, L. H., et al. (1998). Elevated anxiety and antidepressant-like responses in serotonin 5-HT$_{1A}$ receptor mutant mice. *Proceedings of the National Academy of Sciences of the United States of America, 95,* 15049–15054.

Hollander, E., DeCaria, C. M., Nitescu, A., Gully, R., Suckow, R. F., Cooper, T. B., et al. (1992). Serotonergic function in obsessive–compulsive disorder: Behavioral and neuroendocrine responses to oral m-chlorophenylpiperazine and fenfluramine in patients and healthy volunteers. *Archives of General Psychiatry, 49,* 21–28.

Horton, R. W. (1992). The neurochemistry of depression: Evidence derived from studies of post-mortem brain tissue. *Molecular Aspects of Medicine, 13,* 191–203.

Hoyer, D., Clarke, D. E., Fozard, J. R., Hartig, P. R., Martin, G. R., Mylecharane, E. J., et al. (1994). International Union of Pharmacology classification of receptors for 5-hydroxytryptamine. *Pharmacological Reviews, 46,* 157–203.

Hoyer, D., Hannon, J. P., & Martin, G. R. (2002). Molecular, pharmacological and functional diversity of 5-HT receptors. *Pharmacology, Biochemistry, and Behavior, 71,* 533–554.

Hoyer, D., & Martin, G. (1997). 5-HT receptor classification and nomenclature: Towards a harmonization with the human genome. *Neuropharmacology, 36,* 419–428.

Hoyer, D., Pazos, A., Probst, A., & Palacios, J. M. (1986). Serotonin receptors in the human brain: II. Characterisation and autoradiographic localisation of 5-HT$_{1C}$ and 5-HT$_2$ recognition sites. *Brain Research, 376,* 97–107.

Invernizzi, R. W., Cervo, L., & Samani, R. (1998). 8-Hydroxy-2-(Di-N-propylamino) tetralin, a selective serotonin-1A receptor agonist, blocks haloperidol-induced catalepsy by an action on raphe nuclei medianus and dorsalis. *Neuropharmacology, 27,* 515–518.

Jacobs, B. L., & Azmitia, E. C. (1992). Structure and function of the brain serotonin system. *Physiological Review, 72,* 165–229.

Jorgensen, H., Knigge, U., Kjaer, A., & Warberg, J. (1999). Adrenocorticotropic hormone secretion in rats induced by stimulation with serotonergic compounds. *Journal of Neuroendocrinology, 11,* 283–290.

Kahn, R. S., Van Praag, H. M., Weltzer, S., Asnis, G., & Barr, G. (1988). Serotonin and anxiety revisited. *Biological Psychiatry, 23,* 189–208.

Kane, J. M., Carson, W. H., Saha, A. R., McQuade, R. D., Ingenito, G. G. Zimbroff, D. L., et al. (2002). Efficacy and safety of aripiprazole and haloperidol versus placebo in patients with schizophrenia and schizoaffective disorder. *Journal of Clinical Psychiatry, 63,* 763–771.

Kapur, S., & Remington, G. (1996). Serotonin–dopamine interaction and its relevance to schizophrenia. *American Journal of Psychiatry, 153,* 466–476.

Kapur, S., & Seeman, P. (2001). Does fast dissociation from the dopamine D$_2$ receptor explain the action of atypical antipsychotics?: A new hypothesis. *American Journal of Psychiatry, 158,* 360–369.

Kapur, S., Zipursky, R. B., & Remington, G. (1999). Comparison of the 5-HT$_2$ and D$_2$ receptor occupancy of clozapine, risperidone, and olanzapine in schizophrenia: Clinical and theoretical implications. *American Journal of Psychiatry, 156,* 286–293.

Korsgaard, S., Gerlach, J., & Christensson, E. (1985). Behavioral aspects of serotonin–dopamine interaction in the monkey. *European Journal of Pharmacology, 118,* 245–252.

Laporte, A. M., Kidd, E., Verge, D., Gozlan, H., & Hamon, M. (1992). Autoradiographic mapping of central 5-HT$_3$ receptors. In A. M. Hamon (Ed.), *Central and peripheral 5-HT3 receptors* (pp. 157–187). London: Academic Press.

Lebert, F., Pasquier, F., & Petit, H. (1994). Behavioral effects of trazodone in Alzheimer's disease. *Journal of Clinical Psychiatry, 55,* 536–538.

Lebert, F., Stekke, W., Hasenbroekx, C., & Pasquier, F. (2004). Frontotemporal dementia: A randomised, controlled trial with trazodone. *Dementia and Geriatric Cognitive Disorders, 17,* 355–359.

Leysen, J. E., Gommeren, W., Heylen, L., Luyten, W. H., Van de Weyer, I., Vanhoenacker, P., et al. (1996). Alniditan, a new 5-hydroxytryptamine1D agonist and migraine-abortive agent: Ligand-binding properties of human 5-hydroxytryptamine1D alpha, human 5-hydroxytryptamine1D beta, and calf 5-hydroxytryptamine1D receptors investigated with [$^3$H]5-hydroxytryptamine and [$^3$H]alniditan. *Molecular Pharmacology, 50,* 1567–1580.

Linnolia, M., Virkkunen, M., & Higley, G. (1993). Impulse control disorders. *International Clinical Psychopharmacology, 8*(Suppl. 1), 53–56.

Lowther, S., De Paermentier, F., Crompton, M. R., Katona, C. L., & Horton, R. W. (1994). Brain 5-HT$_2$ receptors in suicide victims: Violence of death, depression and effects of antidepressant treatment. *Brain Research, 642,* 281–289.

Mann, J. J., Malone, K. M., Diehl, D. J., Perel, J., Cooper, T. B., & Mintun, M. A. (1996a). Demonstration *in vivo* of reduced serotonin responsivity in the brain of untreated depressed patients. *American Journal of Psychiatry, 153,* 174–182.

Mann, J. J., Malone, K. M., Diehl, D. J., Perel, J., Nichols, T. E., & Mintun, M. A. (1996b). Positron emission tomographic imaging of serotonin activation effects on prefrontal cortex in healthy volunteers. *Journal of Cerebral Blood Flow and Metabolism, 16,* 418–426.

Mann, J. J., McBride, P. A., Brown, R. P., Linnolia, M., Leon, A. C., De Meo, M., et al. (1992). Relationship between central and peripheral serotonin indexes in depressed and suicidal psychiatric inpatients. *Archives of General Psychiatry, 49*, 442–446.

Mann, J. J., McBride, P. A., & Stanley, M. (1986). Postmortem serotonergic and adrenergic receptor binding to frontal cortex: Correlations with suicide. *Psychopharmacological Bulletin, 22*, 647–649.

Marazziti, D., Marracci, S., Palego, L., Rotondo, A., Mazzanti, C., Nardi, I., et al. (1994). Localisation and gene expression of serotonin1A receptors in human brain postmortem. *Brain Research, 658*, 55–59.

Mega, M. S., & Cummings, J. L. (1994). Frontal–subcortical circuits and neuropsychiatric disorders. *Journal of Neuropsychiatry and Clinical Neurosciences, 6*, 358–370.

Meltzer, H. Y. (1992, May). The importance of serotonin–dopamine interactions in the action of clozapine. *British Journal of Psychiatry, 17*(Suppl.), 22–29.

Meltzer, H. Y., Perline, R., Tricou, B. J., Lowy, M., & Robertson, A. (1984). Effect of 5-hydroxytryptophan on serum cortisol levels in major affective disorders: II. Relation to suicide, psychosis, and depressive symptoms. *Archives of General Psychiatry, 41*, 379–387.

Millan, M. J., Dekeyne, A., & Gobert, A. (1998). Serotonin (5-HT)2C receptors tonically inhibit dopamine (DA) and noradrenaline (NA), but not 5-HT, release in the frontal cortex *in vivo. Neuropharmacology, 37*, 953–955.

Miller, L. A. (1992). Impulsivity, risk taking, and the ability to synthesize fragmented information after frontal lobectomy. *Neuropsychologia, 30*, 69–79.

Mobini, S., Chiang, T. J., Ho, M. Y., Bradshaw, C. M., & Szabadi, E. (2000). Effects of central 5-hydroxytryptamine depletion on sensitivity to delayed and probabilistic reinforcement. *Psychopharmacology (Berlin), 152*, 390–397.

Moeller, F. G., Barratt, E. S., Dougherty, D. M., Schmitz, J. M., & Swann, A. C. (2001). Psychiatric aspects of impulsivity. *American Journal of Geriatric Psychiatry, 158*, 1783–1793.

Monferini, E., Gaetani, P., Rodriguez y Baena, R., Giraldo, E., Parenti, M., Zoccheti, A., et al. (1993). Pharmacological characterization of the 5-HT receptor coupled to adenylyl cyclase stimulation in human brain. *Life Sciences, 52*, 61–65.

Moretti, R., Torre, P., Antonello, R. M., Cazzato, G., & Bava, A. (2003). Frontotemporal dementia: Paroxetine as a possible treatment of behavior symptoms: A randomized, controlled, open 14-month study. *European Neurology, 49*, 13–19.

Mullins, U. L., Gianutsos, G., & Eison, A. S. (1999). Effects of antidepressants on 5-HT$_7$ receptor regulation in the rat hypothalamus. *Neuropsychopharmacology, 21*, 352–367.

New, A. S., Hazlett, E. A., Buchsbaum, M. S., Goodman, M., Reynolds, D., Mitropoulou, V., et al. (2002). Blunted prefrontal cortical 18-fluorodeoxyglucose positron emission tomography response to meta-chlorophenylpiperazine in impulsive aggression. *Archives of General Psychiatry, 59*, 621–629.

New, A. S., Trestman, R. F., Mitropoulou, V., Goodman, M., Koenigsberg, H. H., Silverman, J., et al. (2004). Low prolactin response to fenfluramine in impulsive aggression. *Journal of Psychiatry Research, 38*, 223–230.

Nyth, A. L., & Gottfries, C. G. (1990). The clinical efficacy of citalopram in treatment of emotional disturbances in dementia disorders. *British Journal of Psychiatry, 157*, 894–901.

O'Doherty, J. P., Dayan, P., Friston, K., Critchley, H., & Dolan, R. J. (2003). Temporal difference models and reward-related learning in the human brain. *Neuron, 38*, 329–337.

Park, S. B., Coull, J. T., McShane, R. H., Young, A. H., Sahakian, B. J., Robbins, T. W., et al. (1994). Tryptophan depletion in normal volunteers produces selective impairments in learning and memory. *Neuropharmacology, 33*, 575–588.

Parks, C. L., Robinson, P. S., Sibille, E., Shenk, T., & Toth, M. (1998). Increased anxiety of mice lacking the serotonin 1A receptor. *Proceedings of the National Academy of Sciences of the United States of America, 95*, 10734–10739.

Paul, S. M., Rehavi, M., Skolnick, P., & Goodwin, F. K. (1980). Demonstration of specific "high affinity" binding sites for [$^3$H]imipramine on human platelets. *Life Sciences, 26*, 953–959.

Pauwels, P. J. (1997). 5-HT$_{1B/D}$ receptor antagonists. *General Pharmacology, 29*, 293–303.

Pazos, A., Cortes, R., & Palacios, J. M. (1985). Quantitative autoradiographic mapping of serotonin receptors in the rat brain. *Brain Research, 346*, 241–249.

Peroutka, S. J., & Snyder, S. H. (1979). Multiple serotonin receptors: Differential binding of [$^3$H]5-hydroxytryptamine, [$^3$H]lysergic acid diethylamide and [$^3$H]spiroperidol. *Molecular Pharmacology, 16*, 687–699.

Pigott, T. A., Hill, J. L., Grady, T. A., L'Heureux, F., Bernstein, S., Rubenstein, C. S., et al. (1993). A comparison of the behavioral effects of oral versus intravenous mCPP administration in OCD patients and the effect of metergoline prior to i.v. mCPP. *Biological Psychiatry, 33*, 3–14.

Procter, A. W., Qurne, M., & Francis, P. T. (1999). Neurochemical features of frontotemporal dementia. *Dementia and Geriatric Cognitive Disorders, 10*, 80–84.

Radja, F., Laporte, A. M., Daval, G., Verge, D., Gozlan, H., & Hamon, M. (1991). Autoradiography of serotonin receptor subtypes in the central nervous system. *Neurochemistry International, 18*, 1–15.

Raisman, R., Sechter, D., Briley, M. S., Zarifian, E., & Langer, S. Z. (1981). High-affinity $^3$H-imipramine binding in platelets from untreated and treated depressed patients compared to healthy volunteers. *Psychopharmacology (Berlin), 75*, 368–371.

Rogers, R. D., Blackshaw, A. J., Middleton, H. C.,

Matthews, K., Hawtin, K., Crowley, C., et al. (1999). Tryptophan depletion impairs stimulus–reward learning while methylphenidate disrupts attentional control in healthy young adults: Implications for the monoaminergic basis of impulsive behaviour. *Psychopharmacology (Berlin)*, 146, 482–491.

Rogers, R. D., Everitt, B. J., Baldacchino, A., Blackshaw, A. J., Swainson, R., Wynne, K., et al. (1999). Dissociable deficits in the decision-making cognition of chronic amphetamine abusers, opiate abusers, patients with focal damage to prefrontal cortex, and tryptophan-depleted normal volunteers: Evidence for monoaminergic mechanisms. *Neuropsychopharmacology*, 20, 322–339.

Rolls, E. (1999). *The brain and emotion*. Oxford, UK: Oxford University Press.

Roth, B. L., Craigo, S. C., Choudhary, M. S., Uluer, A., Monsma, F. J., Jr., Shen, Y., et al. (1994). Binding of typical and atypical antipsychotic agents to 5-hydroxytryptamine-6 and 5-hydroxytryptamine-7 receptors. *Journal of Pharmacology and Experimental Therapeutics*, 268, 1403–1410.

Roy, A., Virkkunen, M., & Linnolia, M. (1990). Serotonin in suicide, violence and alcoholism. In E. F. Coccaro & D. L. Murphy (Eds.), *Serotonin in major psychiatric disorders* (pp. 185–208). Washington, DC: American Psychiatric Press.

Sasaki-Adams, D. M., & Kelley, A. E. (2001). Serotonin–dopamine interactions in the control of reinforcement and motor behavior. *Neuropsychopharmacology*, 25, 440–452.

Seibyl, J. P., Krystal, J. H., Price, L. H., Woods, S. W., D'Amico, C., Heninger, G. R., et al. (1991). Effects of ritanserin on the behavioral, neuroendocrine, and cardiovascular responses to meta-chlorophenylpiperazine in healthy human subjects. *Psychiatry Research*, 38, 227–236.

Sheehan, D. V., Raj, B. A., Trehan, R. R., & Knapp, E. L. (1993). Serotonin in panic disorder and social phobia. *International Clinical Psychopharmacology*, 8(Suppl. 2), 63–77.

Soloff, P. H., Kelly, T. M., Strotmeyer, S. J., Malone, K. M., & Mann, J. J. (2003). Impulsivity, gender, and response to fenfluramine challenge in borderline personality disorder. *Psychiatry Research*, 119, 11–24.

Sparks, D. L., & Markesbery, W. R. (1991). Altered serotonergic and cholinergic synaptic markers in Pick's disease. *Archives of Neurology*, 48, 796–799.

Swartz, J. R., Miller, B. L., Lesser, I. M., & Darby, A. L.

(1997). Frontotemporal dementia: Treatment response to serotonin selective reuptake inhibitors. *Journal of Clinical Psychiatry*, 58, 212–216.

Tanaka, S. C., Doya, K., Okada, G., Ueda, K., Okamoto, Y., & Yamawaki, S. (2004). Prediction of immediate and future rewards differentially recruits cortico-basal ganglia loops. *Nature Neuroscience*, 7, 887–893.

Tarter, R. E., Kirisci, L., Reynolds, M., & Mezzich, A. (2004). Neurobehavior disinhibition in childhood predicts suicide potential and substance use disorder by young adulthood. *Drug and Alcohol Dependence*, 76(Suppl.), S45–S52.

Ugedo, L., Grenhoff, J., & Svensson, T. H. (1989). Ritanserin, a $5\text{-HT}_2$ receptor antagonist, activate midbrain dopamine neurons by blocking serotonergic inhibition. *Psychopharmacology*, 98, 45–50.

Van de Kar, L. D., Javed, A., Zhang, Y., Serres, F., Raap, D. K., & Gray, T. S. (2001). $5\text{-HT}_{2A}$ receptors stimulate ACTH, corticosterone, oxytocin, renin, and prolactin release and activate hypothalamic CRF and oxytocin-expressing cells. *Journal of Neuroscience*, 21, 3572–3579.

Van Praag, H. M. (1982). Depression, suicide and metabolism of serotonin in the brain. *Journal of Affective Disorders*, 4, 275–290.

Walsh, S. L., & Cunningham, K. A. (1997). Serotonergic mechanisms involved in the discriminative stimulus, reinforcing and subjective effects of cocaine. *Psychopharmacology*, 130, 41–58.

Wang, G. J., Volkow, N. D., Logan, J., Fowler, J. S., Schlyer, D., MacGregor, R. R., et al. (1995). Evaluation of age-related changes in serotonin $5\text{-HT}_2$ and dopamine $D_2$ receptor availability in healthy human subjects. *Pharmacology Letters*, 14, 249–253.

Woolley, M. L., Bentley, J. C., Sleight, A. J., Marsden, C. A., & Fone, K. C. (2001). A role for $5\text{-HT}_6$ receptors in retention of spatial learning in the Morris water maze. *Neuropharmacology*, 41, 210–219.

Yakel, J. L., Shao, X. M., & Jackson, M. B. (1990). The selectivity of the channel coupled to the 5-HT3 receptor. *Brain Research*, 533, 46-52.

Yoshimoto, K., Yayama, K., Sorimachi, Y., Tani, J., Ogata, M., Nishimura, A., et al. (1996). Possibility of $5\text{-HT}_3$ receptor involvement in alcohol dependence: A microdialysis study of nucleus accumbens dopamine and serotonin release in rats with chronic alcohol consumption. *Alcoholism, Clinical, and Experimental Research*, 20, 311A–319A.

# CHAPTER 10

# Oiling the Gears of the Mind

## ROLES FOR ACETYLCHOLINE IN THE MODULATION OF ATTENTION

*Serena Amici*
*Adam L. Boxer*

Attention is a basic component of brain function on which many neural processes depend. One of the earliest and best definitions of attention was provided by William James in 1890: "Everyone knows what attention is. It is the taking possession of the mind in clear and vivid form of what seems several simultaneous objects or trains of thought" (Cohen, Aston-Jones, & Gilzenrat, 2004, p. 403). Over the past century, the construct of attention has been operationalized in many ways to allow for explorations of its psychological, physiological, anatomical, neurochemical and genetic mechanisms. Based on these explorations, a restatement of James's definition that reflects modern principles of cognitive neuroscience might be as follows: "Attention is the emergent property of the cognitive system that allows it to successfully process some sources of information to the exclusion of others, in the service of achieving some goals to the exclusion of others" (Cohen et al., 2004, p. 71). This definition implies that attention depends on multiple aspects of brain function that act in parallel to allow each of us to achieve our goals efficiently, with minimal waste of cognitive resources. When attention is impaired under conditions of disease or altered brain physiology, many brain processes continue to operate, but often in a slower or more disorganized fashion.

The measurement of attentional processes has been facilitated by the recognition that common mechanisms underlie *overt* shifts of attention, or changes in the direction of gaze through saccadic eye movements to focus on a particular stimulus (see Kaufer, Chapter 4, this volume, on eye movement control by the frontal lobes), and *covert* shifts of attention, in which a stimulus is focused upon without an accompanying eye movement (Corbetta et al., 1998). Attention is influenced by external signals during cognitively demanding tasks ("signal-driven" or "bottom-up" modulation of detection), as well as by intrinsic knowledge- or practice-based executive influences ("cognitive" or "top-down" modulation of detection; Sarter, Hasselmo, Bruno, & Givens, 2005). Importantly, both bottom-up and top-down modulation of attention is mediated by release of acetylcholine (ACh) from basal forebrain neurons that project to regions throughout the cerebral cortex, particularly in the medial frontal lobes. Voluntary, top-down modulation of attention involves a direct stimulation of basal forebrain cholinergic, and possibly brainstem cholinergic, neurons by structures within the frontal lobes (Figure 10.1).

Important roles for ACh in modulating attention have long been recognized from the behavioral effects of alkaloids such as musca-

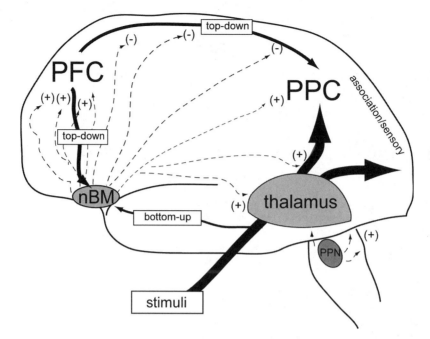

FIGURE 10.1. Frontal lobe: Cholinergic circuits that mediate attention. The prefrontal cortex (PFC) sends glutamatergic projections to the nucleus basalis of Meynert (nBM), the major source of cholinergic inputs to the cerebral cortex. Voluntary, "top-down" shifts of attention are mediated by this PFC–nBM pathway, as well as by direct intracortical connections to other brain regions, such as posterior parietal cortex (PPC) and occipital lobe, which contain neurons with primary sensory and association functions. Reciprocal cholinergic projections to the medial PFC form a feed-forward loop that futher promote attention. ACh release from nBM neurons (dashed lines) suppresses ("–" signs) intracortical information transfer (thin arrows) and promotes information transfer through thalamocortical circuits ("+" signs). Most of ACh's direct effects on the thalamus are mediated by projections from the pedunculopontine nucleus (PPN), which also project to the superior colliculus in the dorsal midbrain and promotes overt shifts of attention (saccadic eye movements). Difficult tasks or unusual stimuli can also directly activate ACh release from the nBM ("bottom-up"). Data from Sarter et al. (2005).

rine, atropine, and nicotine. These agents interfere with or augment ACh's central nervous system (CNS) actions and have profound effects on attention in both animals and normal or diseased humans (Robbins, Milstein, & Dalley, 2004). Studies of neurodegenerative disorders, such as Alzheimer's disease and dementia with Lewy bodies, that lead to profound deficits in attention, have demonstrated that loss of CNS Ach explains a significant component of patients' cognitive deficits.

The role of ACh in mediating different aspects of attention has progressively come into focus at multiple levels of analysis. At the systems level, ACh helps to recruit multiple brain regions involved in attentional processes (Bentley, Husain, & Dolan, 2004; Bentley, Vuilleumier, Thiel, Driver, & Dolan, 2003; Fan,

2005). This may occur through changes in neural synchrony at a macroscopic level by promoting 40-Hz oscillations of brain activity that synchronize brain regions involved in attention. Modeling studies based on classical tests of attention suggest that ACh may signal *expected* uncertainty, whereas other neurotransmitters, such as norepinephrine, signal *unexpected* uncertainty, thus potentially playing different roles in "top-down" and "bottom-up" modulation of attention (Yu & Dayan, 2005). Consistent with these models, *in vivo* microdialysis experiments have also demonstrated that extracellular Ach levels increase in frontal lobe structures during attention-demanding tasks. At the cellular level, ACh induces changes in intrinsic electrical properties and synaptic physiology of neurons. These

ACh-induced changes in neuronal physiology have different effects on intracortical and thalamocortical connectivity. They inhibit intracortical information processing, while promoting thalamocortical transfer of information. Advances in molecular physiology have led to cloning of the genes for ACh receptors, transporters, and metabolic enzymes. Evidence from the dopamine (DA) receptor system suggests that genetic heterogeneity within ACh receptor and transporter genes may explain differential attentional performance in individual subjects.

This chapter summarizes the current state of knowledge about the roles of the frontal lobes and ACh in mediating different aspects of attention.

## ANATOMY OF CHOLINERGIC CONNECTIONS TO THE FRONTAL LOBES

ACh acts as an excitatory neurotransmitter in the peripheral nervous system, but in the CNS, it plays a neuromodulatory role. At the neuromuscular junction, presynaptic release of ACh from motor neurons directly depolarizes postsynaptic muscle fibers leading to muscle contraction at specific sites, a direct excitatory effect, with a rapid onset and offset. In contrast, ACh release in the cerebral cortex often occurs from axonal varicosities that do not form direct synapses with other neurons. The neurotransmitter is free to diffuse to multiple synaptic sites in the vicinity of its release, thus leading to a more prolonged effect that modulates the synaptic activity of glutamate and γ-aminobutyric acid (GABA), the primary cortical excitatory and inhibitory neurotransmitters. Depending on the type of neuron, and its pattern of ACh receptor and ion channel expression, ACh can have either excitatory or inhibitory effects.

Cholinergic neurons contain the synthetic enzyme choline acetyltransferase (ChAT), as well as the vesicular ACh transporter, both of which can be visualized presynaptically in cortical cholinergic projections using immunocytochemical techniques (Mesulam, 2004). The majority of cholinergic inputs to the cortex arise from the basal forebrain, of which the nucleus basalis of Meynert (nBM, also known as the Ch4 cell group) constitutes the largest group of cortically projecting cells. Cholinergic innervation of the striatum is primarily intrinsic, arising from ChAT positive interneurons.

The thalamus and brainstem receive cholinergic innervation from the pedunculopontine nucleus (PPN) and lateral dorsal nuclei (also known as the Ch5 and Ch6 cell groups). Although not initially thought to be important for mediating attention, new evidence of direct modulation of thalamic (Mooney et al., 2004) and superior collicular (Sparks, 2002) neurons' electrophysiological responses suggests that brainstem cholinergic neurons may promote attention through increased information transfer through the thalamus, and by promoting overt shifts of attention in the superior colliculus.

## PHYSIOLOGY OF ACh IN THE CEREBRAL CORTEX

A role for acetylcholine in the modulation of cortical neurons was first demonstrated by Krnjevic and Phillis (1963). They showed an increased firing of neocortical neurons during the infusion of ACh and other cholinergic agents. Later studies focused on cholinergic modulation of intrinsic electrophysiological properties of cortical neurons and its role in neural networks. These studies used a cortical slice preparation for recording extracellular and intracellular polarization. An increase in firing of cortical neurons was seen in response to ACh application. The increased firing rate of cortical neurons induced by Ach was found to be related to direct depolarizing effects of ACh. ACh causes a depolarization of 3–5 mV in pyramidal cells (Barkai & Hasselmo, 1994) and an even larger depolarization in interneurons (McQuiston & Madison, 1999; Reece & Schwartzkroin, 1991). This effect is likely to be mediated primarily by postsynaptic, muscarinic receptor activation (Andrade, 1991).

Secondary to its effects on intrinsic membrane potentials and firing rates, ACh modulates the presynaptic release of glutamate, and GABA and glutamate. Muscarinic receptors activation can suppress the release of GABA and glutamate in different brain regions: somatosensory cortex (Hasselmo & Cekic, 1996), primary visual cortex (Brocher, Artola, & Singer, 1992), piriform cortex (Hasselmo & Bower, 1993), and hippocampus (Valentino & Dingledine, 1981). Muscarinic suppression of synaptic potentials occurs also in prefrontal cortex (Vidal & Changeux, 1993), along with a presynaptic nicotinic enhancement of neurotransmitter release at glutamatergic synapses

(Gray, Rajan, Radcliffe, Yakehiro, & Dani, 1996). Interestingly, evidence of muscarinic suppression of neurotransmitter release occurred in 100% of the cells, whereas nicotinic enhancement occurred in only 14% of the cells.

In addition to its synaptic effects, ACh also leads to activity-dependent enhancement of neuronal responses, due to afterdepolarization effects on neurons, which promote bursting. After exposure to ACh neurons are more prone to spike again, altering the response of a network (Andrade, 1991). In layer IV of the cerebral cortex, muscarinic cholinergic receptors play important roles in modulating both long- and short-term synaptic plasticity plasticity. Cortical long-term potentiation (LTP) and long-term depression (LTD) of synaptic transmission are strongly influenced by pharmacological modulation of ACh (Bear & Singer, 1986; Kirkwood, Rozas, Kirkwood, Perez, & Bear, 1999), and reorganization of cortical representation of sensory information is facilitated by manipulations that increase ACh levels (Kilgard & Merzenich, 1998).

## PHYSIOLOGY OF ACh
## IN FRONTAL–SUBCORTICAL CIRCUITS

Much of the processing performed by the frontal lobe is accomplished by neural circuits that include the basal ganglia. Two primary cholinergic pathways exist in frontal–subcortical circuits: (1) afferent cholinergic projection neurons from the nBM to the frontal cortex, and (2) cholinergic interneurons within the striatum that receive large numbers of afferents from the thalamus and minor afferents form the cortex (Carpenter, 1981; Graybiel, 1998). These neurons synapse with GABA-ergic striatal output neurons. The basal ganglia cholinergic neurons are thought to play important modulatory roles for reinforcement learning. The PPN and dorsolateral tegmentum send afferents to the thalamus and may thus secondarily influence these circuits (Reese, Garcia-Rill, & Skinner, 1995).

The cholinergic synapses in the basal ganglia demonstrate a specific regional pattern of ACh receptor expression. Muscarinic $M_1$, $M_2$, and $M_4$ receptors are localized in the striatum (Levey, Kitt, Simonds, Price, & Brann, 1991). $M_1$ and $M_4$ are more dense in the neostriatum and nucleus accumbens. The $M_2$ receptor is localized in caudate putamen and nucleus accumbens. $M_3$ and $M_4$ receptors are present in the subthalamic nucleus (Chesselet & Delfs, 1996). Striatal ACh neurons receive three major afferents: from intrinsic, medium-size spiny neurons, from extrinsic dopaminergic neurons of the mesencephalic tegmentum, and from extrinsic glutamatergic neurons of the intralaminar thalamus. Neuronal nicotinic receptors are abundant in the striatum and substantia nigra (Perry, Court, Johnson, Piggott, & Perry, 1992), and nicotinic receptor activation modulates DA neurons and glutamatergic neurons within these structures (Dalack, Healy, & Meador-Woodruff, 1998). In this manner, ACh facilitates DA release from the striatum (Di Chiara & Morelli, 1993). ACh and DA exert opposite influences on stratopallidal and on striatonigral neurons by affecting different receptor subtypes ($D_1/D_2$; $M_1/M_4$; Di Chiara, Morelli, & Consolo, 1994). In turn blockade of the N-methyl-D-aspartate (NMDA) subtype of glutamate receptor decreases ACh release, and NMDA receptor activation increases ACh release.

## DIRECT EFFECTS OF ACh
## ON FRONTAL LOBE NEURONS

ACh has a role in modulating attention mediated by the frontal cortex. Two types of evidence from rodent models exist: (1) Lesions made with a selective immunotoxin for cholinergic neurons in the nBM mimic the effects of less specific lesions of the frontal lobe (McGaughy, Everitt, Robbins, & Sarter, 2000); and (2) microdialysis experiments reveal that ACh is released from the frontal cortex of the awake behaving rat (Passetti, Dalley, O'Connell, Everitt, & Robbins, 2000; Sarter & Bruno, 1997). Specific correlation between demands on attentional capacity and cortical ACh efflux is related to an increases in "background noise" (McGaughy & Sarter, 1995).

At the cellular level, ACh mediates the conditioned responses of cortical neurons and thus contributes to the enhanced processing of behaviorally significant stimuli (Pirch, 1993; Pirch, Rigdon, Rucker, & Turco, 1991). Local administration of Ach increases stimulation-elicited neuronal activity in the medial prefrontal cortex of rats (Andrade, 1991) and behavior-elicited neuronal activity in the orbitofrontal cortex of primates (Aou, Oomura, & Nishino, 1983). Pirch (1993) investigated the role of ACh in the conditioning of frontal cortical units. Sensory stimuli were paired with medial forebrain bundle stimulation, yielding an augmented discharge of these cortical neurons in response to the stimuli following training. Infusions of GABA or procaine into the basal forebrain result in the inhibition of cortical effects of Ach on the frontal cortex.

## TONIC VERSUS PHASIC EFFECTS OF CORTICAL ACh RELEASE

ACh is released into the cortex in two temporal patterns. Slow, tonic effects of ACh on cortical neurons globally enhance the processing of information, making subjects more receptive to sensory stimuli. Cortical Ach levels correlate with circadian rhythms, which provides the best evidence of tonic effects of Ach release on attention (Marrosu et al., 1995) Furthermore, cholinergic neuron activation in the basal forebrain increases wakefulness and suppression of rapid eye movement (REM) sleep, and is turn mediated by basal forebrain and thalamic neuronal activity in response to signals from brainstem cholinergic cells (Steriade, Datta, Pare, Oakson, & Curro Dossi, 1990).

The amplification of sensory information requires a more precise, phasic, stimulus-bound release of neurotransmitter. Richardson and DeLong (1991) stressed the significance of brief, phasic changes in basal forebrain neuronal activity as a result of the presentation of behaviorally significant stimuli and reward (Maho, Hars, Edeline, & Hennevin, 1995). They also proposed that the power of individual stimuli to activate the cortical ACh is a function of their "arousal" value. These phasic effects of ACh are restricted to defined sets of cortical neurons and local circuits (Robbins & Everitt, 1982; Steriade & Buzsaki, 1990).

## FROM STIMULUS AMPLIFICATION TO ATTENTION

The role of cortical cholinergic inputs in the detection and selection of stimuli and associations for processing (i.e., attentional functions) is apparent from the potent effects of basal forebrain lesions on the performance of animals in procedures taxing various aspects of attention support (Chiba, Bucci, Holland, & Gallagher, 1995). Sarter and Bruno (1997) tested the effects of selective lesions of the

cholinergic neurons of the basal forebrain on sustained attention and vigilance. They infused a potent immunotoxin (192IgG-saporin) into the basal forebrain, which caused a selective lesion of cholinergic neurons projecting to the cortex, but not those projecting to the amygdalae. The result was impairment in the animals' ability to detect visual signals of various lengths. The animals' ability to reject correctly nonsignal trials was not affected, supporting the exclusive role of cortical ACh in the detection of signals. Also the animals' ability to retrieve and execute the response rules was spared.

The selectivity of the effects of manipulations of cortical cholinergic afferents on behavioral vigilance suggests that these effects were not due to secondary, nonspecific changes in the animals' behavior. The effects of the noradrenergic system on sustained attention support this hypothesis. Although cortical norepinephrine (NE) levels were decreased by over 90% following 6-hydroxydopamine infusions into the dorsal noradrenergic bundle, the animals' performance remained unaffected (Ruland, Ronis, Bruno, & Sarter, 1995). Yu and Dayan (2005) conducted a meta-analysis of data from different attentional tasks using a computational model designed to simulate the effects of changes in ACh and NE levels. They noted independent but complementary effects of ACh and NE on attention in classic tasks such as the Attention Network Test (ANT). Specifically ACh signaled *expected* uncertainty, whereas NE signaled *unexpected* uncertainty. At times, the predicted effects of depletion of these neurotransmitters were antagonistic, such that effects of ACh depletion were ameliorated by NE depletion. These data support an independent and central role of ACh in amplifying certain types of sensory information.

## DEPENDENCE OF ATTENTIONAL ABILITIES ON THE INTEGRITY OF THE AGGREGATE OF CORTICAL CHOLINERGIC INPUTS

Cholinergic deafferentation throughout the neocortex is necessary to induce significant impairments in attentional functions. For example, the effects of the loss of cortical cholinergic afferents on behavioral vigilance, as assessed by a visual vigilance task, are not primarily due to a loss of cholinergic inputs to the visual cortex. Intracortical infusions of the immunotoxin

192IgG-saporin into the primary and secondary visual cortex did not produce a robust change in performance in this task (Sarter, Hasselmo, Bruno, & Givens, 2005). This finding supports the view that sustained attention does not primarily reflect the efficacy of perceptual processes. Because the perceptual demands of this task requires stimulus discrimination not involving spatial frequencies, manipulations in primary or secondary visual cortex functions would not be expected to produce major effects (Pasternak, Tompkins, & Olson, 1995). In this context, it is important to note that the presentation of signals of various lengths is intended to tax more effectively attentional capacity and not perceptual functions (Parasuraman & Mouloua, 1987).

Ongoing studies aimed at defining the critical amount and location of cortical cholinergic inputs for maintaining intact attentional abilities use intracortical infusions of 192IgG-saporin to disconnect specific cortical areas from their cholinergic inputs. The available data provide the basis for the working hypothesis that a minimum loss of approximately 50% of cortical cholinergic inputs in the anterior half of the cortex is required to yield impairments in behavioral vigilance (Sarter & Bruno, 1997).

## CORTICAL ACh AND ATTENTION: AFFERENT CONTROL OF CHOLINERGIC ACTIVITY AND THE SPECIFICITY OF ACh-MEDIATED CORTICAL PROCESSING

The cholinergic system is unlikely to "know" about the specific cortical input to be amplified and, in anatomical terms, is not organized to selectively activate individual cortical target neurons. In other words, the cholinergic system is not "prewired" for all possible stimuli; therefore, it is thought that the preparation for enhanced cortical processing of sensory inputs and associations is global (Mesulam, 1990). Although it may be trivial to note that the attentional functions of cortical ACh that emerge from the collective amplifying effects are not independent of the subjects' global behavioral state, the relationships between the role of cortical ACh in circadian rhythms and patterns of wakefulness versus those responsible for the processing of sensory inputs and associations are largely unknown. One possibility is that these two components of cortical

cholinergic function might be attributed to different afferent networks, that is, the ascending projections from brainstem nuclei to the basal forebrain and thalamus may regulate sleep and wakefulness, whereas the attention-mediating effects of cortical ACh may be triggered by the regulation of activity of basal forebrain cholinergic neurons by mesolimbic, cortical, and amygdaloid afferents (Chiba et al., 1995). In general functional terms, the limbic and cortical networks that converge on the basal forebrain provide information about the behavioral significance of stimuli based on previous experience, motivation, and behavioral context (Wilson & Rolls, 1993).

Evidence suggests that attention-associated changes in cortical ACh release vary with attentional demands over a time course of minutes (Sarter et al., 1996). If generally true, effects of ACh on higher cortical function operate in a more tonic that phasic manner. The hypothesis that increases in cortical ACh release remain relatively stable over the period of time during which demands on attentional abilities are presented is supported by the finding that acetylcholinesterase inhibitors partly ameliorate the attentional impairments due to partial basal forebrain lesions (Muir, Dunnett, Robbins, & Everitt, 1992; Muir, Everitt, & Robbins, 1995) or to degenerative cell loss (Giacobini, 1994). However, the relative ineffectiveness of systemically administered cholinesterase inhibitors in boosting attention in other experimental paradigms suggests that, under some conditions, pharmacological approaches that further dissociate postsynaptic muscarinic receptor stimulation from presynaptic cholinergic activity may interfere with optimal information processing (Sarter & Bruno, 1994).

## FUNCTIONAL NEUROIMAGING STUDIES OF ACh AND ATTENTION IN HUMANS

Functional magnetic resonance imaging (fMRI) studies have explored the association between attention and the cholinergic system using acetylcholinesterase inhibitors such as physostigmine and muscarinic ACh receptor blockers such as scopolamine. Furey and colleagues (1997) found improvement in stimulus processing in healthy volunteers using the cholinesterase inhibitor physostigmine. In this study the effects of enhancing cholinergic neurotransmission on a visual working memory task for faces were explored. Increased blood oxygenation level–dependent (BOLD) activity in the extrastriate cortex, particularly during the encoding portion of the task was observed, suggesting that information processing is enhanced by cholinergic neurotransmission. The same group explored the effects of decreased ACh signaling at muscarinic receptors on auditory conditioning with fMRI by administering scopolamine to subjects performing the task. Experience-dependent activations in human auditory cortex were blocked after scopolamine treatment (Thiel, Bentley, & Dolan, 2002). In a follow-up study, the same paradigm was used to investigate effects of cholinergic enhancement on conditioning-related auditory cortical responses (Thiel, Friston, & Dolan, 2002). Contrary to expectations, it was found that physostigmine reduced the conditioning-specific activity by increasing activations to irrelevant stimuli. In summary, these studies suggest that blockade of cholinergic neurotransmission reduces processing of relevant stimuli, whereas too much, or poorly regulated, cholinergic neurotransmission increases processing of irrelevant stimuli. This latter finding likely explains the lack of efficacy of cholinesterase inhibitors in many experimental and clinical situations.

Cholinergic projections may modulate attention- and emotion-related activity in distinct parts of extrastriate and frontoparietal cortices (Bentley et al., 2003). Attention and emotional processing can independently activate the fusiform gyri in subjects treated with physostigmine. However this medication decreased activation in the posterolateral occipital cortex during the attention task. Physostigmine also modulated responses to emotional stimuli depending on whether they were task-irrelevant (in orbitofrontal and intraparietal cortices) or task-relevant (in dorsolateral and medial prefrontal cortices).

The same researchers explored the effect of physostigmine on attention using an fMRI task that presented simple visual stimuli and spatial stimuli that required a shift of attention. The visual control task activated primary visual cortex and lateral occipital cortices in both placebo- and physostigmine-treated subjects (Bentley et al., 2004). A treatment effect was seen in primary visual cortex, with physostigmine reducing stimulus-evoked BOLD activity compared to placebo. In the spatial

attention task, a direct comparison of physostigmine- and placebo-treated subjects showed that these regions were differentially modulated by cholinergic enhancement with physostigmine: Extrastriate cortex and prefrontal cortex showed enhanced activity, whereas dorsomedial parietal cortex showed reduced differential activity after cortical ACh levels were increased with physostigmine (Figure 10.2). This is of interest because dorsomedial parietal cortex activity is thought to reflect a default mode in which the brain is awaiting new stimuli, whereas the regions activated in the frontal and extrastriate cortex are involved in processing visual stimuli and programming shifts of attention (Corbetta, Kincade, & Shulman, 2002). Physostigmine enhanced the degree of activation in both hemi-

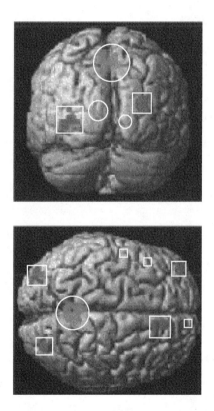

FIGURE 10.2. Effects of increasing cortical ACh levels with physostigmine on cortical activity during a visual attention task. Surface rendering of regions show activity during delay periods of attention versus control tasks after treatment with placebo (circles) or physostigmine (squares). From Bentley et al. (2004). Copyright 2004 by Elsevier. Reprinted by permission.

spheres, most significantly in the extrastriate region ipsilateral to the visual hemifield to which a stimulus was presented. Thus, cholinergic modulation of visual cortex occurs with presentation of both simple stimuli in the striate cortex and attention-demanding tasks in extrastriate cortex and premotor cortex. These studies suggest that physostigmine reduces the degree of occipital activity associated with attention, and that this hypercholinergic state is associated with heightened processing of irrelevant information. Taken together, these data are highly consistent with data obtained in animal experiments and support a model by which ACh acts in both a task-driven (top-down modulation) and a stimulus-driven (bottom-up modulation) manner to enhance attention (Sarter, Givens, & Bruno, 2001).

# REFERENCES

Andrade, R. (1991). Cell excitation enhances muscarinic cholinergic responses in rat association cortex. *Brain Research, 548,* 81–93.

Aou, S., Oomura, Y., & Nishino, H. (1983). Influence of acetylcholine on neuronal activity in monkey orbitofrontal cortex during bar press feeding task. *Brain Research, 275,* 178–182.

Barkai, E., & Hasselmo, M. E. (1994). Modulation of the input/output function of rat piriform cortex pyramidal cells. *Journal of Neurophysiology, 72,* 644–658.

Bear, M. F., & Singer, W. (1986). Modulation of visual cortical plasticity by acetylcholine and noradrenaline. *Nature, 320,* 172–176.

Bentley, P., Husain, M., & Dolan, R. J. (2004). Effects of cholinergic enhancement on visual stimulation, spatial attention, and spatial working memory. *Neuron, 41,* 969–982.

Bentley, P., Vuilleumier, P., Thiel, C. M., Driver, J., & Dolan, R. J. (2003). Cholinergic enhancement modulates neural correlates of selective attention and emotional processing. *NeuroImage, 20,* 58–70.

Brocher, S., Artola, A., & Singer, W. (1992). Agonists of cholinergic and noradrenergic receptors facilitate synergistically the induction of long-term potentiation in slices of rat visual cortex. *Brain Research, 573,* 27–36.

Carpenter, M. B. (1981). Anatomy of the corpus striatum and brain stem integrating system. In V. B. Brooks (Ed.), *Handbook of physiology: Section 1. The nervous system II* (pp. 947–955). Bethesda, MD: American Physiological Society.

Chesselet, M. F., & Delfs, J. M. (1996). Basal ganglia and movement disorders: An update. *Trends in Neurosciences, 19,* 417–422.

Chiba, A. A., Bucci, D. J., Holland, P. C., & Gallagher, M. (1995). Basal forebrain cholinergic lesions disrupt increments but not decrements in conditioned stimulus processing. *Journal of Neuroscience, 15,* 7315–7322.

Cohen, J. D., Aston-Jones, G., & Gilzenrat, M. S. (2004). A systems-level perspective on attention and cognitive control. In M. I. Posner (Ed.), *Cognitive neuroscience of attention* (pp. 71–90). New York: Guilford Press.

Corbetta, M., Akbudak, E., Conturo, T. E., Snyder, A. Z., Ollinger, J. M., Drury, H. A., et al. (1998). A common network of functional areas for attention and eye movements. *Neuron, 21,* 761–773.

Corbetta, M., Kincade, J. M., & Shulman, G. L. (2002). Neural systems for visual orienting and their relationships to spatial working memory. *Journal of Cognitive Neuroscience, 14,* 508–523.

Dalack, G. W., Healy, D. J., & Meador-Woodruff, J. H. (1998). Nicotine dependence in schizophrenia: Clinical phenomena and laboratory findings. *American Journal of Psychiatry, 155,* 1490–1501.

Di Chiara, G., & Morelli, M. (1993). Dopamine–acetylcholine–glutamate interactions in the striatum: A working hypothesis. *Advances in Neurology, 60,* 102–106.

Di Chiara, G., Morelli, M., & Consolo, S. (1994). Modulatory functions of neurotransmitters in the striatum: ACh/dopamine/NMDA interactions. *Trends in Neurosciences, 17,* 228–233.

Fan, J., McCandliss, B. D., Fossella, J., Flombaum, J. I., & Posner, M. I. (2005). The activation of attentional networks. *NeuroImage, 26*(2), 471–479.

Furey, M. L., Pietrini, P., Haxby, J. V., Alexander, G. E., Lee, H. C., Vanmeter, J., et al. (1997). Cholinergic stimulation alters performance and task-specific regional cerebral blood flow during working memory. *Proceedings of the National Academy of Sciences of the United States of America, 94,* 6512–6516.

Giacobini, E. (1994). Therapy for Alzheimer's disease: Symptomatic or neuroprotective? *Molecular Neurobiology, 9,* 115–118.

Gray, R., Rajan, A. S., Radcliffe, K. A., Yakehiro, M., & Dani, J. A. (1996). Hippocampal synaptic transmission enhanced by low concentrations of nicotine. *Nature, 383,* 713–716.

Graybiel, A. M. (1998). The basal ganglia and chunking of action repertoires. *Neurobiology of Learning and Memory, 70,* 119–136.

Hasselmo, M. E., & Bower, J. M. (1993). Acetylcholine and memory. *Trends in Neurosciences, 16,* 218–222.

Hasselmo, M. E., & Cekic, M. (1996). Suppression of synaptic transmission may allow combination of associative feedback and self-organizing feedforward connections in the neocortex. *Behavioural Brain Research, 79,* 153–161.

James, W. (1890). *Principles of psychology.* New York: Holt.

Kilgard, M. P., & Merzenich, M. M. (1998). Cortical map reorganization enabled by nucleus basalis activity. *Science, 279,* 1714–1718.

Kirkwood, A., Rozas, C., Kirkwood, J., Perez, F., & Bear, M. F. (1999). Modulation of long-term synaptic depression in visual cortex by acetylcholine and norepinephrine. *Journal of Neuroscience, 19,* 1599–1609.

Krnjevic, K., & Phillis, J. W. (1963). Acetylcholine-sensitive cells in the cerebral cortex. *Journal of Physiology, 166,* 296–327.

Levey, A. I., Kitt, C. A., Simonds, W. F., Price, D. L., & Brann, M. R. (1991). Identification and localization of muscarinic acetylcholine receptor proteins in brain with subtype-specific antibodies. *Journal of Neuroscience, 11,* 3218–3226.

Maho, C., Hars, B., Edeline, J. W., & Hennevin, E. (1995). Conditioned changes in the basal forebrain: Relations with learning-induced cortical plasticity. *Psychobiology, 23,* 10–25.

Marrosu, F., Portas, C., Mascia, M. S., Casu, M. A., Fa, M., Giagheddu, M., et al. (1995). Microdialysis measurement of cortical and hippocampal acetylcholine release during sleep–wake cycle in freely moving cats. *Brain Research, 671,* 329–332.

McGaughy, J., Everitt, B. J., Robbins, T. W., & Sarter, M. (2000). The role of cortical cholinergic afferent projections in cognition: Impact of new selective immunotoxins. *Behavioural Brain Research, 115,* 251–263.

McGaughy, J., & Sarter, M. (1995). Behavioral vigilance in rats: Task validation and effects of age, amphetamine, and benzodiazepine receptor ligands. *Psychopharmacology (Berlin), 117,* 340–357.

McQuiston, A. R., & Madison, D. V. (1999). Muscarinic receptor activity induces an afterdepolarization in a subpopulation of hippocampal CA1 interneurons. *Journal of Neuroscience, 19,* 5703–5710.

Meredith, G. E., & Wouterlood, F. G. (1990). Hippocampal and midline thalamic fibers and terminals in relation to the choline acetyltransferase-immunoreactive neurons in nucleus accumbens of the rat: A light and electron microscopic study. *Journal of Comparative Neurology, 296*(2), 204–221.

Mesulam, M. M. (1990). Large-scale neurocognitive networks and distributed processing for attention, language, and memory. *Annals of Neurology, 28,* 597–613.

Mesulam, M. M. (2004). The cholinergic innervation of the human cerebral cortex. *Progress in Brain Research, 145,* 67–78.

Mooney, D. M., Zhang, L., Basile, C., Senatorov, V. V., Ngsee, J., Omar, A., et al. (2004). Distinct forms of cholinergic modulation in parallel thalamic sensory pathways. *Proceedings of the National Academy of Science, 101*(1), 320–324.

Muir, J. L., Dunnett, S. B., Robbins, T. W., & Everitt, B. J. (1992). Attentional functions of the forebrain cholinergic systems: Effects of intraventricular hemicholinium, physostigmine, basal forebrain lesions and intracortical grafts on a multiple-choice serial reaction time task. *Experimental Brain Research, 89,* 611–622.

Muir, J. L., Everitt, B. J., & Robbins, T. W. (1995). Reversal of visual attentional dysfunction following lesions of the cholinergic basal forebrain by physostigmine and nicotine but not by the 5-HT$_3$ receptor antagonist, ondansetron. *Psychopharmacology (Berlin), 118,* 82–92.

Parasuraman, R., & Mouloua, M. (1987). Interaction of signal discriminability and task type in vigilance decrement. *Perception and Psychophysics, 41,* 17–22.

Passetti, F., Dalley, J. W., O'Connell, M. T., Everitt, B. J., & Robbins, T. W. (2000). Increased acetylcholine release in the rat medial prefrontal cortex during performance of a visual attentional task. *European Journal of Neuroscience, 12,* 3051–3058.

Pasternak, T., Tompkins, J., & Olson, C. R. (1995). The role of striate cortex in visual function of the cat. *Journal of Neuroscience, 15,* 1940–1950.

Perry, E. K., Court, J. A., Johnson, M., Piggott, M. A., & Perry, R. H. (1992). Autoradiographic distribution of [$^3$H]nicotine binding in human cortex: Relative abundance in subicular complex. *Journal of Chemical Neuroanatomy, 5,* 399–405.

Pirch, J., Rigdon, G., Rucker, H., & Turco, K. (1991). Basal forebrain modulation of cortical cell activity during conditioning. *Advances in Experimental Medicine and Biology, 295,* 219–231.

Pirch, J. H. (1993). Basal forebrain and frontal cortex neuron responses during visual discrimination in the rat. *Brain Research Bulletin, 31,* 73–83.

Reece, L. J., & Schwartzkroin, P. A. (1991). Effects of cholinergic agonists on two non-pyramidal cell types in rat hippocampal slices. *Brain Research, 566,* 115–126.

Reese, N. B., Garcia-Rill, E., & Skinner, R. D. (1995). The pedunculopontine nucleus—auditory input, arousal and pathophysiology. *Progress in Neurobiology, 47,* 105–133.

Richardson, R. T., & De Long, M. R. (1991). Functional implications of tonic and phasic activity changes in nucleus basalis neurons. In R. T. Richardson (Ed.), *Activation to acquisition: Functional aspects of the basal forebrain cholinergic system* (pp. 135–166). Boston: Birkhauser.

Robbins, T. W., & Everitt, B. J. (1982). Functional studies of the central catecholamines. *International Review of Neurobiology, 23,* 303–365.

Robbins, T. W., Milstein, J. A., & Dalley, J. W. (2004). Neuropharmacology of attention. In M. I. Posner (Ed.), *Cognitive neuroscience of attention* (pp. 283–293). New York: Guilford Press.

Ruland, S., Ronis, V., Bruno, J. P., & Sarter, M. (1995). Effects of lesions of the dorsal noradrenergic bundle on behavioral vigilance. *Society for Neuroscience Abstracts, 21,* 1944.

Sarter, M., & Bruno, J. P. (1994). Cognitive functions of cortical ACh: Lessons from studies on trans-synaptic modulation of activated efflux. *Trends in Neurosciences, 17,* 217–221.

Sarter, M., & Bruno, J. P. (1997). Cognitive functions of

cortical acetylcholine: Toward a unifying hypothesis. *Brain Research: Brain Research Reviews, 23*, 28–46.

Sarter, M., Bruno, J. P., Givens, B., Moore, H., McGaughty, J., & McMahon, K. (1996). Neuronal mechanisms mediating drug-induced cognition enhancement: Cognitive activity as a necessary intervening variable. *Brain Research: Cognitive Brain Research, 3*, 329–343.

Sarter, M., Givens, B., & Bruno, J. P. (2001). The cognitive neuroscience of sustained attention: Where top-down meets bottom-up. *Brain Research: Brain Research Reviews, 35*, 146–160.

Sarter, M., Hasselmo, M. E., Bruno, J. P., & Givens, B. (2005). Unraveling the attentional functions of cortical cholinergic inputs: Interactions between signal-driven and cognitive modulation of signal detection. *Brain Research: Brain Research Reviews, 48*, 98–111.

Sparks, D. L. (2002). The brainstem control of saccadic eye movements. *Nature Reviews: Neuroscience, 3*, 952–964.

Steriade, M., & Buzsaki, G. (1990). Parallel activation of thalamic and cortical neurons by brainstem and forebrain cholinergic system. In M. Steriade & D. Biesold (Eds.), *Brain cholinergic system* (pp. 3–62). Oxford, UK: Oxford University Press.

Steriade, M., Datta, S., Pare, D., Oakson, G., & Curro

Dossi, R. C. (1990). Neuronal activities in brain-stem cholinergic nuclei related to tonic activation processes in thalamocortical systems. *Journal of Neuroscience, 10*, 2541–2559.

Thiel, C. M., Bentley, P., & Dolan, R. J. (2002). Effects of cholinergic enhancement on conditioning-related responses in human auditory cortex. *European Journal of Neuroscience, 16*, 2199–2206.

Thiel, C. M., Friston, K. J., & Dolan, R. J. (2002). Cholinergic modulation of experience-dependent plasticity in human auditory cortex. *Neuron, 35*, 567–574.

Valentino, R. J., & Dingledine, R. (1981). Presynaptic inhibitory effect of acetylcholine in the hippocampus. *Journal of Neuroscience, 1*, 784–792.

Vidal, C., & Changeux, J. P. (1993). Nicotinic and muscarinic modulations of excitatory synaptic transmission in the rat prefrontal cortex *in vitro. Neuroscience, 56*, 23–32.

Wilson, F. A., & Rolls, E. T. (1993). The effects of stimulus novelty and familiarity on neuronal activity in the amygdala of monkeys performing recognition memory tasks. *Experimental Brain Research, 93*, 367–382.

Yu, A. J., & Dayan, P. (2005). Uncertainty, neuromodulation, and attention. *Neuron, 46*, 681–692.

# CHAPTER 11

# The Mesocortical Dopaminergic System

*Antonello Bonci*
*Susan Jones*

Midbrain dopaminergic (DA-ergic) neurons of the ventral tegmental area (VTA) and substantia nigra pars compacta (SNc) play a central role in behaviors ranging from movement control to higher cognitive functions, including motivation, reward, learning, and memory. In addition, altered DA-ergic function is implicated in pathological conditions such as Parkinson's disease, dementias, drug addiction, schizophrenia, depression, and eating disorders. Despite more than 30 years of multidisciplinary studies of the physiology, pharmacology, and pathology of midbrain dopamine (DA) nuclei and their projections, the exact role that DA plays in these disorders is still poorly understood. For example, the initial evidence linking DA and drug addiction came from studies showing that acute exposure to many drugs of abuse increases extracellular DA levels (Di Chiara & Imperato, 1988; Robinson & Berridge, 1993). Since then, scientists have taken new "snapshots" of DA levels and of DA receptor activity at several time points related to both acute and chronic drug exposure. However, too many frames are still missing for us to be able to make sense of the sequence of events linking DA to addiction.

The midbrain DA nuclei A8 (retrorubral), A9 (SNc), and A10 (VTA), contain 70–80% of brain DA (Grillner & Mercuri, 2002). Although DA neurons of the SNc and the VTA are anatomically, physiologically, and pharmacologically similar, they are functionally independent. The A10 VTA DA neurons consist of a group of loosely defined nuclei, including parabrachial, paranigral, rostral and caudal linear, and interfascicular nuclei (Kalivas, 1993). This medial group of midbrain DA nuclei project predominantly to limbic and cortical regions, so they are commonly referred to as mesolimbic and mesocortical systems, respectively, and are collectively referred to as the mesocorticolimbic DA system. This chapter focuses on the mesocortical neurons, since our main goal is to summarize our current knowledge about the anatomy and physiology of the mesocortical DA system.

## INTRINSIC CIRCUITRY OF THE VTA

Traditionally, the VTA was thought to consist of two main neuronal populations: the DA neurons (or primary neurons), representing the majority of cells, and γ-aminobutyric acid (GABA)-ergic neurons (or secondary cells), acting merely as local circuit neurons that synapse onto DA neurons (Johnson & North, 1992; Lacey, Mercuri, & North, 1989) (Figure 11.1). Recent studies, however, have suggested that the VTA in fact contains at least three main neuronal populations on the basis of their electrophysiological (intrinsic conductances), pharmacological (response to DA, opioids, and serotonin), and biochemical (presence of tyrosine hydroxylase) properties (Cameron, Wessendorf, & Williams, 1997; Margolis et al., 2003). For this reason, VTA neurons are

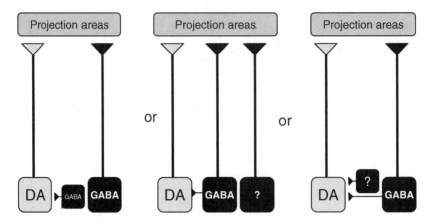

FIGURE 11.1. Schematic representation of the three types of neurons present in the VTA, namely, the primary (DA), secondary (GABA), and tertiary.

now called primary, secondary and tertiary. Whereas primary neurons of the VTA are still considered to be DA-ergic, and secondary neurons are GABA-ergic, the exact biochemical identity of the "tertiary neurons" is still under investigation.

## PHYSIOLOGICAL PROPERTIES OF VTA NEURONS

When compared to GABA-ergic neurons within the VTA, DA neuron action potentials have a longer duration (> 1 msec) and a larger after-hyperpolarization. DA neurons also have a time-dependent, hyperpolarization-activated, nonselective cation conductance (Mercuri, Bonci, Calabresi, Stefani, & Bernardi, 1995) that distinguishes them from GABA-ergic neurons, but not from tertiary neurons (Cameron et al., 1997; Margolis et al., 2003).

*In vivo*, VTA DA neurons exhibit two main patterns of firing activity: single-spike firing, often irregular, and burst firing (Grace & Bunney, 1984a, 1984b; Overton & Clark, 1997; Tepper, Martin, & Anderson, 1995) (Figure 11.2). When spikes of DA neurons are clustered into bursts, the increase in extracellular DA in the projection areas is much greater than that observed for regularly spaced trains of action potential at the same average frequency, due to supralinear summation (Bean & Roth, 1991; Gonon, 1988; Suaud-Chagny, Chergui, Chouvet, & Gonon, 1992). One possible explanation is that DA release outpaces DA uptake (Cragg & Rice, 2004; Wightman & Zimmerman, 1990). *In vivo*, DA neurons can also fire in a pacemaker mode, and this is thought to produce persistent release of relatively small amounts of DA (Overton & Clark, 1997).

Behavioral studies in rodents and primates have demonstrated that DA neurons respond in a phasic manner to novel, unexpected stimuli, such as rewards, as well as to conditioned cues

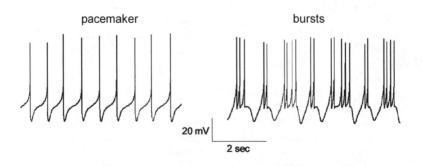

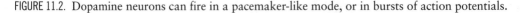

FIGURE 11.2. Dopamine neurons can fire in a pacemaker-like mode, or in bursts of action potentials.

that signal rewards (Schultz, 2002). These studies suggest that burst firing of VTA DA neurons encodes the occurrence of nonspecific, unexpected stimuli, or salient stimuli with a positive valence. Thus, highly processed information is being transmitted by DA neurons to the forebrain as phasic bursts of activity, and these patterns of activity might facilitate the expression of various physiological and pathological behaviors related to motivation.

With the exception of *in vivo* burst firing patterns, the physiological features of DA neurons are also readily observed *in vitro* with use of a brain slice preparation, suggesting that many physiological properties result from intrinsic Na$^+$, Ca$^{2+}$, and K$^+$ conductances in DA neurons (Grace & Onn, 1989; Overton & Clark, 1997; White, 1996). *In vitro*, DA neurons typically fire in a regular "pacemaker" pattern at 1–5 Hz, and evidence suggests that the irregular and burst firing patterns observed *in vivo* are dependent on afferent excitatory input. Burst firing patterns similar to those observed *in vivo* can be reproduced *in vitro* by bath application of N-methyl-D-aspartate (NMDA) (Komendantov, Komendantova, Johnson, & Canavier, 2004; Seutin, Johnson, & North, 1994). Furthermore, an increase in burst firing is also produced (or facilitated in the presence of NMDA) by the bath application of the calcium-activated, small K$^+$ conductance (I$_{SKCa2}$$^+$) blocker, apamin (Komendantov et al., 2004; Nedergaard, Flatman, & Engberg, 1993; Paul, Keith, & Johnson, 2003; Ping & Shepard, 1996; Seutin, Johnson, & North, 1993).

Identifying the potential importance of bursting activity of DA neurons, leading to increased DA release, in mediating addictive behaviors has been the object of a significant amount of research (reviewed in Berridge & Robinson, 2003; Wise, 2004).

## PROJECTIONS TO AND FROM THE VTA

Several lines of evidence suggest that within the VTA, the mesolimbic and mesocortical DA neurons form two anatomically distinct projection pathways (Albanese & Minciacchi, 1983; Berger, Thierry, Tassin, & Moyne, 1976; Deniau, Thierry, & Feger, 1980; Fallon, 1981; Lindvall, Bjorklund, & Divac, 1978; Palkovits et al., 1979; Simon, Scatton, & Le Moal, 1979; Slopsema, van der Gugten, & de Bruin, 1982;

Swanson, 1982). The mesolimbic projections of VTA DA neurons are primarily directed to the nucleus accumbens (NAcc), olfactory tubercle, amygdala, and septum, whereas mesocortical projections are mainly to frontal cortex, cingulate cortex, and perirhinal cortex (Fallon & Loughlin, 1985, 1987; Swanson, 1982) (Figure 11.3). VTA DA neurons also project to other neocortical areas (Berger, Gaspar, & Verney, 1991; Berger, Verney, Febvret, Vigny, & Helle, 1985) as well as to the cerebellum (Ikai et al., 1992), hypothalamus, hippocampus, ventral pallidum, locus coeruleus, and dorsal raphe (Fallon & Moore, 1978; Faull & Mehler, 1978; Gasbarri, Campana, Pacitti, Hajdu, & Tombol, 1991; Gerfen, Staines, Arbuthnott, & Fibiger, 1982; Kilpatrick, Starr, Fletcher, James, & MacLeod, 1980; Kizer, Palkovits, & Brownstein, 1976; Klitenick, Deutch, Churchill, & Kalivas, 1992; Simon, Le Moal, Stinus, & Calasa, 1979), and the dorsolateral geniculate nucleus (Papadopulous & Parnavelas, 1990).

The notion that GABA-ergic neurons in the VTA are exclusively exerting their physiological actions as local interneurons has been challenged by recently rediscovered evidence. Although previous studies suggested that non-DA neurons projected to the prefrontal cortex (PFC) (Albanese & Minciacchi, 1983; Ferron, Thierry, Le Douarin, & Glowinski, 1984; Swanson, 1982; Thierry, Deniau, Herve, & Chevalier, 1980), these studies did not receive proper attention for several years. Results from more recent studies drew new interest to this issue (Carr & Sesack, 2000a; Steffensen, Svingos, Pickel, & Henriksen, 1998; Van Bockstaele & Pickel, 1995), and provided further anatomical and electrophysiological evidence that a subpopulation of GABA-containing neurons in the VTA project to the NAcc and to the PFC. GABA-ergic projection neurons in the VTA also send a significant projection to the visual cortex (Dinopaulos & Parnevalas, 1991) (Figure 11.4). Other, less anatomically conspicuous projections of non-DA VTA neurons innervate the hypothalamus, the central gray, the locus coeruleus, the lateral habenula, the raphe, and several cerebellar nuclei (dorsal and interposed nuclei and cortex of the cerebellum) (Kalivas, 1993) (Figure 11.3).

Taken together, these studies suggest that although attention has largely focused on mesocorticolimbic projections of VTA DA neurons, VTA DA and GABA neurons send diffuse pro-

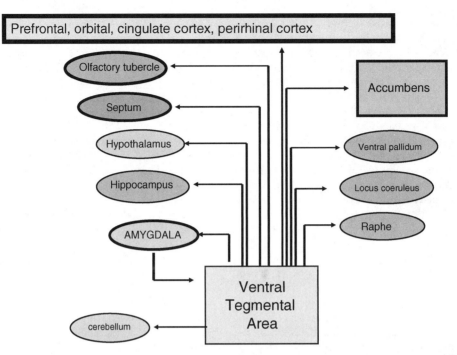

FIGURE 11.3. Schematic representation of the dopaminergic projections from the VTA.

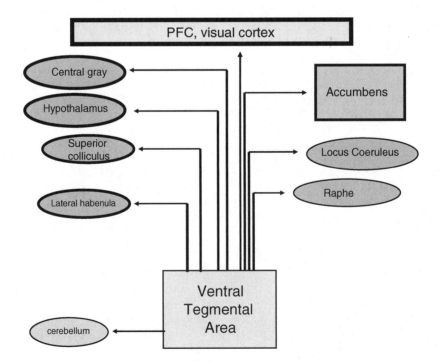

FIGURE 11.4. Schematic representation of the nondopaminergic projections from the VTA.

jections throughout the central nervous system. Furthermore, the DA-ergic and GABA-ergic projections overlap anatomically on the primary brain regions that control "behavioral planning" and goal-directed behaviors, such as the PFC and NAcc. It is tempting to speculate that simultaneous activation of DA- and GABA-ergic neurons would increase coherent release of both neurotransmitters, thus contributing to increase the signal-to-noise ratio and possibly improve the specificity of behavioral responses. On the other hand, DA and GABA projection neurons might be recruited under different behavioral conditions, dependent on the afferent input to VTA neuronal populations.

## AFFERENT CONTROL OF THE VTA

The activity of VTA DA-ergic neurons is under the physiological control of several neurotransmitter systems (Grillner & Mercuri, 2002; Kalivas, 1993; White, 1996) (Figure 11.5). These include GABA, from local GABA-releasing cells and from GABA-ergic projections from the basal ganglia; glutamate, from several brain regions including PFC, hippocampus, amygdala, and pontine nuclei via both direct and indirect projections; ascending biogenic amine systems, including noradrenaline from locus coeruleus and serotonin from the raphe nuclei; acetylcholine from pontine nuclei; and various neuropeptides (Phillipson, 1979). Importantly, DA itself is released somatodendritically within the VTA (Beckstead, Grandy, Wickman, & Williams, 2004). The balance of afferent input to the VTA and the activation of different neurotransmitter receptors on different VTA neurons determines the overall output activity of VTA DA neurons. Furthermore, these afferent inputs are possible targets for addictive drugs, as well as for current pharmacological therapies in psychiatric disorders, including schizophrenia and depression. Here, we focus on afferent control by the two major neurotransmitter systems in the brain, GABA (inhibitory) and glutamate (excitatory), as well as by the biogenic amines DA and serotonin, whose receptors are considered important in disorders of mesocorticolimbic function such as addiction, schizophrenia, and depression.

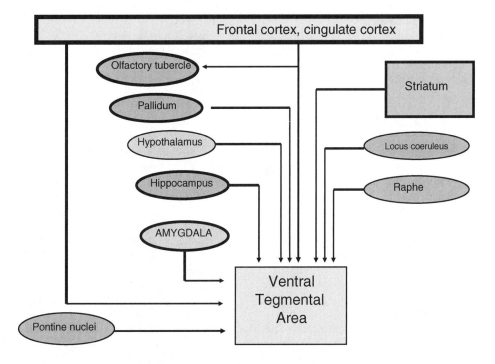

FIGURE 11.5. Schematic representation of the afferent projections to the VTA.

## γ-Aminobutyric Acid

GABA is released both from local GABA-ergic neurons intrinsic to the VTA and from extrinsic GABA-ergic projections to the VTA from basal ganglia nuclei, notably from the NAcc and from the ventral pallidum (Kalivas, 1993; White, 1996). GABA-ergic synapses are found on both DA and non-DA neurons in the VTA (Kalivas, 1993). Both $GABA_A$ and $GABA_B$ receptors are present in the VTA (Kalivas, 1993; Okada, Matsushita, Kobayashi, & Kobayashi, 2004). $GABA_A$ receptor subtypes are found in DA and non-DA neurons; therefore, $GABA_A$ receptor agonists have complex effects on DA neuronal activity via both direct inhibitory and indirect disinhibitory mechanisms (Kalivas, 1993). $GABA_B$ receptor agonists cause hyperpolarization of DA neurons via activation of $K^+$ conductances (Lacey, Mercuri, & North, 1988), and reduce voltage-gated $Ca^{2+}$ currents (Cardozo & Bean, 1995). Electrical stimulation of GABA-ergic afferents to VTA DA cells elicits inhibitory postsynaptic potentials (IPSPs) mediated by both $GABA_A$ receptors and $GABA_B$ receptors (Johnson & North, 1992). The $GABA_B$ receptor agonist baclofen also decreases glutamatergic synaptic transmission onto DA neurons, but not onto non-DA neurons (Bonci & Malenka, 1999).

Intrinsic and extrinsic sources of GABA are likely to serve distinct physiological roles in their regulation of DA neuronal activity. Extrinsic sources come from projection targets for VTA DA neurons and are possibly engaged in long-loop feedback (Kalivas, 1993; White, 1996). Local circuit GABA-ergic neurons show high firing rates *in vivo*, whereas *in vitro* they either fire at high frequency or are silent. It is likely that local GABA-ergic neurons provide tonic inhibition of DA neuronal activity, such that one mechanism of activating DA neurons is through a process of disinhibition. It is tempting to speculate that VTA GABA-ergic neurons might play a role in coordinating the firing patterns of populations of DA neurons (Komendantov et al., 2004). Furthermore, it has been suggested that some level of $GABA_A$ receptor activation within the VTA might help to optimize the efficiency of burst firing of DA neurons, by slightly hyperpolarizing them (Komendantov et al., 2004). Thus, local levels of GABA in the VTA are likely to play a key role in determining the output of VTA DA and GABA projection neurons to their common targets, and might be required to coordinate simultaneous coherent release of DA and GABA in target regions, or to select the balance in favor of one or the other.

## Glutamate

The PFC sends monosynaptic excitatory projections to VTA DA neurons (Carr & Sesack, 2000b; Sesack & Pickel, 1992), and lesions of the PFC cause a decrease in excitatory amino acid levels in the VTA (Christie, Bridge, James, & Beart, 1985). Electrical stimulation of the frontal cortex (medial PFC [mPFC] or cingulate cortex) causes burst firing of VTA DA neurons in anesthetized rats (Gariano & Groves, 1988; Tong, Overton, & Clark, 1995), and inactivation of the PFC or administration of a general glutamate receptor antagonist interferes with DA neuron burst firing patterns (Grenhoff, Tung, & Svensson, 1988; Svensson & Tung, 1989). Interestingly, PFC glutamatergic projections form synapses only with DA neurons that project back to the PFC, and not with DA neurons that project to the NAcc (Carr & Sesack, 2000b). Together, these data suggest that an important excitatory feedback loop between the PFC and the VTA DA neurons regulates DA neuron activity and DA release in PFC.

It has been suggested that PFC excitatory efferents also regulate VTA–NAcc DA neurons, possibly through a polysynaptic projection via the pedunculopontine tegmentum (PPT). Excitatory inputs to the midbrain come from the PPT (Charara, Smith, & Parent, 1996; Futami, Takakusaki, & Kitai, 1995; Scarnati, Campana, & Pacitti, 1984), although these might predominantly innervate SNc rather than VTA DA neurons (Futami et al., 1995; Scarnati et al., 1984; White, 1996). Stimulation of the PPT induces burst firing in midbrain DA neurons in anesthetized rats (SNc DA neurons—Lokwan, Overton, Berry, & Clark, 1999; VTA DA neurons—Floresco, West, Ash, Moore, & Grace, 2003). The VTA also receives excitatory input from the amygdala (Fudge & Haber, 2000; Shinonaga, Takada, & Mizuno, 1992; Vankova, Arluison, Leviel, & Tramu, 1992; Wallace, Magnuson, & Gray, 1992), the bed nucleus of the stria terminalis (Georges & Aston-Jones, 2002), the hypothalamus preoptic area (Nauta, Smith, Faull, & Domesick, 1978), and from other areas of neocortex, including the cingulate cortex (Hurley, Herbert,

Moga, & Saper, 1991; Wyss & Sripanid-kulchai, 1984). Hippocampal glutamatergic output also regulates the activity of VTA DA neuron populations through a polysynaptic input via the NAcc (Floresco, Todd, & Grace, 2001).

VTA DA neurons have synaptic ionotropic and metabotropic glutamate receptors. Electrical stimulation of afferent input to VTA DA neurons *in vitro* evokes excitatory synaptic depolarizations mediated by NMDA and non-NMDA glutamate receptors, as well as slow excitatory and slow inhibitory synaptic potentials mediated by metabotropic glutamate receptors (Bonci, Grillner, Siniscalchi, Mercuri, & Bernardi, 1991; Fiorillo & Williams, 1998; Johnson & North, 1992; Mereu, Costa, Armstrong, & Vicini, 1991; Shen & Johnson, 1997). Paired or repetitive stimulation of glutamatergic synapses onto DA neurons produces synaptic depression, but it produces facilitation in non-DA neurons. DA neurons exhibit long-lasting forms of synaptic plasticity, including long-term potentiation (LTP) (Bonci & Malenka, 1999) and long-term depression (LTD) (Jones, Kornblum, & Kauer, 2000; Thomas, Malenka, & Bonci, 2000). Non-DA neurons do not exhibit LTP but do exhibit LTD. Thus, excitatory synapses on VTA DA neurons can be bidirectionally modulated, and this synaptic plasticity in the VTA might represent a neural substrate for learning processes involving midbrain DA systems. Up- and down-regulation of glutamatergic synaptic transmission onto VTA DA neurons might also have direct consequences for DA neuron action potential firing patterns and DA release.

*In vivo* data suggest that PFC-driven NMDA receptor activation appears to underlie burst firing, because *in vivo* administration of an NMDA receptor antagonist (but not an α-amino-3-hydroxy-5-methyl-4-isoxazolepropionic acid [AMPA] receptor antagonist) decreases the occurrence of burst firing of VTA and SNc DA neurons in anesthetized rats (Chergui et al., 1993). Burst firing of DA neurons can be induced by NMDA receptor agonists *in vivo* (Chergui et al., 1993) and *in vitro* (Komendantov et al., 2004; Mereu et al., 1997; Seutin et al., 1994). The role of non-NMDA receptors is equivocal, but they appear to be less effective at inducing burst firing (Chergui et al., 1993; Christoffersen & Meltzer, 1995; Suaud-Chagny et al., 1992). Infusion of glutamate receptor agonists (glutamate, quisqualate,

NMDA, kainate) into the VTA increases DA neuron firing rates and causes increased DA levels in the NAcc (Suaud-Chagny et al., 1992; Westerink, Kwint, & de Vries, 1996), and in PFC (Takahata & Moghaddam, 1998).

Thus, glutamate from many different sources concerned with behavioral planning and high order cognitive processing converge on VTA DA and GABA cells, and influence DA neuronal activity via different glutamate receptor subtypes. Glutamatergic inputs probably determine DA neuron output and DA release, and plasticity at these synapses might contribute to learning processes in reward and motivation. The interaction of glutamate receptors with DA pathways are proposed to be perturbed in a number of brain disorders, including addiction and schizophrenia (Ungless, Whistler, Malenka, & Bonci, 2001).

## Dopamine

Dopamine itself causes hyperpolarization and decreased firing of midbrain DA neurons (but not GABA-ergic neurons) both *in vivo* and *in vitro* (for review, see Johnson & North, 1992; White, 1996). DA is released from DA cell somata and dendrites (Adell & Artigas, 2004), because there is no extrinsic DA projection to the VTA. The inhibitory autoreceptors are present on DA cell distal dendrites, and the inhibitory DA autoreceptor is likely to be the $D_2$ subtype, because autoreceptor function is lost in $D_2$-null mice (Mercuri et al., 1997), whereas DA neuron firing rates are not different in $D_3$-null mice, suggesting that $D_3$ receptors do not autoregulate DA neuron activity (Koeltzow et al., 1998). DA $D_2$ receptors reduce voltage-gated $Ca^{2+}$ currents (Cardozo & Bean, 1995) and block the induction of LTD in VTA DA neurons (Thomas et al., 2000), suggesting that $D_2$ receptors exert a variety of effects on DA neurons depending on the functional state of the cells.

$D_1$-type DA receptors are present on terminals of GABA afferents to the VTA, but probably are not present on VTA DA cells (Ciliax et al., 2000; Khan et al., 2000). $D_1$ receptors augment GABA release from GABA-ergic afferents to VTA and facilitate $GABA_B$ receptor-mediated IPSPs, with no effect on $GABA_A$ IPSPs, although DA $D_1$ receptors inhibit GABA release following chronic cocaine and morphine exposure (Bonci & Williams, 1996; Cameron & Williams, 1993). Furthermore, microdialysis studies have reported that $D_1$ receptors increase glutamate release in the VTA (Kalivas & Duffy, 1995). In conclusion, DA exerts a variety of effects within the VTA: It increases $GABA_B$ responses via presynaptic $D_1$ receptor activation; it inhibits DA neuron firing via $D_2$-type autoreceptor activation; and it inhibits LTD via $D_2$ receptors. These apparently conflicting effects might all contribute to increase the signal-to-noise ratio, thus improving the stringency and efficiency of DA release. In fact, by activating $D_1$ receptors (which increase GABA release) and $D_2$ receptors (which hyperpolarize DA cells) DA will decrease the probability of tonic DA release. On the other hand, inhibiting LTD might improve the expression of LTP and of tight bursts of activity that lead to a more efficient and temporally coherent DA release.

## Serotonin

A dense serotoninergic (5-HT-ergic) projection to the VTA comes from the raphe nuclei and innervates both DA and non-DA neurons in the midbrain (see De Matteo, De Blasi, Di Giulio, & Esposito, 2001, for review). Due to the diversity of serotonin (5-HT) receptor subtypes, the effects of 5-HT on VTA neuronal activity are complex and have been difficult to characterize. Such complexity was first suggested in a study by Cameron and colleagues (1997) in which 5-HT was shown to depolarize both DA and GABA-ergic neurons, and to hyperpolarize tertiary neurons.

$5\text{-HT}_{2A}$ receptors are present on DA neurons and, sparsely, on non-DA neurons (Doherty & Pickel, 2000; Nocjar, Roth, & Pehek, 2002) and $5\text{-HT}_2$ receptors on DA neurons could mediate direct depolarization and increase spontaneous firing rates of DA neurons (Pessia, Jiang, North, & Johnson, 1994). Conversely, $5\text{-HT}_{2C}$ receptor messenger ribonucleic acid (mRNA) expression appears to be restricted to local GABA-ergic neurons in the midbrain (Eberle-Wang, Mikeladze, Uryu, & Chesselet, 1997) and $5\text{-HT}_{2C}$ receptor agonists increase the firing rate of non-DA neurons and decrease the firing rate of DA neurons in vivo, an effect that is reversed by $5\text{-HT}_{2C}$ receptor antagonists (Di Giovanni, Di Matteo, La Grutta, & Esposito, 2001; Di Matteo et al., 2001). $5\text{-HT}_{2C}$ receptor antagonists can promote burst firing of DA neurons and may facilitate DA release in terminal regions (Di Matteo et al., 2001), indicating

an important tonic inhibitory role for $5\text{-HT}_{2C}$ receptors over VTA DA neuron output.

5-HT is proposed to act at presynaptic $5\text{-HT}_{1B}$ receptors on GABA-ergic terminals in the VTA to inhibit GABA release (Yan & Yan, 2001), inhibiting $GABA_B$ receptor–mediated IPSPs (Cameron & Williams, 1994, 1995; Johnson, Mercuri, & North, 1992), which may contribute to disinhibition of DA neurons and possibly to increased DA release in terminal regions (Yan & Yan, 2001). The effect of 5-HT on $GABA_B$ receptor-mediated IPSPs is absent in $5\text{-HT}_{1B}$ receptor knockout mice (Morikawa, Manzoni, Crabbe, & Williams, 2000). Finally, 5-HT inhibits evoked glutamatergic excitatory postsynaptic currents (EPSCs) in VTA DA and non-DA neurons via an unidentified 5-HT receptor subtype (Bonci & Malenka, 1999; Jones & Kauer, 1999).

The 5-HT-ergic innervation of the VTA and presence of multiple 5-HT receptor subtypes in the VTA suggest an important role for 5-HT in VTA physiology, but the complexity of direct and indirect effects of different 5-HT receptor subtypes on VTA DA neurons, GABA neurons, and on the terminals of afferent inputs to the VTA makes it difficult to provide a conclusive picture of 5-HT-ergic function in the VTA. It will be important to shed further light on this because of the therapeutic potential of 5-HT-ergic receptors in brain disorders, including depression and addiction.

## PHYSIOLOGICAL CONSEQUENCES OF DA RELEASED IN THE PFC

To understand the consequences of DA released from VTA DA neurons on PFC activity, it is necessary to review the physiology of the PFC neurons. In vivo, the membrane potential of PFC neurons oscillates between two states: a down state, which is mainly determined by the intrinsic conductances of the PFC neurons, and an up state, which represents a depolarized state from which the neuron can fire action potentials (Figure 11.6). The spontaneous transitions between up and down states have been observed in vivo in both anesthetized and nonanesthetized animals (Cowan & Wilson, 1994; Lewis & O'Donnell, 2000; Steriade et al., 1993; Wilson & Groves, 1981).

What effect does DA, released by VTA DA projection neurons, have on PFC neuronal ac-

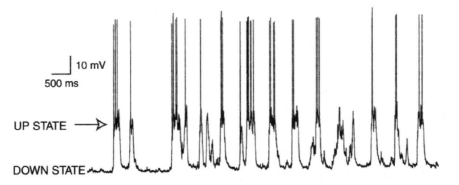

FIGURE 11.6. Cortical neurons oscillate between down states and up states, depending on the amount of the excitatory stimulation. From O'Donnell (2003). Reprinted by permission of author.

tivity? DA $D_1$- and $D_2$-like receptors have been detected on both PFC pyramidal neurons and interneurons in rodents (Benes & Beretta, 2001). $D_1$-like receptor mRNA and binding sites exceed the signal measured for $D_2$ receptors (Farde, Halldin, Stone-Elander, & Sedvall, 1987; Gaspar, Bloch, & Le Moine, 1995; Goldman-Rakic, Lidow, Smiley, & Williams, 1992; Lidow, Goldman-Rakic, Gallager, & Rakic, 1991). Primate studies have shown that $D_1$-like receptors are primarily located on the dendritic spines and shafts of pyramidal neurons, and on both dendrites and axon terminals of GABA-ergic interneurons (Bergson, Mrzljak, Lidow, Goldman-Rakic, & Levenson, 1995), indicating that the effects of DA on PFC pyramidal neurons, via $D_1$ receptor activation, are both direct, modulating the firing activity of PFC neurons, and also indirect, tuning the release of GABA onto them.

Intra-VTA stimulation, leading primarily to DA release, might produce a variety of effects on PFC neurons, depending on whether PFC neurons are in the up or in the down state (for a comprehensive review, see O'Donnell, 2003; Seamans & Yang, 2004). One hypothesis is that DA $D_1$ receptor activation sustains and stabilizes up states by activating NMDA receptors, as well as yet unidentified ionic conductances (Wang & O'Donnell, 2001). An elegant study by Lewis and O'Donnell (2000) showed that *in vivo* stimulation of VTA with trains of pulses resembling VTA DA neuron burst firing evoked a sustained depolarization of PFC neurons that had very similar temporal and spatial features to an up state. Such an effect was also observed with chemical activation of VTA and was reduced by ad-

ministration of a $D_1$ antagonist (Lewis & O'Donnell, 2000).

The effect of $D_2$ receptor activation on the activity of PFC neurons is less clear. In general, the few reports available have pictured $D_2$ receptor activation as exerting an inhibitory action onto PFC neurons (Cepeda et al., 1999). However, $D_2$ receptors might act in concert with $D_1$ receptors to facilitate PFC neuronal firing, similar to what has been observed in the NAcc shell (Hopf, Cascini, Gordon, Diamond, & Bonci, 2003).

Furthermore, *in vivo* data suggest that PFC field potential oscillations—an indirect measure of synchronized up–down states among groups of cortical PFC neurons—are suppressed by inactivation of the VTA (Peters, Barnhardt, & O'Donnell, 2004). Taken together, these data suggest that activation of the VTA has two main consequences in the PFC: promoting up states, and reducing weak and incoherent synaptic inputs. As mentioned before, DA release during burst firing of VTA neurons is significantly increased compared to the amount of DA released during tonic activity, due to the supralinear relationship between firing frequency and DA release (Bean & Roth, 1991; Gonon, 1988; Suaud-Chagny et al., 1992). From a behavioral perspective, it is reasonable to speculate that high DA levels in the PFC during salient or novel stimuli sustain up states to allow synchronized cortical neurons to produce a specific behavioral output. In conclusion, it is likely that clusters of synchronized PFC neurons represent the basic matrix that encodes the expression of PFC-dependent behaviors, and that mesocortical DA plays an important role in this synchronicity.

## DA IN THE PFC:
## FROM COGNITIVE FUNCTIONS TO SCHIZOPHRENIA

The PFC plays an important role in attention processes, choice of appropriate responses, spatial learning, temporal planning and sequencing of motor actions, planning of future behaviors based on previously acquired information, and working memory (Castner, Goldman-Rakic, & Williams, 2004; Goldman-Rakic, Castner, Svensson, Siever, & Williams, 2004). There is evidence that disruption of DA receptor activity in the dorsolateral PFC is associated with profound working memory alterations, in agreement with evidence that DA receptor malfunction underlies comparable working memory deficits in schizophrenia (Castner et al., 2004), originally called *dementia praecox* (Kraepelin, 1909). This is particularly important, since a working memory dysfunction is the most prominent cognitive deficit observed in patients with schizophrenia (Park, Puschel, Sauter, Rentsch, & Hell, 1999), and it has proven to be a very important predictive measure for relapse and prognosis in patients with schizophrenia (Green, 1996; Liddle, 2000; Lysaker, Bell, Bioty, & Zito, 1996; McGurk & Meltzer, 2000; Meltzer, Park, & Kessler, 1999; Sevy & Davidson, 1995). The original hypothesis that correlated DA receptor dysfunction to the deficit in working memory observed in patients with schizophrenia came from the fact that DA receptor antagonists alleviate some of the symptoms that these patients experience (Seeman, 2002), whereas elevated DA levels increase positive symptoms of schizophrenia (Angrist, Peselow, Rubinstein, Wolkin, & Rotrosen, 1985). Studies have provided evidence that $D_1$ rather than $D_2$ receptors in the PFC are the most promising target in the treatment of PFC-dependent cognitive dysfunctions (Abi-Dargham et al., 2002; Arnsten, Cai, Murphy, & Goldman-Rakic, 1994; Castner, Williams, & Goldman-Rakic, 2000; Sawaguchi & Goldman-Rakic, 1991; reviewed in Castner et al., 2004).

## DA IN THE PFC AND ADDICTIVE BEHAVIORS

Although the PFC has not been studied as extensively as other regions of the brain, such as the VTA and Nacc, in relation to addictive behaviors, there is evidence that the PFC is involved in mediating some aspects of drug addiction. As described below, confusion over the precise role of the PFC arises from the fact that distinct drugs of abuse have different or no effects on a range of addictive behaviors when directly injected into the PFC.

Human studies support a role for the PFC in addictive behaviors. fMRI studies in humans have shown that the mPFC is activated by cocaine (Breiter et al., 1996) and during cocaine withdrawal (Volkow et al., 1991; Volkow, Ding, Fowler, & Wang, 1996) and cocaine craving (Childress, McElgin, Mozley, Reveich, & O'Brien, 1996; Childress, Mozley, Fitzgerald, Reivich, & O'Brien, 1999; Grant et al., 1996; Maas et al., 1998). Addictive behaviors have been modeled in animal studies by researchers in an attempt to understand the role of DA in the PFC in modulating such behaviors. Among popular animal models of addiction, we mention conditioned place preference (CPP), drug self-administration, and intracranial self-stimulation (ICSS).

To teach a rodent to learn CPP, drugs are paired with a specific environment, usually one that is abundant in visual or auditory stimuli, while a control (e.g., saline exposure) is paired with a different environment and a different set of sensory cues. There is evidence that intra-PFC injections of cocaine, but not other drugs of abuse such as amphetamine and morphine, induce CPP (Bals-Kubik, Ableitner, Herz, & Shippenberg, 1993; Carr & White, 1986; Hemby, Jones, Justice, & Neill, 1990; Olmstead & Franklin, 1997), whereas the opposite is true when the same drugs are injected into the NAcc (Hemby, Jones, Justice, & Neill, 1992; Olmstead & Franklin, 1997; Van der Kooy, Mucha, O'Shaughnessy, & Bucenieks, 1982; White, Messier, & Carr, 1985). There is still confusion over whether these effects in the PFC are DA-dependent (Hemby, Jones, Neill, & Justice, 1992). Along the same lines, rodents can learn to self-administer drugs directly into discrete brain areas, including the VTA and NAcc. There is evidence that cocaine and DA, but not other drugs of abuse, are self-administered into the PFC, and such an effect is abolished by a specific $D_2$ antagonist (Goeders & Smith, 1983, 1986, 1993). Interestingly, $D_1$ receptor antagonists do not inhibit cocaine and DA self-administration, suggesting two possibilities: $D_2$ but not $D_1$ receptors modulate this behavior, or $D_1$ receptors might be necessary but not sufficient to modulate it.

ICSS is performed by the animal after the operator implants a stimulating electrode into a specific brain area. If the rodent experiences the stimulation as rewarding, it will learn a simple behavior such as lever-pressing to achieve the stimulation. Several studies have shown that ICSS via electrodes implanted into the PFC is performed by rodents (Routtenberg & Sloan, 1972; for review, see Tzschentke, 2001). However, as for other addictive behaviors, the role of DA in sustaining ICSS of PFC is only partially understood.

Interestingly, bidirectional modifications of DA activity in the PFC underlie temporally discrete aspects of addictive behaviors. For example, a decrease in PFC DA-ergic activity has been described in rats predisposed to rapid acquisition of amphetamine self-administration, whereas the opposite has been observed in the NAcc (Piazza et al., 1991; Piazza & Le Moal, 1996). Interestingly, spontaneous and naloxone-precipitated withdrawal from morphine increase significantly DA levels in the mPFC (Bassareo, Tanda, & Di Chiara, 1995) but decrease it in the NAcc (Hildebrand, Nomikos, Hertel, Schilstrom, & Svensson, 1998).

In general, there seem to be consensus on the hypothesis that chronic exposure to drugs of abuse results in deficits in behaviors executed by the mPFC (Jentsch & Taylor, 1999; Tzschentke, 2001). In particular, such cognitive deficits would express themselves as inappropriate responses following exposure to the drugs of abuse, so that both conditioned and unconditioned responses might trigger a sequence of events leading to drug taking, with the subject losing the ability to inhibit such impulsive behaviors (Tzschentke, 2001). Human studies have revealed that decision making and attention levels can be impaired in chronic drug abusers (Jentsch & Roth, 1999; McKetin & Mattick, 1998; O'Malley, Adamse, Heaton, & Gawin, 1992; Rogers et al., 1999; Rosselli & Ardila, 1996).

## SUMMARY AND CONCLUSIONS

Our idea of DA as being merely a "reward" molecule has evolved over the past 10 years. It is now clear that DA is a major player in a series of attention-dependent and cognitive tasks, and DA might more accurately be described as a "learning" molecule. Through this brief overview of the anatomy and physiology of the mesocortical system, we hope to convey to the reader one simple take-home message: DA plays a role in a wide variety of physiological and pathological behaviors, but we are still far from having a complete understanding of how DA modulates such behaviors.

This incomplete understanding cannot be attributed to an inattention to DA-ergic function: On January 1, 2005, the word "dopamine" yielded about 92,000 results on PubMed. More than 30 years of multidisciplinary research into DA-ergic function and dysfunction has indeed generated an enormous amount of information about mesocortical and other DA pathways. In our opinion, the following priority questions regarding mesocortical pathways need to be investigated in future studies:

1. What is the precise localization and functional significance of DA receptor subtypes in the VTA and PFC? DA receptor agonist and antagonists are still far from selective for one subtype of DA receptor, which has made this difficult to address unequivocally.
2. What are the patterns of dopamine release in the PFC under different states of DA neuronal activity?
3. How do the normal physiological patterns of activity of DA neurons, and associated patterns of DA release, relate to behavior? Many physiological effects of DA have been described, but others are still in need of further study, and the relationship of these effects to behavior needs to be established.
4. What is the complete sequence of events in mesocortical pathways that underlie key behaviors that involve DA? DA plays different roles in modulating behaviors depending on the time point, for example, induction versus expression and consolidation of a given behavior, and the pictures are incomplete.

A better understanding of these issues will provide a sound basis for evaluating the mechanisms contributing to mesocortical disease states, and for designing novel approaches to manage and treat these disorders.

## ACKNOWLEDGMENTS

We thank Marcus Cavness, Tara Crowder, and Anjlee Mahajan for proofreading the manuscript. We also thank Patricio O'Donnell for allowing us to use a figure from his review (O'Donnell, 2003).

# REFERENCES

Abi-Dargham, A., Mawlawi, O., Lombardo, I., Gil, R., Martinez, D., Huang, Y., et al. (2002). Prefrontal dopamine D1 receptors and working memory in schizophrenia. *Journal of Neuroscience, 22,* 3708–3719.

Adell, A., & Artigas, F. (2004). The somatodendritic release of dopamine in the ventral tegmental area and its regulation by afferent transmitter systems. *Neuroscience and Biobehavioral Reviews, 28*(4), 415–431.

Albanese, A., & Minciacchi, D. (1983). Organization of the ascending projections from the ventral tegmental area, a multiple fluorescent retrograde tracer study in the rat. *Journal of Comparative Neurology, 216*(4), 406–20.

Angrist, B., Peselow, E., Rubinstein, M., Wolkin, A., & Rotrosen, J. (1985). Amphetamine response and relapse risk after depot neuroleptic discontinuation. *Psychopharmacology, 85,* 277–283.

Arnsten, A. F. T., Cai, J. X., Murphy, B. L., & Goldman-Rakic, P. S. (1994). Dopamine $D_1$ receptor mechanisms in the cognitive performance of young adult and aged monkeys. *Psychopharmacology, 116,* 143–151.

Bals-Kubik, R., Ableitner, A., Herz, A., & Shippenberg, T. S. (1993). Neuroanatomical sites mediating the motivational effects of opioids as mapped by the conditioned place preference paradigm in rats. *Journal of Pharmacology and Experimental Therapeutics, 264,* 489–495.

Bassareo, V., Tanda, G., & Di Chiara, G. (1995). Increase of extracellular dopamine in the medial prefrontal cortex during spontaneous and naloxone-precipitated opiate abstinence. *Psychopharmacology (Berlin), 122*(2), 202–205.

Bean, A. J., & Roth, R. H. (1991). Extracellular dopamine and neurotensin in rat prefrontal cortex *in vivo*: Effects of median forebrain bundle stimulation frequency, stimulation pattern and dopamine autoreceptors. *Journal of Neuroscience, 11,* 2694–2702.

Beckstead, M. J., Grandy, D. K., Wickman, K., & Williams, J. T. (2004). Vesicular dopamine release elicits an inhibitory postsynaptic current in midbrain dopamine neurons. *Neuron, 42*(6), 939–946.

Benes, F. M., & Berretta, S. (2001). GABAergic interneurons, implications for understanding schizophrenia and bipolar disorder. *Neuropsychopharmacology, 25*(1), 1–27.

Berger, B., Gaspar, P., & Verney, C. (1991). Dopaminergic innervation of the cerebral cortex: Unexpected differences between rodents and primates. *Trends in Neurosciences, 14*(1), 21–27.

Berger, B., Thierry, A. M., Tassin, J. P., & Moyne, M. A. (1976). Dopaminergic innervation of the rat prefrontal cortex: A fluorescence histochemical study. *Brain Research, 106*(1), 133–145.

Berger, B., Verney, C., Febyret, A., Vigny, A., & Helle, K. B. (1985). Postnatal ontogenesis of the dopaminergic innervation in the rat anterior cingulate cortex (area 24): Immunocytochemical and catecholamine fluorescence histochemical analysis. *Brain Research, 353*(1), 31–47.

Bergson, C., Mrzljak, L., Lidow, M. S., Goldman-Rakic, P. S., & Levenson, R. (1995) Characterization of subtype-specific antibodies to the human $D_5$ dopamine receptor: Studies in primate brain and transfected mammalian cells. *Proceedings of the National Academy of Sciences of the United States of America, 92,* 3468–3472.

Berridge, K. C., & Robinson, T. E. (2003). Parsing reward. *Trends in Neurosciences, 26*(9), 507–513.

Bonci, A., Grillner, P., Siniscalchi, A., Mercuri, N. B., & Bernardi, G. (1997). Glutamate metabotropic receptor agonists depress excitatory and inhibitory transmission on rat mesencephalic principal neurons. *European Journal of Neuroscience, 9*(11), 2359–2369.

Bonci, A., & Malenka, R. C. (1999). Properties and plasticity of excitatory synapses on dopaminergic and GABAergic cells in the VTA. *Journal of Neuroscience, 19,* 3723–3730.

Bonci, A., & Williams, J. T. (1996). A common mechanism mediates long-term changes in synaptic transmission after chronic cocaine and morphine. *Neuron, 16*(3), 631–639.

Breiter, H., Gollub, R., Weisskoff, R., Kennedy, W., Kantor, H., Gastfriend, D., et al. (1996). Activation of human brain reward circuitry by cocaine observed using fMRI. *Abstracts—Society for Neuroscience, 22,* 758.6.

Cameron, D. L., Wessendorf, M. W., & Williams, J. T. (1997). A subset of ventral tegmental area neurons is inhibited by dopamine, 5-hydroxytryptamine and opioids. *Neuroscience, 77*(1), 155–166.

Cameron, D. L., & Williams, J. T. (1993). Dopamine $D_1$ receptors facilitate transmitter release. *Nature, 366,* 344–347.

Cameron, D. L., & Williams, J. T. (1994). Cocaine inhibits GABA release in the VTA through endogenous 5-HT. *Journal of Neuroscience, 11*(1), 6763–6767.

Cameron, D. L., & Williams, J. T. (1995). Opposing roles for dopamine and serotonin at presynaptic receptors in the ventral tegmental area. *Clinical and Experimental Pharmacology and Physiology, 22*(11), 841–845.

Cardozo, D. L., & Bean, B. P. (1995). Voltage-dependent calcium channels in rat midbrain dopamine neurons: Modulation by dopamine and GABAB receptors. *Journal of Neurophysiology, 74*(3), 1137–1148.

Carr, D. B., & Sesack, S. R. (2000a). GABA-containing neurons in the rat ventral tegmental area project to the prefrontal cortex. *Synapse, 38*(2), 114–23.

Carr, D. B., & Sesack, S. R. (2000b). Projections from the rat prefrontal cortex to the ventral tegmental area: Target specificity in the synaptic associations with mesoaccumbens and mesocortical neurons. *Journal of Neuroscience, 20,* 3864–3873.

Carr, G. D., & White, N. M. (1986). Anatomical disassociation of amphetamine's rewarding and aversive effects, an intracranial microinjection study. *Psychopharmacology, 89*, 340–346.

Castner, S. A., Goldman-Rakic, P. S., & Williams, G. V. (2004). Animal models of working memory: Insights for targeting cognitive dysfunction in schizophrenia. *Psychopharmacology (Berlin), 174*(1), 111–125.

Castner, S. A., Williams, G. V., & Goldman-Rakic, P. S. (2000). Reversal of antipsychotic-induced working memory deficits by short-term dopamine $D_1$ receptor stimulation. *Science, 287*, 2020–2022.

Cepeda, C., Li, Z., Cromwell, H. C., Altemus, K. L., Crawford, C. A., Nansen, E. A., et al. (1999). Electrophysiological and morphological analyses of cortical neurons obtained from children with catastrophic epilepsy, dopamine receptor modulation of glutamatergic responses. *Developmental Neuroscience, 21*(3–5), 223–235.

Charara, A., Smith, Y., & Parent, A. (1996). Glutamate inputs from the pedunculopontine nucleus to midbrain dopaminergic neurons in primates. *Journal of Comparative Neurology, 364*, 254–266.

Chergui, K., Charlety, P. J., Akaoka, H., Saunier, C. F., Brunet, J. L., Buda, M., et al. (1993). Tonic activation of NMDA receptors causes spontaneous burst discharge of rat midbrain dopamine neurons *in vivo*. *European Journal of Neuroscience, 5*, 137–144.

Childress, A. R., McElgin, W., Mozley, D., Reivich, M., & O'Brien, C. P. (1996). Brain correlates of cue-induced and opiate craving. *Society for Neuroscience Abstracts, 22*, 365.5.

Childress, A. R., Mozley, P. D., Fitzgerald, J., Reivich, M., & O'Brien, C. P. (1999). Limbic activation during cue-induced cocaine craving. *American Journal of Psychiatry, 156*, 11–18.

Christie, M. J., Bridge, S., James, L. B., & Beart, P. M. (1985). Excitotoxic lesions suggest an aspartatergic projection from rat medial prefrontal cortex to ventral tegmental area. *Brain Research, 333*, 169–172.

Christoffersen, C. L., & Meltzer, L. T. (1995). Evidence for *N*-methyl-D-aspartate and AMPA subtypes of the glutamate receptor on substantia nigra dopamine neurons: Possible preferential role for N-methyl-D-aspartate receptors. *Neuroscience, 67*(2), 373–381.

Ciliax, B. J., Nash, N., Heilman, C., Sunahara, R., Hartney, A., Tiberi, M., et al. (2000). Dopamine $D_5$ receptor immunolocalization in rat and monkey brain. *Synapse, 37*, 125–145.

Cowan, R. L., & Wilson, C. J. (1994). Spontaneous firing patterns and axonal projections of single corticostriatal neurons in the rat medial agranular cortex. *Journal of Neurophysiology, 71*(1), 17–32.

Cragg, S. J., & Rice, M. E. (2004). DAncing past the DAT at a DA synapse. *Trends in Neurosciences, 27*(5), 270–277.

Deniau, J. M., Thierry, A. M., & Feger, J. (1980). Electrophysiological identification of mesencephalic ventromedial tegmental (VMT) neurons projecting to

the frontal cortex, septum and nucleus accumbens. *Brain Research, 189*(2), 315–326.

Di Chiara, G., & Imperato, A. (1988). Drugs abused by humans preferentially increase synaptic dopamine concentrations in the mesolimbic system of freely moving rats. *Proceedings of the National Academy of the Sciences of the United States of America, 85*(14), 5274–5278.

Di Giovanni, G., Di Matteo, V., La Grutta, V., & Esposito, E. (2001). m-Chlorophenylpiperazine excites non-dopaminergic neurons in the rat substantia nigra and ventral tegmental area by activating serotonin-2C receptors. *Neuroscience, 103*(1), 111–116.

Di Matteo, V., De Blasi, A., Di Giulio, C., & Esposito, E. (2001). Role of 5-HT(2C) receptors in the control of central dopamine function. *Trends in Pharmacological Sciences, 22*(5), 229–232.

Dinopoulos, A., & Parnavelas, J. G. (1991). The development of ventral tegmental area (VTA) projections to the visual cortex of the rat. *Neuroscience Letters, 134*(1), 12–6.

Doherty, M. D., & Pickel, V. M. (2000). Ultrastructural localization of the serotonin 2A receptor in dopaminergic neurons in the ventral tegmental area. *Brain Research, 864*(2), 176–185.

Eberle-Wang, K., Mikeladze, Z., Uryu, K., & Chesselet, M. F. (1997). Pattern of expression of the serotonin2C receptor messenger RNA in the basal ganglia of adult rats. *Journal of Comparative Neurology, 384*(2), 233–247.

Fallon, J. H. (1981). Collateralization of monoamine neurons, mesotelencephalic dopamine projections to caudate, septum and frontal cortex. *Journal of Neuroscience, 1*(12), 1361–1368.

Fallon, J. H., & Loughlin, S. E. (1985). The substantia nigra. In G. Paxinos & J. Watson (Eds.), *The rat central nervous system: A handbook for neuroscientist* (pp. 353–374). New York: Academic Press.

Fallon, J. H., & Loughlin, S. E. (1987). Monoamine innervation of the cerebral cortex and a theory of the role of monoamines in cerebral cortex and basal ganglia. In E. G. Jones & A. Peters (Eds.), *Cerebral cortex* (Vol. 6, pp. 41–127). New York: Plenum Press.

Fallon, J. H., & Moore, R. Y. (1978). Catecholamine innervation of the basal forebrain: IV. Topography of the dopamine projection to the basal forebrain and neostriatum. *Journal of Comparative Neurology, 180*(3), 545–580.

Farde, L., Halldin, C., Stone-Elander, S., & Sedvall, G., (1987). PET analysis of human dopamine receptor subtypes using 11C-SCH 23390 and 11C-raclopride. *Psychopharmacology, 92*, 278–284.

Faull, R. L., & Mehler, W. R. (1978). The cells of origin of nigrotectal, nigrothalamic and nigrostriatal projections in the rat. *Neuroscience, 3*(11), 989–1002.

Ferron, A., Thierry, A. M., Le Douarin, C., & Glowinski, J. (1984). Inhibitory influence of the mesocortical dopaminergic system on spontaneous activity or excitatory response induced from the thalamic mediodorsal nucleus in the rat medial prefrontal cortex. *Brain Research, 302*(2), 257–265.

Fiorillo, C. D., & Williams, J. T. (1998). Glutamate mediates an inhibitory postsynaptic potential in dopamine neurons. *Nature, 394*, 78–82.

Floresco, S. B., Todd, C. L., & Grace, A. A. (2001). Glutamatergic afferents from the hippocampus to the nucleus accumbens regulate activity of ventral tegmental area dopamine neurons. *Journal of Neuroscience, 21*, 4915–4922.

Floresco, S. B., West, A. R., Ash, B., Moore, H., & Grace, A. A. (2003). Afferent modulation of dopamine neuron firing differentially regulates tonic and phasic dopamine transmission. *Nature Neuroscience, 6*(9), 968–973.

Fudge, J. L., & Haber, S. N. (2000). The central nucleus of the amygdala projection to dopamine subpopulations in primates. *Neuroscience, 97*(3), 479–94.

Futami, T., Takakusaki, K., & Kitai, S. T. (1995). Glutamatergic and cholinergic inputs from the pedunculopontine tegmental nucleus to dopamine neurons in the substantia nigra pars compacta. *Neuroscience Research, 21*, 331–342.

Gariano, R. F., & Groves, P. M. (1988). Burst firing induced in midbrain dopamine neurons by stimulation of the medial prefrontal and anterior cingulate cortices. *Brain Research, 462*, 194–198.

Gasbarri, A., Campana, E., Pacitti, C., Hajdu, F., & Tombol, T. (1991). Organization of the projections from the ventral tegmental area of Tsai to the hippocampal formation in the rat. *J. Hirnforsch, 32*(4), 429–437.

Gaspar, P., Bloch, B., & Le Moine, C. (1995). $D_1$ and $D_2$ receptor gene expression in the rat frontal cortex, cellular localization in different classes of efferent neurons. *European Journal of Neuroscience, 7*(5), 1050–1063.

Georges, F., & Aston-Jones, G. (2002). Activation of ventral tegmental area cells by the bed nucleus of the stria terminalis: A novel excitatory amino acid input to midbrain dopamine neurons. *Journal of Neuroscience, 22*(12), 5173–5187.

Gerfen, C. R., Staines, W. A., Arbuthnott, G. W., & Fibiger, H. C. (1982). Crossed connections of the substantia nigra in the rat. *Journal of Comparative Neurology, 207*(3), 283–303.

Goeders, N. E., & Smith, J. E. (1983). Cortical dopaminergic involvement in cocaine reinforcement. *Science, 221*, 773–775.

Goeders, N. E., & Smith, J. E. (1986). Reinforcing properties of cocaine in the medial prefrontal cortex, primary action on presynaptic dopaminergic terminals. *Pharmacology, Biochemistry, and Behavior, 25*(1), 191–199.

Goeders, N. E., & Smith, J. E. (1993). Intracranial cocaine self-administration into the medial prefrontal cortex increases dopamine turnover in the nucleus accumbens. *Journal of Pharmacology and Experimental Therapeutics, 265*(2), 592–600.

Goldman-Rakic, P. S., Lidow, M. S., Smiley, J. F., & Williams, M. S. (1992). The anatomy of dopamine in monkey and human prefrontal cortex. *Journal of Neural Transmission, 36*(Suppl.), 163–177.

Goldman-Rakic, P. S., Castner, S. A., Svensson, T. H., Siever, L. J., & Williams, G. V. (2004). Targeting the dopamine D1 receptor in schizophrenia: Insights for cognitive dysfunction. *Psychopharmacology (Berlin), 174*(1), 3–16.

Gonon, F. G. (1988). Non-linear relationship between impulse flow and dopamine released by rat midbrain dopaminergic neurons as studied by *in vivo* electrochemistry. *Neuroscience, 24*, 19–28.

Grace, A. A., & Bunney, B. S. (1984a). The control of firing pattern in nigral dopamine neurons, burst firing. *Journal of Neuroscience, 4*(11), 2877–90.

Grace, A. A., & Bunney, B. S. (1984b). The control of firing pattern in nigral dopamine neurons, single spike firing. *Journal of Neuroscience, 4*(11), 2866–2876.

Grace, A. A., & Onn, S. P. (1989). Morphology and electrophysiological properties of immunocytochemically identified rat dopamine neurons recorded *in vitro*. *Journal of Neuroscience, 9*(10), 3463–3481.

Grant, S., London, E. D., Newlin, D. B., Villemagne, V. L., Liu, X., Contoreggi, C., et al. (1996). Activation of memory circuits during cue-elicited cocaine craving. *Proceedings of the National Academy of the Sciences of the United States of America, 93*, 2040–12045.

Green, M. F. (1996). What are the functional consequences of neurocognitive deficits in schizophrenia? *American Journal of Psychiatry, 153*, 321–330.

Grenhoff, J., Tung, C. S., & Svensson, T. H. (1988). The excitatory amino acid antagonist kynurenate induces pacemaker-like firing of dopamine neurons in rat VTA *in vivo*. *Acta Physiologica Scandinavica, 134*, 567–568.

Grillner, P., & Mercuri, N. B. (2002). Intrinsic membrane properties and synaptic inputs regulating the firing activity of the dopamine neurons. *Behavioural Brain Research, 130*(1–2), 149–169.

Hemby, S. E., Jones, G. H., Justice, J. B., Jr., & Neill, D. B. (1990). Neuropharmacological assessment of cocaine-induced conditioned place preference using intra-cranial microinjections. *Abstracts—Society for Neuroscience, 16*, 243.6.

Hemby, S. E., Jones, G. H., Justice, J. B., Jr., & Neill, D. B. (1992). Conditioned locomotor activity but not conditioned place preference following intra-accumbens infusions of cocaine. *Psychopharmacology (Berlin), 106*(3), 330–336.

Hemby, S. E., Jones, G. H., Neill, D. B., & Justice, J. B., Jr. (1992). 6-Hydroxydopamine lesions of the medial prefrontal cortex fail to influence cocaine-induced place conditioning. *Behavioural Brain Research, 49*(2), 225–230.

Hildebrand, B. E., Nomikos, G. G., Hertel, P., Schilstrom, B., & Svensson, T. H. (1998). Reduced dopamine output in the nucleus accumbens but not in the medial prefrontal cortex in rats displaying a mecamylamine-precipitated nicotine withdrawal syndrome. *Brain Research*, 779(1–2), 214–225.

Hopf, F. W., Cascini, M. G., Gordon, A. S., Diamond, I., & Bonci, A. (2003). Cooperative activation of dopamine D1 and D2 receptors increases spike firing of nucleus accumbens neurons via G-protein beta-gamma subunits. *Journal of Neuroscience*, 23(12), 5079–5087.

Hurley, K. M., Herbert, H., Moga, M. M., & Saper, C. B. (1991). Efferent projections of the infralimbic cortex of the rat. *Journal of Comparative Neurology*, 308(2), 249–276.

Ikai, Y., Takada, M., Shinonaga, Y., & Mizuno, N. (1992). Dopaminergic and non-dopaminergic neurons in the ventral tegmental area of the rat project, respectively, to the cerebellar cortex and deep cerebellar nuclei. *Neuroscience*, 51(3), 719–728.

Jentsch, J. D., & Roth, R. H. (1999). The neuropsychopharmacology of phencyclidine, from NMDA receptor hypofunction to the dopamine hypothesis of schizophrenia. *Neuropsychopharmacology*, 20(3), 201–225.

Jentsch, J. D., & Taylor, J. R. (1999). Impulsivity resulting from frontostriatal dysfunction in drug abuse: Implications for the control of behavior by reward-related stimuli. *Psychopharmacology (Berlin)*, 146(4), 373–390.

Johnson, S. W., Mercuri, N. B., & North, R. A. (1992). 5-hydroxytryptamine1B receptors block the GABAB synaptic potential in rat dopamine neurons. *Journal of Neuroscience*, 12(5), 2000–2006.

Johnson, S. W., & North, R. A. (1992). Two types of neurone in the rat VTA and their synaptic inputs. *Journal of Physiology*, 450, 455–468.

Jones, S., & Kauer, J. A. (1999). Amphetamine depresses excitatory synaptic transmission via serotonin receptors in the ventral tegmental area. *Journal of Neuroscience*, 19, 9780–9787.

Jones, S., Kornblum, J. L., & Kauer, J. A. (2000). Amphetamine blocks long term synaptic depression in the VTA. *Journal of Neuroscience*, 20, 5575–5580

Kalivas, P. W. (1993). Neurotransmitter regulation of dopamine neurons in the ventral tegmental area. *Brain Research: Brain Research Reviews*, 18, 75–113.

Kalivas, P. W., & Duffy, P. (1995). $D_1$ receptors modulate glutamate transmission in the ventral tegmental area. *Journal of Neuroscience*, 15(7, Pt. 2), 5379–5388.

Khan, Z. U., Gutierrez, A., Martin, R., Penafiel, A., Rivera, A., & de la Calle, A. (2000). Dopamine $D_5$ receptors of rat and human brain. *Neuroscience*, 100, 689–699.

Kilpatrick, I. C., Starr, M. S., Fletcher, A., James, T. A., & MacLeod, N. K. (1980). Evidence for a GABAergic nigrothalamic pathway in the rat: I. Behavioural and biochemical studies. *Experimental Brain Research*, 40(1), 45–54.

Kizer, J. S., Palkovits, M., & Brownstein, M. J. (1976). The projections of the A8, A9 and A10 dopaminergic cell bodies: Evidence for a nigral–hypothalamic–median–eminence dopaminergic pathway. *Brain Research*, 108(2), 363–370.

Klitenick, M. A., Deutch, A. Y., Churchill, L., & Kalivas, P. W. (1992). Topography and functional role of dopaminergic projections from the ventral mesencephalic tegmentum to the ventral pallidum. *Neuroscience*, 50(2), 371–386.

Koeltzow, T. E., Xu, M., Cooper, D. C., Hu, X. T., Tonegawa, S., Wolf, M. E., et al. (1998). Alterations in dopamine release but not dopamine autoreceptor function in dopamine $D_3$ receptor mutant mice. *Journal of Neuroscience*, 18(6), 2231–2238.

Komendantov, A. O., Komendantova, O. G., Johnson, S. W., & Canavier, C. C. (2004). A modeling study suggests complementary roles for GABAA and NMDA receptors and the SK channel in regulating the firing pattern in midbrain dopamine neurons. *Journal of Neurophysiology*, 91(1), 346–357.

Kraepelin, E. (1909). Dementia praecox and paraphrenia. In R. M. Barclay (Trans.), *Kraepelin's textbook of psychiatry* (8th ed., p. 1919). Edinburgh: Livingstone.

Lacey, M. G., Mercuri, N. B., & North, R. A. (1988). On the potassium conductance increase activated by GABAB and dopamine $D_2$ receptors in rat substantia nigra neurones. *Journal of Physiology*, 401, 437–453.

Lacey, M. G., Mercuri, N. B., & North, R. A. (1989). Two cell types in rat substantia nigra zona compacta distinguished by membrane properties and the actions of dopamine and opioids. *Journal of Neuroscience*, 9(4), 1233–1241.

Lewis, B. L., & O'Donnell, P. (2000). Ventral tegmental area afferents to the prefrontal cortex maintain membrane potential "up" states in pyramidal neurons via D(1) dopamine receptors. *Cerebral Cortex*, 10(12), 1168–1175.

Liddle, P. F. (2000). Cognitive impairment in schizophrenia, its impact on social functioning. *Acta Psychiatrica Scandinavica: Supplement*, 400, 11–16.

Lidow, M. S., Goldman-Rakic, P. S., Gallager, D. W., & Rakic, P. (1991). Distribution of dopaminergic receptors in the primate cerebral cortex, quantitative autoradiographic analysis using [$^3$H]raclopride, [$^3$H]spiperone and [$^3$H]SCH23390. *Neuroscience*, 40(3), 657–671.

Lindvall, O., Bjorklund, A., & Divac, L. (1978). Organization of catecholamine neurons projecting to the frontal cortex in the rat. *Brain Research*, 142(1), 1–24.

Lokwan, S. J., Overton, P. G., Berry, M. S., & Clark, D. (1999). Stimulation of the pedunculopontine tegmental nucleus in the rat produces burst firing in A9 dopamine neurons. *Neuroscience*, 92, 245–254.

Lysaker, P. H., Bell, M. D., Bioty, S., & Zito, W. S. (1996) Performance on the Wisconsin Card Sorting Test as a predictor of rehospitalization in schizophrenia. *Journal of Nervous Mental and Disease*, 184, 319–321.

Maas, L. C., Lukas, S. E., Kaufman, M. J., Weiss, R. D., Daniels, S. L., Rogers, V. W., et al. (1998). Functional magnetic resonance imaging of human brain activation during cue-induced cocaine craving. *American Journal of Psychiatry, 155,* 124–126.

Margolis, E. B., Hjelmstad, G. O., Bonci, A., & Fields, H. L. (2003). Kappa-opioid agonists directly inhibit midbrain dopaminergic neurons. *Journal of Neuroscience, 23*(31), 9981–9986.

McGurk, S. R., & Meltzer, H. Y. (2000). The role of cognition in vocational functioning in schizophrenia. *Schizophrenia Research, 45,* 175–184.

McKetin, R., & Mattick, R. P. (1998). Attention and memory in illicit amphetamine users, comparison with non-drug-using controls. *Drug and Alcohol Dependence, 50*(2), 181–184.

Meltzer, H. Y., Park, S., & Kessler, R. (1999) Cognition, schizophrenia and the atypical antipsychotic drugs. *Proceedings of the National Academy of Sciences of the United States of America, 96,* 13591–13593.

Mercuri, N. B., Bonci, A., Calabresi, P., Stefani, A., & Bernardi, G. (1995). Properties of the hyperpolarization-activated cation current Ih in rat mid brain dopaminergic neurons. *European Journal of Neuroscience, 7*(3), 462–469.

Mercuri, N. B., Saiardi, A., Bonci, A., Picetti, R., Calabresi, P., Bernardi, G., et al. (1997). Loss of autoreceptor function in dopaminergic neurons from dopamine $D_2$ receptor deficient mice. *Neuroscience, 79*(2), 323–327.

Mereu, G., Costa, E., Armstrong, D. M., & Vicini, S. (1991). Glutamate receptor subtypes mediate excitatory synaptic currents of dopamine neurons in midbrain slices. *Journal of Neuroscience, 11*(5), 1359–1366.

Mereu, G., Lilliu, V., Casula, A., Vargiu, P. F., Diana, M., Musa, A., et al. (1997). Spontaneous bursting activity of dopaminergic neurons in midbrain slices from immature rats, role of NMDA receptors. *Neuroscience, 77,* 1029–1036.

Morikawa, H., Manzoni, O. J., Crabbe, J. C., & Williams, J. T. (2000). Regulation of central synaptic transmission by 5-HT(1B) auto- and heteroreceptors. *Molecular Pharmacology, 58*(6), 1271–1278.

Nauta, W. J., Smith, G. P., Faull, R. L., & Domesick, V. B. (1978). Efferent connections and nigral afferents of the nucleus accumbens septi in the rat. *Neuroscience, 3*(4–5), 385–401.

Nedergaard, S., Flatman, J. A., & Engberg, I. (1993). Nifedipine- and omega-conotoxin-sensitive $Ca^{2+}$ conductances in guinea pig substantia nigra pars compacta neurons. *Journal of Physiology, 466,* 727–747.

Nocjar, C., Roth, B. L., & Pehek, E. A. (2002). Localization of 5-HT(2A) receptors on dopamine cells in subnuclei of the midbrain A10 cell group. *Neuroscience, 111*(1), 163–176.

O'Donnell, P. (2003). Dopamine gating of forebrain neural ensembles. *European Journal of Neuroscience, 17*(3), 429–435.

Okada, H., Matsushita, N., Kobayashi, K., & Kobayashi, K. (2004). Identification of GABAA receptor subunit variants in midbrain dopaminergic neurons. *Journal of Neurochemistry, 89*(1), 7–14.

Olmstead, M. C., & Franklin, K. B. J. (1997). The development of a conditioned place preference to morphine, effects of microinjections into various CNS sites. *Behavioral Neuroscience, 111*(6), 1324–1334.

O'Malley, Adamse, M., Heaton, R. K., & Gawin, F. H. (1992). Neuropsychological impairment in chronic cocaine abusers. *American Journal of Drug and Alcohol Abuse, 18*(2), 131–144.

Overton, P. G., & Clark, D. (1997). Burst firing in midbrain dopaminergic neurons. *Brain Research: Brain Research Reviews, 25*(3), 312–334.

Palkovits, M., Zaborszyk, L., Brownstein, M. J., Fekete, M. I., Herman, J. P., & Kanyicska, B. (1979). Distribution of norepinephrine and dopamine in cerebral cortical areas of the rat. *Brain Research Bulletin, 4*(5), 593–601.

Papadopoulos, G. C., & Parnavelas, J. G. (1990). Distribution and synaptic organization of serotoninergic and noradrenergic axons in the lateral geniculate nucleus of the rat. *Journal of Comparative Neurology, 294*(3), 345–355.

Park, S., Puschel, J., Sauter, B. H., Rentsch, M., & Hell, D. (1999). Spatial working memory deficits and clinical symptoms in schizophrenia, a 4-month follow-up study. *Biological Psychiatry, 46,* 392–400.

Paul, K., Keith, D. J., & Johnson, S. W. (2003). Modulation of calcium-activated potassium small conductance (SK) current in rat dopamine neurons of the ventral tegmental area. *Neuroscience Letters, 348*(3), 180–184.

Pessia, M., Jiang, Z. G., North, R. A., & Johnson, S. W. (1994). Actions of 5-hydroxytryptamine on ventral tegmental area neurons of the rat *in vitro. Brain Research, 654*(2), 324–330.

Peters, Y., Barnhardt, N. E., & O'Donnell, P. (2004). Prefrontal cortical up states are synchronized with ventral tegmental area activity. *Synapse, 52*(2), 143–152.

Phillipson, O. T. (1979). Afferent projections to the ventral tegmental area of Tsai and interfascicular nucleus, a horseradish peroxidase study in the rat. *Journal of Comparative Neurology, 187*(1), 117–143.

Piazza, P. V., & Le Moal, M. L. (1996). Pathophysiological basis of vulnerability to drug abuse, role of an interaction between stress, glucocorticoids and dopaminergic neurons. *Annual Review of Pharmacology and Toxicology, 36,* 359–378.

Piazza, P. V., Rouge-Pont, F., Deminiere, J. M., Kharoubi, M., Le Moal, M., & Simon, H. (1991). Dopaminergic activity is reduced in the prefrontal cortex and increased in the nucleus accumbens of rats predisposed to develop amphetamine self-administration. *Brain Research, 567*(1), 169–174.

Ping, H. X., & Shepard, P. D. (1996). Apamin-sensitive Ca(2+)-activated K+ channels regulate pacemaker activity in nigral dopamine neurons. *NeuroReport*, 7(3), 809–814.

Robinson, T. E., & Berridge, K. C. (1993). The neural basis of drug craving, an incentive–sensitization theory of addiction. *Brain Research: Brain Research Reviews*, 18, 247–291.

Rogers, R. D., Everitt, B. J., Baldacchino, A., Blackshaw, A. J., Swainson, R., Wynne, K., et al. (1999). Dissociable deficits in the decision-making cognition of chronic amphetamine abusers, opiate abusers, patients with focal damage to prefrontal cortex and tryptophan-depleted normal volunteers, evidence for monoaminergic mechanisms. *Neuropsychopharmacology*, 20(4), 322–339.

Rosselli, M., & Ardila, A. (1996). Cognitive effects of cocaine and polydrug abuse. *Journal of Clinical and Experimental Neuropsychology*, 18(1), 122–135.

Routtenberg, A., & Sloan, M. (1972). Self-stimulation in the frontal cortex of *Rattus norvegicus*. *Behavioral Biology*, 7(4), 567–572.

Sawaguchi, T., & Goldman-Rakic, P. S. (1991). $D_1$ dopamine receptors in prefrontal cortex, involvement in working memory. *Science*, 251, 947–950.

Sawaguchi, T., & Goldman-Rakic, P. S. (1994). The role of $D_1$-dopamine receptor in working memory, local injections of dopamine antagonists into the prefrontal cortex of rhesus monkeys performing an oculomotor delayed-response task. *Journal of Neurophysiology*, 71, 515–528.

Scarnati, E., Campana, E., & Pacitti, C. (1984). Pedunculopontine-evoked excitation of substantia nigra neurons in the rat. *Brain Research*, 304(2), 351–361.

Schultz, W. (2002). Getting formal with dopamine and reward. *Neuron*, 36(2), 241–263.

Seamans, J. K., & Yang, C. R. (2004). The principal features and mechanisms of dopamine modulation in the prefrontal cortex. *Progress in Neurobiology*, 74(1), 1–58.

Seeman, P. (2002). Atypical antipsychotics, mechanism of action. *Canaian Journal of Psychiatry*, 47, 27–38.

Sesack, S. R., & Pickel, V. M. (1992). Prefrontalcortical efferents in the rat synapse on unlabeled targets of catecholamine terminals in the nucleus accumbens septi and on dopamine neurons in the VTA. *Journal of Comparative Neurology*, 320, 145–160.

Seutin, V., Johnson, S. W., & North, R. A. (1993). Apamin increases NMDA-induced burst-firing of rat mesencephalic dopamine neurons. *Brain Research*, 630(1–2), 341–344.

Seutin, V., Johnson, S. W., & North, R. A. (1994). Effect of dopamine and baclofen on NMDA-induced burst firing in rat VTA neurons. *Neuroscience*, 58, 201–206.

Sevy, S., & Davidson, M. (1995). The cost of cognitive impairment in schizophrenia. *Schizophrenia Research*, 17, 1–3.

Shen, K. Z., & Johnson, S. W. (1997). A slow excitatory postsynaptic current mediated by G protein coupled metabotropic glutamate receptors in rat ventral teg-

mental dopamine neurons. *European Journal of Neuroscience*, 9, 48–54.

Shinonaga, Y., Takada, M., & Mizuno, N. (1992). Direct projections from the central amygdaloid nucleus to the globus pallidus and substantia nigra in the cat. *Neuroscience*, 51(3), 691–703.

Simon, H., Le Moal, M., Stinus, L., & Calas, A. (1979). Anatomical relationships between the ventral mesencephalic tegmentum—a 10 region and the locus coeruleus as demonstrated by anterograde and retrograde tracing techniques. *Journal of Neural Transmission*, 44(1–2), 77–86.

Simon, H., Scatton, B., & Le Moal, M. (1979). Definitive disruption of spatial delayed alternation in rats after lesions in the ventral mesencephalic tegmentum. *Neuroscience Letters*, 15(2–3), 319–324.

Slopsema, J. S., van der Gugten, J., & de Bruin, J. P. (1982). Regional concentrations of noradrenaline and dopamine in the frontal cortex of the rat, dopaminergic innervation of the prefrontal subareas and lateralization of prefrontal dopamine. *Brain Research*, 250(1), 197–200.

Steffensen, S. C., Svingos, A. L., Pickel, V. M., & Henriksen, S. J. (1998). Electrophysiological characterization of GABAergic neurons in the ventral tegmental area. *Journal of Neuroscience*, 18(19), 8003–8015.

Steriade, M., Nunez, A., & Amzica, F. (1993). A novel slow (< 1 Hz) oscillation of neocortical neurons *in vivo*: Depolarizing and hyperpolarizing components. *Journal of Neuroscience*, 13(8), 3252–65.

Suaud-Chagny, M. F., Chergui, K., Chouvet, G., & Gonon, F. (1992). Relationship between dopamine release in the rat nucleus accumbens and the discharge activity of dopaminergic neurons during local *in vivo* application of amino acids in the ventral tegmental area. *Neuroscience*, 49, 63–72.

Svensson, T. H., & Tung, C. S. (1989). Local cooling of prefrontal cortex induces pacemaker-like firing of dopamine neurons in rat VTA *in vivo*. *Acta Physiologica Scandinavica*, 136, 135–136.

Swanson, L. W. (1982). The projections of the ventral tegmental area and adjacent regions: A combined fluorescent retrograde tracer and immunofluorescence study in the rat. *Brain Research Bulletin*, 9(1–6), 321–353.

Takahata, R., & Moghaddam, B. (1998). Glutamatergic regulation of basal and stimulus-activated dopamine release in the prefrontal cortex. *Journal of Neurochemistry*, 71(4), 1443–1449.

Tepper, J. M., Martin, L. P., & Anderson, D. R. (1995). GABAA receptor-mediated inhibition of rat substantia nigra dopaminergic neurons by pars reticulata projection neurons. *Journal of Neuroscience*, 15(4), 3092–3103.

Thierry, A. M., Deniau, J. M., Herve, D., & Chevalier, G. (1980). Electrophysiological evidence for nondopaminergic mesocortical and mesolimbic neurons in the rat. *Brain Research*, 201(1), 210–214.

Thomas, M. J., Malenka, R. C., & Bonci, A. (2000).

Modulation of long-term depression by dopamine in the mesolimbic system. *Journal of Neuroscience, 20,* 5581–5586.

Tong, Z. Y., Overton, P. G., & Clark, D. (1995). Chronic administration of (+)-amphetamine alters the reactivity of midbrain dopaminergic neurons to prefrontal cortex stimulation in the rat. *Brain Research, 674*(1), 63–74.

Tzschentke, T. M. (2001). Pharmacology and behavioral pharmacology of the mesocortical dopamine system. *Progress in Neurobiology, 63*(3), 241–320.

Ungless, M. A., Whistler, J., Malenka R. C., & Bonci A. (2001). Single cocaine exposure *in vivo* induces long-term potentiation in dopamine neurons. *Nature, 411,* 583–587.

Van Bockstaele, E. J., & Pickel, V. M. (1995). GABA-containing neurons in the ventral tegmental area project to the nucleus accumbens in rat brain. *Brain Research, 682*(1–2), 215–221.

van der Kooy, D., Mucha, R. F., O'Shaughnessy, M., & Bucenieks, P. (1982). Reinforcing effects of brain microinjections of morphine revealed by conditioned place preference. *Brain Research, 243*(1), 107–117.

Vankova, M., Arluison, M., Leviel, V., & Tramu, G. (1992). Afferent connections of the rat substantia nigra pars lateralis with special reference to peptide-containing neurons of the amygdalo-nigral pathway. *Journal of Chemical Neuroanatomy, 5*(1), 39–50.

Volkow, N. D., Ding, Y. S., Fowler, J. S., & Wang, G. J. (1996). Cocaine addiction, hypothesis derived from imaging studies with PET. *Journal of Addictive Diseases, 15,* 55–71.

Volkow, N. D., Fowler, J. S., Wolf, A. P., Hitzemann, F., Dewey, S., Bendriem, B., et al. (1991). Changes in brain glucose metabolism in cocaine dependence and withdrawal. *American Journal of Psychiatry, 148,* 621–626.

Wallace, D. M., Magnuson, D. J., & Gray, T. S. (1992). Organization of amygdaloid projections to brainstem dopaminergic, noradrenergic and adrenergic cell groups in the rat. *Brain Research Bulletin, 28*(3), 447–454.

Wang, J., & O'Donnell, P. (2001). D(1) dopamine receptors potentiate NMDA-mediated excitability increase in layer V prefrontal cortical pyramidal neurons. *Cerebral Cortex, 11*(5), 452–462.

Westerink, B. H., Kwint, H. F., & deVries, J. B. (1996). The pharmacology of mesolimbic dopamine neurons, a dual-probe microdialysis study in the ventral tegmental area and nucleus accumbens of the rat brain. *Journal of Neuroscience, 16*(8), 2605–2611.

White, F. J. (1996). Synaptic regulation of mesocortico-limbic dopamine neurons. *Annual Review of Neuroscience, 19,* 405–436.

White, N. M., Messier, C., & Carr, G. D. (1985). Operationalizing and measuring the organizing influence of drugs on behaviour. In M. A. Bozarth (Ed.), *Methods of assessing the reinforcing properties of abused drugs* (pp. 591–618). New York: Springer.

Wightman, R. M., & Zimmerman, J. B. (1990). Control of dopamine extracellular concentration in rat striatum by impulse flow and uptake. *Brain Research: Brain Research Reviews, 15*(2), 135–144.

Wilson, C. J., & Groves, P. M. (1981). Spontaneous firing patterns of identified spiny neurons in the rat neostriatum. *Brain Research, 220*(1), 67–80.

Wise, R. A. (2004). Dopamine, learning and motivation. *Nature Reviews: Neuroscience, 5*(6), 483–494.

Wyss, J. M., & Sripanidkulchai, K. (1984). The topography of the mesencephalic and pontine projections from the cingulate cortex of the rat. *Brain Research, 293*(1), 1–15.

Yan, Q. S., & Yan, S. E. (2001). Serotonin-1B receptor-mediated inhibition of [(3)H]GABA release from rat ventral tegmental area slices. *Journal of Neurochemistry, 79*(4), 914–922.

# PART IV

## FUNCTIONAL AND STRUCTURAL
## IMAGING APPROACHES

# CHAPTER 12

# Structural Imaging of the Frontal Lobes

*Howard Rosen*
*David Dean*

The last 30 years have seen a revolution in our ability to examine noninvasively examine the structure of the living human brain. With the advent of computed tomography (CT) scanning in the mid-1970s, researchers working with humans acquired the ability to correlate immediately clinical abnormalities and the location of lesions in the brain. Subsequent years have seen the development of newer, more sensitive methods of visualizing the brain's structure, along with increasingly efficient and sophisticated approaches for analysis. These changes have led to major advances in the diagnosis of neurological disease and in our understanding of brain function, including the functions of the frontal lobes. Our goal in this chapter is to review briefly the methods of examining brain structure and to introduce the reader to some of the relevant terminology. Rather than focusing on the many specific research findings regarding the frontal lobes, we place a particular emphasis on the various techniques used to analyze structural imaging data, including their strengths and weaknesses, and provide examples of the ways they have been used to study the frontal lobes.

## IMAGING MODALITIES

The two most common methods for structural brain imaging are CT scanning and magnetic resonance imaging (MRI). The physics behind these methods are beyond the scope of this chapter. Straightforward explanations for non-physicists are available (Greenberg & Adams, 1999; Horowitz, 1995). Here, we briefly discuss these methods in terms of their relative strengths and weaknesses.

## Magnetic Resonance Imaging

Most structural imaging used for research today is obtained using MRI, which produces brain images using strong magnetic fields and radio frequencies. MR images can be obtained at very high resolution, now below 1 mm. This, combined with the signal characteristics in different tissues, allows MRI to differentiate between tissue types in the brain, such as gray matter and white matter. MRI is also very sensitive to even very small brain lesions, which are associated with edema (accumulation of water). While most current MRI is performed using 1.5 T (tesla) magnets, newer machines using 3 T and 4 T magnets are now in use at many centers, and magnets of even higher field strength are beginning to be used. With higher field strength comes better signal to noise ratio and higher resolution, although such images are also more susceptible to artifacts induced by the idiosyncrasies and variations in tissue content in the human body. Figure 12.1 depicts these types of susceptibility artifacts. In this case, the images are from a 1.5 T scanner using a magnetization-prepared rapid gradient echo (MP-RAGE) and echo-planar imaging sequence. In addition to field strength, advances

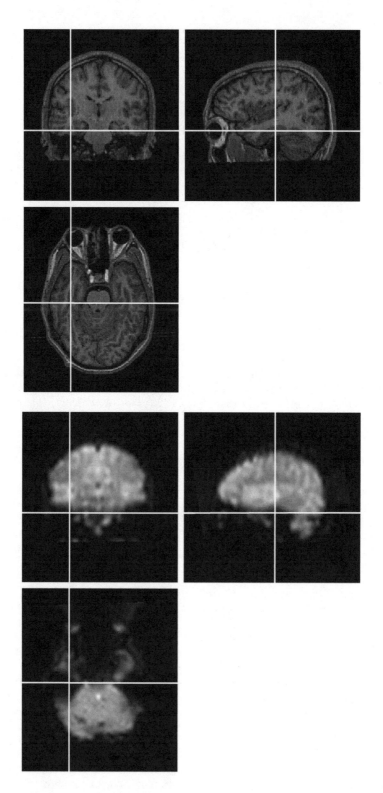

FIGURE 12.1. Orthogonal views of MRIs obtained from the same individual with T1-weighted (top) and EPI (echo-planar imaging; bottom) sequences. The crosshairs are on the same location in the head in both images. Magnetic susceptibility artifacts are exaggerated in the EPI image, so that clearly present brain regions on the T1 image are not seen on the EPI image. Courtesy of Simona Brambati, University of California, San Francisco.

in MRI acquisition techniques allow MRI to be sensitive to blood flow in large vessels (Wetzel & Bongartz, 1999), perfusion of small vessels (Cha, 2003; Detre et al., 1994), cerebrospinal fluid (CSF) flow (Levy, 1999), and diffusion of water through brain tissue (Mori, 2002).

## Computed Tomography

CT scanning involves the use of standard X-rays to create images of the brain. Compared with MRI, these images are usually lower in resolution, less sensitive to lesions, and the contrast between gray matter and white matter is relatively poor. However, CT scans are relatively inexpensive and quick; a complete scan can be obtained in 15 minutes. Because CT scanning is an older, more commonly available and less expensive technology than MRI, CT scans are routinely available for almost any patient with neurological disease. CT scans are also more sensitive to minerals in tissue (e.g., calcium or iron, which produce no signal on MRI) and to the presence of recent bleeding. CT scans are also safe for patients with metal implants that could move or heat up in a magnetic field, and for patients with pacemakers or other implanted physiological devices that could malfunction.

## SPECIFIC ANALYTIC APPROACHES

### Case Series

The vast majority of structural imaging data in the brain has come from associations between lesion locations and behavior, ranging from clinically observed abnormalities to impairments documented on neuropsychological or other directed testing. Many important observations on frontal lobe function have been gleaned from single patients or small case series. For instance, the importance of the orbital and ventromedial prefrontal regions in regulation of emotion and social behavior was first highlighted in the modern era by a single case (Eslinger & Damasio, 1986), and subsequently supported by small group studies of patients with ventral frontal lesions (Hornak, Rolls, & Wade, 1996; Saver & Damasio, 1991). Single cases or small case series have also been recently used to bolster arguments about the role of the frontal lobes processes such as autonomic functioning (Critchley et al., 2003), performance monitoring (Swick & Turken, 2002),

self-conscious thought (Beer, Heerey, Keltner, Scabini, & Knight, 2003), theory of mind (Stone, Baron-Cohen, & Knight, 1998), and working memory (Thompson-Schill et al., 2002). Because these studies begin with a lesion location and proceed to analyze the behavioral consequences, these techniques have been referred to as "lesion-defined" (Bates et al., 2003).

## Lesion Overlap Methods

Many lesions are quite large and may encompass several brain regions with different functions; accordingly, they may be associated with many behavioral deficits. Methods that overlap lesion locations in groups of patients with behaviors of interest can refine the localization for a behavioral deficit. Because these approaches start with a behavior of interest and seek to localize the associated lesion, they have been termed "behavior-defined" (Bates et al., 2003). For example, Stuss and colleagues (2000) recently used this method to supplement a more basic lesion–behavioral analysis. They examined performance on the Stroop test in 51 patients whose lesion locations were classified as being in the right or left frontal regions (or both), or in nonfrontal locations. This "lesion-defined" component of their study revealed that patients with frontal lesions were slower at the Stroop test, and left frontal lesions produced more impairment than right frontal lesions. To learn more, they used a template that divided the frontal lobes into subregions such as lateral, polar, and superior and inferior medial regions. These templates were superimposed on drawings of patients' lesions to classify each of these regions as involved or uninvolved in each case. Using this "behavior-defined" approach, they divided patients into good and poor performers, and found that poor performance on the incongruent condition of the Stroop task was specifically associated with bilateral superior medial and right posteromedial frontal lesions, consistent with the putative role of these regions in maintaining consistent activation of the intended response. Similar lesion overlap analyses using templates have been done by other groups to identify regions associated with autonomic function (Tranel & Damasio, 1994), various aspects of language (Kertesz, Harlock, & Coates, 1979; Naeser et al., 1998), and complex motor function (Kertesz & Ferro, 1984).

By dividing the template into several a priori discrete regions, these studies limited the impact of variability across patients, because a lesion only had to affect one of the regions to a prespecified degree to be counted, rather than having to overlap precisely with other patients' lesions in that region. Using regions of an a priori size and shape in a template limits the precision with which a behavior can be localized. For example, a template that contains only a lateral frontal region cannot discriminate the effects of lesions affecting the superior versus middle frontal gyrus. As the number of patients in a study grows, the chances that multiple patients with a given behavior will have overlapping lesions in smaller and smaller regions grows as well. Thus, in large-enough studies, lesions can be overlapped without reference to any predefined regions of interest to localize their behavior. Such studies would use templates without predefined regions of interest, as depicted in Figure 12.2. The only limit on the precision of this type of analysis is the image resolution and the accuracy with which lesions are represented. This type of approach has

been used to define lesions associated with various types of behavior, including speech production deficits associated with insular lesions, by using paper templates (Dronkers, 1996) and collecting behaviors associated with medial frontal lesions by using electronic templates (Anderson, Damasio, & Damasio, 2005).

Typical template-based measures for lesion analysis treat behavioral deficits in a binary fashion, and do not make use of the fact that some patients have more severe deficits in the behavior than others. Bates and colleagues (2003) have recently described a technique called voxel-based lesion–symptom mapping (VLSM), which involves digitizing lesion reconstructions made on templates and analyzing behavioral effects of lesion location at every pixel. Behavioral scores for those with a lesion at that pixel are compared with scores for patients with no lesions at that pixel to create a $t$ score. Pixels with significant $t$ scores provide a map of the regions that account for behavior. This approach allows researchers to use the whole range of values for continuous variables, rather than relying on a designation of patients as impaired or intact (Bates et al., 2003). VLSM has been used to identify lesion locations in the left inferolateral frontal and left middle and inferior temporal gyri (Baldo et al., 2005) that account for performance on the Wisconsin Card Sorting Task.

These examples illustrate how lesion–behavior analyses have become increasingly sophisticated, allowing more refined localization of the neuroanatomical underpinnings of specific cognitive or behavioral functions. These advances have been paralleled by increasingly sophisticated analyses of more subtle changes seen in neurodegenerative, psychiatric, and genetic disorders, as we describe below.

## METHODS FOR ANALYZING ATROPHY

Clinical, pathological, and functional imaging data have demonstrated that particular neurodegenerative processes, psychiatric disorders and genetic disorders have proclivities for specific brain regions (Braak et al., 1999; Bunney, Potkin, & Bunney, 1995; Drevets, 2000; Kuhl et al., 1982; Mann & South, 1993; Mann, South, Snowden, & Neary, 1993; Mayberg, 1994; Vonsattel et al., 1985). In contrast to lesions occurring from tumors and strokes,

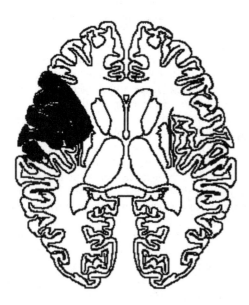

FIGURE 12.2. Single "slice" from a brain template used to represent lesion location in a standardized way relative to normal brain structures. Here, a perisylvian brain lesion is depicted. Courtesy of Nina Dronkers, Center for Aphasia and Related Disorders, VA Northern California Health Care System, Martinez.

changes in the brain occurring with these types of pathology are difficult to "localize" with the naked eye, because these processes manifest themselves in structural images mainly as brain atrophy whose borders cannot be grossly appreciated. Disease-related atrophy also can be superimposed on age-related atrophy which must be accounted for; however, quantification of these changes has potential utility for diagnosis, and for following disease progression and further delineating brain–behavior relationships. As with more focal lesions, many approaches are available to quantify these changes, each with its advantages and pitfalls.

## Visual Ratings

Probably the simplest method of quantifying brain atrophy involves visual ratings. These methods are fast and flexible, in that they can provide semiquantitative data on images in any format (printed or digital) and may be applied to any structure that can be seen. Typically, the degree of atrophy is rated by one or two raters on a semiquantitative scale (e.g., 0, *no atrophy* to 3, *severe atrophy*). Methods of this type have reasonable reliability and good correlation with more quantitative assessments (Fazekas et al., 2002; Wahlund, Julin, Lindqvist, & Scheltens, 1999). These methods have been used most commonly to study the temporal lobes. Temporal rating scales have been used in several studies to differentiate individuals with dementia from normal individuals (Wahlund et al., 1999) and to rate the severity of dementia (Galton et al., 2001). When applied to the frontal lobes, these methods are less reliable, but ratings done by a single individual appear to be consistent (Scheltens, Pasquier, Weerts, Barkhof, & Leys, 1997). At least one study has used frontal visual ratings from MRI to study patients with frontotemporal dementia (FTD; Rosso et al., 2001).

Although they are fast and require no special software, visual rating scales have many pitfalls. In regions where landmarks are difficult to identify, reliability across raters can be disappointing (Scheltens et al., 1997). The methods depend entirely on the skill and experience of the raters and yield only ordinal, rather than continuous, data, limiting their sensitivity to subtle effects. They are also very sensitive to the orientation and placement of the image slices; a region sliced obliquely rather than perpendicularly looks larger.

## Simple Linear Measures

Simple linear measures are a solution to an important problem associated with visual rating methods, in that they provide truly quantitative data. In most cases, easily identifiable landmarks provide the basis of measurement, which improves interrater reliability. To accomplish this, trained users identify two landmarks in the brain, and the software (or a ruler, or calipers on printed films) can be used calculate the absolute distance between those two points. This simple approach has been used extensively for the measurement of medial temporal lobe (MTL) structures (Denihan, Wilson, Cunningham, Coakley, & Lawlor, 2000; Erkinjuntti et al., 1993; Frisoni et al., 1994, 1995; Frisoni, Beltramello, Geroldi, et al., 1996; Frisoni, Beltramello, Weiss, et al., 1996; Gao et al., 2003; Jobst, Smith, Barker, et al., 1992; Jobst, Smith, Szatmari, et al. 1992; Pasquier, Bail, Lebert, Pruvo, & Petit, 1994; Pasquier et al., 1997). As with visual ratings, these techniques are sensitive to the orientation of the image. If measurements are to be done on printed images, the images need to be acquired with a standard orientation and slicing, because the hard copy CT scans cannot be reoriented after they are acquired. Recent studies have successfully applied linear measurement methods using calipers and printed images to MRI scans (Frisoni, Beltramello, Weiss, et al., 1996; Gao et al., 2003, 2004), with highly reproducible results and minimal training required (Gao et al., 2003). Images available in digital format can be manipulated and reoriented into a standard orientation for analysis.

Linear measurement methods for nontemporal structures, including the frontal lobe, have been established. Barr, Heinze, Dobben, Valvassori, and Sugar (1978) defined a linear measure called the "bicaudate index", which is defined as the ratio of the width of both lateral ventricles at the level of the heads of the caudate nuclei to the width of the brain at the same level. This method was able to discriminate patients with Huntington's disease from patients with cerebral atrophy and normal controls. Frisoni and colleagues (Frisoni, Beltramello, Geroldi, et al., 1996; Frisoni, Beltramello, Weiss, et al., 1996) have defined a more comprehensive set of linear measures that include the identification of three planes: the bicommissural plane, the brainstem axis plane, and the temporal lobe plane. Using these planes, they can make a set of eight linear measurements: the bifrontal index (same as the bicaudate index described earlier), interhemispheric fissure width, interuncal distance, minimum MTL width, hippocampal height, cranial width, choroid fissure width, and temporal horn width. Although this approach is complicated, test–retest reliability for these measures are high, and they have been useful in the diagnosis of Alzheimer's disease (AD), as well as detecting different patterns of regional brain atrophy between patients with AD and FTD (Frisoni, Beltramello, Geroldi, et al., 1996; Frisoni, Beltramello, Weiss, et al., 1996).

The manual labor and computing resources required for this approach are minimal, which enables these measures to be made on very large samples of subjects. In addition, these measurements are not dependent on complex algorithms and imaging software, making the data comparable across research centers and thereby enabling research centers to pool their data into a common research study. For example, Bosscher and Scheltens (2001) reviewed of 10 studies from 1992 to 2000 and were able to compile data from a total of 450 patients with AD and 515 control subjects. However, the drawbacks of these simple measures are that they provide a limited amount of information and are not practical for whole-brain analyses. Given the recent advances in computer technology and comprehensive image analysis methodologies, many promising options beyond linear measurements are currently available.

## Volumetric Methods: Region-of-Interest Tracing

Manual tracing of a region of interest (ROI) to obtain an absolute tissue volume is considered to be the anatomical "gold standard" to which other volumetric approaches are compared. Like linear measurements, manual tracing of ROIs is a conceptually straightforward and easy approach to understand. Most commonly, these methods measure volumes in specific regions by assessing the surface area within that region in each brain slice over successive slices to create a volume. Typically, images are analyzed in digital format, so that all images are usually digitally preprocessed to prepare them for ROI tracing. To do this, raw MR images must first be reoriented to a standard orientation and resampled, allowing regions to be assessed from the same point of view in every individual. The most commonly used standard

space is the one defined by Talairach and Tournoux (1988), originally created for stereotactically based neurosurgery. The Talairach grid is a coordinate system that places the brain into a rectangular grid system anchored to the location of the anterior commissure (AC), the posterior commissure (PC), and the outer boundaries of the brain (Talairach & Tournoux, 1988). This system requires that images be spatially transformed and resampled, so that the line connecting the anterior and posterior commissures (AC–PC line) is aligned horizontally and along the main horizontal plane of the Talairach reference system, and the interhemispheric fissure is aligned to match the central vertical plane of this system. Usually, the T1-weighted images are used for this purpose, because they are highest in resolution. Figure 12.3 shows a T1-weighted brain image with the Talairach grid superimposed for reference. Frequently, a tissue classification algorithm is then applied to generate a tissue-classified image, or "segmented image," which allows the tracing algorithms to generate tissue-specific volumes (e.g., gray matter and white matter). Once the images are preprocessed, a trained operator must go through the image slice by slice, with an unambiguous definition of the ROI, and trace out the brain region on each two-dimensional (2D) slice.

Research groups have established protocols for the parcellation of the cerebral cortex using sulcal landmarks and anatomical conventions (Caviness, Verne, & Meyer, 1996; Crespo-Facorro et al., 1999, 2000b; Kim et al., 2000; Rademacher, Galaburda, Kennedy, Filipek, & Caviness, 1992). The primary consideration in this process is to define regions that most accurately reflect the underlying functional anatomy of the cortex. Cognitive neuroscientists are interested in how brain functions map onto the structure of the cortex, and therefore require precise and consistent ROI definitions. Seminal work by Rademacher and colleagues (1992) established a thorough parcellation protocol for the entire cerebral cortex, which resulted in a total of 47 ROIs, 11 from the frontal lobe, 16 from the temporal lobe, 7 from the parietal lobe, 6 from the occipital lobe, and 7 from medial paralimbic cortices. Subsequent work has presented implementations of manually tracing these regions with the support of computer software, along with reliability data (Caviness et al., 1996; Crespo-Facorro et al., 1999, 2000b; Kim et al., 2000).

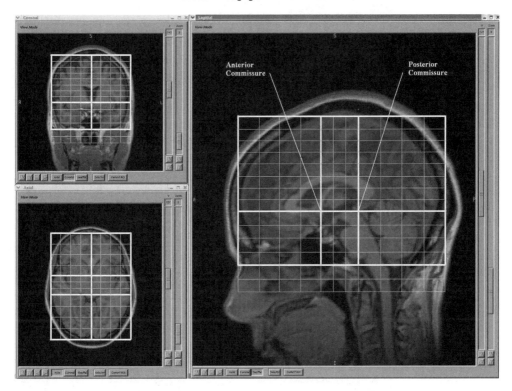

FIGURE 12.3. T1-weighted MRI in three orthogonal 2D views with Talairach grid superimposed. Heavier grid lines indicate the grid boundaries aligned with specific points in the image to fit the grid onto the brain.

ROI analyses have been done for practically every patient population and for almost every region of the cortex. For instance, regional volumes in the prefrontal cortex have been correlated with working memory performance in aging and AD populations (Salat, Kaye, & Janowsky 2001, 2002), and many groups have used manual tracing to examine regional brain volumes in schizophrenic populations (Buchanan et al., 2004; Crespo-Facorro et al., 2000; Gur et al., 2004; Gur, Turetsky, Bilker, & Gur, 1999). Emotion comprehension deficits in patients with FTD have been associated with atrophy in the right amygdala and right orbitofrontal cortex using these types of measurements (Rosen, Perry, et al., 2002). These studies are among the many examples of how these methods can be used to characterize specific diseases and to enhance our understanding of brain–behavior relationships.

Both image preprocessing and manual tracing protocols have become efficient and user-friendly through the use of software designed specifically for these methods, much of which is freely available. The image preprocessing pipeline of reorientation, resampling, and segmentation of the raw MR images has become almost fully automated, minimizing the operator time required for these steps. And although manual tracing is quite a laborious, time-consuming endeavor, appropriate tracing software can be very helpful with this task (Magnotta et al., 2002). Programs that offer the ability to visualize 2D slices in the three orthogonal planes (coronal, axial, and sagittal), and a 3D rendering of the brain simultaneously have been developed, greatly facilitating the tracing process (Figure 12.4).

Despite the strengths of the manual tracing approach, there are also some disadvantages. A great amount of variability in sulcal patterns of the cerebral cortex can make it difficult to identify landmarks reliably with a simple ROI definition. Thus, this approach demands the training of users and the establishment of interrater and intrarater reliability. Users need to become familiar with the tracing software and must then learn to trace a brain region accurately ac-

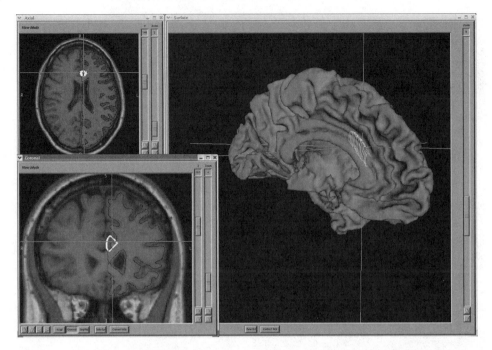

FIGURE 12.4.  2D coronal and axial sections through a T1-weighted MRI, and a 3D rendering of the surface of the left hemisphere. The white tracings depict a partial ROI drawn around the left anterior cingulate gyrus.

cording to a specific protocol. Therefore, in addition to potential reliability problems, this approach can be rather time-consuming and labor-intensive. This approach initially demands not only a significant amount of time to train users but also the manual labor required to perform slice-by-slice traces on numerous MRIs.

## Image Segmentation

Degenerative diseases are often considered to affect primarily gray matter. However, evidence emerging over the last few years has shown that white matter changes can be quite prominent in some neurodegenerative processes (Dickson et al., 2002) and some developmental processes (Barnea-Goraly et al., 2003; Klingberg et al., 2000). Thus, some research questions examining structural changes in the brain benefit from assessment of white matter and gray matter changes separately, which requires generation of tissue-classified, or "segmented," images from the raw MR images, where each voxel is labeled with a specific tissue type. Though many computational algorithms have been applied to solve and automate this pro-

cess, they typically require that the raw MR images be reoriented to a standard anatomical space, such as the one defined by Talairach and Tournoux (1988). As detailed below, segmentation algorithms can use T1, T2, and proton density MR images to provide a better estimate of local tissue types, requiring that they be moved into the same space as, or "coregistered" to, the T1 image. Placing the images into standard space allows comparison of the images to template images, so that the likely locations of gray, white, and CSF pixels can be incorporated into the classification algorithm.

Once the raw MR images have been reoriented and coregistered, the resampled images are then used to generate a segmented (tissue-classified) image. First, samples from each of the three tissue types (gray matter, white matter, and CSF) are identified on the coregistered images. These tissue samples are then used as "training classes" to generate a linear discriminant function, which is then used to classify the remaining voxels in the image (Cohen et al., 1992; Harris et al., 1999). Once the segmented image is generated (Figure 12.5), it can be visually inspected to check for image quality.

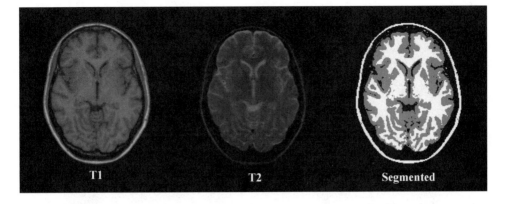

FIGURE 12.5. T1- and T2-weighted images, along with a segmented image that categorically designates pixels as gray matter, white matter, and CSF.

Alternative methods have been developed that use a variety of computational techniques, including automated training class selection (Cocosco, Zijdenbos, & Evans, 2003; Harris et al., 1999), expectation-maximization algorithms (Schroeter, Vesin, Langenberger, & Meuli, 1998; Van Leemput, Maes, Vandermeulen, & Suetens, 1999b, 2003; Wells, Grimson, Kikinis, & Jolesz, 1996), standardized template images (Kamber, Shinghal, Collins, Francis, & Evans, 1995; Van Leemput et al., 1999a, 1999b, 2003; Warfield, Kaus, Jolesz, & Kikinis, 2000), genetic algorithms (Schroeter et al., 1998), Markov random fields (Van Leemput et al., 1999a), and artificial neural networks (Zijdenbos, Forghani, & Evans, 2002).

## Volumetric Methods: Semiautomated Approaches

To minimize the manual labor required for measuring brain volumes, many research groups have implemented semiautomated volumetric methods. By reducing the dependence on human operators for tracing, this approach is made quicker and less susceptible to problems of rater bias and rater drift (Tisserand, Van Boxtel, Gronenschild, & Jolles, 2001; Tisserand et al., 2002).

These techniques are critically dependent on spatial transformation of images into standardized space. Whereas ROI volumetric studies use standardized views to help raters consistently identify landmarks for tracing, semiautomated methods are based on automatic identification of ROIs based on their alignment with the portion of the grid that represents that ROI in the standard anatomical space. Again, the most commonly used system is the Talairach coordinate system. With this approach, ROIs are determined a priori by assigning each of the "Talairach boxes" in the Talairach grid to one ROI or another. If a box includes gray matter from two regions, one possibility is to assign it to the region that contributes the majority of the tissue to that box. Another possibility would be to split the box and have it contribute partially to both regions. Figure 12.6 depicts a brain parcellated into sublobar regions using this method.

The operator-dependent aspect of this approach consists of realigning the brains to the Talairach grid. As described earlier, this requires a trained operator to align the AC-PC plane with the horizontal axis of the grid, and to align the interhemispheric fissure with the vertical axis. After reorienting the brain, the six outer boundaries of the brain (anterior, posterior, superior, inferior, left, and right) must also be identified, either manually or automatically. This enables the Talairach grid to be adapted to each individual brain, thereby correcting for differences in overall head size and shape.

Andreasen and colleagues (1994, 1996) have presented a valid, reliable, and efficient procedure for estimating regional brain volumes based on the Talairach atlas. They defined 12 ROIs: the frontal lobe, temporal lobe, parietal lobe, occipital lobe, as well as cerebellar and subcortical regions on both the left and right hemisphere. They supplemented the traditional Talairach grid with additional boxes to include the cerebellum and validated their methods by showing that the volumes generated corre-

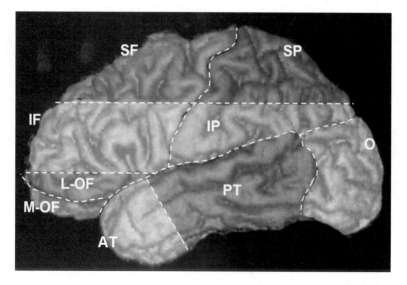

FIGURE 12.6. Results of parcellation of the brain into sublobar volumes using the SABRE method. Courtesy of Brian Levine, L. C. Campbell Cognitive Neurology Research Unit, Sunnybrook and Women's, University of Toronto.

spond with the "gold standard" of manually traced volumes. Other research groups have continued to develop this methodology, most notably by delineating subregions within the frontal lobe and prefrontal cortex (Dade et al., 2004; Kovacevic et al., 2002; Tisserand et al., 2001, 2002).

This approach has been successfully applied to schizophrenia (Andreasen et al., 1994; Quarantelli et al., 2002), pediatric populations (Kaplan et al., 1997), aging populations (Goldszal et al., 1998; Resnick et al., 2000; Tisserand et al., 2001, 2002), and dementia (Kovacevic et al., 2002). Andreasen and colleagues (1994) showed a relative decrease in brain tissue volume in the frontal lobes of patients with schizophrenia. Tisserand and colleagues (2001) produced volumes indicating that the medial prefrontal and dorsolateral prefrontal cortices are more profoundly affected by the aging process than the orbitoprefrontal cortex. They also presented data consistent with previous literature that reductions in total brain volume and prefrontal volumes, but not cerebellar volumes, are associated with advancing age (Tisserand et al., 2001).

However, despite the strengths of this approach, a major disadvantage is that it may be too crude for smaller brain regions, such as the caudate nucleus or subregions of the prefrontal cortex (Goldszal et al., 1998; Kaplan et al.,

1997; Resnick et al., 2000; Tisserand et al., 2002). Ultimately, when comparing these semiautomated methods with manual tracing, there is a trade-off of accuracy for time and labor. Manual tracing requires that raters be trained to have a good understanding of neuroanatomy; then inter- and intrarater reliability must be established. When deciding among volumetrics methods, one must balance the accuracy that comes with manual tracing against the speed with which data can be processed. For a reasonably large ROI in a large data set comprising many brains, a semiautomated approach may be a better option.

## Morphometric Methods

### Voxel-Based Morphometry

Despite their accuracy and simplicity, volumetric methods have limitations. In addition to being labor-intensive, volumetric approaches constrain the potential for anatomical findings. In large ROIs, which are only represented by a single number (e.g., left frontal gray matter volume), potential effects in only a portion of the region may be diluted by the lack of effect in other parts. In addition, because they are time-consuming, ROI analyses often do not encompass the whole brain, so that potential effects outside the ROI can be missed. Morphometric approaches address these issues, in that they allow the analysis of effects across the entire brain at a very high resolution. In addition, they are accomplished almost entirely by computer algorithms, making them relatively immune to problems of inter- and intrarater variability.

One of the earliest morphometric methods to receive extensive use was voxel-based morphometry (VBM). The technique is conceptually simple and provides a good model from which to understand other morphometric techniques. Figure 12.7 depicts the steps necessary to perform VBM. The technique begins with spatial transformation of each subject's brain into a standard anatomical space, either Talairach space or a similar reference system. This allows the assumption that changes in a particular voxel (volume element—a pixel in three dimensions) in the analysis space corresponds to a particular anatomical structure. Spatial transformation proceeds through an initial gross transformation, where the subject's brain is moved into the location of a target brain and resized to that target's rough size and shape (as described earlier for the Talairach transformation). The first steps of this transfor-

mation are linear (all changes are applied uniformly across the brain in that dimension) and are said to represent an affine transformation (usually consisting of 12 parameters: translation, rotation, resizing, and shear correction in three dimensions each). The affine transformation is often followed by more detailed fitting of local structure in the subject's brain to the target brain. Because these may affect some parts of the brain more than others (say, the right frontal lobe more than the left), this component of spatial transformation is nonlinear. In VBM, a key methodological point is to allow a rough transformation of a subject's brain into the target space, but not to allow such a highly detailed transformation that all the effects of interest (e.g., disease-related atrophy) are corrected.

Spatial transformation is followed by segmentation of the subject's image into gray, white, and CSF compartments (the principles of which were described earlier). Most commonly, the gray matter image, which is a high contrast image depicting gray matter structures and the empty space around them, is used. The gray matter image is then smoothed with an image filter, which averages the value at each

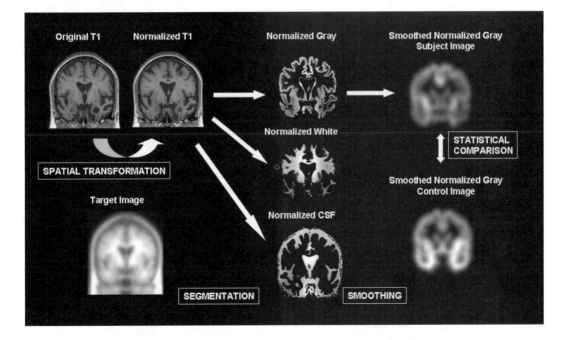

FIGURE 12.7. Preprocessing steps required to perform basic VBM. For simplicity, some details are omitted. Text in boxes represent processing steps, whereas nonboxed text is used to label images produced by the process.

voxel with the values at voxels immediately around it. The distance is defined by the size of the filter, with 12 mm being a common size. In the smoothed image, voxels that previously had high intensities, indicating that they were all gray matter, now have lower intensities, particularly if they were surrounded by many low-intensity pixels. This is more common in regions of brain atrophy. These smoothed images are then entered into an analysis to look for effects of interest. In the most commonly used program, Statistical Parametric Mapping (SPM) (www.fil.ion.ucl.ac.uk/spm), each voxel in the image is treated as a dependent variable in a linear regression analysis, with subject variables such as disease state, or cognitive or behavioral features, as independent variables. Contrasts of interest can be specified to find the voxels significantly associated with the behavioral feature of interest. The result is that effects can be detected anywhere in the brain, with the lower limit of resolution being determined by the image resolution and the size of the smoothing filter. Since this is being done with hundreds of voxels across the brain, it is necessary to correct the $p$ values to account for this, by using an estimate of the number of comparisons based the image resolution and filter size.

VBM has been used to examine structural abnormalities associated with normal aging (Good et al., 2001), as well as many neurological and psychiatric disorders characterized by frontal dysfunction, including AD (Boxer et al., 2003; Testa et al., 2004), FTD (Boccardi et al., 2005; Rosen, Gorno-Tempini, et al., 2002), progressive supranuclear palsy (Price et al., 2004), corticobasal degeneration (Grossman et al., 2004), Huntington's disease (Kassubek, Juengling, Ecker, & Landwehrmeyer, 2004), schizophrenia (Giuliani, Calhoun, Pearlson, Francis, & Buchanan, 2005), bipolar disorder (Adler, Levine, DelBello, & Strakowski, 2005) and autism (Abell et al., 1999). Most of these studies have compared the group of interest with age-matched healthy controls to reveal regions of atrophy associated with the condition being studied. Figure 12.8 gives an example of VBM findings in several neurodegenerative syndromes. More recently, researchers have begun to examine regional structural changes associated with specific behavioral features using VBM. For example, Grossman and colleagues (2004) examined the neuroanatomical correlates of naming difficulties in patients with

neurodegenerative disease and has shown that naming deficits are correlated with decreased tissue content in distinct but overlapping brain regions in patients with neurodegenerative disease. Rosen and colleagues (2005) recently examined the neuroanatomical correlates of behavioral disorders in dementia and showed that different types of behavioral abnormalities are associated with different regions of tissue loss in the medial prefrontal cortex. Tissue loss was best correlated with disinhibition in the subgenual cingulate cortex, with apathy in the ventromedial superior frontal gyrus, and with aberrant motor behavior in the dorsal anterior cingulate cortex and adjacent supplementary motor area (see Figure 12.9). These data are consistent with existing ideas about the ventral and medial frontal regions having important emotional functions, and the more dorsal medial frontal regions having cognitive and motoric functions (Vogt, Berger, & Derbyshire, 2003). In the case of apathy and disinhibition, both regions might have been included in a ventromedial frontal ROI in a different study, obscuring the fact that these regions have different behavioral associations.

VBM represents an important advance in structural imaging analysis, because it can identify regional associations in any part of the brain without a priori assumptions, and it is quick and relatively uninfluenced by operator bias. The price one pays for this is that the performance of so many comparisons across the entire brain requires a high statistical threshold to consider the results significant. If one has a priori assumptions about the regions that may be involved with a particular assumption, they can be combined with a morphometric analysis to limit the multiple-comparisons problem (Vogt et al., 2003). VBM has also been criticized on methodological grounds, because it does not differentiate between tissue that has disappeared and tissue that has moved out of place because of tissue loss in other brain regions (Bookstein, 2001). This may particularly be a problem with periventricular structures, such as the caudate nucleus and thalamus. Thus, findings in which this could be a factor should be cautiously interpreted.

### Deformation-Based Morphometry

VBM is based on a rough transformation of a subject's brain into a target space, which can be particularly problematic if white matter

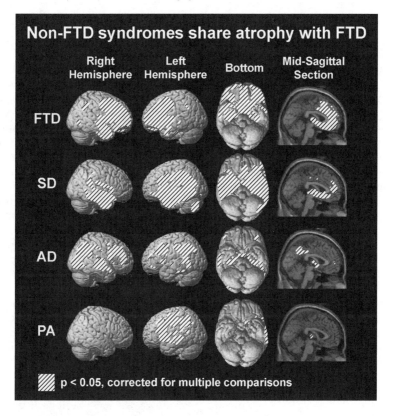

FIGURE 12.8. Maps of statistically significant differences resulting from the comparison of structural images in different dementia syndromes with control images. Patterns of frontal involvement differ according to the clinical syndrome, with FTD particularly affecting medial and lateral frontal regions, AD affecting the lateral frontal regions and parietal, and PA affecting mainly the left lateral frontoparietal (perisylvian) region. FTD, frontotemporal dementia; SD, semantic dementia; AD, Alzheimer's disease; PA, progressive nonfluent aphasia.

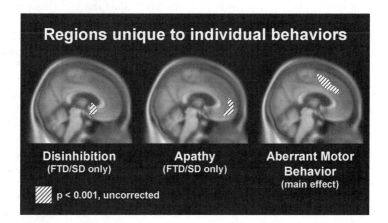

FIGURE 12.9. Maps of statistically significant correlations between brain tissue loss and behavioral dysfunction. Regions representing a main effect were significant across patients with several types of dementia syndromes, whereas regions indicated as "FTD/SD only" showed the correlation specifically in this subgroup. FTD, frontotemporal dementia; SD, semantic dementia.

volume loss causes changes in the location of overlying gray matter. Newer methods, such as deformation-based morphometry (DBM), are available due to increased computational power. DBM allows a much more precise transformation of a subject's brain into a target space by using millions of parameters in the nonlinear phase, rather than the hundreds used in VBM. These methods give rise to a voxel-by-voxel map, called a Jacobian matrix, of the transformation parameters that were required to morph a subject's brain to match a brain template. The Jacobian matrix contains an indirect but precise record of the original brain's shape and size. Researchers who use DBM perform these high-dimensional warps on the subject images using a common target space, and then use the Jacobian matrices to identify tissue changes that correlate with features of interest.

DBM is computationally demanding and requires several hours to process a brain; therefore, this method has been used less commonly to study structural changes in clinical populations. Recently, it has been used to track the progress longitudinally of cerebral atrophy in patients with AD (Janke et al., 2001), and to study the patterns of atrophy in semantic dementia (Studholme, Cardenas, Blumenfeld, et al., 2004), progressive supranuclear palsy (Paviour et al., 2004), and schizophrenia (Gaser, Volz, Kiebel, Riehemann, & Sauer, 1999). Using DBM to compare 20 patients with semantic dementia with 20 control subjects, Studholme and colleagues (Studholme, Cardenas, Blumenfeld, et al., 2004; Studholme, Cardenas, Song, et al., 2004) demonstrated that patients with semantic dementia had significant tissue contraction in the left temporal pole, as well as the hippocampus, occipito-temporal gyrus, and parahippocampal gyrus (Studholme, Cardenas, Blumenfeld, et al., 2004; Studholme, Cadenas, Song, et al., 2004). This finding is consistent with our understanding that regions of the left hemisphere, particularly in the temporal lobe, are involved with language functions. Gaser and colleagues (1999) demonstrated the effectiveness of DBM by performing a whole-brain analysis on a set of scans obtained from 85 patients with schizophrenia and 75 healthy controls. By analyzing the deformation fields produced by a nonlinear registration process, they observed that the patients with schizophrenia had significantly reduced tissue volumes in the thalamus and superior temporal gyrus bilaterally, as well as the left superior frontal gyrus, left precentral gyrus, and right middle frontal gyrus (Gaser et al., 1999).

These examples demonstrate how DBM can be useful for identifying patterns of tissue loss that are characteristic of various neurological diseases. Since the warps performed in DBM are much more detailed, they can more accurately differentiate changes occurring in white matter from those in gray matter. DBM, like VBM, is also attractive because it is a fully automated technique that is insensitive to user bias, and does not require predefined ROIs. Ultimately, these methods may provide a more refined view of subtle differences in brain anatomy and will likely gain popularity as increased computer power becomes more widely available.

In addition to computational demands, the attempt to match precisely every feature in a given brain to a target brain gives rise to questions of validity, because the variation among individuals' minor sulci is considerable. Although any brain can be arbitrarily reshaped to match any other brain, there is no way to be certain that the histologically defined Brodmann's areas have been perfectly aligned. This problem establishes a limit of accuracy that must be considered with any analysis based on gross structure.

### Boundary-Shift Integral

A third morphometric technique that has become popular in structural imaging, the boundary-shift integral (BSI), is a quantitative measure of brain atrophy used to evaluate longitudinal changes in an individual subject. This technique is based on precise coregistration of images collected over time, so that subtle changes in anatomical boundaries can be quantified. The great benefit offered by BSI is that the problem of anatomical variability among individuals is avoided, because each subject is used as his or her own control.

This technique is based on the identification of tissue surfaces (or boundaries) from the signal intensities in the image (Fox & Freeborough, 1997; Freeborough & Fox, 1997). The BSI calculates how much the surface of a given cerebral structure has moved over time. The movement of the structure's surface can be summated in three dimensions to provide a direct measure of volume change. This measure of cerebral volume loss has been shown to correlate strongly with clinical measures of cognitive decline in patients with AD (Fox, Scahill, Crum, & Rossor, 1999). The use of robust longitudinal measures such as the BSI can help neuroscientists detect the onset of neurodegenerative disease, track the disease progression, as well as help to differentiate various forms of dementia from each other and from normal aging. Many studies have shown that this technique can be used to differentiate reliably between patients with AD and normal controls based on global and regional atrophy rates (Barnes et al., 2004; Ezekiel et al., 2004; Fox & Freeborough 1997; Fox, Freeborough, & Rossor, 1996; O'Brien et al., 2001; Rusinek et al., 2003; Schott et al., 2003, 2005). The BSI has also been utilized to track patterns of cerebral atrophy in patients with frontotemporal lobar degeneration (Janssen et al., 2005). As potential treatments become available for patients with dementia, BSI may be a robust and reliable measure of their efficacy (Fox, Cousens, Scahill, Harvey, & Rossor, 2000; Schott et al., 2005).

## STRUCTURAL IMAGING OF WHITE MATTER

### Measurement of White Matter Signal Hyperintensity

In addition to examining and measuring gray matter changes, recent advances have been made in the imaging of white matter changes. For example, white matter hyperintensities (WMHs) are abnormalities usually identified on T2-weighted MRIs (Figure 12.10) and associated with cognitive impairment, and to some degree, vascular disease (DeCarli et al., 1995; DeCarli, Fletcher, et al., 2005; de Groot et al., 2000, 2001; Hachinski, Potter, & Merskey, 1987; Longstreth et al., 1996; Ylikoski et al., 1993). Although the etiology of these WMHs is still somewhat uncertain, much evidence suggests an ischemic mechanism of pathology, which is supported by the presence of vascular fibrosis and lipohyalinosis in postmortem tissue (DeCarli, Fletcher, et al., 2005). However, there is also evidence of demyelination, possibly caused by arterial changes and breakdown of the ventricular lining, as the primary cause of these signal abnormalities (Fazekas et al., 1993; Scheltens et al., 1995). Despite this uncertainty, it has been well established that the development of WMHs is significantly associated with advancing age. In addition, WMHs have been associated with a history of stroke, hypertension, diabetes, ischemic heart disease, and claudication (Kertesz et al., 1988; Streifler et al., 2003).

Similar to volumetric methods developed for examining gray matter, Meyer and colleagues (1999) have established a comprehensive protocol for the parcellation of cerebral white matter using MRI. This protocol divides the major white matter tracts of the human brain into three main compartments: outer radiate fibers, intermediate sagittal fibers, and deep bridging fibers. These three compartments are further

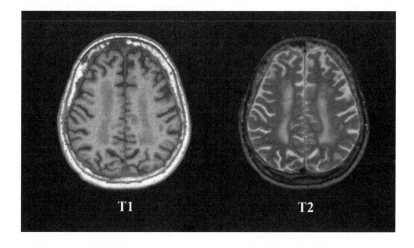

FIGURE 12.10. T1- and T2-weighted images in a patient with a moderate-to-severe degree of subcortical white matter signal hyperintensity.

subdivided to enable the measurement of specific white matter tracts. Methods of this type have been used to determine which axonal systems are critical for particular cognitive and behavioral functions. For example, WMH in the dorsolateral prefrontal cortex (DLPFC) have been shown to be significantly more common in late-life depression—a finding with specific implications for the understanding and treatment of depression in elderly populations (Thomas et al., 2003). Increasingly sophisticated approaches to measurement of WMH allow a better understanding of the etiology of these changes. For instance, automated analysis of WMH location on a voxel-by-voxel basis has revealed new information about the patterns of WMH. Many researchers make a distinction between two types of WMH: periventricular (PVWMH) and deep (DWMH), based on anatomical location. However, DeCarli, Massaro, and colleagues (2005) suggest that these categorical distinctions are arbitrary, and instead support the notion of a "single vascular watershed area that extends from the CSF ventricular surface to the central white matter" (DeCarli, Fletcher, et al., 2005, p. 54). Ultimately, when examining frontal lobe function, particularly in elderly populations, one must consider white matter changes that may be contributing to cognitive and behavioral deficits.

## Diffusion Tensor Imaging

Advanced imaging technologies, such as diffusion tensor imaging (DTI), are currently being developed to enhance our ability to examine and quantify white matter changes. DTI is a type of image that can be acquired with an MR scanner, but it is characteristically different than typical MR sequences, in which the strength of the magnetic field ($B_0$) is kept as homogenous as possible. Any signal inhomogeneity that exists during image acquisition must be corrected for during image preprocessing, because the received signal intensity is directly proportional to the magnetic field strength. However, with DTI, a magnetic field gradient is purposefully introduced. This field gradient can be controlled and allows researchers to make diffusion measurements (Mori, 2002).

The key to understanding how DTI works lies in the distinction between isotropic and *an*isotropic diffusion. Isotropic diffusion refers to the state in which molecules are diffusing equally in all directions. Anisotropic diffusion, on the other hand, refers to the state in which molecules are diffusing more in a particular direction than in other directions. This anisotropic diffusion, in which there is coherent molecular motion, can also be called "flow." Anisotropic diffusion and isotropic diffusion have different effects on the MR signal, which enables diffusion measurements to be acquired. In certain biological structures, such as muscle or axonal fibers, there is an ordered arrangement of cells that causes the diffusion of water to be significantly greater along the axis of those fibers. In healthy white matter, there tends to be an extensive number of neuronal axons, all traveling in the same direction, which means that this tissue will have a high degree of anisotropic diffusion in a particular direction (Basser, Mattiello, & LeBihan, 1994; Beaulieu & Allen, 1994; Henkelman, Stanisz, Kim, & Bronskill, 1994; Makris et al., 1997; Moseley et al., 1990; Pierpaoli, Jezzard, Basser, Barnett, & Di Chiro, 1996; Ulug & van Zijl, 1999). Therefore, diffusion measurements can provide information concerning the type of matter present in a given voxel, as well as its orientation.

Thus, DTI is a valuable technology for the study of white matter. Information concerning the orientation of tissue is unique to DTI and enables the 3D reconstruction of white matter tracts in the brain. DTI has been used to visualize several cortical association tracts, including the anterior (ATR) and posterior (PTR) thalamic radiations, and the uncinate (UNC), superior longitudinal (SLF), inferior longitudinal (ILF), and inferior frontal–occipital (IFO) fasciculi; these findings showed good qualitative agreement with anatomical knowledge of these structures (Mori, Kaufmann, et al., 2002). Figure 12.11 depicts the identification of the SLF with these methods. The effects of disease processes on white matter tracts can be examined with DTI, and has been done so with cases of birth defects, developmental disorders, brain tumors, and chronic stroke (Mori, Fredericksen, et al., 2002; Pierpaoli et al., 2001; Werring et al., 2000; Wieshmann et al., 2000). A recent study involving elderly subjects found that depression correlated significantly with lower fractional anisotropy values in the right superior frontal gyrus, even after controlling for age, sex, hypertension, and heart disease (Taylor et al., 2004).

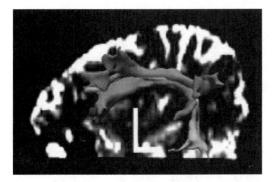

FIGURE 12.11. Depiction of the superior longitudinal fasciculus using DTI-based white matter fiber tracking. Courtesy of Roland Henry, Department of Radiology, University of California, San Francisco.

DTI, like all MRI technologies, is noninvasive and provides a unique ability to visualize neuronal projections that connect various regions of the brain. DTI can be a vital imaging tool for understanding the complex functional connectivity of the healthy human brain, as well as various disease processes that impact these connections. Current limitations of DTI are that the raw images used to perform DTI analysis are low-resolution and prone to artifacts (Mori, 2002).

## REFERENCES

Abell, F., Krams, M., Ashburner, J., Passingham, R., Friston, K., Frackowiak, R., et al. (1999). The neuroanatomy of autism: A voxel-based whole brain analysis of structural scans. *NeuroReport*, *10*(8), 1647–1651.

Adler, C. M., Levine, A. D., DelBello, M. P., & Strakowski, S. M. (2005). Changes in gray matter volume in patients with bipolar disorder. *Biological Psychiatry*, *58*(2), 151–157.

Anderson, S. W., Damasio, H., & Damasio, A. R. (2005). A neural basis for collecting behaviour in humans. *Brain*, *128*(1), 201–212.

Andreasen, N. C., Flashman, L. A., Flaum, M., Arndt, S., Swayze, V. W., II, O'Leary, D. S., et al. (1994). Regional brain abnormalities in schizophrenia measured With magnetic resonance imaging. *Journal of the American Medical Association*, *272*(22), 1763–1769.

Andreasen, N. C., Rajarethinam, R., Cizadlo, T., Arndt, S., Swayze, V. W., II, Flashman, L. A., et al. (1996). Automatic atlas-based volume estimation of human brain regions from MR images. *Journal of Computer Assisted Tomography*, *20*(1), 98–106.

Baldo, J. V., Dronkers, N. F., Wilkins, D., Ludy, C., Raskin, P., & Kim, J. (2005). Is problem solving dependent on language? *Brain and Language*, *92*(3), 240–250.

Barnea-Goraly, N., Eliez, S., Hedeus, M., Menon, V., White, C. D., Moseley M., et al. (2003). White matter tract alterations in fragile X syndrome: Preliminary evidence from diffusion tensor imaging. *American Journal of Medical Genetics*, *118*(1), 81–88.

Barnes, J., Scahill, R. I., Boyes, R. G., Frost, C., Lewis, E. B., Rossor, C. L., et al. (2004). Differentiating AD from aging using semiautomated measurement of hippocampal atrophy rates. *NeuroImage*, *23*(2), 574–581.

Barr, A., Heinze, W., Dobben, G., Valvassori, G., & Sugar, O. (1978). Bicaudate index in computerized tomography of Huntington disease and cerebral atrophy. *Neurology*, *28*(11), 1196–1200.

Basser, P. J., Mattiello, J., & LeBihan, D. (1994). Estimation of the effective self-diffusion tensor from the NMR spin echo. *Journal of Magnetic Resonance, Series B*, *103*(3), 247–254.

Bates, E., Wilson, S. M., Saygin, A. P., Dick, F., Sereno, M. I., Knight, R. T., et al. (2003). Voxel-based lesion-symptom mapping. *Nature Neuroscience*, *6*(5), 448–450.

Beaulieu, C., & Allen, P. S. (1994). Determinants of anisotropic water diffusion in nerves. *Magnetic Resonance in Medicine*, *31*(4), 394–400.

Beer, J. S., Heerey, E. A., Keltner, D., Scabini, D., & Knight, R. T. (2003). The regulatory function of self-conscious emotion: Insights from patients with orbitofrontal damage. *Journal of Personality and Social Psychology*, *85*(4), 594–604.

Boccardi, M., Sabattoli, F., Laakso, M. P., Testa, C., Rossi, R., Beltramello, A., et al. (2005). Frontotemporal dementia as a neural system disease. *Neurobiology of Aging*, *26*(1), 37–44.

Bookstein, F. L. (2001). "Voxel-based morphometry" should not be used with imperfectly registered images. *NeuroImage*, *14*(6), 1454–1462.

Bosscher, L., & Scheltens, P. (2001). MRI of the medial temporal lobe for the diagnosis of Alzheimer's disease practice. In N. Qizibash, L. Schneider, H. Brodaty, P. Tariot, J. Kaye, H. Chui, et al. (Eds.), *Evidence-based dementia practice* (pp. 154–161). Oxford, UK: Blackwell.

Boxer, A. L., Kramer, J. H., Du, A.-T., Schuff, N., Weiner, M. W., Miller, B. L., et al. (2003). Focal right inferotemporal atrophy in AD with disproportionate visual constructive impairment. *Neurology*, *61*, 1485–1491.

Braak, E., Griffing, K., Arai, K., Bohl, J., Bratzke, H., & Braak, H. (1999). Neuropathology of Alzheimer's disease: What is new since A. Alzheimer? *European Archives of Psychiatry and Clinical Neuroscience*, *249*(Suppl. 3), 14–22.

Buchanan, R. W., Francis, A., Arango, C., Miller, K., Lefkowitz, D. M., McMahon, R. P., et al. (2004). Morphometric assessment of the heteromodal association cortex in schizophrenia. *American Journal of Psychiatry, 161*(2), 322–331.

Bunney, B. G., Potkin, S. G., & Bunney, W. E., Jr. (1995). New morphological and neuropathological findings in schizophrenia: A neurodevelopmental perspective. *Clinical Neuroscience, 3*(2), 81–88.

Caviness, J., Verne, S., & Meyer, J. (1996). MRI-based topographic parcellation of human neocortex: An anatomically specified method with. . . . *Journal of Cognitive Neuroscience, 8,* 566.

Cha, S. (2003). Perfusion MR imaging: Basic principles and clinical applications. *Magnetic Resonance Imaging Clinics of North America, 11*(3), 403–413.

Cocosco, C. A., Zijdenbos, A. P., & Evans, A. C. (2003). A fully automatic and robust brain MRI tissue classification method. *Medical Image Analysis, 7*(4), 513–527.

Cohen, G., Andreasen, N. C., Alliger, R., Arndt, S., Kuan, J., Yuh, W. T. C., et al. (1992). Segmentation techniques for the classification of brain tissue using magnetic resonance imaging. *Psychiatry Research: Neuroimaging, 45*(1), 33–51.

Crespo-Facorro, B., Kim, J.-J., Andreasen, N. C., O'Leary, D. S., & Magnotta, V. (2000a). Regional frontal abnormalities in schizophrenia: A quantitative gray matter volume and cortical surface size study. *Biological Psychiatry, 48*(2), 110–119.

Crespo-Facorro, B., Kim, J.-J., Andreasen, N. C., O'Leary, D. S., Wiser, A. K., Bailey, J. M., et al. (1999). Human frontal cortex: An MRI-based parcellation method. *NeuroImage, 10*(5), 500–519.

Crespo-Facorro, B., Kim, J.-J., Andreasen, N. C., Spinks, R., O'Leary, D. S., Bockholt, H. J., et al. (2000). Cerebral cortex: A topographic segmentation method using magnetic resonance imaging. *Psychiatry Research: Neuroimaging, 100*(2), 97–126.

Critchley, H. D., Mathias, C. J., Josephs, O., O'Doherty, J., Zanini, S., Dewar, B. K., et al. (2003). Human cingulate cortex and autonomic control: Converging neuroimaging and clinical evidence. *Brain, 126*(10), 2139–2152.

Dade, L. A., Gao, F. Q., Kovacevic, N., Roy, P., Rockel, C., O'Toole, C. M., et al. (2004). Semiautomatic brain region extraction: A method of parcellating brain regions from structural magnetic resonance images. *NeuroImage, 22*(4), 1492–1502.

DeCarli, C., Fletcher, E., Ramey, V., Harvey, D., & Jagust, W. J. (2005). Anatomical mapping of white matter hyperintensities (WMH): Exploring the relationships between periventricular WMH, deep WMH, and total WMH burden. *Stroke, 36*(1), 50–55.

DeCarli, C., Massaro, J., Harvey, D., Hald, J., Tullberg, M., Au, R., et al. (2005). Measures of brain morphology and infarction in the Framingham Heart Study: Establishing what is normal. *Neurobiology of Aging, 26*(4), 491–510.

DeCarli, C. M., Murphy, D. G. M. M., Tranh, M. B., Grady, C. L. P., Haxby, J. V. P., Gillette, J. A. M., et al. (1995). The effect of white matter hyperintensity

volume on brain structure, cognitive performance, and cerebral metabolism of glucose in 51 healthy adults. *Neurology, 45*(11), 2077–2084.

de Groot, J. C., de Leeuw, F.-E., Oudkerk, M., Hofman, A., Jolles, J., & Breteler, M. M. B. (2001). Cerebral white matter lesions and subjective cognitive dysfunction: The Rotterdam Scan Study. *Neurology, 56*(11), 1539–1545.

de Groot, J. C., de Leeuw, F.-E., Oudkerk, M., van Gijn, J., Hofman, A., Jolles, J., et al. (2000). Cerebral white matter lesions and cognitive function: The Rotterdam Scan Study. *Annals of Neurology, 47*(2), 145–151.

Denihan, A., Wilson, G., Cunningham, C., Coakley, D., & Lawlor, B. A. (2000). CT measurement of medial temporal lobe atrophy in Alzheimer's disease, vascular dementia, depression and paraphrenia. *International Journal of Geriatric Psychiatry, 15*(4), 306–312.

Detre, J. A., Zhang, W., Roberts, D. A., Silva, A. C., Williams, D. S., Grandis, D. J., et al. (1994). Tissue specific perfusion imaging using arterial spin labeling. *NMR in Biomedicine, 7*(1–2), 75–82.

Dickson, D. W., Bergeron, C., Chin, S. S., Duyckaerts, C., Horoupian, D., Ikeda, K., et al. (2002). Office of Rare Diseases neuropathologic criteria for corticobasal degeneration. *Journal of Neuropathology and Experimental Neurology, 61*(11), 935–946.

Drevets, W. C. (2000). Functional anatomical abnormalities in limbic and prefrontal cortical structures in major depression. *Progress in Brain Research, 126,* 413–431.

Dronkers, N. F. (1996). A new brain region for coordinating speech articulation. *Nature, 384,* 159–161.

Erkinjuntti, T., Lee, D. H., Gao, F., Steenhuis, R., Eliasziw, M., Fry, R., et al. (1993). Temporal lobe atrophy on magnetic resonance imaging in the diagnosis of early Alzheimer's disease. *Archives of Neurology, 50*(3), 305–310.

Eslinger, P., & Damasio, A. (1986). Preserved motor learning in Alzheimer's disease: Implications for anatomy and behaviour. *Journal of Neuroscience, 6,* 3006–3009.

Ezekiel, F. B. A., Chao, L. P., Kornak, J. P., Du, A.-T. M. D., Cardenas, V. P., et al. (2004). Comparisons between global and focal brain atrophy rates in normal aging and Alzheimer disease: Boundary shift integral versus tracing of the entorhinal cortex and hippocampus. *Alzheimer Disease and Associated Disorders, 18*(4), 196–201.

Fazekas, F., Barkhof, F., Wahlund, L. O., Pantoni, L., Erkinjuntti, T., Scheltens, P., et al. (2002). CT and MRI rating of white matter lesions. *Cerebrovascular Disease, 13*(Suppl. 2), 31–36.

Fazekas, F., Kleinert, R., Offenbacher, H., Schmidt, R., Kleinert, G., Payer, F., et al. (1993). Pathologic correlates of incidental MRI white matter signal hyperintensities. *Neurology, 43*(9), 1683–1689.

Fox, N. C., Cousens, S., Scahill, R., Harvey, R. J., &

Rossor, M. N. (2000). Using serial registered brain magnetic resonance imaging to measure disease progression in Alzheimer disease: Power calculations and estimates of sample size to detect treatment effects. *Archives of Neurology, 57*(3), 339–344.

Fox, N. C., & Freeborough, P. A. (1997). Brain atrophy progression measured from registered serial MRI: Validation and application to Alzheimer's disease. *Journal of Magnetic Resonance Imaging, 7*(6), 1069–1075.

Fox, N. C., Freeborough, P. A., & Rossor, M. N. (1996). Visualisation and quantification of rates of atrophy in Alzheimer's disease. *Lancet, 348,* 94–97.

Fox, N. C., Scahill, R. I., Crum, W. R., & Rossor, M. N. (1999). Correlation between rates of brain atrophy and cognitive decline in AD. *Neurology, 52*(8), 1687–1689.

Freeborough, P. A., & Fox, N. C. (1997). The boundary shift integral: An accurate and robust measure of cerebral volume changes from registered repeat MRI. *IEEE Transactions on Medical Imaging, 16*(5), 623–629.

Frisoni, G. B., Beltramello, A., Geroldi, C., Weiss, C., Bianchetti, A., & Trabucchi, M. (1996). Brain atrophy in frontotemporal dementia. *Journal of Neurology, Neurosurgery, and Psychiatry, 61*(2), 157–165.

Frisoni, G. B., Beltramello, A., Weiss, C., Geroldi, C., Bianchetti, A., & Trabucchi, M. (1995). Usefulness of simple measures of temporal lobe atrophy in probable Alzheimer's disease. *Dementia, 7,* 15–22.

Frisoni, G. B., Beltramello, A., Weiss, C., Geroldi, C., Bianchetti, A., & Trabucchi, M. (1996). Linear measures of atrophy in mild Alzheimer disease. *American Journal of Neuroradiology, 17*(5), 913–923.

Frisoni, G. B., Bianchetti, A., Geroldi, C., Trabucchi, M., Beltramello, A., & Weiss, C. (1994). Measures of medial temporal lobe atrophy in Alzheimer's disease. *Journal of Neurology, Neurosurgery, and Psychiatry, 57*(11), 1438–1439.

Galton, C. J., Gomez-Anson, B., Antoun, N., Scheltens, P., Patterson, K., Graves, M., et al. (2001). Temporal lobe rating scale: Application to Alzheimer's disease and frontotemporal dementia. *Journal of Neurology, Neurosurgery, and Psychiatry, 70*(2), 165–173.

Gao, F. Q., Black, S. E., Leibovitch, F. S., Callen, D. J., Lobaugh, N. J., & Szalai, J. P. (2003). A reliable MR measurement of medial temporal lobe width from the Sunnybrook Dementia Study. *Neurobiology of Aging, 24*(1), 49–56.

Gao, F. Q., Black, S. E., Leibovitch, F. S., Callen, D. J., Rockel, C. P., & Szalai, J. P. (2004). Linear width of the medial temporal lobe can discriminate Alzheimer's disease from normal aging: The Sunnybrook Dementia Study. *Neurobiology of Aging, 25*(4), 441–448.

Gaser, C., Volz, H.-P., Kiebel, S., Riehemann, S., & Sauer, H. (1999). Detecting structural changes in whole brain based on nonlinear deformations—application to schizophrenia research. *NeuroImage, 10*(2), 107–113.

Giuliani, N. R., Calhoun, V. D., Pearlson, G. D., Francis, A., & Buchanan, R. W. (2005). Voxel-based morphometry versus region of interest: A comparison of two methods for analyzing gray matter differences in schizophrenia. *Schizophrenia Research, 74*(2–3), 135–147.

Goldszal, A. F., Davatzikos, C., Pham, D. L., Yan, M. X. H., Bryan, R. N., & Resnick, S. M. (1998). An image-processing system for qualitative and quantitative volumetric analysis of brain images. *Journal of Computer Assisted Tomography, 22*(5), 827–837.

Good, C. D., Johnsrude, I. S., Ashburner, J., Henson, R. N., Friston, K. J., & Frackowiak, R. S. (2001). A voxel-based morphometric study of ageing in 465 normal adult human brains. *NeuroImage, 14*(1, Pt. 1), 21–36.

Greenberg, J. O., & Adams, R. D. (1999). *Neuroimaging: A companion to Adams and Victor's* Principles of Neurology. New York: McGraw-Hill Professional.

Grossman, M., McMillan, C., Moore, P., Ding, L., Glosser, G., Work, M., et al. (2004). What's in a name?: Voxel-based morphometric analyses of MRI and naming difficulty in Alzheimer's disease, frontotemporal dementia and corticobasal degeneration. *Brain, 127*(3), 628–649.

Gur, R. E., Kohler, C., Turetsky, B. I., Siegel, S. J., Kanes, S. J., Bilker, W. B., et al. (2004). A sexually dimorphic ratio of orbitofrontal to amygdala volume is altered in schizophrenia. *Biological Psychiatry, 55*(5), 512–517.

Gur, R. E., Turetsky, B. I., Bilker, W. B., & Gur, R. C. (1999). Reduced gray matter volume in schizophrenia. *Archives of General Psychiatry, 56*(10), 905–911.

Hachinski, V. C., Potter, P., & Merskey, H. (1987). Leuko-araiosis. *Archives of Neurology, 44*(1), 21–23.

Harris, G., Andreasen, N. C., Cizadlo, T., Bailey, J. M., Bockholt, H. J., Magnotta, V. A., et al. (1999). Improving tissue classification in MRI: A three-dimensional multispectral discriminant analysis method with automated training class selection. *Journal of Computer Assisted Tomography, 23*(1), 144–154.

Henkelman, R. M., Stanisz, G. J., Kim, J. K., & Bronskill, M. J. (1994). Anisotropy of NMR properties of tissues. *Magnetic Resonance in Medicine, 32*(5), 592–601.

Hornak, J., Rolls, E. T., & Wade, D. (1996). Face and voice expression identification in patients with emotional and behavioural changes following ventral frontal lobe damage. *Neuropsychologia, 34*(4), 247–261.

Horowitz, A. L. (1995). *MRI physics for radiologists: A visual approach.* New York: Springer-Verlag.

Janke, A. L., de Zubicaray, G., Rose, S. E., Griffin, M., Chalk, J. B., & Galloway, G. J. (2001). 4D deformation modeling of cortical disease progression in Alzheimer's dementia. *Magnetic Resonance in Medicine, 46*(4), 661–666.

Janssen, J. C., Schott, J. M., Cipolotti, L., Fox, N. C.,

Scahill, R. I., Josephs, K. A., et al. (2005). Mapping the onset and progression of atrophy in familial frontotemporal lobar degeneration. *Journal of Neurology, Neurosurgery, and Psychiatry, 76*(2), 162–168.

Jobst, K., Smith, A., Barker, C., Wear, A., King, E., Smith, A., et al. (1992). Association of atrophy of the medial temporal lobe with reduced blood flow in the posterior parietotemporal cortex in patients with a clinical and pathological diagnosis of Alzheimer's disease. *Journal of Neurology, Neurosurgery, and Psychiatry, 55*(3), 190–194.

Jobst, K. A., Smith, A. D., Szatmari, M., Jaskowski, A., King, E., Smith, A., et al. (1992). Detection in life of confirmed Alzheimer's disease using a simple measurement of medial temporal lobe atrophy by computed tomography. *Lancet, 340,* 1179–1183.

Kamber, M., Shinghal, R., Collins, D. L., Francis, G. S., & Evans, A. C. (1995). Model-based 3-D segmentation of multiple sclerosis lesions in magnetic resonance brain images. *IEEE Transactions on Medical Imaging, 14*(3), 442–453.

Kaplan, D. M., Liu, A. M. C., Abrams, M. T., Warsofsky, I. S., Kates, W. R., White, C. D., et al. (1997). Application of an automated parcellation method to the analysis of pediatric brain volumes. *Psychiatry Research: Neuroimaging, 76*(1), 15–27.

Kassubek, J., Juengling, F. D., Ecker, D., & Landwehrmeyer, G. B. (2004). Thalamic atrophy in Huntington's disease co-varies with cognitive performance: A morphometric MRI analysis. *Cerebral Cortex, 15*(6), 846–853.

Kertesz, A., Black, S. E., Tokar, G., Benke, T., Carr, T., & Nicholson, L. (1988). Periventricular and subcortical hyperintensities on magnetic resonance imaging: "Rims, caps, and unidentified bright objects." *Archives of Neurology, 45*(4), 404–408.

Kertesz, A., & Ferro, J. M. (1984). Lesion size and location in ideomotor apraxia. *Brain, 107*(3), 921–933.

Kertesz, A., Harlock, W., & Coates, R. (1979). Computer tomographic localization, lesion size, and prognosis in aphasia and nonverbal impairment. *Brain and Language, 8*(1), 34–50.

Kim, J.-J., Crespo-Facorro, B., Andreasen, N. C., O'Leary, D. S., Zhang, B., Harris, G., et al. (2000). An MRI-based parcellation method for the temporal lobe. *NeuroImage, 11*(4), 271–288.

Klingberg, T., Hedehus, M., Temple, E., Salz, T., Gabrieli, J. D., Moseley, M. E., et al. (2000). Microstructure of temporo-parietal white matter as a basis for reading ability: Evidence from diffusion tensor magnetic resonance imaging. *Neuron, 25*(2), 493–500.

Kovacevic, N., Lobaugh, N. J., Bronskill, M. J., Levine, B., Feinstein, A., & Black, S. E. (2002). A robust method for extraction and automatic segmentation of brain images. *NeuroImage, 17*(3), 1087–1100.

Kuhl, D. E., Phelps, M. E., Markham, C. H., Metter, E. J., Riege, W. H., & Winter, J. (1982). Cerebral metabolism and atrophy in Huntington's disease determined by [18]FDG and computed tomographic scan. *Annals of Neurology, 12*(5), 425–434.

Levy, L. M. (1999). MR imaging of cerebrospinal fluid flow and spinal cord motion in neurologic disorders of the spine. *Magnetic Resonance Imaging Clinics of North America, 7*(3), 573–587.

Longstreth, W. T., Manolio, T. A., Arnold, A., Burke, G. L., Bryan, N., Jungreis, C. A., et al. (1996). Clinical correlates of white matter findings on cranial magnetic resonance imaging of 3,301 elderly people: The Cardiovascular Health Study. *Stroke, 27*(8), 1274–1282.

Magnotta, V. A., Harris, G., Andreasen, N. C., O'Leary, D. S., Yuh, W. T. C., & Heckel, D. (2002). Structural MR image processing using the 2 toolbox. *Computerized Medical Imaging and Graphics, 26*(4), 251–264.

Makris, N., Worth, A. J., Sorensen, A. G., Papadimitriou, G. M., Wu, O., Reese, T. G., et al. (1997). Morphometry of *in vivo* human white matter association pathways with diffusion-weighted magnetic resonance imaging. *Annals of Neurology, 42*(6), 951–962.

Mann, D. M., & South, P. W. (1993). The topographic distribution of brain atrophy in frontal lobe dementia. *Acta Neuropathologica, 85*(3), 334–340.

Mann, D. M. A., South, P. W., Snowden, J. S., & Neary, D. (1993). Dementia of frontal lobe type: Neuropathology and immunohistochemistry. *Journal of Neurology, Neurosurgery, and Psychiatry, 56,* 605–614.

Mayberg, H. S. (1994). Frontal lobe dysfunction in secondary depression. *Journal of Neuropsychiatry and Clinical Neurosciences, 6*(4), 428–442.

Meyer, J. W., Makris, N., Bates, J. F., Caviness, J., Verne, S., & Kennedy, D. N. (1999). MRI-based topographic parcellation of human cerebral white matter: I. Technical foundations. *NeuroImage, 9*(1), 1–17.

Mori, S. (2002). Principles, methods, and applications of diffusion tensor imaging. In A. W. Toga & J. C. Mazziotta (Eds.), *Brain mapping: The methods.* San Diego, CA: Academic Press.

Mori, S., Fredericksen, K., van Zijl, P. C. M., Stieltjes, S., Kraut, M. A., et al. (2002). Brain white matter anatomy of tumor patients evaluated with diffusion tensor imaging. *Annals of Neurology, 51*(3), 377–380.

Mori, S., Kaufmann, W. E., Davatzikos, C., Stieltjes, B., Amodei, L., Fredericksen, K., et al. (2002). Imaging cortical association tracts in the human brain using diffusion-tensor-based axonal tracking. *Magnetic Resonance in Medicine, 47*(2), 215–223.

Moseley, M., Cohen, Y., Kucharczyk, J., Mintorovitch, J., Asgari, H., Wendland, M., et al. (1990). Diffusion-weighted MR imaging of anisotropic water diffusion in cat central nervous system. *Radiology, 176*(2), 439–445.

Naeser, M. A., Baker, E. H., Palumbo, C. L., Nicholas, M., Alexander, M. P., Samaraweera, R., et al. (1998).

Lesion site patterns in severe, nonverbal aphasia to predict outcome with a computer-assisted treatment program. *Archives of Neurology, 55*(11), 1438–1448.

O'Brien, J. T., Paling, S., Barber, R., Williams, E. D., Ballard, C., McKeith, I. G., et al. (2001). Progressive brain atrophy on serial MRI in dementia with Lewy bodies, AD, and vascular dementia. *Neurology, 56*(10), 1386–1388.

Pasquier, F., Bail, L., Lebert, F., Pruvo, J. P., & Petit, H. (1994). Determination of medial temporal lobe atrophy in early Alzheimer's disease with computed tomography. *Lancet, 343,* 861–862.

Pasquier, F., Hamon, M. L., Lebert, F., Jacob, B., Pruvo, J.-P., & Petit, H. (1997). Medial temporal lobe atrophy in memory disorders. *Journal of Neurology, 244*(3), 175–181.

Paviour, D. C., Schott, J. M., Stevens, J. M., Revesz, T., Holton, J. L., Rossor, M. N., et al. (2004). Pathological substrate for regional distribution of increased atrophy rates in progressive supranuclear palsy. *Journal of Neurology, Neurosurgery, and Psychiatry, 75*(12), 1772–1775.

Pierpaoli, C., Barnett, A., Pajevic, S., Chen, R., Penix, L., Virta, A., et al. (2001). Water diffusion changes in Wallerian degeneration and their dependence on white matter architecture. *NeuroImage, 13*(6), 1174–1185.

Pierpaoli, C., Jezzard, P., Basser, P., Barnett, A., & Di Chiro, G. (1996). Diffusion tensor MR imaging of the human brain. *Radiology, 201*(3), 637–648.

Price, S., Paviour, D., Scahill, R., Stevens, J., Rossor, M., Lees, A., et al. (2004). Voxel-based morphometry detects patterns of atrophy that help differentiate progressive supranuclear palsy and Parkinson's disease. *NeuroImage, 23*(2), 663–669.

Quarantelli, M., Larobina, M., Volpe, U., Amati, G., Tedeschi, E., Ciarmiello, A., et al. (2002). Stereotaxy-based regional brain volumetry applied to segmented MRI: Validation and results in deficit and nondeficit schizophrenia. *NeuroImage, 17*(1), 373–384.

Rademacher, J., Galaburda, A. M., Kennedy, D. N., Filipek, P. A., & Caviness, V. S. (1992). Human cerebral cortex: Localization, parcellation, and morphometry with magnetic resonance imaging. *Journal of Cognitive Neuroscience, 4*(4), 352–374.

Resnick, S. M., Goldszal, A. F., Davatzikos, C., Golski, S., Kraut, M. A., Metter, E. J., et al. (2000). One-year age changes in MRI brain volumes in older adults. *Cerebral Cortex, 10*(5), 464–472.

Rosen, H. J., Allison, S. C., Schauer, G. F., Gorno-Tempini, M. L., Weiner, M. W., & Miller, B. L. (2005). Neuroanatomical correlates of behavioural disorders in dementia. *Brain, 128,* 2612–2625.

Rosen, H. J., Gorno-Tempini, M. L., Goldman, W. P., Perry, R. J., Schuff, N., Weiner, M., Feiwell, R., et al. (2002). Patterns of brain atrophy in frontotemporal dementia and semantic dementia. *Neurology, 58*(2), 198–208.

Rosen, H. J., Perry, R. J., Murphy, J., Kramer, J. H., Mychack, P., Schuff, N., et al. (2002). Emotion comprehension in the temporal variant of frontotemporal dementia. *Brain, 125*(10), 2286–2295.

Rosso, S. M., Roks, G., Stevens, M., de Koning, I., Tanghe, H. L. J., Kamphorst, W., et al. (2001). Complex compulsive behaviour in the temporal variant of frontotemporal dementia. *Journal of Neurology, 248*(11), 965–970.

Rusinek, H., De Santi, S., Frid, D., Tsui, W.-H., Tarshish, C. Y., Convit, A., et al. (2003). Regional brain atrophy rate predicts future cognitive decline: 6-year longitudinal MR imaging study of normal aging. *Radiology, 229*(3), 691–696.

Salat, D. H., Kaye, J. A., & Janowsky, J. S. (2001). Selective preservation and degeneration within the prefrontal cortex in aging and Alzheimer disease. *Archives of Neurology, 58*(9), 1403–1408.

Salat, D. H., Kaye, J. A., & Janowsky, J. S. (2002). Greater orbital prefrontal volume selectively predicts worse working memory performance in older adults. *Cerebral Cortex, 12*(5), 494–505.

Saver, J. L., & Damasio, A. R. (1991). Preserved access and processing of social knowledge in a patient with acquired sociopathy due to ventromedial frontal damage. *Neuropsychologia, 29*(12), 1241–1249.

Scheltens, P., Pasquier, F., Weerts, J. G., Barkhof, F., & Leys, D. (1997). Qualitative assessment of cerebral atrophy on MRI: Inter- and intra-observer reproducibility in dementia and normal aging. *European Neurology, 37*(2), 95–99.

Scheltens, P. M., Barkhof, F. M., Leys, D. M., Wolters, E. C., Ravid, R. P., & Kamphorst, W. M. (1995). Histopathologic correlates of white matter changes on MRI in Alzheimer's disease and normal aging. *Neurology, 45*(5), 883–888.

Schott, J. M., Fox, N. C. Frost, C., Scahill, R. I., Janssen, J. C., Chan, D., et al. (2003). Assessing the onset of structural change in familial Alzheimer's disease. *Annals of Neurology, 53*(2), 181–188.

Schott, J. M., Price, S. L., Frost, C., Whitwell, J. L., Rossor, M. N., & Fox, N. C. (2005). Measuring atrophy in Alzheimer disease: A serial MRI study over 6 and 12 months. *Neurology, 65*(1), 119–124.

Schroeter, P., Vesin, J.-M., Langenberger, T., & Meuli, R. (1998). Robust parameter estimation of intensity distributions for brain magnetic resonance images. *IEEE Transactions on Medical Imaging, 17*(2), 172–186.

Stone, V. E., Baron-Cohen, S., & Knight, R. T. (1998). Frontal lobe contributions to theory of mind. *Journal of Cognitive Neuroscience, 10*(5), 640–656.

Streifler, J. Y., Eliasziw, M., Benavente, O. R., Alamowitch, S., Fox, A. J., Hachinski, V., et al. (2003). Development and progression of leuko-araiosis in patients with brain ischemia and carotid artery disease. *Stroke, 34*(8), 1913–1916.

Studholme, C., Cardenas, V., Blumenfeld, R., Schuff, N., Rosen, H. J., Miller, B., et al. (2004). Deformation tensor morphometry of semantic dementia with quantitative validation. *NeuroImage, 21*(4), 1387–1398.

Studholme, C., Cardenas, V., Song, E., Ezekiel, F., Maudsley, A., & Weiner, W. (2004). Accurate template-based correction of brain MRI intensity distortion with application to dementia and aging. *IEEE Transactions on Medical Imaging, 23*(1), 99–110.

Stuss, D. T., Levine, B., Alexander, M. P., Hong, J., Palumbo, C., Hamer, L., et al. (2000). Wisconsin Card Sorting Test performance in patients with focal frontal and posterior brain damage: Effects of lesion location and test structure on separable cognitive processes. *Neuropsychologia, 38*(4), 388–402.

Swick, D., & Turken, A. U. (2002). Dissociation between conflict detection and error monitoring in the human anterior cingulate cortex. *Proceedings of the National Academy of Sciences of the United States of America, 99*(25), 16354–16359.

Talairach, J., & Tournoux, P. (1988). *Co-planar stereotaxic atlas of the human brain.* New York: Thieme.

Taylor, W. D., MacFall, J. R., Payne, M. E., McQuoid, D. R., Provenzale, J. M., Steffens, D. C., et al. (2004). Late-life depression and microstructural abnormalities in dorsolateral prefrontal cortex white matter. *American Journal of Psychiatry, 161*(7), 1293–1296.

Testa, C., Laakso, M. P., Sabattoli, F., Rossi, R., Beltramello, A., Soininen, H., et al. (2004). A comparison between the accuracy of voxel-based morphometry and hippocampal volumetry in Alzheimer's disease. *Journal of Magnetic Resonance Imaging, 19*(3), 274–282.

Thomas, A. J., Perry, R., Kalaria, R. N., Oakley, A., McMeekin, W., & O'Brien, J. T. (2003). Neuropathological evidence for ischemia in the white matter of the dorsolateral prefrontal cortex in late-life depression. *International Journal of Geriatric Psychiatry, 18*(1), 7–13.

Thompson-Schill, S. L., Jonides, J., Marshuetz, C., Smith, E. E., D'Esposito, M., Kan, I. P., et al. (2002). Effects of frontal lobe damage on interference effects in working memory. *Cognitive Affective, and Behavioral Neuroscience, 2*(2), 109–120.

Tisserand, D. J., Pruessner, J. C., Sanz Arigita, E. J., van Boxtel, M. P. J., Evans, A. C., Jolles, J., et al. (2002). Regional frontal cortical volumes decrease differentially in aging: An MRI study to compare volumetric approaches and voxel-based morphometry. *NeuroImage, 17*(2), 657–669.

Tisserand, D. J., Van Boxtel, M. P. J., Gronenschild, E., & Jolles, J. (2001). Age-related volume reductions of prefrontal regions in healthy individuals are differential. *Brain and Cognition, 47*, 182–185.

Tranel, D., & Damasio, H. (1994). Neuroanatomical correlates of electrodermal skin conductance responses. *Psychophysiology, 31*(5), 427–438.

Ulug, A. M., & van Zijl, P. C. M. (1999). Orientation-independent diffusion imaging without tensor diagonalization: Anisotropy definitions based on physical attributes of the diffusion ellipsoid. *Journal of Magnetic Resonance Imaging, 9*(6), 804–813.

Van Leemput, K., Maes, F., Vandermeulen, D., & Suetens, P. (1999a). Automated model-based bias field correction of MR images of the brain. *IEEE Transactions on Medical Imaging, 18*(10), 885–896.

Van Leemput, K., Maes, F., Vandermeulen, D., & Suetens, P. (1999b). Automated model-based tissue classification of MR images of the brain. *IEEE Transactions on Medical Imaging, 18*(10), 897–908.

Van Leemput, K., Maes, F., Vandermeulen, D., & Suetens, P. (2003). A unifying framework for partial volume segmentation of brain MR images. *IEEE Transactions on Medical Imaging, 22*(1), 105–119.

Vogt, B. A., Berger, G. R., & Derbyshire, S. W. (2003). Structural and functional dichotomy of human midcingulate cortex. *European Journal of Neuroscience, 18*(11), 3134–3144.

Vonsattel, J.-P., Myers, R. H., Stevens, T. J., Ferrante, R. J., Bird, E. D., & Richardson, E. P. (1985). Neuropathological classification of Huntington's disease. *Journal of Neuropathology and Experimental Neurology, 44*, 559–577.

Wahlund, L. O., Julin, P., Lindqvist, J., & Scheltens, P. (1999). Visual assessment of medical temporal lobe atrophy in demented and healthy control subjects: Correlation with volumetry. *Psychiatry Research, 90*(3), 193–199.

Warfield, S. K., Kaus, M., Jolesz, F. A., & Kikinis, R (2000). Adaptive, template moderated, spatially varying statistical classification. *Medical Image Analysis, 4*(1), 43–55.

Wells, W. M., III, Grimson, W. E. L., Kikinis, R., & Jolesz, F. A. (1996). Adaptive segmentation of MRI data. *IEEE Transactions on Medical Imaging, 15*(4), 429–442.

Werring, D. J., Toosy, A. T., Clark, C. A., Parker, G. J., Barker, G. J., Miller, D. H., et al. (2000). Diffusion tensor imaging can detect and quantify corticospinal tract degeneration after stroke. *Journal of Neurology, Neurosurgery, and Psychiatry, 69*(2), 269–272.

Wetzel, S., & Bongartz, G. (1999). MR angiography: Supra-aortic vessels. *European Radiology, 9*(7), 1277–1284.

Wieshmann, U. C., Symms, M. R., Parker, G. J. M., Clark, C. A., Lemieux, L., Barker, G. J., et al. (2000). Diffusion tensor imaging demonstrates deviation of fibres in normal appearing white matter adjacent to a brain tumour. *Journal of Neurology, Neurosurgery, and Psychiatry, 68*(4), 501–503.

Ylikoski, R., Ylikoski, A., Erkinjuntti, T., Sulkava, R., Raininko, R., & Tilvis, R. (1993). White matter changes in healthy elderly persons correlate with attention and speed of mental processing. *Archives of Neurology, 50*(8), 818–824.

Zijdenbos, A. P., Forghani, R., & Evans, A. C. (2002). Automatic "pipeline" analysis of 3-D MRI data for clinical trials: Application to multiple sclerosis. *IEEE Transactions on Medical Imaging, 21*(10), 1280–1291.

# CHAPTER 13

## Unifying Prefrontal Cortex Function

### EXECUTIVE CONTROL, NEURAL NETWORKS, AND TOP-DOWN MODULATION

*Adam Gazzaley*
*Mark D'Esposito*

The function of the frontal lobes has historically been shrouded in mystery and misconception, with the earliest functional assessment based solely on observations of the behavioral consequences of frontal lobe injury. This began in 1848, when Phineas Gage, a 25-year-old railroad construction foreman, suffered extensive frontal lobe damage as an iron tamping bar was driven through his head by an explosion at a construction site (Harlow, 1868). Prior to this accident, Gage was described as a religious, family-loving, honest and hardworking man. The injury that he miraculously survived resulted in a dramatic change in his personality and what was considered to be a preservation of his cognitive abilities. He became "fitful, irreverent, indulging at times in the grossest profanity, . . . impatient of restraint or advice when it conflicts with his desires, . . . obstinate, . . . devising many plans of operation, which are no sooner arranged than they are abandoned in turn for others appearing more feasible" (Harlow, 1868). Interpretations of observations such as these, coupled with early findings that damage to the frontal lobes does not translate into gross changes in

intelligence (Hebb, 1945), suggested a principle role of the frontal lobes in personality and emotion.

With the advent of sophisticated neuropsychological testing in the mid-20th century (Benton, 1968; Luria, 1966; Milner, 1963), our understanding of frontal lobe function expanded to include cognitive abilities encapsulated under the rubric of "executive functions." This label encompasses a diverse collection of processes, including divided and sustained attention, working memory, flexibility of thought, set shifting, motor sequencing, planning, and the regulation of goal-directed behavior (Hecaen & Albert, 1978; Lezak, 1995). For the last two decades, elucidation of the role of the frontal lobes in cognition, particularly the prefrontal cortex (PFC), has been a major focus of cognitive neuroscience research, with an emphasis on detailed psychological and anatomical parcellation of these processes. Evidence for PFC involvement in both cognition and emotion now rests securely on detailed physiological and lesion studies on experimental animals and neuropsychological, electrophysiological, and functional imaging studies on humans.

Although decades of research have greatly advanced our knowledge of the involvement of the PFC in diverse mental processes, functional segregation has in some respects perpetuated the mystery of its function. For instance, the rift between the PFC role in emotion and cognition, perhaps established with the case of Phineas Gage, has largely persisted in modern cognitive neuroscience.[1] Emotion and cognition are usually dissociated conceptually and on the basis of anatomical localization, with the orbitofrontal PFC coupled to emotion and the dorsolateral PFC linked to cognition (Berlin, Rolls, & Kischka, 2004; Dias, Robbins, & Roberts, 1996; Hecaen & Albert, 1978; Otani, 2002). Even within the domains of emotion and cognition there is a pervasive tendency for increasingly detailed parcellation of function to discrete anatomical sites within the PFC. As an example, numerous studies of working memory have focused on whether anatomical segregation exists on the basis of subcomponent processes (e.g., maintenance vs. manipulation of information) or stimulus category (e.g., spatial vs. verbal information) localized to either ventrolateral versus dorsolateral PFC or the left versus right hemisphere (for reviews, see D'Esposito et al., 1998; Goldman-Rakic, 1996). This practice has been stimulated in recent years by the development of high-resolution functional neuroimaging, such as functional magnetic resonance imaging (fMRI).

Although this approach has clearly been informative and has contributed greatly to our understanding of the intricacies of PFC organization, to attain a global view of PFC function it is critical to identify common, underlying operational features and neural mechanisms that transcend such borders. Once general organizing principles are established, they can then be placed within the anatomical and functional architecture of the PFC. We propose that this objective has been most advanced by theoretical and empirical accounts of PFC *control processes*, with a structural and functional basis on *neural networks* and an underlying neural mechanism of *top-down modulation*. Our goal in this chapter is to establish a unifying model of PFC influence on cognition and emotion based on a framework of executive control, neural networks, and top-down modulation. We then consider this model from a clinical perspective by relating it to the "frontal lobe syndrome" that occurs in patients with PFC dysfunction.

## EXECUTIVE CONTROL

The rationale to search for a unifying theory of PFC function is that despite anatomical specialization, there may be a common function that underlies PFC involvement in seemingly diverse mental processes. This may be expected solely on the basis of an underlying evolutionary drive for PFC development in humans—demand for increasingly sophisticated control of the environment. Indeed, a unifying PFC function may be control, the *executive control*[2] of mental processes whose primary operative sites are localized elsewhere in the brain. From an evolutionary perspective, control is a natural extension of the motor system from which the PFC evolved, and as the "highest" level of the motor system this control might be expected to extend far beyond the regulation of body movements. In fact, executive control can be viewed to encompass higher-level influences over *sensory input*, *internal states* (both emotion and cognition), and *motor output*. By exerting influence over these domains, humans have evolved increasingly more sophisticated control over interactions with both the natural world and each other.[3] This control permits the goal-directed override of primitive and inflexible reactions to environmental stimuli, what Mesulam (2002) refers to as the "default mode." Thus, an underlying function of the PFC may be the control and dynamic integration of the *external* and *internal* environment.

The control of *sensory input* involves the selective focus of limited cognitive resources on features of the external environment that are relevant, and ignoring those elements that are irrelevant. This is essentially the control of cortical representations, or symbolic codes of information from any sensory modality: visual, auditory, tactile, and olfactory. Such control is indispensable for processes such as selective attention, working memory (WM) encoding, and long-term memory (LTM) encoding. Control of *internal state* entails PFC influence over both emotive and cognitive features of the internal milieu, such as affect and autonomic tone (*emotion*), as well as generating and maintaining representations in the absence of external stimuli, also known as thinking (*cognition*). The emotive control component encompasses processes such as fear extinction, impulsivity, and addictive tendencies, whereas cognitive control includes WM maintenance and manipulation, mental imagery, introspection, organization, and planning. As will be discussed, there is extensive interaction between these features of internal state control, leading to complex processes such as social conduct and decision making. Control of *motor output* comprises regulation of all body movements, with eye movements and reach being the most extensively studied.

Perhaps the most influential theory of executive control is Baddeley's (1986) model of working memory. Based on behavioral studies of healthy young subjects, Baddeley proposed that WM involves a central executive system that actively regulates the distribution of limited attentional resources and coordinates information within verbal and spatial memory buffers. This concept of the central executive system was based on Norman and Shallice's analogous supervisory attentional system, which is proposed to control cognitive processing when novel tasks are involved or existing habits must be overridden (Shallice, 1988). Many other authors have attributed a similar operational role to the PFC: contingent en-

coding (Mesulam, 2002), dynamic filtering (Shimamura, 1997), and adaptive encoding (Curtis & D'Esposito, 2003; Duncan, 2001; Knight, Staines, Swick, & Chao, 1999; Miyashita, 2004; Petrides, 1994). However, several notable theories also assign the PFC a role in the actual storage and representation of information (structured event complex: Graffman, 2002; connectionist model: Burnod, 1991), and those that are a hybrid of processing and representational models (Goldman-Rakic, 1998; Miller & Cohen, 2001). We have organized the evidence from neuropsychological studies of patients with frontal lobe injury and functional neuroimaging studies of healthy young adults within the framework of a PFC control model (Table 13.1).

Neuropsychological studies of patients with focal PFC lesions have revealed deficits in a wide range of measures that can be viewed to represent executive control of sensory input, internal state, and motor output (Table 13.1). It is important to note that several studies cross these categories and/or it is unclear which cate-

**TABLE 13.1. Lesion–Behavior and Neuroimaging Studies of PFC Involvement in Executive Control in Humans**

| Sensory input | Internal: cognition | Internal: emotion | Motor output |
|---|---|---|---|
| | Lesion–behavior studies | | |
| Selective attention: (Stroop)[1-3] (Flanker)[4] (Negative priming)[5] Perceptual attention set shifting[6] | WM[12] (DRT)[7-11] WM and LTM (CVLT)[13] (Tower of London)[14] Set shifting (WCST)[15] Organization[16] (verbal fluency)[17,18] Planning[14] Non-emotion-based decision making[19] | Social perception[20,21] Regret[22] Impulsivity[23] Self-conscious emotion[24] Empathy[25] Emotional intelligence[26] Emotional processing[27] Aggression[28] Reward-related decision making[29,30] Emotional imagery[31] | Memory-guided saccades[32] Reflexive saccade suppression[33,34] Motor response suppression[35]: (Go/no-go)[36,37] Motor monitoring[38,39] |
| | Neuroimaging studies | | |
| Selective attention[40]: (Stroop)[41,42] Divided attention[43] Episodic memory retrieval[44] Selective attention of emotional stimuli[45] Perceptual decision making ^[46] | WM maintenance (DRT)[47-49] WM manipulation (DRT)[50] WM monitoring[51] WM (n-back task)[52] Mental imagery[53,54] Set shifting (WCST)[55,56] | Social appropriateness[57] Aggression imagery[58] Reward-related decision making[59] Risk-related decision making[60] | Memory-guided saccades[61] Reflexive saccade suppression[62,63] Motor response suppression[64,65]: (Stop task)[66] (Go/no-go)[67,68] |

*Note.* This is not a comprehensive list, but it is meant to illustrate the evidence for a PFC role across the broad scope of control processes. It is important to note that for the neuroimaging studies, it is almost universal that brain regions in addition to the PFC are activated during the task. Parenthetical text indicates specific cognitive tasks. WM, working memory; LTM, long-term memory; DRT, delayed-response task; CVLT, California Verbal Learning Test; WCST, Wisconsin Card Sorting Task. References corresponding to superscript numerals are listed at the end of the chapter.

gory is the most appropriate. For example, when using the lesion–behavior experimental approach, it is difficult to determine whether delayed-response task (DRT) deficits are based on impairments in sensory control (WM encoding) or internal state control (WM maintenance), and whether deficits in the Stroop task are the result of deficiencies in sensory or motor control. Additionally, as research continues to emphasize the integration between orbito-frontal/emotional and dorsolateral/cognitive processes, the classification of internal state into cognitive and emotional domains becomes increasingly arbitrary, especially for higher-order processes such as decision making (Hornak et al., 2004; Manes et al., 2002) and social perception (Mah, Arnold, & Grafman, 2004).

PFC lesion studies in humans have been reported relatively infrequently, primarily due to the clinical observation that few patients have selective lesions confined to the PFC. Those patients with lesions restricted to the PFC typically include diverse etiologies, such as strokes within the middle or anterior cerebral artery territory, focal cerebral trauma, tumor resection, or epileptic patients following frontal lobe excisions. Aside from difficulties in interpreting disparity in etiology, extent of dysfunction, and time course of neural changes, the impact that compensatory plasticity has on these studies is unclear. Nevertheless, when significant and reproducible deficits are documented in patients with focal PFC lesions, the results are compelling. For example, a meta-analysis of studies spanning the years 1960–1997 has revealed consistent impairment on DRTs, thus establishing the necessity of the PFC for successful WM performance (D'Esposito & Postle, 1999). To overcome limitations of the lesion–behavior design in human subjects, technological advances in transcranial magnetic stimulation (TMS) now permit the generation of a transient, "virtual lesion" restricted to precise and spatially limited cortical targets (Pascual-Leone, Walsh, & Rothwell, 2000). Consistent with the chronic lesion–behavior studies discussed, TMS has revealed that transient functional disruption of the dorsolateral PFC results in WM deficits (Grafman et al., 1994; Mottaghy et al., 2000), and has great potential of elucidating the brain–behavior relationship for other control processes.

The recent advent of functional neuroimaging studies on healthy individuals with positron emission tomography (PET) and fMRI has complemented physiology studies in humans using event-related potentials (ERP), and in many ways has revolutionized our approach to assessing PFC involvement in control processes. It has enabled the study of physiology in the intact human PFC with high anatomical–spatial resolution. This has permitted the detailed parcellation of functions to PFC subdivisions, and when coupled with event-related designs, has allowed the dissection of subcomponent stages of cognitive processes. Review of these studies reveals an overwhelming consensus for PFC involvement in all varieties of control processes (Table 13.1). It is important to note, however, that unlike lesion studies, functional neuroimaging, and indeed all physiological measurements on intact systems, only support inferences about the *engagement* of a particular brain region by a cognitive process and not its *necessity* for these processes (Sarter, Bernston, & Caciioppo, 1996). However, when these results are combined with lesion–behavior data, they provide convincing evidence for the essential role that the human PFC has in the executive control of sensory input, internal state, and motor output.

Also, numerous lesion–behavior and physiology studies have been performed on experimental animals, offering converging evidence of PFC involvement in comparable models of executive control (Table 13.2). Two of these studies that represent landmark contributions to the field are the behavioral observations of Jacobsen (1935) that monkeys with bilateral prefrontal lesions are impaired on DRTs, and the results of single-cell recordings in the PFC by Fuster and Alexander (1971), revealing that lateral PFC neurons exhibit sustained, elevated levels of activity during the delay period of a DRT. These studies firmly established the role of the PFC in working memory, and the many elegant animal studies that followed have enabled an assessment of PFC physiology on a neuronal level that is not practical in human subjects.

## NEURAL NETWORKS

Although the studies referenced in Tables 13.1 and 13.2 provide evidence for the engagement and necessity of the PFC in cognition and emotion, they do not necessarily support our claim that these are control processes. A core element

**TABLE 13.2. Lesion–Behavior and Physiological Studies of PFC Involvement in Executive Control in Experimental Animals**

| Sensory input | Internal: cognition | Internal: emotion | Motor output |
|---|---|---|---|
| | **Lesion–behavior studies** | | |
| Perceptual attention set shifting[69, 70] | WM (DRT)[72, 73] | Affect processing[69, 76] | Memory-guided saccades[81] |
| Sustained attention[71] | Set shifting (WCST-analog)[74, 75] | Fear/anxiety[77–80] | Reaching[82] |
| | | | Response suppression[35] (go/no-go)[83] |
| | | | Perseveration[84, 85] |
| | **Physiological studies** | | |
| Focused attention[86, 87] | WM maintenance (DRT)[89–92] | Reward-related decision making[96–100] | Memory-guided saccades[102] |
| Sustained attention[88] | Anticipation[93–95] | Motivation[101] | Motor preparation[103] |
| | | | Response suppression[104] (go/no-go)[105, 106] |

*Note.* This is not a comprehensive list, but it is meant to illustrate the evidence for a PFC role across the broad scope of control processes. WM, working memory; LTM, long-term memory; DRT, delayed-response task; CVLT, California Verbal Learning Test. References corresponding to superscript numerals are listed at the end of the chapter.

of an operational model of PFC control is that processes and representations being controlled are primarily localized to other brain regions. Although, on some level, this is a matter of debate (Wood & Grafman, 2003), it seems to be a logical conclusion for sensory and motor control. It is well established that sensory and motor representations are predominantly the domain of primary sensory–motor and unimodal association regions optimally organized to encode such representations, and functional neuroimaging studies reveal coactivation of these distant regions along with the PFC during all of these processes. Furthermore, frontal lobe lesions are not associated with primary deficits of motility or sensation. As we discuss below, this argument can be extended to internal state control. Accepting this premise leads to a fundamental question: Is there a system by which the PFC can influence sensory input, internal states, and motor output? A model of executive control must possess a structural and functional framework for long-range influence, and it is likely that the bases of such control processes are distributed *neural networks*.

Complex cognitive processes are not localized to brain regions functioning in isolation, but rather are emergent properties of intricate neural connections subserving dynamic interactions between brain regions, or "neural networks" (Fuster, 2003; Gazzaley & D'Esposito, in press; Mesulam, 1981, 1990). The extensive reciprocal connections between the PFC and

virtually all cortical and subcortical structures situate the PFC in a unique neuroanatomical position to monitor and manipulate diverse cognitive and affective processes (Barbas, 2000; Goldman-Rakic & Friedman, 1991). Tract-tracing studies in experimental animals have revealed long-range reciprocal connections between the PFC and the parietal, temporal, cingulate, and insula cortex, the limbic system (hypothalamus, amygdala, and hippocampus), and extensive subcortical connections with the striatum, globus pallidus, substantia nigra, and mediodorsal nucleus of the thalamus (Cavada & Goldman-Rakic, 1989; Ilinsky, Jouandet, & Goldman-Rakic, 1985; Morecraft, Geula, & Mesulam, 1992; Ongur, An, & Price, 1998; Petrides & Pandya, 1984, 1999, 2002; Selemon & Goldman-Rakic, 1985, 1988; Ungerleider, Gaffan, & Pelak, 1989; Webster, Bachevalier, & Ungerleider, 1994). Several of the more well-defined pathways have also been described in humans with postmortem dissection (Heimer, 1983) and, more recently, with *in vivo* diffusion tensor MRI (Makris et al., 2004).

These anatomically defined networks establish the structural basis by which the PFC exerts control over diverse cognitive and affective processes; however, there is also accumulating functional evidence of PFC networks and their role in control processes. Traditionally, most functional imaging studies have utilized univariate analyses, permitting only the independent assessment of activity within each brain region in isolation. However, there has been a steady development of multivariate approaches to analyzing neuroimaging data in a manner more directly in alignment with the network model of the cognition (Friston, Frith, Liddle, & Frackowiak, 1993; Friston, Phillips, Chawla, & Buchel, 2000; Lin et al., 2003; McIntosh, 1998; Penny, Stephan, Mechelli, & Friston, 2004; Rissman, Gazzaley, & D'Esposito, 2004; Sun, Miller, & D'Esposito, 2004). Multivariate analyses generate functional and effective connectivity maps of interacting brain regions, thus emphasizing the role of brain regions within the context of co-varying anatomically connected regions and the cognitive processes being performed. Several groups, including our own laboratory, have begun to establish the presence of functional interactions between the PFC and posterior cortical regions during executive control processes, such as attention (Rowe, Friston, Frackowiak, & Passingham, 2002), WM (Gazzaley, Rissman, & D'Esposito, 2004; McIntosh, Grady, Haxby, Ungerleider, & Horwitz, 1996), and visual imagery (Mechelli, Price, Friston, & Ishai, 2004). We expect this trend to dominate the future of functional neuroimaging and to solidify the existence of neural networks as the structural and functional basis of PFC executive control.

It is important to recognize that PFC neural networks are not nebulous, web-like communications between the PFC and the rest of the brain that are equivalently engaged in all mental processes. On the contrary, the existence of precise and dissociable networks between distinct PFC subregions and specific distant brain regions establishes the basis for the diversity of PFC control. For example, the orbitofrontal PFC, unlike the dorsolateral PFC, is extensively interconnected with the hypothalamus and the amygdala (Morecraft et al., 1992; Ongur et al., 1998), underlying its distinctive role in controlling visceral correlates of emotion (Barbas, Saha, Rempel-Clower, & Ghashghaei, 2003). It has long been established in experimental animals that electrical stimulation of the orbitofrontal cortex and neighboring paralimbic regions regulates respiratory rate, heart rate, vascular tone, and gastric secretions (Kaada, Pribrahm, & Epstein, 1949; Pool & Ransohoff, 1949). Additionally, inhibitory control by the PFC over amygdala-based fear processes is considered to be responsible for fear extinction, the ability to adapt to changing situations by suppressing previously learned fears (Sotres-Bayon, Bush, & LeDoux, 2004). Autonomic and emotional control networks then further interact with other PFC control networks, such as sensory and motor networks subserved by pathways between the PFC and posterior association sensory cortices and premotor cortex, respectively; this in turn influences complex processes of decision making, reward, motivation, social interactions, and attention (Bechara, 2004; Bechara, Damasio, Tranel, & Damasio, 1997; Bechara, Tranel, & Damasio, 2000; Blair & Cipolotti, 2000; Compton, 2003; Compton et al., 2003; Crone, Somsen, Van Beek, & Van Der Molen, 2004; Mesulam, 2002).

Neural networks are dynamic interactions between brain regions, and as such are under the influence of the local neurochemical environment of constituent nodes. There is an extensive literature on the role of ascending modulatory neurotransmitter systems, including dopamine, norepinephrine, serotonin, and acetylcholine in the regulation of PFC function (Arnsten & Robbins, 2002; Goldman-Rakic, Lidow, & Gallager, 1990). Although research on the behavioral influence of these neuromodulatory transmitters and their influence on activity levels within the PFC (Arnsten & Robbins, 2002) has advanced, only recently have studies evaluated their impact on PFC networks by measuring neurochemically induced regulation of functional connectivity (Coull, Buchel, Friston, & Frith, 1999; Honey et al., 2003; Williams et al., 2002). Furthering our understanding of the structural and functional basis of PFC control requires elucidation of network interaction regulation by these ascending transmitter systems.

## TOP-DOWN MODULATION

If neural networks serve as the structural–functional basis of executive control, what is the neural mechanism by which such control is exerted? There is accumulating evidence that the PFC mediates its influence over diverse mental processes by modulating the magnitude of neural activity in distant brain regions via the long-range projections described. This mechanism of control, known as *top-down modulation*, has been most extensively characterized for visual processing. It rests on the concept that human interaction with the environment involves an integration of externally driven information that demands attention based on stimulus salience or novelty (bottom-up processes) and internally driven goal-directed decisions concerning stimuli or stored representations (top-down modulation). Electrophysiology and neuroimaging studies have revealed that top-down modulation involves control of the magnitude of neural activity in posterior visual cortical regions during goal-directed visual processing, both when a stimulus is present (e.g., selective attention and memory encoding: sensory control—Bar, 2003; Gazzaley, Cooney, McEvoy, Knight, & D'Esposito, 2005; Pessoa, Kastner, & Ungerleider, 2003; Treue & Martinez Trujillo, 1999; Wojciulik, Kanwisher, & Driver, 1998) and when a stimulus is absent (e.g., mental imagery, WM maintenance, and visual anticipation: internal state control—Fuster, 1990; Ishai, Haxby, & Ungerleider, 2002; Kastner, Pinsk, De Weerd, Desimone, & Ungerleider, 1999; Miller, Li, & Desimone, 1993). Comparable descriptions of top-down modulation of activity magnitude has been described for the auditory (Hillyard, Hink, Schwent, & Picton, 1973), olfactory (Zelano et al., 2005), and somatosensory (Seminowicz, Mikulis, & Davis, 2004) systems. Employing a combination of fMRI and ERP recordings, we have recently discovered that top-down modulation of activity in the visual association cortex also involves modulation of the speed of neural processing (Gazzaley, Cooney, McEvoy, et al., 2005). This is expressed as a shorter time to reach maximal synchronized activity when attention is directed toward a specific stimulus in a goal-directed manner (i.e., WM encoding).

Inherent to the concept of stimulus-present top-down modulation is the notion that neural activity is modulated relative to a level of activity generated by the bottom-up perceptual influences of a stimulus, and this level of activity may be differentially enhanced or suppressed if the stimulus is, respectively, attended to or ignored. Despite this logic, modulation relative to a stimulus-present neutral baseline has rarely been evaluated, and comparisons are usually between attend and ignore tasks, or relative to a resting baseline without visual stimulation (O'Craven, Downing, & Kanwisher, 1999; Pinsk, Doniger, & Kastner, 2004; Rees, Frith, & Lavie, 1997; Vuilleumier, Armony, Driver, & Dolan, 2001; Wojciulik et al., 1998). This makes it difficult to interpret whether top-down influences reflect enhancement or suppression of activity. However, evidence of both

enhancement and suppression relative to a passive baseline has been revealed with ERP studies of selective spatial attention (Luck & Hillyard, 1995; Luck et al., 1994) and our fMRI–ERP study of selective WM encoding (Gazzaley, Cooney, McEvoy, et al., 2005). We feel it is likely that top-down modulation and parallel mechanisms of *enhancement* and *suppression* of neural activity mediate all control processes discussed in this chapter. It is well documented that the nervous system utilizes interleaved inhibitory and excitatory mechanisms throughout the neuroaxis (e.g., spinal reflexes, cerebellar outputs, and basal ganglia movement control networks). It is thus not surprising that the PFC would utilize enhancement and suppression to control cognition and affect, providing a powerful contrast for sculpting these neural processes (Knight et al., 1999; Shimamura, 1997).

Evidence that the PFC mediates control via top-down modulation is largely based on data from physiology and neuroimaging studies, revealing simultaneous engagement of PFC regions while control is required and posterior cortical activity is being modulated (Corbetta & Shulman, 2002; Hopfinger, Buonocore, & Mangun, 2000; Rainer, Asaad, & Miller, 1998; Ungerleider, Courtney, & Haxby, 1998). As already discussed, these correlational data only support the engagement of the PFC in a cognitive process and are thus indirect evidence that the PFC actually mediates control via top-down modulation. An optimal experimental design to assess directly the mechanism of PFC control involves the disruption of PFC afferents and physiological recordings of distant brain regions while the subject is engaged in a control task. Several studies have implemented such a lesion–physiology design on experimental animals and humans. These studies support the conclusion that top-down modulation, utilizing both enhancement and suppression, is a mechanism of PFC control over diverse mental processes (Table 13.3). Although clinical experience with patients with PFC lesions reveals behavioral deficits encompassing all domains of executive control (see the section on frontal lobe syndrome), the majority of research utilizing the lesion–physiology design has focused on sensory control. Thus, the *modulatory control hypothesis* of PFC function remains a fertile area for future research.

Research on experimental animals provided the first direct electrophysiological evidence of a PFC role in modulating activity in sensory

**TABLE 13.3. Studies That Directly Assess PFC-Mediated Top-Down Modulation Using the Lesion–Physiology Design**

| Sensory input | Internal: cognition | Internal: behavior | Motor output |
|---|---|---|---|
| | | Enhancement | |
| Monkeys/cooling/DRT/ single-cell/visual-IT[107] | Monkeys/cooling/ DRT/single cell/ visual-IT[107] | | Humans/TBI/reach/ ERP[111] |
| Monkeys/callusotomy/ memory recall/single cell/ visual-IT[108] | | | Humans/lesions/finger movements/ERP[112] |
| Humans/lesions/SA/ERP/ visual[109] | | | |
| Humans/lesions/SA/ERP/ auditory[110] | | | |
| | | Suppression | |
| Humans/lesions/SA/ERP/ auditory[110, 113] | | Humans/lesions/ aversive stimuli/ ERP/somatosensory and auditory[116] | |
| Humans/lesions/DRT/ERP/ auditory[11] | | | |
| Rats/electrolytic lesions/ DRT/single cell/ perirhinal[114] | | | |
| Rats/lesions/foraging/single cell/hippo place cells[115] | | | |

*Note.* Categorization is to the four domains of executive control and indicates if the results attribute an enhancement or suppression role to PFC modulation. The study description is subjects/lesions/task/physiological marker/region or modality. DRT, delayed-response task; TBI, traumatic brain injury; SA, selective attention; ERP, event-related potential; IT, inferotemporal cortex; hippo, hippocampus. References corresponding to superscript numerals are listed at the end of the chapter.

cortices. It was observed that cooling the PFC in cats results in increased amplitudes of evoked electrophysiological responses recorded from the primary cortex for all sensory modalities (Skinner & Yingling, 1977). Conversely, stimulation of specific regions of the thalamus that surround the sensory relay thalamic nuclei (i.e., nucleus reticularis thalami) results in modality-specific suppression of activity in primary sensory cortex (Yingling & Skinner, 1977). Thus, these findings suggest the presence of an inhibitory pathway from PFC that regulates the flow of sensory information via thalamic relay nuclei. This prefrontal–thalamic inhibitory system provides a mechanism for modality-specific suppression of irrelevant inputs at an early stage of sensory processing.

In nonhuman primates, PFC-mediated top-down modulation during an executive control task was studied by coupling single-cell recordings and cortical cooling in monkeys (Fuster, Bauer, & Jervey, 1985). This experiment revealed that PFC cooling results in both augmentation and diminution of spontaneous and task-specific activity in inferotemporal neurons during the encoding (stimulus-present modulation) and delay period (stimulus-absent modu-

lation) of a visual DRT, suggesting the presence of both enhancing and suppressive PFC influences. Furthermore, cooling was accompanied by WM performance deficits, thus establishing a link between PFC-mediated top-down modulation and cognition. These findings have been complemented by the elegant callosal lesion–physiology study of Tomita, Ohbayashi, Nakahara, Hasegawa, and Miyashita (1999), which revealed that top-down enhancement signals from the PFC to inferior temporal cortex during visual memory recall are mediated not by subcortical pathways, but frontotemporal corticocortical projections, and that this modulatory influence is necessary for successful memory recall. This supports the assertion that representations are stored in posterior sensory regions, and top-down signals from the PFC trigger the activation of these memory representations (Miyashita, 2004). Coupled with the results of lesion–behavior studies (Hasegawa, Fukushima, Ihara, & Miyashita, 1998) and functional neuroimaging studies (Lee et al., 2002; Ranganath, Johnson, & D'Esposito, 2003), these results establish a role of PFC-mediated top-down modulation in LTM. Recent lesion–physiology studies in rodents have also revealed the presence of modulatory PFC influences on the activity of hippocampal place cells (Kyd & Bilkey, 2003) and perirhinal neurons during a spatial DRT (Zironi, Iacovelli, Aicardi, Liu, & Bilkey, 2001).

In humans, combined lesion–ERP studies have provided evidence of PFC-dependent top-down enhancement of visual association cortex activity occurring in the first few hundred milliseconds of the visual processing for selectively attended stimuli (Barcelo, Suwazono, & Knight, 2000). Moreover, electrophysiological alterations accompanying PFC lesions were associated with deficits in visual detection ability. Comparable findings of PFC-mediated ERP enhancement and performance dependence have been obtained during a selective attention auditory task (Knight, Hillyard, Woods, & Neville, 1981). There is also evidence in humans that the PFC exhibits suppressive control over distant cortical regions. For example, ERP studies in patients with focal PFC damage have revealed that auditory (Knight, Scabini, & Woods, 1989) and somatosensory (Yamaguchi & Knight, 1990) evoked responses are enhanced, suggesting disinhibition of sensory flow to these regions. These suppressive influences have also been extended to emotionally salient stimuli, as was recently demonstrated by enhanced ERPs recorded in response to mildly aversive stimuli in patients with orbitofrontal lesions (Rule, Shimamura, & Knight, 2002). Furthermore, there is evidence that PFC-mediated suppression extends to selectively ignored auditory stimuli (Chao & Knight, 1998; Knight et al., 1981).

It is likely that such parallel enhancement–suppression control entails large-scale neural networks (Knight, 1997), including an inhibitory PFC–thalamic gating network and a direct excitatory PFC projection to specific cortical regions. Alternatively, suppression might entail long-range excitatory prefrontal–cortical projections that then activate local inhibitory neurons (Carr & Sesack, 1998), or perhaps involves the withdrawal of excitatory influences by the reallocation of resources. For a review of computational models of inhibitory control, see Houghton and Tipper (1996). Clearly, more empirical research is needed to further our understanding of the mechanisms of top-down enhancement and suppression, as well as to place these modulatory control mechanisms within the framework of PFC functional architecture and associated neural networks. One exciting new route of development is the use of TMS to induce transient cortical disruptions of the PFC while activity in distant brain regions is recorded with either PET (Mottaghy et al., 2000; Paus, Castro-Alamancos, & Petrides, 2001) or ERP (Evers, Bockermann, & Nyhuis, 2001) during task performance.

## FRONTAL LOBE SYNDROME

Two aspects of the behavioral manifestations of frontal lobe lesions, prominent in clinical reports since the first descriptions of Phineas Gage's personality transformation, are the diversity of symptoms within a patient and the variability of symptoms between patients. The *frontal lobe syndrome* is not a uniform entity, but a constellation of behavioral alterations that present and evolve in different patterns in patients with PFC lesions. It includes difficulty holding information in mind, distractibility, poor organization and planning, emotional blunting and lability, perseveration,[4] utilization behavior, social inappropriateness, and the loss of judgment, insight, and initiative (Mesulam, 2002). This diversity is a consequence of the interaction among three factors: (1) the variety of etiologies associated with PFC dysfunction (stroke, frontotemporal dementia [FTD], tumor, aneurysm, traumatic brain injury, epilepsy, attention-deficit/hyperactivity disorder [ADHD], schizophrenia, and perhaps normal aging); (2) the different anatomical localizations, neurochemical alterations, and rate of progression of these conditions; and (3) the wide range of control processes mediated by the PFC. For example, orbitofrontal PFC neurodegeneration accompanying FTD frequently presents gradually with emotional dysregulation and socially inappropriate behavior (see Miller, Chapter 1, this volume), whereas dorsolateral PFC lesions from middle cerebral artery strokes lead to acute executive function deficits (Ferreira et al., 1998). As discussed, this clinical disparity is the product of structurally and functionally dissociable neural networks mediating distinct control processes. Thus, the subtleties of the frontal lobe syndrome may be interpreted by exploring the interactions between pathology, executive control processes, and neural networks.

Clinical evaluation of patients with behavioral deficits suggesting neurological disease frequently involves extensive neuropsychological assessment to aid in diagnosis and prognosis. The battery of tests utilized to evaluate frontal lobe dysfunction is quite varied in an attempt to capture the breadth of potential behavioral alterations (see Kramer & Quintania, Chapter 18, this volume). Clinician review of the pattern of deficits displayed by a patient is often used to establish the anatomical localization of a lesion based on the functional anatomy of the frontal lobes.[5] We propose a complementary approach when evaluating the pattern of deficits in such patients: the organization of signs and symptoms within the framework of a modulatory control model. Despite the diverse manifestations of the frontal lobe syndrome, it is possible to sort associated behavioral alterations within categories of sensory, internal state, and motor control with dissociable enhancement and suppressive mechanisms (Table 13.4). It is our hope that this organization will contribute to the understanding of pathological processes, PFC function, and ultimately to the development of pharmacological treatments optimized to treat deficiencies of different control process.

We propose that deficits of top-down enhancement result in an inability to attend to environmental stimuli (sensory control), failure to maintain relevant information in mind, difficulty in planning and organization (internal state: cognition control), emotional blunting and apathy (internal state: affective control), and deficits in initiating movements (motor control). On the other hand, deficits in top-down suppression lead to increased distractibility (sensory control and internal state: cognition control), emotional lability and social disinhibition (internal state: affective control), and perseveration and utilization behavior (motor control). A condition might be also be accompanied by an excessive degree of top-down modulation, such as the illusions (sensory control) or hallucinations of schizophrenia (internal state control: cognition) and the obsessions of obsessive–compulsive disorder (internal state control: cognition). Alterations in enhancement and suppression may occur in numerous patterns reflecting the neurochemi-

**TABLE 13.4. Signs and Symptoms of the Frontal Lobe Syndrome Organized within the Modulatory Control Model**

|  | Sensory input | Internal: cognition | Internal: affect | Motor output |
|---|---|---|---|---|
| Executive control function | Selective attention WM encoding LTM encoding | WM maintenance Mental imagery Planning | Emotion | Reach control Eye movements |
| Enhancement deficit Signs and symptoms | Difficulty in attending and remembering | Inability to hold information in mind Poor planning Poor organization | Emotional blunting | Movement initiation deficit |
| Neuropsychological test | CVLT, DRT | DRT, WCST, Tower of London, verbal fluency |  |  |
| Suppression deficit Signs and symptoms | Distractibility | Distractibility | Emotional lability Social disinhibition | Perseveration Utilization behavior Motor sequencing deficit |
| Neuropsychological test | CVLT, DRT, Stroop | Tasks with distractors |  | Go/no-go |

*Note.* DRT, delayed-response task; CVLT, California Verbal Learning Test; WM, working memory; LTM, long-term memory; WCST, Wisconsin Card Sorting Task.

cal and anatomical heterogeneity of the pathological processes that generate a frontal lobe syndrome.

The categories identified in Table 13.4 are not mutually exclusive. For example, utilization behavior, which occurs in patients with frontal lobe dysfunction (e.g., ADHD; Nicpon, Wodrich, & Kurpius, 2004), FTD (Miller, Chapter 1, this volume), and focal frontal lesions (Lhermitte, 1983), refers to the appropriate use of an object in an inappropriate context (e.g., opening an umbrella in a confined indoor space) and is a component of the so-called "environmental dependency syndrome" (Lhermitte, 1986). This syndrome includes an assortment of uncontrolled actions that presumably have their basis in excessive influence by external stimuli. However, although it is apparent that utilization behavior is a manifestation of a suppression deficit, it is unclear whether it reflects a deficit in sensory and/or motor control. Additionally, as already mentioned, neuropsychological tests such as the Stroop task (see Kramer & Quitania, Chapter 18, this volume) that assess inhibitory deficits in these patients, exhibit this same limitation in precisely dissociating sensory and motor control deficits. These processes may be resolved via the coupling of cognitive paradigms with event-related functional neuroimaging to study sensory and motor control processes in isolation (Gazzaley, Cooney, McEvoy, et al., 2005).

The frontal lobe syndrome is not the exclusive domain of neurological and psychiatric conditions; elements of it are present at both ends of the life spectrum, in *childhood* and *old age*. During child development, the protracted emergence of control processes is presumably based on the relatively late maturation of the frontal lobes that continues throughout childhood into adolescence. This includes processes such as dendritic arborization, myelination, and synaptogenesis, as well as three growth spurts demarcated by electroencephalogram (EEG) and functional imaging studies (birth–2 years, 7–9 years, and 16–19 years) (Anderson, Levin, & Jacobs, 2002). At the other end of life, older adults experience a wide range of cognitive deficits, often within the domain of executive control processes (Craik & Salthouse, 2000). For example, there is an emerging behavioral literature on an age-associated failure to ignore distracting information and its impact on WM performance in older adults, referred to as the *inhibitory deficit hypothesis* of

cognitive aging (Hasher & Zacks, 1988). In an extension of this hypothesis, we have recently generated fMRI data revealing that age-related WM impairment is associated with selective physiological deficits in the suppression of irrelevant information during WM encoding, with preserved enhancement of relevant information (Gazzaley, Cooney, Rissman, & D'Esposito, 2005). These data support the mechanistic dissociation of top-down enhancement and suppression processes. Others have documented structural alterations of the frontal lobes that may account for executive control deficits (Raz et al., 1997); the *frontal lobe hypothesis* of cognitive aging is an arena of active debate (Greenwood, 2000; West, 1996).

Interestingly, the development of a frontal lobe syndrome does not actually require the presence of a lesion in any of the cortical regions that constitute PFC control networks. A frontal lobe syndrome frequently emerges as a consequence of multifocal white matter disease or metabolic encephalopathy (Ishihara, Nishino, Maki, Kawamura, & Murayama, 2002; Mesulam, 2002; Wolfe, Linn, Babikian, Knoefel, & Albert, 1990). Additionally, the accumulation of white matter lesions as a result of small vessel disease, regardless of location, is associated with frontal hypometabolism and executive dysfunction (Reed et al., 2004; Tullberg et al., 2004). By hindering communication within the network, white matter disease produces comparable executive control deficits, without directly damaging any cortical network nodes; thus, it offers strong support for the network model of modulatory control described in this chapter. This may be a potential underlying basis for the cognitive deficits that occur in normal aging and vascular dementia (Gunning-Dixon & Raz, 2003; Wolfe et al., 1990).

## CONCLUSIONS

The search for a unifying theory of PFC function has been a major focus of cognitive neuroscience research, with the power to inform both basic science and clinical objectives. In this chapter, we have presented a synthesis of the literature supporting a unifying role of the PFC in executive control. This control extends to both cognition and emotion via influence on sensory input, internal state (both cognitive and affective), and motor output. The structural–functional bases of PFC executive control are distributed neural networks, with complexity manifest by neurochemical and anatomical heterogeneity of PFC circuits. The neural mechanism of this control is top-down modulation of the speed and magnitude of activity in distant brain regions, characterized by parallel processes of enhancement and suppression. Dysfunctional PFC control by either structural or neurochemical alterations results in a frontal lobe syndrome that can be organized within the framework of this modulatory control model. This model has generated numerous testable hypotheses whose empirical support will be essential for the establishment a unifying physiological basis of PFC function, as well as the development of new treatments for patients with cognitive deficits from PFC dysfunction.

## NOTES

1. There has been an emerging effort to integrate emotion and cognition in the context of the PFC and its interactions with other regions (Compton, 2003; Gray, Braver, & Raichle, 2002; Holland & Gallagher, 2004).
2. Executive control should be differentiated from "executive function," which often refers exclusively to cognitive and not affective processes.
3. Clearly, we still have a long way to evolve in both of these regards.
4. Perseveration is the uncontrollable repetition of a particular response.
5. Structural imaging is frequently unhelpful when assessing behavioral changes in cognitive neurology patients.

## REFERENCES

Anderson, V., Levin, H. S., & Jacobs, R. (2002). Executive functions after frontal lobe injury: A developmental perspective. In D. T. Stuss & R. T. Knight (Eds.), *Principles of frontal lobe function* (pp. 504–527). Oxford, UK: Oxford University Press.

Arnsten, A. F. T., & Robbins, T. W. (2002). Neurochemical modulation of prefrontal cortical function in humans and animals. In D. T. Stuss & R. T. Knight (Eds.), *Principles of frontal lobe function* (pp. 51–84). Oxford, UK: Oxford University Press.

Baddeley, A. (1986). *Working memory.* Oxford, UK: Oxford University Press.

Bar, M. (2003). A cortical mechanism for triggering top-down facilitation in visual object recognition. *Journal of Cognitive Neuroscience, 15*(4), 600–609.

Barbas, H. (2000). Connections underlying the synthesis of cognition, memory, and emotion in primate prefrontal cortices. *Brain Research Bulletin, 52*(5), 319–330.

Barbas, H., Saha, S., Rempel-Clower, N., & Ghashghaei, T. (2003). Serial pathways from primate prefrontal cortex to autonomic areas may influence emotional expression. *BMC Neuroscience, 4*(1), 25.

Barcelo, F., Suwazono, S., & Knight, R. T. (2000). Prefrontal modulation of visual processing in humans. *Nature Neuroscience, 3*(4), 399–403.

Bechara, A. (2004). The role of emotion in decision-making: Evidence from neurological patients with orbitofrontal damage. *Brain and Cognition, 55*(1), 30–40.

Bechara, A., Damasio, H., Tranel, D., & Damasio, A. R. (1997). Deciding advantageously before knowing the advantageous strategy. *Science, 275,* 1293–1295.

Bechara, A., Tranel, D., & Damasio, H. (2000). Characterization of the decision-making deficit of patients with ventromedial prefrontal cortex lesions. *Brain, 123*(11), 2189–2202.

Benton, A. (1968). Differential behavioral effects in frontal lobe disease. *Neuropsychologia, 28,* 171–179.

Berlin, H. A., Rolls, E. T., & Kischka, U. (2004). Impulsivity, time perception, emotion and reinforcement sensitivity in patients with orbitofrontal cortex lesions. *Brain, 127*(5), 1108–1126.

Blair, R. J., & Cipolotti, L. (2000). Impaired social response reversal: A case of "acquired sociopathy." *Brain, 123*(6), 1122–1141.

Burnod, Y. (1991). Organizational levels of the cerebral cortex: An integrated model. *Acta Biotheoretica, 39*(3–4), 351–361.

Carr, D. B., & Sesack, S. R. (1998). Callosal terminals in the rat prefrontal cortex: Synaptic targets and association with GABA-immunoreactive structures. *Synapse, 29*(3), 193–205.

Cavada, C., & Goldman-Rakic, P. S. (1989). Posterior parietal cortex in rhesus monkey: II. Evidence for segregated corticocortical networks linking sensory and limbic areas with the frontal lobe. *Journal of Comparative Neurology, 287*(4), 422–445.

Chao, L. L., & Knight, R. T. (1998). Contribution of human prefrontal cortex to delay performance. *Journal of Cognitive Neuroscience, 10*(2), 167–177.

Compton, R. J. (2003). The interface between emotion and attention: A review of evidence from psychology and neuroscience. *Behavioral and Cognitive Neuroscience Reviews, 2*(2), 115–129.

Compton, R. J., Banich, M. T., Mohanty, A., Milham, M. P., Herrington, J., Miller, G. A., et al. (2003). Paying attention to emotion: An fMRI investigation of cognitive and emotional stroop tasks. *Cognitive, Affective, and Behavioral Neuroscience, 3*(2), 81–96.

Corbetta, M., & Shulman, G. L. (2002). Control of goal-directed and stimulus-driven attention in the brain. *Nature Reviews: Neuroscience, 3*(3), 201–215.

Coull, J. T., Buchel, C., Friston, K. J., & Frith, C. D. (1999). Noradrenergically mediated plasticity in a human attentional neuronal network. *NeuroImage*, *10*(6), 705–715.

Craik, F. I., & Salthouse, T. A. (2000). *Handbook of aging and cognition II*. Mahwah, NJ: Erlbaum.

Crone, E. A., Somsen, R. J., Van Beek, B., & Van Der Molen, M. W. (2004). Heart rate and skin conductance analysis of antecendents and consequences of decision making. *Psychophysiology*, *41*(4), 531–540.

Curtis, C. E., & D'Esposito, M. (2003). Persistent activity in the prefrontal cortex during working memory. *Trends in Cognitive Science*, *7*(9), 415–423.

D'Esposito, M., Aguirre, G. K., Zarahn, E., Ballard, D., Shin, R. K., & Lease, J. (1998). Functional MRI studies of spatial and nonspatial working memory. *Brain Research: Cognitive Brain Research*, *7*(1), 1–13.

D'Esposito, M., & Postle, B. R. (1999). The dependence of span and delayed-response performance on prefrontal cortex. *Neuropsychologia*, *37*(11), 1303–1315.

Dias, R., Robbins, T. W., & Roberts, A. C. (1996). Dissociation in prefrontal cortex of affective and attentional shifts. *Nature*, *380*, 69–72.

Duncan, J. (2001). An adaptive coding model of neural function in the prefrontal cortex. *Nature Reviews: Neuroscience*, *2*, 820–829.

Evers, S., Bockermann, I., & Nyhuis, P. W. (2001). The impact of transcranial magnetic stimulation on cognitive processing: An event-related potential study. *Neuroreport*, *12*(13), 2915–2918.

Ferreira, C. T., Verin, M., Pillon, B., Levy, R., Dubois, B., & Agid, Y. (1998). Spatio-temporal working memory and frontal lesions in man. *Cortex*, *34*(1), 83–98.

Friston, K., Phillips, J., Chawla, D., & Buchel, C. (2000). Nonlinear PCA: characterizing interactions between modes of brain activity. *Philosophical Transactions of the Royal Society of London, Series B, Biological Sciences*, *355*, 135–146.

Friston, K. J., Frith, C. D., Liddle, P. F., & Frackowiak, R. S. (1993). Functional connectivity: The principal-component analysis of large (PET) data sets. *Journal of Cerebral Blood Flow and Metabolism*, *13*(1), 5–14.

Fuster, J. M. (1990). Inferotemporal units in selective visual attention and short-term memory. *Journal of Neurophysiology*, *64*(3), 681–697.

Fuster, J. M. (2003). *Cortex and mind: Unifying cognition*. New York: Oxford University Press.

Fuster, J. M., & Alexander, G. E. (1971). Neuron activity related to short-term memory. *Science*, *173*, 652–654.

Fuster, J. M., Bauer, R. H., & Jervey, J. P. (1985). Functional interactions between inferotemporal and prefrontal cortex in a cognitive task. *Brain Research*, *330*(2), 299–307.

Gazzaley, A., Cooney, J., McEvoy, L. K., Knight, R. T., & D'Esposito, M. (2005). Top-down enhancement and suppression of the magnitude and speed of neural activity. *Journal of Cognitive Neuroscience*, *17*(3), 507–517.

Gazzaley, A., Cooney, J. W., Rissman, J., & D'Esposito, M. (2005). Top-down suppression on deficit underlies working memory impairment in normal aging. *Nature Neuroscience*, *8*, 1298–1300.

Gazzaley, A., & D'Esposito, M. (in press). Neural networks: An empirical neuroscience approach toward understanding cognition. *Cortex*.

Gazzaley, A., Rissman, J., & D'Esposito, M. (2005). Functional connectivity during working memory maintenance. *Cognitive Affective, and Behavioral Neuroscience*, *4*, 580–599.

Goldman-Rakic, P. S. (1996). The prefrontal landscape: Implications of functional architecture for understanding human mentation and the central executive. *Philosophical Transactions of the Royal Society of London, Series B, Biological Sciences*, *351*, 1445–1453.

Goldman-Rakic, P. S. (1998). The prefrontal landscape: Implications of functional architecture for understanding human mentation and central executive. In A. C. Roberts, T. W. Robbins, & L. Weiskrantz (Eds.), *The prefrontal cortex: Executive and cognitive functions* (pp. 87–102). Oxford, UK: Oxford University Press.

Goldman-Rakic, P. S., & Friedman, H. R. (1991). The circuitry of working memory revealed by anatomy and metabolic imaging. In H. Levin, H. Eisenberg, & A. Benton (Eds.), *Frontal lobe function and dysfunction* (pp. 72–91). New York: Oxford University Press.

Goldman-Rakic, P. S., Lidow, M. S., & Gallager, D. W. (1990). Overlap of dopaminergic, adrenergic, and serotoninergic receptors and complementarity of their subtypes in primate prefrontal cortex. *Journal of Neuroscience*, *10*, 2125–2138.

Graffman, J. (2002). The structured event complex and the human frontal cortex. In D. Stuss & R. T. Knight (Eds.), *Principles of frontal lobe function* (pp. 292–310). Oxford, UK: Oxford University Press.

Grafman, J., Pascual-Leone, A., Alway, D., Nichelli, P., Gomez-Tortosa, E., & Hallett, M. (1994). Induction of a recall deficit by rapid-rate transcranial magnetic stimulation. *NeuroReport*, *5*(9), 1157–1160.

Gray, J. R., Braver, T. S., & Raichle, M. E. (2002). Integration of emotion and cognition in the lateral prefrontal cortex. *Proceedings of the National Academy of the Sciences of the United States of America*, *99*(6), 4115–4120.

Greenwood, P. M. (2000). The frontal aging hypothesis evaluated. *Journal of the International Neuropsychological Society*, *6*(6), 705–726.

Gunning-Dixon, F. M., & Raz, N. (2003). Neuroanatomical correlates of selected executive functions in middle-aged and older adults: A prospective MRI study. *Neuropsychologia*, *41*(14), 1929–1941.

Harlow, J. M. (1868). Recovery from the passage of an iron bar through the head. *Proceedings of the Massachusetts Medical Society*, *2*, 725–728.

Hasegawa, I., Fukushima, T., Ihara, T., & Miyashita, Y. (1998). Callosal window between prefrontal cortices:

Cognitive interaction to retrieve long-term memory. *Science, 281,* 814–818.

Hasher, L., & Zacks, J. M. (1988). Working memory, comprehension and aging: A review and a new view. In G. H. Bower (Ed.), *The psychology of learning and motivation* (Vol. 22, pp. 193–225). New York: Academic Press.

Hebb, D. O. (1945). Man's frontal lobes: A critical review. *Archives of Neurology and Psychiatry, 54,* 10–24.

Hecaen, H., & Albert, M. L. (1978). *Human neuropsychology.* New York: Wiley.

Heimer, L. (1983). *The human brain and spinal cord: Functional neuroanatomy and dissection guide.* New York: Springer-Verlag.

Hillyard, S. A., Hink, R. F., Schwent, V. L., & Picton, T. W. (1973). Electrical signs of selective attention in the human brain. *Science, 182,* 177–179.

Holland, P. C., & Gallagher, M. (2004). Amygdala-frontal interactions and reward expectancy. *Current Opinion in Neurobiology, 14*(2), 148–155.

Honey, G. D., Suckling, J., Zelaya, F., Long, C., Routledge, C., Jackson, S., et al. (2003). Dopaminergic drug effects on physiological connectivity in a human cortico–striato–thalamic system. *Brain, 126*(8), 1767–1781.

Hopfinger, J. B., Buonocore, M. H., & Mangun, G. R. (2000). The neural mechanisms of top-down attentional control. *Nature Neuroscience, 3*(3), 284–291.

Hornak, J., O'Doherty, J., Bramham, J., Rolls, E. T., Morris, R. G., Bullock, P. R., et al. (2004). Reward-related reversal learning after surgical excisions in orbito-frontal or dorsolateral prefrontal cortex in humans. *Journal of Cognitive Neuroscience, 16*(3), 463–478.

Houghton, G., & Tipper, S. P. (1996). Inhibitory mechanisms of neural and cognitive control: Applications to selective attention and sequential action. *Brain and Cognition, 30*(1), 20–43.

Ilinsky, I. A., Jouandet, M. L., & Goldman-Rakic, P. S. (1985). Organization of the nigrothalamocortical system in the rhesus monkey. *Journal of Comparative Neurology, 236*(3), 315–330.

Ishai, A., Haxby, J. V., & Ungerleider, L. G. (2002). Visual imagery of famous faces: Effects of memory and attention revealed by fMRI. *NeuroImage, 17*(4), 1729–1741.

Ishihara, K., Nishino, H., Maki, T., Kawamura, M., & Murayama, S. (2002). Utilization behavior as a white matter disconnection syndrome. *Cortex, 38*(3), 379–387.

Jacobsen, C. F. (1935). Functions of frontal association areas in primates. *Archives of Neurology and Psychiatry, 33,* 558–560.

Kaada, B., Pribrahm, K., & Epstein, J. A. (1949). Respiratory and vascular responses in monkeys from the temporal pole, insula, orbital surface and cingulate gyrus. *Journal of Neurophysiology, 12,* 348–356.

Kastner, S., Pinsk, M. A., De Weerd, P., Desimone, R., & Ungerleider, L. G. (1999). Increased activity in human visual cortex during directed attention in the absence of visual stimulation. *Neuron, 22*(4), 751–761.

Knight, R. T. (1997). Distributed cortical network for visual attention. *Journal of Cognitive Neuroscience, 9*(1), 75–91.

Knight, R. T., Hillyard, S. A., Woods, D. L., & Neville, H. J. (1981). The effects of frontal cortex lesions on event-related potentials during auditory selective attention. *Electroencephalography and Clinical Neurophysiology, 52*(6), 571–582.

Knight, R. T., Scabini, D., & Woods, D. L. (1989). Prefrontal cortex gating of auditory transmission in humans. *Brain Research, 504*(2), 338–342.

Knight, R. T., Staines, W. R., Swick, D., & Chao, L. L. (1999). Prefrontal cortex regulates inhibition and excitation in distributed neural networks. *Acta Psychologica (Amsterdam), 101*(2–3), 159–178.

Kyd, R. J., & Bilkey, D. K. (2003). Prefrontal cortex lesions modify the spatial properties of hippocampal place cells. *Cerebral Cortex, 13*(5), 444–451.

Lee, A. C., Robbins, T. W., Smith, S., Calvert, G. A., Tracey, I., Matthews, P., et al. (2002). Evidence for asymmetric frontal-lobe involvement in episodic memory from functional magnetic resonance imaging and patients with unilateral frontal-lobe excisions. *Neuropsychologia, 40*(13), 2420–2437.

Lezak, M. D. (1995). *Neuropsychological assessment* (3rd ed.). New York: Oxford University Press.

Lhermitte, F. (1983). "Utilization behaviour" and its relation to lesions of the frontal lobes. *Brain, 106,* 237–255.

Lhermitte, F. (1986). Human autonomy and the frontal lobes: Part II. Patient behavior in complex and social situations: The "environmental dependency syndrome." *Annals of Neurology, 19*(4), 335–343.

Lin, F. H., McIntosh, A. R., Agnew, J. A., Eden, G. F., Zeffiro, T. A., & Belliveau, J. W. (2003). Multivariate analysis of neuronal interactions in the generalized partial least squares framework: Simulations and empirical studies. *NeuroImage, 20*(2), 625–642.

Luck, S. J., & Hillyard, S. A. (1995). The role of attention in feature detection and conjunction discrimination: An electrophysiological analysis. *International Journal of Neuroscience, 80*(1–4), 281–297.

Luck, S. J., Hillyard, S. A., Mouloua, M., Woldorff, M. G., Clark, V. P., & Hawkins, H. L. (1994). Effects of spatial cuing on luminance detectability: Psychophysical and electrophysiological evidence for early selection. *Journal of Experimental Psychology: Human Perception and Performance, 20*(4), 887–904.

Luria, A. R. (1966). *Human brain and psychological processes.* New York: Harper & Row.

Mah, L., Arnold, M. C., & Grafman, J. (2004). Impairment of social perception associated with lesions of the prefrontal cortex. *American Journal of Psychiatry, 161*(7), 1247–1255.

Makris, N., Kennedy, D. N., McInerney, S., Sorensen, A. G., Wang, R., Caviness, V. S., Jr., et al. (2004). Segmentation of subcomponents within the superior longitudinal fascicle in humans: A quantitative, *in vivo,* DT-MRI study. *Cerebral Cortex, 15*(6), 854–869.

Manes, F., Sahakian, B., Clark, L., Rogers, R., Antoun, N., Aitken, M., et al. (2002). Decision-making processes following damage to the prefrontal cortex. *Brain, 125*(3), 624–639.

McIntosh, A. R. (1998). Understanding neural interactions in learning and memory using functional neuroimaging. *Annals of the New York Academy of Sciences, 855,* 556–571.

McIntosh, A. R., Grady, C. L., Haxby, J. V., Ungerleider, L. G., & Horwitz, B. (1996). Changes in limbic and prefrontal functional interactions in a working memory task for faces. *Cerebral Cortex, 6*(4), 571–584.

Mechelli, A., Price, C. J., Friston, K. J., & Ishai, A. (2004). Where bottom-up meets top-down: Neuronal interactions during perception and imagery. *Cerebral Cortex, 14*(11), 1256–1265.

Mesulam, M. (1981). A cortical network for directed attention and unilateral neglect. *Annals of Neurology, 10*(4), 309–325.

Mesulam, M.-M. (2002). The human frontal lobes: Transcending the default mode through contingent encoding. In D. T. Stuss & R. T. Knight (Eds.), *Principles of frontal lobe function* (pp. 8–30). Oxford, UK: Oxford University Press.

Mesulam, M. M. (1990). Large-scale neurocognitive networks and distributed processing for attention, language, and memory. *Annals of Neurology, 28*(5), 597–613.

Miller, E. K., & Cohen, J. D. (2001). An integrative theory of prefrontal cortex function. *Annual Review of Neuroscience, 24,* 167–202.

Miller, E. K., Li, L., & Desimone, R. (1993). Activity of neurons in anterior inferior temporal cortex during a short-term memory task. *Journal of Neuroscience, 13*(4), 1460–1478.

Milner, B. (1963). Effects of different brain regions on card sorting. *Archives of Neurology, 9,* 90–100.

Miyashita, Y. (2004). Cognitive memory: Cellular and network machineries and their top-down control. *Science, 306,* 435–440.

Morecraft, R. J., Geula, C., & Mesulam, M. M. (1992). Cytoarchitecture and neural afferents of orbitofrontal cortex in the brain of the monkey. *Journal of Comparative Neurology, 323*(3), 341–358.

Mottaghy, F. M., Krause, B. J., Kemna, L. J., Topper, R., Tellmann, L., Beu, M., et al. (2000). Modulation of the neuronal circuitry subserving working memory in healthy human subjects by repetitive transcranial magnetic stimulation. *Neuroscience Letters, 280*(3), 167–170.

Nicpon, M. F., Wodrich, D. L., & Kurpius, S. E. (2004). Utilization behavior in boys with ADHD: A test of Barkley's theory. *Devopmental Neuropsychology, 26*(3), 735–751.

O'Craven, K. M., Downing, P. E., & Kanwisher, N. (1999). fMRI evidence for objects as the units of attentional selection. *Nature, 401,* 584–587.

Ongur, D., An, X., & Price, J. L. (1998). Prefrontal cortical projections to the hypothalamus in macaque monkeys. *Journal of Comparative Neurology, 401*(4), 480–505.

Otani, S. (2002). Memory trace in prefrontal cortex: Theory for the cognitive switch. *Biological Reviews of the Cambridge Philosophical Society, 77*(4), 563–577.

Pascual-Leone, A., Walsh, V., & Rothwell, J. (2000). Transcranial magnetic stimulation in cognitive neuroscience—virtual lesion, chronometry, and functional connectivity. *Current Opinion in Neurobiology, 10*(2), 232–237.

Paus, T., Castro-Alamancos, M. A., & Petrides, M. (2001). Cortico-cortical connectivity of the human mid-dorsolateral frontal cortex and its modulation by repetitive transcranial magnetic stimulation. *European Journal of Neuroscience, 14*(8), 1405–1411.

Penny, W. D., Stephan, K. E., Mechelli, A., & Friston, K. J. (2004). Comparing dynamic causal models. *NeuroImage, 22*(3), 1157–1172.

Pessoa, L., Kastner, S., & Ungerleider, L. G. (2003). Neuroimaging studies of attention: From modulation of sensory processing to top-down control. *Journal of Neuroscience, 23*(10), 3990–3998.

Petrides, M. (1994). Frontal lobes and working memory: Evidence from investigations of the effects of cortical excisions in nonhuman primates. In F. Boller & J. Grafman (Eds.), *Handbook of neuropsychology* (Vol. 9, pp. 59–84). Amsterdam: Elsevier.

Petrides, M., & Pandya, D. N. (1984). Projections to the frontal cortex from the posterior parietal region in the rhesus monkey. *Journal of Comparative Neurology, 228*(1), 105–116.

Petrides, M., & Pandya, D. N. (1999). Dorsolateral prefrontal cortex: Comparative cytoarchitectonic analysis in the human and the macaque brain and corticocortical connection patterns. *European Journal of Neuroscience, 11*(3), 1011–1036.

Petrides, M., & Pandya, D. N. (2002). Comparative cytoarchitectonic analysis of the human and the macaque ventrolateral prefrontal cortex and corticocortical connection patterns in the monkey. *European Journal of Neuroscience, 16*(2), 291–310.

Pinsk, M. A., Doniger, G. M., & Kastner, S. (2004). Push–pull mechanism of selective attention in human extrastriate cortex. *Journal of Neurophysiology, 92*(1), 622–629.

Pool, J. L., & Ransohoff, J. (1949). Autonomic effects on stimulating rostral portion of cingulate gyri in man. *Journal of Neurophysiology, 12*(6), 385–392.

Rainer, G., Asaad, W. F., & Miller, E. K. (1998). Selective representation of relevant information by neurons in the primate prefrontal cortex. *Nature, 393,* 577–579.

Ranganath, C., Johnson, M. K., & D'Esposito, M. (2003). Prefrontal activity associated with working memory and episodic long-term memory. *Neuropsychologia, 41*(3), 378–389.

Raz, N., Gunning, F. M., Head, D., Dupuis, J. H., McQuain, J., Briggs, S. D., et al. (1997). Selective aging of the human cerebral cortex observed *in vivo*: Differential vulnerability of the prefrontal gray matter. *Cerebral Cortex, 7*(3), 268–282.

Reed, B. R., Eberling, J. L., Mungas, D., Weiner, M.,

Kramer, J. H., & Jagust, W. J. (2004). Effects of white matter lesions and lacunes on cortical function. *Archives of Neurology, 61*(10), 1545–1550.

Rees, G., Frith, C. D., & Lavie, N. (1997). Modulating irrelevant motion perception by varying attentional load in an unrelated task. *Science, 278,* 1616–1619.

Rissman, J., Gazzaley, A., & D'Esposito, M. (2004). Measuring functional connectivity during distinct stages of a cognitive task. *NeuroImage, 23*(2), 752–763.

Rowe, J., Friston, K., Frackowiak, R., & Passingham, R. (2002). Attention to action: Specific modulation of corticocortical interactions in humans. *NeuroImage, 17*(2), 988.

Rule, R. R., Shimamura, A. P., & Knight, R. T. (2002). Orbitofrontal cortex and dynamic filtering of emotional stimuli. *Cognitive, Affective, and Behavioral Neuroscience, 2*(3), 264–270.

Sarter, M., Bernston, G., & Cacioppo, J. (1996). Brain imaging and cognitive neuroscience: Toward strong inference in attributing function to structure. *American Psychologist, 51,* 13–21.

Selemon, L. D., & Goldman-Rakic, P. S. (1985). Longitudinal topography and interdigitation of corticostriatal projections in the rhesus monkey. *Journal of Neuroscience, 5*(3), 776–794.

Selemon, L. D., & Goldman-Rakic, P. S. (1988). Common cortical and subcortical targets of the dorsolateral prefrontal and parietal cortices in the rhesus monkey: Evidence for a distributed neural network subserving spatially guided behavior. *Journal of Neuroscience, 8,* 4049–4068.

Seminowicz, D. A., Mikulis, D. J., & Davis, K. D. (2004). Cognitive modulation of pain-related brain responses depends on behavioral strategy. *Pain, 112*(1–2), 48–58.

Shallice, T. (1988). *From neuropsychology to mental structure.* Cambridge, UK: Cambridge University Press.

Shimamura, A. P. (1997). The role of the prefrontal cortex in dynamic filtering. *Psychobiology, 28*(2), 207–218.

Skinner, J., & Yingling, C. (1977). Central gating mechanisms that regulate event-related potentials and behavior. In J. Desmedt (Ed.), *Progress in clinical neurophysiology* (Vol. 1, pp. 30–69). Basel, Switzerland: Karger.

Sotres-Bayon, F., Bush, D. E., & LeDoux, J. E. (2004). Emotional perseveration: An update on prefrontal–amygdala interactions in fear extinction. *Learning and Memory, 11*(5), 525–535.

Sun, F. T., Miller, L. M., & D'Esposito, M. (2004). Measuring interregional functional connectivity using coherence and partial coherence analyses of fMRI data. *NeuroImage, 21*(2), 647–658.

Tomita, H., Ohbayashi, M., Nakahara, K., Hasegawa, I., & Miyashita, Y. (1999). Top-down signal from prefrontal cortex in executive control of memory retrieval. *Nature, 401,* 699–703.

Treue, S., & Martinez Trujillo, J. C. (1999). Feature-based attention influences motion processing gain in macaque visual cortex. *Nature, 399,* 575–579.

Tullberg, M., Fletcher, E., DeCarli, C., Mungas, D., Reed, B. R., Harvey, D. J., et al. (2004). White matter lesions impair frontal lobe function regardless of their location. *Neurology, 63*(2), 246–253.

Ungerleider, L. G., Courtney, S. M., & Haxby, J. V. (1998). A neural system for human visual working memory. *Proceedings of the National Academy of Sciences of the United States of America, 95*(3), 883–890.

Ungerleider, L. G., Gaffan, D., & Pelak, V. S. (1989). Projections from inferior temporal cortex to prefrontal cortex via the uncinate fascicle in rhesus monkeys. *Experimental Brain Research, 76*(3), 473–484.

Vuilleumier, P., Armony, J. L., Driver, J., & Dolan, R. J. (2001). Effects of attention and emotion on face processing in the human brain: An event-related fMRI study. *Neuron, 30*(3), 829–841.

Webster, M. J., Bachevalier, J., & Ungerleider, L. G. (1994). Connections of inferior temporal areas TEO and TE with parietal and frontal cortex in macaque monkeys. *Cerebral Cortex, 4*(5), 470–483.

West, R. L. (1996). An application of prefrontal cortex function theory to cognitive aging. *Psychological Bulletin, 120*(2), 272–292.

Williams, D., Tijssen, M., Van Bruggen, G., Bosch, A., Insola, A., Di Lazzaro, V., et al. (2002). Dopamine-dependent changes in the functional connectivity between basal ganglia and cerebral cortex in humans. *Brain, 125*(7), 1558–1569.

Wojciulik, E., Kanwisher, N., & Driver, J. (1998). Covert visual attention modulates face-specific activity in the human fusiform gyrus: fMRI study. *Journal of Neurophysiology, 79*(3), 1574–1578.

Wolfe, N., Linn, R., Babikian, V. L., Knoefel, J. E., & Albert, M. L. (1990). Frontal systems impairment following multiple lacunar infarcts. *Archives of Neurology, 47*(2), 129–132.

Wood, J. N., & Grafman, J. (2003). Human prefrontal cortex: Processing and representational perspectives. *Nature Reviews: Neuroscience, 4*(2), 139–147.

Yamaguchi, S., & Knight, R. T. (1990). Gating of somatosensory input by human prefrontal cortex. *Brain Research, 521*(1–2), 281–288.

Yingling, C. D., & Skinner, J. E. (1977). Gating of thalamic input to cerebral cortex by nucleus reticularis thalami. In J. E. Desmedt (Ed.), *Progress in clinical neurophysiology* (Vol. 1., pp. 70–96). Basel, Switzerland: Karger.

Zelano, C., Bensafi, M., Porter, J., Mainland, J., Johnson, B., Bremner, E., et al. (2005). Attentional modulation in human primary olfactory cortex. *Nature Neuroscience, 8*(1), 114–120.

Zironi, I., Iacovelli, P., Aicardi, G., Liu, P., & Bilkey, D. K. (2001). Prefrontal cortex lesions augment the location-related firing properties of area TE/perirhinal cortex neurons in a working memory task. *Cerebral Cortex, 11*(11), 1093–1100.

## REFERENCES FOR TABLES 13.1–13.3

1. Perret, E. (1974). The left frontal lobe of man and the suppression of habitual responses in verbal categorical behaviour. *Neuropsychologia, 12,* 323–330.
2. Vendrell, P., Junque, C., Jurado, M. A., et al. (1995). The role of prefrontal regions in the Stroop task. *Neuropsychologia, 33,* 341–352.
3. Richer, F., Decary, A., Lapierre, M. F., et al. (1993). Target detection deficits in frontal lobectomy. *Brain and Cognition, 21,* 203–211.
4. Rafal, R., Gershberg, F., Egly, R., et al. (1996). Response channel activation and the lateral prefrontal cortex. *Neuropsychologia, 34,* 1197–1202.
5. Metzler, C., & Parkin, A. J. (2000). Reversed negative priming following frontal lobe lesions. *Neuropsychologia, 38,* 363–379.
6. Owen, A. M., Roberts, A. C., Polkey, C. E., et al. (1991). Extra-dimensional versus intra-dimensional set shifting performance following frontal lobe excisions, temporal lobe excision or amygdalo-hippocampectomy in man. *Neuropsychologia, 29,* 993–1006.
7. Verin, M., Partiot, A., Pillon, B., et al. (1993). Delayed response tasks and prefrontal lesions in man—evidence for self generated patterns of behaviour with poor environmental modulation. *Neuropsychologia, 31,* 1379–1396.
8. Ferreira, C. T., Verin, M., Pillon, B., et al. (1998). Spatio-temporal working memory and frontal lesions in man. *Cortex, 34,* 83–98.
9. D'Esposito, M., & Postle, B. R. (1999). The dependence of span and delayed-response performance on prefrontal cortex. *Neuropsychologia, 37,* 1303–1315.
10. Chao, L. L., & Knight, R. T. (1995). Human prefrontal lesions increase distractibility to irrelevant sensory inputs. *NeuroReport, 6,* 1605–1610.
11. Chao, L. L., & Knight, R. T. (1998). Contribution of human prefrontal cortex to delay performance. *Journal of Cognitive Neuroscience, 10,* 167–177.
12. Baldo, J., & Shimamura, A. (2000). Spatial and color working memory in patients with lateral prefrontal cotex lesions. *Psychobiology, 28,* 156–167.
13. Alexander, M. P., Stuss, D. T., & Fansabedian, N. (2003). California Verbal Learning Test: Performance by patients with focal frontal and non-frontal lesions. *Brain, 126,* 1493–1503.
14. Owen, A. M., Downes, J. J., Sahakian, B. J., et al. (1990). Planning and spatial working memory following frontal lobe lesions in man. *Neuropsychologia, 28,* 1021–1034.
15. Milner, B. (1963). Effects of different brain regions on card sorting. *Archives of Neurology, 9,* 90–100.
16. Dunbar, K., & Sussman, D. (1995). Toward a cognitive account of frontal lobe function: Simulating frontal lobe deficits in normal subjects. In J. Grafman, K. J. Holyoak, & F. Boller (Eds.), *Structure and functions of the human prefrontal cortex* (pp. 289–304). New York: New York Academy of Sciences.
17. Baldo, J. V., & Shimamura, A. P. (1998). Letter and category fluency in patients with frontal lobe lesions. *Neuropsychology, 12,* 259–267.
18. Stuss, D. T., Alexander, M. P., Hamer, L., et al. (1998). The effects of focal anterior and posterior brain lesions on verbal fluency. *Journal of the International Neuropsychological Society, 4,* 265–278.
19. Gomez-Beldarrain, M., Harries, C., Garcia-Monco, J. C., et al. (2004). Patients with right frontal lesions are unable to assess and use advice to make predictive judgments. *Journal of Cognitive Neuroscience, 16,* 74–89.
20. Mah, L., Arnold, M. C., & Grafman, J. (2004). Impairment of social perception associated with lesions of the prefrontal cortex. *American Journal of Psychiatry, 161,* 1247–1255.
21. Rowe, A. D., Bullock, P. R., Polkey, C. E., et al. (2001). "Theory of mind" impairments and their relationship to executive functioning following frontal lobe excisions. *Brain, 124,* 600–616.
22. Camille, N., Coricelli, G., Sallet, J., et al. (2004). The involvement of the orbitofrontal cortex in the experience of regret. *Science, 304,* 1167–1170.
23. Berlin, H. A., Rolls, E. T., & Kischka, U. (2004). Impulsivity, time perception, emotion and reinforcement sensitivity in patients with orbitofrontal cortex lesions. *Brain, 127,* 1108–1126.
24. Beer, J. S., Heerey, E. A., Keltner, D., et al. (2003). The regulatory function of self-conscious emotion: Insights from patients with orbitofrontal damage. *Journal of Personality and Social Psychology, 85,* 594–604.
25. Shamay-Tsoory, S. G., Tomer, R., Berger, B. D., et al. (2003). Characterization of empathy deficits following prefrontal brain damage: The role of the right ventromedial prefrontal cortex. *Journal of Cognitive Neuroscience, 15,* 324–337.
26. Bar-On, R., Tranel, D., Denburg, N. L., et al. (2003). Exploring the neurological substrate of emotional and social intelligence. *Brain, 126,* 1790–1800.
27. Tranel, D., Bechara, A., & Denburg, N. L. (2002). Asymmetric functional roles of right and left ventromedial prefrontal cortices in social conduct, decision-making, and emotional processing. *Cortex, 38,* 589–612.
28. Rueckert, L., & Grafman, J. (1996). Sustained attention deficits and patients with right frontal lesions. *Neuropsychologia, 34,* 953–963.
29. Hornak, J., O'Doherty, J., Bramham, J., et al. (2004). Reward-related reversal learning after surgical excisions in orbito-frontal or dorsolateral prefrontal cortex in humans. *Journal of Cognitive Neuroscience, 16,* 463–478.
30. Bechara, A., Dolan, S., Denburg, N., et al. (2001). Decision-making deficits, linked to a dysfunctional ventromedial prefrontal cortex, revealed in alcohol

and stimulant abusers. *Neuropsychologia, 39,* 376–389.

31. Angrilli, A., Palomba, D., Cantagallo, A., et al. (1999). Emotional impairment after right orbitofrontal lesion in a patient without cognitive deficits. *NeuroReport, 10,* 1741–1746.

32. Pierrot-Deseilligny, C., Rivaud, S., Gaymard, B., et al. (1991). Cortical control of memory-guided saccades in man. *Experimental Brain Research, 83,* 607–617.

33. Pierrot-Deseilligny, C., Muri, R. M., Ploner, C. J., et al. (2003). Decisional role of the dorsolateral prefrontal cortex in ocular motor behaviour. *Brain, 126,* 1460–1473.

34. Walker, R., Husain, M., Hodgson, T. L., et al. (1998). Saccadic eye movement and working memory deficits following damage to human prefrontal cortex. *Neuropsychologia, 36,* 1141–1159.

35. Broersen, L. M., & Uylings, H. B. (1999). Visual attention task performance in Wistar and Lister hooded rats: Response inhibition deficits after medial prefrontal cortex lesions. *Neuroscience, 94,* 47–57.

36. Leimkuhler, M. E., & Mesulam, M. M. (1985). Reversible go–no go deficits in a case of frontal lobe tumor. *Annals of Neurology, 18,* 617–619.

37. Drewe, E. A. (1975). Go–no go learning after frontal lobe lesions in humans. *Cortex, 11,* 8–16.

38. Slachevsky, A., Pillon, B., Fourneret, P., et al. (2003). The prefrontal cortex and conscious monitoring of action: An experimental study. *Neuropsychologia, 41,* 655–665.

39. Slachevsky, A., Pillon, B., Fourneret, P., et al. (2001). Preserved adjustment but impaired awareness in a sensory–motor conflict following prefrontal lesions. *Journal of Cognitive Neuroscience, 13,* 332–340.

40. Pardo, J. V., Fox, P. T., & Raichle, M. E. (1991). Localization of a human system for sustained attention by positron emission tomography. *Nature, 349,* 61–64.

41. Bench, C. J., Frith, C. D., Grasby, P. M., et al. (1993). Investigations of the functional anatomy of attention using the stroop test. *Neuropsychologia, 31,* 907–922.

42. Weiss, E. M., Golaszewski, S., Mottaghy, F. M., et al. (2003). Brain activation patterns during a selective attention test—a functional MRI study in healthy volunteers and patients with schizophrenia. *Psychiatry Research, 123,* 1–15.

43. Loose, R., Kaufmann, C., Auer, D. P., et al. (2003). Human prefrontal and sensory cortical activity during divided attention tasks. *Human Brain Mapping, 18,* 249–259.

44. Wagner, A. D., Desmond, J. E., Glover, G. H., et al. (1998). Prefrontal cortex and recognition memory: Functional-MRI evidence for context-dependent retrieval processes. *Brain, 121*(10), 1985–2002.

45. Lane, R. D., Fink, G. R., Chau, P. M., et al. (1997). Neural activation during selective attention to subjective emotional responses. *NeuroReport, 8,* 3969–3972.

46. Heekeren, H. R., Marrett, S., Bandettini, P. A., et al. (2004). A general mechanism for perceptual decision-making in the human brain. *Nature, 431,* 859–862.

47. Courtney, S. M., Ungerleider, L. G., Keil, K., et al. (1997). Transient and sustained activity in a distributed neural system for human working memory. *Nature, 386,* 608–611.

48. Sakai, K., Rowe, J. B., & Passingham, R. E. (2002). Active maintenance in prefrontal area 46 creates distractor-resistant memory. *Nature Neuroscience, 5,* 479–484.

49. D'Esposito, M., Postle, B. R., & Rypma, B. (2000). Prefrontal cortical contributions to working memory: Evidence from event-related fMRI studies. *Experimental Brain Research, 133,* 3–11.

50. D'Esposito, M., Postle, B. R., Ballard, D., et al. (1999). Maintenance versus manipulation of information held in working memory: An event-related fMRI study. *Brain and Cognition, 41,* 66–86.

51. Wagner, A. D., Maril, A., Bjork, R. A., et al. (2001). Prefrontal contributions to executive control: fMRI evidence for functional distinctions within lateral prefrontal cortex. *NeuroImage, 14,* 1337–1347.

52. Cohen, J. D., Perlstein, W. M., Braver, T. S., et al. (1997). Temporal dynamics of brain activation during a working memory task. *Nature, 386,* 604–608.

53. Ishai, A., Haxby, J. V., & Ungerleider, L. G. (2002). Visual imagery of famous faces: Effects of memory and attention revealed by fMRI. *NeuroImage, 17,* 1729–1741.

54. Mechelli, A., Price, C. J., Friston, K. J., et al. (2004). Where bottom-up meets top-down: Neuronal interactions during perception and imagery. *Cerebral Cortex, 14,* 1256–1265.

55. Nagahama, Y., Fukuyama, H., Yamauchi, H., et al. (1996). Cerebral activation during performance of a card sorting test. *Brain, 119*(5), 1667–1675.

56. Berman, K. F., Ostrem, J. L., Randolph, C., et al. (1995). Physiological activation of a cortical network during performance of the Wisconsin Card Sorting Test: A positron emission tomography study. *Neuropsychologia, 33,* 1027–1046.

57. Berthoz, S., Armony, J. L., Blair, R. J., et al. (2002). An fMRI study of intentional and unintentional (embarrassing) violations of social norms. *Brain, 125,* 1696–1708.

58. Pietrini, P., Guazzelli, M., Basso, G., et al. (2000). Neural correlates of imaginal aggressive behavior assessed by positron emission tomography in healthy subjects. *American Journal of Psychiatry, 157,* 1772–1781.

59. O'Doherty, J., Kringelbach, M. L., Rolls, E. T., et al. (2001). Abstract reward and punishment representations in the human orbitofrontal cortex. *Nature Neuroscience, 4,* 95–102.

60. Fukui, H., Murai, T., Fukuyama, H., et al. (2005). Functional activity related to risk anticipation during performance of the Iowa Gambling Task. *NeuroImage, 24*, 253–259.

61. Brown, M. R., DeSouza, J. F., Goltz, H. C., et al. (2004). Comparison of memory and visually guided saccades using event-related fMRI. *Journal of Neurophysiology, 91*, 873–889.

62. Matsuda, T., Matsuura, M., Ohkubo, T., et al. (2004). Functional MRI mapping of brain activation during visually guided saccades and antisaccades: Cortical and subcortical networks. *Psychiatry Research, 131*, 147–155.

63. Muri, R. M., Heid, O., Nirkko, A. C., et al. (1998). Functional organisation of saccades and antisaccades in the frontal lobe in humans: A study with echo planar functional magnetic resonance imaging. *Journal of Neurology, Neurosurgery, and Psychiatry, 65*, 374–377.

64. de Zubicaray, G. I., Andrew, C., Zelaya, F. O., et al. (2000). Motor response suppression and the prepotent tendency to respond: A parametric fMRI study. *Neuropsychologia, 38*, 1280–1291.

65. Garavan, H., Ross, T. J., & Stein, E. A. (1999). Right hemispheric dominance of inhibitory control: An event-related functional MRI study. *Proceedings of the National Academy of Sciences of the United States of America, 96*, 8301–8306.

66. Rubia, K., Smith, A. B., Brammer, M. J., et al. (2003). Right inferior prefrontal cortex mediates response inhibition while mesial prefrontal cortex is responsible for error detection. *NeuroImage, 20*, 351–358.

67. Menon, V., Adleman, N. E., White, C. D., et al. (2001). Error-related brain activation during a go/no go response inhibition task. *Human Brain Mapping, 12*, 131–143.

68. Liddle, P. F., Kiehl, K. A., & Smith, A. M. (2001). Event-related fMRI study of response inhibition. *Human Brain Mapping, 12*, 100–109.

69. Dias, R., Robbins, T. W., & Roberts, A. C. (1996). Dissociation in prefrontal cortex of affective and attentional shifts. *Nature, 380*, 69–72.

70. Birrell, J. M., & Brown, V. J. (2000). Medial frontal cortex mediates perceptual attentional set shifting in the rat. *Joruanl of Neuroscience, 20*, 4320–4324.

71. Granon, S., Hardouin, J., Courtier, A., et al. (1998). Evidence for the involvement of the rat prefrontal cortex in sustained attention. *Quarterly Journal of Experimental Psychology, B, 51*, 219–233.

72. Jacobsen, C. F. (1936). The functions of the frontal association areas in monkeys. *Comparative Psychology Monographs, 13*, 1–60.

73. Bauer, R. H., & Fuster, J. M. (1976). Delayed-matching and delayed-response deficit from cooling dorsolateral prefrontal cortex in monkeys. *Journal of Comparative Physiological Psychology, 90*, 293–302.

74. Dias, R., Robbins, T. W., & Roberts, A. C. (1996). Primate analogue of the Wisconsin Card Sorting Test: Effects of excitotoxic lesions of the prefrontal cortex in the marmoset. *Behavioral Neuroscience, 110*, 872–886.

75. Joel, D., Weiner, I., & Feldon, J. (1997). Electrolytic lesions of the medial prefrontal cortex in rats disrupt performance on an analog of the Wisconsin Card Sorting Test, but do not disrupt latent inhibition: Implications for animal models of schizophrenia. *Behavioural Brain Research, 85*, 187–201.

76. Izquierdo, A., & Murray, E. A. (2004). Combined unilateral lesions of the amygdala and orbital prefrontal cortex impair affective processing in rhesus monkeys. *Journal of Neurophysiology, 91*, 2023–2039.

77. Shah, A. A., & Treit, D. (2003). Excitotoxic lesions of the medial prefrontal cortex attenuate fear responses in the elevated-plus maze, social interaction and shock probe burying tests. *Brain Research, 969*, 183–194.

78. Deacon, R. M., Penny, C., & Rawlins, J. N. (2003). Effects of medial prefrontal cortex cytotoxic lesions in mice. *Behavioural Brain Research, 139*, 139–155.

79. Morgan, M. A., & LeDoux, J. E. (1999). Contribution of ventrolateral prefrontal cortex to the acquisition and extinction of conditioned fear in rats. *Neurobiology of Learning and Memory, 72*, 244–251.

80. Jinks, A. L., & McGregor, I. S. (1997). Modulation of anxiety-related behaviours following lesions of the prelimbic or infralimbic cortex in the rat. *Brain Research, 772*, 181–190.

81. Funahashi, S., Bruce, C. J., & Goldman-Rakic, P. S. (1993). Dorsolateral prefrontal lesions and oculomotor delayed-response performance: Evidence for mnemonic "scotomas." *Journal of Neuroscience, 13*, 1479–1497.

82. Wallis, J. D., Dias, R., Robbins, T. W., et al. (2001). Dissociable contributions of the orbitofrontal and lateral prefrontal cortex of the marmoset to performance on a detour reaching task. *European Journal of Neuroscience, 13*, 1797–1808.

83. Iversen, S. D., & Mishkin, M. (1970). Perseverative interference in monkeys following selective lesions of the inferior prefrontal convexity. *Experimental Brain Research, 11*, 376–386.

84. Gemmell, C., & O'Mara, S. M. (1999). Medial prefrontal cortex lesions cause deficits in a variable-goal location task but not in object exploration. *Behavioral Neuroscience, 113*, 465–474.

85. Collins, P., Roberts, A. C., Dias, R., et al. (1998). Perseveration and strategy in a novel spatial self-ordered sequencing task for nonhuman primates: effects of excitotoxic lesions and dopamine depletions of the prefrontal cortex. *Journal of Cognitive Neuroscience, 10*, 332–354.

86. DeSouza, J. F., & Everling, S. (2004). Focused at-

tention modulates visual responses in the primate prefrontal cortex. *Journal of Neurophysiology, 91,* 855–862.

87. Everling, S., Tinsley, C. J., Gaffan, D., et al. (2002). Filtering of neural signals by focused attention in the monkey prefrontal cortex. *Nature Neuroscience, 5,* 671–676.

88. Sakai, M., & Hamada, I. (1981). Intracellular activity and morphology of the prefrontal neurons related to visual attention task in behaving monkeys. *Experimental Brain Research, 41,* 195–198.

89. Fuster, J. M., & Alexander, G. E. (1971). Neuron activity related to short-term memory. *Science, 173,* 652–654.

90. Kubota, K., & Niki, H. (1971). Prefrontal cortical unit activity and delayed alternation performance in monkeys. *Journal of Neurophysiology, 34,* 337–347.

91. Funahashi, S., Bruce, C. J., & Goldman-Rakic, P. S. (1989). Mnemonic coding of visual space in the monkey's dorsolateral prefrontal cortex. *Journal of Neurophysiology, 61,* 331–349.

92. Rainer, G., Asaad, W. F., & Miller, E. K. (1998). Selective representation of relevant information by neurons in the primate prefrontal cortex. *Nature, 393,* 577–579.

93. Schlag-Ray, M., & Lindsley, D. B. (1970). Effect of prefrontal lesions on trained anticipatory visual attending in cats. *Physiolgoy and Behavior, 5,* 1033–1041.

94. Liang, H., Bressler, S. L., Ding, M., et al. (2002). Synchronized activity in prefrontal cortex during anticipation of visuomotor processing. *NeuroReport, 13,* 2011–2015.

95. Lecas, J. C. (1995). Prefrontal neurones sensitive to increased visual attention in the monkey. *NeuroReport, 7,* 305–309.

96. Tsujimoto, S., & Sawaguchi, T. (2005). Neuronal activity representing temporal prediction of reward in the primate prefrontal cortex. *Journal of Neurophysiology, 93(6),* 3687–3692.

97. Barraclough, D. J., Conroy, M. L., & Lee, D. (2004). Prefrontal cortex and decision making in a mixed-strategy game. *Nature Neuroscience, 7,* 404–410.

98. Wallis, J. D., & Miller, E. K. (2003). Neuronal activity in primate dorsolateral and orbital prefrontal cortex during performance of a reward preference task. *European Journal of Neuroscience, 18,* 2069–2081.

99. Hikosaka, K., & Watanabe, M. (2000). Delay activity of orbital and lateral prefrontal neurons of the monkey varying with different rewards. *Cerebral Cortex, 10,* 263–271.

100. Watanabe, M. (1996). Reward expectancy in primate prefrontal neurons. *Nature, 382,* 629–632.

101. Watanabe, M., Hikosaka, K., Sakagami, M., et al. (2002). Coding and monitoring of motivational context in the primate prefrontal cortex. *Journal of Neuroscience, 22,* 2391–2400.

102. Funahashi, S., Chafee, M. V., & Goldman-Rakic, P. S. (1993). Prefrontal neuronal activity in rhesus monkeys performing a delayed anti-saccade task. *Nature, 365,* 753–756.

103. Risterucci, C., Terramorsi, D., Nieoullon, A., et al. (2003). Excitotoxic lesions of the prelimbic–infralimbic areas of the rodent prefrontal cortex disrupt motor preparatory processes. *European Journal of Neuroscience, 17,* 1498–1508.

104. Hasegawa, R. P., Peterson, B. W., & Goldberg, M. E. (2004). Prefrontal neurons coding suppression of specific saccades. *Neuron, 43,* 415–425.

105. Sakagami, M., Tsutsui, K., Lauwereyns, J., et al. (2001). A code for behavioral inhibition on the basis of color, but not motion, in ventrolateral prefrontal cortex of macaque monkey. *Journal of Neuroscience, 21,* 4801–4808.

106. Morita, M., Nakahara, K., & Hayashi, T. (2004). A rapid presentation event-related functional magnetic resonance imaging study of response inhibition in macaque monkeys. *Neuroscience Letters, 356,* 203–206.

107. Fuster, J. M., Bauer, R. H., & Jervey, J. P. (1985). Functional interactions between inferotemporal and prefrontal cortex in a cognitive task. *Brain Research, 330,* 299–307.

108. Tomita, H., Ohbayashi, M., Nakahara, K., et al. (1999). Top-down signal from prefrontal cortex in executive control of memory retrieval. *Nature, 401,* 699–703.

109. Barcelo, F., Suwazono, S., & Knight, R. T. (2000). Prefrontal modulation of visual processing in humans. *Nature Neuroscience, 3,* 399–403.

110. Knight, R. T., Hillyard, S. A., Woods, D. L., et al. (1981). The effects of frontal cortex lesions on event-related potentials during auditory selective attention. *Electroencephalography and Clinical Neurophysiology, 52,* 571–582.

111. Wiese, H., Stude, P., Nebel, K., et al. (2004). Impaired movement-related potentials in acute frontal traumatic brain injury. *Clinical Neurophysiology, 115,* 289–298.

112. Singh, J., & Knight, R. T. (1990). Frontal lobe contribution to voluntary movements in humans. *Brain Research, 531,* 45–54.

113. Knight, R. T., Scabini, D., & Woods, D. L. (1989). Prefrontal cortex gating of auditory transmission in humans. *Brain Research, 504,* 338–342.

114. Zironi, I., Iacovelli, P., Aicardi, G., et al. (2001). Prefrontal cortex lesions augment the location-related firing properties of area TE/perirhinal cortex neurons in a working memory task. *Cerebral Cortex, 11,* 1093–1100.

115. Kyd, R. J., & Bilkey, D. K. (2003). Prefrontal cortex lesions modify the spatial properties of hippocampal place cells. *Cerebral Cortex, 13,* 444–451.

116. Rule, R. R., Shimamura, A. P., & Knight, R. T. (2002). Orbitofrontal cortex and dynamic filtering of emotional stimuli. *Cognitive, Affective, and Behavioral Neuroscience, 2,* 264–270.

# CHAPTER 14

# Insight into Frontal Lobe Function
# from Functional Neuroimaging Studies
# of Episodic Memory

*W. Dale Stevens*
*Cheryl L. Grady*

From early neuropsychological investigation of patients with frontal lobe lesions to the most recent evidence emerging in experimental cognitive neuroscience, it is now clear that the human frontal lobes play an integral role in episodic memory. The concepts of "frontal lobe functions" and "episodic memory" have been dynamic, evolving concepts over time, and the methods used to investigate different aspects of human cognition have changed as well. This progress has led to a modification of traditional concepts of episodic memory, and has influenced the emergence of new cognitive and neuroanatomical models of the role of the human frontal lobes in episodic memory. Perspectives on neurocognitive specialization and integration have been the emerging theme in defining the diverse nature of this role.

Traditionally, neuropsychological findings relating to frontal lobe involvement in episodic memory were based on studies of patients with frontal lobe lesions (Wheeler, Stuss, & Tulving, 1997). Although this approach laid the foundation for subsequent research, limitations in what can be learned from the impaired cognitive functions of neurological patients are numerous. This is partly a consequence of the fact that it is difficult to dissociate deficits of encoding versus retrieval in patients with brain dam-

age. Moreover, alteration of function in the injured or recovering brain may not be generalizable to "normal" functioning in the healthy brain. More recently, neuroimaging techniques have allowed for new strategies of addressing specific questions. Positron emission tomography (PET) is a neuroimaging technique that has been used extensively to provide insight into the underlying neural and functional correlates of these cognitive processes. Other techniques, such as functional magnetic resonance imaging (fMRI) and electrophysiological measures of event-related potentials (ERPs), have advantages that improve upon the major limitations of PET, such as better spatial and temporal resolution, respectively. Although ERPs provide valuable information about neural activity with millisecond temporal resolution, limited spatial resolution for identifying the locus of the neural generators of ERP components limits its utility as a brain mapping technique. Conversely, fMRI renders indirect information about neural activation via hemodynamic measures with excellent spatial specificity but reduced temporal resolution. Nonetheless, advances in techniques and experimental designs in fMRI studies, such as event-related fMRI (efMRI), and newer hybrid or "mixed" fMRI designs, have increased the utility of this neuroimaging technique. The efMRI technique may currently be the most promising investigative approach for defining and mapping the frontal lobe functions involved in episodic memory.

The concept of "episodic memory" (EM), originally defined as the conscious recollection of events from one's past (Tulving, 1972), has evolved since its inception in 1972. Wheeler and colleagues (1997) defined two different ways in which the term has been applied to related, yet fundamentally different concepts. The first of these defines a *kind of memory system*. This system is responsible for one's conscious recollection of personal experiences and events (autobiographical memory). It is thought to be responsible for (and specifically evolved for) the ability of humans to experience "mental time travel" (Wheeler et al., 1997). Furthermore, the system itself is not limited to experiences of the past, but serves to allow one to anticipate one's subjective future through mental projection. The second way in which EM has been described is as a *type of memory performance or task*. Many examples of standard tests of EM defined in this way permeate the cognitive neuroscience literature. This laboratory-based type of memory performance is characterized by the production of a recall, recognition, or recollective judgment of some sort, based on previous acquisition of declarative or propositional information (Wheeler et al., 1997). Recent neuroimaging data suggest that these two cognitively distinct phenomena—autobiographical and laboratory-based EM—are associated with different neural activation in the prefrontal cortex (PFC) (for review, see Gilboa, 2004). This chapter focuses on data relevant to the latter aspect of EM; a full treatment of imaging approaches to frontal lobe involvement in autobiographical memory appears in McKinnon, Svoboda, and Levine (Chapter 15, this volume).

To delineate further the meaning of EM that is to be adopted in this discussion, it is necessary to identify another distinction. EM may be defined in terms of its distinction from semantic memory (Tulving, 1972), in that these two forms of memory differ in the type of awareness with which they are associated. Autonoetic, or "self-knowing" awareness, and noetic, or simply "knowing" awareness, are associated with episodic and semantic memory, respectively (Tulving, 1983; for a detailed discussion, see Wheeler et al., 1997). Some neuro-

imaging studies of EM have set out to assess explicitly the level and/or quality of such awareness accompanying the memory decision. This has typically been achieved by requiring experimental participants to render a "remember" or "know" judgment (Tulving, 1985) corresponding to autonoetic and noetic recollection, respectively. Differences in activity associated with these distinct forms of memory have been identified in ERP studies during both encoding (Mangels, Picton, & Craik, 2001) and retrieval (Duzel, Yonelinas, Mangun, Heinze, & Tulving, 1997), as well as in fMRI studies at encoding (Henson, Rugg, Shallice, Josephs, & Dolan, 1999; Ranganath et al., 2003) and retrieval (Bunge, Burrows, & Wagner, 2004; Dobbins, Simons, & Schacter, 2004; Eldridge, Knowlton, Furmanski, Bookheimer, & Engel, 2000; Henson, Rugg, et al., 1999; Wheeler & Buckner, 2004). Nevertheless, many of the data underlying conclusions about EM within the literature are from tasks that make no such distinctions.

## NEUROCOGNITIVE SPECIALIZATION AND INTEGRATION

The human frontal lobes comprise a large anatomically and functionally diverse set of structures. Scientific exploration of the frontal lobes has focused on functional and anatomical differentiation and integration across frontal regions. The primary goal of much neuroimaging research in this field has been to determine the nature of this functional specialization, should it exist, and to identify potential neuroantomically discrete regions, or integrated networks of regions, associated with such functional specialization.

In keeping with the highly complex anatomical connectivity of frontal regions, and between frontal and posterior regions of the brain (for a review, see Kaufer & Lewis, 1999), it is unlikely that any neuroantomically discrete frontal region operates in isolation to produce a particular cognition or behavior (Fuster, 1997). However, differing schools of thought on the nature and extent of neurocognitive specialization have emerged within the neuroimaging research community. For example, disagreement has persisted between theories of brain function that stress discrete regional specialization and those emphasizing integration across regions (McIntosh, 2004). Consistent with the former, frontal regions have been identified wherein activation has been proposed to be a necessary neural component of a some given aspect of EM (for a detailed review, see Fletcher & Henson, 2001). Traditional univariate parametric statistical approaches, which contrast conditions of interest against a chosen baseline and/or other conditions of interest, are used to demonstrate neurocognitive specialization of this form. Consistent with integration theory, frontal regions have also been identified (Della-Maggiore et al., 2000; McIntosh et al., 1994; McIntosh, Nyberg, Bookstein, & Tulving, 1997) for which the functional relevance of activation presumably depends upon the status of regions with which they are connected (i.e., function depends upon a "neural context"; McIntosh, 2004). Studies stressing neural integration, networks, or neural context tend to employ multivariate statistical assessment of distributed, whole-brain neural activation (Friston, Frith, Fracowiak, & Turner, 1995; Gonzalez-Lima & McIntosh, 1994; McIntosh, Bookstein, Haxby, & Grady, 1996; McIntosh, Chau, & Protzner, 2004). Thus, when interpreting and integrating findings across neuroimaging studies, it is necessary to consider the theoretical bias and statistical approach of the researcher.

The various models of neurocognitive specialization within the frontal lobes for EM functions can be broadly categorized within two general organizational domains. The first pertains to a *localization* dissociation—either a right–left lateralization of function, or bilaterally distributed organization of function. The second pertains to the particular cognitive *form* of the dissociation either a content specific dissociation (e.g., verbal vs. nonverbal), or a process-specific dissociation (e.g., encoding vs. retrieval).

With all of the forgoing as a context, this chapter reviews and assesses various frameworks and perspectives put forth, or suggested by the data, within the neuroimaging literature regarding neurocognitive specialization and integration of the frontal lobes associated with EM. First, we review current models of functional *lateralization* within the frontal lobes, considering both *process-specific* and *content-specific* asymmetry, as well as the potential coexistence of these dissociations. Thereafter, we review other process-specific models of functional organization of the frontal lobes in EM that do not strictly adhere to a pattern of

asymmetrical left–right lateralization, beginning with a *preretrieval* versus *postretrieval* (retrieval processes) dissociation, followed by a *state-related* versus *item-related* dissociation.

## LATERALIZATION

Various methods of investigating the human frontal lobes have revealed asymmetrical lateralization of various cognitive functions (Gazzaniga, 2000). For example, it has long been known that language is almost exclusively left lateralized. Neuroimaging techniques have revealed that the cognitive processes of EM are no exception to lateralized functional organization. However, the nature of this lateralization remains a contentious issue. The debate persists among three general perspectives: (1) *process-specific* lateralization, (2) *content-specific* lateralization, and (3) nonlateralization (or bilaterally distributed localization of function). This section includes a discussion of the former two perspectives, whereas the latter is discussed in subsequent sections.

### Process-Specific Lateralization

Findings from PET studies were the first to substantiate specific forms of frontal lobe involvement in EM that had been foreshadowed in the frontal lobe lesion literature (Schacter, 1987; Tulving, 1985). The most salient and persistent finding across multiple PET studies indicated process-specific lateralization of functions involved in EM. In a number of PET studies, activity associated with encoding appeared to be primarily left lateralized, whereas activity associated with episodic retrieval appeared to be right lateralized. This phenomenon led to the "HERA" model of memory: "hemispheric encoding/retrieval asymmetry" (Nyberg, Cabeza, & Tulving, 1996; Tulving, Kapur, Craik, Moscovitch, & Houle, 1994). Perhaps the most compelling argument for right PFC involvement in episodic retrieval was one based on a summary of 26 previous PET studies (Nyberg et al., 1996). Of these 26 studies, 25 demonstrated a preferential right PFC involvement in EM retrieval. Data from other PET studies have supported the HERA model as well (e.g., Grady et al., 1995; Ragland et al., 2000).

More recent studies using other neuroimaging techniques also have supported the general

HERA dissociation. An fMRI study indicated that both encoding and retrieval elicited bilateral PFC activity when compared to baseline, but increased activity for encoding on the left, and for retrieval on the right, when the two conditions were contrasted directly (Mottaghy et al., 1999). Data from other fMRI studies have supported the HERA model as well (e.g., Heun et al., 1999; Kavcic, Zhong, Yoshiura, & Doty, 2003; McDermott, Buckner, Petersen, Kelley, & Sanders, 1999), as have studies using visual-field tachistoscopy (Blanchet et al., 2001), and repetitive transcranial magnetic stimulation (rTMS) (Rossi et al., 2004)—a technique involving transient interference applied to a discrete region of the brain, often producing a temporary circumscribed "functional lesion."

Although some recent research has revealed that the left PFC may be equally involved in retrieval processes as the right PFC (see "Retrieval Processes" for a full discussion of frontal activity during retrieval), the majority of data concerning PFC involvement in encoding suggests that these functions are—as HERA would suggest—primarily left lateralized (but see alternate theories discussed under "Content-Specific Lateralization" below). PET studies of encoding of *verbal* stimuli have unanimously demonstrated preferentially left-lateralized activation in PFC. Kapur and colleagues (1994) found increased activity in left inferior PFC (Brodmann's areas, or BAs, 45, 46, 47, 10) during a semantic (deep) encoding task, relative to a perceptual (shallow) encoding task, associated with increased recognition performance. Similarly, in a subsequent study, Kapur and colleagues (1996) reported increased left-lateralized activation in anterior and inferior (BA 45, 46) and midfrontal (BA 6, 44) PFC during intentional encoding of word pairs, associated with increased recognition performance (compared to simply reading word pairs), which they attributed to semantic and rehearsal processes, respectively. A number of other PET studies have identified left inferior PFC activity associated with verbal encoding as well (Fletcher, Shallice, & Dolan, 1998; Fujii et al., 2002; Petersson, Reis, Castro-Caldas, & Ingvar, 1999; Ragland et al., 2000).

Some PET and blocked fMRI data suggest left PFC involvement in encoding of *nonverbal* stimuli as well. Two PET studies demonstrated preferentially left-lateralized activation of PFC areas during encoding of nonverbal stimuli. A study by Grady, McIntosh, Rajah, Beig, and Craik (1999) identified a distributed neural network of cortical regions, including left PFC, with increased activation during both shallow and deep encoding of pictures. In another PET study that examined encoding of pictures and sentences, network analysis revealed a group of regions, including left PFC (dorsolateral BA 8), with increased activity during encoding compared to retrieval, regardless of stimulus type (Nyberg et al., 2000). Two PET studies also reported left inferior frontal activation during encoding of faces (Bernstein, Beig, Siegenthaler, & Grady, 2002; Haxby et al., 1996). In the first of two blocked fMRI studies by Iidaka and colleagues (Iidaka, Sadato, Yamada, & Yonekura, 2000), activation was reported to be primarily left lateralized within dorsolateral PFC and bilateral within ventrolateral PFC (BA 45/47) for verbal material, whereas encoding of checkerboard patterns elicited widespread bilateral activation within the middle frontal gyrus. However, using conjunction analysis, the authors identified "a common network" including the left dorsolateral PFC involved in encoding regardless of stimulus type. A second study demonstrated common left dorsolateral PFC activation during encoding of semantically unrelated concrete images and abstract images as well (Iidaka et al., 2001). Finally, in a blocked fMRI study, a common group of regions was found to be activated during encoding of both words and unfamiliar faces during semantic encoding tasks (living–nonliving and male–female judgments for words and unfamiliar faces, respectively), including bilateral dorsolateral PFC (BA 44/45) and, most saliently, left ventrolateral PFC (BA 47; Leube, Erb, Grodd, Bartels, & Kircher, 2001). The authors also reported increased left-lateralized versus right-lateralized PFC activity for encoding of words versus faces, respectively, in a "laterality analysis." These results suggest the coexistence of a process-specific dissociation of left-lateralized encoding regardless of content, and a simultaneous content-specific left–right dissociation for verbal processing versus face processing, respectively, within the PFC.

Unlike PET and blocked fMRI, efMRI studies of encoding allow the researcher to investigate neural activity during encoding of individual stimulus events, and group these events post hoc based on subsequent memory performance. This allows a direct investigation of the potential differential effects of encoding processes on subsequent retrieval success or quality—referred to as "subsequent memory effects." Consistent with the findings of blocked studies, efMRI studies have unanimously demonstrated preferentially left-lateralized PFC activity during encoding of *verbal* material. Wagner, Schacter, and colleagues (1998) were among the first to identify greater activation in left inferior PFC areas associated with semantic encoding of words that were later confidently recalled (confident hits) than for words that were later forgotten (misses). This general finding of left PFC activation associated with subsequent memory success for words has recently been corroborated (Chee, Goh, Lim, Graham, & Lee, 2004).

Numerous researchers have set out to differentiate the factors and/or component processes of verbal encoding associated with subregions of the left PFC. Fletcher, Shallice, and Dolan (2000) reported increased activation of left ventrolateral PFC during encoding of word pairs that were distantly versus closely semantically related (e.g., *Net . . . Ship* vs. *King . . . Queen*, respectively). They argued that this finding supports the notion that the left ventrolateral PFC supports successful encoding as a function of the formation of meaningful semantic associations. Otten and colleagues conducted a series of studies addressing the differential roles of left PFC regions in semantic processing during encoding as well (Otten, Henson, & Rugg, 2001, 2002; Otten & Rugg, 2001a, 2001b). Although left ventrolateral PFC was the most consistently activated region during encoding, the pattern of left-lateralized activation varied depending on the specific task demands, with increased activation for an animacy decision task (living–nonliving?) compared to an alphabetical task (Otten et al., 2001) and a syllable judgment task (odd or even number of syllables?) (Otten & Rugg, 2001a). This suggests the possibility that there might not be areas of the left PFC invariably involved in encoding; rather, varying task demands during encoding may elicit different forms of semantic processing that differentially support effective encoding of verbal information into memory. However, another efMRI study demonstrated left-lateralized PFC, primarily in a ventrolateral region, associated with both a deep encoding task (semantic—pleasant–unpleasant) and shallow encoding task (alphabetical judgment), with increased activity for the former (Fletcher, Stephenson,

Carpenter, Donovan, & Bullmore, 2003). Another study reported that left ventrolateral PFC activation may be more predictive of subsequent *recognition* of verbal material, as opposed to subsequent *recall* of information (Maril, Simons, Mitchell, Schwartz, & Schacter, 2003). The authors further argued that observed left dorsolateral PFC activation, predictive of subsequent recall, may be related to semantic integration of multiple items/elements during encoding, as required by their particular task.

Finally, some studies have directly investigated the neural correlates of intentional and incidental encoding of verbal information. In a study by Reber and colleagues (2002), participants were presented with words during the study phase, each followed by a cue instructing them to either intentionally remember (R) or forget (F) the word. Because activity in left inferior PFC was increased for R trials but did not correlate with subsequent retrieval success, the authors argued that this region is involved in intentional encoding operations regardless of level of successful encoding into memory. However, another study found nearly an opposite correlation between activity in this region and cognitive functions (Buckner, Wheeler, & Sheridan, 2001). In this efMRI study, participants were imaged during a recognition task for previously presented words among new words (foils), then given a surprise recognition test for these foils. Activation within two areas along the left inferior frontal gyrus (dorsal: BA 44/6; ventral: BA 44/45/47) was increased for those foils from the initial recognition test that were subsequently recognized. Thus, in contrast to the findings of the previous study, the left ventrolateral PFC was shown to be involved in incidental encoding, and predictive (rather than nonpredictive) of subsequent retrieval success. The authors argued that incidental encoding occurs during retrieval tasks, supporting successful formation of memories as effectively as intentional encoding, and that this may have implications for the interpretation of studies attempting to investigate encoding versus retrieval per se by contrasting these two conditions.

All of these studies implicate the left PFC (primarily ventrolateral) in verbal encoding processes, although various hypotheses concerning the differential contributions of left PFC regions to encoding have been put forth (see Fletcher & Henson, 2001). Conversely, studies rarely identified right-lateralized PFC activation specifically attributed to encoding processes. The picture is somewhat more complicated, however, regarding PFC involvement in encoding of *nonverbal* content, as revealed by conflicting conclusions across efMRI studies. Nonetheless, as for verbal content, the process-specific HERA distinction of preferentially left-lateralized encoding processes has held for encoding of nonverbal content in several studies as well. A study by Fletcher and colleagues (2002) investigated the effects of both content (words and abstract figures) and task (meaning- and form-based judgments) on the lateralization of function during encoding. Encoding of the abstract figures elicited more right inferior PFC activation, compared to word encoding, but there were no differences between verbal and nonverbal encoding in left PFC. Thus, although additional right-lateralized PFC regions were recruited in the processing of abstract images, equivalent left PFC activation during the two encoding tasks suggests that common regions are involved in encoding of both words and abstract images. In another efMRI study, subjects made a natural–artificial judgment in regard to pictures presented in one of four spatially distinct quadrants during encoding, and were later tested for both recognition of old objects among distracters and spatial location of the objects at the time of encoding (Cansino, Maquet, Dolan, & Rugg, 2002). Regions that showed increased activation during encoding associated with increased accuracy of subsequent source judgment included left PFC: two regions in anterior superior frontal gyrus (BA 8/9), as well as dorsal inferior frontal gyrus (BA 6/44)—an area previously associated with subsequent accuracy of semantically processed words (Otten et al., 2001; Otten & Rugg, 2001a, Wagner, Schacter, et al., 1998). In a number of other efMRI studies, it has been argued that left-lateralized activation associated with encoding of pictures may relate to the degree to which the cognitive processing of these pictures can be verbalized or semantic in nature (see "Content-Specific Lateralization" below).

In addition to the HERA model, other models of process-specific lateralization have been proposed. For example, the production-monitoring hypothesis (Cabeza, Locantore, & Anderson, 2003) proposes a left–right process-specific dissociation of another form: The left PFC is preferentially involved in semantically guided production of information, whereas the right PFC is preferentially involved in the monitoring and verification of information. Another process-specific dissociation model suggests preferential activity in the left PFC for "refreshing" (short-term recall of information) and in the right PFC for "noting" (short-term recognition) (Johnson, Raye, Mitchell, Greene, & Anderson, 2003). These authors also proposed a simultaneous content-specific dissociation between verbal and nonverbal material; thus, they argued that the functioning of the PFC can simultaneously adhere to both process- and content-specific organization. Other process-specific models of EM encoding and retrieval that do not adhere specifically to lateralization of function (e.g., pre- and post-retrieval processes) are discussed below.

### Content-Specific Lateralization

As neuroimaging techniques have evolved, there has been an accumulation of studies supporting a content-specific left–right lateralization of function rather than the process view of HERA. As alluded to earlier, encoding of nonverbal material elicits both right and left PFC activity, whereas verbal encoding elicits only left PFC activity, and a number of investigators have emphasized this left–right dissociation between verbal and nonverbal material. A PET study by Lee, Robbins, Pickard, and Owen (2000) demonstrated that left lateral PFC activation was greater for verbal stimuli, whereas right lateral PFC activation was greater for nonverbal stimuli, during both encoding and retrieval. A subsequent fMRI study by this group (Lee et al., 2002) reached similar conclusions. Wagner, Poldrack, and colleagues (1998) also proposed a content-specific lateralization, in which inferior PFC activation was left lateralized for verbal stimuli, and right lateralized for nonverbal stimuli (e.g., abstract visual textures), across both encoding and retrieval tasks. Another study reported an increase in right dorsolateral PFC activation associated with increased subsequent memory for complex photographs, although brain scans covered a very limited portion of the PFC (Brewer, Zhao, Desmond, Glover, & Gabrieli, 1998). Miller, Kingstone, and Gazzaniga (2002) argued that converging data from neuroimaging and split-brain patient studies indicate that for encoding, lateralization of function depends on recruitment of posterior cortical regions involved in processing of the specific types of content (stimuli), which are organized by content-specific lateralization. Thus, for example, the right PFC is more involved in encoding of faces, because face processing is primarily right lateralized in posterior cortical regions. Conversely, PFC activity during encoding of verbal information relies on left lateralized frontal–posterior cortical interactions. Other studies have reported increased activity during encoding in the right PFC for nonverbal material versus left PFC for verbal material in ventrolateral (Kirchhoff, Wagner, Maril, & Stern, 2000) and dorsolateral (McDermott et al., 1999; Opitz, Mecklinger, & Friederici, 2000) regions.

Two studies (Golby et al., 2001; Kelley et al., 1998) supported a view that during memory encoding, the degree of "verbalizability" across a continuum determined the degree of left–right frontal lateralization, from most to least verbal, respectively. Kelley and colleagues (1998) identified dorsal PFC activation on the left for words, on the right for faces, and bilaterally for "nameable objects." Similarly, Golby and colleagues (2001) first demonstrated the verbalizability of different stimuli (scenes, faces, and abstract patterns), then showed that activity in the inferior PFC during encoding was left lateralized for words, right lateralized for abstract patterns (nonverbalizable material), and bilateral for scenes and faces (intermediately verbalizable stimuli). However, it is important to note that encoding of faces has been shown to produce primarily left-lateralized activity as well (Bernstein et al., 2002; Haxby et al., 1996), suggesting again that PFC organization might involve both process- and material-specific lateralization.

Although it has been argued that findings such as these just described stand in contrast to the HERA model, a recent elaboration (or reformulation) of the HERA model contests that this is not the case (Habib, Nyberg, & Tulving, 2003). The authors argued that an encoding–retrieval *asymmetry* implies greater PFC activity on the left for encoding, and on the right for retrieval, when the two tasks are compared directly, with all other experimental parameters, including stimulus content–type, held constant. Furthermore, it was argued that process-specific and content-specific dissociations are not mutually exclusive; rather, HERA can, and does, coexist with other laterally asymmetrical functional dissociations, including, for example, verbalizability. Therefore, Habib and colleagues (2003) argued that studies such as those we just described are not relevant to the HERA model. For example, studies in which neural activity during encoding only is contrasted across various stimulus types, indicating content-specific PFC lateralization, do not speak to a left–right asymmetry for *encoding* versus *retrieval* at all. The authors, therefore, asserted that the HERA model, which differentiates *between* encoding and retrieval, remains valid regardless of content-specific lateralization *within* either encoding or retrieval.

## RETRIEVAL PROCESSES

"Retrieval" of information from EM is likely best characterized not as a single function, but as a coordinated set of functions, or processes. Many terms have been invoked to describe the various component processes of episodic retrieval. Diverse, often contradictory, conclusions by researchers attempting to link process-specific neural activations within the frontal lobes to functions of episodic retrieval in general may reflect the confounding of these heterogeneous subfunctions. It has been suggested that various retrieval processes involving the frontal lobes can be classified into two general categories (Rugg & Henson, 2002): (1) *preretrieval processes*, which operate in support of an attempt to retrieve information in response to a cue; and (2) *postretrieval processes*, which operate on the products of a retrieval attempt prior to a memory decision. The actual process of retrieval per se bridging these two processes may be the activation of memory traces in posterior cortical regions, initiated by the preretrieval processes, and yielding the products to be subjected to the postretrieval processes. Various subprocesses have been identified and referred to by various researchers (for a detailed review, see Rugg & Wilding, 2000). Subcomponents of preretrieval processing may be *retrieval mode* (Tulving, 1983), *retrieval effort* (Rugg & Wilding, 2000), and *retrieval orienting* (Buckner, Koutstaal, Schacter, Wagner, & Rosen, 1998b; Dobbins, Rice, Wagner, & Schacter, 2003; Dobbins et al., 2004; Rugg & Wilding, 2000). The primary postretrieval process is *retrieval monitoring* (Henson, Rugg, et al., 1999; Moscovitch & Winocur, 2002; Rugg, Henson, & Robb, 2003). In the following discussion, we begin with the concept of "retrieval success"—a phenomenon that initially was very frequently investigated, producing considerable insight that generated subsequent hypotheses about specific component processes involved. Then, we provide a more detailed definition of the pre- and postretrieval processes listed earlier, and a brief review of the data associated with their proposed neural correlates.

## Retrieval Success

"Retrieval success" refers to an instance when a retrieval attempt produces a correct response (defined as a "hit" in most tests of episodic retrieval). The term "ecphory," originally proposed by Semon (as cited in Rugg & Wilding, 2000), refers to the process whereby a retrieval cue, either externally or internally generated, prompts the activation of the pre- and postretrieval processes described previously, and results in the successful retrieval of a memory trace related to a specific episode. In reference to the definition of ecphory, we posit here that an important distinction should be made: The term "ecphory" is often used heterogeneously to describe either (1) the *subjective experience* of recollection or successful episodic retrieval of some memory trace(s) in response to a retrieval effort (regardless of whether the memory traces are actually relevant or not), (2) the *objective act* of correctly endorsing an item as recollected, when it was in fact previously encountered (retrieval of a "correct" memory trace), or (3) both. Therefore, the terms "subjective ecphory" and "objective ecphory" are hereby introduced and defined as the first and second phenomena, respectively. Subjective ecphory, then, accompanies any confident endorsement of a retrieval product (i.e., a confident positive decision), which can occur in the case of both hits and false alarms; it is the cognitive phenomenon of retrieving memory traces, regardless of whether they are true or false relative to the retrieval cue or nature of the retrieval attempt. Therefore, the neural correlates of subjective ecphory could be identified by contrasting activation common to confident hits and confident false alarms with all other response types. Objective ecphory occurs (in concert with subjective ecphory) only in the selective case in which a confident endorsement is objectively correct, which occurs only in the case of hits; it is the cognitive phenomenon of retrieving appropriate (i.e., correct) memory

traces relative to the retrieval cue or nature of the retrieval attempt. Therefore, the *independent* neural correlates of objective ecphory, should they exist, could be identified by contrasting confident hits with confident false alarms. It is important to note that many of the findings related to retrieval success reviewed here make no such distinction, and thus, as a corollary of contrasting hits with correct rejections, identify confounded activation associated with both subjective and objective ecphory.

Whereas postretrieval processing in general operates on the products of retrieval attempts regardless of their content, retrieval success implies the production of the correct memory trace. To identify neural correlates specific to retrieval success per se, one must make the distinction between activations directly related to retrieval success and activations related indirectly as a function of other processes that promote or increase the likelihood of retrieval success. Therefore, one approach would be to contrast a condition of retrieval success with various types of retrieval failure (i.e., false alarms and misses) as well as nonretrieval (i.e., correct rejections).

A review of studies identifying neural activity associated with retrieval success requires a reiteration of the distinction between noetic and autonoetic reexperiencing associated with semantic and episodic retrieval, respectively. In recognition studies that require only a new–old (often force-choice alternative) response, for example, there is no measure of the magnitude or quality of the retrieval experience. Thus, there is the possibility of episodic retrieval being confounded with semantic processes. However, some experimental paradigms attempt to control for this confound by requiring an indication of the quality (remember–know) or magnitude (high–low confidence) of the recollection. Studies reporting neural correlates of retrieval success—both with and without a measure of subjective level of reexperiencing—are reviewed below.

A number of studies contrasting hits with correct rejections have demonstrated an increase in anterior PFC (i.e., BA 10) activation associated with hits, predominantly right PFC (Buckner et al., 1998b), with some left-lateralized activation (Rugg, Fletcher, Chua, & Dolan, 1999). Similarly, efMRI studies have consistently indicated an increase in right anterior PFC activity in association with hits

(Buckner et al., 1998a), although bilateral anterior PFC activation has been reported (McDermott, Jones, Petersen, Lageman, & Roediger, 2000; Rugg et al., 2003).

Different results were demonstrated in an efMRI study by Ranganath, Johnson, and D'Esposito (2000), in which increases in left dorsolateral PFC (BA 9) and right inferior PFC activity (BA 47) were associated with hits relative to correct rejections. For the same contrast, another efMRI study indicated an increase in bilateral anterior PFC (BA 10) and left ventral/dorsolateral PFC (BA 45/47/46) (Konishi, Wheeler, Donaldson, & Buckner, 2000).

The conclusions of one efMRI study stand in direct contrast to the general pattern of mainly anterior PFC activity associated with retrieval success. Herron, Henson, and Rugg (2004) varied the relative probability of old and new items, by manipulating the new–old ratio of items during a recognition test for previously studied words. They found that activation in the typical PFC regions that have been implicated in retrieval success—anterior, dorsolateral, and ventrolateral PFC—varied with the ratio of new–old items throughout the task, showing a complete crossover interaction in some cases. They concluded that perhaps only a limited subset of brain regions—*including no PFC regions*—traditionally associated with retrieval success per se are *necessarily* involved.

Looking at retrieval success by comparing activity during the presentation of "old," or previously encountered stimuli, to that seen during presentation of "new" stimuli fails to account for the quality of the retrieval experience (noetic vs. autonoetic), or level of subjective ecphory, allowing the potential for contamination by implicit memory processes. Some studies have attempted to account for these additional factors by requiring participants to indicate not only whether an item was old or new, but also to rate their subjective ecphory with a "remember" (autonoetic) or "know" (noetic) response. Using this approach, Henson, Rugg, and colleagues (1999) conducted two studies wherein a subjective index of the retrieval experience was measured. In one study in which subjects were required to respond with remember (R), know (K), or new (N), correct R and K responses were associated with increased left PFC activation relative to correct N responses. Furthermore, correct R responses were associated with increased activation in anterior left PFC relative to correct K responses. Conversely, correct K responses elicited greater activation in right lateral and medial PFC relative to correct R and N responses (see "Postretrieval Processes" below). In the second study, confidence (high vs. low) in the response decision was assessed with each new–old response (i.e., high-new, low-new, low-old, and high-old) (Henson, Rugg, Shallice, & Dolan, 2000). Unfortunately, the new–old comparison was collapsed across confidence levels due to an insufficient number of some individual response types, so level of subjective retrieval experiencing was not reflected in the new–old contrast. The authors observed results similar to those of previous studies, with increased activation in bilateral anterior PFC (BA 10) for old versus new responses.

In another efMRI study (Eldridge et al., 2000), participants were required to give a new or old response to test items, and in the case of an old response, to make remember (R) or know (K) judgments. Contrasting remember versus know responses revealed increased activity in left dorsolateral PFC (BA 8/9) and right inferior PFC (BA 6/44). Interestingly, K items, compared to R items, were again associated with right PFC, but in a slightly more anterior location (BA 9/10) to that identified by Henson, Rugg, and colleagues (1999).

Finally, two more recent studies observed primarily left-lateralized PFC activity associated with retrieval success, as well as for increased subjective recollective experiencing. One study contrasted test trials wherein subjects recalled an item (R), failed to recall an item (N), or experienced a "feeling of knowing" (FOK)—an intermediate level of reexperiencing that occurred when a subject failed to recall an item, yet felt it might be recognized on a later test (Maril et al., 2003). A consistent pattern of activation in the left PFC, including inferior (BA 45/47) and dorsal regions (BA46/9), was reported for R trials compared to FOK trials, which in turn showed stronger activation than N trials. Thus, the authors reported a pattern of left-lateralized PFC regions wherein activation was positively correlated with the degree of subjective reexperiencing. Similarly, Wheeler and Buckner (2004) contrasted R and K trials, and observed primarily left-lateralized PFC activation associated with R trials, including left middle frontal gyrus (BA 6/8).

Thus, the inclusion of information about the nature or quality of retrieval success, although again producing varying results across studies, has contributed to elaboration of the potential subprocesses involved. The most consistent finding across these studies was increased left-hemisphere PFC activity associated with an "increase in autonoetic quality." Conversely, the opposite pattern was typically observed for the right PFC, wherein increased activity (often in dorsolateral regions) was associated with a "decrease in autonoetic quality." Insights as to the relevant subprocesses suggested by these observations are discussed further below.

This brief review of the literature reporting neural activation associated with retrieval success reveals consensus on only general patterns across studies. This may be a consequence of the confounding of a number of dissociable neurocognitive processes and experiences. First, early studies may have confounded implicit (semantic) retrieval experiences with episodic retrieval, as discussed earlier. Second, the nature of all aforementioned studies did not allow for any direct distinction between sustained state-related and transient item-related neurocognitive functions or related neural activation (see "State- and Item-Related Activity" below). Finally, neural correlates of retrieval success can be parsed into activation associated with a number of dissociable preretrieval and postretrieval processes (discussed below).

## Preretrieval Processes

Preretrieval processes involve those controlled neurocognitive functions that operate in support of a retrieval attempt, and potentially involve the maintenance of an internally or externally generated retrieval cue, as well as guidance or orientation of the intensity, scope, and form of the retrieval attempt. These processes are thought to be engaged at the onset of a retrieval attempt and remain engaged until a memory decision is rendered, regardless of the products of this attempt (or lack thereof) or type of decision ultimately rendered. These general cognitive processes have been more explicitly defined and investigated as component processes referred to as *retrieval mode*, *retrieval effort*, and *retrieval orientation*.

### Retrieval Mode

The concept of retrieval mode, first introduced by Tulving (1983), is defined here as a hypothetical tonically maintained cognitive state that may be a prerequisite for successful episodic retrieval, and that is thought to be the fundamental preretrieval process of the PFC. Many studies have identified activations within regions of the PFC postulated to be related to retrieval mode, using PET (e.g., Grady, McIntosh, Beig, & Craik, 2001; Lepage, Ghaffar, Nyberg, & Tulving, 2000; Nyberg et al., 1995), ERP (e.g., Duzel et al., 1999), and fMRI (e.g., Cabeza, Dolcos, Graham, & Nyberg, 2002; Velanova et al., 2003). Assuming this definition of retrieval mode, properties of its underlying neural correlates must logically follow: (1) Activation must coincide temporally with the onset and duration of engagement in an episodic retrieval task; and (2) activation must remain constant across differential classes of stimuli (retrieval cues) and decisions/responses, but should reveal differential activation across differential task demands (e.g., episodic vs. nonepisodic retrieval). The essential principle in this case is that neural activations specific to retrieval mode should be consistently apparent when an episodic retrieval task is contrasted with a task that is identical in every way, with the exception that it does not involve episodic retrieval. This implies as well that retrieval mode activation, which is invoked anytime a retrieval attempt is made, is independent of activation associated with the product of that retrieval attempt. Therefore, activations common to all types of retrieval cues and all types of responses (i.e., hits, misses, correct rejections, and false alarms), contrasted with a nonretrieval task that is otherwise identical, would identify neural activity associated with retrieval mode.

Early reports of data suggesting neural activity related to retrieval mode were from PET studies (Kapur et al., 1995; Nyberg et al., 1995, 2000), and later from studies using ERP (Duzel et al., 1999; Herron & Wilding, 2004; Johnson, Kreiter, Zhu, & Russo, 1998), or fMRI (Donaldson, Petersen, Ollinger, & Buckner, 2001; Velanova et al., 2003). A multistudy analysis of PET data identified five areas of PFC, three right and two left, with activity indicative of retrieval mode (Lepage et al., 2000). The criteria for inclusion in this analysis were studies that afforded a contrast of conditions involving (1) a retrieval task associated with a high episodic retrieval rate, (2) a retrieval task with a low episodic retrieval rate, and 3) a comparison/baseline condition with no retrieval task required or allowed. Areas associated with retrieval mode, then, were those producing activity common to conditions (1) and (2), and greater than in condition (3).

Across the studies in this analysis, bilateral frontal poles (BA 10), bilateral frontal operculum (BA 47/45), and right dorsolateral PFC (BA 8/9) showed this pattern of activation associated with retrieval mode.

ERP studies also have found PFC activity associated with retrieval mode, particularly in the right anterior PFC. Duzel and colleagues (1999) compared an episodic retrieval task to a semantic retrieval task, and identified a sustained positive ERP in right anterior frontal regions that they attributed to retrieval mode. Similarly, a positive-going right-lateralized ERP was attributed to retrieval mode in two subsequent studies (Morcom & Rugg, 2002; Herron & Wilding, 2004). In these experiments, intermixed trials of episodic or semantic retrieval tasks were each preceded by a task cue, indicating which task the subject was required to perform upon presentation of the retrieval cue. Thus, two events—a task cue (instruction) followed by a retrieval cue (new or old word)—made up each trial. The characteristic ERP signal was observed during the "preparatory" response to the task-cue (instruction), but only on the second and subsequent consecutive presentations of an episodic trial (when two or more episodic trials occurred consecutively). The authors argued that it may take at least two trials for retrieval-mode neural activity to engage. Therefore, the ERP data across several studies suggest a right-lateralized locus for retrieval mode, at least when episodic retrieval is contrasted with semantic retrieval.

Finally, several fMRI studies have identified PFC activation associated with retrieval mode. Cabeza and colleagues (2002) compared an episodic retrieval task with a working memory task, and found increased activation during the episodic retrieval task in bilateral anterior PFC (BA 10). A study by Donaldson and colleagues (2001) identified primarily left-lateralized PFC activation associated with retrieval mode, including inferior and middle frontal gyrus, medial frontal gyrus, and bilateral operculum, and Velanova and colleagues (2003) found increased activation in left inferior PFC and right frontal–polar PFC during an episodic retrieval task. However, the results of these latter two studies were based on activation during a recognition task contrasted with a fixation baseline (a series of rest periods in which subjects were not engaged in any form of cognitive task), which is not an ideal control task for identifying retrieval mode (discussed in detail in "State- and Item-Related Activity" below).

Nevertheless, it is interesting to note that Velanova and colleagues identified right anterior frontal activity associated with retrieval mode, as found in ERP and PET studies.

### Retrieval Effort

"Retrieval effort" is a concept that may be broadly defined as the degree of demand on cognitive resources imposed by a particular retrieval attempt (Rugg & Wilding, 2000). The neural correlates of retrieval effort might be activity that fluctuated solely as a function of the task difficulty, or demand on cognitive resources of a particular task. One region of dorsolateral PFC, BA 9/46, has been implicated in a number of studies (Moscovitch & Winocur, 2002) as an area where activation is related to complexity of the task. This region also has been directly implicated as an area involved in retrieval effort (Rugg & Henson, 2002). A blocked fMRI study contrasted episodic retrieval task conditions following shallow or deep encoding tasks, under the assumption that retrieval after shallow encoding would be more difficult. The authors concluded that greater activity in the left dorsolateral PFC in the retrieval task condition following shallow encoding was related to increased retrieval effort (Buckner et al., 1998b). Conversely, another blocked study (PET) found no overall differences in PFC activation during retrieval between items that had been presented during either a deep or shallow encoding task (Grady et al., 2001). In this study, an area of right anterior PFC was consistently activated during recognition, regardless of the previous encoding condition, suggesting the involvement of this area in retrieval mode. However, an analysis of functional connectivity revealed that this right anterior PFC area interacted in a network of regions for which activity was negatively correlated with retrieval success, indicating an effect of retrieval effort. Grady and colleagues (2001) reasoned that these results demonstrate a dual role of this anterior PFC region in visual recognition: (1) a general increase in activity during retrieval, as compared to a low-level control task, related to retrieval mode, and (2) a negative correlation between its functional connectivity and individual differences in performance accuracy, indicative of an effect of retrieval effort.

To identify the neural correlates of retrieval effort, one must contrast the activity elicited by retrieval cues of the same material–type, which differ only in their relative level of difficulty. However, it may be hard to assess the level of difficulty of a retrieval effort elicited by a particular retrieval cue. Behavioral measures such as response latencies (reaction times) and accuracy rates may provide estimates for degree of difficulty of the retrieval task (e.g., Grady et al., 2001). Another approach would be to contrast conditions of varying difficulty separately for different response types (i.e., hits, misses, correct rejections, and false alarms). Then, the effects of retrieval effort on the processing of retrieval cues could be distinguished from fluctuations due to various products of retrieval associated with different response types during postretrieval processing. However, it may in practice be difficult to distinguish between differences in neural activity related to variable task difficulty and differences due to the resultant increased retrieval monitoring, or retrieval orientation, discussed below.

### Retrieval Orientation

A third and final proposed preretrieval process, retrieval orientation (Johnson, 1992; Rugg & Wilding, 2000), refers to "the specific form of the processing that is applied to a retrieval cue" (Rugg & Wilding, 2000, p. 108). This implies a distinction between the requirement of the task and the retrieval cue itself. Therefore, physically identical retrieval cues may result in different preretrieval processing, depending on the demands of the task (e.g., requiring recognition vs. source judgments). In their "working with memory model," Moscovitch and Winocur (2002) argue that the dorsolateral PFC may be involved in setting the goals of the task, which may be analogous to retrieval orientation. Thus, retrieval orientation may be thought of as the difference in preretrieval processing as a function of the particular strategy employed.

Various conclusions have been reached about the neural correlates of retrieval orientation across studies. A blocked fMRI study in which instructions were varied for an episodic retrieval task indicated modulation of right PFC activation (Wagner, Desmond, Glover, & Gabrieli, 1998). In another blocked fMRI study, in addition to making a new–old judgment during an episodic retrieval task, subjects were required to make a source judgment (Rugg et al., 1999). Greater activity was found in left frontal polar PFC (BA 10), left inferior frontal gyrus (BA 45/47), and bilateral frontal

operculum during the source judgment task, compared to item memory.

An ERP study demonstrated an increase in left frontal activity for new words in an episodic recognition task when it was preceded by a shallow (alphabetic judgment) as opposed to a deep (sentence generation) encoding task (Rugg, Allan, & Birch, 2000). Another ERP experiment found evidence for a left-lateralized modulation of activity dependent on retrieval orientation (Herron & Wilding, 2004). Although the authors reported common right-lateralized anterior frontal activity associated with two different episodic retrieval task-cues when contrasted with semantic task-cues (see "Retrieval Mode" section), there were differences in left frontal activity between these two episodic task-cues (spatial location, or type of semantic judgment at time of encoding), reflecting the different retrieval orientation sets.

efMRI studies have generally indicated differences in left PFC for varying task demands. Increased activation in left anterior and ventrolateral PFC (BAs 10, 45, 47) was found for episodic retrieval of source information compared to simple item recall (Fan, Snodgrass, & Bilder, 2003). Similarly, increased activation in left-lateralized PFC regions was associated with an episodic retrieval task requiring source information compared to temporal information (a recency judgment; Dobbins et al., 2003). A study by Ranganath and colleagues (2000) assessed the effects of requiring varying degrees of contextual retrieval by having participants respond old or new, or give a source judgment in response to presentations of pictures of objects. Prefrontal areas showing differential activity for source versus old–new judgments included an increase in left anterior PFC (BA 10). As suggested by Moscovitch and Winocur (2002), anterior PFC might be responsible for maintaining the activation of the retrieval cue. Accordingly, others have noted that this area may be preferentially involved when a high degree of perceptual detail is required within the task (Rugg et al., 1999). Alternatively, such activation may be related to retrieval orienting as well.

For most, if not all, of the aforementioned cases, it is difficult to determine whether the differences in activation observed are attributable to a difference in retrieval orientation, or whether this difference is best described as one of varying demand on cognitive resources, relating to retrieval effort, if indeed the two are different phenomena. Nonetheless, differing retrieval task demands, whether qualitative (orientation) or quantitative (effort), tend to result most consistently in modulations of left PFC activity.

## Postretrieval Processes

Postretrieval processes are those neurocognitive functions that operate on the *products* of a retrieval attempt and ultimately result in a memory decision. The most commonly studied postretrieval process, *retrieval monitoring*, is thought to involve those cognitive functions that operate on the product(s) of a retrieval effort prior to a memory decision. The role of this monitoring function may be to evaluate the products of retrieval attempts, comparing information from retrieved memory traces with the retrieval cue, and evaluating the validity of these products in terms of what is known about the world. Right-lateralized PFC activity has consistently been identified as a correlate of retrieval monitoring in neuroimaging studies. PET studies comparing blocks of high-density repeated retrieval cues, when presumably more retrieval monitoring would be engaged, to blocks of zero-density repeated retrieval cues demonstrated increases in right PFC (Rugg et al., 1998), and specifically in right dorsolateral PFC (Allan, Dolan, Fletcher, & Rugg, 2000). In an efMRI study, a recognition task included words presented at study (old), novel words (new), and semantically related lures (Cabeza, Rao, Wagner, Mayer, & Schacter, 2001). Old and lure trials combined, contrasted with new items, were associated with increased activity in bilateral dorsolateral PFC, which the authors attributed to increased retrieval monitoring. Another efMRI study attempted to manipulate the degree of retrieval monitoring by contrasting item recognition with a "judgment of frequency task," which is presumably more dependent on monitoring of familiarity than simple recognition (Dobbins et al., 2004). The judgment of frequency condition revealed increased activity in right dorsolateral and frontal polar PFC regions when contrasted with simple recognition.

In the first of three retrieval studies addressing this issue by Henson, Rugg, and colleagues (1999), participants were required to respond in one of three ways—new, remember, or know. An increase in activation was observed in the right dorsolateral PFC (BA 46) for K responses as contrasted with R responses. The authors speculated that this region's activation reflects its involvement in retrieval monitoring. This conclusion follows from the assumption that the level of uncertainty, and lack of confidence accompanying a K response, would be higher than for a R response, and would therefore be correlated with a higher degree of retrieval monitoring. In a second study, Henson, Shallice, and Dolan (1999) found that retrieval of the spatiotemporal context present when words were studied resulted in increased activation in a right dorsolateral PFC region compared to simple word recognition. Finally, a third study (Henson et al., 2000) required subjects to make one of four choices in response to test items, indicating new or old and a judgment of their level of confidence in their decision (high or low) as well. Increased activation in the right dorsolateral PFC (BA 46) was associated specifically with low confidence as compared to high confidence when collapsed across new and old items, supporting their hypothesis that the right dorsolateral PFC (BA 46) area reflects the activity of retrieval monitoring as a function of confidence.

## STATE- AND ITEM-RELATED ACTIVITY

The final dissociation of frontal lobe function during EM that we discuss is the distinct forms of neural activity associated with two different types of cognitive processes: state- and item-related activity. "State-related activity" refers to sustained neural activation that persists over time within a given task-relevant cognitive set. An example is the initiation of a particular pattern of neural activation associated with the cognitive state known as retrieval mode (Tulving, 1983). "Item-related activity" refers to transient neural activation related to a specific event- or item-type, such as that associated with a correct recollection during a recognition memory task.

The ability of neuroimaging techniques to distinguish state- and item-related neural activity has been one of the key ways the technology has advanced most recently. Characterization of the hemodynamic response (HDR) as measured by PET or blocked fMRI produces a single mean activation recorded over some time interval. As such, it is not possible to obtain a direct estimate of neural activity related to any one specific trial, response, or item type. efMRI (Dale & Buckner, 1997; Josephs, Turner, & Friston, 1997; Zarahn, Aguirre, & D'Esposito, 1997) allows quantification of particular individual trial or event types, because presentation of trial types can be completely randomized. However, traditional efMRI studies still overlook the fact that activation can potentially be fractionated into its component neural causes; hence, state-related activity may still be confounded with item-related activity, or ignored altogether.

Further developments have produced the mixed block/event-related fMRI (mixed-efMRI) design (Chawla, Rees, & Friston, 1999; Donaldson et al., 2001). In this approach, alternating blocks of experimental trials of a particular cognitive task type, and blocks of some cognitive baseline or comparison task, are presented. Within the task blocks, trials are presented in a standard stochastic event-related distribution (Friston, Zarahn, Josephs, Henson, & Dale, 1999). By this means, it is then possible statistically to parse neural activity in the brain into sustained state-related neural activity associated with a particular task, and transient item-related activity associated with a particular trial type per se. A small number of recent studies have begun to apply mixed-efMRI designs to the investigation of EM. The following section begins with a brief review of the studies that have investigated EM retrieval, followed by those that have investigated EM encoding.

## Retrieval

The first study to apply a mixed-efMRI design to the investigation of EM was by Donaldson and colleagues (2001), who identified three different types of activity: (1) regions displaying sustained state-related activation associated with a word recognition task (relative to a fixation control block), (2) regions displaying transient item-related activity dissociating different trial types (e.g., hits vs. correct rejections), and (3) regions displaying both transient and sustained activity. The identification of different brain areas displaying transient activity, sustained activity, or both, may be consistent with the concept of neural context, in that some regions appeared to be contributing to several different cognitive operations differentially (even simultaneously) depending on the relevant activity of other regions.

In this mixed-efMRI study (Donaldson et al., 2001), the contrast of hits versus correct rejections revealed increased item-related activity associated with hits in left PFC regions, including two left middle frontal gyrus regions. The bilateral frontal operculum regions showed sustained task-related activity, as well as additional transient fluctuations of item-related activation, demonstrating that areas of the PFC can be simultaneously involved in more than one neurocognitive process. The sustained state-related activation that the authors attributed to retrieval mode involved increases in PFC regions only, including left inferior and middle frontal regions, left medial frontal gyrus, and bilateral frontal operculum. However, because the baseline chosen for this contrast was a series of rest periods in which subjects were not engaged in any form of cognitive task, some of this state-related activity was possibly due to perceptual or other cognitive functions engaged during the retrieval task, and not related to retrieval mode per se.

In a second mixed-efMRI study that investigated state- versus item-related retrieval activation was conducted by Velanova and colleagues (2003), two different retrieval conditions—high control versus low control—were elicited by exposing subjects to two different encoding tasks—a list of words intentionally encoded during multiple exposures, and a list of words semantically encoded with a pleasant–unpleasant judgment during only one exposure. Transient activation within the left anterior PFC (BA 10/46) associated with hits regardless of condition (i.e., both high and low control conditions) was reported. Another transient effect—increased activation of left ventrolateral PFC (BA 45/47) and more posterior inferior PFC (BA 44)—was observed for all items (new and old) in the high-control compared to the low-control condition, consistent with the idea that these regions may be specifically involved in semantic processing. Right BA 10 demonstrated a sustained increase in activity during the high-control condition and no difference from baseline throughout the low-control condition. Thus, the authors demonstrated dissociable contributions of various PFC regions, arguing for a sustained right anterior PFC involvement in retrieval mode, and more posterior left inferior PFC regions involved in transient semantic retrieval processes on a trial-by-trial basis.

Although these two mixed-efMRI studies of EM retrieval are not completely without methodological shortcomings, they provide an excellent model for continued research into the nature of state- and item-related neurocognitive processes within the PFC. Furthermore, the results have supported some earlier interpretations of the dissociable roles of various PFC regions, while extending these findings and possibly reconciling discrepant conclusions from past studies (e.g., is the right anterior PFC [BA 10] involved transiently in retrieval success or tonically in retrieval mode?).

## Encoding

Although it has been less often proposed throughout the literature than EM retrieval, there is no reason to assume that EM encoding might not be associated with both sustained state-related and transient item-related processes. Perhaps, in cases of intentional and/or effortful encoding tasks, a cognitive set equivalent to an "encoding mode" may be engaged. To investigate related hypotheses concerning various aspects of EM, two studies have employed mixed-efMRI designs (Otten et al., 2002; Reynolds, Donaldson, Wagner, & Braver, 2004). In a study by Otten and colleagues (2002), subjects were scanned during alternating task blocks wherein words were to be classified by either an animacy judgment (living–nonliving) or a syllable judgment (odd–even number of syllables) for the duration of each block. Sustained state-related activation during encoding was found in the left superior frontal gyrus for the animacy task, and in the left middle frontal gyrus for the syllable task, regardless of subsequent recognition accuracy. However, an analysis of the sustained state-related activation during the animacy task revealed that increased activity in the left inferior PFC (BA 45/47) was associated with increased retrieval accuracy on the subsequent recognition test. Furthermore, an overlapping region of left inferior PFC was involved in an interaction, such that the state-related subsequent memory effects were greater for the animacy task than for the syllable task. This result extends the idea that the left ventrolateral PFC is involved in semantic processing during encoding, by suggesting that this process may involve a sustained cognitive state within which variable item-related processing may operate, and for which increased activity is associated with improved memory encoding.

Regions demonstrating item-related activation positively correlated with subsequent recognition performance included left ventrolateral PFC (BA 45/47) during the animacy task, and more posterior/dorsal regions of left inferior PFC (BA 9/44) for the syllable task. Again, for the animacy task, an interaction analysis revealed regions with relatively greater subsequent memory effects than for the syllable task in a left inferior PFC region overlapping/ adjacent to that identified by the within-task contrast. Thus, beyond the efficacy of encoding related to the sustained cognitive set discussed earlier, encoding success appears to rely to some extent on transient increases in activation on a trial-by-trial basis as well.

Another mixed-efMRI study set out to investigate the hypothesis that two potentially dissociable processes may compete to recruit a region in the left inferior PFC to different ends, under various circumstances (Reynolds et al., 2004). The authors proposed that the left inferior PFC may be involved in both instantiation of an appropriate semantic task set and transient biasing toward task relevant semantic processing. Furthermore, they argued that these task-level and item-related computations might actually compete for resources, or interfere with one another. To test this hypothesis, subjects were scanned during an encoding task wherein they were presented with words and required to make a size or semantic judgment in response to a cue presented prior to each word. In some blocks (single-task condition), the task remained the same for each trial, whereas in other blocks (task-switch condition), the task changed or stayed the same randomly from trial to trial. It was hypothesized that the task-switch condition would place a higher demand on monitoring of the relevant task set to be employed from trial to trial. The analysis that modeled sustained state-related activity, with the effects of transient item-related activations statistically removed (Donaldson et al., 2001), did not reveal any significant effects. However, regions including a large portion of the left inferior PFC met predetermined event-related criteria, indicating effects of both the task-switching manipulation and subsequent recognition accuracy. Increased activity in this region was associated with subsequently recognized words compared to forgotten words, and increased activation in this region was also associated with the task for which, on average, subsequent recognition accuracy was worse (i.e., task switching > single task). Thus, the authors concluded that activation in this same region of left inferior PFC was indicative of both item-related processing correlated with successful encoding, and task-related processing detrimental to successful encoding.

## CONCLUSIONS

In this chapter we have reviewed the different theoretical approaches taken to understanding frontal lobe function during EM, and the neuroimaging evidence to support these theories. Although there is considerable evidence to support these theories, we have argued that the different models need not be mutually exclusive (e.g., both *process-specific* and *content-specific* lateralization of function may well coexist across the frontal lobes). The best evidence to date indicates that different regions in left PFC mediate encoding, whereas retrieval processes involve bilaterally distributed PFC regions. In terms of preretrieval processes, some consistent findings have emerged in regards to:

1. *Retrieval mode*—although no single region of PFC has been invariably activated across all EM retrieval tasks in all studies, the right anterior PFC has been most often associated with retrieval tasks across variable task demands, stimulus types, and response decisions.
2. *Retrieval effort*—it has proven difficult to identify some variable that manipulates retrieval effort per se. Variable cognitive demands on retrieval attempts may be more usefully examined as the variation in the particular retrieval strategy employed, referred to as retrieval orientation.
3. *Retrieval orientation*—manipulation of retrieval task demands has most consistently resulted in modulation of left PFC regions.

However, it may be that there is no universally invariable retrieval mode state, dissociable from retrieval orientation, engaged across all EM retrieval attempts. Rather, participants may adopt a cognitive set that represents a "dynamic retrieval mode," with variable functional connections engaged among a subset of PFC regions depending on the nature of the retrieval attempt and particular task demands. In terms of postretrieval monitoring, the most consistent evidence to date indicates a region of right dorsolateral PFC involved in this process. The interaction of all preretrieval processes and postretrieval monitoring must somehow culmi-

nate and produce sufficient information upon which to base a retrieval decision, but this final process is not well understood.

Finally, the mixed-efMRI design has afforded researchers the ability to parse neural activation associated with neurocognitive functions directly into component state- and item-related processes (Donaldson, 2004). The findings from mixed design studies have extended our knowledge by resolving previously ambiguous conclusions. There is now some direct evidence (Velanova et al., 2003) to support previous claims that the right anterior PFC is involved in sustained retrieval mode. As well, these studies have added further converging data to support the well-established hypothesis that the left inferior PFC is crucially involved in semantic encoding. The novel insights that this approach has produced include the identification of dissociable sustained state-related and transient item-related processes involving this region during encoding, and that these processes may operate in competition with one another, possibly competing to recruit common PFC resources. The mixed-efMRI design should play a prominent role in future investigation of the component processes of the PFC in EM encoding and retrieval.

## REFERENCES

Allan, K., Dolan, R. J., Fletcher, P. C., & Rugg, M. D. (2000) The role of the right anterior prefrontal cortex in episodic retrieval. *NeuroImage, 11*, 217–227.

Bernstein, L. J., Beig, S., Siegenthaler, A. L., & Grady, C. L. (2002). The effect of encoding strategy on the neural correlates of memory for faces. *Psychology and Aging, 17*, 7–23.

Blanchet, S., Desgranges, B., Denise, P., Lechevalier, B., Eustache, F., & Faure, S. (2001). New questions on the hemispheric encoding/retrieval asymmetry (HERA) model assessed by divided visual-field tachistoscopy in normal subjects. *Neuropsychologia, 39*, 502–509.

Brewer, J. B., Zhao, Z., Desmond, J. E., Glover, G. H., & Gabrieli, J. D. (1998). Making memories: Brain activity that predicts how well visual experience will be remembered. *Science, 281*, 1185–1187.

Buckner, R. L., Koutstaal, W., Schacter, D. L., Dale, A. M., Rotte, M., & Rosen, B. R. (1998a). Functional-anatomic study of episodic retrieval: II. Selective averaging of event-related fMRI trials to test the retrieval success hypothesis. *NeuroImage, 7*, 163–175.

Buckner, R. L., Koutstaal, W., Schacter, D. L., Wagner, A. D., & Rosen, B. R. (1998b). Functional-anatomic study of episodic retrieval using fMRI: I. Retrieval effort versus retrieval success. *NeuroImage, 7,* 151–162.

Buckner, R. L., Wheeler, M. E., & Sheridan, M. A. (2001). Encoding processes during retrieval tasks. *Journal of Cognitive Neuroscience, 13,* 406–415.

Bunge, S. A., Burrows, B., & Wagner, A. D. (2004). Prefrontal and hippocampal contributions to visual associative recognition: Interactions between cognitive control and episodic retrieval. *Brain and Cognition, 56,* 141–52.

Cabeza, R., Dolcos, F., Graham, R., & Nyberg, L. (2002). Similarities and differences in the neural correlates of episodic memory retrieval and working memory. *NeuroImage, 16,* 317–330.

Cabeza, R., Locantore, J. K., & Anderson, N. D. (2003). Lateralization of prefrontal activity during episodic memory retrieval: Evidence for the production-monitoring hypothesis. *Journal of Cognitive Neuroscience, 15,* 249–259.

Cabeza, R., Rao, S. M., Wagner, A. D., Mayer, A. R., & Schacter, D. L. (2001). Can medial temporal lobe regions distinguish true from false?: An event-related functional MRI study of veridical and illusory recognition memory. *Proceedings of the National Academy of Sciences of the United States of America, 98,* 4805–4810.

Cansino, S., Maquet, P., Dolan, R. J., & Rugg, M. D. (2002). Brain activity underlying encoding and retrieval of source memory. *Cerebral Cortex, 12,* 1048–1056.

Chawla, D., Rees, G., & Friston, K. J. (1999). The physiological basis of attentional modulation in extrastriate visual areas. *Nature Neuroscience, 2,* 671–676.

Chee, M. W., Goh, J. O., Lim, Y., Graham, S., & Lee, K. (2004). Recognition memory for studied words is determined by cortical activation differences at encoding but not during retrieval. *NeuroImage, 22,* 1456–1465.

Dale, A. M., & Buckner, R. L. (1997). Selective averaging of rapidly presented individual trials using fMRI. *Human Brain Mapping, 5,* 17–22.

Della-Maggiore, V., Sekuler, A. B., Grady, C. L., Bennett, P. J., Sekuler, R., & McIntosh, A. R. (2000). Corticolimbic interactions associated with performance on a short-term memory task are modified by age. *Journal of Neuroscience, 20,* 8410–8416.

Dobbins, I. G., Rice, H. J., Wagner, A. D., & Schacter, D. L. (2003). Memory orientation and success: Separable neurocognitive components underlying episodic recognition. *Neuropsychologia, 41,* 318–333.

Dobbins, I. G., Simons, J. S., & Schacter, D. L. (2004). fMRI evidence for separable and lateralized prefrontal memory monitoring processes. *Journal of Cognitive Neuroscience, 16,* 908–920.

Donaldson, D. I. (2004). Parsing brain activity with fMRI and mixed designs: What kind of a state is neuroimaging in? *Trends in Neurosciences, 27,* 442–444.

Donaldson, D. I., Petersen, S. E., Ollinger, J. M., & Buckner, R. L. (2001). Dissociating state and item components of recognition memory using fMRI. *NeuroImage, 13*(1), 129–142.

Duzel, E., Cabeza, R., Picton, T. W., Yonelinas, A. P., Scheich, H., Heinze, H. J., et al. (1999). Task-related and item-related brain processes of memory retrieval. *Proceedings of the National Academy of Sciences of the United States of America, 96,* 1794–1799.

Duzel, E., Yonelinas, A. P., Mangun, G. R., Heinze, H. J., & Tulving, E. (1997). Event-related brain potential correlates of two states of conscious awareness in memory. *Proceedings of the National Academy of Sciences of the United States of America, 94,* 5973–5978.

Eldridge, L. L., Knowlton, B. J., Furmanski, C. S., Bookheimer, S. Y., & Engel, S. A. (2000). Remembering episodes: A selective role for the hippocampus during retrieval. *Nature Neuroscience, 3*(11), 1149–1152.

Fan, J., Snodgrass, J. G., & Bilder, R. M. (2003). Functional magnetic resonance imaging of source versus item memory. *NeuroReport, 14,* 2275–2281.

Fletcher, P. C., & Henson, R. N. (2001). Frontal lobes and human memory: Insights from functional neuroimaging. *Brain, 124,* 849–881.

Fletcher, P. C., Palomero-Gallagher, N., Zafiris, O., Fink, G. R., Tyler, L. K., & Zilles, K. (2002). The influence of explicit instructions and stimulus material on lateral frontal responses to an encoding task. *NeuroImage, 17,* 780–791.

Fletcher, P. C., Shallice, T., & Dolan, R. J. (1998). The functional roles of prefrontal cortex in episodic memory: I. Encoding. *Brain, 121,* 1239–1248.

Fletcher, P. C., Shallice, T., & Dolan, R. J. (2000). "Sculpting the response space"—an account of left prefrontal activation at encoding. *NeuroImage, 12,* 404–417.

Fletcher, P. C., Stephenson, C. M., Carpenter, T. A., Donovan, T., & Bullmorel, E. T. (2003). Regional brain activations predicting subsequent memory success: An event-related fMRI study of the influence of encoding tasks. *Cortex, 39,* 1009–1026.

Friston, K. J., Frith, C. D., Fracowiak, R. S. J., & Turner, R. (1995). Characterizing dynamic brain responses with fMRI: A multivariate approach. *NeuroImage, 2,* 166–172.

Friston, K. J., Zarahn, E., Josephs, O., Henson, R. N., & Dale, A. M. (1999). Stochastic designs in event-related fMRI. *NeuroImage, 10,* 607–619.

Fujii, T., Okuda, J., Tsukiura, T., Ohtake, H., Suzuki, M., Kawashima, R., et al. (2002). Encoding-related brain activity during deep processing of verbal materials: A PET study. *Neuroscience Research, 44,* 429–438.

Fuster, J. M. (1997). *The prefrontal cortex: Anatomy, physiology, and neuropsychology of the frontal lobe* (3rd ed.). Philadelphia: Lippincott-Raven.

Gazzaniga, M. S. (2000). Cerebral specialization and interhemispheric communication: Does the corpus callosum enable the human condition? *Brain, 123,* 1293–1326.

Gilboa, A. (2004). Autobiographical and episodic memory—one and the same?: Evidence from prefrontal activation in neuroimaging studies. *Neuropsychologia, 42,* 1336–1349.

Golby, A. J., Poldrack, R. A., Brewer, J. B., Spencer, D., Desmond, J. E., Aron, A. P., et al. (2001). Material-specific lateralization in the medial temporal lobe and prefrontal cortex during memory encoding. *Brain, 124,* 1841–1854.

Gonzalez-Lima, F., & McIntosh, A. R. (1994). Structural equation modeling and its application to network analysis in functional brain imaging. *Human Brain Mapping, 2,* 2–22.

Grady, C. L., McIntosh, A. R., Beig, S., & Craik, F. I. (2001). An examination of the effects of stimulus type, encoding task, and functional connectivity on the role of right prefrontal cortex in recognition memory. *NeuroImage, 14,* 556–571.

Grady, C. L., McIntosh, A. R., Horwitz, B., Maisog, J. M., Ungerleider, L. G., Mentis, M. J., et al. (1995). Age-related reductions in human recognition memory due to impaired encoding. *Science, 269,* 218–221.

Grady, C. L., McIntosh, A. R., Rajah, M. N., Beig, S., & Craik, F. I. (1999). The effects of age on the neural correlates of episodic encoding. *Cerebral Cortex, 9,* 805–814.

Habib, R., Nyberg, L., & Tulving, E. (2003). Hemispheric asymmetries of memory: The HERA model revisited. *Trends in Cognitive Sciences, 7,* 241–245.

Haxby, J. V., Ungerleider, L. G., Horwitz, B., Maisog, J. M., Rapoport, S. I., & Grady, C. L. (1996). Storage and retrieval of new memories for faces in the intact human brain. *Proceedings of the National Academy of Sciences of the United States of America, 93,* 922–927.

Henson, R. N., Rugg, M. D., Shallice, T., & Dolan, R. J. (2000). Confidence in recognition memory for words: Dissociating right prefrontal roles in episodic retrieval. *Journal of Cognitive Neuroscience, 12,* 913–923.

Henson, R. N., Rugg, M. D., Shallice, T., Josephs, O., & Dolan, R. J. (1999). Recollection and familiarity in recognition memory: An event-related functional magnetic resonance imageing study. *Journal of Neuroscience, 19*(10), 3962–3972.

Henson, R. N., Shallice, T., & Dolan, R. J. (1999). Right prefrontal cortex and episodic memory retrieval: A functional MRI test of the monitoring hypothesis. *Brain, 122,* 1367–1381.

Herron, J. E., Henson, R. N., & Rugg, M. D. (2004). Probability effects on the neural correlates of retrieval success: An fMRI study. *NeuroImage, 21,* 302–310.

Herron, J. E., & Wilding, E. L. (2004). An electrophysiological dissociation of retrieval mode and retrieval orientation. *NeuroImage, 22,* 1554–1562.

Heun, R., Klose, U., Jessen, F., Erb, M., Papassotiropoulos, A., Lotze, M., et al. (1999). Functional MRI of cerebral activation during encoding and retrieval of words. *Human Brain Mapping, 8,* 157–169.

Iidaka, T., Sadato, N., Yamada, H., Murata, T., Omori, M., & Yonekura, Y. (2001). An fMRI study of the functional neuroanatomy of picture encoding in younger and older adults. *Cognitive Brain Research, 11,* 1–11.

Iidaka, T., Sadato, N., Yamada, H., & Yonekura, Y. (2000). Functional asymmetry of human prefrontal cortex in verbal and non-verbal episodic memory as revealed by fMRI. *Cognitive Brain Research, 9,* 73–83.

Johnson, M. K. (1992). MEM—mechanisms of recollection. *Journal of Cognitive Neuroscience, 4,* 268–280.

Johnson, M. K., Raye, C. L., Mitchell, K. J., Greene, E. J., & Anderson, A. W. (2003). FMRI evidence for an organization of prefrontal cortex by both type of process and type of information. *Cerebral Cortex, 13,* 265–273.

Johnson, R., Jr., Kreiter, K., Zhu, J., & Russo, B. (1998). A spatio-temporal comparison of semantic and episodic cued recall and recognition using event-related brain potentials. *Cognitive Brain Research, 7,* 119–136.

Josephs, O., Turner, R., & Friston, K. (1997). Event-related fMRI. *Human Brain Mapping, 5,* 243–248.

Kapur, S., Craik, F. I., Jones, C., Brown, G. M., Houle, S., & Tulving, E. (1995). Functional role of the prefrontal cortex in retrieval of memories: A PET study. *NeuroReport, 6,* 1880–1884.

Kapur, S., Craik, F. I., Tulving, E., Wilson, A. A., Houle, S., & Brown, G. M. (1994). Neuroanatomical correlates of encoding in episodic memory: levels of processing effect. *Proceedings of the National Academy of Sciences of the United States of America, 91,* 2008–2011.

Kapur, S., Tulving, E., Cabeza, R., McIntosh, A. R., Houle, S., & Craik, F. I. (1996). The neural correlates of intentional learning of verbal materials: A PET study in humans. *Cognitive Brain Research, 4,* 243–249.

Kaufer, D. I., & Lewis, D. A. (1999). Frontal lobe anatomy and cortical connectivity. In B. L. Miller & J. L. Cummings (Eds.), *The human frontal lobes: Functions and disorders* (pp. 27–44). New York: Guilford Press.

Kavcic, V., Zhong, J., Yoshiura, T., & Doty, R. W. (2003). Frontal cortex, laterality, and memory: Encoding versus retrieval. *Acta Neurobiologiae Experimentalis, 63,* 337–350.

Kelley, W. M., Miezin, F. M., McDermott, K. B., Buckner, R. L., Raichle, M. E., Cohen, N. J., et al. (1998). Hemispheric specialization in human dorsal frontal cortex and medial temporal lobe for verbal and nonverbal memory encoding. *Neuron, 20,* 927–936.

Kirchhoff, B. A., Wagner, A. D., Maril, A., & Stern, C. E. (2000). Prefrontal–temporal circuitry for episodic encoding and subsequent memory. *Journal of Neuroscience, 20,* 6173–6180.

Konishi, S., Wheeler, M. E., Donaldson, D. I., & Buckner, R. L. (2000). Neural correlates of episodic retrieval success. *NeuroImage, 12,* 276–286.

Lee, A. C., Robbins, T. W., Pickard, J. D., & Owen, A. M. (2000). Asymmetric frontal activation during episodic memory: The effects of stimulus type on encoding and retrieval. *Neuropsychologia, 38,* 677–692.

Lee, A. C., Robbins, T. W., Smith, S., Calvert, G. A., Tracey, I., Matthews, P., et al. (2002). Evidence for asymmetric frontal-lobe involvement in episodic memory from functional magnetic resonance imaging and patients with unilateral frontal-lobe excisions. *Neuropsychologia, 40,* 2420–2437.

Lepage, M., Ghaffar, O., Nyberg, L., & Tulving, E. (2000). Prefrontal cortex and episodic memory retrieval mode. *Proceedings of the National Academy of Sciences of the United States of America, 97,* 506–511.

Leube, D. T., Erb, M., Grodd, W., Bartels, M., & Kircher, T. T. (2001). Differential activation in parahippocampal and prefrontal cortex during word and face encoding tasks. *NeuroReport, 12,* 2773–2777.

Mangels, J. A., Picton T. W., & Craik, F. (2001). Attention and successful episodic encoding: An event-related potential study. *Cognitive Brain Research, 11,* 77–95.

Maril, A., Simons, J. S., Mitchell, J. P., Schwartz, B. L., & Schacter, D. L. (2003). Feeling-of-knowing in episodic memory: En event-related fMRI study. *NeuroImage, 18,* 827–836.

McDermott, K. B., Buckner, R. L., Petersen, S. E., Kelley, W. M., & Sanders, A. L. (1999). Set- and code-specific activation in frontal cortex: An fMRI study of encoding and retrieval of faces and words. *Journal of Cognitive Neuroscience, 11,* 631–640.

McDermott, K. B., Jones, T. C., Petersen, S. E., Lageman, S. K., & Roediger, H. L. (2000). Retrieval success is accompanied by enhanced activation in anterior prefrontal cortex during recognition memory: An event-related fMRI study. *Journal of Cognitive Neuroscience, 12,* 965–976.

McIntosh, A. R. (2004). Contexts and catalysts: A resolution of the localization and integration of function in the brain. *Neuroinformatics, 2,* 175–182.

McIntosh, A. R., Bookstein, F. L., Haxby, J. V., & Grady, C. L. (1996). Spatial pattern analysis of functional brain images using partial least squares. *NeuroImage, 3,* 143–57.

McIntosh, A. R., Chau, W. K., & Protzner, A. B. (2004). Spatiotemporal analysis of event-related fMRI data using partial least squares. *NeuroImage, 23,* 764–775.

McIntosh, A. R., Grady, C. L., Ungerleider, L. G., Haxby, J. V., Rapoport, S. I., & Horwitz, B. (1994). Network analysis of cortical visual pathways mapped with PET. *Journal of Neuroscience, 14,* 655–666.

McIntosh, A. R., Nyberg, L., Bookstein, F. L., & Tulving, E. (1997). Differential functional connectivity of prefrontal and medial temporal cortices during episodic memory retrieval. *Human Brain Mapping, 5,* 323–327.

Miller, M. B., Kingstone, A., & Gazzaniga, M. S. (2002). Hemispheric encoding asymmetry is more apparent than real. *Journal of Cognitive Neuroscience, 14,* 702–708.

Morcom, A. M., & Rugg, M. D. (2002). Getting ready to remember: The neural correlates of task set during recognition memory. *NeuroReport, 13,* 149–152.

Moscovitch, M., & Winocur, G. (2002). The frontal cortex and working with memory. In D. T. Stuss & R. T. Knight (Eds.), *Principles of frontal lobe function* (pp. 188–298). New York: Oxford University Press.

Mottaghy, F. M., Shah, N. J., Krause, B. J., Schmidt, D., Halsband, U., Jancke, L., et al. (1999). Neuronal correlates of encoding and retrieval in episodic memory during a paired-word association learning task: A functional magnetic resonance imaging study. *Experimental Brain Research, 128,* 332–342.

Nyberg, L., Cabeza, R., & Tulving, E. (1996). PET studies of encoding and retrieval: The HERA model. *Psychonomic Bulletin and Review, 3,* 135–148.

Nyberg, L., Persson, J., Habib, R., Tulving, E., McIntosh, A. R., Cabeza, R., et al. (2000). Large scale neurocognitive networks underlying episodic memory. *Journal of Cognitive Neuroscience, 12,* 163–173.

Nyberg, L., Tulving, E., Habib, R., Nilsson, L. G., Kapur, S., Houle, S., et al. (1995). Functional brain maps of retrieval mode and recovery of episodic information. *NeuroReport, 7,* 249–252.

Opitz, B., Mecklinger, A., & Friederici, A. D. (2000). Functional asymmetry of human prefrontal cortex: Encoding and retrieval of verbally and nonverbally coded information. *Learning and Memory, 7,* 85–96.

Otten, L. J., Henson, R. N., & Rugg, M. D. (2001). Depth of processing effects on neural correlates of memory encoding: Relationship between findings from across- and within-task comparisons. *Brain, 124,* 399–412.

Otten, L. J., Henson, R. N., & Rugg, M. D. (2002). State-related and item-related neural correlates of successful memory encoding. *Nature Neuroscience, 5,* 1339–1344.

Otten, L. J., & Rugg, M. D. (2001a). Task-dependency of the neural correlates of episodic encoding as measured by fMRI. *Cerebral Cortex, 11,* 1150–1160.

Otten, L. J., & Rugg, M. D. (2001b). When more means less: Neural activity related to unsuccessful memory encoding. *Current Biology, 11,* 1528–1530.

Petersson, K. M., Reis, A., Castro-Caldas, A., & Ingvar, M. (1999). Effective auditory–verbal encoding activates the left prefrontal and the medial temporal lobes: A generalization to illiterate subjects. *NeuroImage, 10,* 45–54.

Ragland, J. D., Gur, R. C., Lazarev, M. G., Smith, R. J., Schroeder, L., Raz, J., et al. (2000). Hemispheric activation of anterior and inferior prefrontal cortex during verbal encoding and recognition: A PET study of healthy volunteers. *NeuroImage, 11,* 624–633.

Ranganath, C., Johnson, M. K., & D'Esposito, M. (2000). Left anterior prefrontal activation increases with demands to recall specific perceptual information. *Journal of Neuroscience, 20*(22), RC108.

Ranganath, C., Yonelinas, A. P., Cohen, M. X., Dy, C. J., Tom, S. M., & D'Esposito, M. (2003). Dissociable correlates of recollection and familiarity within the medial temporal lobes. *Neuropsychologia, 42*, 2–13.

Reber, P. J., Siwiec, R. M., Gitelman, D. R., Parrish, T. B., Mesulam, M. M., & Paller, K. A. (2002). Neural correlates of successful encoding identified using functional magnetic resonance imaging. *Journal of Neuroscience, 22*, 9541–9548.

Reynolds, J. R., Donaldson, D. I., Wagner, A. D., & Braver, T. S. (2004). Item- and task-level processes in the left inferior prefrontal cortex: Positive and negative correlates of encoding. *NeuroImage, 21*, 1472–1483.

Rossi, S., Miniussi, C., Pasqualetti, P., Babiloni, C., Rossini, P. M., & Cappa, S. F. (2004). Age-related functional changes of prefrontal cortex in long-term memory: A repetitive transcranial magnetic stimulation study. *Journal of Neuroscience, 24*, 7939–7944.

Rugg, M. D., Allan, K., & Birch, C. S. (2000). Electrophysiological evidence for the modulation of retrieval orientation by depth of study processing. *Journal of Cognitive Neuroscience, 12*, 664–678.

Rugg, M. D., Fletcher, P. C., Allan, K., Frith, C. D., Frackowiak, R. S., & Dolan, R. J. (1998). Neural correlates of memory retrieval during recognition memory and cued recall. *NeuroImage, 8*, 262–273.

Rugg, M. D., Fletcher, P. C., Chua, P. M.-L., & Dolan, R. J. (1999). The role of the prefrontal cortex in recognition memory and memory for source: An fMRI study. *NeuroImage, 10*, 520–529.

Rugg, M. D., & Henson, R. N. (2002). Episodic memory retrieval: An (event-related) functional neuroimaging perspective. In A. M. Park, E. L. Wilding, & T. J. Bussey (Eds.), *The cognitive neuroscience of memory*. East Sussex, UK: Psychology Press.

Rugg, M. D., Henson, R. N., & Robb, W. G. (2003). Neural correlates of retrieval processing in the prefrontal cortex during recognition and exclusion tasks. *Neuropsychologia, 41*, 40–52.

Rugg, M. D., & Wilding, E. L. (2000). Retrieval processing and episodic memory. *Trends in Cognitive Sciences, 4*(3), 108–115.

Schacter, D. L. (1987). Memory, amnesia, and frontal lobe dysfunction. *Psychobiology, 15*, 21–38.

Tulving, E. (1972). Episodic and semantic memory. In E. Tulving & W. Donaldson (Eds.), *Organization of memory*. New York: Plenum Press.

Tulving, E. (1983). *Elements of episodic memory*. New York: Oxford University Press.

Tulving, E. (1985). Memory and consciousness. *Canadian Psychology, 26*, 1–12.

Tulving, E., Kapur, S., Craik, F. I., Moscovitch, M., & Houle, S. (1994). Hemispheric encoding/retrieval asymmetry in episodic memory: Positron emission tomography findings. *Proceeding of the National Academy of Sciences of the United States of America, 91*, 2016–2020.

Velanova, K., Jacoby, L. L., Wheeler, M. E., McAvoy, M. P., Petersen, S. E., & Buckne, R. L. (2003). Functional–anatomic correlates of sustained and transient processing components engaged during controlled retrieval. *Journal of Neuroscience, 23*, 8460–8470.

Wagner, A. D., Desmond, J. E., Glover, G. H., & Gabrieli, J. D. (1998). Prefrontal cortex and recognition memory: Functional-MRI evidence for context-dependent retrieval processes. *Brain, 121*, 1985–2002.

Wagner, A. D., Poldrack, R. A., Eldridge, L. L., Desmond, J. E., Glover, G. H., & Gabrieli, J. D. (1998). Material-specific lateralization of prefrontal activation during episodic encoding and retrieval. *NeuroReport, 9*, 3711–3717.

Wagner, A. D., Schacter, D. L., Rotte, M., Koutstaal, W., Maril, A., Dale, A. M., et al. (1998). Building memories: Remembering and forgetting of verbal experiences as predicted by brain activity. *Science, 281*, 1188–1191.

Wheeler, M. E., & Buckner, R. L. (2004) Functional–anatomic correlates of remembering and knowing. *NeuroImage, 21*, 1337–1349.

Wheeler, M. A., Stuss, D. T., & Tulving, E. (1997). Toward a theory of episodic memory: The frontal lobes and autonoetic consciousness. *Psychological Bulletin, 121*, 331–354.

Zarahn, E., Aguirre, G., & D'Esposito, M. (1997). A trial-based experimental design for fMRI. *NeuroImage, 6*, 122–138.

# CHAPTER 15

# The Frontal Lobes and Autobiographical Memory

*Margaret C. McKinnon*
*Eva Svoboda*
*Brian Levine*

Consider the following experiment. Subjects complete a questionnaire ostensibly concerned with their eating preferences and personality. The experimenter later informs them that computer analysis has determined that they became ill after eating a certain food as a child. Half the subjects are told the food was deviled eggs; the other half are told it was dill pickles. Many of the subjects came to believe this false memory, and subjects in each group demonstrated a bias against selecting the eggs or pickles, even though they were randomly assigned to groups (Bernstein, Laney, Morris, & Loftus, 2005). Memory researcher Elizabeth Loftus recently demonstrated this effect with actor Alan Alda, host of *Scientific American Frontiers*, who turned his nose up at deviled eggs when offered them during a picnic with members of Loftus's group.

As illustrated in this example, autobiographical memory is reconstructive rather than fixed (Bartlett, 1932; Burgess & Shallice, 1996a). The plastic, multifaceted nature of autobiographical memory implies the active, simultaneous reactivation of elements similar to those that were activated during the initial experience. Although autobiographical retrieval of episodes may occur spontaneously to a specific cue, such as an odor, they are more commonly accessed through generative retrieval strategies. These strategies are mediated by executive control operations associated with the frontal lobes, including initiating, guiding, and organizing a memory search, as well as monitoring its recovered content (Luria, 1980; Moscovitch, 1992; Stuss & Benson, 1986).

In this chapter, we review and integrate research on the frontal lobes (more specifically, the prefrontal cortex lying anterior to primary motor cortex) and autobiographical memory. Following a brief review of the conceptual underpinnings of autobiographical memory and assessment techniques, we review research on autobiographical memory according to various domains of function. We follow with sections describing autobiographical memory in psychiatric disorders and functional retrograde amnesia. Our emphasis is on studies of patients with brain disease. When available, evidence from functional neuroimaging is included.

## CONCEPTUAL UNDERPINNINGS OF AUTOBIOGRAPHICAL MEMORY

A surprisingly small proportion of memory research has been directed toward the study of memory for information and experiences pertaining to one's own life, or autobiographical memory. Although memory processes more amenable to laboratory-based study, such as encoding, retention, and retrieval contribute to everyday functioning, autobiographical memory is additionally implicated in one's protracted self-awareness across time and self-identity (Tulving, 2001). Like other memory domains, autobiographical memory is not unitary; researchers have identified contrasting autobiographical memory systems and processes in healthy people that can be affected differentially by brain damage (Conway & Fthenaki, 2000). Such complexity has contributed to the number of different, but often complementary, theories of autobiographical memory we review here.

Tulving's (1972, 1985a) conception of human memory, in which episodic and semantic memory are mediated by independent memory systems, has been both influenced by studies of autobiographical memory (particularly in patients with loss of episodic autobiographical memory) and influential to students of autobiographical memory. Episodic memory entails the conscious recollection of a temporally and spatially specific event from one's personal past, including event details, sensory–perceptual details, thoughts, and feelings. It is supported by autonoetic consciousness, a uniquely human capacity that is strongly associated with the prefrontal cortex (Wheeler, Stuss, & Tulving, 1997). Autonoetic consciousness mediates mental time travel and facilitates awareness of the self as a continuous entity across time (Tulving, 2001). Semantic memory comprises both public (world knowledge) and personal factual information, such as identity and trait information, historical data, and the facts supporting awareness of personal past events, including knowledge that an event has occurred. Unlike episodic memory, semantic memory is time-independent and less reliant on prefrontal function. In this sense, the distinction between public and personal semantic memory is merely heuristic; it does not imply separate neurocognitive processes.

The episodic–semantic distinction also illuminates the development of autobiographical memory in early childhood. Childhood amnesia refers to the normal inability to recall specific events occurring prior to approximately 4 years of age (Bruce, Dolan, & Phillips-Grant, 2000). The offset of childhood amnesia corresponds to increases in a number of frontally mediated processes, including children's ability to perform source memory tasks (Gopnik & Graf, 1988), to reliably recall event details such as time and place (Fivush & Hamond, 1990; Hudson & Fivush, 1991), to perform tests of working memory and executive functioning

(Case, 1974; Case, Kurland, & Goldberg, 1982; Wheeler et al., 1997), and to maintain a consistent representation of the self across time (Povinelli, Landau, & Perilloux, 1996). These changes coincide further with regressive cortical gray matter and progressive white matter changes that may increase signal-to-noise ratio in prefrontal systems interconnectivity and mediate the development of circuits shaped by environmental stimulation and input from other cortical areas (for a review, see Levine, 2004). Although children are undoubtedly able to learn and retain information prior to age 4, many memory theorists regard this as semantic in nature (Wheeler et al., 1997).

In another formulation of autobiographical memory, Conway and colleagues (Conway & Fthenaki, 2000; Conway, Pleydell-Pearce, & Whitecross, 2001) define a self-memory system with three levels of autobiographical memory knowledge: lifetime periods representing personal eras (e.g., time spent in university) and general knowledge of others, locations, activities, and goals; general events, either repeated (e.g., a Passover Seder), extended (e.g., college orientation week), or sets of associated events ("minihistories"; e.g., learning to ride a horse); and event-specific knowledge comprising specific-event, imagery, and sensory details of a memory. Conway (2001) restricts the term "episodic memory" to recent experiences (within the past 24 hours) that involve highly specific sensory–perceptual details. These experiences are not transferred to autobiographical memory unless anchored to broader and more stable general autobiographical knowledge. Information retrieved from autobiographical memory is integrated with the broader, more stable frameworks of repeated events and life periods, which are accessed first during autobiographical memory retrieval (Conway & Bekerian, 1987).

As is apparent in Conway's model, autobiographical memory retrieval is reliant upon retrieval of sensory–perceptual information, with visual imagery playing a prominent role (Conway, 2001; Rubin & Greenberg, 1998). According to Brewer (1986), single instances of an event can give rise to either imaginal components of personal memory involving strong visual imagery, or nonimaginal components involving an autobiographical fact stored as an abstract, nonimage representation (e.g., a proposition). Long-term visual representations in turn reactivate nonvisual percepts, conceptual knowledge, and emotions related to the event as they are placed within a spatial and temporal context. Accordingly, the literature on retrograde amnesia contains case studies of remote memory loss following posterior neocortical damage affecting access to visual material (O'Connor, Butters, Miliotis, Eslinger, & Cermak, 1992; Ogawa et al., 1992; Rubin & Greenberg, 1998). This does not exclude the possibility of autobiographical memory deficits arising from damage to other brain regions; rather, it highlights the notion that participants may fail a task (e.g., autobiographical memory) for more than one reason (e.g., retrieval deficit; failure of visual imagery) stemming from damage to different brain regions (e.g., prefrontal, occipital lobes) (Rosenbaum, McKinnon, Levine, & Moscovitch, 2004).

Other authors have emphasized the separation between events that people experienced or perceived and those about which people merely thought. For example, in her reality monitoring framework, Johnson (1988; Johnson & Raye, 1981) concludes that whereas memories for experienced events are rich in sensory details and in temporal, spatial, and contextual elements, memories for imagined events contain detailed references to mentally based elements such as thoughts and feelings. In line with this view, participants assign higher ratings for visual details, sound, smell, taste, realism, location, setting spatial arrangement of objects and people, and temporality for real compared to imagined events (Johnson, Foley, Suengas, & Raye, 1988), suggesting that sensory stimuli play an important role in episodic recollection.

More recent studies have focused on the contribution of emotions to autobiographical memory recollection. Regions of the prefrontal cortex are intimately connected to limbic regions involved in emotional processing and are themselves implicated in diverse social cognition tasks recruiting emotion, such as moral reasoning (Greene, Sommerville, Nystrom, Darley, & Cohen, 2001; Moll et al., 2002), emotional comprehension (Rosen et al., 2002), theory of mind (Fletcher et al., 1995; Stuss, Gallup, & Alexander, 2001), and humor (Shammi & Stuss, 1999). These findings suggest a role for the prefrontal cortex in emotional autobiographical memory. We explore this topic in greater detail throughout this review.

It should be apparent from the foregoing that autobiographical memory cannot be re-

duced to a single memory system or process. It emerges from interaction between episodic and semantic mnemonic processes, as well as domain-specific (e.g., visual imagery) and domain-general (e.g., working memory) resources. It therefore engages a distributed network of brain regions (Conway, Pleydell-Pearce, Whitecross, & Sharpe, 2002; Maguire, 2001; Svoboda, McKinnon, & Levine, 2006). Indeed, there are few major cortical regions or subcortical structures that have not been implicated in autobiographical memory. Nonetheless, prefrontal cortices figure prominently in autobiographical memory. Figure 15.1 depicts the results of a recent meta-analysis surveying 23 functional neuroimaging studies of autobiographical memory. A core network of regions (defined by activation in more than half of the studies) included the ventrolateral and medial prefrontal cortex, lateral and medial temporal regions, the temporoparietal cortex, posterior cingulate/retrosplenial regions, and the cerebellum. The lateral and orbital prefrontal cortices were also noted among secondary regions (defined by activation in at least five studies).

## ASSESSING AUTOBIOGRAPHICAL MEMORY

Interest in the analysis of autobiographical memory dates back to Freud and Galton. Freud (1982) was interested primarily in remote memory, stemming from his conviction that neuroses were grounded in childhood events. More formal assessment of autobiographical memory began with Galton (1879, 1907) and is mirrored in many of the current techniques used to study autobiographical memory. The heterogeneity of assessment techniques reflects the complexity of autobiographical memory. Unlike standard memory assessment, autobiographical memoranda are inherently idiosyncratic and by definition cannot be presented in a controlled environment. Assessment of any psychological construct is always an approximation, but this is even more the case for autobiographical memory. Any study of autobiographical memory must therefore represent a compromise between experimental control and real-life relevance.

Clinical interviews may also involve autobiographical recall of personally experienced episodes and general knowledge of current events. For example, patients with brain trau-

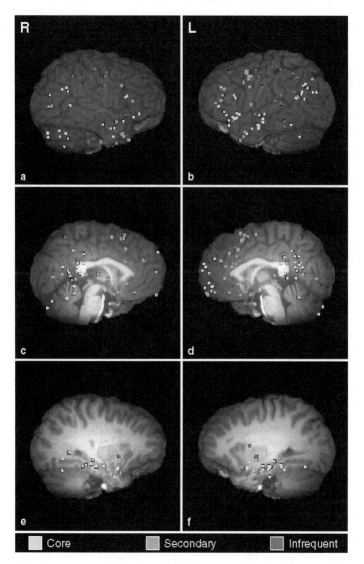

FIGURE 15.1. Significant peaks of activation reported across imaging studies of autobiographical memory. Activations in core, secondary and infrequently reported regions are depicted across right (left column) and left (right column) lateral, medial, and lateral subcortical planes.

ma are often asked, "What's the last thing you remember?" with little regard for their understanding of this question. In a typical behavioral study of autobiographical memory, participants are asked to list or describe events that happened in their past (Crovitz & Schiffman, 1974; Kopelman, Wilson, & Baddeley, 1990; Levine, Svoboda, Hay, Winocur, & Moscovitch, 2002). Several standardized measures of autobiographical memory have emerged in recent years. For example, the most commonly used standardized, commercially available test

of autobiographical memory, the Autobiographical Memory Interview (AMI) (Kopelman et al., 1990) assesses autobiographical memory through a structured interview concerning lifetime semantic autobiographical memory. Episodic autobiographical memory is probed through free recall of events and scored according to a 0- to 3-point system for specificity and richness.

More recent behavioral testing methods have emphasized the careful separation of episodic and semantic memory (Levine et al.,

2002; Moscovitch, Yaschyshyn, Ziegler, & Nadel, 2000; Piolino, Desgranges, et al., 2003). For example, our Autobiographical Interview and accompanying text-based scoring method have been used to separate elements of episodic and semantic autobiographical memory. In other measures of autobiographical memory, distinctions among elements of autobiographical memory are made at the time of testing (Johnson et al., 1988; Kopelman, 1994). In the case of the AMI, this is done using different interviews not necessarily matched for psychometric characteristics. By contrast, the Autobiographical Interview involves only one test; separation of detail types is done at the scoring stage. The Autobiographical Interview also incorporates different levels of cueing to support retrieval. This method is distinct from other, more recent autobiographical memory assessment tools (e.g., Piolino, Belliard, Desgranges, Perron, & Eustace, 2003; Piolino, Desgranges, et al., 2003; Piolino, Desgranges, Benali, & Eustache, 2002), where little cueing is given to facilitate recall and scoring is based on rating scales. The Autobiographical Interview, however, is more cumbersome in that it requires transcription of the interview and training of the scorer.

In retrograde amnesia following traumatic brain injury and in studies involving electroconvulsive shock therapy, extended periods of episodic memory loss have been reported across the hours (Grossi, Trojano, Grasso, & Orsini, 1988), days (Russell & Nathan, 1946), weeks (Dusoir, Kapur, Byrnes, McKinstry, & Hoare, 1990; Kapur et al., 1994), and years (Squire, Slater, & Chace, 1975; Teuber, 1968) preceding neural insult. Similarly, animal studies have pointed toward a time-limited effect of acute brain insult, with amnestic periods of several days (Laurent-Demir & Jaffard, 1997) and weeks (Thornton, Rothblat, & Murray, 1997) duration reported. It is therefore often necessary to separate recent from remote memories. Autobiographical memory assessment tools, however, differ widely in their quantification of the period of time spanning a "new" memory. By some definitions, new or recent memories are thought to extend back as far as 5 years, as evidenced in studies investigating temporal gradients of episodic recall in amnesics (Bayley, Hopkins, & Squire, 2003; Graham & Hodges, 1997; Nestor, Graham, Bozeat, Simons, & Hodges, 2002). Other authors date new episodic memories to brief retention intervals measured in minutes or hours, with the broader concept of autobiographical memory spanning retention intervals measured in weeks, months, years, decades, and across the lifespan (Conway, 2001).

In functional neuroimaging research, methods for evoking autobiographical memories have been adapted according to the methodological constraints of the imaging platform. Autobiographical memory paradigms for neuroimaging studies can be broadly classified as uncued or cued. In uncued techniques, participants are asked simply to retrieve an autobiographical memory (Andreasen et al., 1995, 1999; Gemar, Kapur, Segal, Brown, & Houle, 1996). Within cued techniques, events may be based on arbitrary word cues (i.e., a revision of the Galton technique, Conway et al., 1999; Crovitz & Schiffman, 1974; Graham, Lee, Brett, & Patterson, 2003; Nyberg, Forkstam, Petersson, Cabeza, & Ingvar, 2002). These methods, which have been used extensively to investigate the distribution of autobiographical memories across the lifespan (Nyberg et al., 2002; Rubin, Rahhal, & Poon, 1998; Rubin & Schulkind, 1997), provide a greater degree of standardization relative to uncued methods, but the generation of autobiographical memories is not guaranteed. Both cued and uncued methods are expected to engage considerable executive processes.

More specific retrieval cues may be culled from interviews conducted prior to scanning, the most common method for studying autobiographical memory with functional neuroimaging (e.g., Maguire & Mummery, 1999; Piefke, Weiss, Zilles, Markowitsch, & Fink, 2003; Ryan et al., 2001). Although the prescan interview technique has been criticized due to the possibility of reencoding of the episode (Conway et al., 2002), there is evidence that this is not the case (Maguire, 2001; Ryan et al., 2001). Gilboa, Winocur, Grady, Hevenor, and Moscovitch (2004) created cues without interviewing subjects by collecting photographs from subjects' spouses that had not been recently viewed, so that subjects saw the photographs for the first time in the scanner. Similarly, in a study conducted in our laboratory (Levine et al., 2004), highly specific audio retrieval cues were selected at random from a pool harvested by subjects using portable audio recorders in the months preceding the scan (and not listened to in advance of the scan).

In summary, there is significant heterogeneity in autobiographical assessment techniques, with associated heterogeneity in the results arising from these techniques. Therefore, a major challenge in interpreting autobiographical memory research is the separation of method variance from other factors. Clearly, episodic and semantic contributions to remote memory need to be separated. Public knowledge, as assessed, for example, with famous faces and events, should not be confused with personal episodic memory. Although this may seem obvious, contamination of personal episodic memory data by semantic memory (personal or public) can be insidious (Moscovitch & Nadel, 1998; Nadel & Moscovitch, 1997; Steinvorth, Levine, & Corkin, 2005). To compensate for the variability inherent to autobiographical memory, multiple memories should be sampled for each time period and, when possible, large N samples should be employed. Researchers and clinicians need to be mindful of the effects of various cueing methods on autobiographical retrieval, preferably manipulating these to contrast cued versus uncued retrieval.

## EXECUTIVE AND COGNITIVE CONTROL OPERATIONS

The reconstructive nature of autobiographical recollection includes specification of retrieval search parameters monitored in response to an internally or externally generated cue that itself is prone to ongoing modification (Burgess & Shallice, 1996b; Conway & Fthenaki, 2000a; Norman & Bobrow, 1979). On laboratory memory tasks, patients with prefrontal damage are prone to intrusions, perseverations, and source confusion (Petrides, 1989; Schacter, 1987; Stuss & Benson, 1986). In comparison to these tasks, cues for autobiographical memory retrieval are often less specific, placing greater demands on executive search and retrieval operations. Accordingly, older adults, who are likely to have executive dysfunction relative to younger adults, show impoverished access to episodic details (Levine et al., 2002; Piolino et al., 2002). One explanation for this finding is an age-related reduction of "resolving power" within autobiographical retrieval, causing search operations to terminate at the level of nonspecific generic or semantic representations (e.g., general events; Conway, 2001; see also Cohen, 2000; Craik & Grady, 2002).

Preliminary data from our laboratory suggest that this effect is even greater for patients with frontotemporal lobar dementia (FTLD) and focal prefrontal damage, particularly when such damage encroaches upon the ventral prefrontal regions, which are intimately connected to the medial temporal lobe (MTL) and involved in retrieval cue specification (Fletcher & Henson, 2001).

Performance on tests of executive functioning is related to autobiographical memory retrieval (Della Sala, Laiacona, Spinnler, & Trivelli, 1993; Kopelman, 1991; Kopelman & Kapur, 2001). For example, Della Sala and his colleagues (1993) assessed autobiographical memory performance in patients with focal frontal damage; autobiographical memory impairment correlated strongly with executive dysfunction in these patients. By contrast, Kopelman (1989) found that performance on the AMI correlated only weakly with tests of prefrontally mediated executive function in patients with Korsakoff's syndrome and Alzheimer's dementia (AD), possibly due to the contribution of MTL damage in these patients. In other studies of patients with nonfocal frontal damage, including AD and epilepsy, researchers have reported a correlation between episodic memory recall and phonological verbal fluency, considered a test of executive functioning (Barnett, Newman, Richardson, Thompson, & Upton, 2000; Greene, Hodges, & Baddeley, 1995); personal semantic recall has also been correlated with performance on this measure (Barnett et al., 2000), as well as with working memory (Greene et al., 1995).

The executive contribution to autobiographical memory retrieval may be examined by applying retrieval support such as structured cueing, which may compensate for executive deficits (e.g., Baddeley & Wilson, 1986; Craik & McDowd, 1987). There are very limited data addressing this question. Sagar, Sullivan, and Corkin (1991) found that nonspecific cueing was effective in eliminating group differences among patients with AD, and younger and older adults for recent, but not remote, memories. It may be that more structured probing was necessary to access the difficult-to-retrieve remote memories. We found that relatively highly structured cueing in the Autobiographical Interview increased episodic recall in both younger and older adults (Levine et al., 2002). It did not, however, alter the age-related bias toward semantic details in older adults. If anything, cueing accentuated this effect. Using the same test, preliminary data from our laboratory show a similar effect for patients with FTLD (Levine, 2004). In patients with focal prefrontal lesions, however, cueing was effective in reducing deficits, as long as the lesion was in the ventral prefrontal sector. Patients with focal dorsolateral prefrontal cortical (PFC) damage, like older adults and patients with FTLD, responded to cueing by increasing their production of extraneous information (Levine, 2004), likely due to monitoring deficits (Fletcher & Henson, 2001). Clearly, the effects of cueing depend on the type of cue and the patients' characteristics. If the cue is not specific enough, or if the patient lacks the capacity to engage effectively with the cue, cueing may increase retrieval output, but the additional retrieved information will lack specificity. On the other hand, patients with amnesia due to diencephalic and medial temporal damage show little change in their recall from cueing due to more complete inaccessibility to remote autobiographical episodes (Moscovitch et al., 2000; Rosenbaum et al., 2004).

These findings have implications for interpretation of patients with temporal lobe damage who may have concomitant frontal systems dysfunction. Research in patients with semantic dementia (or temporal lobe variant frontotemporal lobar dementia) has found reverse temporal gradients, whereby remote memories are disproportionately impaired relative to recent memories (Graham & Hodges, 1997; Nestor et al., 2002). Considering the fact that remote memories are more difficult to retrieve than recent memories, this finding could be explained by strategic retrieval deficits that may be amenable to cueing. Accordingly, we have shown that reverse gradients in two patients with semantic dementia are reversed when structured cueing is provided (McKinnon, Miller, Black, Moscovitch, & Levine, 2006; see also Moss, Kopelman, Cappelletti, De Mornay Davies, & Jaldow, 2003). In a separate study, remote memory was improved through the use of nonverbal cues (compensating for patients' linguistic deficits; Westmacott, Leach, Freedman, & Moscovitch, 2001; but see Graham, Kropelnicki, Goldman, & Hodges, 2003).

Few data address lateralization effects on autobiographical memory in patients with prefrontal damage. From research on laboratory materials, including early functional neuroimaging research, one might predict a preferential role for the right prefrontal cortex (Stuss et al., 1994; Tulving, Kapur, Craik, Moscovitch, & Houle, 1994). Some support for this hypothesis is drawn from patients with episodic autobiographical memory loss (e.g., Levine et al., 1998) and an early functional neuroimaging study of autobiographical memory (Fink et al., 1996). Yet subsequent studies of autobiographical memory have found predominantly left prefrontal activation, particularly along the medial prefrontal wall (Maguire, 2001; Svoboda et al., 2006). Other functional neuroimaging studies involving self-reference and complex, reconstructive retrieval of laboratory stimuli engage these same left prefrontal regions (Buckner, Koutstaal, Schacter, Wagner, & Rosen, 1998; Cabeza, Anderson, Kester, Lennartsson, & McIntosh, 2001; Craik et al., 1999; Kelley et al., 2002; Nolde, Johnson, & D'Esposito, 1998; Raye, Johnson, Mitchell, Nolde, & D'Esposito, 2000).

In comparing functional neuroimaging studies of laboratory and autobiographical memory, Gilboa (2004) noted that mundane laboratory stimuli require greater monitoring processes (mediated by right PFC) to distinguish targets from distracters, whereas retrospectively identified autobiographical events are already established in the autobiographical memory network and therefore require little monitoring. Accordingly, the only studies showing significant right dorsolateral prefrontal activation in response to autobiographical memory were those involving *prospective* collection of everyday events (Cabeza et al., 2004; Levine et al., 2004).

Activation in the ventrolateral PFC is also more frequent in the left hemisphere in functional neuroimaging studies of autobiographical memory (Svoboda et al., 2006). Ventrolateral prefrontal activity has been associated with strategic retrieval, verification, and selection of information from posterior cortical association areas (Fletcher & Henson, 2001; Henson, Shallice, & Dolan, 1999; Petrides & Pandya, 2002), all tasks relevant to autobiographical memory retrieval. Activity in ventrolateral cortex is also observed when participants are required to maintain search results online (D'Esposito, Postle, Ballard, & Lease, 1999; Wagner, Maril, Bjork, & Schacter, 2001), a process central to successful retrieval of an autobiographical event. Activity in the ventrolateral region may be material-specific, with the left hemisphere engaged by verbal retrieval (as is nearly always the case for autobiographical tasks) and the right hemisphere engaged by the retrieval of images (see Petrides, 2002).

## SEPARATION OF EPISODIC FROM SEMANTIC AUTOBIOGRAPHICAL MEMORY

Although amnesia for remote events can affect both semantic and episodic autobiographical memory, effects are greater for episodic memory (Cermak, 1985; Kapur, 1999), especially when the PFC is affected. Many case studies of retrograde amnesia with disproportionate effects on episodic autobiographical memory involve patients with prefrontal damage, although not exclusively so (Kapur, 1999; Levine et al., 2002). Early studies of episodic and semantic autobiographical memory in groups with mixed prefrontal etiology involved primarily patients with alcoholic Korsakoff's syndrome (Kopelman, 1989, 1991), involving volume loss in the PFC and cingulate gyrus, as well as the mamillary bodies, thalamus, and cerebellum. Such patients have dense anterograde amnesia, but data concerning retrograde memory (i.e., predating the onset of the illness) are mixed, likely due to method variance. Baddeley and Wilson (1986) used the cue-word technique and did not examine retrograde semantic memory. Episodic sparing in a study by Zola-Morgan, Cohen, and Squire (1983) focused on very remote memories, 30–40 years in age, whereas retrograde semantic impairment was noted for more recent time periods. Two studies documenting impairment of episodic and semantic autobiographical memory used the AMI (Kopelman, 1986, 1989). Butters and Cermak (1986) came to a similar conclusion using autobiographical material from a patient's autobiography, written 2 years prior to disease onset.

As noted earlier, patients with frontal damage due to FTLD and focal prefrontal lesions show episodic autobiographical impairment, with relative sparing of personal semantic memory (Levine, 2004; McKinnon et al., 2006; Piolino, Desgranges, et al., 2003; Thomas-Anterion, Jacquin, & Laurent, 2000), as do normal older adults (Levine et al., 2002; Piolino et al., 2002). Here, episodic, but not semantic, recall appears highly reliant on the integrity of prefrontal lobe structures. Interestingly, a similar pattern of overgeneralized, highly semanticized recall has been observed in several groups of patients with psychiatric disorders that involve altered PFC function, such as schizophrenia (Riutort, Cuervo, Danion, Peretti, & Salame, 2003), posttraumatic stress disorder (McNally, Lasko, Macklin, & Pitman, 1995; McNally, Litz, Prassas, Shin, & Weathers, 1994; Meesters, Merckelbach, Tisserand, van den Hoorn, & Huygens, 1998; Rubin, Feldman, & Beckham, 2004), and depression (Hermans et al., 2004). In semantic dementia, personal semantic memory appears spared, possibly due to the temporal and spatial context provided by intact components of episodic recall that bolsters recall of related personal (but not general) semantic information (Snowden, Griffiths, & Neary, 1994, 1996; Westmacott & Moscovitch, 2003). Accordingly, it is important that current assessment techniques provide a reliable method of separating episodic and personal semantic components of recall. Otherwise, contamination by personal semantic information may inflate indices of episodic memory (Steinvorth et al., 2005).

The episodic–semantic distinction within autobiographical memory has also been examined in functional neuroimaging studies of healthy adults (Addis, Moscovitch, Crawley, & McAndrews, 2004; Graham, Lee, et al., 2003; Levine et al., 2004; Maguire & Frith, 2003; Maguire & Mummery, 1999). Overall, these studies have revealed more similarities than differences in PFC recruitment across these two autobiographical conditions. Although both episodic and autobiographical memory conditions are associated with anteromedial prefrontal activation (likely due to self-related information processing; see below), this has been greater for the personal episodic condition (Levine et al., 2004; Maguire & Frith, 2003; Maguire & Mummery, 1999), probably due to the connectivity of this region to medial temporal regions via the cingulum bundle. In contrast, Addis and colleagues (2004) found differences only with a lowered threshold, possibly due to method variance: This study compared single-occurrence memories to those that had occurred 10 or more times, whereas the other studies adopted a less stringent comparison, including autobiographical factual information in the semantic condition.

# SELF-AWARENESS

Self-referential processing can also be considered a key element of autobiographical memory. Indeed, self-referential processes may provide a basis for the development of autobiographical memory over time (Howe & Courage, 1997), are central to the social and directive function of autobiographical memory (Conway, 2003), and are fundamental to the human capacity for episodic memory (Tulving, 2002). According to Conway and Fthenaki (2000), the self-memory system is a superordinate, goal-based control system that is both informed by autobiographical knowledge and guides future behavior and the retrieval of events in accordance with currently activated goals (the "working self"). In this view, the self is considered both stable and adaptable on the basis of being shaped by previous incidents and general self-knowledge while coordinating the reconstruction of personal memories. Considerable data link self-related information processing to the PFC (Kelley et al., 2002; Stuss & Levine, 2002).

PFC damage appears requisite to amnestic syndromes in which self-awareness is clearly disrupted, most notably in cases of confabulation and reduplicative paramnesia (Alexander, Stuss, & Benson, 1979; Baddeley & Wilson, 1986; Moscovitch & Melo, 1997; Stuss, Alexander, Lieberman, & Levine, 1978). Put briefly, confabulation is the unintentional recollection of erroneous information that can be either plausible or completely bizarre. In either case, the patient is unaware of or unconcerned about the memory deficits and will hold his or her views with absolute conviction. Confabulation is most frequently reported for episodic information (Della Barba, 1993), although it has also been reported for semantic information (Moscovitch & Melo, 1997). In amnesics, confabulation is typically associated with damage to the ventromedial frontal region, PFC, and basal forebrain (Gilboa & Moscovitch, 2002; Schnider & Ptak, 1999), although damage to these regions does not necessarily imply the presence of confabulation.

Studies of patients with prefrontal damage provide support for the predominant explanation of confabulation as a symptom of impaired search and memory processes during memory retrieval (Gilboa & Moscovitch, 2002; Moscovitch, 1989). Executive dysfunction stemming from disinhibition, lack of self-monitoring, and decreased awareness, accompanied by an underlying memory impairment, is thought to lead to confabulation (DeLuca & Diamond, 1995; Moscovitch & Melo, 1997; Schnider, von Daniken, & Gutbrod, 1996). Without the proper functioning of such search and monitoring mechanisms, memories and their fragments may be retrieved out of context, out of order, or be overly influenced by the immediate social or physical environment. The ability to differentiate real events from thought content or imagined events may also be impaired. Consistent with this view, several researchers have reported that performance improvements on measures of executive functioning are associated with reduced confabulation in tests of patients with prefrontal damage, including the ventral PFC (Kapur & Coughlan, 1980; Papagno & Baddeley, 1997); other studies show an association between severity of executive dysfunction and extent of confabulation (DeLuca & Cicerone, 1991; Fischer, Alexander, D'Esposito, & Otto, 1995) following aneurysm of the anterior communicating artery. Notably, Moscovitch and Melo (1997) found that confabulating and nonconfabulating patients did not differ in degree of memory impairment, suggesting that amnesia is not sufficient, but may be necessary, for confabulation to be observed. They also documented confabulation for both episodic and semantic memory when increased retrieval demands were matched across these two conditions, indicating that previous findings of confabulation for episodic, but not semantic, autobiographical material (Della Barba, 1993) may be related to differential demands on strategic retrieval operations.

Other paramnestic syndromes associated with prefrontal damage can be regarded as disorders of temporally extended self-awareness. For example, Baddeley and Wilson (1986) reported the case of a patient with no concept of the link between his past and his present, who denied that he was the groom in photographs of his own wedding. The reduplicative paramnesias, including Capgras syndrome, are considered to arise from an inability to reconcile feelings of "warmth and intimacy" within episodic memory with perceptual or cognitive information (Stuss, 1991; Stuss, Picton, & Alexander, 2001). For example, upon returning home after a long absence due to a traumatic brain injury causing right frontotemporal damage, a patient encountered his teenage children grown, a new automobile, and his wife's new hairstyle. Unable to resolve the conflict between the two "versions" of his family, and lacking monitoring processes normally supported by the right PFC, the patient subsequently developed the delusion that his family had been duplicated (Alexander et al., 1979)

As noted earlier, functional neuroimaging studies of self-awareness have revealed activation in medial prefrontal regions (Brodmann's areas [BAs] 9, 10, usually on the left) when self-referential or internally oriented processing is manipulated (Craik et al., 1999; Fossati et al., 2003; Frith & Frith, 1999; Gusnard, Akbudak, Shulman, & Raichle, 2001; Johnson et al., 2002; Kelley et al., 2002; Zysset, Huber, Ferstl, & von Cramon, 2002). These same regions have been implicated in neuroimaging studies of autobiographical memory (see Figure 15.1; e.g., Addis et al., 2004; Conway et al., 1999; Levine et al., 2004). Indeed, activity in this region appears to distinguish autobiographical memory from laboratory-based episodic memory imaging studies (Gilboa, 2004).

Although functional neuroimaging studies of autobiographical memory have clearly implicated the PFC in self-related information processing within autobiographical memory, further work is needed to account for regional variability in these processes. For example, the robust left medial prefrontal activation observed in relation to self-reference and autobiographical memory in these studies would not have been predicted based on patient data, which stress ventral and right-lateralized locations in self-referential processing (Miller, Mychack, Seeley, Rosen, & Boone, 2001). Unilateral damage along the medial prefrontal wall is rare, and bilateral damage here causes severe deficits in arousal and initiation of behavior, possibly obscuring more subtle lesion effects. On the other hand, the functional neuroimaging findings may signal coactivation with connected posteromedial temporal lobe regions engaged by mnemonic stimuli rather than regional processing *necessary* for the task.

## FRONTOTEMPORAL INTERACTIONS

The synergistic interaction of the PFC and medial temporal regions for laboratory mnemonic tasks (Simons & Spiers, 2003) holds for autobiographical memory (Kopelman, 1991; Levine et al., 1998; Maguire, Henson, Mummery, & Frith, 2001). The MTL/hippocampal complex mediates the binding of mnemonic information into memory traces, whereas the PFC is involved in the activation and retrieval processing of these traces. When patients with frontal and temporal damage are compared directly on unstructured tests of episodic and semantic autobiographical memory, both groups show impairment, although the magnitude of deficit is greater in patients with bilateral prefrontal damage, likely due to the absence of appropriate cues to guide recall (Kopelman, Stanhope, & Kingsley, 1999).

As mentioned earlier, structured cueing may selectively reduce the memory deficit observed in patients with prefrontal, but not temporal lobe, damage. Specifically, Eslinger (1998) found that whereas a patient with bilateral prefrontal cortical damage was able to benefit from rigorous cueing of personal semantic and episodic memories, several amnestic patients with unilateral and bilateral temporal amnesia showed no such benefit.

Further evidence for the role of frontotemporal interactions in autobiographical memory can be derived from the case study literature on isolated (focal) retrograde amnesia (Kapur, 1999; Kopelman, 2000). Based on a review of this literature, Markowitsch (1995) hypothesized that the right uncinate fasciculus, connecting the anterior temporal with the ventral prefrontal cortex, is critical to autobiographical episodic memory retrieval. Evidence in support of this hypothesis was garnered from patients with large lesions. More specific support came from patient M. L., who could not recollect a single event from his preinjury past following recovery from a severe traumatic brain injury (Levine et al., 1998). Additionally, his anterograde memory, while relatively spared, had an impersonal quality, verified by impoverished "remember" responses on tests of delayed anterograde memory, which reflect impaired autonoetic consciousness (Gardiner, 1988; Tulving, 1985b). Upon examination with high-resolution structural magnetic resonance imaging (MRI), a prominent right ventral prefrontal lesion affecting the frontal projections of the uncinate fasciculus was discovered. Accordingly, M. L. showed right frontopolar hypoactivation in response to an anterograde episodic retrieval task in comparison to healthy controls and other matched patients with traumatic brain injury. In a follow-up study (Svoboda et al., 2005),

M. L.'s anterograde deficit was confirmed through quantitative autobiographical memory assessment (Levine et al., 2002). Interestingly, he demonstrated marked impairment of emotional recollection of autobiographical events relative to controls, suggesting disconnection of regions involved in emotional processing (e.g., right amygdala).

## EMOTION

Autobiographical remembering is inherently personal and is characterized by varying gradients of emotional content, yet most studies of autobiographical memory to date have not accounted separately for feeling states, such as joy or sadness, associated with the retrieval of emotional events from memory. Emotion is known to enhance recall of stimuli presented in the laboratory (Cahill et al., 1996; Canli, Zhao, Brewer, Gabrieli, & Cahill, 2000; Hamann, Cahill, McGaugh, & Squire, 1997; Hamann, Ely, Grafton, & Kilts, 1999). Within autobiographical memory, emotion has mostly been studied in the context of "flashbulb" memories, memories involving a high level of surprise and that are very arousing (e.g., the assassination of JFK—Brown & Kulik, 1977; Weaver, 1993).

The orbitofrontal cortex is involved in emotional processing (Damasio et al., 2000; Rolls, 2002) and shares extensive connections with other limbic regions, including the amygdala (Morecraft, Geula, & Mesulam, 1992) and MTL regions involved in recognition memory (Aggleton & Brown, 1999). To our knowledge, there are no studies directly investigating the effects of emotion on autobiographical memory in patients with prefrontal damage. Flashbulb memory has been assessed in older adults, who have mild prefrontal volume loss (Raz, 2000). The results, however, are conflicting, with some showing preservation (Davidson & Glisky, 2002; Gerdy, Multhaup, & Ivey, 2003) and others not (Cohen, Conway, & Maylor, 1994), probably due to method variance. Using the Autobiographical Interview, St.-Jacques and Levine (2006) showed enhanced richness for emotional autobiographical memory in both younger and older adults, but the overall pattern of an age-related bias towards semantic details remained.

Functional MRI (fMRI) studies of autobiographical memories unselected for emotion show secondary activation in the orbital PFC, bilaterally, but more so in the right hemisphere (e.g., Andreasen et al., 1995; Niki & Luo, 2002; Nyberg et al., 2002) . The extent of orbitofrontal contributions to memory and to emotion processes involved in autobiographical remembering as probed by fMRI is likely underestimated as a result of susceptibility artifact in this region due to its proximity to the nasal cavity and sphenoidal sinuses (Binder & Price, 2001).

When emotional events are probed directly with fMRI, bilateral or right-lateralized activation is observed, contrasting with the primarily left-lateralized findings from standardized autobiographical memory studies. The additional recruitment of right-hemisphere brain regions in emotional reexperiencing is consistent with other findings across numerous domains suggesting preferential right-hemisphere involvement in emotional processing (Shammi & Stuss, 1999; Stuss, Gallup, et al., 2001; Winner, Brownell, Happe, Blum, & Pincus, 1998; Winston, Strange, O'Doherty, & Dolan, 2002).

Activation in specific regions unique to emotional autobiographical memory studies primarily involved areas associated with emotional processing, including the insular and amygdalar cortices (Fink et al., 1996). Activation has also been reported in the orbitofrontal cortex in response to recall of happy (Markowitsch, Vandekerckhovel, Lanfermann, & Russ, 2003; Piefke et al., 2003) and of sad events (Markowitsch et al., 2003). This pattern of activation is consistent with the role of the orbitofrontal cortex in the representation of both positive and negative affective aspects of stimuli, and in the modulation of behavior in response to reward-related and punishment-related stimuli (Rolls, 2002).

Deactivation was also reported in most of the emotional autobiographical memory retrieval studies. The bulk of reported deactivation occurred in regions associated with cognitive processing (e.g., working memory, attention), including the lateral prefrontal and parietal cortex (Fink et al., 1996; Gemar et al., 1996; Levine, Turner, Graham, & Hevenor, in preparation). Deactivation in these cognitive regions may be related to the relatively automatic and less resource-demanding nature of recollecting emotional autobiographical memories, or to cognitive activity in the reference condition (e.g., neutral autobiographical memory retrieval, rest). However, these studies also activated many of the same regions as reported earlier for standard autobiographical retrieval tasks, suggesting that, in addition to emotion-related patterns of activation and deactivation, emotional autobiographical memory retrieval engages many of the same prefrontal regions involved in domain-general processing as does retrieval of everyday memories.

## AUTOBIOGRAPHICAL MEMORY IN PSYCHIATRIC DISORDERS

Overgeneralization of autobiographical memory has been reported in a number of psychiatric disorders involving altered PFC function. Specifically, in a pattern similar to that reported for older adults and patients with PFC syndromes, patients with psychiatric disorders involving altered PFC function (Bremner et al., 1997; Kapur & Remington, 1996; Mayberg et al., 1990), including schizophrenia (Riutort et al., 2003), PTSD (McNally et al., 1994, 1995; Meesters et al., 1998; Rubin et al., 2004) and depression (Barnhofer, Kuehn, & de Jong-Meyer, 2005; Burnside, Startup, Byatt, Rollinson, & Hill, 2004; Hermans et al., 2004; Iqbal, Birchwood, Hemsley, Jackson, & Morris, 2004; Mackinger et al., 2004; Mansell & Lam, 2004; Nandrino, Pezard, Poste, Reveillere, & Beaune, 2002), show a pattern of autobiographical memory recall that is characterized by iterative retrievals of overgeneral categorical or semantic memories.

Although the directionality of disease–memory effects have not been firmly established in these populations (see, e.g., Gibbs & Rude, 2004), there is reason to believe that alterations in PFC function may lead to autobiographical memory retrieval deficits similar to those observed in other populations with prefrontal deficits. For example, alterations in neuronal function in prefrontal and limbic regions, including the amygdala, hippocampus, orbital and medial PFC, superior prefrontal and inferior parietal cortex, and cingulate cortex, have been observed in posttraumatic stress disorder (PTSD) (Bremner et al., 1997, 1999; Driessen et al., 2004; Lanius et al., 2001; Liberzon et al., 1999; Osuch et al., 2001; Pissiota et al., 2002; Rauch et al., 1996, 2000; Shin et al., 1997, 1999). Decreased functioning of cognitive regions (e.g., dorsolateral PFC) associated with working memory and monitoring resources required for memory retrieval, cou-pled with overactivity of emotional processing regions (e.g., orbitofrontal cortex) associated with arousal and anxiety may reduce the likelihood of successful episodic recall in these populations. Moreover, research indicating that these patients are vulnerable to the encoding of false memories (Bremner, Krystal, Charney, & Southwick, 1996; Bremner, Shobe, & Kihlstrom, 2000) suggests further alterations in memory encoding and in source monitoring in these populations, mediated by abnormal prefrontal brain function (Clancy, Schacter, McNally, & Pitman, 2000; Qin et al., 2003).

## FUNCTIONAL RETROGRADE AMNESIA

Cases of functional retrograde amnesia are marked by severe remote memory loss in the absence of significant anterograde amnesia, and without any known brain injuries or disease (e.g., Markowitsch et al., 1997; Schacter, Wang, Tulving, & Freedman, 1982). Many of these patients have a significant premorbid psychiatric history and one or more precipitating factors for their amnesia (e.g., death of a loved one), with the onset of retrograde amnesia typically associated with a loss of personal identity (e.g., fugue; Kritchevsky, Chang, & Squire, 2004). In some cases, memory impairment is permanent, but in other cases, such as transient global amnesia, it resolves spontaneously (Kritchevsky, Squire, & Zouzounis, 1988).

Although altered PFC functioning has been proposed as a mechanism contributing to retrograde amnesia in these cases, the exact nature of this influence and the mediation of other brain regions is not yet firmly established (De Renzi, 2002; De Renzi, Lucchelli, Muggia, & Spinnler, 1997). For example, Kopelman (2000; 2002; see also Markowitsch, 2000) proposed a model suggesting that social and psychiatric factors associated with functional retrograde amnesia interact with the PFC to inhibit the retrieval of autobiographical memories in this disorder. Here, extreme arousal, depression, or past learning experiences of transient amnesia are thought to inhibit prefrontal control and executive systems involved in the retrieval of retrograde autobiographical memories. Anterograde learning, however, remains intact by virtue of intact medial temporal or diencephalic functioning that is invulnerable to this input.

Several case studies involving functional imaging methods have reported hypofrontality under positron emission tomographic (PET) imaging in patients with functional retrograde amnesia (Costello, Fletcher, Dolan, Frith, & Shallice, 1998; Glisky et al., 2004; Markowitsch et al., 1997; Starkstein, Sabe, & Dorrego, 1997; Stracciari, Ghidoni, Guarino, Poletti, & Pazzaglia, 1994) while attempting to recall memories acquired prior to the onset of retrograde amnesia. Fujiwara and colleagues (in press) recently reported enhanced activation in anterior prefrontal regions during recall of pre- versus postamnesia episodes; the authors attribute increases in activation in this region during recall of old memories to the greater retrieval effort required for amnestic memories. Although these studies point toward a prominent contribution of the PFC in autobiographical memory deficits involving functional amnesia, it is worth noting that altered function is observed in other brain regions in this disorder, including the temporal and parietal lobes (De Renzi & Lucchelli, 1993; Fujiwara et al., in press; Nakamura et al., 2002; Sellal, Manning, Seegmuller, Scheiber, & Schoenfelder, 2002; Stracciari et al., 1994).

Finally, other attempts to tie PFC function to functional retrograde amnesia using tests of neuropsychological function have proven somewhat inconclusive. Although correlations between functional retrograde amnesia and prefrontally mediated executive functions have been observed (Glisky et al., 2004; Kritchevsky et al., 2004), in some cases, this relation was observed within the context of extant correlations with other measures surveying functions mediated by nonprefrontal brain regions (e.g., Kritchevsky et al., 2004). Taken together, however, the results of the imaging and behavioral studies suggest that altered PFC function may play a role in functional retrograde amnesia with either reduced prefrontal functioning due to anxiety triggered by environmental stressors (Kopelman, 2000, 2002; Markowitsch, 2000) or increased prefrontal activation in regions associated with retrieval effort (Fujiwara et al., in press).

## CONCLUSIONS

Our review of the current theoretical and empirical literature surrounding autobiographical memory indicates that the PFC plays a prominent role in the recollection of memories unselected for emotional content, as well as in emotional memory retrieval. We have emphasized the influence of diverse behavioral and neuroimaging methods in revealing this contribution, with current assessment techniques focused on the careful application of retrieval support to compensate for prefrontal dysfunction, separation of different components of memory (e.g., episodic and semantic), and cueing as a method of eliciting recall.

Consistent with the view that autobiographical memory arises from the interaction of multiple memory systems and brain regions engaging domain-specific and domain-general resources, prefrontal contributions to autobiographical memory are multifaceted, engaging diverse cortical regions. For example, dorsal and ventral lateral prefrontal regions implicated in neuroimaging studies of autobiographical memory appear to mediate preferentially executive and cognitive control operations involved in memory recall. Accordingly, numerous tests of executive function correlate with autobiographical memory performance. Moreover, patients with damage to these regions show intrusions, preseverations, and source confusions on tests of autobiographical memory, along with impoverished access to specific episodic representations; retrieval support may selectively reduce these deficits by compensating for impaired search and retrieval processes.

Confabulation or reduplicative paramnesia are disorders of autobiographical memory stemming from deficits of self-awareness and impaired search and monitoring processes accompanying frontal lobe insult. Medial prefrontal regions are commonly activated in neuroimaging studies of autobiographical memory and appear involved in self-referential aspects of memory retrieval. Additional prefrontal cortical regions, most prominently the orbitofrontal cortex, appear requisite for retrieval of highly emotional events, being activated across neuroimaging studies of emotional memories and memories unselected for emotional content. Recall of emotional autobiographical memories appears to selectively activate regions involved in emotional memory (e.g., orbifrontal cortex) and deactivate regions involved in cognitive processing (e.g., lateral frontal cortex). Selective preservation of orbitofrontal cortex, relative to dorsolateral PFC, in older adults results in enhanced episodic richness of emotional memories compared to memory for events unselected for emotional content. By contrast, emotional recollection appears selectively impaired in patients with ventral prefrontal lesions.

PFC contributions to autobiographical memory occur in synergistic interaction with the operation of the MTL, where the MTL/hippocampal complex mediates the binding of mnemonic information into memory traces, and the PFC is involved in the activation and retrieval processing of these traces. Accordingly, retrieval supports may enhance autobiographical recall in patients with damage to PFC, but are unsuccessful in ameliorating retrieval deficits in patients with damage to MTL/hippocampal regions.

Altered prefrontal function in psychiatric disorders, including PTSD, schizophrenia, and depression, leads to a pattern of autobiographical recall characterized by iterative retrieval of overgeneral or categoric memories; this pattern is similar to that observed in patients with other frontal lobe syndromes (FTLD, cognitive aging) and in patients with focal frontal lesions. Altered prefrontal function may also play a role in functional retrograde amnesia involving severe remote memory loss in the absence of significant anterograde amnesia, and without any known brain injuries or disease. Both reduced prefrontal functioning due to anxiety triggered by environmental stressors and increased prefrontal activation in regions associated with retrieval effort has been observed in this disorder.

Finally, the study of prefrontal contributions to autobiographical memory has enhanced our understanding of the component structure of memory. In retrograde amnesia, both semantic and episodic components of autobiographical memory are affected, but the effects are greater for episodic memory, especially when the PFC is affected. The pattern of memory impairment observed in these patients appears related to the extent of neural damage and the type of memory assessment tool administered. In functional neuroimaging studies of older adults, differences in activation have been observed across single-occurrence memories and those that occurred multiple times, as well as memories with differing episodic and semantic content. Differential activation in these studies is likely related to the engagement of these differential components of autobiographical recall, as well as method variance.

As illustrated in Elizabeth Loftus's experiment, autobiographical memory is an essentially reconstructive process. It ultimately recruits multiple brain regions and cognitive processes in service of its construction. We have reviewed here the contribution of the PFC to autobiographical memory. Autobiographical memory is essential to self-identity and allows for the transmission of human culture and history. Future work aimed at revealing the temporal sequencing and interactivity of prefrontal and posterior regions will guide our understanding of autobiographical memory and its component and integrative structure.

## REFERENCES

Addis, D. R., Moscovitch, M., Crawley, A. P., & McAndrews, M. P. (2004). Recollective qualities modulate hippocampal activation during autobiographical memory retrieval. *Hippocampus, 14*(6), 752–762.

Aggleton, J. P., & Brown, M. W. (1999). Episodic memory, amnesia, and the hippocampal-anterior thalamic axis. *Behavioural and Brain Sciences, 22*(3), 425–444; discussion, 444–489.

Alexander, M. P., Stuss, D. T., & Benson, D. F. (1979). Capgras syndrome: A reduplicative phenomenon. *Neurology, 29*, 334–339.

Andreasen, N. C., O'Leary, D. S., Cizadlo, T., Arndt, S., Rezai, K., Watkins, G. L., et al. (1995). Remembering the past: Two facets of episodic memory explored with positron emission tomography. *American Journal of Psychiatry, 152*, 1576–1585.

Andreasen, N. C., O'Leary, D. S., Paradiso, S., Cizadlo, T., Arndt, S., Watkins, G. L., et al. (1999). The cerebellum plays a role in conscious episodic memory retrieval. *Human Brain Mapping, 8*, 226–234.

Baddeley, A., & Wilson, B. (1986). Amnesia, autobiographical memory, and confabulation. In D. C. Rubin (Ed.), *Autobiographical memory* (pp. 225–252). Cambridge, UK: Cambridge University Press.

Barnett, M. P., Newman, H. W., Richardson, J. T., Thompson, P., & Upton, D. (2000). The constituent structure of autobiographical memory: Autobiographical fluency in people with chronic epilepsy. *Memory, 8*(6), 413–424.

Barnhofer, T., Kuehn, E. M., & de Jong-Meyer, R. (2005). Specificity of autobiographical memories and basal cortisol levels in patients with major depression. *Psychoneuroendocrinology, 30*(4), 403–411.

Bartlett, F. C. (1932). *Remembering: A study in experimental and social psychology.* New York: Cambridge University Press.

Bayley, P. J., Hopkins, R. O., & Squire, L. R. (2003). Successful recollection of remote autobiographical memories by amnesic patients with medial temporal lobe lesions. *Neuron, 38*(1), 135–144.

Bernstein, D. M., Laney, C., Morris, E. K., & Loftus, E. F. (2005). False memories about food can lead to food avoidance. *Social Cognition, 23*(1), 11–34.

Binder, J., & Price, C. J. (2001). Functional neuroimaging of language. In R. Cabeza & A. Kingstone (Eds.), *Handbook of functional neuroimaging of cognition* (pp. 187–252). Cambridge, MA: MIT Press.

Bremner, J. D. (1999). Neural correlates of memories of childhood sexual abuse in women with and without posttraumatic stress disorder. *American Journal of Psychiatry, 156*(11), 1787–1795.

Bremner, J. D., Innis, R. B., Ng, C. K., Staib, L. H., Salomon, R. M., Bronen, R. A., et al. (1997). Positron emission tomography measurement of cerebral metabolic correlates of yohimbine administration in combat-related posttraumatic stress disorder. *Archives of General Psychiatry, 54*(3), 246–254.

Bremner, J. D., Krystal, J. H., Charney, D. S., & Southwick, S. M. (1996). Neural mechanisms in dissociative amnesia for childhood abuse: Relevance to the current controversy surrounding the "false memory syndrome." *American Journal of Psychiatry, 153*(Suppl. 7), 71–82.

Bremner, J. D., Shobe, K. K., & Kihlstrom, J. F. (2000). False memories in women with self-reported childhood sexual abuse: An empirical study. *Psychological Science, 11*(4), 333–337.

Brewer, W. F. (1986). What is autobiographical memory? In D. C. Rubin (Ed.), *Autobiographical memory* (pp. 25–49). New York: Cambridge University Press.

Brown, R., & Kulik, J. (1977). Flashbulb memories. *Cognition, 5*, 73–99.

Bruce, D., Dolan, A., & Phillips-Grant, K. (2000). On the transition from childhood amnesia to the recall of personal memories. *Psychological Science, 11*(5), 360–364.

Buckner, R. L., Koutstaal, W., Schacter, D. L., Wagner, A. D., & Rosen, B. R. (1998). Functional–anatomic study of episodic retrieval using fMRI: I. Retrieval effort versus retrieval success. *NeuroImage, 7*(3), 151–162.

Burgess, P. W., & Shallice, T. (1996a). Confabulation and the control of recollection. *Memory, 4*(4), 359–411.

Burgess, P. W., & Shallice, T. (1996b). Response suppression, initiation, and strategy use following frontal lobe lesions. *Neuropsychologia, 34*, 263–273.

Burnside, E., Startup, M., Byatt, M., Rollinson, L., & Hill, J. (2004). The role of overgeneral autobiographical memory in the development of adult depression following childhood trauma. *British Journal of Clinical Psychology, 43*(4), 365–376.

Butters, N., & Cermak, L. S. (1986). A case study of the forgetting of autobiographical knowledge: Implications for the study of retrograde amnesia. In D. C. Rubin (Ed.), *Autobiographical memory* (pp. 253–272). Cambridge, UK: Cambridge University Press.

Cabeza, R., Anderson, N. D., Kester, J., Lennartsson, E. R., & McIntosh, A. R. (2001). Involvement of prefrontal regions on episodic retrieval: Evidence for a generate–recognize asymmetry model. *Brain and Cognition, 47*, 62–66.

Cabeza, R., Prince, S. E., Daselaar, S. M., Greenberg, D. L., Budde, M., Dolcos, F., et al. (2004). Brain activity during episodic retrieval of autobiographical and laboratory events: An fMRI study using a novel photo paradigm. *Journal of Cognitive Neuroscience, 16*(9), 1583–1594.

Cahill, L., Haier, R. J., Fallon, J., Alkire, M. T., Tang, C., Keator, D., et al. (1996). Amygdala activity at encoding correlated with long-term, free recall of emotional information. *Proceedings of the National Academy of Sciences of the United States of America, 93*(15), 8016–8021.

Canli, T., Zhao, Z., Brewer, J., Gabrieli, J. D., & Cahill, L. (2000). Event-related activation in the human amygdala associates with later memory for individual emotional experience. *Journal of Neuroscience, 20*(19), RC99.

Case, R. (1974). Mental strategies, mental capacity and instruction: A neo-Piagetian perspective. *Journal of Experimental Child Psychology, 18*, 382–397.

Case, R., Kurland, M., & Goldberg, J. (1982). Operational efficiency and the growth of short-term memory span. *Journal of Experimental Child Psychology, 33*, 386–404.

Cermak, L. S. (1985). The episodic–semantic distinction in amnesia. In L. R. Squire & N. Butters (Eds.), *Neuropsychology of memory* (pp. 55–62). New York: Guilford Press.

Clancy, S. A., Schacter, D. L., McNally, R. J., & Pitman, R. K. (2000). False recognition in women reporting recovered memories of sexual abuse. *Psychological Science, 11*(1), 26–31.

Cohen, G. (2000). Hierarchical models in cognition: Do they have psychological reality? *European Journal of Cognitive Psychology, 12*(1), 1–36.

Cohen, G., Conway, M. A., & Maylor, E. A. (1994). Flashbulb memories in older adults. *Psychology and Aging, 9*(3), 454–463.

Conway, M. A. (2001). Sensory–perceptual episodic memory and its context: Autobiographical memory. *Philosophical Transactions of the Royal Society of London, Series B, Biological Sciences, 356*, 1375–1384.

Conway, M. A. (2003). Commentary: Cognitive-affective mechanisms and processes in autobiographical memory. *Memory, 11*(2), 217–224.

Conway, M. A., & Bekerian, D. A. (1987). Organization in autobiographical memory. *Memory and Cognition, 15*(2), 119–132.

Conway, M. A., & Fthenaki, A. (2000). Disruption and loss of autobiographical memory. In L. Cermak (Ed.), *Handbook of neuropsychology: Memory and its disorders* (2nd ed., pp. 257–288). Amsterdam: Elsevier.

Conway, M. A., Pleydell-Pearce, C. W., & Whitecross,

S. E. (2001). The neuroanatomy of autobiographical memory: A slow cortical potential study of autobiographical memory retrieval. *Journal of Memory and Language, 45,* 493–524.

Conway, M. A., Pleydell-Pearce, C. W., Whitecross, S., & Sharpe, H. (2002). Brain imaging autobiographical memory. *Psychology of Learning and Motivation, 41,* 229–264.

Conway, M. A., Turk, D. J., Miller, S. L., Logan, J., Nebes, R. D., Meltzer, C. C., et al. (1999). A positron emission tomography (PET) study of autobiographical memory retrieval. *Memory, 7*(5–6), 679–702.

Costello, A., Fletcher, P. D., Dolan, R. J., Frith, C. D., & Shallice, T. (1998). The origins of forgetting in a case of isolated retrograde amnesia following a hemorrhage: Evidence from functional neuroimaging. *Neurocase, 4,* 437–466.

Craik, F. I. M., & Grady, C. L. (2002). Aging, memory, and frontal lobe functioning. In D. T. Stuss & R. Knight (Eds.), *Principles of frontal lobe function* (pp. 528–540). New York: Oxford University Press.

Craik, F. I. M., & McDowd, J. M. (1987). Age differences in recall and recognition. *Journal of Experimental Psychology: Learning, Memory, and Cognition, 13*(3), 474–479.

Craik, F. I. M., Moroz, T. M., Moscovitch, M., Stuss, D. T., Winocur, G., Tulving, E., et al. (1999). In search of the self: A positron emission tomography study. *Psychological Science, 10,* 27–35.

Crovitz, H. F., & Schiffman, H. (1974). Frequency of episodic memories as a function of their age. *Bulletin of the Psychonomic Society, 4,* 517–518.

Damasio, A. R., Grabowski, T. J., Bechara, A., Damasio, H., Ponto, L. L., Parvizi, J., et al. (2000). Subcortical and cortical brain activity during the feeling of self-generated emotions. *Nature Neuroscience, 3*(10), 1049–1056.

Davidson, P. S. R., & Glisky, E. L. (2002). Is flashbulb memory a special instance of source memory?: Evidence from older adults. *Memory, 10*(2), 99–111.

Della Barba, G. (1993). Confabulation: Knowledge and recollective experience. *Cognitive Neuropsychology, 10,* 1–20.

Della Sala, S., Laiacona, M., Spinnler, H., & Trivelli, C. (1993). Autobiographical recollection and frontal damage. *Neuropsychologia, 31*(8), 823–839.

DeLuca, J., & Cicerone, K. D. (1991). Confabulation following aneurysm of the anterior communicating artery. *Cortex, 27*(3), 417–423.

DeLuca, J., & Diamond, B. J. (1995). Aneurysm of the anterior communicating artery: A review of the neuroanatomical and neuropsychological sequelae. *Journal of Clinical and Experimental Neuropsychology, 17,* 100–121.

De Renzi, E. (2002). What does psychogen mean? *Cortex, 38,* 678–681.

De Renzi, E., & Lucchelli, F. (1993). Dense retrograde amnesia, intact learning capability and abnormal forgetting rate: A consolidation deficit? *Cortex, 29*(3), 449–466.

De Renzi, E., Lucchelli, F., Muggia, S., & Spinnler, H. (1997). Is memory loss without anatomical damage tantamount to a psychogenic deficit?: The case of pure retrograde amnesia. *Neuropsychologia, 35*(6), 781–794.

D'Esposito, M., Postle, B. R., Ballard, D., & Lease, J. (1999). Maintenance versus manipulation of information held in working memory: An event-related fMRI study. *Brain and Cognition, 41*(1), 66–86.

Driessen, M., Beblo, T., Mertens, M., Piefke, M., Rullkoetter, N., Silva-Saavedra, A., et al. (2004). Posttraumatic stress disorder and fMRI activation patterns of traumatic memory in patients with borderline personality disorder. *Biological Psychiatry, 55*(6), 603–611.

Dusoir, H., Kapur, N., Byrnes, D., McKinstry, S., & Hoare, R. (1990). The role of diencephalic pathology in human memory disorder: Evidence from a penetrating paranasal brain injury. *Brain, 113,* 1695–1706.

Eslinger, P. J. (1998). Autobiographical memory after temporal lobe lesions. *Neurocase, 4*(6), 481–495.

Fink, G. R., Markowitsch, H. J., Reinkemeier, M., Bruckbauer, T., Kessler, J., & Heiss, W. (1996). Cerebral representation of one's own past: Neural networks involved in autobiographical memory. *Journal of Neuroscience, 16*(13), 4275–4282.

Fischer, R. S., Alexander, M. P., D'Esposito, M., & Otto, R. (1995). Neuropsychological and neuroanatomical correlates of confabulation. *Journal of Clinical and Experimental Neuropsychology, 17*(1), 20–28.

Fivush, R., & Hamond, N. R. (1990). Autobiographical memory across the preschool years: Toward reconceptualizing childhood amnesia. In R. Fivush & J. A. Hudson (Eds.), *Knowing and remembering in young children: Emory Symposia in Cognition* (Vol. 3, pp. 223–248). Cambridge, UK: Cambridge University Press.

Fletcher, P. C., Happe, F., Frith, U., Baker, S. C., Dolan, R. J., Frackowiak, R. S., et al. (1995). Other minds in the brain: A functional imaging study of "theory of mind" in story comprehension. *Cognition, 57*(2), 109–128.

Fletcher, P. C., & Henson, R. N. (2001). Frontal lobes and human memory: Insights from functional neuroimaging. *Brain, 124*(5), 849–881.

Fossati, P., Hevenor, S. J., Graham, S. J., Grady, C., Keightley, M. L., Craik, F., et al. (2003). In search of the emotional self: An FMRI study using positive and negative emotional words. *American Journal of Psychiatry, 160*(11), 1938–1945.

Freud, S. (1982). An early memory from Goethe's autobiography. In U. Neisser (Ed.), *Memory observed: Remembering in natural contexts* (pp. 64–72). New York: Freeman.

Frith, C. D., & Frith, U. (1999). Interacting minds—a biological basis. *Science, 286,* 1692–1695.

Fujiwara, E., Brand, M., Kracht, L., Kessler, J., Diebel, A., Netz, J., et al. (in press). Functional retrograde amnesia: A multiple case study. *Cortex.*

Galton, F. (1879). Psychometric experiments. *Brain, 2,* 149–162.

Galton, F. (1907). *Inquiries into human faculty and its development.* London: Dent.

Gardiner, J. M. (1988). Functional aspects of recollective experience. *Memory and Cognition, 16,* 309–313.

Gemar, M. C., Kapur, S., Segal, Z. V., Brown, G. M., & Houle, S. (1996). Effects of self-generated sad mood on regional cerebral activity: A PET study in normal subjects. *Depression, 4*(2), 81–88.

Gerdy, J., Multhaup, K. S., & Ivey, P. (2003, March). *Flashbulb memories in older and younger adults.* Poster presented at the annual meeting of the Southeastern Psychological Association, New Orleans, LA.

Gibbs, B. R., & Rude, S. S. (2004). Overgeneral autobiographical memory as depression vulnerability. *Cognitive Therapy and Research, 28*(4), 511–526.

Gilboa, A. (2004). Autobiographical and episodic memory—one and the same?: Evidence from prefrontal activation in neuroimaging studies. *Neuropsychologia, 42*(10), 1336–1349.

Gilboa, A., & Moscovitch, M. (2002). The cognitive neuroscience of confabulation: A review and a model. In A. D. Baddeley, M. D. Kopelman, & B. A. Wilson (Eds.), *The handbook of memory disorders* (2nd ed., pp. 315–342). Chichester, UK: Wiley.

Gilboa, A., Winocur, G., Grady, C. L., Hevenor, S. J., & Moscovitch, M. (2004). Remembering our past: Functional neuroanatomy of recollection of recent and very remote personal events. *Cerebral Cortex, 14,* 1214–1225.

Glisky, E. L., Ryan, L., Reminger, S., Hardt, O., Hayes, S. M., & Hupbach, A. (2004). A case of psychogenic fugue: I understand, *aber ich verstehe nichts. Neuropsychologia, 42*(8), 1132–1147.

Gopnik, A., & Graf, P. (1988). Knowing how you know: Young children's ability to identify and remember the sources of their beliefs. *Child Development, 59*(5), 1366–1371.

Graham, K. S., & Hodges, J. R. (1997). Differentiating the roles of the hippocampal complex and the neocortex in long-term memory storage: Evidence from the study of semantic dementia and Alzheimer's disease. *Neuropsychology, 11*(1), 77–89.

Graham, K. S., Kropelnicki, A., Goldman, W. P., & Hodges, J. R. (2003). Two further investigations of autobiographical memory in semantic dementia. *Cortex, 39*(4–5), 729–750.

Graham, K. S., Lee, A. C. H., Brett, M., & Patterson, K. (2003). The neural basis of autobiographical and semantic memory: New evidence from three PET studies. *Cognitive, Affective and Behavioral Neuroscience, 3*(3), 234–254.

Greene, J. D., Hodges, J. R., & Baddeley, A. D. (1995). Autobiographical memory and executive function in early dementia of Alzheimer type. *Neuropsychologia, 33*(12), 1647–1670.

Greene, J. D., Sommerville, R. B., Nystrom, L. E., Darley, J. M., & Cohen, J. D. (2001). An fMRI investigation of emotional engagement in moral judgment. *Science, 293,* 2105–2108.

Grossi, D., Trojano, L., Grasso, A., & Orsini, A. (1988). Selective "semantic amnesia" after closed-head injury: A case report. *Cortex, 24,* 457–464.

Gusnard, D. A., Akbudak, E., Shulman, G. L., & Raichle, M. E. (2001). Medial prefrontal cortex and self-referential mental activity: Relation to a default mode of brain function. *Proceedings of the National Academy of Sciences of the United States of America, 98*(7), 4259–4264.

Hamann, S. B., Cahill, L., McGaugh, J. L., & Squire, L. R. (1997). Intact enhancement of declarative memory for emotional material in amnesia. *Learning and Memory, 4*(3), 301–309.

Hamann, S. B., Ely, T. D., Grafton, S. T., & Kilts, C. D. (1999). Amygdala activity related to enhanced memory for pleasant and aversive stimuli. *Nature Neuroscience, 2*(3), 289–293.

Henson, R. N. A., Shallice, T., & Dolan, R. J. (1999). Right prefrontal cortex and episodic memory retrieval: A functional MRI test of the monitoring hypothesis. *Brain, 122,* 1367–1381.

Hermans, D., Van den Broeck, K., Belis, G., Raes, F., Pieters, G., & Eelen, P. (2004). Trauma and autobiographical memory specificity in depressed inpatients. *Behaviour Research and Therapy, 42*(7), 775–789.

Howe, M. L., & Courage, M. L. (1997). The emergence and early development of autobiographical memory. *Psychological Review, 104*(3), 499–523.

Hudson, J. A., & Fivush, R. (1991). As time goes by: Sixth graders remember a kindergarten experience. *Applied Cognitive Psychology, 5*(4), 347–360.

Iqbal, Z., Birchwood, M., Hemsley, D., Jackson, C., & Morris, E. (2004). Autobiographical memory and post-psychotic depression in first episode psychosis. *British Journal of Clinical Psychology, 43*(1), 97–104.

Johnson, M. K. (1988). Reality monitoring: An experimental phenomenological approach. *Journal of Experimental Psychology: General, 117,* 390–394.

Johnson, M. K., Foley, M. A., Suengas, A. G., & Raye, C. L. (1988). Phenomenal characteristics of memories for perceived and imagined autobiographical events. *Journal of Experimental Psychology: General, 117*(4), 371–376.

Johnson, M. K., & Raye, C. L. (1981). Reality monitoring. *Psychological Review, 88,* 67–85.

Johnson, S. C., Baxter, L. C., Wilder, L. S., Pipe, J. G., Heiserman, J. E., & Prigatano, G. P. (2002). Neural correlates of self-reflection. *Brain, 125*(8), 1808–1814.

Kapur, N. (1999). Syndromes of retrograde amnesia: A conceptual and empirical synthesis. *Psychological Bulletin, 125*(6), 800–825.

Kapur, N., & Coughlan, A. K. (1980). Confabulation and frontal lobe dysfunction. *Journal of Neurology, Neurosurgery, and Psychiatry, 43*(5), 461–463.

Kapur, N., Scholey, K., Moore, E., Barker, S., Mayes, A., Brice, J., et al. (1994). The mammillary bodies revisited: Their role in human memory functioning. In L. Cermak (Ed.), *Neuropsychological explorations of memory and cognition: Essays in honor of Nelson Butters* (pp. 159–189). New York: Plenum Press.

Kapur, S., & Remington, G. (1996). Serotonin–dopamine interaction and its relevance to schizophrenia. *American Journal of Psychiatry, 153*(4), 466–476.

Kelley, W. M., Macrae, C. N., Wyland, C. L., Caglar, S., Inati, S., & Heatherton, T. F. (2002). Finding the self?: An event-related fMRI study. *Journal of Cognitive Neuroscience, 14*, 785–794.

Kopelman, M. D. (1986). The cholinergic neurotransmitter system in human memory and dementia: A review. *Quarterly Journal of Experimental Psychology, 38A*, 535–573.

Kopelman, M. D. (1989). Remote and autobiographical memory, temporal context memory and frontal atrophy in Korsakoff and Alzheimer patients. *Neuropsychologia, 27*(4), 437–460.

Kopelman, M. D. (1991). Frontal dysfunction and memory deficits in the alcoholic Korsakoff syndrome and Alzheimer-type dementia. *Brain, 114*, 117–137.

Kopelman, M. D. (1994). The Autobiographical Memory Interview (AMI) in organic and psychogenic amnesia. *Memory, 2*(2), 211–235.

Kopelman, M. D. (2000). Focal retrograde amnesia and the attribution of causality: An exceptionally critical review. *Cognitive Neuropsychology, 17*(7), 585–621.

Kopelman, M. D. (2002). Disorders of memory. *Brain, 125*(10), 2152–2190.

Kopelman, M. D., & Kapur, N. (2001). The loss of episodic memories in retrograde amnesia: Single-case and group studies. *Philosophical Transactions of the Royal Society of London, Series B: Biological Sciences, 356*, 1409–1421.

Kopelman, M. D., Stanhope, N., & Kingsley, D. (1999). Retrograde amnesia in patients with diencephalic, temporal lobe or frontal lesions. *Neuropsychologia, 37*, 939–958.

Kopelman, M. D., Wilson, B. A., & Baddeley, A. D. (1990). *The Autobiographical Memory Interview*. Bury, St. Edmunds, UK: Thames Valley Test Company.

Kritchevsky, M., Chang, J., & Squire, L. R. (2004). Functional amnesia: Clinical description and neuropsychological profile of 10 cases. *Learning and Memory, 11*(2), 213–226.

Kritchevsky, M., Squire, L. R., & Zouzounis, J. A. (1988). Transient global amnesia: Characterization of anterograde and retrograde amnesia. *Neurology, 38*(2), 213–219.

Lanius, R. A., Williamson, P. C., Densmore, M., Boksman, K., Gupta, M. A., Neufeld, R. W., et al. (2001). Neural correlates of traumatic memories in posttraumatic stress disorder: A functional MRI investigation. *American Journal of Psychiatry, 158*(11), 1920–1922.

Laurent-Demir, C., & Jaffard, R. (1997). Temporally extended retrograde amnesia for spatial information resulting from afterdischarges induced by electrical stimulation of the dorsal hippocampus in mice. *Psychobiology, 25*, 133–140.

Levine, B. (2004). Autobiographical memory and the self in time: Brain lesion effects, functional neuroanatomy, and lifespan development. *Brain and Cognition, 55*(1), 54–68.

Levine, B., Black, S. E., Cabeza, R., Sinden, M., Mcintosh, A. R., Toth, J. P., et al. (1998). Episodic memory and the self in a case of isolated retrograde amnesia. *Brain, 121*, 1951–1973.

Levine, B., Svoboda, E., Hay, J., Winocur, G., & Moscovitch, M. (2002). Aging and autobiographical memory: Dissociating episodic from semantic retrieval. *Psychology and Aging, 17*, 677–689.

Levine, B., Turner, G. R., Graham, S. J., & Hevenor, S. J. *Emotional re-experiencing in the human brain: An fMRI study of flashbulb memory.* Manuscript in preparation.

Levine, B., Turner, G. R., Tisserand, D. J., Hevenor, S. J., Graham, S. J., & McIntosh, A. R. (2004). The functional neuroanatomy of episodic and semantic autobiographical remembering: A prospective functional fMRI study. *Journal of Cognitive Neuroscience, 16*(9), 1633–1646.

Liberzon, I., Taylor, S. F., Amdur, R., Jung, T. D., Chamberlain, K. R., Minoshima, S., et al. (1999). Brain activation in PTSD in response to trauma-related stimuli. *Biological Psychiatry, 45*(7), 817–826.

Luria, A. R. (1980). *Higher cortical functioning in man.* New York: Basic Books.

Mackinger, H. F., Leibetseder, M. F., Kunz-Dorfer, A. A., Fartacek, R. R., Whitworth, A. B., & Feldinger, F. F. (2004). Autobiographical memory predicts the course of depression during detoxification therapy in alcohol dependent men. *Journal of Affective Disorders, 78*(1), 61–65.

Maguire, E. A. (2001). Neuroimaging studies of autobiographical event memory. *Philosophical Transactions of the Royal Society of London, Series B, Biological Sciences, 356*, 1441–1451.

Maguire, E. A., & Frith, C. D. (2003). Lateral asymmetry in the hippocampal response to the remoteness of autobiographical memories. *Journal of Neuroscience, 23*(12), 5302–5307.

Maguire, E. A., Henson, R. N. A., Mummery, C. J., & Frith, C. D. (2001). Activity in prefrontal cortex, not hippocampus, varies parametrically with the increasing remoteness of memories. *NeuroReport* [Special Issue], *12*(3), 441–444.

Maguire, E. A., & Mummery, C. J. (1999). Differential modulation of a common memory retrieval network revealed by positron emission tomography. *Hippocampus, 9*(1), 54–61.

Mansell, W., & Lam, D. (2004). A preliminary study of autobiographical memory in remitted bipolar and unipolar depression and the role of imagery in the specificity of memory. *Memory, 12*(4), 437–446.

Markowitsch, H. J. (1995). Anatomical basis of memory disorders. In M. S. Gazzaniga (Ed.), *The cognitive neurosciences* (pp. 765–779). Cambridge, MA: MIT Press.

Markowitsch, H. J. (2000). Repressed memories. In E. Tulving (Ed.), *Memory, consciousness, and the brain: The Tallinn conference* (pp. 319–330). Philadelphia: Psychology Press/Taylor & Francis.

Markowitsch, H. J., Calabrese, P., Fink, G. R., Durwen, H. F., Kessler, J., Harting, C., et al. (1997). Impaired episodic memory retrieval in a case of probable psychogenic amnesia. *Psychiatry Research, 74,* 119–126.

Markowitsch, H. J., Vandekerckhovel, M. M., Lanfermann, H., & Russ, M. O. (2003). Engagement of lateral and medial prefrontal areas in the ecphory of sad and happy autobiographical memories. *Cortex, 39*(4–5), 643–665.

Mayberg, H. S., Starkstein, S. E., Sadzot, B., Preziosi, T., Andrezejewski, P. L., Dannals, R. F., et al. (1990). Selective hypometabolism in the inferior frontal lobe in depressed patients with Parkinson's disease. *Annals of Neurology, 28*(1), 57–64.

McKinnon, M. C., Miller, B., Black, S., Moscovitch, M., & Levine, B. (2006). *Autobiographical memory in semantic dementia: Implications for theories of limbic-neocortical interaction in remote memory.* Manuscript under revision.

McNally, R. J., Lasko, N. B., Macklin, M. L., & Pitman, R. K. (1995). Autobiographical memory disturbance in combat-related posttraumatic stress disorder. *Behaviour Research and Therapy, 33*(6), 619–630.

McNally, R. J., Litz, B. T., Prassas, A., Shin, L. M., & Weathers, F. W. (1994). Emotional priming of autobiographical memory in post-traumatic stress disorder. *Cognition and Emotion, 8*(4), 351–367.

Meesters, C., Merckelbach, H., Tisserand, D., van den Hoorn, M., & Huygens, K. (1998). Trauma and autobiographical memory in adolescents. *Kind en Adolescent, 19*(2), 274–282.

Miller, B. L., Mychack, P., Seeley, W. W., Rosen, H. J., & Boone, K. (2001). Neuroanatomy of the self: Evidence from patients with fronto-temporal dementia. *Neurology, 57,* 817–821.

Moll, J., de Oliveira-Souza, R., Eslinger, P. J., Bramati, I. E., Mourao-Miranda, J., Andreiuolo, P. A., et al. (2002). The neural correlates of moral sensitivity: A functional magnetic resonance imaging investigation of basic and moral emotions. *Journal of Neuroscience, 22*(7), 2730–2736.

Morecraft, R. J., Geula, C., & Mesulam, M. M. (1992). Cytoarchitecture and neural afferents of orbitofrontal cortex in the brain of the monkey. *Journal of Comparative Neurology, 323*(3), 341–358.

Moscovitch, M. (1989). Confabulation and the frontal systems: Strategic versus associative retrieval in neuropsychological theories of memory. In H. L. Roediger & F. I. M. Craik (Eds.), *Varieties of memory and consciousness: Essays in honor of Endel Tulving* (pp. 133–160). Hillsdale, NJ: Erlbaum.

Moscovitch, M. (1992). Memory and working-with-memory: A component process model based on modules and central systems. *Journal of Cognitive Neuroscience, 4,* 257–267.

Moscovitch, M., & Melo, B. (1997). Strategic retrieval and the frontal lobes: Evidence from confabulation and amnesia. *Neuropsychologia, 35*(7), 1017–1034.

Moscovitch, M., & Nadel, L. (1998). Consolidation and the hippocampal complex revisited: In defense of the multiple-trace model. *Current Opinion in Neurobiology, 8*(2), 297–300.

Moscovitch, M., Yaschyshyn, T., Ziegler, M., & Nadel, L. (2000). Remote episodic memory and retrograde amnesia: Was Endel Tulving right all along? In E. Tulving (Ed.), *Memory, consciousness, and the brain: The Tallinn conference* (pp. 331–345). Philadelphia: Psychology Press/Taylor & Francis.

Moss, H. E., Kopelman, M., Cappelletti, M., De Mornay Davies, P., & Jaldow, E. (2003). Lost for words or loss of memories?: Autobiographical memory in semantic dementia. *Cognitive Neuropsychology, 20*(8), 703–732.

Nadel, L., & Moscovitch, M. (1997). Memory consolidation, retrograde amnesia and the hippocampal complex. *Currrent Opinion in Neurobiology, 7*(2), 217–227.

Nakamura, H., Kunori, Y., Mori, K., Nakaaki, S., Yoshida, S., & Hamanaka, T. (2002). Two cases of functional focal retrograde amnesia with impairment of object use. *Cortex, 38*(4), 613–622.

Nandrino, J. L., Pezard, L., Poste, A., Reveillere, C., & Beaune, D. (2002). Autobiographical memory in major depression: A comparison between first-episode and recurrent patients. *Psychopathology, 35*(6), 335–340.

Nestor, P. J., Graham, K. S., Bozeat, S., Simons, J. S., & Hodges, J. R. (2002). Memory consolidation and the hippocampus: Further evidence from studies of autobiographical memory in semantic dementia and frontal variant frontotemporal dementia. *Neuropsychologia, 40*(6), 633–654.

Niki, K., & Luo, J. (2002). An fMRI study on the time-limited role of the medial temporal lobe in long-term topographical autobiographic memory. *Journal of Cognitive Neuroscience, 14*(3), 500–507.

Nolde, S. F., Johnson, M. K., & D'Esposito, M. (1998). Left prefrontal activation during episodic remembering: An event-related fMRI study. *NeuroReport, 9*(15), 3509–3514.

Norman, D. A., & Bobrow, D. G. (1979). Descriptions: An intermediate stage in memory retrieval. *Cognitive Psychology, 11,* 107–123.

Nyberg, L., Forkstam, C., Petersson, K. M., Cabeza, R., & Ingvar, M. (2002). Brain imaging of human memory systems: Between-systems similarities and within-system differences. *Cognitive Brain Research, 13*(2), 281–292.

O'Connor, M., Butters, N., Miliotis, P., Eslinger, P., & Cermak, L. S. (1992). The dissociation of anterograde and retrograde amnesia in a patient with herpes encephalitis. *Journal of Clinical and Experimental Neuropsychology, 14*(2), 159–178.

Ogawa, T., Sekino, H., Uzura, M., Sakamoto, T., Taguchi, Y., Yamaguchi, Y., et al. (1992). Comparative study of magnetic resonance and CT scan imaging in cases of severe head injury. *Acta Neurochirurgica: Supplementum, 55*, 8–10.

Osuch, E. A., Benson, B., Geraci, M., Podell, D., Herscovitch, P., McCann, U. D., et al. (2001). Regional cerebral blood flow correlated with flashback intensity in patients with posttraumatic stress disorder. *Biological Psychiatry, 50*(4), 246–253.

Papagno, C., & Baddeley, A. (1997). Confabulation in a dysexecutive patient: Implications for models of retrieval. *Cortex, 33*(4), 743–752.

Petrides, M. (1989). Frontal lobes and memory. In F. Boller & J. Grafman (Eds.), *Handbook of neuropsychology* (Vol. 3, pp. 75–90). Amsterdam: Elsevier.

Petrides, M. (2002). The mid-ventrolateral prefrontal cortex and active mnemonic retrieval. *Neurobiology of Learning and Memory, 78*, 528–538.

Petrides, M., & Pandya, D. N. (2002). Association pathways of the prefrontal cortex and functional observations. In D. T. Stuss & R. T. Knight (Eds.), *Principles of frontal lobe function* (pp. 31–50). New York: Oxford University Press.

Piefke, M., Weiss, P. H., Zilles, K., Markowitsch, H. J., & Fink, G. R. (2003). Differential remoteness and emotional tone modulate the neural correlates of autobiographical memory. *Brain, 126*(3), 650–668.

Piolino, P., Belliard, S., Desgranges, B., Perron, M., & Eustace, F. (2003). Autobiographical memory and autonoetic consciousness in a case of semantic dementia. *Cognitive Neuropsychology, 20*, 619–639.

Piolino, P., Desgranges, B., Belliard, S., Matuszewski, V., Lalevee, C., De la Sayette, V., et al. (2003). Autobiographical memory and autonoetic consciousness: Triple dissociation in neurodegenerative diseases. *Brain, 126*(10), 2203–2219.

Piolino, P., Desgranges, B., Benali, K., & Eustache, F. (2002). Episodic and semantic remote autobiographical memory in ageing. *Memory, 10*(4), 239–257.

Pissiota, A., Frans, O., Fernandez, M., von Knorring, L., Fischer, H., & Fredrikson, M. (2002). Neurofunctional correlates of posttraumatic stress disorder: A PET symptom provocation study. *European Archives of Psychiatry Clinical Neuroscience, 252*(2), 68–75.

Povinelli, D. J., Landau, K. R., & Perilloux, H. K. (1996). Self-recognition in young children using delayed versus live feedback: Evidence of a developmental asynchrony. *Child Development, 67*(4), 1540–1554.

Qin, J., Mitchell, K. J., Johnson, M. K., Krystal, J. H., Southwick, S. M., Rasmusson, A. M., et al. (2003). Reactions to and memories for the September 11, 2001 terrorist attacks in adults with posttraumatic stress disorder. *Applied Cognitive Psychology, 17*(9), 1081–1097.

Rauch, S. L., van der Kolk, B. A., Fisler, R. E., Alpert, N. M., Orr, S. P., Savage, C. R., et al. (1996). A symptom provocation study of posttraumatic stress disorder using positron emission tomography and script-driven imagery. *Archives of General Psychiatry, 53*(5), 380–387.

Rauch, S. L., Whalen, P. J., Shin, L. M., McInerney, S. C., Macklin, M. L., Lasko, N. B., et al. (2000). Exaggerated amygdala response to masked facial stimuli in posttraumatic stress disorder: A functional MRI study. *Biological Psychiatry, 47*(9), 769–776.

Raye, C. L., Johnson, M. K., Mitchell, K. J., Nolde, S. F., & D'Esposito, M. (2000). fMRI investigations of left and right PFC contributions to episodic remembering. *Psychobiology, 28*(2), 197–206.

Raz, N. (2000). Aging of the brain and its impact on cognitive performance: Integration of structural and functional findings. In F. I. M. Craik & T. A. Salthouse (Eds.), *The handbook of aging and cognition* (2nd ed., pp. 1–90). Mahwah, NJ: Erlbaum.

Riutort, M., Cuervo, C., Danion, J. M., Peretti, C. S., & Salame, P. (2003). Reduced levels of specific autobiographical memories in schizophrenia. *Psychiatry Research, 117*(1), 35–45.

Rolls, E. T. (2002). The functions of the orbitofrontal cortex. In D. T. Stuss & R. T. Knight (Eds.), *Principles of frontal lobe function* (pp. 354–375). New York: Oxford University Press.

Rosen, H. J., Perry, R. J., Murphy, J., Kramer, J. H., Mychack, P., Schuff, N., et al. (2002). Emotion comprehension in the temporal variant of frontotemporal dementia. *Brain, 125*(10), 2286–2295.

Rosenbaum, R. S., McKinnon, M. C., Levine, B., & Moscovitch, M. (2004). Visual imagery deficits, impaired strategic retrieval, or memory loss: Disentangling the nature of an amnesic person's autobiographical memory deficit. *Neuropsychologia, 42*(12), 1619–1635.

Rubin, D. C., Feldman, M. E., & Beckham, J. C. (2004). Reliving, emotions, and fragmentation in the autobiographical memories of veterans diagnosed with PTSD. *Applied Cognitive Psychology, 18*(1), 17–35.

Rubin, D. C., & Greenberg, D. L. (1998). Visual memory-deficit amnesia: A distinct amnesic presentation and etiology. *Proceedings of the National Academy of Sciences of the United States of America, 95*(9), 5413–5416.

Rubin, D. C., Rahhal, T. A., & Poon, L. W. (1998). Things learned in early adulthood are remembered best. *Memory and Cognition, 26*(1), 3–19.

Rubin, D. C., & Schulkind, M. D. (1997). The distribution of autobiographical memories across the lifespan. *Memory and Cognition, 25*(6), 859–866.

Russell, R. W., & Nathan, P. W. (1946). Traumatic amnesia. *Brain, 69*, 280–300.

Ryan, L., Nadel, L., Keil, K., Putnam, K., Schnyer, D., Trouard, T., et al. (2001). Hippocampal complex and retrieval of recent and very remote autobiographical memories: Evidence from functional magnetic resonance imaging in neurologically intact people. *Hippocampus, 11*(6), 707–714.

Sagar, H. J., Sullivan, E. V., & Corkin, S. (1991). Autobiographical memory in normal ageing and dementia. *Behavioural Neurology, 4*(4), 235–248.

Schacter, D. L. (1987). Memory, amnesia, and frontal lobe dysfunction. *Psychobiology, 15,* 21–36.

Schacter, D. L., Wang, P. L., Tulving, E., & Freedman, M. (1982). Functional retrograde amnesia: A quantitative case study. *Neuropsychologia, 20*(5), 523–532.

Schnider, A., & Ptak, R. (1999). Spontaneous confabulators fail to suppress currently irrelevant memory traces. *Nature Neuroscience, 2*(7), 677–681.

Schnider, A., von Daniken, C., & Gutbrod, K. (1996). The mechanisms of spontaneous and provoked confabulations. *Brain, 119*(4), 1365–1375.

Sellal, F., Manning, L., Seegmuller, C., Scheiber, C., & Schoenfelder, F. (2002). Pure retrograde amnesia following a mild head trauma: A neuropsychological and metabolic study. *Cortex, 38*(4), 499–509.

Shammi, P., & Stuss, D. T. (1999). Humour appreciation: A role of the right frontal lobe. *Brain, 122*(4), 657–666.

Shin, L. M., Kosslyn, S. M., McNally, R. J., Alpert, N. M., Thompson, W. L., Rauch, S. L., et al. (1997). Visual imagery and perception in posttraumatic stress disorder: A positron emission tomographic investigation. *Archives of General Psychiatry, 54*(3), 233–241.

Shin, L. M., McNally, R. J., Kosslyn, S. M., Thompson, W. L., Rauch, S. L., Alpert, N. M., et al. (1999). Regional cerebral blood flow during script-driven imagery in childhood sexual abuse-related PTSD: A PET investigation. *American Journal of Psychiatry, 156*(4), 575–584.

Simons, J. S., & Spiers, H. J. (2003). Prefrontal and medial temporal lobe interactions in long-term memory. *Nature Reviews: Neuroscience, 4*(8), 637–648.

Snowden, J. S., Griffiths, H. L., & Neary, D. (1996). Semantic–episodic memory interactions in semantic dementia: Implications for retrograde memory function. *Cognitive Neuropsychology, 13,* 1101–1127.

Snowden, J. S., Griffiths, H. L., & Neary, D. (1994). Semantic dementia: Autobiographical contribution to preservation of meaning. *Cognitive Neuropsychology, 11*(3), 265–288.

Squire, L. R., Slater, P. C., & Chace, P. M. (1975). Retrograde amnesia: Temporal gradient in very long term memory following electroconvulsive therapy. *Science, 187,* 77–79.

St.-Jacques, P. L., & Levine, B. (2006). *Aging and autobiographical memory for emotional and neutral events.* Manuscript submitted for publication.

Starkstein, S., Sabe, L., & Dorrego, M. F. (1997). Severe retrograde amnesia after a mild closed head injury. *Neurocase, 3,* 105–109.

Steinvorth, S., Levine, B., & Corkin, S. (2005). Medial temporal lobe structures are needed to re-experience remote autobiographical memories: Evidence from H. M. and W. R. *Neuropsychologia, 43*(4), 479–496.

Stracciari, A., Ghidoni, E., Guarino, M., Poletti, M., & Pazzaglia, P. (1994). Post-traumatic retrograde amnesia with selective impairment of autobiographical memory. *Cortex, 30*(3), 459–468.

Stuss, D. T. (1991). Self, awareness, and the frontal lobes: A neuropsychological perspective. In J. Strauss & G. R. Goethals (Eds.), *The self: Interdisciplinary approaches* (pp. 255–277). New York: Springer-Verlag.

Stuss, D. T., Alexander, M. P., Lieberman, A., & Levine, H. (1978). An extraordinary form of confabulation. *Neurology, 28,* 1166–1172.

Stuss, D. T., Alexander, M. P., Palumbo, C. L., Buckle, L., Sayer, L., & Pogue, J. (1994). Organizational strategies of patients with unilateral or bilateral frontal lobe injury in word list learning tasks. *Neuropsychology, 8,* 355–373.

Stuss, D. T., & Benson, D. F. (1986). *The frontal lobes.* New York: Raven.

Stuss, D. T., Gallup, G. G., & Alexander, M. P. (2001). The frontal lobes are necessary for "theory of mind." *Brain, 124*(2), 279–286.

Stuss, D. T., & Levine, B. (2002). Adult clinical neuropsychology: Lessons from studies of the frontal lobes. *Annual Review of Psychology, 53,* 401–433.

Stuss, D. T., Picton, T. W., & Alexander, M. P. (2001). Consciousness, self-awareness and the frontal lobes. In S. P. Salloway, P. F. Malloy, & J. D. Duffy (Eds.), *The frontal lobes and neuropsychiatric illness* (pp. 101–109). Washington, DC: American Psychiatric Publishing.

Svoboda, E., Lobaugh, N. J., Stainsz, G., Kanagasabai, S., Skocic, J., Turner, G., et al. (2005). Autonoetic consciousness in retrograde amnesic patients M. L.: Functional neuroanatomy. *Journal of the International Neuropsychological Society, 11*(Suppl. S1), 135.

Svoboda, E., McKinnon, M. C., & Levine, B. (2006). *The functional neuroanatomy of autobiographical memory: A meta-analysis of neuroimaging studies.* Manuscript under revision.

Teuber, H. L. (1968). Disorders of memory following penetrating missile wounds of the brain. *Neurology, 18*(3), 287–288.

Thomas-Anterion, C., Jacquin, K., & Laurent, B. (2000). Differential mechanisms of impairment of remote memory in Alzheimer's and frontotemporal dementia. *Dementia and Geriatric Cognitive Disorders, 11*(2), 100–106.

Thornton, J. A., Rothblat, L. A., & Murray, E. A. (1997). Rhinal cortex removal produces amnesia for preoperatively learned discrimination problems but fails to disrupt postoperative acquisition and retention in rhesus monkeys. *Journal of Neuroscience, 17*(21), 8536–8549.

Tulving, E. (1972). Episodic and semantic memory. In E. Tulving & W. Donaldson (Eds.), *Organization of memory* (pp. 382–403). New York: Academic Press.

Tulving, E. (1985a). How many memory systems are there? *American Psychologist, 40,* 385–398.

Tulving, E. (1985b). Memory and consciousness. *Canadian Psychology, 26*, 1–12.

Tulving, E. (2001). Episodic memory and common sense: How far apart? *Philosophical Transactions of the Royal Society of London, Series B, Biological Sciences, 356*, 1505–1515.

Tulving, E. (2002). Episodic memory: From mind to brain. *Annual Review of Psychology, 53*, 1–25.

Tulving, E., Kapur, S., Craik, F. I. M., Moscovitch, M., & Houle, S. (1994). Hemispheric encoding/retrieval asymmetry in episodic memory: Positron emission tomography findings. *Proceedings of the National Academy of Sciences of the United States of America, 91*, 2016–2020.

Wagner, A. D., Maril, A., Bjork, R. A., & Schacter, D. L. (2001). Prefrontal contributions to executive control: fMRI evidence for functional distinctions within lateral prefrontal cortex. *NeuroImage, 14*(6), 1337–1347.

Weaver, C. A. (1993). Do you need a "flash" to form a flashbulb memory? *Journal of Experimental Psychology: General, 122*(1), 39–46.

Westmacott, R., Leach, L., Freedman, M., & Moscovitch, M. (2001). Different patterns of autobiographical memory loss in semantic dementia and medial temporal lobe amnesia: A challenge to consolidation theory. *Neurocase, 7*(1), 37–55.

Westmacott, R., & Moscovitch, M. (2003). The contribution of autobiographical significance to semantic memory. *Memory and Cognition, 31*(5), 761–774.

Wheeler, M. A., Stuss, D. T., & Tulving, E. (1997). Toward a theory of episodic memory: The frontal lobes and autonoetic consciousness. *Psychological Bulletin, 121*, 331–354.

Winner, E., Brownell, H., Happe, F., Blum, A., & Pincus, D. (1998). Distinguishing lies from jokes: Theory of mind deficits and discourse interpretation in right hemisphere brain-damaged patients. *Brain and Language, 62*(1), 89–106.

Winston, J. S., Strange, B. A., O'Doherty, J., & Dolan, R. J. (2002). Automatic and intentional brain responses during evaluation of trustworthiness of faces. *Nature Neuroscience, 5*(3), 277–283.

Zola-Morgan, S., Cohen, N. J., & Squire, L. R. (1983). Recall of remote episodic memory in amnesia. *Neuropsychologia, 21*(5), 487–500.

Zysset, S., Huber, O., Ferstl, E., & von Cramon, D. Y. (2002). The anterior frontomedian cortex and evaluative judgment: An fMRI study. *NeuroImage, 15*(4), 983–991.

# CHAPTER 16

# Planning and the Brain

*Jordan Grafman*

The human frontal lobes play an important role in many aspects of human behavior, including those processes concerned with higher level functioning. A prominent example of such a process is a plan. Plans are a ubiquitous part of human activity. A "plan" can be defined as a structured event series that generally contains one or more goals. Plans range from the short term and motoric (e.g., planning a sequence of key presses) (Pascual-Leone et al., 1993) to the long term and cognitive (e.g., deciding on the steps required for air-traffic controllers to land a specific airplane) (Suchman, 1987). How plans are developed and executed has been the focus of study in artificial intelligence (AI) (Allen, Kautz, Pelavin, & Tenenberg, 1991; Hammond, 1994), cognitive science (Friedman & Scholnick, 1997; Hoc, 1988), and neuropsychology (Owen, 1997). In their prescient book on planning, Miller, Galanter, and Pribram (1960) revealed the difficulty that neuropsychology might have identifying which brain structures would be concerned with planning as defined by contemporary computer science terminology, eventually admitting, "The relation between computers and the brain was a battle the authors fought with one another until the exasperation became unbearable" (p. 197). The responsibility for this difficulty may partly lie in the different methods used to investigate planning by each discipline. Besides their differences, each discipline's methods had particular weaknesses. For example, Langley and Drummond (1990) decried the nonexperimental basis of much of the AI literature on planning. They argued for the development of

testable hypotheses that can be experimentally addressed, for example,

> "What are the resources required to generate a plan?"
> "In reacting to an unexpected event, how much sampling of the environment is done?"
> "What is the ratio of deliberation to execution (and upon what does that ratio depend)?"
> "How do subjects modify stored plans versus constructing entirely new plans?"

Many AI and cognitive researchers have also noted the similarity between plans and other knowledge structures, such as story grammars, themes, action sets, cases, schemas, and scripts (Schank & Abelson, 1977). All of these knowledge structures represent sequentially structured information that must be sustained in some active state over time for processing (Kolodner, 1993).

In this chapter, I survey the cognitive neuroscience study of planning. I primarily draw upon results of studies that explicitly tested planning, although I refer to data from a few studies that investigated script and story processing. My goal in this review is not to describe the important role that objects, scenes, lexical knowledge, and motor actions have in constructing and executing a plan, but to provide a description of the cognitive components of plan-specific knowledge that can be mapped to brain. My bias is that the crucial components of plan-specific knowledge are primarily stored in the prefrontal cortex, with plan execution assisted by motor processes stored in the basal ganglia and frontal lobes (Grafman, 1989, 1994, 1995; Grafman & Hendler, 1991). Before reviewing the cognitive neuroscience investigation of planning, I briefly discuss the cognitive and computational science foundations that provide the groundwork for my claims about which plan-specific components of knowledge are distinctively stored in the human prefrontal cortex.

## COGNITIVE AND COMPUTATIONAL FOUNDATIONS

"Planning" has been described as the process of formulating an abstract sequence of operations intended for achieving some goal (Hayes-Roth & Hayes-Roth, 1979; Scholnick & Friedman, 1987). The *representation* of this sequence is called a plan (Wilensky, 1983). A plan can be represented internally (in the planner's mind) or externally (e.g., a blueprint, a travel route). There are two predominant views of planning within cognitive psychology: *successive refinement models* and *opportunistic models*. Successive refinement models propose that planning is a top-down, hierarchical process, much like a computer program, that controls the order in which a series of operations can be performed (Miller et al., 1960; Newell & Simon, 1972; Sacerdoti, 1975). Opportunistic models propose that planning is a data-driven process that can operate concurrently at several different levels of abstraction, with decisions at any level affecting subsequent decisions at both higher and lower levels (Hayes-Roth & Hayes-Roth, 1979). Both views may be correct.

The view of planning as successive refinement had its beginning in the work of Miller and colleagues (1960), who proposed that a plan is "any hierarchical process in the organism that can control the order in which a sequence of operations can be performed" (p. 16). These plans usually include hierarchically organized subplans, which can include further subplans, down to the level of motor action (Das, Kar, & Parrila, 1996). At *each* level or subplan, the planner executes a TOTE (test–operate–test–exit) unit, where the planner *tests* to see if a goal is satisfied. If it is not, he or she *operates* to achieve the goal, *tests* the efficacy of the operation, and then if the goal is met, *exits*. Upon exiting, the planner moves to the next step in the sequence (Scholnick &

Friedman, 1987). This hierarchical, top-down view of planning is evident in many cognitive models, including planning as problem solving within the SOAR (state, operator, and result) architecture (Rosenbloom, Laird, & Newell, 1993), Schank and Abelson's (1977) view of plans as a general mechanisms underlying the formation of scripts, and in views of planning drawn from AI (e.g., Fikes & Nilsson, 1971; Sacerdoti, 1975).

An alternative to the hierarchical, successive refinement models of planning is *opportunistic models*, such as that proposed by Hayes-Roth and Hayes-Roth (1979). They proposed that at each point in the planning process, a planner's current decision affects the opportunities available and the decisions that must be made later in the development of a plan. Thus, plans grow incrementally as each new decision is incorporated into, and revises, previous decisions, creating a multidirectional, flexible, planning process. Thus, decisions can be made at any level of abstraction at any point in the planning process. In some domains and planning situations, this process will begin at a high level of abstraction, and the plan will develop in an orderly, top-down expansion of goals and subgoals, much like in planning by successive refinement. In other domains and planning situations, however, this process will begin as a series of concrete local decisions, and the planning process will move between highly abstract decisions and concrete local decisions, often without an overall framework for the decision-making process (Pea & Hawkins, 1987). This basic model of opportunistic planning has influenced many cognitive psychologists studying planning in adults and in children (Baker-Sennett, Matusov, & Rogoff, 1993; Dreher & Oerter, 1987; Pea & Hawkins, 1987).

Both successive refinement and opportunistic planning have been supported empirically, and both appear to explain some central aspect of human planning. Successive refinement models capture the top-down, goal-directed characteristics of human planning (Anderson, 1983) but would lead to the conclusion that young children, who consistently find the use of hierarchies and the process of sequencing difficult, cannot plan (Das et al., 1996). This conclusion has been challenged by the results of developmental studies showing that children do plan, and are often quite good at it (see Freidman, Scholnick, & Cocking, 1987, for an excellent review of the development of planning). Opportunistic planning, in turn, has

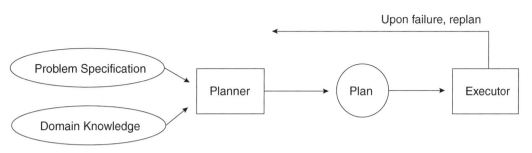

FIGURE 16.1. The total planning framework. Unlike opportunistic planning models, the "total-order" planning framework provides the planning agent with all necessary knowledge from which he or she is expected to produce a complete, fully specified plan *before any actions are taken*.

been criticized for making "distractibility" a central aspect of human planning, overlooking a great deal of evidence suggesting that human behavior is controlled by organized structures (Anderson, 1983). It appears that both views are necessary to describe accurately the process of planning. When factors such as age, cortical damage, knowledge of the planning domain, and constraints placed upon planning efficiency by the human cognitive system are examined, it is clear that both successive refinement and opportunistic planning play a role.

Improvements to the analysis and design of total-order planning algorithms (see Figure 16.1) continue to appear in the literature (Blum & Furst, 1997). More recently, however, AI research has focused on *integrating* planning and execution operations, with new information becoming known to the agent in the course of action. This work on "reactive" or "dynamic-world" planning often uses techniques entirely different from those in the traditional AI planning literature (Chapman, 1991). Reactive planning implies a "least commitment" strategy that allows plans to be more easily modified as planning progresses, similar to opportunistic planning. For example, knowledge that

there are no newspaper stands beyond the security checkpoint can be integrated into the plan in Figure 16.2 by inserting an arrow from "Buy Newspaper" to "Go through Security Checkpoint." In contrast, more reasoning and replanning will normally be required to correct a sequential plan relative to new information: The system will have to change ordering decisions to which it has already committed, and will have to reason afresh about the validity of the new plan. The trade-offs for the efficiencies of partial-order representations are that more memory and, in some cases, more complex algorithms are also required. Figure 16.3 summarizes many of the key variables that need to be considered in the design of planning experiments.

## COGNITIVE NEUROSCIENCE PERSPECTIVES

Studies of patients with neurological disorders, as well as the implementation of planning designs in functional neuroimaging experiments, have increased steadily over the last 20 years. In general, most cognitive neuroscience (CN) studies have tested subjects in well-structured scenarios, where an explicit goal is explained to

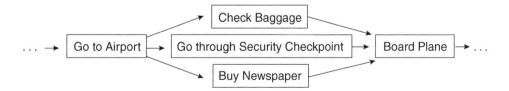

FIGURE 16.2. A partially ordered plan. An action at the tail of an arrow must be executed some time before the action of the head of that arrow, but these are the only constraints on execution order. In this partial plan, Check Baggage, Go Through Security Checkpoint, and Buy Newspaper may be executed in any order.

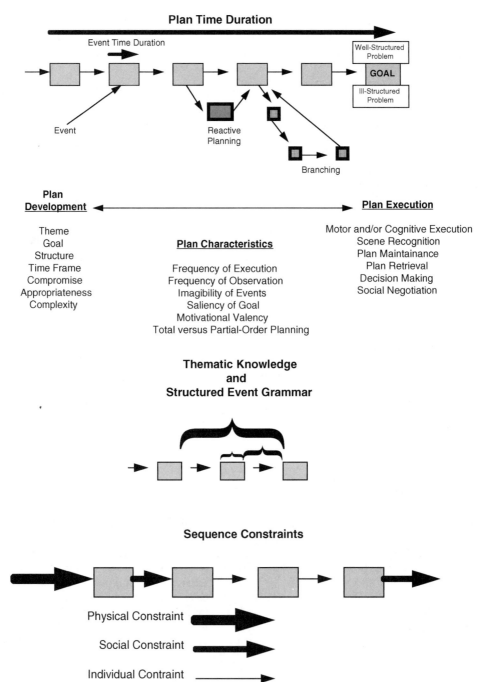

FIGURE 16.3. A cognitive view of a plan. Based on the discussion of cognitive and computational planning models, it is possible to construct a framework for the CN investigation of planning. This framework indicates the complexities facing investigators attempting to disambiguate the cause of planning failures in patients or brain activation profiles in normal subjects performing a planning task. Plans have a number of cognitive components that can be seen here. Each plan, as well as plan event, has a characteristic time

the subject, who then attempts to plan how to achieve the goal before (in some cases) executing the plan (Owen, Downes, Sahakian, Polkey, & Robbins, 1990; Owen, Doyon, Petrides, & Evans, 1996). On occasion, ill-structured problems are presented to the subject, who then has to develop the goals of the activity, as well as the plan to achieve those goals. In addition, ill-structured problems make it more likely that some form of reactive planning (changing the structure of the plan online) will be required during execution of the plan (Spector & Grafman, 1994). A limitation of many CN planning studies is the time domain within which the plan may be developed and executed, and the planning problem itself is often artificial. In observing the planning and execution of real-life activities, in rare instances the time scale can be as long as several hours. Although planning problems may also be reflected in the performance of simple, everyday tasks such as brushing one's teeth or making coffee (Schwartz, Reed, Montgomery, Palmer, & Mayer, 1991), the focus of this chapter is on higher-level cognitive plans.

The majority of paradigms used in CN planning studies are those evaluating subject route finding, Tower task performance, and performance in simulated or real-life scenarios. In each of these paradigms, subjects are first usually asked to assemble in their mind the required actions they need to make to achieve the instructed goal (planning time), which is fol-

lowed by the execution of the task (planning execution). Most often, subject response times and accuracy scores are used to derive inferences about planning failures. In general, patients with frontal lobe lesions and those with subcortical disorders (e.g., Parkinson's disease [PD]) affecting the basal ganglia are the most impaired on a variety of planning paradigms. Many other CN studies use tasks that require processing similar to what a subject might do in constructing and executing a plan, including script event generation and verification studies, whose results we believe are relevant for understanding which brain regions store plan representations.

Route finding and learning tasks concerned with examining planning ability require that subjects clearly perceive the geometric properties of the route, and that they have the motor and attention skills necessary to perform the task. To plan how to navigate through a complex maze, the subject must identify the sequence of proper turns, encode the path as a plan, and commit the plan to memory. The plan execution phase begins as soon as the path is encoded. Patients with prefrontal cortex lesions are often able to navigate well-known routes, but they are particularly impaired in learning new routes or in utilizing old routes to adapt to a new route (Karnath & Wallesch, 1992; Karnath, Wallesch, & Zimmerman, 1991). Flitman, Cooper, and Grafman (1997) have used $O^{15}$ positron emission tomography

---

duration; event order is generally in a left-to-right direction, although most plans have some level of branching or recursiveness. The number of component plan events can vary across plans. Plans can be based on well- or ill-structured problems. The key features of plan development are somewhat different from those of plan execution, although some overlap is apparent. The general characteristics of plans have to do with conditions for their retrievability and instantiation. Frequency, imagability, saliency, and motivation are relevant characteristics of any form of knowledge representation including plan-level knowledge. Total-order plans are those that do not allow any deviation from the plan path. Partial-order plans allow for opportunistic deviations and the ability to rejoin the plan path at a juncture close to where one left it. To understand the overall meaning of a plan, conceptual and semantic knowledge must be distilled and integrated across individual plan events—each of which has its own semantic and conceptual value. Reactive planning involves the unexpected *introduction of another plan event in the main plan path*, whereas branching is the process whereby the main plan path is appended with a subsidiary path that returns to the main plan path *at the point where one left it*. Well-structured problems have an explicit goal that can induce the plan path selection. Ill-structured problems require the formation of goals *and* multiple plan paths. Note that the sequential structure of plan events depends to some extent on whether the transition from one plan event to another is characterized by physical (to take a shower, one must step into the shower stall), social (in the United States, the population generally showers once per day in the morning, before eating breakfast and leaving for work), or individual constraints (individuals having their own idiosyncratic sequence in carrying out a plan). This latter constraint or, viewed from a different perspective, ability, allows for the most flexible and inventive of human behaviors.

(PET) to demonstrate that the right prefrontal cortex is particularly active during the retrieval of an encoded route compared to times when a subject is simply traversing a seen maze. The anterior cingulate cortex was also active during task performance, indicating that subjects actively planned their route and then monitored their chosen path. These findings suggest that subjects tend to navigate mazes by using an opportunistic (rather than a "look-ahead") strategy, which depends more on the immediate maze environment and perceptual–spatial processing, whereas the retrieval of a complete cognitive plan for traversing the maze requires prefrontal cortex mediation.

Tower-type tasks are composed of three or more pegs, with a number of disks sitting on the pegs (see Figure 16.4). There is usually a beginning state and a goal state. To achieve the goal state, subjects have to move the disks and place them on the other pegs according to the rules of the particular Tower task adapted (the most commonly used tasks in the CN literature are the Towers of Hanoi [ToH], London [ToL], and Toronto). In general, on Tower tasks, the more moves required to achieve a goal state, the more difficult the problem appears to the subject. Ward and Allport (1997), using five-disk ToL problems, found that planning actions online was limited by subject difficulty in evaluating and selecting one course of action or one subgoal chunk from the set of competing actions at each step in the course of plan execution, with increased premove preparation time re-

lated to the number of competing alternative choices. Dehaene and Changuex (1997) used a connectionist model to simulate performance on the ToL task. They postulated that planning requires working memory units, plan units that cause novel activation patterns among lower-level operation units generating a plan, and reward units that evaluate the correct or incorrect status of a plan. Each additional *indirect* move added up to 110 cycles to the stimulation! Although humans appear able to chunk an entire action series, Dehaene and Changuex's model was unable to do so. When they disturbed the plan units in their model, it effectively disconnected the operation network from the reward network, making it difficult for the model to judge the relevance of individual ToL moves to achieving the overall plan. The "lesioned" model also predicted that patients might find it difficult to select a move, although they would be able to verify whether a move shown to them would be correct.

PET functional neuroimaging studies identify a large set of brain areas that are activated during performance of the ToL by normal subjects. However, when performance on the easy ToL problems was subtracted from the harder ToL problem brain activation profile, only right Brodmann's area 10 and left Brodmann's area 9, along with premotor cortex, remain significantly activated (Baker et al., 1996). Morris, Ahmed, Syed, and Toone (1993), using single-photon emission computer tomography (SPECT), found left prefrontal activation re-

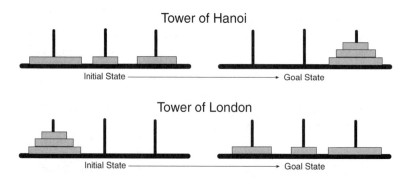

FIGURE 16.4. The Towers of Hanoi and London are illustrated. While each has three pegs, the number, size, and color of the disks may vary. Both tasks require that subjects move the disks across the pegs to achieve a goal state. Each task only allows for one disk to be moved at a time. The ToH task does not allow for a larger disk to be put on top of a smaller disk. The ToL task must be solved in the minimum number of moves or the subject must begin to execute the plan anew.

lated to ToL performance with the more difficult problems (as indicated by greater subject
planning time and number of moves) inducing
greater the left frontal activation. If normal
subjects are given feedback on their ToL performance during PET functional neuroimaging, additional activation can be seen in orbitofrontal and medial caudate brain regions
(Elliott, Frith, & Dolan, 1997). Depressed patients performing the ToL during PET scanning
fail to show activation in ventromedial cortex
or striatum, and show no increase in activation
from easy to difficult problems (Baker et al.,
1997; Elliott, Baker, et al., 1997).

Goel and Grafman (1995) confirmed that
patients with prefrontal cortex lesions are impaired on the ToH task. They noted, however,
that the deficit was apparent when patients had
to overcome a prepotent strategy and make a
counterintuitive move (regardless of problem
difficulty). This finding suggested that patients
with frontal lobe lesions could initiate a plan
similar to controls but had difficulty branching
out from the main plan path (see also Morris,
Miotto, Feigenbaum, Bullock, & Polkey,
1997). Task-switching capability is important
for developing and executing plans when opportunistic shifting between subgoals is necessary. Rogers and colleagues (1998) found that
patients with left frontal lobe lesions showed
increased time costs associated with predictable switches between tasks when there was
interference between the tasks, and when available task cues were relatively weak and arbitrary.

Shallice and Burgess (1991, 1996) pioneered
the objective study of patients with frontal lobe
lesions as they execute real-life plans. These patients performed normally on many standard
cognitive tasks evaluating perception, language, and episodic memory. The real-life tasks
involved shopping and similar activities that
needed to be performed within a time limit.
The patients were able to remember each task
and its different rules of engagement. Impaired
plan execution and goal attainment was observed when the patients failed to divide their
time appropriately on each of a set of tasks.
Some patients appeared unable to reactivate,
after a delay, a previously generated intention
to perform a task when they were not directly
signaled by a stimulus in the environment.
Shallice and Burgess speculated that an internal
marker may be set for stored plans, whereas for
new plans or plan development, the marker(s)

may be more fragile and subject to interference
when patients have frontal lobe brain damage.
They termed this deficit a "strategy application
disorder." Goldstein, Bernard, Fenwick, Burgess, and McNeil (1993) evaluated a patient
with a unilateral left frontal lesion who performed normally on standard neuropsychological tests and learned the rules to a multiple errands task designed by Shallice and Burgess.
The patient's errors were characteristic of a
planning failure and included deficits in executing multiple errands, inefficiency (e.g., he could
have bought all the goods he needed from one
store at one time; instead, he returned to the
store more than once), rule breaking (he left the
neighborhood to purchase some goods), disinhibition, and post hoc rationalizations for his
inappropriate behaviors.

Bechara, Damasio, Damasio, and Anderson
(1994) found that patients with ventromedial
frontal lobe lesions performing a gambling task
tended to choose from the high-risk, quick payoff cards rather than the low paying but better
long-term-risk cards. They hypothesized that
these patients had a dissociation between
knowledge of the ramifications of their strategic plan and somatic input that would have
alerted them to the negative consequences of
their chosen plan. Goel, Grafman, Tajik, Gana,
and Danto (1997) examined patients with
frontal lobe lesions on a realistic financial planning task and found that patients were impaired at the global level of planning but had
normal local level performance; that is, patients with frontal lobe lesions had difficulty in
organizing and structuring their plan development space. They were able to begin planning
but were unable to divide their cognitive efforts
adequately among each planning phase. They
spent too much time planning for events that
would occur in closer chronological proximity
to the plan development time. Patients expressed consternation that there were no right
or wrong answers, nor obvious termination
points in their planning task, and tended to terminate the testing session before they specified
all their plan details or satisfied the task goals.
Interestingly, the patients did not attempt (as
did controls) to negotiate some apparent constraints imposed by the investigators. The patients' planning failures were attributed to difficulty in generalizing from particular events,
failure to shift between mental sets, poor judgment regarding the adequacy and completeness
of the plan, and inadequate access to structured

event complexes (i.e., memory for plan-level attributes such as thematic knowledge, plan grammars, etc.).

Scripts are knowledge structures that resemble plans and contain information pertinent to carrying out an action sequence, including characterizations of the events, the temporal order of events, and thematic information. Script tasks typically ask participants to sort events, to make decisions about a set of events they are shown (e.g., whether they are in the correct order or belong to the same script), or to carry out a typical script in real time. CN research on *script* processing (Sirigu et al., 1995a, 1995b, 1996, 1998) indicates that patients with prefrontal cortex lesions have selective difficulty generating (or sorting) an appropriate script event sequence, particularly when the events come from less familiar scripts. Functional neuroimaging findings indicate significant right prefrontal cortex activation when subjects make script event sequence decisions, whereas the left prefrontal cortex is more active when subjects judge whether a single event is a member of a particular script (Partiot, Grafman, Sadato, Flitman, & Wild, 1996). Nichelli and colleagues (1995) demonstrated that normal subjects also activate right prefrontal cortex when determining the moral of a story. In addition, when normal subjects mentally generate nonemotional script events, they activate lateral prefrontal and posterior temporal cortices, but when they mentally generate emotional scripts, they activate ventromedial prefrontal and anterior temporal cortices (Partiot, Grafman, Sadato, Wachs, & Hallett, 1995).

In summary, patients with frontal lobe lesions unambiguously demonstrate difficulty in developing and/or executing a plan. Patients with subcortical lesions in structures that receive frontal lobe projections (e.g., those with Parkinson's disease) may have a similar, but more mild, planning problem (Berns & Sejnowski, 1998; Grafman et al., 1992; Morris et al., 1988; Pascual-Leone et al., 1993; Wallesch et al., 1990). Patients with lesions outside the area of the frontal lobe–basal ganglia–cerebellum axis may fail on planning tasks, not because of an essential deficit to plan-level processes but because of, for example, cognitive deficits in spatial perception or language comprehension. Category-specific plan impairment may also be observed with ventromedial frontal lobe lesions affecting so-cial cognitive or emotionally arousing plans more than nonsocial, unemotional cognitive plans (partially due to damage to, or dissociation of ventromedial cortex from, the autonomic nervous system; Bechara et al., 1994). Planning processes requiring the structural analysis of plans may be more compromised by left prefrontal lesions, whereas the temporal and dynamic aspects of plans may be more compromised by right prefrontal lesions.

## CONCLUSIONS

The major representation of plan-level knowledge in the human brain appears to be in the prefrontal cortex. The failures in planning associated with prefrontal cortex lesions include problems in both top-down and bottom-up plan development, in the development and execution of novel plans, in the analogical mapping of plans, in parallel processing, in opportunistic/partial-order planning, in time management, in both development and execution of a complete plan event sequence, in discriminating between relevant and irrelevant events, in both well- and ill-structured planning, in accessing category-specific plans, and in the adequate successive refinement of plans.

The cognitive processing deficits that appear responsible for these planning failures include representational degradation (e.g., making low-frequency plans more difficult to retrieve), difficulty in inhibiting prepotent plans and other action units (disinhibition), deficits in thematic induction (which can hinder plan retrieval), plan grammar deficits (leading to failures in following a sequential path), and modality-specific failure in plan development and retrieval (distinguishing between verbal–propositional, visual, and real-time representation of plan behavior), and impaired opportunistic, partial-order processing. Patients with frontal lobe lesions may exhibit one or more of these deficits.

Animal and human research suggests that neural networks in the prefrontal cortex are specialized for sustaining information processing over long periods of time even in the absence of stimulus-specific input (Cohen et al., 1997; Courtney, Ungerleider, Keil, & Haxby, 1997; Fuster, 1995; Goldman-Rakic, 1996; Miller, Erickson, & Desimone, 1996). These observations indicate that the neural mechanisms required to support plan-level processing (which by definition would need to occur over long periods of time and to be sustained in the absence of stimulus-specific behavior) are available in the prefrontal cortex. The prefrontal cortex, however, is a large structure, and in addition to possessing the general processing capability to handle many aspects of plan-level behavior, including processing multiple plans simultaneously (Lingard & Richards, 1998), the findings I have reviewed also suggest some specificity in the topographical representation of several of the cognitive processes responsible for plans (see Figure 16.5).

In this chapter I have argued that the prefrontal cortex is crucial for mediating planning functions that are extended in time and comprise a set of sequential events. It is currently possible to make some claims about the role of several prefrontal cortex regions in planning functions. For this purpose, I have divided the prefrontal cortex into left and right sectors, medial and lateral sectors, dorsal and ventral sectors, and anterior and posterior sectors.

Wood and Grafman (2003) have proposed assigning different representational forms of the structured event complex to each of these areas, and I can use that same schema for describing planning functions because we believe that plans are just one form of a structured event complex. There is evidence that the left prefrontal cortex focuses on the specific features of individual events (including features and meanings) that make up a plan, whereas the right prefrontal cortex mediates the integration of information across events (including the acquisition of meaning and features at the macroplan level, e.g., themes and morals). I have hypothesized that the medial prefrontal cortex stores key features of predictable, overlearned cognitive plans that have a contingent relationship with sensorimotor processes and are rarely modified. Lateral prefrontal cortex would store key features of plans that are frequently modified to adapt to special circumstances. Ventral prefrontal cortex is concerned with social-category-specific plans that often have an emo-

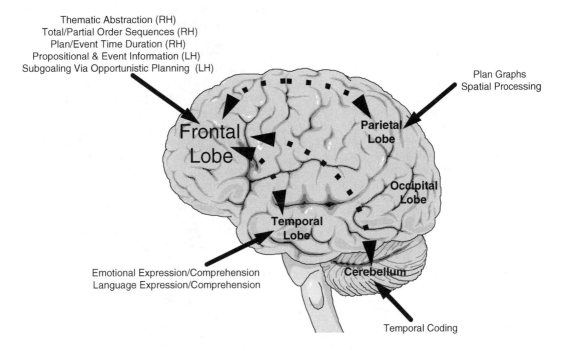

Thematic Abstraction (RH)
Total/Partial Order Sequences (RH)
Plan/Event Time Duration (RH)
Propositional & Event Information (LH)
Subgoaling Via Opportunistic Planning (LH)

Plan Graphs
Spatial Processing

Frontal Lobe

Parietal Lobe

Occipital Lobe

Temporal Lobe

Cerebellum

Emotional Expression/Comprehension
Language Expression/Comprehension

Temporal Coding

FIGURE 16.5. Mapping planning processes to brain. This cartoon figure of the brain indicates that many plan-level processes are most likely stored and subserved by prefrontal cortex. There is some evidence that indicates which hemisphere (RH, right hemisphere; LH, left hemisphere) is predominant in mediating a particular planning process (see text). Plan-level knowledge in the prefrontal cortex must be linked or bound to information-processing components stored in other brain areas (as shown in the figure) in order for a complete characterization of the plan to be formed. Presumably, the hippocampus and other memory structures contribute to this linkage.

tional component. Dorsal prefrontal cortex is concerned more with aspects of plans representing mechanistic activities without a social component (e.g., repairing a food processor). Finally, anterior prefrontal cortex tends to represent plans of long duration that comprise many events, whereas posterior prefrontal cortex tends to represent plans and actions of short duration and fewer events (e.g., a simple association). Since no single prefrontal cortex region would represent all features or components of a plan, specific plans would tend to evoke selected patterns of prefrontal cortex activation. Any region could participate in plan processing, depending on the type of plan, with the different plan (and cortical) subcomponents being differentially weighted in importance (and activation) based on the kind of plan, the moment-by-moment demands of the plan, and previous experience with the plan. For example, the left anterior ventromedial prefrontal cortex would be expected to represent a long, multievent sequence of social interactions (i.e., a social plan), with specialized processing of the meaning and features of single events within the event sequence making up the plan, including the computation of their temporal and sequential dependencies and primary meaning. This view differs from that of Newman, Carpenter, Varma, and Just (2003), who assign different processes to each hemisphere. For example, based on functional neuroimaging and computational modeling of ToL performance, they hypothesize that the right prefrontal cortex is more involved in the generation of a plan, and the left prefrontal cortex is more involved in the execution of a plan. My view is that either hemisphere can initiate and guide plan execution, but only specific features of the plans would be encoded and stored in subregions within each hemisphere.

The prefrontal cortex is connected to many other brain regions and, in particular, the basal ganglia may play an important role in learning and executing overlearned cognitive plans. I suspect that over time the execution of a routine plan would rely more and more on the simpler sensorimotor components of the activity rather than the associated, complex cognitive knowledge contained in the plan. This would result in the recruitment of selected basal ganglia structures to help mediate the sensorimotor activity. In turn this would result in decreased activation in the prefrontal cortex, because the cognitive components of the plan

would not be explicitly relied upon for its execution. This reduction of prefrontal cortex resources as a plan is routinely repeated and allows for the same resources in the prefrontal cortex to be utilized cognitively to focus on another plan allowing for multitasking behavior. Many of the subregions within the prefrontal cortex are monosynaptically connected to subcortical structures such as the amygdala and nucleus accumbens that mediate the retrieval of affective input and its binding to cognitive processes, so I suspect that social plans and other plans of personal relevance to the person would be infused with emotional cues that bias the development and execution of the plan.

One of the main take-home messages of this chapter is that brains do not represent plans per se. Plans are our descriptions of certain activities we perform. But the plan itself relies upon activating a variety of representations and processes that may be commonly activated by other stimuli (e.g., stories) and are stored in a distributed manner in frontal lobe brain regions. Given that conceptualization, it is my belief that future CN research should focus on how event sequences in general are parsed (Zacks & Tversky, 2001) and stored, whether there is unique information that can be abstracted *across* a sequence of events, whether event sequences are organized by category and frequency, more explicit depiction and modeling of the plan-level cognitive processes referred to in this review (e.g., plan grammars), and more precise mapping of plan-related cognitive components to sectors within the human prefrontal cortex and basal ganglia using combined patient and functional neuroimaging studies to acquire evidence. Ignored in this chapter but of importance to understanding planning is how individual differences influence planning development and execution. For example, how do sex differences impact performance (Unterrainer et al., 2005)? Are there genetic factors or polymorphisms that influence level of plan performance (e.g., Foltynie et al., 2004)? Are there particular molecules or transmitters that play a key role in motivating the development and execution of plans (e.g., Phillips, Ahn, & Floresco, 2004)?

Human CN research is in a position to deliver crucial evidence regarding both the cognitive architecture and the neural topography of plans. By being able to represent and execute plans, we are able to integrate events from the past, present, and future into a single plan-level memory unit (Grafman, 1995; Haith, Benson, Roberts, & Pennington, 1994). Planning enables us to outsmart others and to cope with a changing environment while achieving a myriad of goals (Nichelli et al., 1994). There should be no doubt that the elaboration of planning abilities enabled humans to overcome evolutionary obstacles and to achieve superiority in certain environments. I am also convinced that the evolution of plan representations/processes preceded and later motivated the development of other cognitive abilities, such as the language and thematic knowledge needed to explain and cognitively shape the new ability to remember structured event sequences. Thus, the ability to plan is of primary importance to the human endeavor, and its significance to a complete understanding of the human brain is ensured.

## ACKNOWLEDGMENTS

My funding is provided by the National Institutes of Health Intramural Research Program. Portions of this chapter were adapted from Grafman, Spector, and Rattermann (2005). I would like to thank my wife, Sarah, and my son, Daniel, for their support during the writing of this chapter.

## REFERENCES

Allen, J. F., Kautz, H. A., Pelavin, R. N., Tenenberg, J. D. (Eds.). (1991). *Reasoning about plans*. San Mateo, CA: Morgan Kaufmann.

Anderson, J. (1983). *The architecture of cognition*. Cambridge, MA: Harvard University Press.

Baker, R., Baker, S. C., Rogers, R. D., O'Leary, D. A., Paykel, E. S., Frith, C. D., et al. (1997). Prefront al dysfunction in depressed patients performing a complex planning task: A study using positron emission tomography. *Psychological Medicine, 27,* 931–942.

Baker, S. C., Rogers, R. D., Owen, A. M., Frith, C. D., Dolan, R. J., Frackowiak, R. S. J., et al. (1996). Neural systems engaged by planning: A PET study of the Tower of London task. *Neuropsychologia, 34,* 515–526.

Baker-Sennett, J., Matusov, E., & Rogoff, B. (1993). Planning as developmental process. *Advances in Child Development and Behavior, 24,* 253–281.

Bechara, A., Damasio, A. R., Damasio, H., Anderson, S. W. (1994). Insensitivity to future consequences following damage to human prefrontal cortex. *Cognition, 50,* 7–15.

Berns, G. S., & Sejnowski, T. J. (1998). A computational model of how the basal ganglia produces se-

quences. *Journal of Cognitive Neuroscience, 10,* 108–121.

Blum, A., & Furst, M. (1997). Fast planning through planning graph analysis. *Artificial Intelligence, 90,* 281–300.

Chapman D. (1991). *Vision, instruction, and action*. Cambridge, MA: MIT Press.

Cohen, J. D., Perlstein, W. M., Braver, T. S., Nystrom, L. E., Noll, D. C., Jonides, J., et al. (1997). Temporal dynamics of brain activation during a working memory task. *Nature, 386,* 604–608.

Courtney, S. M., Ungerleider, L. G., Keil, K., & Haxby, J. V. (1997). Transient and sustained activity in a distributed neural system for human working memory. *Nature, 386,* 608–611.

Das, J. P., Kar, B. C., & Parrila, R. K. (1996). *Cognitive planning: The psychological basis of intelligent behavior*. New Delhi: Sage.

Dehaene, S., & Changeux, J.-P. (1997). A hierarchical neuronal network for planning behavior. *Proceedings of the National Academy of Sciences of the United States of America, 94,* 13293–13298.

Dreher, M., & Oerter, R. (1987). Action planning competencies during adolescence and early adulthood. In S. L. Friedman, E. K. Scholnick, & R. R. Cocking (Eds.), *Blueprints for thinking: The role of planning in cognitive development* (pp. 321–355). Cambridge, UK: Cambridge University Press.

Elliott, R., Baker, S. C., Rogers, R. D., O'Leary, D. A., Paykel, E. S., Frith, C. D., et al. (1997). Prefrontal dysfunction in depressed patients performing a complex planning task: A study using positron emission tomography. *Psychological Medicine, 27,* 931–942.

Elliott, R., Frith, C. D., & Dolan, R. J. (1997). Differential neural response to positive and negative feedback in planning and guessing tasks. *Neuropsychologia, 35,* 1395–1404.

Fikes, R., & Nilsson, N. J. (1971). STRIPS: A new approach to the application of theorem proving to problem solving. *Artificial Intelligence, 2,* 189–208.

Flitman, S., Cooper, V., & Grafman, J. (1997). PET imaging of maze processing. *Neuropsychologia, 35,* 409–420.

Phillips, A.G., Ahn, S., & Floresco, S. B. (2004). Magnitude of dopamine release in medial prefrontal cortex predicts accuracy of memory on a delayed response task. *Journal of Neuroscience, 24,* 547–553.

Foltynie, T., Goldberg, T. E., Lewis, S. G., Blackwell, A. D., Kolachana, B. S., Weinberger, D. R., et al. (2004). Planning ability in Parkinson's disease is influenced by the COMT val158met polymorphism. *Movement Disorders, 19,* 885–891.

Friedman, S. L., & Scholnick, E. K. (Eds.). (1997). *The developmental psychology of planning*. Mahwah, NJ: Erlbaum.

Friedman, S. L., Scholnick, E. K., & Cocking, R. R. (Eds.). (1987). *Blueprints for thinking: The role of planning in cognitive development*. Cambridge, UK: Cambridge University Press.

Fuster, J. M. (1995). Memory and planning: Two temporal perspectives of frontal lobe function. *Advances in Neurology, 66,* 9–20.

Goel, V., & Grafman, J. (1995). Are the frontal lobes implicated in planning functions: Re-interpreting data from the Tower of Hanoi. *Neuropsychologia, 33,* 623–642.

Goel, V., Grafman, J., Tajik, J., Gana, S., & Danto, D. (1997). A study of the performance of frontal patients in a financial planning task. *Brain, 120,* 1805–1822.

Goldman-Rakic, P. (1996). The prefrontal landscape: Implications of functional architecture for understanding human mentation and the central executive. *Philosophical Transactions of the Royal Society of London, Series B, Biological Sciences, 351,* 1445–1453.

Goldstein, L. H., Bernard, S., Fenwick, P. B. C., Burgess, P. W., & McNeil, J. (1993). Unilateral frontal lobectomy can produce strategy application disorder. *Journal of Neurology, Neurosurgery, and Psychiatry, 56,* 274–276.

Grafman, J. (1989). Plans, actions, and mental sets: The role of the frontal lobes. In E. Perecman (Ed.), *Integrating theory and practice in clinical neuropsychology* (pp. 93–138). Hillsdale, NJ: Erlbaum.

Grafman, J. (1994). Neuropsychology of higher cognitive processes. In D. Zaidel (Ed.), *Handbook of perception and cognition (neuropsychology)* (Vol. 15, pp. 159–181). San Diego, CA: Academic Press.

Grafman, J. (1995). Similarities and distinctions among models of prefrontal cortical functions. In J. Grafman, K. J. Holyoak, & F. Boller (Eds.), *Structure and function of the human prefrontal cortex* (pp. 337–368). New York: New York Academy of Sciences.

Grafman, J., & Hendler, J. (1991). Planning and the brain. *Behavioral and Brain Sciences, 14,* 563–564.

Grafman, J., Litvan, I., Massaquoi, S., Stewart, M., Sirigu, A., & Hallett, M. (1992). Cognitive planning deficit in patients with cerebellar atrophy. *Neurology, 42,* 1493–1496.

Grafman, J., Spector, L., & Rattermann, M. J. (2005). Planning and the brain. In R. Morris & G. Ward (Eds.), *The cognitive psychology of planning* (pp. 181–198). Hove, UK: Psychology Press.

Haith, M. M., Benson, J. B., Roberts, R. J., Jr., & Pennington, B. F. (Eds.). (1994). *The development of future-oriented processes.* Chicago: University of Chicago Press.

Hammond, K. (Ed.). (1994). *Proceedings of the Second International Conference on Artificial Intelligence Planning Systems.* Menlo Park, CA: AAAI Press.

Hayes-Roth, B., & Hayes-Roth, F. (1979). A cognitive model of planning. *Cognitive Science, 3,* 275–310.

Hoc, J.-M. (1988). *Cognitive psychology of planning.* London: Academic Press.

Karnath, H. O., & Wallesch, C. W. (1992). Inflexibility of mental planning: A characteristic disorder with prefrontal lobe lesions? *Neuropsychologia, 30,* 1011–1016.

Karnath, H. O., Wallesch, C. W., & Zimmermann, P. (1991). Mental planning and anticipatory processes with acute and chronic frontal lobe lesions: A comparison of maze performance in routine and nonroutine situations. *Neuropsychologia, 29,* 271–290.

Kolodner, J. (1993). *Case-based reasoning.* San Mateo, CA: Kaufmann.

Langley, P., & Drummond, M. (1990). Toward an experimental science of planning. In *Proceedings of the 1990 DARPA Workshop on Innovative Approaches to Planning, Scheduling and Control* (pp. 109–114). San Mateo, CA: Kaufmann.

Lingard, A. R., & Richards, E. B. (1998). Planning parallel actions. *Artificial Intelligence, 99,* 261–324.

Miller, E. K., Erickson, C. A., & Desimone, R. (1996). Neural mechanisms of visual working memory in prefrontal cortex of the macaque. *Journal of Neuroscience, 16,* 5154–5167.

Miller, G. A., Galanter, E., & Pribram, K. (1960). *Plans and the structure of behavior.* New York: Holt, Rinehart & Winston.

Morris, R. G., Ahmed, S., Syed, G. M., & Toone, R. K. (1993). Neural correlates of planning ability: Frontal lobe activation during the Tower of London test. *Neuropsychologia, 31,* 1367–1378.

Morris, R. G., Downes, J. J., Sahakian, B. J., Evenden, J. L., Heald, A., & Robbins, T. W. (1988). Planning and spatial working memory in Parkinson's disease. *Journal of Neurology, Neurosurgery, and Psychiatry, 51,* 757–766.

Morris, R. G., Miotto, E. C., Feigenbaum, J. D., Bullock, P., & Polkey, C. E. (1997). The effect of goal–subgoal conflict on planning ability after frontal- and temporal-lobe lesions in humans. *Neuropsychologia, 35,* 1147–1157.

Newell, A., & Simon, H. A. (1972). *Human problem solving.* Englewood Cliffs, NJ: Prentice-Hall.

Newman, S. D., Carpenter, P. A., Varma, S., & Just, M. A. (2003). Frontal and parietal participation in problem solving in the Tower of London: fMRI and computational modeling of planning and high-level perception. *Neuropsychologia, 41,* 1668–1682.

Nichelli, P., Grafman, J., Pietrini, P., Alway, D., Carton, J. C., & Miletich, R. (1994). Brain activation in chess playing. *Nature, 369,* 191.

Nichelli, P., Grafman, J., Pietrini, P., Clark, K., Lee, K. Y., & Miletich, R. (1995). Where the brain appreciates the moral of a story. *NeuroReport, 6,* 2309–2313.

Owen, A. M. (1997). Cognitive planning in humans: Neuropsychological, neuroanatomical and neuropharmacological perspectives. *Progress in Neurobiology, 53,* 431–450.

Owen, A. M., Downes, J. J., Sahakian, B. J., Polkey, C. E., & Robbins, T. W. (1990). Planning and spatial working memory following frontal lobe lesions in man. *Neuropsychologia, 28,* 1021–1034.

Owen, A. M., Doyon, J., Petrides, M., & Evans, A. C. (1996). Planning and spatial working memory: A positron emission tomography study in humans. *European Journal of Neuroscience, 8,* 353–364.

Partiot, A., Grafman, J., Sadato, N., Flitman, S., & Wild, K. (1996). Brain activation during script event processing. *NeuroReport, 7,* 761–766.

Partiot, A., Grafman, J., Sadato, N., Wachs, J., & Hallett, M. (1995). Brain activation during the generation of non-emotional and emotional plans. *NeuroReport, 6,* 1269–1272.

Pascual-Leone, A., Grafman, J., Clark, K., Stewart, M., Massaquoi, S., Lou, J.-L, et al. (1993). Procedural learning in Parkinson's disease and cerebellar degeneration. *Annals of Neurology, 34,* 594–602.

Pea, R. D., & Hawkins, J. (1987). Planning in a chore-scheduling task. In S. L. Friedman, E. K. Scholnick, & R. R. Cocking (Eds.), *Blueprints for thinking: The role of planning in cognitive development* (pp. 273–302). Cambridge, UK: Cambridge University Pres.

Rogers, R. D., Sahakian, B. J., Hodges, J. R., Polkey, C. E., Kennard, C., & Robbins, T. W. (1998). Dissociating executive mechanisms of task control following frontal lobe damage and Parkinson's disease. *Brain, 121,* 815–842.

Rosenbloom, P. S., Laird, J. E., & Newell, A. (Eds.). (1993). *The SOAR papers: Research on integrated intelligence.* Cambridge, MA: MIT Press.

Sacerdoti, E. D. (1975). The nonlinear nature of plans. In *Proceedings of the Fourth International Joint Conference on Artificial Intelligence* (pp. 206–214). San Mateo, CA: Kaufmann.

Schank, R. C., & Abelson, R. P. (1977). *Scripts, plans, goals, and understanding.* Hillsdale, NJ: Erlbaum.

Scholnick, E.K., & Friedman, S. L. (1987). The planning construct in the psychological literature. In S. L. Friedman, E. K. Scholnick, & R. R. Cocking (Eds.), *Blueprints for thinking: The role of planning in cognitive development* (pp. 3–38). Cambridge, UK: Cambridge University Press.

Schwartz, M. F., Reed, E. S., Montgomery, M., Palmer, C., & Mayer, N. H. (1991). The quantitative description of action disorganization after brain damage: A case study. *Cognitive Neuropsychology, 8,* 381–414.

Shallice, T., & Burgess, P. (1996). The domain of supervisory processes and temporal organization of behaviour. *Philosophical Transactions of the Royal Society of London, Series B, 351,* 1405–1412.

Shallice, T., & Burgess, P. W. (1991). Deficits in strategy application following frontal lobe damage in man. *Brain, 114,* 727–741.

Sirigu, A., Cohen, L., Zalla, T., Pradat-Diehl, P., Van Eeckhout, P., Grafman, J., et al. (1998). Distinct prefrontal regions for processing sentence syntax and story grammar. *Cortex, 34,* 771–778.

Sirigu, A., Zalla, T., Pillon, B., Grafman, J., Agid, Y., & Dubois, B. (1995a). Selective impairments in managerial knowledge following prefrontal cortex damage. *Cortex, 31,* 301–316.

Sirigu, A., Zalla, T., Pillon, B., Grafman, J., Dubois, B., & Agid, Y. (1995b). Planning and script analysis following pre-frontal lobe lesions. In J. Grafman, K. J. Holyoak, & F. Boller (Eds.), Structure and function of the human prefrontal cortex. *New York Academy of Sciences, 769,* 277–288.

Sirigu, A., Zalla, T., Pillon, B., Grafman, J., Dubois, B., & Agid, Y. (1996). Encoding of sequence and boundaries of scripts following prefrontal lesions. *Cortex, 32,* 297–310.

Spector, L., & Grafman, J. (1994). Planning, neuropsychology, and artificial intelligence: Cross fertilization. In F. Boller & J. Grafman (Eds.), *Handbook of neuropsychology* (Vol. 9, pp. 377–392). Amsterdam: Elsevier Science.

Suchman, L. A. (1987). *Plans and situated actions.* Cambridge, UK: Cambridge University Press.

Unterrainer, J. M., Ruff, C. C., Rahm, B., Kaller, C. P., Spreer, J., Schwarzwald, R., et al. (2005). The influence of sex differences and individual task performance on brain activation during planning. *NeuroImage, 24,* 586–590.

Wallesch, C.-W., Karnath, H. O., Papagno, C., Zimmermann, P., Deuschl, G., & Lucking, C. H. (1990). Parkinson's disease patient's behavior in a covered maze learning task. *Neuropsychologia, 28,* 839–849.

Ward, G., & Allport, A. (1997). Planning and problem-solving using the five-disk Tower of London task. *Quarterly Journal of Experimental Psychology, 50A,* 49–78.

Wilensky, R. (1983). *Planning and understanding: A computational approach to human reasoning.* Reading, MA: Addison-Wesley.

Wood, J. N., & Grafman, J. (2003). Human prefrontal cortex: Processing and representational perspectives. *Nature Reviews: Neuroscience, 4,* 139–147.

Zacks, J. M., & Tversky, B. (2001). Event structure in perception and conception. *Psychological Bulletin, 127,* 3–21.

# CHAPTER 17

# Principles of Motor Control by the Frontal Lobes as Revealed by the Study of Voluntary Eye Movements

*Adam L. Boxer*

The study of eye movement control provides many advantages over the study of other movement systems for understanding the basic neural mechanisms of motor control. Three sets of muscles move the eyes primarily in one Cartesian plane, which makes the oculomotor system considerably simpler to understand than other motor systems that use multiple sets of muscles to move limbs through three-dimensional space. Particularly, the voluntary control of movement initiation and cessation, or how the brain decides to initiate a movement, is being progressively elucidated down to the single-cell level. A growing body of evidence suggests that principles of motor control gleaned from studying oculomotor function are likely to be applicable to the study of other, more complex movements, such as reaching movements with the arms and hands (Cisek & Kalaska, 2005). Because the direction of gaze often indicates the visual stimuli to which a subject attends, the study of eye movement control is also producing important insights into the mechanisms of visual attention and other higher-order cognitive processes (Corbetta et al., 1998). As cognitive neuroscientists progressively delineate the relationships between brain activity and behavior, the wealth of knowledge about basic oculomotor physiology that has accumulated over the past 30 years will serve as an important basis for developing computational neurophysiological models of human behavior (Schall, 2004).

Much of what is known about eye movement control has been learned from combined eye movement and single-cell electrophysiological recordings from awake, behaving monkeys. Monkeys can be trained to complete complicated oculomotor tasks, and the identical tasks can be performed in humans, usually producing similar results. Phylogenetically, the brain regions that control eye movements are well conserved among monkeys, humans, and lower vertebrates. The emergence of powerful functional neuroimaging technologies, such as functional magnetic resonance imaging (fMRI) and event-related potentials (ERPs) that can measure brain activity in human subjects (or monkeys) while performing eye movement tasks, has confirmed that there are similar patterns of brain activity in monkeys and humans while performing similar eye movement tasks (Koyama et al., 2004). In addition, studies of human subjects with focal brain lesions (from strokes or tumors) provide additional support for models of eye movement control that are based on electrophysiological data from monkeys (Pierrot-Deseilligny, Milea, & Muri, 2004).

Two types of eye movements are studied most often in human and nonhuman primates: saccades and smooth pursuit. Saccades are rapid shifts of gaze that serve to maintain an image on the fovea, the area of the retina with the highest visual acuity. Saccades can be *reflexive*, such as the rapid shifts of gaze that occur without conscious input as a subject views a face or reads a page, or *voluntary*, such as when a subject chooses to look toward a specific stimulus from a group of distracters.

Smooth pursuit allows for continuous, undistorted vision of objects moving across the visual field by matching the velocity of eye movements with the velocity of a target. Computationally, saccades are less complex than smooth pursuit, and much of the neural circuitry necessary to produce accurate saccades is located in the brainstem. In contrast, smooth pursuit likely requires a more complicated neural network, and more processing in cortical, basal ganglia, brainstem, and cerebellar regions for proper functioning (Krauzlis, 2004). Consistent with the relative simplicity of saccades, these eye movements are found in simple vertebrates such as fish and rodents, whereas only higher vertebrates are capable of smooth pursuit. Although the computational mechanisms that produce saccades and smooth pursuit are different, higher-order aspects of their control are likely to be similar, particularly the decisions to initiate a movement, choose a target, or stop a movement. Because the generation of saccades can be largely automatic and independent of cortical structures, study of "top-down" control of saccades can be used to model cognitive aspects of motor control (Stuphorn & Schall, 2002).

Multiple regions within the frontal cortex and subcortical nuclei are involved in the generation of eye movements. These brain regions form critical nodes in the neural networks responsible for oculomotor control; however, it is uncertain to what degree each computation is carried out within frontal lobe structures as opposed to being an emergent property of frontal–parietal, frontal–subcortical, or frontal–brainstem circuits. For saccades, it is believed that the frontal lobe oculomotor regions are most important for voluntary saccades, whereas accurate reflexive saccades can be generated with little input from the frontal lobes (Pierrot-Deseilligny et al., 2004). Data from both monkeys and humans support roles for the frontal lobes in both movement perception and representation (Rizzolatti & Luppino, 2001), as well as the planning and execution of movements. This chapter reviews the role of frontal lobe structures involved in the planning and execution of eye movements, with an emphasis on the insights gained into higher-order aspects of cognitive function, such as decision making.

## ANATOMY OF EYE MOVEMENT CONTROL: NODES AND CIRCUITS

In the frontal lobes, three regions are most involved in eye movement control: the frontal eye fields (FEFs), the supplementary eye fields (SEFs), and the dorsolateral prefrontal cortex (DLPFC; see Figure 17.1). These frontal eye movement control regions are strongly connected to regions in the dorsal parietal lobe involved in eye movement control, particularly in the vicinity of the lateral intraparietal sulcus (LIP), the basal ganglia, and brainstem structures. In the brainstem, the superior colliculus (SC) plays a dominant role in organizing many aspects of eye movement control through its connections with other nuclei in the dorsal midbrain (for vertical eye movements) and pons (for horizontal eye movements). Neurons in the cerebellum are critical for maintaining smooth pursuit eye movements and may help to refine certain types of saccades. The connections and circuitry of brainstem control of eye movement are well described elsewhere (Sparks, 2002).

Thus, the frontal, parietal, basal ganglia, and brainstem neurons involved in eye movement control form critical nodes within the neural circuits that produce saccades and smooth pursuit. Two lines of evidence suggest that accurate voluntary eye movements are an emergent property of this brain network. First, electrophysiological recordings in monkeys, and to a lesser extent, functional imaging experiments in humans, show similar patterns of activity during eye movement tasks in multiple brain regions, suggesting that neural computations occur in parallel or in a distributed fashion over this eye movement network. Second, studies of human patients with brain lesions that interrupt the connections between eye movement control regions but spare the actual nodes themselves clearly demonstrate that disconnection of these nodes can abolish normal voluntary eye movement control. This section delineates the most important nodes and connections for the control of voluntary saccades (Figure 17.2).

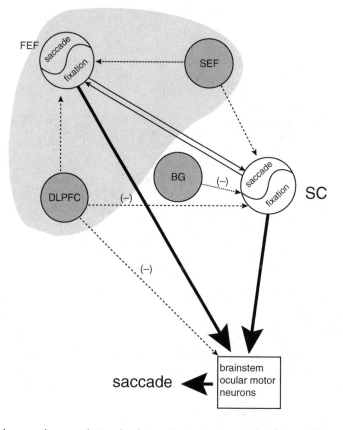

FIGURE 17.1. A simple neural network involved in voluntary saccade initiation. The structures that are most important for deciding to initiate a voluntary saccade are the frontal eye field (FEF) and superior colliculus (SC). These regions are tightly connected and show parallel patterns of activity prior to a voluntary saccade. Within the FEF and SC are both saccade-related and fixation-related neurons having reciprocal patterns of activity that allow these regions to quickly and sensitively react to the presence of a new visual stimulus. The activity of these decision-making neurons is monitored by neurons within the supplementary eye field (SEF) that sense errors, and can exert an instructive influence on FEF and SC neurons. Likewise, neurons the activity of neurons in the DLPFC imparts an instructive influence on the SC and FEF to generate the correct preparatory set for voluntary saccade initiation. The basal ganglia (BG), producing output through the SNr, also help to suppress reflexive saccade activity that may interfere with voluntary saccades.

## Frontal Eye Field

The frontal eye field (FEF) is located in the rostral bank of the arcuate sulcus in macaque monkeys (Stuphorn & Schall, 2002). In humans, high-resolution fMRI studies have localized the FEF to the anterior wall of the precentral sulcus, near the caudal end of the superior frontal sulcus, a region homologous to the location of the FEF in monkeys (Rosano et al., 2002). The FEF can be further subdivided into two regions, one involved in the generation of saccades, which is located in the upper portion of the anterior wall of the precentral sulcus, and a smooth pursuit–related area, which is found deeper along the anterior wall, extending in some subjects to the fundus or deep posterior wall. Using histopathological markers from postmortem specimens, these regions have been demonstrated to be structurally similar to other regions of motor cortex (Rosano, Sweeney, Melchitzky, & Lewis, 2003). Based on electrical stimulation studies of human subjects prior to brain surgery, the saccade-generating portion of the FEF is found 1–2 cm anterior to primary motor cortical regions involved in finger and hand movements, a region in close agreement to that identified in

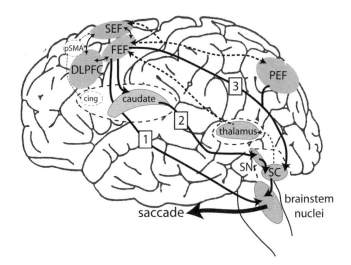

FIGURE 17.2. Brain regions involved in saccade control. In the frontal lobes, the frontal eye field (FEF) is a critical node for initiation of voluntary saccades. It receives inputs from the parietal eye fields (PEFs) and thalamus, which provide visual information. The supplementary eye field (SEF) monitors and supervises FEF activity, and the dorsolateral prefrontal cortex (DLPFC) likely exerts a direct modulatory influence on the FEF, as well as on downstream structures in the brainstem. Other regions in the medial frontal lobes, including the pre–supplementary motor area (pSMA) and anterior cingulate (cing), may also exert modulatory influences on the FEF via the SEF and DLPFC. There are three main pathways from the FEF to the primary and secondary motor neurons in the brainstem nuclei that generate saccades: (1) a direct connection between the FEF and the brainstem oculomotor nuclei; (2) a pathway through the caudate eye field and substantia nigra pars reticulata (SNr), which helps to suppress saccades; and (3) a direct connection between the FEF and superior colliculus (SC), which is finely tuned for saccade programming and can generate reflexive saccades independently of the FEF.

fMRI studies (Yamamoto et al., 2004). Similarly, cortical stimulation experiments in humans confirm that the smooth pursuit region is located more posteriorly than the saccade region (Blanke & Seeck, 2003).

The FEF receives connections that convey both visuosensory information and motor information to its neurons. Importantly, regions within the FEF receive information from both the ventral visual stream (the "what" pathway) and the dorsal visual stream (the "where" pathway; Schall, Morel, King, & Bullier, 1995). The neurons of the FEF that receive connections from the ventral stream generate shorter saccades than those innervated by dorsal stream neurons. This is consistent with the expected size of saccades necessary to explore visually a small object or face (in detail) versus those necessary to characterize distant aspects of a subject's spatial environment. The FEF also receives information from the SEF, the DLPFC, the thalamus, and the substantia nigra pars reticulata (SNr). These inputs can positively

and negatively modulate the activity of neurons within the FEF (discussed below).

In addition to, and as part of, their roles in generating saccades, the neurons of the FEF represent the behavioral relevance of objects within the visual field; thus, the activity over portions of the FEF can be said to represent a visual salience map (Thompson & Bichot, 2005). After presentation of a visual stimulus, over time, activity within the FEF evolves to represent the behavioral significance of the stimulus. This behavioral significance can be read out as a saccade to the novel stimulus, but it may also be represented as a covert shift of attention without an actual eye movement.

### Supplementary Eye Fields

The supplementary eye field (SEF) is located on the medial surface of the superior frontal gyrus, in the dorsal aspect of the paracentral sulcus. The SEF receives connections from the FEF, the DLPFC, and the anterior cingulate cortex. The

SEF is involved in programming sequences of saccades or combined saccade–body movements and likely has important preparatory roles in more complex eye movements (Isoda & Tanji, 2003). Functional imaging studies in humans suggest that the SEF is activated prior to both simple and more complex saccade tasks (Gagnon, O'Driscoll, et al., 2002), suggesting that it may have a supervisory role over neurons in the FEF (Schall, Stuphorn, & Brown, 2002).

## Dorsolateral Prefrontal Cortex

The dorsolateral prefrontal cortex (DLPFC) is involved in multiple aspects of saccade programming, including making decisions to initiate voluntary saccades and maintaining spatial working memory for target locations (Funahashi, Chafee, & Goldman-Rakic, 1993; Pierrot-Deseilligny, Muri, Rivaud-Pechoux, Gaymard, & Ploner, 2002; Pierrot-Deseilligny et al., 2003). Recent monkey data also support a role for these and nearby regions in mental rehearsal of eye movements, prior to actual saccade initiation (Cisek & Kalaska, 2004). The regions of the DLPFC that are most important for control of eye movements are located in the middle frontal gyrus in Brodmann's areas 46 and 9. Subjects with brain lesions involving the DLPFC have difficulty in suppressing unwanted reflexive saccades and in generating predictive saccades to targets presented in a predictable sequence in time and space (Pierrot-Deseilligny et al., 2003). The suppression of unwanted reflexive saccades likely involves a direct inhibitory projection from DLPFC neurons to the brainstem saccade-generating circuitry, including the SC (Condy, Rivaud-Pechoux, Ostendorf, Ploner, & Gaymard, 2004). Experiments with monkeys suggest that there are neurons in the vicinity of the DLPFC whose activity signals the suppression of a reflexive saccade or the command "Don't look" (Hasegawa, Peterson, & Goldberg, 2004). Activity from these neurons may be crucial for the DLPFC's ability to help select one behaviorally relevant saccade over a range of other visually salient targets.

Transcranial magnetic stimulation, when applied to the DLPFC 3 seconds after presentation of the locations to be remembered, significantly alters the amplitude of subsequent memory-guided saccades in normal humans (Nyffeler et al., 2002), confirming roles for this structure in spatial working memory first identified in nonhuman primates (Constantinidis, Franowicz, Goldman-Rakic, 2001).

## Superior Colliculus

Although the superior colliculus (SC) is not part of the frontal lobes, it plays a central role in saccade programming and has multiple recurrent connections with the frontal lobe eye movement control regions. This is evident in electrophysiological studies of saccade and smooth pursuit initiation, which demonstrate similar patterns of neural activity in the FEF and SC. Studies in nonhuman primates suggest that in normal subjects, most of the control of saccades by the frontal eye movement regions is mediated by the SC (Sparks, 2002). Under conditions of SC damage, other cortical and brainstem regions can partially compensate for the lost SC functions; however, saccades are much less accurate in time and space.

Neurons that have saccade-related activity in the intermediate and deep layers of the SC are arranged topographically and fire bursts of activity before an eye movement, be it a saccade or smooth pursuit (Krauzlis & Dill, 2002). The location of SC neurons within this topographic map (in polar coordinates) determines the saccade amplitude and direction, and not the firing rate of the cells. There is a rostrocaudal gradient in the SC, such that activation of rostral cells generates small-amplitude eye movements, and activation of caudal cells generates larger-amplitude saccades. Electrical stimulation of the rostral pole of the SC inhibits saccades, consistent with an important role for this region in maintaining fixation on a target. These neurons have monosynaptic excitatory inputs to neurons in the brainstem that inhibit eye movements (Leigh & Kennard, 2004). Upward saccades are represented medially and downward saccades, laterally, within the SC (Sparks, 2002). Neurons that are downstream of these signals, in midbrain and pontine oculomotor nuclei, have firing rates that directly correlate with the speed and amplitude of saccades.

The SC forms a critical node in the network for incorporating reward information into the generation of eye movements. Via a basal ganglia circuit, which includes the oculomotor portions of the caudate nucleus, with projections to the SNr, the SC integrates information regarding the reward value of saccades to specific locations (Hikosaka, Takikawa, & Kawagoe, 2000). Impairments in memory-guided and predictive saccades in neurodegenerative diseases with basal ganglia damage may in part arise from damage to this circuit (Leigh & Kennard, 2004). Nicotinic cholinergic inputs from the pedunculopontine nucleus to the SC may also have important effects on attention and motivation for saccades through a stimulatory effect on the SC (Kobayashi, Saito, & Isa, 2001). Decreased attention and visual search efficiency (Daffner, Scinto, Weintraub, Guinessey, & Mesulam, 1992; Mosimann, Felblinger, Ballinari, Hess, & Muri, 2004), and difficulties with saccade programming (Shafiq-Antonacci, Maruff, Masters, & Currie, 2003) in Alzheimer's disease may be in part explained by damage to this cholinergic circuit.

# EXPERIMENTAL PARADIGMS THAT REVEAL THE ROLES OF THE FRONTAL LOBES IN VOLUNTARY EYE MOVEMENT CONTROL

Two of the most commonly used oculomotor tasks that have been used to investigate top-down control of motor functions by the frontal lobe are the countermanding task (Logan, Cowan, & Davis, 1984) and the antisaccade task (Hallet, 1978). Both tasks require suppression of a reflexive response to shift gaze to a novel visual stimulus and have been extensively studied in both human subjects and monkeys. Functional imaging technology has revealed similar patterns of brain activation in humans to those obtained from single-unit records in monkeys, suggesting that insights gained in nonhuman primate models can be readily applied to the understanding of human behavior in these tasks.

## The Countermanding Task

The countermanding task tests a subject's ability to control the initiation of a movement in a reaction time task by infrequently presenting a stop signal. This is comparable to a "go/no-go" task performed with patients at the bedside (e.g., Dubois, Slachevsky, Litvan, & Pillon, 2000). An oculomotor version of this task has been implemented in both monkeys and humans, and both species perform similarly (Hanes & Carpenter, 1999; Stuphorn & Schall, 2002). Combined oculomotor and electrophysiological recordings from the FEF, SEF, and SC have provided much insight into the neural computational mechanisms of movement initiation and error monitoring.

### Task Components

As implemented by Hanes, Schall, and coworkers in 1999, a subject gazes at a central fixation spot, and after a variable interval, the fixation spot disappears and a target appears to the right or to the left of the target (Figure 17.3) (Stuphorn & Schall, 2002). The subject then makes a saccade to the target (and, if the subject is a monkey, receives a reward such as a sip of juice). On some trials, called "stop signal trials," the central fixation spot reappears after the target appears, after a variable delay called the "stop signal delay." On the stop signal trials, the subject is instructed not to make a saccade to the target. If he or she is successful, then the saccade is cancelled (and again, if the subject is a monkey, there is an additional reward). If the subject is unable to cancel the saccade, usually due to the short latency of the stop signal, then there is no reward. After a large number of randomly interleaved trials (no stop signal, stop signal with different latencies), a unique "stop signal reaction time" (SSRT) can be calculated for each individual subject. For monkeys, this averages around 100 milliseconds. Humans have slightly longer SSRTs (Hanes & Carpenter, 1999). Recently, a smooth pursuit version of the countermanding task implemented in monkeys was found to have similar characteristics at the cellular level in the FEF and SC (Kornylo, Dill, Saenz, & Krauzlis, 2003).

### Race Model

Performance on the countermanding task can be accounted for by a model in which two competing processes drive the decision to shift gaze toward the target: One process will initiate the saccade; the other will hold gaze on the central fixation point (Figure 17.4). There is a race between these two processes: Whichever process accumulates enough of a signal (evidence) to cross a threshold value will win the race. The rate of accumulated evidence is influenced by

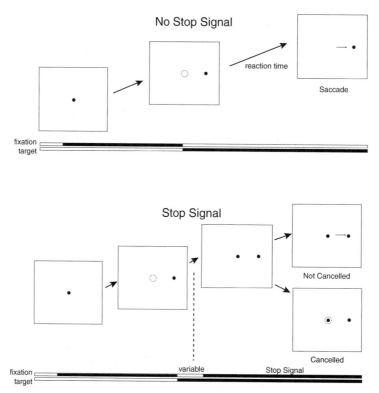

FIGURE 17.3. The countermanding task. A subject gazes at a central fixation spot, and after a variable interval, the fixation spot disappears and a target appears to the right or to the left of the target. The subject then makes a saccade to the target (no stop signal). On some trials, called "stop signal trials," the central fixation spot reappears after the target appears, after a variable delay called the "stop signal delay." On the stop signals trials, the subject is instructed not to make a saccade to the target. If successful, then the saccade is cancelled.

upstream processes that contribute to this decision-making process. In addition, the threshold to initiate or cancel a saccade may be modified depending on the behavioral context for the movement. This model is consistent with psychophysical studies demonstrating that reaction times for such tasks are stochastic (Schall, 2003).

### FEF Neural Activity Resembles the Race Model

Schall and colleagues (2002) hypothesized that the activity of single neurons within the primate FEF might be sufficient to initiate saccades, and if so, the activity of these movement-related neurons should resemble that predicted by the race model. Neurons should discharge differently when a saccade is initiated than when a saccade is withheld, and the difference in activity must occur by the time

the movement has been canceled (i.e., within the SSRT). Consistent with this hypotheses, single-unit recordings from movement-related neurons in FEF showed activity and began to grow toward a threshold but decayed back to baseline in successfully canceled countermanding trials (Figure 17.5A) (Hanes, Patterson, & Schall, 1998). Also consistent with the model, this activity occurred before the SSRT had elapsed. Moreover, fixation-related neurons showed an inverse pattern of activity; their firing rate increased around the time of the SSRT in successfully canceled trials (Figure 17.5B). There was no qualitative difference between activity in single neurons associated with movements executed without, or in spite of, a stop signal, consistent with notion that stop and go processes are independent. Thus, the activity of single neurons within the FEF embodies the decision-making process predicted by

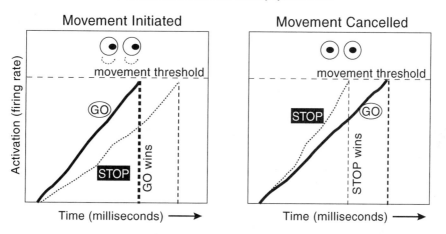

FIGURE 17.4. A race or accumulator model for movement initiation. Based on reaction time data for tasks such as the countermanding task, it has been proposed that the decision to initiate a movement involves a competition between two processes: a GO process that will initiate a movement and a STOP process that will cancel the movement. Both processes operate simultaneously and accumulate evidence (activation) at different rates. Whichever accumulates the greatest amount of evidence first will cross the threshold for movement initiation first and "win" the race. If the GO process accumulates evidence faster than the STOP process, a movement will be initiated. If the STOP process accumulates evidence faster than the GO process, the movement will be cancelled. There is a theoretical time limit at which the STOP process will never have enough time to accumulate the necessary information to reach the threshold, which is reflected in a psychophysical parameter: the stop signal reaction time (SSRT; see text).

psychophysiologically based models of the countermanding task.

### The SEF Serves a Supervisory Role

As with most psychophysical tasks, subjects can improve their performance on the countermanding task with practice, until they reach the latency threshold set by the SSRT, which is a characteristic value for each individual subject. To improve performance, subjects must be able to monitor correct versus incorrect (noncanceled stop signal trials) responses and then adjust their responses accordingly. This implies that there are brain region(s) whose activity should reflect accuracy and potentially instructive influences on the countermanding task. Stuphorn and coworkers (2000) found that neurons within the SEF had the expected patterns of activity that would be consistent with a supervisory role over FEF neurons involved in controlling gaze shifts on the countermanding task. They found specific neurons in the SEF whose activity reflected noncanceled stop signal trials (errors). Error-related neurons in the SEF had activity that was time-locked to saccade onset, and reflected whether a saccade

was made on a no-stop signal trial (correct response) or on a stop signal trial (error) (Stuphorn, Taylor, & Schall, 2000) (Figure 17.6). Other neurons within the SEF showed firing patterns consistent with a role in representing conflict between a programmed saccade and a stop signal. Finally, there were neurons whose activity was related to the presence of a reward after a successful response. These latter neurons' responses are consistent with greater innervation of the SEF by dopaminergic neurons than cells in the FEF. These findings are consistent with a growing body of literature that suggests the SEF is involved in supervisory control and reprogramming other components of the saccade-generating circuitry to adapt to new circumstances (e.g., the expectation of a stop signal) (Carpenter, 2004).

### Functional Imaging Support for Homologous Brain Activations in Monkeys and Humans

Curtis, Cole, Rao, and D'Esposito (2004) implemented the countermanding task in normal human volunteers using event-related fMRI and found patterns of blood oxygenation level–

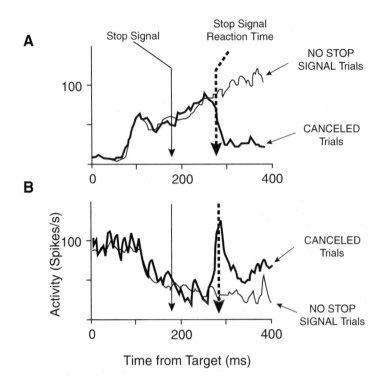

FIGURE 17.5. Relationship between FEF activity and canceling a movement. (A) Activity of a saccade neuron in FEF in trials in which the movement was produced but would have been canceled if the stop signal had been presented (thin line) is compared with activity on trials when the planned saccade was cancelled because the stop signal appeared (thick line). The time of the stop signal is indicated by the solid vertical arrow. The time needed to cancel the planned movement, the stop signal reaction time, is indicated by the dashed vertical arrow. The activity when the movement was canceled decayed immediately before the SSRT. (B) Comparison of the activity of a fixed neuron in FEF when saccades were initiated or canceled. From Stuphorn and Schall (2002). Copyright 2002 by John Wiley & Sons, Inc. Reprinted by permission.

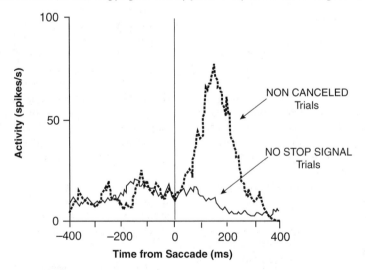

FIGURE 17.6. Example of an error neuron in the SEF. Neural activity following initiation of rightward eye movements in trials without a stop signal (thin solid line) is compared with activity on trials in which the saccade was not canceled despite the stop signal (thick dotted line). The neuron became active after the erroneous saccade. From Stuphorn and Schall (2002). Copyright 2002 by John Wiley & Sons, Inc. Reprinted by permission.

dependent (BOLD) signal changes highly consistent with the electrophysiological results from monkeys. This study found greater activation of the FEF on stop signal trials, regardless of whether the saccade was successfully canceled. Consistent with the monkey-derived evidence for a supervisory role for the SEF in the countermanding task, BOLD signal changes in the SEF distinguished between successful and unsuccessful countermanding trials.

### Studies in Humans with Altered Brain Function

The available evidence using the countermanding task suggests that humans and monkeys engage homologous brain regions when canceling a planned eye movement. Because there is strong evidence for involvement of the FEF and SEF, this task may be useful in assessing populations of subjects with frontal lobe dysfunction. Although not extensively studied in diseased populations, the countermanding task may provide a sensitive measure of cortical disinhibition in subjects with impaired frontal lobe function, such as adults with attention-deficit/hyperactivity disorder. These subjects are impaired on the task and are more sensitive to changes in the position of the stop signal than are normal adults (Armstrong & Munoz, 2003). The countermanding task is also sensitive to medications that alter cortical function and alertness. For example, inhalation of a surgical anesthetic (sevoflurane) increases the SSRT in a dose-

dependent manner (Nouraei, De Pennington, Jones, & Carpenter, 2003).

## The Antisaccade Task

The antisaccade task has two components: suppression of a reflexive saccade toward a target, and programming of a new saccade in the opposite direction. In part due to its ease of performance at the bedside, this task has been used extensively in both normal humans and diseased populations to investigate aspects of voluntary motor control. As with the countermanding task, electrophysiological studies in monkeys have provided much insight into the computational mechanisms that lead to successful task performance.

### Task Components

In this task, a subject gazes at a central fixation spot, the spot disappears, and a target appears, usually to the left or to the right of center. The subject is directed to "look away" from the target, and to instead look at a spot on the opposite side of the center. To increase the difficulty of the task, a gap, or delay, is often introduced between disappearance of the fixation point and appearance of the target. In addition, the antisaccade trials may be randomly interleaved with "prosaccade" trials in which the subject is directed to look at the targets (Figure 17.7).

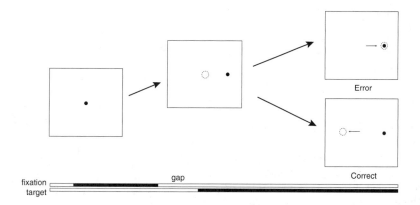

FIGURE 17.7. The antisaccade task. A subject gazes at a central fixation spot; then the spot disappears, and a target appears, usually to the left or to the right of center. The subject is directed to "look away" from the target, and to instead look at a spot on the opposite side. If the suject is unable to suppress a reflexive prosaccade toward the target, an error is made.

## Electrophysiological Correlates of Antisaccades in Awake Behaving Monkeys

Two neural computations must be successfully performed to generate a correct antisaccade. Suppression of a reflexive prosaccade toward the target relies heavily on frontal lobe structures, whereas programming a saccade in the opposite direction of the stimulus may involve both frontal and parietal eye movement regions. Because the first component of the antisaccade task is better understood, this discussion focuses primarily on reflexive saccade suppression.

Similar to the countermanding task, an accumulator, or race model, has been proposed to account for the reaction times of subjects performing the antisaccade task (Munoz & Everling, 2004). Recordings from both the FEF and SC show that there is reciprocal activity of fixation-related neurons and saccade-related neurons just prior to the saccades that occur during this task, whether they are directed correctly, away from the target, or incorrectly, towards the target. Both types of neurons have direct outputs to the brainstem oculomotor circuitry that generates each actual saccade. During the gap period between the offset of the central fixation stimulus and the onset of the peripheral target, the baseline level of activity of the saccade-related neurons increases and that of the fixation neurons decreases in anticipation of a possible target appearing in either visual field. For a prosaccade, the onset of the visual stimulus in the receptive field of a saccade neuron (e.g., for a left FEF or SC cell, onset of a target in the right visual field), leads to a rapid buildup of activity, presumably driven by greater input from the visual cortex or thalamus. For a correct antisaccade to occur, there must be inhibition of saccade neurons in the FEF and SC before the target appears, so that summation of the pretarget and target-related neural activity does not trigger a saccade (Everling & Munoz, 2000). Thus, it is the neural activity before the onset of the visual stimulus that is critical for successful antisaccade performance. This pattern of activity just prior to initiation of a saccade has been termed the "preparatory set" and is in part generated by a strong top-down modulation of the FEF and SC by other brain regions.

It is likely that multiple neural mechanisms contribute to generating the preparatory set for antisaccades. Importantly, for many neurons in the FEF and SC, the amount of activity that accompanies antisaccades is less than that accompanying prosaccades, which suggests that the increase in saccade neuron activity due to the visual response to appearance of the target is not sufficient to generate antisaccades (Everling & Munoz, 2000). This observation raises a number of possible mechanisms by which top-down modulation of saccade control operates to suppress reflexive saccades in the antisaccade task. One possibility is that the threshold level of activity necessary to activate reflexive saccades downstream of the FEF and SC is very briefly increased during antisaccades, so that the early visual stimulus-induced increase in saccade neuron activity is not able to activate the brainstem saccade machinery, but the later saccade in the opposite direction is able to do so. An alternative possibility is that the activity of saccade and fixation neurons in the FEF and SC is modulated, or augmented, by neurons from other brain regions. For example, neurons in the SEF have been shown to have visual and motor responses that are increased on antisaccade trials (Schlag-Rey, Amador, Sanchez, & Schlag, 1997) and could summate with FEF and SC activity to drive correct antisaccades.

Inhibition of saccade-related neurons in the FEF and SC is a critical component of successful antisaccade performance. A number of brain regions, including the SEF, DLPFC, and basal ganglia, might potentially generate inhibitory signals that suppress the reflexive saccade generating signals at the level of the FEF and SC. Input from these modulatory brain regions could directly increase activity of fixation neurons in the FEF and other regions, which in turn laterally inhibit the FEF and SC saccade neurons, or alternatively, these inhibitory regions might act downstream of the FEF and SC, to directly inhibit the brainstem oculomotor machinery.

In addition to possible stimulatory roles of the SEF on antisaccade generation, SEF neurons may also inhibit the FEF and SC during the preparatory set prior to an antisaccade. This hypothesis is supported by increased fixation-related neuron activity in the SEF prior to target presentation, with decreased activity of these same neurons when a direction error is made (Schlag-Rey et al., 1997).

Neurons in the SNr, acting as the output of a basal ganglia circuit, might also help to suppress saccade-related activity in the SEF and FEF during the antisaccade task (Hikosaka, Takikawa, & Kawagoe, 2000). However, a recent analysis of brain lesions in human patients with saccade impairments suggests that this basal ganglia circuit is less important for reflexive saccade suppression than other brain regions (Condy et al., 2004). These authors found that patients with subcortical lesions that involved the basal ganglia or thalamus, but spared the subcortical white matter tracts exiting the frontal lobes, do not lead to impairments on the antisaccade task. Lesions that included the anterior limb or genu of the internal capsule led to antisaccade impairments. This supports the existence of a frontal lobe brainstem circuit for suppression of reflexive prosaccades during the antisaccade task. The DLPFC is likely to play multiple, important roles in generating the preparatory set for the antisaccade task, including coding the location of the stimulus, as well as the required response to the stimulus (Funahashi, Chafee, & Goldman-Rakic, 1993). Other nearby neurons may also signal regions to which the subject must not look (Hasegawa, Peterson, & Goldberg, 2004).

## Functional Imaging Experiments in Humans

fMRI, ERP, and magnetoencephalography (MEG) studies of subjects performing the antisaccade task have demonstrated similar patterns of brain activation as those identified in monkeys. Using interleaved pro- and antisaccades, event-related fMRI experiments have demonstrated increased BOLD activity during the preparatory, pretarget phase of the antisaccade task in the SEF, FEF, and DLPFC on antisaccade trials relative to prosaccade trials (Connolly, Goodale, Menon, & Munoz, 2002; DeSouza, Menon, & Everling, 2003). One study reported that BOLD activity in the pre–supplementary motor area, which is contiguous with the SEF, predicted correct and incorrect antisaccades (Curtis & D'Esposito, 2003). Similar to the fMRI results, ERP studies have shown presaccade activations in lateral and medial frontal regions on the antisaccade task and a version of the countermanding task (Matthews, Flohr, & Everling, 2002). Only the antisaccade task was associated with activation of the parietal lobes, consistent with their proposed role in programming a novel saccade trajectory to look away from the target.

## Studies in Normal Adults and Development

A large body of normative data exist on the antisaccade task in humans. In over 2,000 young Greek army recruits, normative values for the antisaccade task have been determined and related to demographic, psychosocial, and cognitive measures. As with other reaction time tests, there is a speed–accuracy trade-off, such that 40% of the variance of error rate could be explained by decreased response latency on error trials. In addition, the effect of subtle modifications in task parameters has been studied in the same group (Smyrnis et al., 2002, 2003). The ability to perform antisaccades accurately develops in late childhood (Fischer, Biscaldi, & Gezeck, 1997; Fukushima, Hatta, & Fukushima, 2000; Klein, 2001; Klein & Foerster, 2001; Munoz, Broughton, Goldring, & Armstrong, 1998) and declines in normal elderly subjects in parallel to other cognitive measures of frontal lobe function (Klein, Fischer, Hartnegg, Heiss, & Roth, 2000).

## Lesion Studies

Early studies in patients with frontal lobe lesions showed that the antisaccade task is exquisitely sensitive to frontal lobe damage (Guitton, Buchtel, & Douglas, 1985). As mentioned earlier, the anatomy of antisaccade dysfunction has been elucidated in subjects with focal brain lesions and shown to involve a DLPFC–internal capsule–SC brainstem circuit, in which damage to any component of the circuit results in difficulty in reflexive saccade suppression (Condy et al., 2004; Pierrot-Deseilligny et al., 2003).

## Attention-Deficit/Hyperactivity Disorder and Tourette's Syndrome

Antisaccade function is abnormal in attention-deficit/hyperactivity disorder in both children (Mostofsky, Lasker, Cutting, Denckla, & Zee, 2001) and adults (Feifel, Farber, Clementz, Perry, & Anllo-Vento, 2004). In contrast, subjects with Tourette's syndrome have enhanced ability to perform this task, possibly consistent with subjects' necessity to suppress unwanted movements (Munoz, Le Vasseur, & Flanagan, 2002).

## Schizophrenia

A large number of studies have described the prominent antisaccade abnormalities associated with schizophrenia (reviewed in Hutton & Kennard, 1998). The antisaccade task is exquisitely sensitive to first-episode schizophrenia and correlates with disease severity and working memory impairments (Nieman et al., 2000). Antisaccade impairments are also found in first-degree relatives of patients with schizophrenia, suggesting that they may serve as a marker of an endophenotype or genetic risk factor for schizophrenia (Thaker et al., 2000). More recently, antisaccade performance has been used as an outcome measure in trials of therapeutic agents for this disease (Depatie et al., 2002; Ettinger et al., 2003; Wonodi et al., 2004).

### Dementia

Impairment on the antisaccade task is a sensitive marker of human immunodeficiency virus (HIV) dementia (Johnston, Miller, & Nath, 1996) and is present in subjects with Alzheimer's disease (Abel, Unverzagt, & Yee, 2002; Shafiq-Antonacci, Maruff, Masters, & Currie, 2003). In these subjects, antisaccade performance is correlated with the overall degree of cognitive impairment, as measured by tests such as the Mini-Mental State Exam. Antisaccade impairment is also associated with the presence of dementia in subjects with Parkinson's disease but not in cognitively normal patients with Parkinson's disease (Mosimann et al., 2005).

## CONCLUSION

Studies of the voluntary control of eye movements, particularly saccades, are revealing important principles about the mechanisms of motor control by the frontal lobes. There is convergent evidence from studies in nonhuman primates and humans performing simple voluntary saccade paradigms, such as the countermanding and antisaccade tasks, that the same brain regions and patterns of activity are involved in deciding to initiate or cancel an eye movement in both species. Data from human subjects with focal brain lesions or neurodegenerative syndromes suggest that the integrity of these circuits is necessary for accurate voluntary saccade initiation. Because these simple tasks are highly sensitive to disease, further understanding of the mechanisms that operate to control saccade generation in these oculomotor paradigms may allow for future development of computational models of oculomotor function that can be examined to better understand the effects of disease and medications on the frontal lobes. In this way, computational models of oculomotor control may facilitate the development and testing of novel therapies for frontal lobe dysfunction.

## REFERENCES

Abel, L. A., Unverzagt, F., & Yee, R. D. (2002). Effects of stimulus predictability and interstimulus gap on saccades in Alzheimer's disease. *Dementia and Geriatric Cognitive Disorders, 13,* 235–243.

Armstrong, I. T., & Munoz, D. P. (2003). Inhibitory control of eye movements during oculomotor countermanding in adults with attention-deficit hyperactivity disorder. *Experimental Brain Research, 152,* 444–452.

Blanke, O., & Seeck, M. (2003). Direction of saccadic and smooth eye movements induced by electrical stimulation of the human frontal eye field: effect of orbital position. *Experimental Brain Research, 150,* 174–183.

Carpenter, R. H. (2004). Supplementary eye field: Keeping an eye on eye movement. *Current Biology, 14,* R416–R418.

Cisek, P., & Kalaska, J. F. (2004). Neural correlates of mental rehearsal in dorsal premotor cortex. *Nature, 431,* 993–996.

Cisek, P., & Kalaska, J. F. (2005). Neural correlates of reaching decisions in dorsal premotor cortex: Specification of multiple direction choices and final selection of action. *Neuron, 45,* 801–814.

Condy, C., Rivaud-Pechoux, S., Ostendorf, F., Ploner, C. J., & Gaymard, B. (2004). Neural substrate of antisaccades: Role of subcortical structures. *Neurology, 63,* 1571–1578.

Connolly, J. D., Goodale, M. A., Menon, R. S., & Munoz, D. P. (2002). Human fMRI evidence for the neural correlates of preparatory set. *Nature Neuroscience, 5,* 1345–1352.

Constantinidis, C., Franowicz, M. N., & Goldman-Rakic, P. S. (2001). The sensory nature of mnemonic representation in the primate prefrontal cortex. *Nature Neuroscience, 4,* 311–316.

Corbetta, M., Akbudak, E., Conturo, T. E., Snyder, A. Z., Ollinger, J. M., Drury, H. A., et al. (1998). A common network of functional areas for attention and eye movements. *Neuron, 21,* 761–773.

Curtis, C. E., Cole, M. W., Rao, V. Y., & D'Esposito, M. (2004). Canceling planned action: An fMRI Study of countermanding saccades. *Cerebral Cortex, 15,* 1281–1289.

Curtis, C. E., & D'Esposito, M. (2003). Success and failure suppressing reflexive behavior. *Journal of Cognitive Neuroscience, 15,* 409–418.

Daffner, K. R., Scinto, L. F., Weintraub, S., Guinessey, J. E., & Mesulam, M. M. (1992). Diminished curiosity in patients with probable Alzheimer's disease as measured by exploratory eye movements. *Neurology, 42,* 320–328.

Depatie, L., O'Driscoll, G. A., Holahan, A. L., Atkinson, V., Thavundayil, J. X., Kin, N. N., et al. (2002). Nicotine and behavioral markers of risk for schizophrenia: A double-blind, placebo-controlled, cross-over study. *Neuropsychopharmacology*, 27, 1056–1070.

DeSouza, J. F., Menon, R. S., & Everling, S. (2003). Preparatory set associated with pro-saccades and anti-saccades in humans investigated with event-related FMRI. *Journal of Neurophysiology*, 89, 1016–1023.

Dubois, B., Slachevsky, A., Litvan, L., & Pillon, B. (2000). The FAB: A Frontal Assessment Battery at bedside. *Neurology*, 55, 1621–1626.

Ettinger, U., Kumari, V., Zachariah, E., Galea, A., Crawford, T. J., Corr, P. J., et al. (2003). Effects of procyclidine on eye movements in schizophrenia. *Neuropsychopharmacology*, 28, 2199–2208.

Everling, S., & Munoz, D. P. (2000). Neuronal correlates for preparatory set associated with pro-saccades and anti-saccades in the primate frontal eye field. *Journal of Neuroscience*, 20, 387–400.

Feifel, D., Farber, R. H., Clementz, B. A., Perry, W., & Anllo-Vento, L. (2004). Inhibitory deficits in ocular motor behavior in adults with attention-deficit/hyperactivity disorder. *Biological Psychiatry*, 56, 333–339.

Fischer, B., Biscaldi, M., & Gezeck, S. (1997). On the development of voluntary and reflexive components in human saccade generation. *Brain Research*, 754, 285–297.

Fukushima, J., Hatta, T., & Fukushima, K. (2000). Development of voluntary control of saccadic eye movements: I. Age-related changes in normal children. *Brain and Development*, 22, 173–180.

Funahashi, S., Chafee, M. V., & Goldman-Rakic, P. S. (1993). Prefrontal neuronal activity in rhesus monkeys performing a delayed anti-saccade task. *Nature*, 365, 753–756.

Gagnon, D., O'Driscoll, G. A., Petrides, M., & Pike, G. B. (2002). The effect of spatial and temporal information on saccades and neural activity in oculomotor structures. *Brain*, 125, 123–139.

Guitton, D., Buchtel, H. A., & Douglas, R. M. (1985). Frontal lobe lesions in man cause difficulties in suppressing reflexive glances and in generating goal-directed saccades. *Experimental Brain Research*, 58, 455–472.

Hallet, P. E. (1978). Primary and secondary saccades to goals defined by instructions. *Vision Research*, 18, 1279–1296.

Hanes, D. P., & Carpenter, R. H. (1999). Countermanding saccades in humans. *Vision Research*, 39, 2777–2791.

Hanes, D. P., Patterson, W. F., II, & Schall, J. D. (1998). Role of frontal eye fields in countermanding saccades: Visual, movement, and fixation activity. *Journal of Neurophysiology*, 79, 817–834.

Hasegawa, R. P., Peterson, B. W., & Goldberg, M. E. (2004). Prefrontal neurons coding suppression of specific saccades. *Neuron*, 43, 415–425.

Hikosaka, O., Takikawa, Y., & Kawagoe, R. (2000). Role of the basal ganglia in the control of purposive saccadic eye movements. *Physiological Reviews*, 80, 953–978.

Hutton, S., & Kennard, C. (1998). Oculomotor abnormalities in schizophrenia: A critical review. *Neurology*, 50, 604–609.

Isoda, M., & Tanji, J. (2003). Contrasting neuronal activity in the supplementary and frontal eye fields during temporal organization of multiple saccades. *Journal of Neurophysiology*, 90, 3054–3065.

Johnston, J. L., Miller, J. D., & Nath, A. (1996). Ocular motor dysfunction in HIV-1-infected subjects: A quantitative oculographic analysis. *Neurology*, 46, 451–457.

Klein, C. (2001). Developmental functions for saccadic eye movement parameters derived from pro- and antisaccade tasks. *Experimental Brain Research*, 139, 1–17.

Klein, C., Fischer, B., Hartnegg, K., Heiss, W. H., & Roth, M. (2000). Optomotor and neuropsychological performance in old age. *Experimental Brain Research*, 135, 141–154.

Klein, C., & Foerster, F. (2001). Development of pro-saccade and antisaccade task performance in participants aged 6 to 26 years. *Psychophysiology*, 38, 179–189.

Kobayashi, Y., Saito, Y., & Isa, T. (2001). Facilitation of saccade initiation by brainstem cholinergic system. *Brain and Development*, 23(Suppl. 1), S24–S27.

Kornylo, K., Dill, N., Saenz, M., & Krauzlis, R. J. (2003). Cancelling of pursuit and saccadic eye movements in humans and monkeys. *Journal of Neurophysiology*, 89, 2984–2999.

Koyama, M., Hasegawa, I., Osada, T., Adachi, Y., Nakahara, K., & Miyashita, Y. (2004). Functional magnetic resonance imaging of macaque monkeys performing visually guided saccade tasks: Comparison of cortical eye fields with humans. *Neuron*, 41, 795–807.

Krauzlis, R., & Dill, N. (2002). Neural correlates of target choice for pursuit and saccades in the primate superior colliculus. *Neuron*, 35, 355–363.

Krauzlis, R. J. (2004). Recasting the smooth pursuit eye movement system. *Journal of Neurophysiology*, 91, 591–603.

Leigh, R. J., & Kennard, C. (2004). Using saccades as a research tool in the clinical neurosciences. *Brain*, 127, 460–477.

Logan, G. D., Cowan, W. B., & Davis, K. A. (1984). On the ability to inhibit simple and choice reaction time responses: A model and a method. *Journal of Experimental Psychology: Human Perception and Performance*, 10, 276–291.

Matthews, A., Flohr, H., & Everling, S. (2002). Cortical activation associated with midtrial change of instruction in a saccade task. *Experimental Brain Research*, 143, 488–498.

Mosimann, U. P., Felblinger, J., Ballinari, P., Hess, C. W., & Muri, R. M. (2004). Visual exploration behaviour during clock reading in Alzheimer's disease. *Brain*, *127*, 431–438.

Mosimann, U. P., Muri, R. M., Burn, D. J., Felblinger, J., O'Brien, J. T., & McKeith, I. G. (2005). Saccadic eye movement changes in Parkinson's disease dementia and dementia with Lewy bodies. *Brain*, *128*, 1267–1276.

Mostofsky, S. H., Lasker, A. G., Cutting, L. E., Denckla, M. B., & Zee, D. S. (2001). Oculomotor abnormalities in attention deficit hyperactivity disorder: A preliminary study. *Neurology*, *57*, 423–430.

Munoz, D. P., Broughton, J. R., Goldring, J. E., & Armstrong, I. T. (1998). Age-related performance of human subjects on saccadic eye movement tasks. *Experimental Brain Research*, *121*, 391–400.

Munoz, D. P., & Everling, S. (2004). Look away: The anti-saccade task and the voluntary control of eye movement. *Nature Reviews: Neuroscience*, *5*, 218–228.

Munoz, D. P., Le Vasseur, A. L., & Flanagan, J. R. (2002). Control of volitional and reflexive saccades in Tourette's syndrome. *Progress in Brain Research*, *140*, 467–481.

Nieman, D. H., Bour, L. J., Linszen, D. H., Goede, J., Koelman, J. H., Gersons, B. P., et al. (2000). Neuropsychological and clinical correlates of antisaccade task performance in schizophrenia. *Neurology*, *54*, 866–871.

Nouraei, S. A., De Pennington, N., Jones, J. G., & Carpenter, R. H. (2003). Dose-related effect of sevoflurane sedation on higher control of eye movements and decision making. *British Journal of Anaesthesia*, *91*, 175–183.

Nyffeler, T., Pierrot-Deseilligny, C., Felblinger, J., Mosimann, U. P., Hess, C. W., & Muri, R. M. (2002). Time-dependent hierarchical organization of spatial working memory: A transcranial magnetic stimulation study. *European Journal of Neuroscience*, *16*, 1823–1827.

Pierrot-Deseilligny, C., Milea, D., & Muri, R. M. (2004). Eye movement control by the cerebral cortex. *Current Opinion in Neurology*, *17*, 17–25.

Pierrot-Deseilligny, C., Muri, R. M., Ploner, C. J., Gaymard, B., Demeret, S., & Rivaud-Pechoux, S. (2003). Decisional role of the dorsolateral prefrontal cortex in ocular motor behaviour. *Brain*, *126*, 1460–1473.

Pierrot-Deseilligny, C., Muri, R. M., Rivaud-Pechoux, S., Gaymard, B., & Ploner, C. J. (2002). Cortical control of spatial memory in humans: The visuooculomotor model. *Annals of Neurology*, *52*, 10–19.

Rizzolatti, G., & Luppino, G. (2001). The cortical motor system. *Neuron*, *31*, 889–901.

Rosano, C., Krisky, C. M., Welling, J. S., Eddy, W. F., Luna, B., Thulborn, K. R., et al. (2002). Pursuit and saccadic eye movement subregions in human frontal eye field: A high-resolution fMRI investigation. *Cerebral Cortex*, *12*, 107–115.

Rosano, C., Sweeney, J. A., Melchitzky, D. S., & Lewis, D. A. (2003). The human precentral sulcus: Chemo-

architecture of a region corresponding to the frontal eye fields. *Brain Research*, *972*, 16–30.

Schall, J. D. (2003). Neural correlates of decision processes: neural and mental chronometry. *Current Opinion in Neurobiology*, *13*, 182–186.

Schall, J. D. (2004). On building a bridge between brain and behavior. *Annual Review of Psychology*, *55*, 23–50.

Schall, J. D., Morel, A., King, D. J., & Bullier, J. (1995). Topography of visual cortex connections with frontal eye field in macaque: Convergence and segregation of processing streams. *Journal of Neuroscience*, *15*, 4464–4487.

Schall, J. D., Stuphorn, V., & Brown, J. W. (2002). Monitoring and control of action by the frontal lobes. *Neuron*, *36*, 309–322.

Schlag-Rey, M., Amador, N., Sanchez, H., & Schlag, J. (1997). Antisaccade performance predicted by neuronal activity in the supplementary eye field. *Nature*, *390*, 398–401.

Shafiq-Antonacci, R., Maruff, P., Masters, C., & Currie, J. (2003). Spectrum of saccade system function in Alzheimer disease. *Archives of Neurology*, *60*, 1272–1278.

Smyrnis, N., Evdokimidis, I., Stefanis, N. C., Avramopoulos, D., Constantinidis, T. S., Stavropoulos, A., et al. (2003). Antisaccade performance of 1,273 men: Effects of schizotypy, anxiety, and depression. *Journal of Abnormal Psychology*, *112*, 403–414.

Smyrnis, N., Evdokimidis, I., Stefanis, N. C., Constantinidis, T. S., Avramopoulos, D., Theleritis, C., et al. (2002). The antisaccade task in a sample of 2,006 young males: II. Effects of task parameters. *Experimental Brain Research*, *147*, 53–63.

Sparks, D. L. (2002). The brainstem control of saccadic eye movements. *Nature Reviews: Neuroscience*, *3*, 952–964.

Stuphorn, V., & Schall, J. D. (2002). Neuronal control and monitoring of initiation of movements. *Muscle and Nerve*, *26*, 326–339.

Stuphorn, V., Taylor, T. L., & Schall, J. D. (2000). Performance monitoring by the supplementary eye field. *Nature*, *408*, 857–860.

Thaker, G. K., Ross, D. E., Cassady, S. L., Adami, H. M., Medoff, D. R., & Sherr, J. (2000). Saccadic eye movement abnormalities in relatives of patients with schizophrenia. *Schizophrenia Research*, *45*, 235–244.

Thompson, K. G., & Bichot, N. P. (2005). A visual salience map in the primate frontal eye field. *Progress in Brain Research*, *147*, 251–262.

Wonodi, I., Adami, H., Sherr, J., Avila, M., Hong, L. E., & Thaker, G. K. (2004). Naltrexone treatment of tardive dyskinesia in patients with schizophrenia. *Journal of Clinical Psychopharmacology*, *24*, 441–445.

Yamamoto, J., Ikeda, A., Satow, T., Matsuhashi, M., Baba, K., Yamane, F., et al. (2004). Human eye fields in the frontal lobe as studied by epicortical recording of movement-related cortical potentials. *Brain*, *127*, 873–887.

# PART V

## NEUROPSYCHOLOGICAL FUNCTIONS

# CHAPTER 18

# Bedside Frontal Lobe Testing

*Joel H. Kramer*
*Lovingly Quitania*

Every clinical assessment of behavior requires a careful review of frontal lobe functions. Nonetheless, several challenges face behavioral neurologists and neuropsychologists in their clinical attempts to assess the frontal lobes. Whereas an assessment of sensorimotor systems is guided by a relatively well understood pattern of brain–behavior relationships, the frontal lobes are incredibly complex, and because of their extensive interconnections with other neural structures, they control or influence a broad range of behaviors. Injury to the frontal lobes can affect initiation of complex motor behavior, attention, executive functioning, working memory, episodic memory, language, emotions, and behavior.

In humans, the frontal lobes comprise almost one third of the cortex and, not surprisingly, are involved in several different functional systems, including initiation and regulation of motor output, sensory processing, cognition, and emotion. For the purposes of this review, we emphasize prefrontal structures, largely dorsolateral prefrontal cortex, orbitofrontal cortex, and ventromedial prefrontal cortex. Prefrontal structures are also extensively linked with other cortical regions and with subcortical structures. Several different subcortical–frontal circuits and their roles in regulating behavior and cognition have been identified (Tekin & Cummings, 2002).

One important issue in bedside frontal lobe testing concerns the relevant cognitive constructs that are assigned to the frontal lobes. There is general agreement that the frontal lobes are important for executive functions, which typically are defined as the capacity to engage in goal-oriented behavior, or as the set of abilities involved in planning, self-monitoring, and purposive action (Lezak, 1995). There is considerably less consensus, however, on how these constructs are best measured. Tasks designed to assess executive skills typically involve a host of other skills that can make test interpretation difficult. For example, the Trail Making Test is a widely used measure of executive skills, because it requires mental flexibility. However, the task involves serially alternating between numbers and letters; thus, it also requires motor speed, visual scanning, attention, working memory, and facility with numbers and letters. Patients can therefore do poorly on this purported measure of executive functioning for reasons quite unrelated to executive ability. On the other hand, the integrity of a patient's frontal lobes can influence performance of a host of nonexecutive tasks. Difficult visuospatial and memory tests, for example, are typically performed better by patients who are adept at planning, organization, and problem solving (Somerville, Tremont, & Stern, 2000). Consequently, careful attention to these aspects of performance can yield important clues about frontal lobe functioning, even on tasks designed to assess other skills.

Taken together, these considerations lead to three conclusions. First, the frontal lobes do not operate in isolation. There are extensive networks between the frontal lobes and other parts of the brain. Prefrontal functioning is particularly sensitive to subcortical injury. Lesions in the midbrain, diencephalon, anterior basal ganglia, and subcortical white matter can all produce symptoms similar to those caused by focal prefrontal cortical lesions, leading some clinicians to replace the term "frontal lobes" with "subcortical–frontal systems." Second, there is no single "frontal lobe" skill or syndrome; the type of neurobehavioral outcome varies as a function of the location and nature of the prefrontal injury. Prefrontal damage can result in seemingly disparate conditions, including withdrawal, disinhibition, apathy, and agitation. Third, no single "frontal lobe" test can reliably identify patients who have frontal lobe injury. Clinicians must rely on a broad range of assessment techniques, which, besides neurobehavioral testing, include clinical observation and informant report to draw accurate inference about prefrontal structures.

This review emphasizes those neurobehavioral domains that are most often disrupted by prefrontal or subcortical–frontal injury and are assessable at the bedside. These include executive functioning, working memory, motor functions, and behavior. Certain practical considerations apply to most of the procedures described. Demographic factors are particularly important to consider when interpreting test performance; these issues have been well summarized by Boone, Ghaffarian, Lesser, Hill-Gutierrez, and Berman (1993). For example, there are large age effects on frontal structures (DeCarli et al., 2005) and functions (Greenwood, 2000; Wecker, Kramer, Wisniewski, Delis, & Kaplan, 2000), and the range of what should be considered "normal" is greater for an older patient than for a younger patient. Similarly, most cognitively oriented tasks are influenced by a patient's education and baseline cognitive abilities. This is particularly true for highly language-based tasks, such as verbal fluency, and for tasks that require problem solving. In fact, tests of frontal lobe function have been shown to correlate with general intellectual capacity (Obonsawin et al., 2002).

In this chapter, we describe the general approach to assessing frontal lobe functions at the bedside based on our experience at the University of California, San Francisco (UCSF) Memory and Aging Center. The tasks were designed to evaluate a patient cohort with neurodegenerative syndromes, some of which have disproportionate involvement of the frontal lobe (e.g., frontotemporal dementia, atypical parkinsonian disorders), and others having greater involvement of more posterior structures (e.g., Alzheimer's disease). We then present the results of some empirical studies that investigate how well these tasks help the clinician make inferences about frontal lobe functioning. These studies include correlations with frontal volumes based on magnetic resonance imaging (MRI) scans, and measuring differences between groups of patients with relatively greater frontal versus nonfrontal disease.

## BEDSIDE FRONTAL LOBE TESTING

### Executive Functioning

Executive functioning globally refers to an individual's ability to engage in goal-oriented behavior. Broadly accepted types of executive abilities include planning, organization, fluency, inhibition, mental flexibility, and abstract reasoning. Neuropsychologists have developed a broad range of tasks designed to measure various aspects of executive abilities, including novel verbal and nonverbal problem-solving tasks, maze tracing, tower tests, card or object sorting, and set shifting. In addition, several batteries for assessing executive functions have been published (e.g., Delis–Kaplan Executive Functioning Test [DKEFS], Cambridge Neuropsychological Test Automated Battery [CANTAB], Frontal Assessment Battery [FAB], Executive Interview [EXIT]). For example, the FAB correlates well with the Mattis Dementia Rating Scale, perseverations, and executive functioning measures, suggesting that this brief questionnaire is sensitive to frontal dysfunction and takes only 10 minutes to administer (Dubois, Slachevsky, Litvan, & Pillon, 2000). The EXIT (Malloy & Richardson, 1994) has been validated as a supplemental instrument to the Mini-Mental State Exam (MMSE) and highly correlates with frontal executive tasks such as fluency and set shifting (Stokholm, Vogel, Gade, & Waldemar, 2005).

Several tasks are available that enable clinicians to evaluate executive abilities quickly and reliably at the bedside.

## Fluency Tasks

Fluency, a widely used neuropsychological task, is known to be sensitive to frontal dysfunction (Baldo & Shimamura, 1998; Reitan & Wolfson, 1994; Tucha, Smely, & Lange, 1999). We assess verbal fluency by asking patients to generate as many words as possible in 1 minute, beginning with specific letters that are not proper nouns. We use two forms of the test, one in which the letters F, A, and S are presented, and a second version in which only the letter D is given. Repetitions and rule violations (e.g., giving responses beginning with a different letter; proper nouns) are also tabulated. Poor word generation on this task in the context of better category fluency is even more specific for frontal involvement, whereas the opposite pattern, with preserved D-words and impaired category fluency, more strongly suggests temporal involvement. A nonverbal analogue to letter fluency is design fluency. We evaluate design fluency by presenting patients with boxes containing five dots, and asking them to generate as many designs as possible in 1 minute that contain four lines that connect dots (see Figure 18.1). As with verbal fluency, the number of repetitions and rule violations are tabulated.

## Mental Flexibility

Measures of mental flexibility typically require patients to shift back and forth between types of stimuli or response sets. Variations of the Trail Making Test are widely used and are among the best validated markers of frontal lobe functioning (Stuss, Bisschop, et al., 2001). In its most widely used format, patients are asked to alternate serially between numbers and letters (see Figure 18.2; DKEFS) (Delis, Kramer, Kaplan, & Holdnack, 2004). We typi-

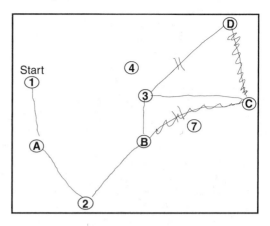

FIGURE 18.2. Example of shifting errors on DKEFS Trail Making Test.

cally have older or more impaired patients alternate serially between numbers and days of the week, and record how long they need to complete the task and how often they make a sequencing error (e.g., 1–Sunday–Monday).

Patients who have difficulty reading, either because of illiteracy or parietal deficits, can be administered Color Trails (Lee & Chan, 2000), a test that requires patients to connect numbered circles rapidly in sequence, alternating between pink and yellow colors. We also assess set shifting using a design fluency task that has two conditions. In each condition, the patient is given 1 minute to generate as many designs as possible that have four straight lines connecting dots. Both conditions use stimulus arrays that contain filled and unfilled dots. In the first condition, however, patients use only the unfilled dots to create designs, whereas in the second condition, they are required to alternate between filled and unfilled dots. Repeated designs and rule violations (e.g., failure to shift) are also recorded (see Figure 18.3).

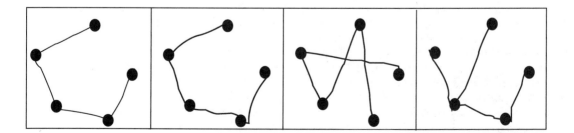

FIGURE 18.1. Example of repetition and rule violation on DKEFS Design Fluency Test.

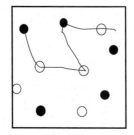

FIGURE 18.3. Example of rule violation on the set-shifting condition.

## Abstract Reasoning

We ask patients to describe conceptual similarities between word pairs ("dog"–"lion"; "table–chair"; "anger–joy") and to interpret proverbs (e.g., "An old ox plows a straight row"; "Shallow brooks are noise"; "A beard well-lathered is half-shaved"). Responses are given credit if they are both abstract and accurate.

## Response Inhibition

Several bedside tasks are available for assessing a patient's ability to suppress either an overlearned response or a response to a salient environmental stimulus. The Stroop test is a widely used instrument that requires inhibition of an overlearned reading response. There are typically at least two conditions, a control task in which patients name the colors of nonlexical color patches, and an interference task in which they name the color of ink in which incongruent color names are printed (e.g., the word "red" printed in green ink). We tabulate the number of correct responses in 60 seconds, and the number of inhibition errors. Another type of response inhibition task involves presenting the patient with a salient stimulus and asking for a competing response (e.g., the examiner asks the patient to point to his or her chin, while the examiner points to his nose, or asks the patient to point to the ceiling, while extending his hand to the patient). Opposite responding tasks similarly require suppressing a response to a salient stimulus (e.g., "When I tap once, you tap twice, but when I tap twice, you tap once").

## Working Memory

Working memory is a functional system that participates in the maintenance, control, and manipulation of information (Baddeley, 1986). We evaluate auditory working memory at the bedside using backward digit span. Patients are orally presented with digit strings ranging from two to eight digits in length, and are required to repeat them in the reverse order. In patients with adequate attention and echoic memory, backward digit span offers an excellent measure of auditory working memory capacity. On the MMSE (Folstein, Robins, & Helzer, 1983), working memory is assessed when the patient carries out serial 7's or spells "world" backward. Other bedside techniques include reciting the months of the year in reverse order.

## Other Cognitive Domains

Although language, spatial ability, and memory are not typically thought of as predominately mediated by the frontal lobes, assessment of these skills at baseline is important for evaluating frontal systems for two reasons. First, diffuse cognitive impairment due to advanced neurodegenerative disease or multifocal injury produces impairment on most "frontal" tasks. Focal frontal pathology is most reliably inferred when a patient's poor performance on frontal tasks occurs in the context of relative preservation of skills mediated predominately by temporal and parietal structures. Second, injury to the frontal lobe can affect performance on a range of "nonfrontal" tasks, and attention to these performance characteristics at the bedside can yield useful diagnostic information. Language changes secondary to frontal injury can include reduced spontaneous speech, agrammaticisms, and labored speech output. Phonemic paraphasic errors can often be heard during conversational speech or on confrontation naming tasks. Repetition tasks, particularly with phonetically complex and linguistically unusual phrases (e.g., "The pastry cook was elated," "Pry the tin lid off") often elicit signs of speech apraxia or articulation problems. We evaluate confrontation naming with a 15-item version of the Boston Naming Test (Mack, Freed, Williams, & Henderson, 1992).

Although word finding difficulties are anatomically non-specific, the presence of severe naming deficits plus loss of word knowledge implicates the anterior temporal lobes, particularly on the left. Assessment of naming is particularly relevant for clinically distinguishing between frontotemporal lobar dementia syndromes (FTLDs). FTLD is a syndrome with several subtypes, two of which are fronto-temporal dementia (FTD) and semantic dementia (SD; Brazis, Masdeu, & Biller, 1996). FTD is characterized by prominent frontal atrophy (Miller & Gearhart, 1999) and manifests initially as decline in social and interpersonal conduct, impairment in regulation of personal conduct, emotional blunting, and loss of insight. SD is associated with prominent atrophy in the anterior temporal lobes and a language disorder characterized by progressive, fluent, empty, spontaneous speech, loss of word meaning, and semantic paraphasias, with near normal visuospatial abilities and autobiographical memory. Both disorders can present with marked personality change and social dysfunction, but the pronounced naming deficit is only observed in SD.

Visuospatial problems are also common in patients with frontal lobe dysfunction, although the types of spatial deficits differ from those found in patients with parietal dysfunction. Copying simpler geometric figures is usually unimpaired, whereas copies of more complex figure are often marked by poor organization and inattention to detail. Episodic memory tasks are also partly mediated by the frontal lobes (Wheeler, Stuss, & Tulving, 1995). Focal frontal injury has a greater impact on immediate recall secondary to poor attention and organization, and relatively less impact on the patient's ability to retain the encoded information over a delay (unlike patients with Alzheimer's disease [AD], who will show a dramatic drop in recall after a delay, regardless of how well they did initially). We routinely assess verbal memory at the bedside using a 9-item list-learning task (Delis, Freeland, Kramer, & Kaplan, 1988), and have shown that hippocampal volumes are the best predictor of delayed recall and recognition memory, whereas frontal lobe volumes are the best predictor of organization during recall and response bias during recognition (Kramer et al., 2005). We evaluated spatial ability and spatial memory by having patients first copy a geometric figure (see Figure 18.4), then recall it 10 minutes later.

## Motor Functions

A significant portion of a bedside neurological exam focuses on the pyramidal and extrapyramidal motor systems. Prefrontal cortex, however, also influences motor behavior. Two ways of assessing prefrontal contributions are measurement of primitive reflexes and complex motor sequences.

### Primitive Reflexes

Primitive reflexes are motor responses that are present during fetal and postnatal central nervous system development when cortical formation and myelination of subcortical structures are not yet complete. Such reflexes become inhibited during normal development but may reemerge in response to cortical damage or disruption of cortical efferents and their connections. Grasp and snout reflexes are two such reflexes that are easily tested during a routine examination. The grasp reflex is elicited by stroking the patient's palm with the index finger, then rubbing the palm and volar aspect of the fingers. For the reflex testing to be most re-

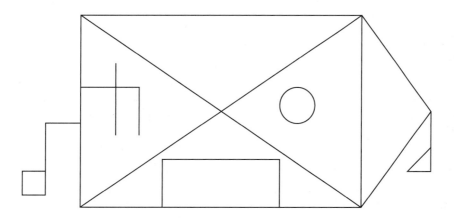

FIGURE 18.4. Example of the modified Rey–Osterrieth design (complex figure).

liable, the patient should be advised not to grab the examiner's fingers. The reflex is positive when the patient's fingers hook around the hand of the examiner. The reflex may be present contralateral to diseased mesial prefrontal cortex (Brodmann's area [BA] 6) (Brazis et al., 1996) or with diffuse bifrontal disease (Wiebers, Dale, Kokmen, & Swanson, 1998).

The snout reflex is elicited if both lips pucker, with elevated protrusion of the lower lip, when pressure is applied to the patient's nasal philtrum. This reflex has been associated with advancing age in healthy subjects but may also reflect disconnectivity of the frontal corticobulbar projections (Walterfang & Velakoulis, 2005).

### Complex Motor Programming

A common test of motor programming involves the use of Luria's hand sequences (Luria, 1966). This task involves three steps: First, the examiner makes a fist, then extends his or her fingers, keeping the palm facing down, concluding with the hand rotated in a 90° angle. This series is repeated 10 times by the patient, and the number of trials necessary to learn the sequence, the number of perseverations, and the fluency of the movements are recorded. We also have patients carry out a graphomotor task in which they repeatedly write out the letter sequence "mn." In addition to eliciting perseverations commonly seen in patients with frontal lobe dysfunction, parkinsonian symptoms and micrographia are also commonly revealed. The rhythm tapping test, an alternative to the hand sequences, is more easily quantifiable by the examiner. Here the patient is asked to tap his or her index finger in a stationary location on a flat surface. The examiner then models different rhythms, which the patient is to follow. The examiner then records whether the patient was unable to keep the pattern of rhythms, and whether the patient deviated from the stationary location. Typically, patients with frontal lobe deficits are found to have difficulties with the switching of rhythm in the complex pattern.

## Behavior

Patients with frontal lobe lesions clinically present with behavioral deficits. These patients are characterized as aloof, apathetic, impulsive, and exhibiting socially inappropriate behavior.

Insight and awareness are diminished with frontal lobe lesions, and stereotypical behaviors, bizarre eating habits, and poor hygiene emerge. These behavior changes are usually evident on clinical exam and are a salient feature of the patient's clinical history. Deficits in social behavior, self-conduct, and emotional processing have been shown to be related to atrophy in the orbitofrontal cortex, as well as nonfrontal structures such as the amygdala and anterior temporal cortex (Rosen et al., 2002). There are also lateralization differences, with behavioral disturbance more strongly associated with right frontal lobe disease.

We have modified the Manchester Behavior Questionnaire (Bathgate, Snowden, Varma, Blackshaw, & Neary, 2001) to survey recent behavioral symptoms based on either informant report or clinical observation. Assessment of social behavior includes symptoms such as altered emotional display, loss of embarrassment, loss of empathy, rudeness, disinhibition, and childishness. Repetitive and compulsive behaviors include rituals, adherence to daily routines, compulsive gaming, and changes in purchasing habits. Eating and vegetative behaviors are reflected in recent weight gain, change in eating habits, craving sweets, increased smoking or drinking, and taking food from others. Environmental dependency is seen as hoarding, excessive touching or handling of objects, echopraxia, echolalia, and utilization behavior. Utilization behavior can often be elicited at the bedside by placing objects within reach of the patient (e.g., pen and paper) to see whether the patient is compelled to use them in a stereotypical fashion.

Several scales are available to clinicians for reviewing and quantifying abnormal behavior at the bedside. The utility of the Neuropsychiatric Inventory (NPI) and NPI-Q (shortened version) for identifying behaviors associated with frontotemporal dementia are well established (Cummings, 1997; Kaufer et al., 2000). The NPI assesses 12 neuropsychiatric disturbances most commonly seen in dementia, as well as their influence on caregiver distress (Miller et al., 1997). Disinhibition, aberrant motor behavior, apathy, and eating disturbance are particularly common in FTLD (Mendez et al., 1996).

Other widely used scales include the Dysexecutive Questionnaire (DEX), the Frontal Behavior Inventory (FBI), and the Frontal Systems Behavior Scale (FrSBe) (Malloy & Grace,

2005). These measures attempt to dissociate the relationships between frontal lesions, personality changes, behavioral decline, and cognitive function. The DEX, a 20-item questionnaire administered to patients, is designed to address everyday signs of dysexecutive symptoms. If the patient has sufficient insight, the DEX provides information about intentionality, interference management, inhibition, planning, and social regulation (Amieva, Phillips, & Della Sala, 2003). The FBI is a 24-item caregiver questionnaire, with 12 items assessing deficit behaviors (apathy, aspontaneity, indifference, inflexibility, concreteness, personal neglect, disorganization, inattention, loss of insight, logopenia, verbal apraxia, and alien hand), and 12 items assessing disinhibition behaviors (perseverations/obsessions, irritability, jocularity, irresponsibility, inappropriateness, impulsivity, restlessness, aggression, hyperorality, hypersexuality, utilization behavior, and incontinence) (Kertesz, Nadkarni, Davidson, & Thomas, 2000; Ready, Ott, Grace, & Cahn-Weiner, 2003). Significant positive and negative behavior and personality changes can be detected with the FBI, and patients with FTD have been shown to have more problems with apathy, indifference, lack of insight, perseverations, and social inappropriateness, in contrast to patients with AD, progressive aphasia, and depression. The FrSBe is a 46-item behavior rating scale, with a self-rating form completed by the patient and a family rating form completed by an informant who has regular contact with the patient (Paul et al., 2005; Stout, Ready, Grace, Malloy, & Paulsen, 2003). The FrSBe yields a total score and classifies subscales measuring apathy, disinhibition, and executive dysfunction.

## EMPIRICAL DATA

We report here on two types of studies that empirically investigate the relationships between bedside cognitive and behavioral measures and the frontal lobes. In the first group of studies, we evaluate how well bedside measures discriminate between FTLD, a group of neurodenegerative conditions primarily affecting either the frontal or anterior temporal lobe, and AD, a neurodegenerative disease with greater involvement of medial temporal structures and temporal–parietal cortex. In the second set of studies, we report on the relationships between bedside cognitive and behavioral measures and frontal lobe volumes.

## Group Differences

Previous reports have shown that several components of our bedside assessment are successful at differentiating between AD and FTLD. Levy, Miller, Cummings, Fairbanks, and Craig (1996) compared 22 patients with FTLD and 30 patients with AD using the NPI. Patients with FTLD had significantly greater total NPI scores than patients with AD, and exhibited more apathy, disinhibition, euphoria, and aberrant motor behavior; these NPI scales accurately assigned 77% of patients with FTLD and 77% of patients with AD to the correct diagnostic group.

We researched how well bedside testing could discriminate between the two most common subtypes of FTLD: FTD and SD. Both disorders are associated with frontotemporal pathology, although FTD has predominately frontal involvement, and SD has predominately temporal involvement. Importantly, both FTD and SD are associated with significant behavioral (Rankin, Baldwin, Pace-Savitsky, Kramer, & Miller, 2005; Rankin, Kramer, & Miller, 2005; Rankin, Kramer, Mychack, & Miller, 2003; Rankin et al., 2004) and cognitive changes, so being able to reliably differentiate between the two is clinically relevant.

We have also previously assessed the ability of our bedside cognitive measures to discriminate between 30 patients with AD, 21 patients with FTD, and 14 patients with SD (Brazis et al., 1996; Kramer et al., 2003). Patients with FTD, SD, and AD were comparable in terms of MMSE score, age, and education. Subjects were administered a brief neuropsychological screen, similar to the one we described previously to assess episodic memory, working memory, executive function, naming, spatial ability, abstract reasoning, and calculations. Both the AD and SD groups were significantly impaired relative to the FTD group on verbal memory, whereas only the AD group was impaired on visual memory. Patients with FTD performed significantly worse on backward digit span and made significantly more executive errors than patients with AD and SD. Patients with SD were more impaired than patients with AD and FTD on confrontation naming. Discriminant function analyses indicated that five variables—Boston Naming Test,

Modified Rey–Osterrieth Recall test, California Verbal Learning Test—Short Form (CVLT-SF) recall, category fluency, and executive errors (the sum of perseverative responses and rule violations summed over several tests)—correctly classified 89.2% of cases.

These previous studies have provided separate analyses of either the behavioral or cognitive changes associated with frontal lobe pathology. Both types of symptoms, however, are typically evaluated in a comprehensive bedside evaluation. We therefore assessed how well a combination of cognitive and behavioral measures could distinguish between AD and FTD. We studied 84 patients with AD (mean age = 73.5, $SD$ = 10) and 35 patients with FTD (mean age = 60.7; $SD$ = 7) who completed our bedside assessment, including the NPI, CVLT-SF, Modified Rey–Osterrieth Recall Test, backward digit span, similarities, modified Trail Making, and Boston Naming tests. The AD group had a slightly lower MMSE score (23.2 vs. 26.2 for the FTD group) but was less impaired than the FTD group when assessed using the Clinical Dementia Rating scale (CDR) sum of box scores (4.6 vs. 6.0 for the FTD group). We selected seven variables from the NPI (presence of agitation, anxiety, apathy, disinhibition, aberrant behavior, irritability) and seven cognitive variables (delayed verbal memory on the CVLT-SF, delayed recall of the Modified Rey test, design copying, backward digit span, similarities, the difference between letter and category fluency, and the 15-item Boston Naming Test.

In the first analysis, all 14 variables were entered into the discriminant function. Overall classification rate was 93.3% of cases, with 95.2% of AD cases correctly classified, and 88.6% of FTD cases correctly classified. A follow-up discriminant function was carried out using a stepwise procedure (Wilks's $\lambda$) to identify the combination of measures that best discriminated. The stepwise method selected three variables: NPI Disinhibition (Wilks's $\lambda$ = .68), delayed free recall from the CVLT-SF (Wilks's $\lambda$ = .36), and the difference between letter and category fluency (Wilks's $\lambda$ = .32). Patients with AD had poorer memory and were disproportionately impaired on category fluency relative to letter fluency. Patients with FTD scored much higher on NPI Disinhibition and did less well on letter fluency relative to category fluency. The final equation using just these three variables correctly classified 88.8%

of the cases, including 91.4% of the AD cases, and 82.9% of the FTD cases.

We studied 35 patients with FTD (mean age = 60.5; MMSE score = 25.0) and 10 patients with SD (mean age = 63.7; MMSE score = 23.3). There were no group differences in age or MMSE scores. We first used univariate analyses to reduce the number of variables to be entered into the discriminant function. Ten variables were initially entered: NPI Apathy, Disinhibition, Aberrant Motor, and Eating subscales, delayed verbal recall from the CVLT-SF, a copy of the Modified Rey Figure test, Boston Naming Test (number correct out of 15), modified Trail Making Test, the difference between letter and category fluency, and number of correct responses on Stroop interference. Entering all 10 variables resulted in 100% classification for both the FTD and SD groups. A follow-up discriminant function using a stepwise procedure selected two variables: Boston Naming Test (Wilks's $\lambda$ = .55) and NPI Apathy (Wilks's $\lambda$ = .27) that alone correctly classified 93.3% of the sample.

The Interpersonal Measure of Psychopathy (IM-P), an 18-item checklist of observed inappropriate behaviors, was completed on 288 patients with dementia by clinicians blind to diagnostic status. Patients with FTLD showed unique abnormal patterns of scores, whereas no other group's behavior differed significantly from controls. Item analysis (e.g., "interrupts interview," "ignores professional boundaries," "discusses personal uniqueness") was most characteristic of patients with FTLD.

## Brain–Behavior Correlations

The results of these studies suggest that a small number of variables easily collected as part of a bedside frontal examination are able to discriminate reliably between FTD, a predominately frontal lobe disorder, and SD and AD, neurodegenerative disorders that disproportionately affect more posterior structures. In the next series of studies, we report on how strongly performance on bedside testing correlates with actual measures of frontal lobe volume.

We generated right and left frontal, temporal, and parietal lobar volumes using the BRAINS2 software package (Magnotta et al., 2002). The T1-weighted images were spatially normalized so that the anterior–posterior axes of the brain can be realigned parallel to the anterior commissure–posterior commissure line and the interhemispheric fissure aligned on the other two axes. Next, the outermost boundaries of the cortex, as well as the anterior commissure and posterior commissure, were identified to warp the Talairach grid onto the current brain. We then realigned the T2- and proton density–weighted images to the spatially normalized T1-weighted image using an automated image registration program (Woods, Dapretto, Sicotte, Toga, & Mazziotta, 1999). We then segmented resampled images into gray matter, white matter, and cerebrospinal fluid (CSF) using the coregistered images and a discriminant analysis method based on automated training class selection (Harris et al., 1999). After generating a brain mask using previously trained artificial neural network (ANN), we calculated lobar volumes using an automated Talairach-based method of regional classification (Woods et al., 1999). The lobar volumes reported here were normalized to correct for differences in overall head size.

Behavioral data for the analyses were drawn from a pool of 99 subjects seen at the Memory and Aging Center. This group comprised 28 normal controls (mean age = 64.4; mean MMSE score = 29.6), 22 patients with AD (mean age = 62.2; mean MMSE score = 24.2), 34 patients with FTD (mean age = 58.6; mean MMSE score = 25.6), and 15 patients with SD (mean age = 61.3; mean MMSE score = 24.9). The actual subject numbers in the individual analyses varied due to missing data. The relationships between cognitive measures and lobar volumes were first determined with bivariate correlations, followed by multiple regression analyses, with all lobar volumes forced into the model.

### Verbal Fluency

Our primary measure of verbal fluency (FAS) was the number of words generated beginning with the letters F, A, and S, and was available for 86 cases. FAS was significantly correlated with five of the six lobar volumes, with the strongest correlation ($r = .45$, $p < .001$). The multiple regression indicated that the MRI measures explained 29.4% of the variance in FAS. Left frontal volume was the only measure that remained in the model ($\beta = .38$, $p < .05$), by itself explaining 19.6% of the variance in FAS.

### Set Shifting

We used the design fluency paradigm as our marker of set shifting. The ability to generate designs while shifting between filled and unfilled dots served as the measure of set shifting, whereas design fluency in the non-shifting condition served as the control. Data were available for 62 subjects. Partial correlations between set shifting and lobar volumes (controlling for design fluency) yielded significant correlations with the left frontal ($r = .43$, $p < .01$) and right frontal ($r = .29$, $p < .05$) lobes. We then carried out hierarchical multiple regression with set shifting as the dependent variable, entering the nonshifting condition into the model first, followed by the lobar volumes. The MRI measures explained an additional 13.6% of the variance above and beyond the 46% explained by the standard design fluency condition. Left frontal volume was the only MRI measure to remain in the model ($\beta = .38$, $p < .05$), by itself adding almost 10% of the variance.

### Abstract Reasoning

We generated a total abstract reasoning score based on three similarities items and three proverb interpretations. Data were available on 78 cases. Correlations with all the lobar volumes were significant, although the largest correlation was with the left frontal lobe ($r = .53$, $p < .001$). Multiple regression indicated that lobar volumes explained 41.9% of the variance in abstract reasoning ($p < .001$). Two lobar volumes remained in the model, left frontal lobe ($\beta = .52$, $p < .01$) and right temporal lobe ($\beta = .42$, $p < .05$).

### Response Inhibition

The Stroop interference paradigm is widely used as a measure of the ability to inhibit prepotent responses. We analyzed data from 74 cases that were administered both the interference condition and a control color-naming condition in which patients named the ink color of nonword letter strings. Partial correlations between the interference condition and lobar volumes controlling for color naming indicated that none of the lobar volumes was significantly correlated with Stroop interference performance. This absence of an effect was borne out with the multiple regression, where lobar volumes were not associated with an increase in the explained variance of the interference condition.

Another approach to measure impaired response inhibition is to study the errors patients make while performing cognitive tasks. Stuss, Murphy, Binns, and Alexander (2003) have argued that a characteristic feature of frontal lesions is an increase in errors that reflects impulsiveness, inattentiveness, stimulus bound-edness, or failure to maintain a cognitive set. To assess directly the neuroanatomical under-pinnings of errors, we tabulated a total error score by summing the number of rule viola-tions on the FAS verbal fluency, design fluency, and Stroop tasks. Rule violations were in-stances in which patients' responses did not conform with task rules (e.g., giving proper nouns on verbal fluency; failure to shift, or drawing designs with the wrong number of lines on design fluency; stimulus-bound errors on Stroop tasks). Error data were available on 54 cases. The mean number of errors was 6.4, with a range of 0–49. Scores were square-root transformed to minimize the skewedness of the distribution. Bivariate correlations showed that errors correlated only with left frontal volume ($r = -.30$, $p < .05$). Multiple regression further supported this finding; left frontal volume was the only significant predictor in the model ($\beta = -.59$, $p < .05$), with the overall model explain-ing 16.6% of the variance in errors.

### Working Memory

Backward digit span served as our index of au-ditory working memory. Data were available on 62 cases. Bivariate correlations indicated significant relationships between backward digit span and parietal volumes, even after partialing out the effects of forward digit span. None of the lobar volumes remained in the model after we controlled for forward digit span in the multiple regression.

### Behavior

We evaluated the lobar contributions to three behaviors indexed by the NPI—disinhibition, apathy, and aberrant motor behavior—in 62 subjects. Our dependent variables were the fre-quency × severity scores, and the MMSE score was used as a covariate to control for degree of cognitive impairment. Disinhibition was most strongly correlated with right temporal ($r = -.56$, $p < .001$), right frontal ($r = -.44$, $p < .001$)

and left frontal ($r = -.30$, $p < .05$). Only right temporal volume was significant in the multi-ple regression ($\beta = -.50$, $p < .01$). Apathy was most strongly correlated with right temporal ($r = -.39$, $p < .01$) and right frontal ($r = -.31$, $p < .05$) volumes, but again, right temporal atro-phy ($\beta = -.26$, $p = .06$) was the best predictor of apathy. Aberrant motor behavior was corre-lated with left frontal ($r = -.29$, $p < .05$), right frontal ($r = -.42$, $p < .001$) and right temporal ($r = -.38$, $p < .01$) lobes. In this instance, al-though the lobar volumes explained an addi-tional 20.6% of the variance ($p < .01$), none of the contributions of the individual lobar vol-umes reached statistical significance.

## DISCUSSION

Evaluating cognition and behavior at the bed-side can be done in an efficient, reliable, and quantitative manner. Brief neuropsychological screening is useful for measuring abilities such as executive function and working memory, which are strongly mediated by the frontal lobes, and abilities such as language, spatial processing, and episodic memory, which are mostly mediated by nonfrontal structures. In-formant interview and careful clinical observa-tion can elicit important information about new behaviors that implicate frontal lobe pa-thology. We propose a bedside frontal lobe evaluation that includes measures of fluency, set shifting, abstract reasoning, response inhi-bition, working memory, list learning, speech output, naming, design copying, motor se-quencing, and the NPI.

A subset of this battery differentiated fairly well between FTD and other neurodegener-ative disorders. Seven cognitive scores and seven domains from the NPI showed fairly good sensitivity and specificity, correctly classi-fying 95.2% of AD cases and 88.6% of FTD cases. Three variables—NPI Disinhibition, CVLT-SF delayed recall, and the difference be-tween letter and category fluency—by them-selves correctly classified 91.4% of the AD cases and 82.9% of the FTD cases. The bedside battery was also successful at discriminating between FTD and SD. Ten variables correctly classified 100% of the FTD cases and 100% of the SD cases. Follow-up analyses indicated that the Boston Naming Test and NPI Apathy were the two most discriminating variables, cor-rectly classifying 93.3% of the cases.

Most neuropsychological tests, particularly those that are brief enough to administer at the bedside, tend to be cognitively heterogeneous and hence require the contributions of multiple brain regions. Verbal fluency, for example, requires not only frontally mediated abilities such as generativity, mental flexibility, and strategic retrieval, but also lexical knowledge, semantic memory, and processing speed. These constraints notwithstanding, we carried out several analyses to identify significant lobar contributions to several bedside tasks. Multiple regressions indicated that the left frontal lobe is the primary predictor of performance on measures of verbal fluency (FAS) and abstract reasoning. In addition, the ability to shift back and forth between stimuli on a design fluency task was also best predicted by left frontal lobe volume, even after controlling for overall design fluency ability. In contrast, Stroop interference, widely considered to be a classic frontal lobe test, was not significantly correlated with frontal lobe volumes. This finding is consistent with other reports suggesting that Stroop interference performance may not be sufficiently sensitive or specific to frontal lobe lesions (Stuss, Floden, Alexander, Levine, & Katz, 2001).

Functional imaging studies with normal patients have repeatedly shown that working memory tasks activate a network that includes dorsolateral prefrontal cortex. In our studies, however, backward digit span did not correlate well with frontal volumes, even after controlling for forward digit span.

Cognitive performance following frontal pathology is often characterized as variable, impulsive, inattentive, and poorly organized. We quantified a component of these features by tabulating the frequency of rule violations and failures to shift set or inhibit prepotent responses. The total number of these types of errors was associated with left frontal atrophy, consistent with previous reports of errors being sensitive to focal frontal lesions (Stuss et al., 2003) and FTD (Kramer et al., 2003).

The behavioral changes seen following frontal injury and degeneration are frequently the family's chief complaint and a major impetus for the bedside frontal lobe evaluation. Our studies with the NPI showed a relationship between right frontal volumes and the presence of disinhibition, apathy, and aberrant motor behavior. However, we also observed a strong relationship between these behaviors and right

temporal volumes. The strong association with right-hemispheric structures is consistent with several reports of greater behavioral disruption following right-sided disease. The lack of a specific relationship with the frontal lobes, however, may be partly attributable to the specific patient cohorts used in the analyses. All of the patients studied had neurodegenerative diseases that rarely localize to a single lobe. Patients with SD, for example, have marked atrophy of ventromedial prefrontal cortex (Rosen et al., 2002), that very likely contributes to their observed changes in behavior and emotion processing. In addition, some of the target behaviors have regional specificity that does not conform well to lobar volumes. Disinhibition, for example, has been shown to be associated with ventromedial prefrontal cortex (Rosen et al., 2002), and apathy is strongly associated with the anterior cingulate (Paul et al., 2005; Rosen et al., 2004). Volumes of the entire frontal lobe may not provide sufficient anatomical specificity to show clear brain–behavior relationships. Similar mechanisms may be at play with the Stroop interference test in light of the opus of functional imaging studies that show anterior cingulate activation on Stroop-like tasks (Peterson et al., 1999). In a similar vein, frontal lobe volumes may be less sensitive to working memory performance than a more focal dorsolateral prefrontal cortex measure (Curtis & D'Esposito, 2004; Gazzaley, Rissman, & D'Esposito, 2004).

None of the information provided by this bedside battery was designed to operate in isolation. There is no single marker of frontal lobe functioning. Patients with nonfrontal or diffuse neuropathology often display deficits on executive and working memory tasks, and can present with significant behavior change. The strength of a battery of bedside frontal tasks is that converging data from multiple sources are available to support hypotheses about frontal lobe functioning. For example, although deficits in phonemic verbal fluency are a strong indicator of left frontal pathology, anatomical inferences are bolstered when category fluency is well preserved. Similarly, problems with set shifting implicate the frontal lobes primarily when the patient is able to carry out the component tasks well. Behavioral disturbance and deficits in executive functioning are more easily linked to the frontal lobes when basic attention, language, memory, and spatial ability are relatively spared.

## REFERENCES

Amieva, H., Phillips, L., & Della Sala, S. (2003). Behavioral dysexecutive symptoms in normal aging. *Brain and Cognition, 53*(2), 129–132.

Baddeley, A. (1986). *Working memory.* Oxford, UK: Clarendon Press.

Baldo, J. V., & Shimamura, A. P. (1998). Letter and category fluency in patients with frontal lobe lesions. *Neuropsychology, 12*(2), 259–267.

Bathgate, D., Snowden, J. S., Varma, A., Blackshaw, A., & Neary, D. (2001). Behaviour in frontotemporal dementia, Alzheimer's disease and vascular dementia. *Acta Neurologica Scandinavica, 103*(6), 367–378.

Boone, K. B., Ghaffarian, S., Lesser, I. M., Hill-Gutierrez, E., & Berman, N. G. (1993). Wisconsin Card Sorting Test performance in healthy, older adults: relationship to age, sex, education, and IQ. *Journal of Clinical Psychology, 49*(1), 54–60.

Brazis, P. W., Masdeu, J. C., & Biller, J. (1996). *Localization in clinical neurology* (3rd ed.). Boston: Little, Brown.

Cummings, J. L. (1997). The Neuropsychiatric Inventory: Assessing psychopathology in dementia patients. *Neurology, 48*(5, Suppl. 6), S10–S16.

Curtis, C. E., & D'Esposito, M. (2004). The effects of prefrontal lesions on working memory performance and theory. *Cognitive, Affective and Behavioral Neuroscience, 4*(4), 528–539.

DeCarli, C., Massaro, J., Harvey, D., Hald, J., Tullberg, M., Au, R., et al. (2005). Measures of brain morphology and infarction in the Framingham Heart Study: Establishing what is normal. *Neurobiology of Aging, 26*(4), 491–510.

Delis, D. C., Freeland, J., Kramer, J. H., & Kaplan, E. (1988). Integrating clinical assessment with cognitive neuroscience: Construct validation of the California Verbal Learning Test. *Journal of Consulting and Clinical Psychology, 56*(1), 123–130.

Delis, D. C., Kramer, J. H., Kaplan, E., & Holdnack, J. (2004). Reliability and validity of the Delis–Kaplan Executive Function System: An update. *Journal of the International Neuropsychological Society, 10*(2), 301–303.

Dubois, B., Slachevsky, A., Litvan, I., & Pillon, B. (2000). The FAB: A Frontal Assessment Battery at bedside. *Neurology, 55*(11), 1621–1626.

Folstein, M. F., Robins, L. N., & Helzer, J. E. (1983). The Mini-Mental State Examination. *Archives of General Psychiatry, 40*(7), 812.

Gazzaley, A., Rissman, J., & D'Esposito, M. (2004). Functional connectivity during working memory maintenance. *Cognitive, Affective and Behavioral Neuroscience, 4*(4), 580–599.

Greenwood, P. M. (2000). The frontal aging hypothesis evaluated. *Journal of the International Neuropsychological Society, 6*(6), 705–726.

Harris, G., Andreasen, N. C., Cizadlo, T., Bailey, J. M., Bockholt, H. J., Magnotta, V. A., et al. (1999). Improving tissue classification in MRI: A three-dimensional multispectral discriminant analysis method with automated training class selection. *Journal of Computer Assisted Tomography, 23*(1), 144–154.

Kaufer, D. I., Cummings, J. L., Ketchel, P., Smith, V., MacMillan, A., Shelley, T., et al. (2000). Validation of the NPI-Q, a brief clinical form of the Neuropsychiatric Inventory. *Journal of Neuropsychiatry and Clinical Neurosciences, 12*(2), 233–239.

Kertesz, A., Nadkarni, N., Davidson, W., & Thomas, A. W. (2000). The Frontal Behavioral Inventory in the differential diagnosis of frontotemporal dementia. *Journal of the International Neuropsychological Society, 6*(4), 460–468.

Kramer, J., Jurik, J., Sha, S. J., Rankin, K. P., Rosen, H. J., Johnson, J. K., et al. (2003). Distinctive neuropsychological patterns in frontotemporal dementia, semantic dementia, and Alzheimer disease. *Cognitive and Behavioral Neurology, 16*(4), 211–218.

Kramer, J., Rosen, H. J., Du, A. T., Schuff, N., Hollgagel, C., Weiner, M., et al. (2005). Dissociations in hippocampal and frontal contributions to episodic memory. *Neuropsychology, 19* 799–805.

Lee, T. M., & Chan, C. C. (2000). Are trail making and color trails tests of equivalent constructs? *Journal of Clinical and Experimental Neuropsychology, 22*(4), 529–534.

Levy, M. L., Miller, B. L., Cummings, J. L., Fairbanks, L. A., & Craig, A. (1996). Alzheimer disease and frontotemporal dementias: Behavioral distinctions. *Archives of Neurology, 53*(7), 687–690.

Lezak, M. (1995). *Neuropsychological assessment* (3rd ed.). New York: Oxford University Press.

Luria, A. (1966). *Higher cortical functions in man.* Andover, Hants, UK: Tavistock.

Mack, W. J., Freed, D. M., Williams, B. W., & Henderson, V. W. (1992). Boston Naming Test: Shortened versions for use in Alzheimer's disease. *Journal of Gerontology, 47*(3), P154–P158.

Magnotta, V. A., Harris, G., Andreasen, N. C., O'Leary, D. S., Yuh, W. T., & Heckel, D. (2002). Structural MR image processing using the BRAINS2 toolbox. *Computerized Medical Imaging and Graphics, 26*(4), 251–264.

Malloy, P., & Grace, J. (2005). A review of rating scales for measuring behavior change due to frontal systems damage. *Cognitive and Behavioral Neurology, 18*(1), 18–27.

Malloy, P. F., & Richardson, E. D. (1994). Assessment of frontal lobe functions. *Journal of Neuropsychiatry and Clinical Neurosciences, 6*(4), 399–410.

Mendez, M. F., Cherrier, M., Perryman, K. M., Pachana, M., Miller, B. L., & Cummings, J. L. (1996). Frontotemporal dementia versus Alzheimer's disease: Differential cognitive features. *Neurology, 47*(5), 1189–1194.

Miller, B. L., & Gearhart, R. (1999). Neuroimaging in the diagnosis of frontotemporal dementia. *Dementia and Geriatric Cognitive Disorders, 10*(Suppl. 1), 71–74.

Miller, B. L., Ikonte, C., Ponton, M., Levy, M., Boone, K., Darby, A., et al. (1997). A study of the Lund–Manchester research criteria for frontotemporal dementia: Clinical and single-photon emission CT correlations. *Neurology, 48*(4), 937–942.

Obonsawin, M. C., Crawford, J. R., Page, J., Chalmers, P., Cochrane, R., & Low, G. (2002). Performance on tests of frontal lobe function reflect general intellectual ability. *Neuropsychologia, 40*(7), 970–977.

Paul, R. H., Brickman, A. M., Navia, B., Hinkin, C., Malloy, P. F., Jefferson, A. L., et al. (2005). Apathy is associated with volume of the nucleus accumbens in patients infected with HIV. *Journal of Neuropsychiatry and Clinical Neurosciences, 17*(2), 167–171.

Peterson, B. S., Skudlarski, P., Gatenby, J. C., Zhang, H., Anderson, A. W., & Gore, J. C. (1999). An fMRI study of Stroop word–color interference: evidence for cingulate subregions subserving multiple distributed attentional systems. *Biological Psychiatry, 45*(10), 1237–1258.

Rankin, K. P., Baldwin, E., Pace-Savitsky, C., Kramer, J. H., & Miller, B. L. (2005). Self awareness and personality change in dementia. *Journal of Neurology, Neurosurgery, and Psychiatry, 76*(5), 632–639.

Rankin, K. P., Kramer, J. H., & Miller, B. L. (2005). Patterns of cognitive and emotional empathy in frontotemporal lobar degeneration. *Cognitive and Behavioral Neurology, 18*(1), 28–36.

Rankin, K. P., Kramer, J. H., Mychack, P., & Miller, B. L. (2003). Double dissociation of social functioning in frontotemporal dementia. *Neurology, 60*(2), 266–271.

Rankin, K. P., Rosen, H. J., Kramer, J. H., Schauer, G. F., Weiner, M. W., Schuff, N., et al. (2004). Right and left medial orbitofrontal volumes show an opposite relationship to agreeableness in FTD. *Dementia and Geriatric Cognitive Disorders, 17*(4), 328–332.

Ready, R. E., Ott, B. R., Grace, J., & Cahn-Weiner, D. A. (2003). Apathy and executive dysfunction in mild cognitive impairment and Alzheimer disease. *American Journal of Geriatric Psychiatry, 11*(2), 222–228.

Reitan, R. M., & Wolfson, D. (1994). A selective and critical review of neuropsychological deficits and the frontal lobes. *Neuropsychology Review, 4*(3), 161–198.

Rosen, H. J., Gorno-Tempini, M. L., Goldman, W. P., Perry, R. J., Schuff, N., Weiner, M., et al. (2002). Patterns of brain atrophy in frontotemporal dementia and semantic dementia. *Neurology, 58*(2), 198–208.

Rosen, H. J., Pace-Savitsky, K., Perry, R. J., Kramer, J. H., Miller, B. L., & Levenson, R. W. (2004). Recognition of emotion in the frontal and temporal variants of frontotemporal dementia. *Dementia and Geriatric Cognitive Disorders, 17*(4), 277–281.

Somerville, J., Tremont, G., & Stern, R. A. (2000). The Boston Qualitative Scoring System as a measure of executive functioning in Rey–Osterrieth Complex Figure performance. *Journal of Clinical and Experimental Neuropsychology, 22*(5), 613–621.

Stokholm, J., Vogel, A., Gade, A., & Waldemar, G. (2005). The executive interview as a screening test for executive dysfunction in patients with mild dementia. *Journal of American Geriatric Society, 53*(9), 1577–1581.

Stout, J. C., Ready, R. E., Grace, J., Malloy, P. F., & Paulsen, J. S. (2003). Factor analysis of the frontal systems behavior scale (FrSBe). *Assessment, 10*(1), 79–85.

Stuss, D. T., Bisschop, S. M., Alexander, M. P., Levine, B., Katz, D., & Izukawa, D. (2001). The Trail Making Test: A study in focal lesion patients. *Psychological Assessment, 13*(2), 230–239.

Stuss, D. T., Floden, D., Alexander, M. P., Levine, B., & Katz, D. (2001). Stroop performance in focal lesion patients: Dissociation of processes and frontal lobe lesion location. *Neuropsychologia, 39*(8), 771–786.

Stuss, D. T., Murphy, K. J., Binns, M. A., & Alexander, M. P. (2003). Staying on the job: The frontal lobes control individual performance variability. *Brain, 126*(11), 2363–2380.

Tekin, S., & Cummings, J. L. (2002). Frontal-subcortical neuronal circuits and clinical neuropsychiatry: An update. *Journal of Psychosomatic Research, 53*(2), 647–654.

Tucha, O. W., Smely, C. W., & Lange, K. W. (1999). Verbal and figural fluency in patients with mass lesions of the left or right frontal lobes. *Journal of Clinical and Experimental Neuropsychology, 21*(2), 229–236.

Walterfang, M., & Velakoulis, D. (2005). Cortical release signs in psychiatry. *Australia and New Zealand Journal of Psychiatry, 39*(5), 317–327.

Wecker, N. S., Kramer, J. H., Wisniewski, A., Delis, D. C., & Kaplan, E. (2000). Age effects on executive ability. *Neuropsychology, 14*(3), 409–414.

Wheeler, M. A., Stuss, D. T., & Tulving, E. (1995). Frontal lobe damage produces episodic memory impairment. *Journal of the International Neuropsychological Society, 1*(6), 525–536.

Wiebers, D. O., Dale, A. J., Kokmen, E., & Swanson, J. W. (1998). *Mayo Clinic examinations in neurology* (7th ed.). St. Louis, MO: Mosby.

Woods, R. P., Dapretto, M., Sicotte, N. L., Toga, A. W., & Mazziotta, J. C. (1999). Creation and use of a Talairach-compatible atlas for accurate, automated, nonlinear intersubject registration, and analysis of functional imaging data. *Human Brain Mapping, 8*(2–3), 73–79.

# CHAPTER 19

# New Approaches to Prefrontal Lobe Testing

## Donald T. Stuss

This chapter addresses the assessment of functions related to the prefrontal region within the frontal lobes. It is proposed in this chapter that the neuropsychological assessment of the prefrontal region of the brain can be divided into four functional categories: (1) *executive cognitive*, (2) *behavioral–emotional self-regulatory*, (3) *energization regulating*, and (4) *metacognitive*. The general frontal regions relating to these four categories are depicted in Figure 19.1.

Several clarifications establish the limits of this review. The reader is first cautioned on the interpretation of the term "categories." It does not designate a functional module, in the Fodorian sense. It reflects a grouping of similar behaviors, all of which have a higher-order, more central relationship to other functions in the brain. These categories are domain-general. Second, although the term "frontal lobes" may be used in the review for sake of simplicity, the em-

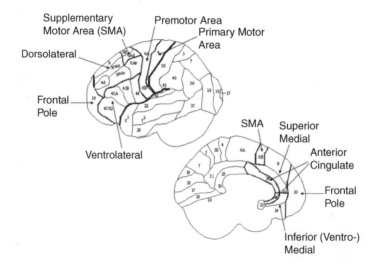

FIGURE 19.1. The cortical maps depicted are divided by rough connectivity patterns. These regions can be grouped into four major categories for neuropsychological assessment: polar, superior medial, inferior medial, and lateral. The anterior cingulate (superior and inferior) are grouped within the superior and inferior medial divisions. The functions of the motor and premotor regions are not discussed in this chapter. The further separation illustrated here (e.g., dorsolateral vs. ventrolateral within the lateral region) is presented as guidelines for future localization research. The axial representations are typical computed tomography plane templates.

phasis is on the prefrontal cortex, and little mention is made of the motor or premotor regions and effects of damage there. Third, there is no attempt to make a direct connection to "executive function" or the "dysexecutive syndrome." These terms are not easily operationalized, and there is inconsistency among authors in the application of these terms. Moreover, executive function is a psychological construct, with no necessary relation to anatomical structure. Test performance purported to measure executive function may be impaired after diffuse brain damage (e.g., traumatic brain injury), inefficient integrative functioning (such as may occur in confusional states), and after damage to many different nonfrontal brain regions. (The latter is likely secondary to impairment in the myriad additional functions required to perform the multifaceted tests often used to test "executive functions." It is also possible that executive dysfunction after damage in nonfrontal brain regions may be due to impairment in network connectivity.) Consequently, deficits on an "executive function" test cannot be automatically interpreted as damage to the frontal lobes (an important concept for those who do research in aging, and use the tests to infer the integrity or nonintegrity of the frontal lobes).

It is nevertheless accepted that executive functions may be best instantiated in the frontal lobes, and in "frontal systems"—those areas with direct connections to the frontal lobes. Because the comparative evidence on how each node in a system is functionally similar or dissimilar has not been completed, the potential role of different nodes in a system is not reviewed.

The four functional distinctions within the frontal lobes are described first, followed by research evidence related to each. Articles referenced are necessarily selective. Because of the focus on frontal/functional distinctions, the articles reviewed are to a great degree based on research in which documentation of lesion location provides such information. The reader is encouraged to check the reference list for a more detailed background and other evidence.

## FOUR FUNCTIONAL DOMAINS WITHIN THE FRONTAL LOBES

The theory of the evolution of cortical architectonics indicates two major functional-anatomical dissociations within the frontal lobes (Pandya & Yeterian, 1996; Sanides, 1970; Stuss & Levine, 2002): a *lateral prefrontal* cortex (LPFC), evolving from a hippocampal, archicortical trend, involved in *spatial and conceptual reasoning* processes; and a *ventral (medial) prefrontal* cortex (VPFC) paleocortical trend, emerging from the caudal orbitofrontal (olfactory) cortex, and closely connected with limbic nuclei involved in *emotional* processing (Nauta, 1971; Pandya & Barnes, 1987), including the acquisition and reversal of stimulus–reward associations (Fuster, 1997; Mishkin, 1964; Rolls, 1996, 2000). These two trends form the two major (*executive cognitive* and *behavioral–emotional self-regulatory*) functional divisions within the frontal lobes. However, two additional dissociations within the prefrontal region seem likely, one (*energization regulating*) based on the evidence of five major frontal–subcortical networks (Alexander, DeLong, & Strick, 1986), and the other (*metacognitive*) suggested by recent research on higher-order integrative functions (for reviews, see Stuss & Alexander, 1999, 2000; Stuss, Picton, & Alexander, 2001). It should be noted that some authors use the term "executive" for all four of these functional domains.

### Executive Cognitive Functions

"Executive cognitive functions" are defined as (and the term is limited to) high-level *cognitive* functions, believed to be mediated primarily by the LPFC, that are involved in the control and direction (e.g., planning, monitoring, energizing, switching, inhibiting) of lower-level, more automatic functions. Much of what is known about executive functions in neuropsychological studies is based on patients with primarily LPFC damage (Goldman-Rakic, 1987; Milner, 1963; Petrides & Milner, 1982; Stuss & Benson, 1986).

### Behavioral–Emotional Self-Regulatory Functions

The VPFC region is involved in *emotional* processing (Nauta, 1971; Pandya & Barnes, 1987), including the acquisition and reversal of stimulus–reward associations (Fuster, 1997; Mishkin, 1964; Rolls, 1996, 2000). An important, and natural, role for the VPFC, because of its involvement in reward processing, is *behavioral self-regulation* required in situations where cognitive analysis, habit, or environmental cues are not sufficient to determine the most adaptive response (Eslinger & Damasio, 1985; Harlow, 1868; Penfield & Evans, 1935).

## Energization Regulating Functions

More superior medial frontal pathology (to dissociate from the orbitofrontal/ventromedial classification, although often the two are concomitant) results in disorders of energization and drive (Stuss, Binns, Murphy, & Alexander, 2002; Stuss, Alexander, et al., 2005), clinically known as apathy or abulia. Disorders of energization have an important impact on self-regulation.

## Metacognitive Processes

The fourth categorization is related to the frontal polar region (possibly more particularly on the right). This frontal region appears to be maximally involved in the most recently studied metacognitive aspects of human nature: integrative aspects of personality, social cognition, autonoetic consciousness, and self-awareness (Shammi & Stuss, 1999; Stuss, Gallup, & Alexander, 2001; Stuss, Picton, & Alexander, 2001; Tulving, 1985). Because they are the most recently evolved, they may be uniquely positioned to integrate the higher-level executive cognitive functions, and emotional or drive-related inputs (Burgess, Simons, Dumontheil, & Gilbert, 2005; Stuss & Alexander, 1999, 2000). They do not appear to be reducible to these functions (Siegal & Varley, 2002; Stuss, Rosenbaum, Malcolm, Christiana, & Keenan, 2005). This bridging of behavioral self-regulatory and executive cognitive functions may be one reason for their role in metacognitive functions. There is some evidence, however, that there are potential dissociations within this domain (Stuss, Rosenbaum, et al., 2005).

## Summary

The first three functional distinctions map onto three of the five parallel but independent frontal–subcortical circuits defined by their distinct major reciprocal subcortical connections (Alexander et al., 1986; Alexander & Crutcher, 1990; Cummings, 1993; Saint-Cyr, Bronstein, & Cummings, 2002): lateral (executive cognitive), lateral orbital (emotional–behavioral), and medial frontal/anterior cingulate (energiza-

tion). It is hypothesized that damage anywhere in each circuit will produce similar deficits (although as noted earlier, the evidence is only partial). Damage in the subcortical segments of these anatomical systems often causes mixed syndromes due to the proximity of the subcortical structures involved in the different circuits.

## NEUROPSYCHOLOGICAL EVIDENCE FOR THE FOUR DOMAINS

### Executive Cognitive Functions

The following tests are used by many clinicians as measures of frontal lobe "executive" functioning: Wisconsin Card Sorting Test (WCST; Stuss et al., 2000); Trail Making Test Part B (Stuss, Bisschop, et al., 2001); and specific measures within verbal fluency tasks (Stuss et al., 1998; Troyer, Moscovitch, Winocur, Alexander, & Stuss, 1998). Because recent research has demonstrated a greater relation to focal LPFC (and also not generally to orbitofrontal–ventromedial pathology; Stuss et al., 2000; Stuss, Bisschop, et al., 2001; Stuss, Floden, Alexander, Levine, & Katz, 2001; Stuss & Levine, 2002; Stuss, Binns, & Alexander, 2003), they fall within the classification of tests of "executive cognitive" processes. These tests do exemplify many of the cautions required for proper interpretation of such tests. The tests are complex and multifactorial, and individuals can fail for many reasons (e.g., Anderson, Damasio, Jones, & Tranel, 1991). Thus, before concluding that there is a relation of performance on such tests with frontal lobe dysfunction, the examiner in interpretation must account for the effect of other processes that could affect performance. Although many clinicians continue to use these tests, it is likely that they will eventually be replaced by more process-specific measures. Efforts in this vein are already under way (see the following text; see also Burgess, Alderman, Evans, Emslie, & Wilson, 1998; Burgess & Shallice, 1996a, 1996b, 1997; Dias, Robbins, & Roberts, 1997).

Little role was proposed historically for the frontal lobes in memory functions. However, it is now clear that strategic aspects of encoding and retrieval in certain memory tests, such as word list learning, are other examples of executive cognitive functions (see Stuss & Alexander, 2005). In memory assessment, it is important to differentiate between basic associative processes of cue–engram interaction (mediated by medial temporal lobe–hippocampal structures) and strategic processes related to the encoding and retrieval of these associations (mediated by LPFC primarily) (Luria, 1973; Moscovitch, 1992; Stuss, Alexander, et al., 1994). Moscovitch and Winocur (1992) very succinctly captured the general role of the frontal lobes in memory by stating that the frontal lobes "work with memory." However, analyses of the different processes involved in some memory tests can unveil the unique contributions of different executive cognitive functions to memory (Alexander, Stuss, & Fansabedian, 2003). The role of the frontal lobes in working memory is in the manipulation and control of information held on-line (Baddeley, 1986). However, it is clear that many different regions of the brain are involved in working memory (D'Esposito & Postle, 2002; Postle, Druzgal, & D'Esposito, 2003).

Word list learning tasks such as the California Verbal Learning Test (CVLT; Delis, Kramer, Kaplan, & Ober, 1987) can yield measures of both basic associative and strategic processes. The latest updates of the Wechsler Instruments have added new tasks stressing manipulation and control (Wechsler, 1997), and even allow for a separate "working memory" composite score. Executive processing in acquiring visuospatial information is less well understood; consequently, measures are lacking that examine learning strategies and working memory manipulation of visuospatial stimuli.

Tests of attention/intention, such as sustained attention, inhibition of irrelevant information (distractibility), monitoring of information, and variability in reaction time (RT) performance also fall within the broad rubric of executive cognitive functions. Indeed, the influential model of Norman and Shallice on frontal lobe functions was once labeled the "supervisory attentional system." Different attentional tests provide the opportunity to assess inhibition and monitoring, using errors and RT as dependent measurements (Godefroy, Lhullier, & Rousseaux, 1994; Godefroy, Lhullier-Lamy, & Rousseaux, 2002; Richer et al., 1993; Richer & LePage, 1996). The right frontal region is important for performance on continuous performance tests, especially when the target complexity is increased (i.e., respond to "O" following "X") (Deutsch, Papanicolaou, Bourbon, & Eisenberg, 1987; Glosser & Goodglass, 1990; Pardo, Fox, & Raichle, 1991; Reuckert & Grafman, 1996; Wilkins,

Shallice, & McCarthy, 1987; Woods & Knight, 1986), and the task is slower rather than faster (Reuckert & Grafman, 1998; Wilkins et al., 1987). The Sustained Attention to Response Task [SART; Robertson, Manly, Andrade, Baddeley, & Yiend, 1997] and the Elevator Counting Test (Robertson, Ward, Ridgeway, & Nimmo-Smith, 1991) are modern neuropsychological tests of these sustained attention abilities.

We (Alexander, Stuss, Shallice, Picton, & Gillingham, 2005; Stuss, Binns, et al., 2002; Stuss, Alexander, et al., 2005) have demonstrated several dissociations of executive cognitive functions within the prefrontal region using different RT tasks (see Figure 19.2). The left lateral frontal region is important for task setting, regardless of type of task. This was demonstrated by deficient criterion setting in a feature integration task (impaired bias, shown by errors that were primarily false positives; Figure 19.2a), and significantly increased errors in the first block of 100 trials in a concentration task requiring rapid stimulus–response matching (Figure 19.2b). Note that the evidence of increased false-positive errors in memory recognition (Alexander et al., 2003) indicates that this central process of task setting is applicable to different tasks, not just RT (Figure 19.2c). The right lateral frontal area has a key role to play in monitoring, with the possibility of different types of monitoring. Only this area within the prefrontal regions revealed an abnormal foreperiod effect, with RT increasing with longer interstimulus interval (ISI) rather than decreasing, suggesting a deficiency in monitoring the occurrence of stimuli over time (Stuss, Alexander, et al., 2005; Figure 19.2d). Damage to the right lateral area also resulted in increased errors of all types in a complex feature integration task, indicating a problem in monitoring the difference between targets and nontargets (Stuss, Binns, et al., 2002). These data suggest different types of monitoring deficits within the right lateral region.

A key impairment found after focal frontal pathology is increased within-subject (intraindividual) variability of performance both within a testing session and across sessions (Stuss et al., 1989; Stuss, Pogue, Buckle, & Bondar, 1994). This fluctuation in top-down control is most visible in more complex tasks; notable trial-to-trial fluctuations in simple tasks such as finger tapping may reflect other issues such as cooperation. The mechanisms

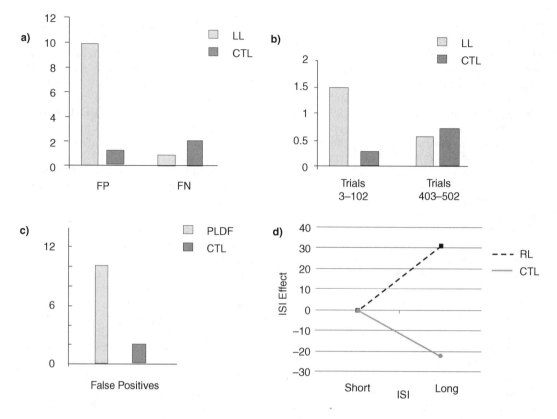

FIGURE 19.2. Results from several different tasks highlighting dissociations of executive cognitive processes in the prefrontal region are illustrated as task setting (a, b, and c) and monitoring (d).

(a) The Left Lateral group (LL) demonstrated a significantly increased number of false positive errors compared to the Control (CTL) group in a feature integration task in which a target was defined by a particular combination of three features, and the distractors shared either zero, one, or two features with the target. FP, false positive; FN, false negative.

(b) The task-setting deficit observed in the LL group is also demonstrated by the significantly higher number of errors committed by this group compared to the CTL group in only the first 100 of 500 trials of a task requiring a button press response to a rapid continuous reaction time (RT) test.

(c) The task-setting deficit was also observed in a word list–learning task, depicted by a significantly higher number of false-positive errors committed by patients with Posterior Left Lateral Frontal pathology (PLDF) on the recognition measure.

(d) In contrast to the task-setting deficit in the LL group, patients with Right Lateral (RL) pathology showed a monitoring deficit. The RL group did not exhibit the standard foreperiod effect of a decreasing reaction time (RT) with an increasing foreperiod, as shown by the CTL group. This was illustrated by the difference in RTs between trials that had either short (3- or 4-second) or long (6- or 7-second) foreperiods (ISI, interstimulus interval). For each group, the short ISI is set at zero and is contrasted to the differences in RT for the long ISI.

behind variability appear to be secondary to deficits in the same attentional mechanisms evidenced by other RT measures: task setting and monitoring (Stuss, Murphy, Binns, & Alexander, 2003). RT tests may provide the most sensitive index of such intraindividual variability, although it can be seen in other tasks, such as memory tasks (Alexander et al., 2003; Murphy,

West, Armilio, Craik, & Stuss, in press; Stuss, Pogue, et al., 1994).

To bridge the gap between laboratory tasks of executive cognitive functions and functional outcome measures of everyday activities, investigators have studied naturalistic actions under controlled conditions. For example, Schwartz and colleagues (1998) developed a Multi-Level

Action Test (MLAT) for assessing rehabilitation potential and outcome in patients who had sustained a traumatic brain injury (TBI). The test was based on a hypothesized disturbance of executive functions after TBI, such as reduced planning, problems in sequencing, working memory, and resistance to interference. The MLAT has not been assessed in patients with focal lesions to the best of my knowledge; indeed, in the patients with TBI, performance was moderately correlated with a measure of functional outcome but not to the presence of frontal lesions. Although naturalistic tasks may reveal executive cognitive deficits, further investigation is required to evaluate the relative contributions of executive cognitive deficit and nonexecutive cognitive impairment to performance on naturalistic tasks. There is considerable overlap in such tests with the behavioral–emotional self-regulatory measures (see below). It is very likely that these more "real-life" measures necessitate the involvement of multiple functional systems. They do bring a functional usefulness, and the relative value of the more "process pure" laboratory tasks and such naturalistic tasks is a very promising area of future research and application.

## Behavioral/Emotional Self-Regulatory Functions

Patients with damage to the inferior medial frontal cortex have difficulty in performing normally in unstructured situations (Eslinger & Damasio, 1985; Levine, 1999; Levine, Black, et al., 1998; Levine, Freedman, Dawson, Black, & Stuss, 1999) and in understanding the emotional consequences of their behavior, despite intact performance on commonly used neuropsychological tests of executive functioning (Bechara, Damasio, Tranel, & Anderson, 1998; Bechara, Damasio, Tranel, & Damasio, 1997; Bechara, Tranel, Damasio, & Damasio, 1996; Stuss & Benson, 1983). Assessment of these abilities tends to be more experimental in nature, and includes gambling tasks (Bechara et al., 1998; Rogers et al., 1999) and naturalistic multiple subgoal tasks (Burgess et al., 1998; Burgess, Veitch, de Lacy Costello, & Shallice, 2000; Goel, Grafman, Tajik, Gana, & Danto, 1997; Levine, Dawson, Boutet, Schwartz, & Stuss, 2000).

Because of the role of the VPFC in emotional processing (basic drives and rewards that inform and direct high-level decision making), tests assessing the acquisition and reversal of stimulus–reward associations can be used

(Fuster, 1997; Mishkin, 1964; Rolls, 2000). This reversal learning (interpreted as affective) is dissociable from the impairment in attentional (extradimensional) set shifting found after LPFC lesions (Dias, Robbins, & Roberts, 1996, 1997), reinforcing the distinction between "executive" attentional and affective/emotional behavioral measures.

The VPFC is also involved in higher-level decision-making tasks involving reward processing in unstructured situations, such as the gambling task developed by Bechara, Damasio, Damasio, and Anderson (1994) that has been suggested as both sensitive and specific to VPFC lesions (Bechara et al., 1998; see also Rogers et al., 1999). However, as with many neuropsychological tests, further evaluation suggests that these tests may also be multifactorial in nature, and the true behavior–anatomy specificity remains to be determined (Bechara et al., 1998; Fellows & Farah, 2005; Manes et al., 2002). Performance on the gambling task has been dissociated from deficits in working memory and inhibition (Bechara et al., 1998).

A broad term to encompass the type of deficits observed on the gambling task is "self-regulatory disorder" (SRD), defined as the inability to regulate behavior according to internal goals and constraints, particularly in less structured situations (Levine, 1999; Levine, Black, et al., 1998; Levine et al., 1999). Shallice and Burgess (1991) quantified the qualitative descriptions with naturalistic, multiple subgoal tasks, and there have been several developments of this task (Burgess et al., 1998, 2000; Levine et al., 2000). A paper-and-pencil laboratory task based on the Six Element Test of the Shallice and Burgess (1991) study, requiring the selection of targets with high payoff to the exclusion of readily available but lesser-valued targets, has been developed. It appears sensitive to focal VPFC damage (particularly on the right) despite preserved performance on other tests described earlier that are sensitive to LPFC damage (Levine, Stuss, et al., 1998). The Behavioral Dyscontrol Scale (Grigsby, Kaye, Baxter, Shetterly, & Hamman, 1998), based on Luria's theory, includes tasks assessing both executive cognitive functions and self-regulatory behaviors.

## Self-Regulation of Energization and Drive

Damage to left or right medial (anterior cingulate and superior) frontal regions results in

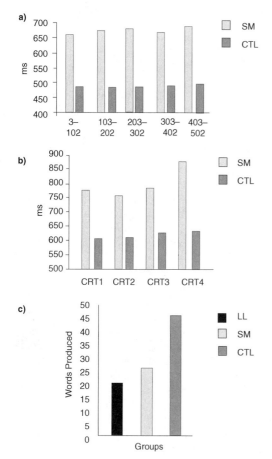

FIGURE 19.3. A deficit in the generation and maintenance of actions or mental processes was revealed in patients with superior medial (SM) pathology. The same impairment is demonstrated in three separate tasks.

(a) The SM group was significantly slower the CTL group on an RT task requiring a button press response to rapidly occurring stimuli for 500 trials (shown separated into five sets of 100 trials).

(b) Patients with SM damage were significantly slower than the CTL group in their correct responses in a choice RT task (four independent conditions) in which subjects were asked to respond to a defined target letter and to withhold response to other letters in four separate blocks of trials.

(c) A similar impairment in energization was illustrated by word generation in a verbal fluency (FAS) task. Patients with SM damage were significantly impaired compared to the CTL group. However, this task may also be sensitive to impairments in other cognitive abilities, such as language, therefore showing deficiencies in other patient groups, such as LL.

poor capacity to generate and maintain actions or mental processes. Patients with damage in this region are slow in RT tasks, particularly if more demanding (Figure 19.3a, 19.3b), are deficient in generating lists of words (particularly in the first 15 seconds—Figure 19.3c), and have problems maintaining a selected target such as in the Stroop interference test (Bench et al., 1993; MacDonald, Cohen, Stenger, & Carter, 2000; Pardo, Pardo, Janer, & Raichle, 1990; Stuss et al., 1998; Stuss, Binns, et al., 2002; Stuss, Bisschop, et al., 2001; Stuss, Floden, et al., 2001). However, tasks such as verbal fluency and the Stroop lack specificity and, depending on administration, may also be sensitive to impairment in executive cognitive functions (Perret, 1974; Vendrell et al., 1995) or other cognitive abilities, such as color naming in the Stroop test (Stuss, Floden, et al., 2001). Thus, patients with LPFC are often impaired on the same tasks (Figure 19.3c). In addition, for executive function tasks, superior medial frontal regions appear "upstream" from lateral frontal cortex, providing energization and drive to organize and sustain action without necessarily providing the content of action. Perhaps the best measure to evaluate impaired energization is demanding RT measures. Choice RT tasks and simple RT tasks demanding concentration demonstrate strongly the effect of pathology in the superior medial regions (Alexander et al., 2005; Stuss, Alexander, et al., 2005).

The general localization of these separable executive processes are summarized in Figure 19.4.

## Metacognitive Processes

The frontal polar region (although there is still question as to how much of this is anterior ventromedial vs. the specific polar Brodmann's area 10) has been related to the highest of human integrative behaviors: theory of mind and self-awareness, humor appreciation, and episodic (autonoetic or self-knowing) memory (Craik et al., 1999; Fink et al., 1996; Frith & Frith, 1999; Goel & Dolan, 2001; Shallice, 2001; Shammi & Stuss, 1999; Stuss, Gallup, et al., 2001; Stuss, Rosenbaum, et al., 2005; Wheeler, Stuss, & Tulving, 1997). Self-awareness implies a metacognitive representation of one's own mental states, beliefs, attitudes, and experiences. This self-reflection is key to understanding the relationship of one's own thoughts and external events, and from

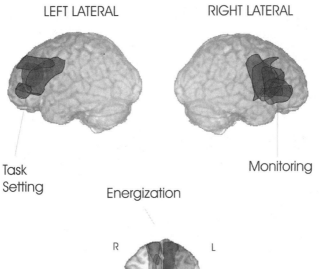

LEFT LATERAL       RIGHT LATERAL

Task
Setting            Monitoring

Energization

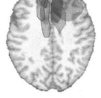

SUPERIOR MEDIAL

FIGURE 19.4. The left and right lateral frontal views and an axial slice depicting a typical superior medial region illustrate the three frontal brain regions related to the three different anterior attentional processes. Left lateral, task setting; right lateral, monitoring; and superior medial, energization.

this self-knowledge to understand the mental states of others. This ability to make inferences about the world, and to empathize with others, allows us to interpret others' actions properly and to make social judgments. Family reports often precisely describe the changes in behavior that have occurred: lack of empathy, unconcern, and inability to appreciate humor that requires self-reflection (appreciation of slapstick humor may be intact).

The neuropsychological assessments in this domain are generally experimental. They include reactions to verbal and cartoon humor (Brownell, Michel, Powelson, & Gardner, 1983; Shammi & Stuss, 1999), visual perspective-taking tasks (Stone, Baron-Cohen, & Knight, 1998; Stuss, Gallup, et al., 2001), and comparison of performance on remember–know memory tasks (Wheeler & Stuss, 2003). It is important to know that, for some individuals, these tasks can be solved on the basis of factual knowledge, not inference. Moreover, the relationship of process to anatomy is not certain,

and it may depend on the differential demands of different tests within the overall "metacognitive" rubric (see Stone et al., 1998). There does appear to be some consistency, however (Frith & Frith, 1999; Shallice, 2001).

## CONSIDERATIONS FOR ASSESSMENT

### Task Difficulty

It was once a dictum that the functions of the frontal lobes were necessary when old information was used in novel ways, or for complex problem solving. But are complex tests necessary to assess frontal lobe functions? The answer itself is a complex one. Some of the functions I have described were revealed with very simple tasks. For example, deficits in energization could be revealed with demanding RT tasks, which themselves were not complex (Alexander et al., 2005).

What are the effects of increasing task complexity? If the task is too complex, the potential dissociations within the frontal regions may be obscured. Thus, in a word list–learning task, the most demanding strategic process (subjective organization, measured by the encoding words together as pairs, regardless of their serial order or category cluster) was impaired by prefrontal lobe damage in virtually all frontal regions (Alexander et al., 2003; Stuss, Alexander, et al., 1994). In a negative priming study with focal frontal lobe lesions, where there were three levels of complexity in identifying the target before responding by moving a joystick to a comparable position as the target on the computer screen, impairment was maximum in the right parietal and right frontal regions—with one exception. At the highest level of complexity (which was in reality quite simple), impairment was observed after damage in all frontal regions identified (Stuss et al., 1999). There is an important corollary of this finding. Perhaps one of the reasons it has been difficult to find processes that are more specific to the frontal lobes, and to uncover clinical behavioral dissociations within the frontal regions, is that the tests used have been *too* complex. Those with a more experimental cognitive approach, sometimes using tests developed for animal research and therefore, of necessity, somewhat less complex, have often been more successful (e.g., Petrides, 1991; Petrides & Milner, 1982).

Thus, the use of complex tasks may depend on which processes are targeted. It is likely that tests will have to be titrated to the appropriate difficulty. For example, in a feature detection and choice response task, errors that were important for separation of the roles of different frontal regions were observed only in the more complex, three-feature detection task (Stuss, Binns, et al., 2002). If the task were not adequately difficult, not enough errors would be elicited to demonstrate the dissociations (Stuss, Alexander, et al., 2005).

### Group and Individual Variability

What should one understand about group variability in evaluating research on the assessment of frontal lobe functions? Group variability may reflect normal variation within a group, or it may indicate inadequate knowledge of group composition and performance. For example, many of our major findings of anatomical–behavioral distinctions within the frontal lobes occurred only after we started using perfor-

mance to group individuals, rather than using a priori classical anatomical distinctions, such as right frontal, left frontal, and bifrontal (see Stuss, Alexander, et al. [2002] for a review, and Stuss, Alexander, et al. [1994] and Stuss et al. [1998] for examples of this approach). Thus, in earlier studies, potential differences may have been obscured. At the same time, potential anatomical–behavioral dissociations may not be found if there is inadequate representation of different frontal regions in the patients being tested. These facts should be considered when reviewing lesion research as a basis for interpretation of findings on neuropsychological tests.

Perhaps the greatest problem in neuropsychological assessment is individual variability in performance. If the frontal lobes do result in such intraindividual variability (Stuss, Murphy, et al., 2003), how can one ever be certain of one's interpretation of test results in patients with frontal lobe damage? There are two key aspects to the response. The first is most obvious; being aware of this finding provides the clinician with an additional tool of assessment. Second, intraindividual variability is not randomness. Intraindividual variability is lawful and can therefore be manipulated and understood (there is a burgeoning literature on such variability, in different populations (Hultsch, MacDonald, Hunter, Levy-Benecheton, & Strauss, 2000; Mirsky, Fantie, & Tatman, 1995; Strauss, MacDonald, Hunter, Moll, & Hultsch, 2002; West, Murphy, Armilio, Craik, & Stuss, 2002).

### SUMMARY

Executive function has assumed too broad a connotation for the adult developed brain (the developing brain may not follow the distinctions outlined). Many use "executive functions" as a general term to encompass all of these higher-level cognitive, behavioral–emotional, energization, and metacognitive processes. Some use descriptors to dissociate the different types of behavior, such as the "cold" and "hot" distinctions within executive function (Metcalfe, 1998), which in reality map onto the two general distinctions of LPFC and VPFC. Others interchange the terms "frontal" and "executive." This review has approached the topic by focusing on the functions related to specific anatomical regions within the frontal lobes. Using this approach, a more precise classification of four prefrontal lobe functional domain general categories based on documented anatomical–behavioral distinctions is possible.

These distinctions are emphasized for several reasons: (1) The term "executive function" has historically been used to relate to the more cognitive abilities, such as planning, switching, and monitoring, which are related to LPFC, and for sake of operational clarity should be retained as such; other important behavioral processes lumped within the larger general term "executive," which depend on other anatomically proximal systems, have been relatively ignored and are usually not considered separately; (2) our proposed distinctions do relate to different anatomical regions and systems with distinct behavioral associations; (3) most importantly, such anatomical–behavioral definitions are essential in understanding the sequelae of frontal lobe damage, and the potential development of new, focused rehabilitation techniques.

There are concerns about the currently available clinical tests for "executive functions," including their lack of specificity, even when they are sensitive (e.g., Trail Making Test: Stuss, Bisschop, et al., 2001). Many of the tests considered "frontal" have weak evidence for their relationship to the frontal lobes; indeed, most of the anatomical validity studies have not considered different regions within the frontal lobes. Although imaging research using these tasks might give some indication of the role of different regions, such data neither inform us of the necessity of these regions for the task nor do they differentiate the different roles related to the different processes required to perform the task. Tasks that differentiate processes more specifically have not yet been transformed into clinical measures with the appropriate normative data. There is a need to follow the current trend to develop new tests that target the aforementioned domains. Although there have been significant advances in recent years, even greater specificity is likely (separation of areas within the general distinctions note, for example, "of the ventrolateral area"). Such tests should be validated in different populations, including their relation to daily functioning and participation in complex activities. Eventual goals in this field of research will be to evaluate the similarities and differences between "executive functions" and the specific

functions of the frontal lobes, and also to investigate in a systematic manner the effect of damage in different nodes in a defined frontal system. Finally, this anatomical–functional division within the frontal lobes should not be viewed as modern phrenology. Although such distinctions can be made (as indicated by the research evidence), these distinctions are to some degree artifactual. Real-life functioning consists of integrative, multisystem networks, and this is the real future of neuropsychological assessment.

## ACKNOWLEDGMENTS

My research reported in this chapter was possible because of research or personnel funding by the Medical Research Council of Canada/Canadian Institutes of Health Research (CIHR), the Reva James Leeds Chair in Neuroscience and Research Leadership to D. Stuss, the JSF McDonnell Foundation, the Posluns Centre for Stroke and Cognition at Baycrest Centre, and the Heart and Stroke Foundation of Ontario Centre for Stroke Recovery. Partial development of concepts was first published in Stuss and Levine (2002). My thanks to S. Gillingham for assistance in figure and manuscript preparation.

## REFERENCES

Alexander, G. E., & Crutcher, M. D. (1990). Neural representations of the target (goal) of visually guided arm movements in three motor areas of the monkey. *Journal of Neurophysiology, 64,* 164–178.

Alexander, G. E., DeLong, M. R., & Strick, P. L. (1986). Parallel organization of functionally segregated circuits linking basal ganglia and cortex. *Annual Review of Neuroscience, 9,* 357–381.

Alexander, M. P., Stuss, D. T., & Fansabedian, N. (2003). California Verbal Learning Test: Performance by patients with focal frontal and non-frontal lesions. *Brain, 126,* 1493–1503.

Alexander, M. P., Stuss, D. T., Shallice, T., Picton, T. W., & Gillingham, S. (2005). Impaired concentration due to frontal lobe damage from two distinct lesion sites. *Neurology, 65,* 572–579.

Anderson, S. W., Damasio, H., Jones, R. D., & Tranel, D. (1991). Wisconsin Card Sorting Test performance as a measure of frontal lobe damage. *Journal of Clinical and Experimental Neuropsychology, 13,* 909–922.

Baddeley, A. (1986). *Working memory.* Oxford, UK: Clarendon Press.

Bechara, A., Damasio, A. R., Damasio, H., & Anderson, S. W. (1994). Insensitivity to future consequences following damage to human prefrontal cortex. *Cognition, 50,* 7–15.

Bechara, A., Damasio, H., Tranel, D., & Anderson, S. W. (1998). Dissociation of working memory from decision making within the human prefrontal cortex. *Journal of Neuroscience, 18,* 428–437.

Bechara, A., Damasio, H., Tranel, D., Damasio, A. R. (1997). Deciding advantageously before knowing the advantageous strategy. *Science, 275,* 1293–1295.

Bechara, A., Tranel, D., Damasio, H., & Damasio, A. R. (1996). Failure to respond automatically to anticipated future outcomes following damage to prefrontal cortex. *Cerebral Cortex, 6,* 215–225.

Bench, C. J., Frith, C. D., Grasby, P. M., Friston, K. J., Paulesu, E., Frackowiak, R. S. J., et al. (1993). Investigations of the functional anatomy of attention using the Stroop test. *Neuropsychologia, 31,* 907–922.

Brownell, H. H., Michel, D., Powelson, J., & Gardner, H. (1983). Surprise but not coherence: Sensitivity to verbal humor in right-hemisphere patients. *Brain and Language, 18,* 20–27.

Burgess, P. W., Alderman, N., Evans, J., Emslie, H., & Wilson, B. A. (1998). The ecological validity of tests of executive function. *Journal of the International Neuropsychological Society, 4,* 547–558.

Burgess, P. W., & Shallice, T. (1996a). Bizarre responses, rule detection and frontal lobe lesions. *Cortex, 32,* 241–259.

Burgess, P. W., & Shallice, T. (1996b). Response suppression, initiation and strategy use following frontal lobe lesions. *Neuropsychologia, 34,* 263–273.

Burgess, P. W., & Shallice, T. (1997). *The Hayling and Brixton tests of dysexecutive syndrome.* London: Harcourt Assessment, Psychological Corporation.

Burgess, P. W., Simons, J. S., Dumontheil, I., & Gilbert, S. J. (2005). The gateway hypothesis of rostral prefrontal cortex (area 10) function. In J. Duncan, L. Phillips, & P. McLeod (Eds.), *Measuring the mind: Speed, control, and age* (pp. 217–248). Oxford, UK: Oxford University Press.

Burgess, P. W., Veitch, E., de Lacy Costello, A., & Shallice, T. (2000). The cognitive and neuroanatomical correlates of multitasking. *Neuropsychologia, 38,* 848–863.

Craik, F. I. M., Moroz, T. M., Moscovitch, M., Stuss, D. T., Winocur, G., Tulving, E., et al. (1999). In search of the self: A positron emission tomography study. *Psychological Science, 10,* 27–35.

Cummings, J. (1993). Frontal–subcortical circuits and human behavior. *Archives of Neurology, 50,* 873–880.

Delis, D. C., Kramer, J. H., Kaplan, E., & Ober, B. A. (1987). *California Verbal Learning Test: Adult version.* San Antonio, TX: Psychological Corporation.

D'Esposito, M., & Postle, B. R. (2002). The neural basis of working memory storage, rehearsal, and control processes: Evidence from patient and functional magnetic resonance imaging studies. In L. R. Squire & D. L. Schacter (Eds.), *Neuropsychology of memory* (3rd ed., pp. 215–224). New York: Guilford Press.

Deutsch, G., Papanicolaou, A. C., Bourbon, W. T., & Eisenberg, H. M. (1987). Cerebral blood flow evidence of right frontal activation in attention demanding tasks. *International Journal of Neuroscience, 36,* 23–28.

Dias, R., Robbins, T. W., & Roberts, A. C. (1996). Dissociation in prefrontal cortex of affective and attentional shifts. *Nature, 380,* 69–72.

Dias, R., Robbins, T. W., & Roberts, A. C. (1997). Dissociable forms of inhibitory control within prefrontal cortex with an analog of the Wisconsin Card Sort Test: Restriction to novel situations and independence from "on-line" processing. *Journal of Neuroscience, 17,* 9285–9297.

Eslinger, P. J., & Damasio, A. R. (1985). Severe disturbance of higher cognition after bilateral frontal lobe ablation: Patient EVR. *Neurology, 35,* 1731–1741.

Fellows, L. K., & Farah, M. J. (2005). Different underlying impairments in decision making following ventromedial and dorsolateral frontal lobe damage in humans. *Cerebral Cortex, 15,* 58–63.

Fink, G. R., Markowitsch, H. J., Reinkemeier, M., Bruckbauer, T., Kessler, J., & Heiss, W. (1996). Cerebral representation of one's own past: Neural networks involved in autobiographical memory. *Journal of Neuroscience, 16,* 4275–4282.

Frith, C. D., & Frith, U. (1999). Interacting minds—a biological basis. *Science, 286,* 1692–1695.

Fuster, J. M. (1997). *The prefrontal cortex: Anatomy, physiology, and neuropsychology of the frontal lobe* (3rd ed.). New York: Raven.

Glosser, G., & Goodglass, H. (1990). Disorders in executive control functions among aphasic and other brain-damaged patients. *Journal of Clinical and Experimental Neuropsychology, 12,* 485–501.

Godefroy, O., Lhullier, C., & Rousseaux, M. (1994). Vigilance and effects of fatigability, practice and motivation on simple reaction time tests in patients with lesions of the frontal lobe. *Neuropsychologia, 32,* 983–990.

Godefroy, O., Lhullier-Lamy, C., & Rousseaux, M. (2002). SRT lengthening: Role of an alertness deficit in frontal damaged patients. *Neuropsychologia, 40,* 2234–2241.

Goel, V., & Dolan, R. J. (2001). The functional anatomy of humor: Segregating cognitive and affective components. *Nature Neuroscience, 4,* 237–238.

Goel, V., Grafman, J., Tajik, J., Gana, S., & Danto, D. (1997). A study of the performance of patients with frontal lobe lesions in a financial planning task. *Brain, 120,* 1805–1822.

Goldman-Rakic, P. S. (1987). Circuitry of primate prefrontal cortex and regulation of behavior by representational memory. In F. Plum & V. Mountcastle (Eds.), *Handbook of physiology: The nervous system* (Vol. 5, pp. 373–417). Bethesda, MD: American Physiological Society.

Grigsby, J., Kaye, K., Baxter, J., Shetterly, S. M., & Hamman, R. F. (1998). Executive cognitive abilities and functional status among community-dwelling older persons in the San Luis Valley Health and

Aging Study. *Journal of the American Geriatrics Society*, 46, 590–596.

Harlow, J. M. (1868). Recovery after severe injury to the head. *Publication of the Massachusetts Medical Society*, 2, 327–346.

Hultsch, D. F., MacDonald, S.W.S, Hunter, M., Levy-Benecheton, J., & Strauss, E. (2000). Intraindividual variability in cognitive performance in older adults: Comparison of adults with mild dementia, adults with arthritis, and healthy adults. *Neuropsychology*, 14, 588–598.

Levine, B. (1999). Self-regulation and autonoetic consciousness. In E. Tulving (Ed.), *Memory, consciousness, and the brain: The Tallinn Conference* (pp. 200–214). Philadelphia: Psychology Press.

Levine, B., Black, S. E., Cabeza, R., Sinden, M., McIntosh, A. R., Toth, J. P., et al. (1998). Episodic memory and the self in a case of retrograde amnesia. *Brain*, 121, 1951–1973.

Levine, B., Dawson, D., Boutet, I., Schwartz, M. L., & Stuss, D. T. (2000). Assessment of strategic self-regulation in traumatic brain injury: Its relationship to injury severity and psychosocial outcome. *Neuropsychology*, 14, 491–500.

Levine, B., Freedman, M., Dawson, D., Black, S. E., & Stuss, D. T. (1999). Ventral frontal contribution to self-regulation: Convergence of episodic memory and inhibition. *Neurocase*, 5, 263–275.

Levine, B., Stuss, D. T., Milberg, W. P., Alexander, M. P., Schwartz, M., & MacDonald, R. (1998). The effects of focal and diffuse brain damage on strategy application: Evidence from focal lesions, traumatic brain injury, and normal aging. *Journal of the International Neuropsychological Society*, 4, 247–264.

Luria, A. R. (1973). *The working brain: An introduction to neuropsychology.* New York: Basic Books.

MacDonald, A. W., III, Cohen, J. D., Stenger, V. A., & Carter, C. S. (2000). Dissociating the role of the dorsolateral prefrontal and anterior cingulate cortex in cognitive control. *Science*, 288, 1835–1838.

Manes, F., Sahakian, B., Clark, L., Rogers, R., Antoun, N., Aitken, M., et al. (2002). Decision making processes following damage to the prefrontal cortex. *Brain*, 125, 624–639.

Metcalfe, J. (1998). Emotional memory: The effects of stress on "cool" and "hot" memory systems. *Psychology of Learning and Motivation*, 38, 187–222.

Milner, B. (1963). Effects of different brain lesions on card sorting: The role of the frontal lobes. *Archives of Neurology*, 9, 100–110.

Mirsky, A. F., Fantie, B. D., & Tatman, J. E. (1995). Assessment of attention across the lifespan. In R. L. Mapou & J. Spector (Eds.), *Clinical neuropsychological assessment: A cognitive approach* (pp. 17–48). New York: Plenum Press.

Mishkin, M. (1964). Perseveration of central sets after frontal lesions in monkeys. In J. M. Warren & K. Akert (Eds.), *The frontal granular cortex and behavior* (pp. 219–241). New York: McGraw-Hill.

Moscovitch, M. (1992). Memory and working-with-memory: A component process model based on modules and central systems. *Journal of Cognitive Neuroscience*, 4, 257–267.

Moscovitch, M., & Winocur, G. (1992). The neuropsychology of memory and aging. In F. I. M. Craik & T. A. Salthouse (Eds.), *The handbook of aging and cognition* (pp. 315–372). Hillsdale, NJ: Erlbaum.

Murphy, K. J., West, R., Armilio, M. L., Craik, F. I. M., & Stuss, D. T. (in press). Word list learning performance in younger and older adults: Intra-individual performance variability and false memory. *Aging, Neuropsychology, and Cognition.*

Nauta, W. J. H. (1971). The problem of the frontal lobe: A reinterpretation. *Journal of Psychiatric Research*, 8, 167–187.

Pandya, D. N., & Barnes, C. L. (1987). Architecture and connections of the frontal lobe. In E. Perecman (Ed.), *The frontal lobes revisited* (pp. 41–72). New York: IRBN Press.

Pandya, D. N., & Yeterian, E. H. (1996). Morphological correlates of human and monkey frontal lobes. In A. R. Damasio, H. Damasio, & Y. Christen (Eds.), *Neurobiology of decision making* (pp. 13–46). New York: Springer.

Pardo, J. V., Fox, P. T., & Raichle, M. E. (1991). Localization of a human system for sustained attention by positron emission tomography. *Nature*, 349, 61–64.

Pardo, J. V., Pardo, P. J., Janer, K. W., & Raichle, M. W. (1990). The anterior cingulate cortex mediates processing selection in the Stroop attentional conflict paradigm. *Proceedings of the National Academy of Sciences of the United States of America*, 87, 256–259.

Penfield, W., & Evans, J. (1935). The frontal lobe in man: A clinical study of maximum removals. *Brain*, 58, 115–133.

Perret, E. (1974). The left frontal lobe of man and the suppression of habitual responses in verbal categorical behavior. *Neuropsychologia*, 12, 323–330.

Petrides, M. (1991). Functional specialization within the dorsolateral frontal-cortex for serial order memory. *Proceedings of the Royal Society of London, Series B: Biological Sciences*, 246, 299–306.

Petrides, M., & Milner, B. (1982). Deficits on subject-ordered tasks after frontal- and temporal-lobe lesions in man. *Neuropsychologia*, 20, 249–262.

Postle, B. R., Druzgal, T. J., & D'Esposito, M. (2003). Seeking the neural substrates of visual working memory storage. *Cortex*, 39, 927–946.

Reuckert, L., & Grafman, J. (1996). Sustained attention deficits in patients with right frontal lesions. *Neuropsychologia*, 34, 953–963.

Reuckert, L., & Grafman, J. (1998). Sustained attention deficits in patients with lesions of posterior cortex. *Neuropsychologia*, 36, 653–660.

Richer, F., Decary, A., Lapierre, M-F., Rouleau, I., Bouvier, G., & Sainthilaire, J. M. (1993). Target detection deficits in frontal lobectomy. *Brain and Cognition*, 21, 203–211.

Richer, F., & LePage, M. (1996). Frontal lesions increase

post-target interference in rapid stimulus streams. *Neuropsychologia, 34,* 509–514.

Robertson, I. H., Manly, T., Andrade, J., Baddeley, B. T., & Yiend, J. (1997). "Oops!": Performance correlates of everyday attentional failures in traumatic brain injured and normal subjects. *Neuropsychologia, 35,* 747–758.

Robertson, I. H., Ward, T., Ridgeway, V., & Nimmo-Smith, I. (1991). *The Test of Everyday Attention.* Bury St. Edmunds, UK: Thames Valley Test Company.

Rogers, R. D., Owen, A. M., Middleton, H. C., Williams, E. J., Pickard, J. D., Sahakian, B. J., et al. (1999). Choosing between small, likely rewards and large, unlikely rewards activates inferior and orbital prefrontal cortex. *Journal of Neuroscience, 19,* 9029–9038.

Rolls, E. T. (1996). The orbitofrontal cortex. *Philosophical Transactions of the Royal Society of London, Series B, 351,* 1433–1444.

Rolls, E. T. (2000). The orbitofrontal cortex and reward. *Cerebral Cortex, 10,* 284–294.

Saint-Cyr, J. A., Bronstein, Y. L., & Cummings, J. L. (2002). Neurobehavioural consequences of neurosurgical treatments and focal lesions of frontal-subcortical circuits. In D. T. Stuss & R. T. Knight (Eds.), *Principles of frontal lobe function* (pp. 408–427). New York: Oxford University Press.

Sanides, F. (1970). Functional architecture of motor and sensory cortices in primates in the light of a new concept of neocortex development. In C. R. Noback & W. Montana (Eds.), *Advances in primatology* (Vol. 1, pp. 137–208). New York: Appleton–Century–Crofts.

Schwartz, M. F., Montgomery, M. W., Buxbaum, L. J., Lee, S. S., Carew, T. G., Coslett, H. B., et al. (1998). Naturalistic action impairment in closed head injury. *Neuropsychology, 12,* 13–28.

Shallice, T. (2001). "Theory of mind" and the prefrontal cortex. *Brain, 124,* 247–248.

Shallice, T., & Burgess, P. W. (1991). Deficits in strategy application following frontal lobe damage in man. *Brain, 114,* 727–741.

Shammi, P., & Stuss, D. T. (1999). Humour appreciation: A role of the right frontal lobe. *Brain, 122,* 657–666.

Siegal, M., & Varley, R. (2002). Neural systems involved in "theory of mind." *Nature Reviews: Neuroscience, 3,* 463–471.

Stone, V. E., Baron-Cohen, S., & Knight, R. T. (1998). Frontal lobe contributions to theory of mind. *Journal of Cognitive Neuroscience, 10,* 640–656.

Strauss, E., MacDonald, S. W. S., Hunter, M., Moll, A., & Hultsch, D. F. (2002). Intraindividual variability in cognitive performance in three groups of older adults: Cross-domain links to physical status and self-perceived affect and beliefs. *Journal of the International Neuropsychological Society, 8,* 893–906.

Stuss, D. T., & Alexander, M. P. (1999). Affectively burnt in: A proposed role of the right frontal lobe. In E. Tulving (Ed.), *Memory, consciousness and the brain: The Tallinn Conference* (pp. 215–227). Philadelphia: Psychology Press.

Stuss, D. T., & Alexander, M. P. (2000). The anatomical basis of affective behavior, emotion and self-awareness: A specific role of the right frontal lobe. In G. Hatano, N. Okada, & H. Tanabe (Eds.), *Affective minds. The 13th Toyota Conference* (pp. 13–25). Amsterdam: Elsevier.

Stuss, D. T., & Alexander, M. P. (2005). Does damage to the frontal lobes produce impairment in memory? *Current Directions in Psychological Science, 14,* 84–88.

Stuss, D. T., Alexander, M. P., Floden, D., Binns, M. A., Levine, B., McIntosh, A. R., et al. (2002). Fractionation and localization of distinct frontal lobe processes: Evidence from focal lesions in humans. In D. T. Stuss & R. T. Knight (Eds.), *Principles of frontal lobe function* (pp. 392–407). New York: Oxford University Press.

Stuss, D. T., Alexander, M. P., Hamer, L., Palumbo, C., Dempster, R., Binns, M., et al. (1998). The effects of focal anterior and posterior brain lesions on verbal fluency. *Journal of the International Neuropsychological Society, 4,* 265–278.

Stuss, D. T., Alexander, M. P., Palumbo, C. L., Buckle, L., Sayer, L., & Pogue, J. (1994). Organizational strategies of patients with unilateral or bilateral frontal lobe injury in word list learning tasks. *Neuropsychology, 8,* 355–373.

Stuss, D. T., Alexander, M. P., Shallice, T., Picton, T. W., Binns, M., MacDonald, R., et al. (2005). Multiple frontal systems controlling response speed. *Neuropsychologia, 43,* 396–417.

Stuss, D. T., & Benson, D. F. (1983). Emotional concomitants of psychosurgery. In K. M. Heilman, & P. Satz (Eds.), *Advances in neuropsychology and behavioral neurology: Vol. 1. Neuropsychology of human emotion* (pp. 111–140). New Yor: Guilford Press.

Stuss, D. T., & Benson, D. F. (1986). *The frontal lobes.* New York: Raven.

Stuss, D. T., Binns, M. A., & Alexander, M. P. (2003). Is the anterior attentional system as complex as the posterior attential system? *Zeitschrift für Neuropsychologie, 14,* 191–201.

Stuss, D. T., Binns, M. A., Murphy, K. J., & Alexander, M. P. (2002). Dissociations within the anterior attentional system: Effects of task complexity and irrelevant information on reaction time speed and accuracy. *Neuropsychology, 16,* 500–513.

Stuss, D. T., Bisschop, S. M., Alexander, M. P., Levine, B., Katz, D., & Izukawa, D. (2001). The Trail Making Test: A study in focal lesion patients. *Psychological Assessment, 13,* 230–239.

Stuss, D. T., Floden, D., Alexander, M. P., Levine, B., & Katz, D. (2001). Stroop performance in focal lesion patients: Dissociation of processes and frontal lobe lesion location. *Neuropsychologia, 39,* 771–786.

Stuss, D. T., Gallup, G. G., & Alexander, M. P. (2001). The frontal lobes are necessary for "theory of mind." *Brain, 124,* 279–286.

Stuss, D. T., & Levine, B. (2002). Adult clinical neuropsychology: Lessons from studies of the frontal lobes. *Annual Review of Psychology, 53,* 401–433.

Stuss, D. T., Levine, B., Alexander, M. P., Hong, J., Palumbo, C., Hamer, L., et al. (2000). Wisconsin Card Sorting Test performance in patients with focal frontal and posterior brain damage: Effects of lesion location and test structure on separable cognitive processes. *Neuropsychologia, 38,* 388–402.

Stuss, D. T., Murphy, K. J., Binns, M. A., & Alexander, M. P. (2003). Staying on the job: The frontal lobes control individual performance variability. *Brain, 126,* 2363–2380.

Stuss, D. T., Picton, T. W., & Alexander, M. P. (2001). Consciousness, self-awareness, and the frontal lobes. In S. P. Salloway, P. F. Malloy, & J. D. Duffy (Eds.), *The frontal lobes and neuropsychiatric illness* (pp. 101–109). Washington, DC: American Psychiatric Press.

Stuss, D. T., Pogue, J., Buckle, L., & Bondar, J. (1994). Characterization of stability of performance in patients with traumatic brain injury: Variability and consistency on reaction time tests. *Neuropsychology, 8,* 316–324.

Stuss, D. T., Rosenbaum, R. S., Malcolm, S., Christiana, W., & Keenan, J. P. (2005). The frontal lobes and self-awareness. In T. E. Feinberg & J. P. Keenan (Eds.), *The lost self: Pathologies of the brain and identity* (pp. 50–64). New York: Oxford University Press.

Stuss, D. T., Stethem, L. L., Hugenholtz, H., Picton, T., Pivik, J., & Richard, M. T. (1989). Reaction time after head injury: Fatigue, divided and focused attention, and consistency of performance. *Journal of Neurology, Neurosurgery, and Psychiatry, 52,* 742–748.

Stuss, D. T., Toth, J. P., Franchi, D., Alexander, M. P., Tipper, S., & Craik, F. I. M. (1999). Dissociation of attentional processes in patients with focal frontal and posterior lesions. *Neuropsychologia, 37,* 1005–1027.

Troyer, A. K., Moscovitch, M., Winocur, G., Alexander, M., & Stuss, D. (1998). Clustering and switching on verbal fluency: The effects of focal frontal- and temporal-lobe lesions. *Neuropsychologia, 36,* 499–504.

Tulving, E. (1985). Memory and consciousness. *Canadian Psychology, 26,* 1–12.

Vendrell, P., Junque, C., Pujol, J., Jurado, M. A., Molet, J., & Grafman, J. (1995). The role of prefrontal regions in the Stroop task. *Neuropsychologia, 33,* 341–352.

Wechsler, D. (1997). *Wechsler Memory Scale* (3rd ed.). Boston: Psychological Corporation.

West, R., Murphy, K. J., Armilio, M. L., Craik, F. I. M., & Stuss, D. T. (2002). Lapses of intention and performance variability reveal age-related increases in fluctuations of executive control. *Brain and Cognition, 49,* 402–419.

Wheeler, M. A., & Stuss, D. T. (2003). Remembering and knowing in patients with frontal lobe injury. *Cortex, 39,* 827–846.

Wheeler, M. A., Stuss, D. T., & Tulving, E. (1997). Toward a theory of episodic memory: The frontal lobes and autonoetic consciousness. *Psychological Bulletin, 121,* 331–354.

Wilkins, A. J., Shallice, T., & McCarthy, R. (1987). Frontal lesions and sustained attention. *Neuropsychologia, 25,* 359–365.

Woods, D. L., & Knight, R. T. (1986). Electrophysiologic evidence of increased distractibility after dorsolateral prefrontal lesions. *Neurology, 36,* 212–216.

# CHAPTER 20

# Language and Frontal Cortex

*Argye E. Hillis*

Although anterior portions of the frontal lobes are critical for a number of cognitive processes that support the understanding and use of language and nonverbal communication, the posterior parts of the frontal lobe have been more directly implicated in language processing per se. In fact, left posterior, inferior frontal lobe (often referred to as "Broca's area") likely has a role in all aspects of language—in comprehension and production of both spoken and written language. In this chapter, I review evidence from lesion studies and functional imaging studies that converges in support the role of Broca's area and surrounding areas in specific components of these language tasks. I focus on processing components for which there is evidence both from functional imaging that posterior frontal regions are engaged in the cognitive process and from lesion studies that the same regions are essential for that process; that is, to confirm that an area of activation observed in a functional imaging task is critical for the component language process, focal damage or dysfunction of that region should result in impairment of that language process.

One caveat is needed before launching into a review of the neuroanatomical regions involved in language. There exists a wealth of evidence that there is a great deal of individual variability in the cytoarchitectural fields, as well as the shape and size of sulci and gyri, of the human brain. Much of the evidence for this individual variability has in fact come from studies of Broca's area, which often (but not always) has been assumed to encompass Brodmann's areas 44 and 45 (pars opercularis and

pars triangularis). Many authors have proposed distinct roles of these two parts of Broca's area, particularly on the basis of functional magnetic resonance imaging (fMRI) studies that show slightly different areas of activation in response to various tasks (Bookheimer, 2002; Paulesu et al., 1997). However, given that morphological studies show that the cytoarchitectonic fields (Brodmann's areas) cannot be reliably predicted from the anatomical boundaries used to define the regions in functional or structural imaging of the intact brain (Rademacher, Caviness, Steinmetz, & Galaburda, 1993; van Essen, Drury, Joshi, & Miller, 1998; Whitaker & Selnes, 1976), no strong claims about the precise location of distinct functions are made here. This limitation is also applicable to functional imaging and lesion studies in which individual subjects' brains are "registered" to a normalized brain atlas or space. In these cases, activation or lesions in the "same" voxel across individuals may in fact be in different gyri, as well as different cytoarchitectonic fields, in various individuals. This fact may account for individual variability in regions of activation in functional imaging in the same task (e.g., Crivello et al., 1995). There is no obvious solution to this problem. The tack that I take in this chapter is to discuss evidence for the role of rather grossly defined areas, such as left posterior, inferior frontal gyrus, or posterior superior frontal gyrus.

To provide a framework for interpreting results of various studies using different language tasks, I briefly discuss models of the cognitive processes underlying basic language tasks, such as sentence production and lexical processing. Then, I review evidence for the essential role of posterior frontal regions for each of the following components of language production: computation of "functional" and "positional" levels of representation in sentence production (including assignment of prefixes and suffixes); access to phonological and orthographic representations of verbs for output; phonological processing required for sublexical phonology–orthography conversion ("phonics") for spelling and orthography–phonology conversion in reading; access to letter-specific motor plans for writing; and access to motor plans required for speech articulation. In addition, evidence indicating a role of posterior frontal regions in comprehension, particularly in syntax processing, is briefly reviewed. It will also be recognized that adequate working memory is critical for both sentence comprehension and production, although data regarding different types of working memory and the neural substrates of each are discussed in Gazzaley and D'Esposito, Chapter 13, this volume.

## LANGUAGE PRODUCTION

One of the most widely accepted models of the cognitive representations and processes underlying sentence production has been described by Garrett (1975, 1980, 1988; see also Levelt, 1993, 1999; schematically depicted in the top three components of Figure 20.1). Briefly, this model specifies several levels of representations that are more or less serially computed to produce a sentence either in writing or speech. The initial representation is the "message level" that specifies the concept to be conveyed—the interface between thought and language (Bock, 1990). This message level is mapped onto the "functional level" representation that specifies the identity and role of open-class morphemes, or "lemmas" (modality-independent representations of nouns, verbs, etc.). Also at the message level, lemmas are assigned grammatical or syntactic roles in the sentence, such as subject/ nominative. From this representation, a "positional level" representation is computed that provides the sentence frame, including the se-

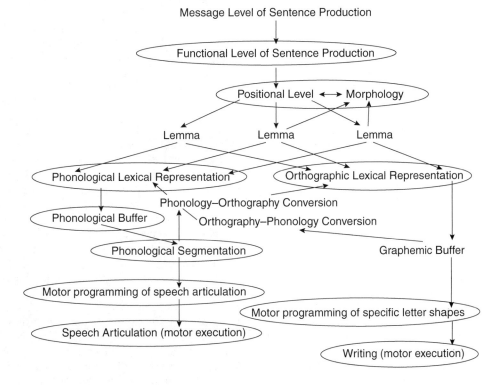

FIGURE 20.1. The cognitive representations and processes underlying spoken and written production of sentences. Circled components are those functions for which there is evidence that the left posterior frontal cortex plays a substantial role.

quence of words and the grammatical morphemes (closed-class words such as functors, and affixes such as prefixes and suffixes). Finally, the phonological or orthographic lexical items are inserted into this positional planning frame to produce the sentence either in writing or in speech.

There are a number of assumptions in this model about accessing specific lexical items. First, it is assumed that lexical access has several stages, beginning with a concept, then accessing a modality-independent "lemma" level representation that specifies the grammatical role and links the concept to a modality-specific phonological or orthographic lexical representation. The phonological representation specifies the learned pronunciation of the word; the orthographic representation specifies the learned spelling of the word. There may in fact be yet another stage of lexical access between the concept and the lemma. For example, to refer to one's own pet as a "collie," it is necessary to access, from one's concept of that particular pet, a lexical–semantic representation that specifies the meaning of the word "collie" that is what makes a collie a collie—the key features of collies and what makes collies different from other types of dogs or animals. This lexical–semantic representation would not include everything one knows about one's own pet collie (e.g., its nature, its name, its likes and dislikes) or even one's own general knowledge about collies (e.g., that many collies live in that person's neighborhood, or that collies with which that person is familiar like to play catch).

From the lexical–semantic representation of collie, one may access a modality-independent "lemma" level of collie (that specifies it as a noun and how it could be used in a sentence), and then a modality-specific (phonological or orthographic) lexical representation. The phonological representation must then be articulated by accessing and executing motor plans. Alternatively, the orthographic representation can be spelled by accessing particular letter shapes and shape-specific motor plans. Because each individual abstract letter identity or "grapheme" in the orthographic representation must be converted to a letter shape with a particular font and case, the orthographic representation must be "held" in a short-term storage system, or graphemic buffer, while each letter shape is accessed and the corresponding motor plan is executed. Whether or not a comparable "phonological buffer" is required for holding the phonological representation while individual phonemes are articulated is less clear, because the word may be articulated as single unit with a particular motor program (see Cohen & Bachoud-Levi, 1995, for discussion). Novel or unfamiliar words may require a phonological buffer for articulation, because production of an unfamiliar word would require executing a sequence of motor programs for each phoneme in the word.

## ROLE OF THE FRONTAL LOBES IN SENTENCE PRODUCTION

Lesions of left posterior, inferior frontal lobe and surrounding areas typically result in agrammatic speech production, characterized by "telegraphic" speech consisting predominantly of content words, with a paucity of functors (grammatical words such as "but," "the," and "before") and of affixes (e.g., -ing, -ed, dis-). Characteristically, sentences are shorter than average, with fewer and simpler syntactic forms (Miceli, Silveri, Romani, & Caramazza, 1989; Thompson & Faroqi-Shah, 2002). This agrammatic speech production can be explained by assuming impairment at the level of assigning functional roles at the "functional level" in the aforementioned model (Caramazza & Miceli, 1991; Martin & Blossom-Stach, 1986), computing a "positional"-level representation of the sentence (Caramazza & Hillis, 1990), or mapping from the functional level to the positional level (Saffran, Schwartz, & Marin, 1980) within Garrett's model of sentence production described earlier. In other cases, agrammatic speech may result from limited short-term storage or working memory required for holding the entire sentence representation or sentence frame while individual words are articulated (Linebarger, Schwartz, Romania, Kohn, & Stephens, 2000). Left posterior frontal regions have been implicated in each of these processes. Functional imaging studies have shown bilateral posterior frontal activation in a variety of working memory tasks (D'Esposito, Postle, Jonides, & Smith, 1999; Rypma & D'Esposito, 1999) in processing of more complex relative to simple grammatical forms (for reviews, see Bookheimer, 2002; Caplan, 2002). Furthermore, lesions in dominant posterior, inferior frontal lobe have resulted in agrammatic speech attributed to impairments in sentence production due to disrupted functional-level processing, verb access, positional-level processing, mapping from functional to positional level, or limited working memory (see Thompson & Faroqi-Shah, 2002, for review).

## ROLE OF LEFT POSTERIOR FRONTAL CORTEX IN VERB NAMING

Several authors have emphasized the role of verb production in formulating grammatical sentences, and have proposed that some cases of agrammatic speech production may result from impaired access to verbs or their argument structures (Fink, Martin, Schwartz, Saffran, & Myers, 1992; Kim & Thompson, 2000; Marshall, Pring, & Chiat, 1998; Mitchum & Berndt, 1994; Thompson & Faroqi-Shah, 2002). Evidence from some positron emission tomography (PET) studies (Perani et al., 1999; Tranel, Damasio, & Damasio, 1997) indicate that left posterior frontal regions may be more important for accessing verbs than nouns, although other PET studies have not confirmed distinct regions of activation for nouns and verbs (Tyler, Russell, Fadili, & Moss, 2001; Warburton et al., 1996). The role of left posterior frontal cortex in verb retrieval has been supported by studies showing that focal lesions of this area impair naming of verbs (particularly action names) relative to nouns (particularly object names) in chronic stroke (Tranel, Adolphs, Damasio, & Damasio, 2001) and acute stroke (Hillis, Tuffiash, Wityk & Barker, 2002). These findings are consistent with chronic lesion studies reporting that patients with "Broca's aphasia" (who generally have left frontal lesions) are more impaired in naming verbs than nouns, whereas patients with Wernicke's aphasia (who generally have more posterior, temporal lesions) show the opposite dissociation (Miceli, Silveri, Villa, & Caramazza, 1984; Zingeser & Berndt, 1988, 1990). Furthermore, repetitive transcranial magnetic stimulation (rTMS) applied over left posterior frontal cortex, causing a temporary "lesion" or dysfunction of that region, interfered with verb more than noun production (Shapiro, Pascual-Leone, Mottaghy, Gangitano, & Caramazza, 2001). Likewise, hypoperfusion—impaired blood flow—in left posterior, inferior frontal cortex resulted in impaired written naming of verbs but spared written naming of nouns and spoken naming of both verbs and nouns in two patients studied within 24 hours of stroke onset (Hillis, Wityk, Barker, & Caramazza, 2003). More importantly, reperfusion of left posterior, inferior frontal cortex resulted in recovery of written naming of verbs in each case, providing stronger evidence that this region is crucial for accessing orthographic representations of verbs.

Taken together, these studies indicate that left posterior frontal cortex is particularly important for accessing modality-specific representations for output, particularly for verbs. Some fMRI studies that have identified activation in the opercular portion of left posterior inferior frontal gyrus during oral naming (semantic or phonemic word fluency) have proposed that this region is critical for accessing lexical representations "through a phonemic/articulatory route" (Paulesu et al., 1997). More posterior regions of the brain, particularly posterior, inferior, and middle temporal gyrus (part of Brodmann's area [BA] 37) have been implicated in accessing modality-independent lexical representations (lemmas) for both nouns and verbs (Hillis et al., 2002, 2005; Price, Winterburn, Giraud, Moore, & Noppeney, 2003). One possible explanation for the observation that frontal lesions affect modality-specific orthographic and phonological representations of verbs more than nouns is that verbs demand more morphological processing in naming tasks (Shapiro & Caramazza, in press). For example, to name the action depicted in a picture of a person walking, it is necessary to access not only the lexical–semantic representation (e.g., translational movement, pedestrian, both feet on ground simultaneously), a lemma, and a lexical representation of [walk], but also to select a morphological form (walk, walks, walking, or walked—all of which would be correct). Several studies have indicated that left posterior frontal cortex may be essential for selection of morphological forms. For instance, rTMS to left posterior frontal cortex in normal subjects interfered with production of the correct form of pseudoverbs (e.g., I *wug*; he *wugs*) but not pseudonouns (e.g., one *wug*; two *wugs*) (Shapiro & Caramazza, 2004). These results suggest the possibility that left posterior, inferior frontal cortex is essential for selecting a lexical representation for a particular morphosyntactic role (e.g., to be used as a verb) in production; it may not be involved in storing or computing lexical representations per se.

## ROLE OF LEFT POSTERIOR, INFERIOR FRONTAL CORTEX IN SPELLING

As reviewed earlier, left posterior, inferior frontal cortex seems to be crucial for accessing lexical representations for modality-specific output, in such a way that verbs are accessed differently from nouns. But lesions in left posterior, inferior frontal cortex are associated with impaired spelling of not only verbs but also nouns and other classes of words. One plausible source of the spelling impairment is disrupted access to, or computation of, modality-specific lexical representations for writing—lexical orthographic representations. Selective impairment in accessing lexical orthographic representations (the stored spelling of words) would be expected to result in (1) poor spelling of words relative to pseudowords (e.g., *shronk*); (2) phonologically plausible spellings of words (e.g., *sope* for "soap"); and (3) worse spelling of low-frequency relative to high-frequency words (Baxter & Warrington, 1987; Beauvois & Dérouesné, 1981; Hatfield & Patterson, 1983; Roeltgen & Heilman, 1984). Spelling of pseudowords to dictation may be accurate, because these can be spelled via sublexical phonology–orthography conversion mechanisms. Several authors have described patients with this pattern of spelling performance, sometimes referred to as "lexical agraphia," resulting from relatively small, acute lesions in posterior frontal cortex (Hillis et al., 2003; Hillis, Chang, Breese, & Heidler, 2004; Rapcsak, Rubens, & Arthur, 1988). However, most patients with lesions in left posterior, inferior frontal cortex are also impaired in phonology–orthography conversion, such that they have poor spelling of pseudowords as well as words, and make few, if any, phonologically plausible spelling errors. In these cases, errors are either omissions or semantically related words. For example, patient RCM (Hillis, Rapp, & Caramazza, 1999) had a pure agraphia characterized by semantic errors (e.g., cup for bowl) in spelling to dictation, written naming, and spontaneous writing, immediately after a small, acute stroke in left posterior, inferior frontal cortex. She had normal comprehension and intact oral naming of most items that elicited semantic errors in written naming. She was unable to spell pseudowords in the acute period. However, she relatively quickly recovered phonology–orthography conversion mechanisms, so that her pseudoword spelling

improved; and she no longer made semantic errors in spelling. Her partially recovered phonology–orthography conversion mechanisms apparently "blocked" semantic errors in writing.

Other patients with lesions in posterior, inferior frontal cortex have disproportionate difficulty spelling pseudowords, indicating a relatively selective impairment in some aspect of phonology–orthography conversion (Marien, Pickuta, Engelborghsa, Martind, & De Deyna, 2001). Based on evidence from functional imaging, it has been hypothesized that posterior, inferior frontal cortex is critical to parsing the phonological input into distinct phonemes (Burton, Blumstein, & Small, 2000) or phoneme discrimination (Demonet, Price, Wise, & Frackowiak, 1994; Zatorre, Evans, Meyer, & Gjedde, 1992; Zatorre, Meyer, Gjedde, & Evans, 1996)—processes that are necessary for sublexical phonology–orthography conversion.

Together, the results indicate that posterior, inferior frontal cortex may include regions that are essential for two separate components of spelling—access to lexical orthographic representations for output and phonological processing for phonology–orthography conversion. Some lesions affect only one or the other of these areas, accounting for the occasional dissociations between word and pseudoword spelling. However, most lesions include both regions, so that both functions are impaired. This proposal would account for the finding that "deep agraphia," characterized by semantic errors in writing words, nouns spelled better than verbs, high-frequency words spelled better than low-frequency words, and inability to spell pseudowords (Bub & Kertesz, 1982), is often associated with lesions in left posterior, inferior frontal cortex and Broca's aphasia.

Functional imaging studies of spelling provide additional evidence that posterior, inferior frontal gyrus is engaged in spelling. For example, Hsieh and Rapp (2004) reported that an fMRI study of a spelling probe task (that required subjects to report whether or not a given word contained a specified letter) in normal subjects resulted in activation of left posterior, inferior frontal gyrus, as well as activation of left angular and fusiform gyri. This task required accessing knowledge of the spelling of words (either stored lexical–orthographic representations or orthographic representations computed from phonology–orthography correspondence) and holding the string of graphemes in short-term storage ("the graphemic buffer"). Activation in left posterior, inferior frontal cortex may have reflected any of these components of spelling, but did not reflect motor components, because writing was not required. Likewise, Beeson and colleagues (2003) reported an fMRI study that revealed activation in left posterior frontal cortex, in addition to left posterior, inferior temporal gyrus (BA 37), during writing of words in a given category relative to writing the alphabet or drawing of circles. They interpreted the posterior frontal activation as reflecting "semantically guided retrieval of lexical representations," and BA 37 activation as reflecting access to orthographic representations. An alternative account of these data is that BA 37 activation reflected access to modality-independent lemmas, whereas left posterior frontal activation reflected access to modality-specific (orthographic or phonological) representations for output.

Other regions of left frontal cortex seem to be important in more peripheral aspects of writing. Converting an abstract orthographic representation to a written response requires access to letter shapes with a particular font and case, or access to letter-shape-specific motor programs. A recent study of patients within 24 hours of stroke onset (Hillis, Chang, et al., 2004) indicated that impairment in this component of the spelling process, manifested by impaired ability to transpose written letters or words into a different case, was strongly associated with damage or dysfunction of left BA 6, just posterior and superior to left posterior, inferior frontal gyrus. Studies of chronic stroke patients have also revealed that impaired access to letter-shape-specific motor plans for writing is associated with posterior, superior frontal lesions (Anderson, Damasio, & Damasio, 1990; Exner, 1881; Rapcsak & Beeson, 2002). Of course, the hand area of dominant motor cortex (precentral gyrus) is also essential for written output, because writing normally requires adequate use of the dominant hand. These motor aspects of writing are reflected in activation of left precentral gyrus and posterior, superior frontal cortex (BAs 6 and 9) in right-handed subjects (Beeson et al., 2003; Hsieh & Rapp, 2004). For instance, activation of left BAs 6 and 9 was observed in writing words or the alphabet compared to drawing circles in the Beeson and colleagues (2003) study, likely reflecting access to letter-shape-specific motor plans.

## ROLE OF LEFT POSTERIOR FRONTAL LOBE IN MOTOR PROGRAMMING OF SPEECH ARTICULATION

Evidence from both functional imaging and lesion studies indicate that left posterior, inferior frontal cortex is essential for motor programming of speech output, as well as motor programming of written output. Paul Broca (1865) was among the first to propose that lesions of posterior, inferior frontal gyrus interfere with speech articulation. More recent studies of patients with impaired motor planning and programming of speech articulation (apraxia of speech) acutely after stroke have shown lesions restricted to left posterior, inferior frontal cortex (Mohr et al., 1978). In contrast, studies show that in chronic stroke patients with persistent apraxia of speech show lesions in this region combination with other regions (Schiff, Alexander, Naeser, & Galaburda, 1983), or lesions that overlap in the precentral gyrus of the anterior insula (Dronkers, 1996). In a recent study of 80 consecutive patients within 24 hours of onset of nonlacunar left-hemisphere stroke, we found that apraxia of speech was most strongly associated with hypoperfusion and/or infarct of left posterior, inferior frontal gyrus, and was not associated with either hypoperfusion or infarct of the anterior insula (Hillis, Work, et al., 2004). The previously reported association between apraxia of speech and lesions involving left anterior insula was attributed to the fact that (1) apraxia of speech persists only after large left middle cerebral artery strokes, and (2) large middle cerebral artery strokes nearly always include the anterior insula. Likewise, recent PET studies show activation in left posterior, inferior frontal gyrus, but not anterior insula, during tasks that require speech articulation, such as word repetition and oral reading (Price et al., 1996, 2003).

## ROLE OF LEFT FRONTAL LOBE IN SENTENCE COMPREHENSION

Although patients with left posterior frontal lesions were once thought to have intact comprehension of language, many studies have demonstrated that patients with such lesions are often impaired in processing sentences with complex syntactic structures (e.g., passive sentences such as, "The boy was kicked by the girl") (Caramazza & Zurif, 1976). Studies of patients with "Broca's aphasia" have demonstrated impairments in comprehending a variety of syntactic structures (Berndt & Caramazza, 1999). However, "asyntactic" comprehension and agrammatic production do not always co-occur, indicating that there is not a common deficit in syntactic processing that underlies both the variety of comprehension deficits and the production deficits (Berndt, Mitchum, & Haendiges, 1996; Caramazza, Capitani, Rey, & Berndt, 2001).

Functional imaging studies also demonstrate activation in left posterior, inferior frontal cortex, along with activation in other regions, during syntax processing in response to sentences (with auditory or visual presentation) (for reviews, see Bookheimer, 2002; Caplan, 2002). Specific components of sentence processing that have been ascribed to this region include grammatical role assignment, "trace deletion" (see Grodzinsky, 2000), processing of complex syntactic forms, integration of syntax and semantics, and phonological working memory needed for syntactic processing (see Caplan, 2002). Several authors have reported evidence from functional imaging or TMS studies that left posterior, inferior frontal cortex is engaged in a variety of morphological processing tasks, including grammatical gender decision in languages such as Italian, German, and Spanish (Heim, Opitz, & Friederici, 2002; Hernandez et al., 2004; Miceli et al., 2002), regular versus irregular past tense (Ullman et al., 1997), or both regular and irregular morphology (de Diego Balaguer, Costa, Sebastián-Galles, Jucandella, & Caramazza, 2004). One lesion study has also implicated this region in processing of locative prepositions (Tranel & Kemmerer, 2004). Some authors have found that ventral and dorsal regions of posterior, inferior frontal cortex have distinct functions in sentence processing. For instance, it has been proposed that the ventral portion of this area is engaged in morphological processing, whereas the dorsal portion is responsible for word-class assignment; the latter appears to be more sensitive to resource demands (Cooke et al., 2002).

## ROLE(S) OF POSTERIOR, INFERIOR FRONTAL GYRUS IN SEMANTIC TASKS

Numerous functional imaging studies have provided evidence that posterior, inferior frontal gyrus, probably centered on BA 47, is acti-

vated in a wide range of semantic tasks, such as semantic priming (Wagner, Koustall, Maril, Schacter, & Buckner, 2000; Wagner, Pare-Blagoev, Clark, & Poldrack, 2001), generating verbs in response to nouns (Petersen, Fox, Posner, Mintun, & Raichle, 1998; Thompson-Schill, Aguirre, D'Esposito, & Farah, 1999), and judging semantic acceptability (Dapretto, Bookheimer, & Mazziota, 1999). These studies indicate that posterior, inferior frontal cortex is engaged in tasks that require evaluation of semantic associations between concepts and phrases or controlled retrieval from semantic memory, although this area is probably not engaged in decoding the meanings of individual words (see Bookheimer, 2002, for review). Others have argued that the activation in this region reflects response selection (Thompson-Schill et al., 1999) rather than semantic processing per se, although the activation associated with response selection may be more posterior and superior to activation observed in some semantic tasks (Bookheimer, 2002). Additional evidence that activation in posterior frontal cortex may reflect some aspect of decision making or response selection is that this region shows activation for "more effortful" decisions relative to "less effortful" decisions, even in nonlanguage tasks such as hue discrimination (Moo, Slotnick, & Hillis, 2002). Consistent with the hypothesis that the role of this region in semantic tasks is in controlled processing, search, or response selection rather than lexical semantics (word meaning), lesions to left posterior, inferior frontal cortex do not interfere with understanding the meaning of individual words even acutely after onset of damage (Hillis et al., 2003).

## A COMMENT ON BROCA'S APHASIA

As reviewed earlier, left posterior, inferior frontal cortex (Broca's area) has been implicated in large number of apparently distinct language processes. There has been converging evidence from lesion studies and functional imaging studies for most of these roles of Broca's area. The majority, but not all, of these processes are engaged in either spoken or written output. There is some evidence, particularly from fMRI, that separate portions of Broca's area are specialized for distinct language processes.

The separate roles of Broca's area can explain the clinical syndrome of Broca's aphasia, as well as evidence that Broca's aphasia is not a theoretical coherent syndrome with a single underlying cause; that is, Broca's aphasia is characterized clinically by effortful, distorted articulation with numerous and varied off-target attempts in production (sometimes called apraxia of speech; McNeil, Doyle, & Wambaugh, 2000); agrammatic sentence production with telegraphic speech and writing composed primarily of nouns; spelling errors; and intact comprehension of simple syntactic structure but impaired comprehension of sentences with complex syntactic structure (Damasio, 1992; Goodglass & Kaplan, 1972; Hillis & Caramazza, 2003). This clinical syndrome has long been attributed to lesions involving Broca's area. However, as elegantly demonstrated by Mohr and colleagues (1978), lesions restricted to Broca's area result in apraxia of speech, but not other components of the syndrome of Broca's aphasia. They argued that the complete syndrome of Broca's aphasia requires damage to a much larger area. The complete syndrome seems to occur when the area of damage (or dysfunction) includes the entire territory of the superior branch of the middle cerebral artery (left posterior, inferior, middle, and superior frontal gyri, precentral gyrus, anterior insula, and anterior pole of the temporal lobe). Occlusion of the superior division of the left middle cerebral artery therefore results in dysfunction of several regions, each with its own role(s) in language comprehension or production. In cases where portions of the territory of the superior branch are spared, their corresponding functions are also spared, explaining the dissociations between various characteristics of Broca's aphasia. Thus, different symptoms of Broca's aphasia have been found to be associated with different anatomical structures in and around posterior, inferior frontal gyrus (Alexander, Naeser, & Palumbo, 1990). This view can also account for the fact that left posterior frontal dysfunction in diseases other than stroke (e.g., progressive nonfluent aphasia in frontotemporal lobar degeneration or corticobasal degeneration) often causes disordered speech and language with some, but not all, features of Broca's aphasia (Hillis, Oh, & Ken, 2004; Neary et al., 1998). Because such diseases do not affect a particular vascular distribution in the brain, the dysfunctional region often overlaps with the region affected by occlusion of the superior division of the left middle cerebral artery.

On a historical note, one of Paul Broca's best described patients, "Tan Tan," had a lesion that encompassed substantially more cortex than what is currently known as Broca's area. Furthermore, his language performance did not conform to what would now be called Broca's aphasia (Selnes & Hillis, 2000). Rather, he apparently had rather poor comprehension, and his speech (at least late in the course of his progressive disease) consisted of a single perseverative utterance: "Tan Tan." These characteristics would now be considered evidence of global aphasia. Nevertheless, Broca was among the first investigators of his time to demonstrate the crucial role of the left posterior frontal lobe in language processing, confirming to the phrenologists their own view of language capacity in the frontal lobes.

## SUMMARY

In summary, left posterior, inferior frontal cortex has diverse roles in both production and comprehension of language. This area appears to be critical for phonological discrimination and segmentation, processing of morphosyntactic structure, and/or working memory functions needed for syntax processing, retrieval of modality-specific lexical forms (especially in particular grammatical categories such as verbs or particular morphological forms) for spoken and written output, motor programming of speech articulation, and selecting letter-specific motor programs for writing. Nearby regions are also engaged in various aspects of semantic tasks, including controlled retrieval from semantic memory and response selection, although they are not critical for decoding the meanings of individual words. The available evidence indicates that these diverse functions are carried out by separate areas within posterior frontal cortex, all supplied by the superior division of the left middle cerebral artery. Thus, impairments of these separate functions frequently co-occur in stroke (due to occlusion of this major artery) but can dissociate in smaller strokes or can recover at different rates and to different degrees after large lesions, as other areas of the brain assume these separate language functions.

## ACKNOWLEDGMENT

Some of the work reported in this chapter was supported by Grant No. NIH RO1 DC05375.

## REFERENCES

Alexander, M. P., Naeser, M. A., & Palumbo, C. (1990). Broca's area aphasias: Aphasia after lesions including the frontal operculum. *Neurology, 40,* 353–362.

Anderson, S. W., Damasio, A. R., & Damasio, H. (1990). Troubled letters but not numbers: Domain specific cognitive impairments following focal damage in frontal cortex. *Brain, 113,* 749–766.

Baxter, D. M., & Warrington, E. K. (1987). Transcoding sound to spelling: Single or multiple sound unit correspondences. *Cortex, 23,* 11–28.

Beauvois, M. F., & Dérouesné, J. (1981). Lexical or orthographic agraphia. *Brain, 104,* 21–49.

Beeson, P. M., Rapczak, S. Z., Plante, E., Chargualaf, J., Chung, A., Johnson, S. C., et al. (2003). The neural substrates of writing: A functional magnetic resonance imaging study. *Aphasiology, 17*(6/7), 647–665.

Berndt, R., & Caramazza, A. (1999). How "regular" is sentence comprehension in Broca's aphasia?: It depends on how you select your patients. *Brain and Language, 67,* 242–247.

Berndt, R., Mitchum, C., & Haendiges, A. (1996). Comprehension of reversible sentences in "agrammatism": A meta-analysis. *Cognition, 58,* 289–308.

Bock, K. (1990). Structure in language. *American Psychologist, 45*(11), 1221–1236.

Bookheimer, S. (2002). Functional MRI of language: New approaches to understanding the cortical organization of semantic processing. *Annual Review of Neurosciences, 25,* 151–188.

Broca, P. (1865). Sur la faculte du langage articule [On the ability of articulated language]. *Paris Bulletin de la Société d'Anthropologie* [Paris Bulletin of the Society of Anthropology], *6,* 337–393.

Bub, D., & Kertesz, A. (1982). Deep agraphia. *Brain and Language, 17,* 146–165.

Burton, M., Blumstein, S., & Small, S. (2000). The role of segmentation in phonological processing: An fMRI investigation. *Journal of Cognitive Neuroscience, 12,* 679–690.

Caplan, D. (2002). The neural basis of syntactic processing: A critical look. In A. E. Hillis (Ed.), *The handbook of adult language disorders: Integrating cognitive neuropsychology, neurology, and rehabilitation* (pp. 331–350). New York: Psychology Press.

Caramazza, A., Capitani, E., Rey, A., & Berndt, R. (2001). Agrammatic Broca's aphasia is not associated with a single pattern of comprehension performance. *Brain and Language, 76,* 158–184.

Caramazza, A., & Hillis, A. (1990). Where do semantic errors come from? *Cortex, 26,* 95–122.

Caramazza, A., & Miceli, G. (1991). Selective impairment of thematic role assignment in sentence processing. *Brain and Language, 41,* 402–436.

Caramazza, A., & Zurif, E. (1976). Dissociation of algorithmic and heuristic processes in language comprehension. *Brain and Language, 3,* 572–582.

Cohen, L., & Bachoud-Levi, A. C. (1995). The role of the output phonological buffer in the control of speech timing: A single case study. *Cortex, 31*(3), 469–486.

Cooke, A., Zurif, E. B., DeVita, C., Alsop D., Koenig, P., Detre J., et al. (2002). Neural basis for sentence comprehension: Grammatical and short-term memory components. *Human Brain Mapping, 15*(2), 80–94.

Crivello, F., Tzourio, N., Poline, J. B., Woods, R. P., Mazziota, J. C., & Mazoyer, B. (1995). Intersubject variability in functional neuroanatomy of silent verb generation: Assessment by a new activation detection algorithm based on amplitude and size information. *NeuroImage, 2*(4), 253–263.

Damasio, A. R. (1992). Aphasia. *New England Journal of Medicine, 326,* 531–539.

Dapretto, M., Bookheimer, S., & Mazziota, J. (1999). Form and content: Dissociating syntax and semantics in sentence comprehension. *Neuron, 24,* 427–432.

de Diego Balaguer, R., Costa, A., Sebastián-Galles, N., Juncadella, M., & Caramazza, A. (2004). Regular and irregular morphology and its relationship with agrammatism: Evidence from two Spanish–Catalan bilinguals. *Brain and Language, 91,* 212–222.

Demonet, J.-F., Price, C., Wise, R., & Frackowiak, R. (1994). A PET study of cognitive strategies in normal subjects during language tasks: Influence of phonetic ambiguity and sequence processing on phoneme monitoring. *Brain, 117,* 671–682.

D'Esposito, M., Aguirre, G. K., Zarahn, E., Ballard, D., Shin R. K., & Lease, J. (1998). Functional MRI studies of spatial and nonspatial working memory. *Brain Research: Cognitive Brain Research, 7*(1), 1–13.

D'Esposito, M., Ballard, D., Aguirre, G. K., & Zarahn, E. (1998). Human prefrontal cortex is not specific for working memory: A functional MRI study. *NeuroImage, 8*(3), 274–282.

D'Esposito, M., Postle, B. R., Jonides, J., & Smith, E. E. (1999). The neural substrate and temporal dynamics of interface effects in working memory as revealed by event-related functional MRI. *Proceedings of the National Academy of Sciences of the United States of America, 96*(13), 7514–7519.

Dronkers, N. F. (1996). A new brain region for coordinating speech articulation. *Nature, 384,* 159–161.

Exner, S. (1881). *Lokalisation des Funcktion der Grosshirnrinde des Menschen.* Wein: Braunmuller.

Fink, R., Martin, N., Schwartz, M., Saffran, E., & Myers, J. (1992). Facilitation of verb retrieval skills in aphasia: A comparison of two approaches. *Clinical Aphasiology, 21,* 263–275.

Garrett, M. F. (1975). The analysis of sentence production. In G. Bower (Ed.), *Psychology of learning and motivation* (Vol. 9, pp. 133–177). New York: Academic Press.

Garrett, M. F. (1980). Levels of processing in sentence production. In B. Butterworth (Ed.), *Language production* (pp. 170–220) London: Academic Press.

Garrett, M. F. (1988). Processes in language production. In N. Frederick (Ed.), *Linguistics: The Cambridge Survey* (Vol. 3, pp. 69–96). Cambridge, UK: Cambridge University Press.

Goodglass H., & Kaplan, E. (1972). *The Boston Diag-*

nostic Aphasia Examination. Philadelphia: Lea & Febiger.

Grodzinsky, Y. (2000). The neurology of syntax: Language use without Broca's area. *Behavioral and Brain Sciences, 23,* 1–71.

Hatfield, F. M., & Patterson, K. E. (1983). Phonological spelling. *Quarterly Journal of Experimental Psychology, 35*A, 451–468.

Heim, S., Opitz, B., & Friederici, A. D. (2002). Broca's area in the human brain is involved in the selection of grammatical gender for language production: Evidence from event-related functional magnetic resonance imaging. *Neuroscience Letters, 328,* 101–104.

Hernandez, A. E., Kotz, S. A., Hofmann, J., Valentin, V. V., Dapretto, M., & Bookheimer, S. Y. (2004). The neural correlates of grammatical gender decisions in Spanish. *NeuroReport, 15*(5), 863–866.

Hillis, A. E., & Caramazza, A. (2003). Aphasia. In L. Nadel (Ed.), *Encyclopedia of cognitive neuroscience* (pp. 469–470). London: Macmillan Reference.

Hillis, A. E., Chang, S., Breese, E., & Heidler, J. (2004). The crucial role of posterior frontal regions in modality specific components of the spelling process. *Neurocase, 10,* 175–187.

Hillis, A. E., Oh, S., & Ken, L. (2004). Deterioration of naming nouns versus verbs in primary progressive aphasia. *Annals of Neurology, 55,* 268–275.

Hillis, A. E., Newhart, M., Heidler, J., Barker, P. B., Herskovits, E., & Degaonkar, M. (2005). The roles of the "visual word form area" in reading. *NeuroImage, 24,* 548–549.

Hillis, A. E., Rapp, B. C., & Caramazza, A. (1999). When a rose is a rose in speaking but a tulip in writing. *Cortex, 35,* 337–356.

Hillis, A. E., Tuffiash, E., Wityk, R. J., & Barker, P. B. (2002). Regions of neural dysfunction associated with impaired naming of actions and objects in acute stroke. *Cognitive Neuropsychology, 19,* 523–534.

Hillis, A. E., Wityk, R., Barker, P. B., & Caramazza, A. (2003). Neural regions essential for writing verbs. *Nature Neuroscience, 6,* 9–20.

Hillis, A. E., Work, M., Breese, E. L., Barker, P. B., Jacobs, M. A., & Maurer, K. (2004). Re-examining the brain regions crucial for orchestrating speech articulation. *Brain, 127,* 1479–1487.

Hsieh, L., & Rapp, B. C. (2004, October). *Functional magnetic resonance imaging of the cognitive components of the spelling process.* Paper presented at the annual meeting of the Academy of Aphasia, Chicago.

Kim, M., & Thompson, C. K. (2000). Verb retrieval in agrammatism. *Brain and Language, 74,* 1–25.

Levelt, W. (1993). Language use in normal speakers and its disorders. In G. Blanken, J. Dittman, H. Grimm, J. C. Marshall, & C.-W. Wallesh (Eds.), *Linguistic disorders and pathologies* (pp. 1–15). Berlin: Walter de Gruyter.

Levelt, W. (1999). Producing spoken language: A blueprint of the speaker. In C. M. Brown & P. Hagoort (Eds.), *The neurocognition of language* (pp. 83–122). New York: Oxford University Press.

Linebarger, M. C., Schwartz, M. F., Romania, J. R.,

Kohn, S. E., & Stephens, D. L. (2000). Grammatical encoding in aphasia: Evidence from a "processing prosthesis." *Brain and Language, 75*(3), 416–427.

Marien, P., Pickuta, B. A., Engelborghsa, S., Martind, J.-J., & De Deyna, P. P. (2001). Phonological agraphia following a focal anterior insulo-opercular infarction. *Neuropsychologia, 39,* 845–855.

Marshall, J., Pring, T., & Chiat, S. (1998). Verb retrieval and sentence production in aphasia. *Brain and Language, 63*(2), 159–183.

Martin, R., & Blossom-Stach, C. (1986). Evidence of a syntactic deficit in a fluent aphasic. *Brain and Language, 28,* 196–234.

McNeil, M. R., Doyle, P. J., & Wambaugh, J. (2000). Apraxia of speech: A treatable disorder of motor planning and programming. In S. E. Nadeau, L. J. Gonzalez Roth, & B. A. Crosson (Eds.), *Aphasia and language: Theory to practice* (pp. 221–265). New York: Guilford Press.

Miceli, G., Silveri, C., Romani, C., & Carramazza, A. (1989). Variation in the pattern of omissions and substitutions of grammatical morphemes in the spontaneous speech of so-called agrammatic patients. *Brain and Language, 36,* 447–492.

Miceli, G., Silveri, C., Villa, G., & Caramazza, A. (1984). On the basis of agrammatic's difficulty in producing main verbs. *Cortex, 20,* 217–220.

Miceli, G., Turriziani, P., Caltagirone, C., Capasso, R., Tomaiuolo, F., & Carramazza, A. (2002). The neural correlates of grammatical gender: An fMRI investigation. *Journal of Cognitive Neuroscience, 14,* 618–628.

Mitchum, C., & Berndt, R. S. (1994). Verb retrieval and sentence construction: Effects of targeted intervention. In M. Riddoch & G. Humphreys (Eds.), *Cognitive neuropsychology and cognitive rehabilitation* (pp. 317–348). Hove, UK: Erlbaum.

Mohr, J. P., Pessin, M. S., Finkelstein, S., Funkenstein, H. H., Duncan, G. W., & Davis, K. R. (1978). Broca aphasia: Pathological and clinical. *Neurology, 28,* 311–324.

Moo, L. R., Slotnick, S. D., & Hillis, A. E. (2002, October). *Left prefrontal activation varies with task difficulty.* Paper presented at the annual meeting of the Society for Neuroscience, Orlando, FL.

Neary, D., Snowden, J.S., Gustafson, L., Passant, U., Stuss, D., Black, S., et al. (1998). Frontotemporal lobar degeneration—a consensus on clinical diagnostic criteria. *Neurology, 51,* 1546–1554.

Paulesu, E., Goldacre, B., Scifo, P., Cappa, S. F., Gilardi, M. C., Castiglioni, I., et al. (1997). Functional heterogeneity of left inferior frontal cortex as revealed by fMRI. *NeuroReport, 8,* 2011–2017.

Perani, D., Cappa, S. F., Schnur, T., Tettamanti, M., Collina, S., Rosa, M. M., et al. (1999). The neural correlates of verb and noun processing: A PET study. *Brain, 122,* 2337–2344.

Petersen, S. E., Fox, P. T., Posner, M. I., Mintun, M., & Raichle, M. E. (1988). Positron emission tomographic studies of the cortical anatomy of single-word processing. *Nature, 331,* 585–589.

Price, C. J., Winterburn, D., Giraud, A. L., Moore, C. J., & Noppeney, U. (2003). Cortical localization of the visual and auditory word form areas: A reconsideration of the evidence. *Brain and Language, 86,* 272–286.

Price, C. J., Wise, R. J., Warburton, E. A., Moore, C. J., Howard, D., & Patterson, K. (1996). Hearing and saying: The functional neuro-anatomy of auditory word processing. *Brain, 119,* 919–931.

Rademacher, J., Caviness, V. S., Steinmetz, H., & Galaburda, A. M. (1993). Topographical variation in the human primary cortices: Implications for neuroimaging, brain mapping, and neurobiology. *Cerebral Cortex, 3,* 313–329.

Rapcsak, S. Z., & Beeson, P. M. (2002). Neuroanatomical correlates of spelling and writing. In A. E. Hillis (Ed.), *Handbook of adult language disorders: Integrating cognitive neuropsychology, neurology, and rehabilitation* (pp. 71–99). Philadelphia: Psychology Press.

Rapcsak, S. Z., Rubens, A. B., & Arthur, S. A. (1988). Lexical agraphia from focal lesion of the left precentral gyrus. *Neurology, 38,* 1119–1123.

Rapp, B., & Hsieh, L. (2001, April). *Functional magnetic resonance imaging of the cognitive components of the spelling process.* Paper presented at the Cognitive Neuroscience Society meeting, San Francisco.

Roeltgen, D. P., & Heilman, K. M. (1984). Lexical agraphia: Further support for the two-system hypothesis of linguistic agraphia. *Brain, 107,* 811–827.

Rypma, B., & D'Esposito, M. (1999). The roles of prefrontal brain regions in components of working memory: Effects of memory load and individual differences. *Proceedings of the National Academy of Sciences of the United States of America, 96*(11), 6558–6563.

Saffran, E., Schwartz, M., & Marin, O. (1980). The word order problem in agrammatism: 2. Production. *Brain and Language, 10,* 263–280.

Schiff, H. B., Alexander, M. P., Naeser, M. A., & Galaburda, A. M. (1983). Aphemia. Clinical–anatomic correlations. *Archives of Neurology, 40,* 720–727.

Selnes, O., & Hillis, A. E. (2000). Patient Tan revisited: A case of atypical global aphasia? *Journal of the History of the Neurosciences, 9,* 233–237.

Shapiro, K., & Caramazza A. (2004). The organization of lexical knowledge in the brain: The grammatical dimension. In M. Gazzaniga (Ed.), *Cognitive neurosciences* (3rd ed., pp. 803–814). Cambridge, MA: MIT Press.

Shapiro, K. A., Pascual-Leone, A., Mottaghy, F. M., Gangitano, M., & Caramazza A. (2001). Grammatical distinctions in the left frontal cortex. *Journal of Cognitive Neuroscience, 13,* 713–720.

Thompson, C. K., & Faroqi-Shah, Y. (2002). Models of sentence production. In A. E. Hillis (Ed.), *The handbook of adult language disorders: Integrating cognitive neuropsychology, neurology, and rehabilitation* (pp. 311–330). New York: Psychology Press.

Thompson-Schill, S., Aguirre, G., D'Esposito, M., & Farah, M. (1999). A neural basis for category and modality specificity of semantic knowledge. *Neuropsychologia, 37,* 671–676.

Tranel, D., Adolphs, R., Damasio, H., & Damasio, A. R. (2001). A neural basis for the retrieval of words for actions. *Cognitive Neuropsychology, 18,* 655–670.

Tranel, D., Damasio, H., & Damasio, A. (1997). On the neurology of naming. In H. Goodglass (Ed.), *Anomia* (pp. 65–90). London: Academic Press.

Tranel, D., & Kemmerer, D. (2004). Neuroanatomical correlates of locative prepositions. *Cognitive Neuropsychology, 21,* 719–749.

Tyler, L. K., Russell, R., Fadili, J., & Moss, H. E. (2001). The neural representation of nouns and verbs: PET studies. *Brain, 124,* 1619–1634.

Ullman, M. T., Corkin, S., Coppola, M., Hickok, G., Growdon, J. H., Koroshetz, W. J., et al. (1997). A neural dissociation within language: Evidence that the mental dictionary is part of declarative memory, and that grammatical rules are processed by the procedural system. *Journal of Cognitive Neuroscience, 9,* 289–299.

Van Essen, D. C., Drury, H. A., Joshi, S., & Miller, M. (1998). Functional and structural mapping of the human cerebral cortex: Solutions are in the surfaces. *Proceedings of the National Academy of Sciences of the United States of America, 95,* 788–795.

Wagner, A., Koustaal, W., Maril, A., Schacter, D., & Buckner, R. (2000). Task-specific repetition priming in left inferior prefrontal cortex. *Cerebral Cortex, 10,* 1176–1184.

Wagner, A. D., Pare-Blagoev, E. J., Clark, J., & Poldrack, R. A. (2001). Recovering meaning: Left prefrontal cortex guides controlled semantic retrieval. *Neuron, 31,* 329–338.

Warburton, E., Wise, R., Price, C., Weiller, C., Hadar, U., Ramsay, S., et al. (1996). Noun and verb retrieval by normal subjects with PET. *Brain, 119,* 159–179.

Whitaker, H. A., & Selnes, O. (1976). Anatomic variations in the cortex: Individual differences and the problem of the localization of language functions. *Annals of the New York Academy of Sciences, 280,* 844–854.

Zatorre, R. J., Evans, A. C., Meyer, E., & Gjedde, A. (1992). Lateralization of phonetic and pitch discrimination in speech processing. *Science, 256,* 846–849.

Zatorre, R. J., Meyer, E., Gjedde, A., & Evans, A. C. (1996). PET studies of phonetic processes in speech perception: Review, replication, and re-analysis. *Cerebral Cortex, 6,* 21–30.

Zingeser, L. B., & Berndt, R. S. (1988). Grammatical class and context effects in a case of pure anomia: Implications for models of language production. *Cognitive Neuropsychology, 5,* 473–516.

Zingeser, L. B., & Berndt, R. S. (1990). Retrieval of nouns and verbs in agrammatism and anomia. *Brain and Language, 39,* 14–32.

# CHAPTER 21

# Self-Representation and the Frontal Lobes

*William W. Seeley*
*Virginia E. Sturm*

The normal human adult experiences the self as unitary, seamless, and continuous through time. Yet the self is no single biological entity. Instead, it is a neural accomplishment built, like all others, from a dynamic set of component processes. To characterize these processes, with all the interacting circuits and neural devices they entail, requires that we sharpen the ways we think and talk about the self. Terminological mainstays such as "self-consciousness," "self-reflection," and "self-awareness" need to be replaced by neurological terms that describe what about its owner a brain is trying to represent. In this spirit, we chose the term *self-representation* for the title of this chapter.

How do our brains build the self as we know it? What is known about self-representation in other species and developing humans? In this chapter, we survey the new cognitive neuroscience of the self, a nascent field just beginning to define its own questions. To illustrate hints of progress, we highlight selected forms of self-representation, their evolution and ontogeny, and the neural architectures that might support them. The frontal lobes are vital to these systems, but we stress that self-representation involves diverse processes within broadly distributed, interacting neural networks. Finally, we point out methodological pitfalls already emerging and suggest avenues for future research.

## PHYLOGENY OF SELF-REPRESENTATION: EVOLUTIONARY PRESSURES AND NEURONAL SPECIALIZATIONS

Nervous systems achieve self-representation at many levels, from mundane biological housekeeping to exalted contemplations of the self's place in human, world, or universal history. Simple representations of the internal milieu evolved in early vertebrates to allow reflexive behaviors that acted on local surroundings to meet ongoing homeostatic demands. Incrementally complex layers of self-representation were then built out of their predecessors to allow more flexible interactions between organisms, their nervous systems (eventually including mental contents), and the environment. To examine this graded evolution is not easy: How can one discern the subjectivity of an iguana? How conscious of its body state is a pelican? A prairie vole? How much mental time travel does an orangutan perform? We may never know for certain, because we require subjective mental state descriptions from these organisms that they are unfit to provide. Furthermore, we cannot address psychological discontinuities or leaps forward in phylogeny when the relevant species are extinct. As Povinelli (1993) observed, "Psychology does not fossilize" (p. 495) and, unlike the bones of the hand, neither does brain architecture. Though certain psychological structures (capacity for imitation and tool use) can be inferred from anthropological evidence, most cannot. Despite these limitations, behavioral and structural commonalities make some form of conscious self-representation likely across mammalian taxa. Even rats possess much of the circuitry that supports interoceptive awareness in humans (Craig, 2002; Critchley, Wiens, Rotshtein, Ohman, & Dolan, 2004; Jasmin, Burkey, Granato, & Ohara, 2004). Yet self-representation in rats differs, in undeniable ways, from our own. At what point in evolution did this fundamental change occur?

In early attempts to grade the phylogeny of self, Gallup observed primates confronted by mirrors and looked for behaviors consistent with self-recognition, such as inspecting body parts only viewable in the mirrors (Gallup, 1970, 1987). Strikingly, orangutans, gorillas (but see Shillito, Gallup, & Beck, 1999), and chimpanzees have all shown mirror self-recognition behaviors not present in monkeys, who often regard their reflections as adversaries (Gallup, 1982; Patterson, 1984). The status of cetaceans is uncertain (Anderson, 1995; Gallup, 1995; Marten & Psarakos, 1995; Reiss & Marino, 2001). To formalize his assessments, Gallup (1987) developed the mark test, in which the examiner covertly discolors a patch of hair on the animal's face and observes whether the animal uses a mirror to direct behaviors toward the mark. In the common chimpanzee, success on the mark test emerges in early adolescence and may decline with advancing age (de Veer, Gallup, Theall, van den Bos, & Povinelli, 2003). Failures could result from an inability to note action–outcome contingencies seen in mirrors or to reason deductively from those contingencies, and it is not straightforward to equate mirror self-recognition with abstract awareness of self (Hauser, Kralik, Botto-Mahan, Garrett, & Oser, 1995; Povinelli, 1993). Nonetheless, this line of research invigorated the study of self-representation and helped create links between comparative and developmental psychology. Gallup (1982) argued from early on that self-recognition grounds attribution of mental states to both the self and others, perhaps through a shared neural architecture.

What selective pressures forged mirror self-recognition competence in apes? Prevailing hypotheses relate to the cognitive demands imposed by arboreal clambering (Povinelli & Cant, 1995), tool-use apprenticeships (Parker, 1997), spatial and temporal fruit resource variability (Potts, 2004), and increasingly complex and fluid social groupings (Joffe & Dunbar, 1997). These challenges would have favored brains that used abstract, recyclable mental representations of objects, including the self. The self, a permanent object (me), would be observable in a mirror and would be the agent (I) of willed actions seen in that mirror. In like fashion, representations of permanent others (her, him, perhaps them) would have conferred predictability and security in competitive social environs. The capacity not only to represent the self but also to reflect on that representation—*awareness of* awareness—may be particularly evolved in humans compared to even our nearest ancestors, though this issue remains debated (Povinelli, 1993; Smith, Shields, & Washburn, 2003). To perform this feat we must abstract from internal stimuli that we are thinking, conscious agents. But it is unclear how unique and privileged this capacity really is, how much it differs from our highly abstract ruminations over relativity, mathematics, or the meaning of art. The ability to travel mentally through time, to conjure lucid images of one's past and future, is thought to be a uniquely human capacity, but this position also lacks empirical grounding or even a clear basis for exploration.

The primate frontal lobe differs from that of other mammals in that it is distinctly larger, more gyriform, and more granular (or isocortical) in architecture (Nauta, 1971; Ongur & Price, 2000). More recently, primate brains have undergone progressive rostral encephalization, hemispheric functional lateralization, and maturational delay, especially among species capable of self-recognition. In addition, two recently identified primate neuroanatomical specializations pertain directly to self-representation.

First, the Lamina I homeostatic afferent pathway carries salient body state information from the spinal cord to the posterior part of the ventromedial thalamus (VMpo). The VMpo is discernible only in primates and is notably more prominent in humans (Craig, 2002). Data processed by the VMpo are fed forward to the ipsilateral dorsal posterior insula, then on to the anterior (especially nondominant) insular and orbital cortices (Craig, Chen, Bandy, & Reiman, 2000; Rolls et al., 2003; Vandenbergh et al., 2005), perhaps to tell us how we feel (Craig, 2002) and support "gut-level" decision making (Bechara, Damasio, & Damasio, 2000). Furthermore, as hinted earlier, we seem to know not only how we feel, but also how we feel about how we feel. This higher-order determination requires an interaction between the interoceptive "here and now" and its potential implications for the future. Crosstalk among efferent limbic, afferent limbic, and prospective memory systems must underlie this type of appraisal.

Second, within the same ancient anterior cingulate (ACC) and frontoinsular (FI) cortices that process autonomic and body state information (Craig, 2003; Critchley, Mathias, & Dolan, 2001b; Critchley et al., 2004), there is a new class of large, spindle-shaped projection neurons seen only in humans and great apes (Nimchinsky et al., 1999; Nimchinsky, Vogt, Morrison, & Hof, 1995; von Economo, 1926). These cells, most recently referred to as von Economo neurons (VENs; Allman, Watson, Tetreault, & Hakeem, 2005), lie clustered within layer 5b of the agranular cortices where they reside. VEN concentration is greater in the right hemisphere and decreases with phyletic distance from humans (Allman, Hakeem, Erwin, Nimchinsky, & Hof, 2001). Whether and how VENs support self-representation in humans is unknown, but they are far newer than the paralimbic regions within which they evolved, suggesting that they confer some new device for handling locally processed information. Could VENs provide the toggle or relay between the visceral "here and now" and the contemplated future?

Observations and questions like these have spawned the field of evolutionary neurology, whose mission it is to address the disease costs imposed by recent neuroevolutionary advances. Some of our most devastating diseases, such as autism and schizophrenia, take hold during critical points in the self's development, the subject to which we now turn.

## ONTOGENY OF SELF-REPRESENTATION: THEMES, LAYERS, AND PARALLELS

From birth, humans iteratively construct the self, beginning with simple body state "building materials" and layering on new skills until we learn to think abstractly about our selves, others, and the complex relations between them (Butterworth, 1995; Neisser, 1993). In this section, we highlight key milestones in self-development and find that they simulate, on many levels, the advances wrought through mammalian brain evolution.

### The First Year of Life

James's (1890) description of the newborn's world as a "blooming, buzzing confusion" of sensory disorganization has been revised through new methods for understanding infant behavior (Harter, 1998). It now appears that we enter the world poised to integrate sensory information into a coherent experience (Meltzoff & Moore, 1997; Rochat, 2001) that sharpens the boundary between self and environment (Rochat, 1998). As newborns cry, they express not only the "paralimbic unpleasantness" of unmet homeostatic needs but also forge connections between their cries and the kinesthetic–proprioceptive, vestibular, tactile, auditory, and visual coherencies they produce (Rochat, 1998). Through this cross-modal perception, infants link together sensorimotor information and build working models of how parallel input streams are related (Meltzoff, 1990). For example, when infants suck on a certain shaped pacifier without seeing it, they will later stare longer at this pacifier than at one shaped differently (Meltzoff & Borton, 1979). Mapping such contingencies allows infants to assemble a body-centered world map that supports navigation and skill learning. Acts of self-exploration accelerate the process, as experimentalist infants spend the bulk of their waking hours touching the mouth and face (Korner & Kraemer, 1972).

In the social realm, cross-modal perception allows infants to detect the composition of others' actions and make models for generating those same actions. Some infants imitate facial expressions within the first hours of life (Meltzoff & Moore, 1983). The social smile, an intentional act that elicits positive reinforcement from others, emerges around 2 months of age and suggests an awareness that actions can influence others (Rochat, 2001; Tronick, 1989). Shortly thereafter, infants learn to discriminate between maternal emotional expressions (Nelson, 1987). Later, capitalizing on this ability, infants associate their own expressive behaviors with internal states, compare their behaviors with those of others, and use these data to transitively infer others' internal states (Meltzoff, 1990). This drive begins early, as indicated by preferences for faces over scrambled facial features (Haith, Bergman, & Moore, 1977; Morton & Johnson, 1991), faces with eyes over those without (Maurer, 1985), and adults looking at them over those with averted gaze (Hains & Muir, 1996). These biases promote the early appreciation of affect.

The second half of the first year of life is marked by increasingly complex understanding of the self, others, and external objects as discrete yet interacting entities (Rochat, 2001). Joint attention, the ability to use gaze and gesture cues to share experiences with others, emerges between 9 and 12 months and develops until 18 months of age (Frith & Frith, 2003). Infants employ this skill to develop incipient theories of mind (Rochat, 2001) and to use others' affective cues to guide behavioral choices (Campos & Stenberg, 1981).

From even the first days of life infants encode, store, and retrieve information about events and are able to remember information over time (Howe, 2004; Howe & Courage, 1997; Howe, Courage, & Edison, 2003). Young infants make unconscious associations between sensory and perceptual experiences (Squire, Knowlton, & Musen, 1993), likely by means of amygdalar and extrahippocampal limbic processing (Siegel, 1999). Primitive forms of explicit memory are thought to emerge late in the first year (Carver, Bauer, & Nelson, 2000; Courage & Howe, 2004), though this question remains debated (Rovee-Collier, 1997).

### The Second Year of Life

The second year of life brings a whirlwind of self-development (Kagan, 1989; Lewis, Sullivan, Stanger, & Weiss, 1989). The ability to pass mirror (Amsterdam, 1972; Papousek & Papousek, 1974) and video (Lewis & Brooks-Gunn, 1985) self-recognition tests emerges between 15 and 24 months of age. Mirror self-recognition tests used are analogous to those of comparative psychology, and, though some have questioned their meaning in toddlers (Howe, 2004), self-recognition remains an important developmental milestone associated with the emergence of other cognitive, emotional, and social skills. Embarrassment, a self-conscious emotion that takes place in the presence of a thinking other, appears only after mirror self-recognition competence can be demonstrated (Lewis et al., 1989; Tangney, 1999). Around 18 months, toddlers begin to use personal pronouns (e.g., "I," "me," "you") in reference to self and others (Bates, 1990; Fay, 1979; Ickes, Reidhead, & Patterson, 1986), indicating the presence of symbolic representations that can be remembered over time (Neisser, 1991). Social standards become internalized, and toddlers may evaluate themselves in reference to others, becoming upset if they perform a novel task less well than adults (Kagan, 1984). They come to understand that people are psychological beings with private, internal worlds; they distinguish behavior from thinking (Bartsch & Wellman, 1995), desire from action (Repacholi & Gopnik, 1997), and reality from pretense (Harris, 1991; Wellman & Estes, 1986).

Memory systems develop dramatically during the second year, and early forms of autobiographical memory provide a foundation for more longitudinal representations of self. These rudimentary autobiographical stores consist of semantic information about physical and personal traits (Snow, 1990). Episodic memory develops, more explicit personal memories are secured, and early life amnesia is replaced by a self-narrative built from experiences anchored in space and time (Howe, 2004).

### Early Childhood (2–4 Years)

Between the ages of 2 and 4, language development provides concrete feedback (Cooley, 1902) and self-relevant information that enhances the self-concept and highlights developmental achievements (Radke-Yarrow, Belmont, Nottelmann, & Bottomly, 1990). Compared with infants, toddlers better comprehend and more often reference their own mental lives. By 2 years of age, they begin to use mental state words (Frith & Frith, 2003), and by age 3, they routinely speak of their thoughts and beliefs (Brown & Dunn, 1991). Three-year-olds know that thinking occurs internally and cannot be seen (Flavell, Green, & Flavell, 1993, 1995), and by age 4, children can reliably pass tests of "theory of mind" (Wellman, Cross, & Watson, 2001).

Toddlerhood also brings modular cognitive representations of self, including separable self-qualities such as physical characteristics and material possessions (Broughton, 1980; Selman, 1980). Steady gains in episodic memory, encoding speed, and memory retention (Courage & Howe, 2004) allow children to organize their experiences into more extended, continuous narratives (Nelson, 1993). A fluid and interconnected network of episodic memories builds a self framework that is more cohesive and longitudinal.

## Childhood (5–11 Years) and Adolescence (12–18 Years)

The childhood and adolescent years bring a greater capacity for abstraction (Case, 1985; Fischer, 1980), allowing previously disjointed self-concepts to become linked, nuanced, and elaborated (Damon & Hart, 1982). Psychological and social (Broughton, 1978) as well as opposing (Case, 1992; Griffin, 1992) self-traits are gradually incorporated, fostering more realistic self-evaluation (Harter, 2003). Socialization and cognitive gains allow evaluation of the self against abstract social standards, which are then internalized to guide behavior and goals (Higgins, 1991). Adolescence heightens awareness of others' opinions, and, in parallel, there is increasing capacity for introspection, the directed examination of internal states as they relate to the imagined past, present, or future (Fischer, Shaver, & Carnochan, 1990). By late adolescence, a nearly mature concept of the self's mental traits and capacities is established.

## FUNCTIONAL AND NEURAL ARCHITECTURES OF SELF-REPRESENTATION

Late-evolving and late-maturing brain regions may support our most sophisticated forms of self-representation, but these capacities are built upon and anchored by our more primitive neural foundations. To review the anatomy of these networks, however, it may help to outline a nomenclature for the psychological constructs under discussion.

Some authors separate the self into a *minimal* self, the immediate experience of one's person unextended in time, and a more longitudinal or *narrative* self, related to one's personal past and future (see Gallagher, 2000, for a review). The minimal self represents data accessible only to its owner: the online impression of the body state and one's conscious stream of imagery and internal dialogue. Damasio (1999) further divides the minimal self into a "proto-self" (body state, unconscious) and "core self" (conscious thought and feeling). The more lon-

gitudinal self, also referred to as the "extended self" (Neisser, 1988) or "autobiographical self" (Damasio, 1999), is made up of elements that follow an individual through time. It provides a sense of continuity and purpose, allowing us to engage in activities that may confer future benefits. We favor the term *longitudinal self* (Seeley & Miller, 2005), because it emphasizes time and continuity, the essential features of the construct, yet leaves room for personal narratives, self-statements or "schemata" (Markus, 1977), episodic memories and projections of the self into the imagined future.

The minimal self provides a platform for the longitudinal self, but each system influences the data handled by the other. For example, the minimal self can bring remembered elements of the longitudinal self into consciousness, but the longitudinal self renders an impression of the self over time, organizing and making sense of the endless accumulation of new experiences. The longitudinal self's readout is iteratively modified and updated by the perceptions of the minimal self, which, conversely, are filtered through the longitudinal self's working model. These designations are, of course, only a shorthand to help us communicate about the self. They do not refer to freestanding biological entities, and what we describe with these terms is sure to reflect a host of component parts. The task at hand is to determine what these parts are, what they do, and how they do what they do, so that our oversimplified nomenclature can be exchanged for more numerous, precise, and evocative terms.

### THE MINIMAL SELF: LIFE IN THE MOMENT

Phylogenetically ancient systems rooted in the brainstem and hypothalamus are the homeostatic bedrock of the minimal self. These networks represent the body and support its most basic needs, all beneath the surface of awareness. Though these systems are crucial to the hierarchical organization of the self, we have chosen to focus our discussion on conscious self-representations that, layered but perceived together, provide the immediate, streaming, and subjective experience of human mental life (James, 1890). These self-representational layers are woven into the larger tapestry our brains create about the world outside. Here we focus on three processing streams the minimal self must organize: interoception, exteroception, and what (for now) we will refer to as *phrenoception*.

## Interoception: Mapping the Body State in Consciousness

The river of body state data that our brains receive is almost always running. Even in a dreamful sleep, biologically relevant information (bladder distention, itch, cold) can enter the flow of consciousness enough to promote wakefulness. Representation of the internal state allows fitness-critical signals to be registered and engaged at need. The system motivates us to solve problems early, before the body falters, even as nonconscious mechanisms address the same homeostatic demand. To provide a simplified example, when the body is in need of water, the serum solute concentration rises and is detected by the anterior hypothalamus, which generates a two-way distress signal. At a nonconscious level, the supraoptic and paraventricular hypothalamic nuclei project to the posterior pituitary, which sends a blood-borne chemical message—arginine vasopressin—to the kidneys, instructing them to retain water. Simultaneously, the hypothalamus communicates directly and indirectly with the thalamus and paralimbic cortex (including the ACC and insula, see Figure 21.1) to bring the situation to mind and promote water-seeking behavior (de Araujo, Kringelbach, Rolls, & McGlone, 2003; Egan et al., 2003; Sewards & Sewards, 2000). As an aside, brain vasopressin 1a receptors are known for their role in mammalian pair bonding (Insel & Young, 2001) and are densely present on layer 5 pyramidal neurons of the ACC, including the newly evolved VENs (Allman et al., 2005). Has emotional attachment evolved from the neural mechanisms for thirst? Is love like water? Perhaps not, but evolution does build new capacities out of existing materials. For infants the thirst and attachment drives are inseparable and addressed by the same action, nursing.

In humans, homeostatic afferent data reaches the dorsal posterior insula (DPI) via the VMpo (see above). This information is then shuttled forward and rerepresented in the anterior insula (AI) of the nondominant hemisphere, providing a substrate for conscious, *evaluative* interoception (Craig, 2002; Critchley et al., 2004). Likely through insular connections to the amygdala, ACC, and orbito-

frontal cortex, body state signals (or their short-circuit analogues) may guide us toward contextually optimized behaviors (Damasio, 1996). Modeling another's interoceptive state, such as a spouse's experience of pain, recruits the same anterior insular regions and the ACC, but not the DPI (Singer et al., 2004). In a rough sense, the ACC and AI are the megaphones into which our bodies can speak when they want to tell us that something important is going on (Figure 21.1, unfilled shapes), whether it is physical or social (Eisenberger & Lieberman, 2004; Ploghaus et al., 1999; Rolls et al., 2003), positive (Bartels & Zeki, 2004; Blood & Zatorre, 2001; Rolls et al., 2003) or negative (Rolls et al., 2003; Singer et al., 2004). The close link between the ACC and AI is apparent from primate anatomical (Carmichael & Price, 1996) and human resting state functional connectivity studies (Beckmann, DeLuca, Devlin, & Smith, 2005 [see Figure 6F therein]). The work of Critchley and his colleagues suggests that the ubiquity of ACC and AI recruitment across task-activation studies may relate more to autonomic processing demands than to the unique task or stimulus features involved (Critchley, Mathias, & Dolan, 2001a; Critchley, Mathias, et al., 2003; Critchley, Tang, Glaser, Butterworth, & Dolan, 2005).

When the adult brain is newly deprived of autonomic feedback by disease, the left ACC and right anterior insula undergo involutional changes (Critchley, Good, et al., 2003), but only minor (if any) emotional changes arise (Critchley et al., 2001b; Heidbreder, Ziegler, Schafferhans, Heidland, & Gruninger, 1984). Conversely, acquired ACC/AI degeneration uncouples nociceptive stimulus detection from its emotional consequences (Seeley, Lomen-Hoerth, & Miller, 2005). Together, these findings suggest that as adults we no longer rely on the periphery for emotional awareness, perhaps because the sensory consequences of outgoing autonomic impulses have been progressively mapped in the insulae. Over time, visceromotor states *to be generated* by the ACC (Critchley, Elliott, Mathias, & Dolan, 2000; Critchley, Mathias, et al., 2003) may be fed forward (directly or via an intermediary circuit) to the anterior insulae as efference copies that are, in turn, sent on to orbitofrontal and anterior temporal regions that integrate stimulus saliency values with context. Thus, the emotomotor and skeletomotor systems bear an elegant similarity. With years of practice, a ten-

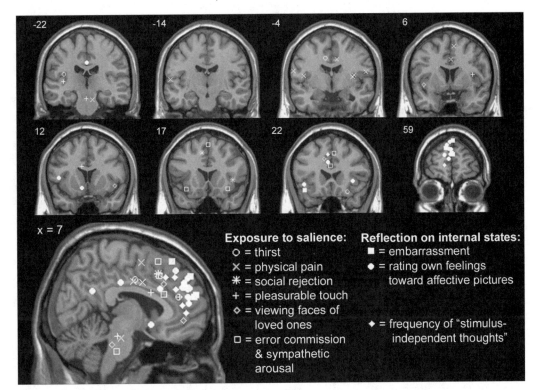

FIGURE 21.1. Functional activations of the minimal self. Tasks in which subjects are exposed to salient stimuli (unfilled shapes) recruit anterior cingulate–pre-supplementary motor area (ACC-pSMA), insular, and frontoinsular cortices, in cooperation with brainstem autonomic control centers. Specific activations relate to thirst (de Araujo et al., 2003; Egan et al., 2003), physical or social pain (Eisenberger, Lieberman, & Williams, 2003; Ploghaus et al., 1999; Rolls et al., 2003), pleasurable touch (Olausson et al., 2002; Rolls et al., 2003), viewing pictures of loved ones (Bartels & Zeki, 2004), and error commission + sympathetic arousal (Critchley et al., 2005). Direct interoceptive stimulation is further accompanied by posterior insula/parietal operculum activation (top row). Tasks that require subjects to reflect on their internal state (filled shapes) recruit the dorsomedial prefrontal cortex (DMPFC) rostral to the ACC-pSMA, at times in concert with cingulate and posterior orbital–insular regions. DMPFC activations are seen during the self-conscious emotion of embarrassment (Berthoz et al., 2002; Takahashi et al., 2004) and ratings of one's own feelings toward affective pictures (Gusnard et al., 2001; Lane et al., 1997; Ochsner et al., 2004). Similar DMPFC activation correlates with the frequency of stimulus-independent thoughts (McGuire, Paulesu, Frackowiak, & Frith, 1996). All significant foci from each study within brainstem, insula/operculum, posterior orbital, and medial frontoparietal regions are projected in Montreal Neurological Institute (MNI) coordinates onto eight coronal images from the MNI template brain. The left side of these images corresponds to the left side of the brain. For illustrative purposes, a sagittal summary image (bottom left) shows activations within 10 mm of the midline.

nis player no longer guides her arm on a forehand with conscious joint position sense (at least, she would do best not to—it takes too much time!). In like fashion, we may train our emotions to use "as if" equivalents (Damasio, 1999), without waiting for the full visceral response set to play out and return to our brains via the spinal cord. Intuitive judgments (like good forehands) need to happen quickly and automatically to be most useful.

## Exteroception: The Body-Centered World Map

Because we live within complex three-dimensional environments, the minimal self must also track the physical extent and location of its owner within the gravitational field. Proprioceptive–kinesthetic, somatic, visual, auditory, and vestibular data are integrated into a spatially refined image and used to construct an egocentric world map. Charted positions of the head, trunk, and limbs facilitate gazing and reaching toward environmental targets. Unlike interoception, whose job is to point us toward homeostatic threats or potential rewards, exteroception allows us to navigate the environment and carry out complex actions that address the homeostatic relevance identified. This exteroceptive system is embedded in a bilateral frontal–cingulo–parietal spatial attentional matrix that draws heavily on the right parietal lobe (Astafiev et al., 2003; Corbetta, 1998; Mesulam, 1981; Vogeley & Fink, 2003).

But what about the saber-toothed tiger? Certainly it is identified via our exteroceptive (visual or auditory) sensors. Indeed so, but knowing that it is dangerous relies on evaluative interoception. The interdependence of the two systems is clear: Objects in the world require a visceral readout of their salience that helps only when translated into skilled action (or inaction) as the situation demands. Thus, the interoceptive minimal self acts as an intermediary between the outside world and the actions we apply to it.

### Phrenoception: Representing Acts of the Mind

Just as visceral and proprioceptive feedback are cortically represented, the brain's own intrinsic spontaneous activities—thoughts—must be projected on the minimal self's screen of consciousness. Spontaneous thoughts are a core feature of the minimal self and have characteristics of both action and perception. Like actions, thoughts are generated using a range of volition (sometimes none at all), marked with a sense of ownership and agency, and subject to feedback control by the sensory consequences of their execution. Like perceptions, spontaneous thoughts have modality-specific features; they are the imagery and inner dialogue that comprise reflection without requisite linkage to the immediate external environment. Though the self-representational problems of agency and ownership relate closely to this "phrenoceptive" system, due to scope limitations they are not discussed further here (for reviews, see Blakemore, 2005; Gallagher, 2000). The important point is that although they may seem more like perceptions (occurring only within

the mind), thoughts bear an underappreciated similarity to actions.

The neural basis of task-unrelated or "stimulus-independent thoughts" (SITS) (Antrobus, 1968) is a daunting frontier, and it is hard to know whether thoughts can ever be entirely spontaneous. Moreover, thoughts do not happen some magical somewhere in the brain; their distributed anatomy depends on the modal features of the image generated. Yet all thoughts share ownership and agency by the self, providing them with a verification stamp (this thought came from and was caused by me) regardless of their image-form. Reflecting on the anatomy of spontaneous thought, Ingvar (1979) noted that the frontal lobes receive disproportionate blood flow during quiet wakefulness and suggested that SITS arise from the frontal lobes. One of the first modern studies to test this hypothesis found that dorsomedial prefrontal cortex (DMPFC) activity was correlated with subjective reports of SITS frequency (see Figure 21.1) (McGuire, Paulesu, Frackowiak, & Frith, 1996). In the 10 years since, the DMPFC has received increasing attention, bolstered by its inclusion within a so-called "default mode network" (DMN) that is deactivated across a range of tasks compared with a resting baseline (Raichle et al., 2001). The DMN includes the DMPFC (Brodmann's areas [BAs] 8/9/10 and the paracingulate region, BA 32), ventromedial PFC (BAs 32/25), posterior cingulate/precuneus (BAs 23/26/29/30/31/7), lateral posterior parietal cortex (BAs 39/40), and the hippocampi, all of which exhibit tight functional connectivity in the undirected human brain (Greicius, Krasnow, Reiss, & Menon, 2003). In keeping with Ingvar's ideas, both SITS and DMN activity are most prominent in unstructured situations and are attenuated by effortful cognitive tasks, which tend to activate the dorsal ACC (BA 24), adjacent pre–supplementary motor area (pSMA, BA 6), and the AI (Greicius et al., 2003; Raichle et al., 2001; Teasdale et al., 1995). Other salient stimuli that activate the ACC–pSMA–AI also deactivate the DMN (for a clear example, see Bartels & Zeki, 2004). The important difference occurs when subjects' assessments are directed inward. Judgments *about* one's current mental or emotional state (Figure 21.1, filled shapes) are less deactivating or even activating to the DMPFC compared with tasks that concern the outside world (Gusnard, Akbudak, Shulman, & Raichle, 2001; Gusnard

& Raichle, 2001; Lane, Fink, Chau, & Dolan, 1997; Ochsner et al., 2004). Induction of self-conscious social emotions, such as guilt and embarrassment (Figure 21.1), activates the same region of the DMPFC (Berthoz, Armony, Blair, & Dolan, 2002; Takahashi et al., 2004), as compared with experiencing primary emotions (anger, sadness, fear, happiness; not shown in Figure 21.1), which activate the ACC, insulae, and brainstem autonomic control sites (Damasio et al., 2000).

The emerging theme is that the DMPFC may help to identify thoughts as originating from or relating to a thinker, whether the thinker is the self or someone else. When subjects infer others' cognitive (Frith & Frith, 1999, 2003; Gallagher et al., 2000) or emotional (Ochsner et al., 2004) states, the activation patterns overlap specifically in the DMPFC. Though few studies have addressed self- and other-focused mental state attribution within the same experiment, those that have show overlapping DMPFC recruitment (Vogeley et al., 2001, 2004). The implication is that mental state attribution to others may indeed be built from the thought–feeling examination capacities we apply to our selves. So-called "metacognitive" or evaluative judgments, like those in which subjects compare statements to internal knowledge about the self or another (Schmitz, Kawahara-Baccus, & Johnson, 2004; Zysset, Huber, Ferstl, & von Cramon, 2002), also activate the DMPFC. Thus, integrating the research streams on body state representation and self-reference, it appears that the transition from the dorsal ACC through the paracingulate cortex and into the DMPFC somehow supports a transition from the emergence of feelings to directed thoughts about them: from interoception to introspection.

A glaring problem with this literature is the lack of carefully designed lesion studies (for an exception, see Bird, Castelli, Malik, Frith, & Husain, 2004) that address the necessity of the DMPFC for these functions. Laterality issues, though relevant, are difficult to dissect for midline structures using functional imaging due to spatial smoothing requirements. Furthermore, in some of the studies just mentioned, apparent activations of the DMPFC may have been driven by *greater deactivations* by cognitive control conditions rather than true activations by self-reflection (see Gusnard, Akbudak, Shulman, & Raichle, 2001, Figure 5, for an example highlighted by the authors).

Nonetheless, researchers report on the DMPFC far more often than other DMN sites that might turn up in this fashion (e.g., posterior cingulate cortex/precuneus), arguing that the DMPFC does in fact contribute to the functions we are describing. Indeed, in the Gusnard and colleagues (2001) study, most of the DMPFC was activated above both the resting baseline and cognitive control conditions.

A point we are quietly making is that body state data, the interoceptive stuff that dominates the minimal self, is manipulated by humans in some very special ways. Not only can we generate thoughts about how we feel, we can hold those thoughts up to the light of our long-term traits, goals, and plans for the future. Most often this window is useful, yet focusing on the past or future is no help when dealing with the saber-toothed tiger. As we next describe, the DMN—so readily deactivated by salient "here and now" stimuli—supports many of the long-term, "there and then" building projects that one had better suspend when homeostasis is imminently threatened.

## LONGITUDINAL SELF: THE SELF ACROSS TIME

If the minimal self describes self-representational acts that occur in the moment, the longitudinal self relates to elements of our extended individual life histories. Patients with global amnesia often illustrate this distinction. For example, the patient K.C. (for a comprehensive review, see Rosenbaum et al., 2005) moves effortlessly from moment to moment, and casual observers may find him quite normal. He makes basic daily decisions about feeding and hygiene and carries on pleasant interpersonal discourse, yet minimal probing reveals that K.C. is unable to travel mentally through time. This capacity, also referred to as "autonoetic consciousness" (Wheeler, Stuss, & Tulving, 1997), is the glue that holds the longitudinal self together. Without it, patients (including K.C.) may still name their own (previous) attributes and specify overlearned facts from their past, but these "memories" ring hollow. In the healthy brain, episodic memories ("Last weekend I helped at a soup kitchen") infuse semantic self-knowledge ("I do volunteer work") with personal significance. With time and experience, facts about the self are organized into enduring self-schemata ("I am a humanitarian") that interact with autonoesis to guide plans for the future (Markus, 1977). For K.C., lesions of the bilateral precuneus, medial temporal structures, and the left lateral frontoparietal lobe have left him confined to the minimal self, never venturing into mental images that flow from his personal past or future.

## The Longitudinal Minimal Self: Disposition and Response Tendencies

As K.C.'s story suggests, certain longitudinal facets of the self endure even when a person cannot conjure episodic proof of past behavior. K.C.'s general personality, a collection of moods, biases, response tendencies, character traits, and habits, has been far less changed by his injury than has his autonoetic awareness. Personality theory is a broad and complex topic with decades of experimental data to ground it. An in-depth review is untenable here. Instead, we briefly point to exciting hints of how genes and the environment might interact with the minimal self's neural architecture to produce a behaviorally consistent longitudinal self in adulthood.

What we are talking about here is how scores of minimal selves behave in the myriad moments that compose a week, a year, or a decade. When aspects of behavior are predictable and recurring, we think of them as traits. Interpersonal warmth, ingenuousness, dominance, persistence, avoidance, and other traits meld together to create persons we recognize as our friends, confidants, allies, lovers, and rivals. Remove these traits and we struggle to recognize persons as the same ones we have known.

Recent functional imaging studies have pursued this melding of the minimal and longitudinal selves, seeking interactions between personality measures collected outside the scanner and neural response patterns observed when subjects perform tasks governed (at least in part) by trait factors. Infants rated as "inhibited," for example, grow up to be adults who show stronger fMRI amygdala activations to novelty than do infants rated "uninhibited" (Schwartz, Wright, Shin, Kagan, & Rauch, 2003). Adults scoring high on trait "persistence" more avidly recruit the dorsal ACC and orbital frontoinsula (the same regions that respond to salience) to maintain task performance as contextual reinforcement wanes (Gusnard et al., 2003). Extending this approach, recent studies have shown how neuromodulatory system genes predict personal traits, perhaps by interacting with the structure and function of relevant brain regions. For instance, the *5-HTTLPR* gene, which helps regulate serotonergic neurotransmission, has a functional polymorphism that skews the likelihood of trait anxiety and alters gray matter volume and functional coupling of the subgenual ACC and amygdala (Pezawas et al., 2005). Approaches such as these promise to push the field forward and untangle the complex interactions among genes, neurodevelopment, environmental factors, and the longitudinal aspects of behavior.

## Self-Semantics, Autobiographical Memory, and the Medial Frontoparietal Surface

Functional imaging research within the past decade has begun to explore how the brain allows us to think about and keep track of who we are. To interpret this line of research is challenging and requires careful attention to methodological details (see Gillihan & Farah, 2005, for a helpful review). One key is to identify the type of self-related data that subjects are required to access in the scanner. For example, in some experiments subjects are asked to rate longitudinal aspects of the self, such as personal preferences or opinions (Seger, Stone, & Keenan, 2004; Zysset et al., 2002), or the self-descriptiveness of personal traits (Craik et al., 1999; Fossati et al., 2004; Johnson et al., 2002; Kelley et al., 2002; Kircher et al., 2000; Schmitz et al., 2004). To reach decisions about presented stimuli, subjects in these experiments may use semantic self-knowledge, related episodic memories, and provoked internal dispositions toward the stimuli and refer these elements back to the self and the stimuli. Thus, these tasks require a straddling of the minimal (how I feel about this trait descriptor right now) and longitudinal (how well that descriptor fits my self-schemata and life history) selves. The most consistent finding from these studies is that directed longitudinal semantic self-evaluation (Figure 21.2, squares) activates the same DMPFC region described previously and highlighted in Figure 21.1. Though less reliably, these self-semantic tasks also recruit medial parietal and posterior cingulate cortices, perhaps due to their episodic memory demands, or in some cases due to the same "lesser deactivation" confound mentioned earlier (see Kelley et al., 2002, for a clear example acknowledged by the authors). Two studies that

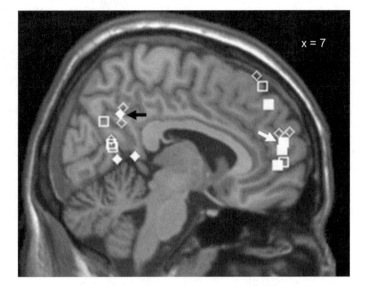

FIGURE 21.2. Functional activations of the longitudinal self. Shown are cluster activation maxima within 10 mm of the midline from regions of interest (ROIs) in the dorsomedial prefrontal (DMPFC: Brodmann's areas [BAs] 8/9/10/32) and precuneus–posterior cingulate (PreCu-PCC: BAs 7/31/30/23/26/29) cortices. Findings from 11 functional imaging studies are projected onto the MNI brain template. In five studies (Craik et al., 1999; Johnson et al., 2002; Kelley et al., 2002; Schmitz et al., 2004; Seger et al., 2004) subjects were asked to rate the self-descriptiveness of traits or opinions (squares), whereas in five others (Fink et al., 1996; Greenberg et al., 2005; Levine et al., 2004; Lou et al., 2004; Maddock et al., 2001), subjects were asked to recall or engage autobiographical episodes (diamonds). Three of five studies in each group reported both DMPFC and PreCu-PCC activations. Filled shapes indicate those foci that were isolated or significantly more prominent (thresholded at a twofold difference in cluster size) for that study. An additional study (Zysset et al., 2002) directly contrasted activations ocurring while subjects made yes–no judgments about their own opinions ("I like New Year's Eve parties") versus episodic memories ("I spent New Year's 2000 at home") and confirmed greater recruitment of the DMPFC for judging opinions (white arrow) and of the PreCu-PCC for episodic retrieval (black arrow).

compared trait judgments about the self versus those about another found greater right lateral frontal participation in self-directed processing (Craik et al., 1999; Schmitz et al., 2004). Two others, however, found no such association despite similar methodologies (Kelley et al., 2002; Seger et al., 2004).

Autobiographical memory is by definition related to the self, and brains cannot (or should not) recall episodes not part of their owner's life. Yet few studies have dissociated self-relevant, time-specific recollection from general retrieval processes within the same group of subjects. Those that have generally support the notion that episodic autobiographical memory recruits the DMPFC more robustly than do general retrieval processes, which involve medial parietal areas, particularly the precuneus and posterior cingulate cortex (Maguire & Mummery, 1999; Zysset

et al., 2002). In additional studies, subjects have been asked to think about (Andreasen et al., 1999; Greenberg et al., 2005; Lou et al., 2004; Maddock, Garrett, & Buonocore, 2001; Nyberg, Forkstam, Peterson, Cabeza, & Ingvar, 2002; Ryan et al., 2001), listen to (Fink et al., 1996; Levine et al., 2004), or judge the self-descriptiveness of specific real-life (Maguire, 2001; Maguire & Mummery, 1999) or recent laboratory (Lou et al., 2004) events. As shown in Figure 21.2, these studies more often show medial parietal activation than do semantic self-evaluation tasks in which episodic memory is not explicitly required. Thus, the DMPFC, which somehow participates in both semantic and episodic self-related memory, may be a node that helps bind the minimal and longitudinal selves together, marking elements of each as originating from or relating to the self.

Lesion studies provide an important complement to functional imaging paradigms by identifying brain regions that not only participate in but also are critical for a given function. Recent lesion analyses of longitudinal self-representation converge to suggest that nondominant frontotemporal connections enable a fluid and organized access to episodic memory (Andelman, Zuckerman-Feldhay, Hoffien, Fried, & Neufeld, 2004; Levine, 2004; Levine et al., 1998) and may help anchor core self-schemata and deeply rooted affiliations (Miller et al., 2001; see Seeley & Miller, 2005, for a review of self-representation disorders in patients with dementia).

## METHODOLOGICAL CHALLENGES AND SUGGESTIONS FOR FUTURE RESEARCH

The optimism conveyed by this chapter is tempered by strong concerns about the pitfalls of studying self-representation. Some of these hazards are better appreciated than others. Animal models will never capture certain qualitative aspects of the self that humans can describe. Functional imaging studies, though compelling and influential, are limited by a lack of understanding for how core networks, especially those implicated in self-representation, behave and interact during "rest." The undirected brain is in fact quite busy representing various aspects of the self. Therefore, block design analyses are ripe for misinterpretation: Those that subtract task activations from a "resting" baseline may underestimate DMN contributions to the task, whereas subtractions from a deactivating cognitive control condition may overestimate DMN contributions. Functional connectivity studies that complement anatomic data from monkeys should foster development of neural network models that are hypothesis-testable. Relationships between traits and brain activation patterns should be cautiously pursued, because they are subject to chicken-and-egg questions about whether traits produce signature activation patterns ("I activate more because I try harder"), or whether patterns produce traits ("I try harder because I activate more"). We suggest that converging research streams that relate or combine functional, structural, lesion-based, cytoarchitectural, and genetic approaches to self-representation have the greatest chance of effecting real progress.

## CONCLUDING REMARKS

The study of self-representation is of not only great intellectual but also biological and medical interest. We evolved the self to make our genes and bodies more fit, more enduring and viable, yet the most devastating neurodevelopmental, psychiatric, and degenerative neurological conditions we face are intimately self-representational and linked to the neural networks described in this chapter. A more sophisticated neurobiology of the self promises new hope for these disorders, in which the self's representational architectures misdevelop, derail, or erode over time.

## REFERENCES

Allman, J. M., Hakeem, A., Erwin, J. M., Nimchinsky, E., & Hof, P. (2001). The anterior cingulate cortex. The evolution of an interface between emotion and cognition. *Annals of the New York Academy of Sciences, 935,* 107–117.

Allman, J. M., Watson, K. K., Tetreault, N. A., & Hakeem, A. Y. (2005). Intuition and autism: A possible role for Von Economo neurons. *Trends in Cognitive Sciences, 9,* 367–373.

Amsterdam, B. (1972). Mirror self-image reactions before age two. *Developmental Psychobiology, 5*(4), 297–305.

Andelman, F., Zuckerman-Feldhay, E., Hoffien, D., Fried, I., & Neufeld, M. Y. (2004). Lateralization of deficit in self-awareness of memory in patients with intractable epilepsy. *Epilepsia, 45*(7), 826–833.

Anderson, J. R. (1995). Self-recognition in dolphins: Credible cetaceans; compromised criteria, controls, and conclusions. *Consciousness and Cognition, 4*(2), 239–43.

Andreasen, N. C., O'Leary, D. S. Paradiso, S., Cizadlo, T., Arndt, S., Watkins, G. L., et al. (1999). The cerebellum plays a role in conscious episodic memory retrieval. *Human Brain Mapping, 8,* 226–234.

Antrobus, J. S. (1968). Information theory and stimulus-independent thought. *British Journal of Psychology, 59,* 423–430.

Astafiev, S. V., Shulman, G. L., Stanley, C. M., Snyder, A. Z., Van Essen, D. C., & Corbetta, M. (2003). Functional organization of human intraparietal and frontal cortex for attending, looking, and pointing. *Journal of Neuroscience, 23*(11), 4689–4699.

Bartels, A., & Zeki, S. (2004). The neural correlates of maternal and romantic love. *NeuroImage, 21*(3), 1155–1166.

Bartsch, K., & Wellman, H. M. (1995). *Children talk about the mind.* New York: Oxford University Press.

Bates, E. (1990). Language about me and you: Pronomial reference and the emerging concept of self. In D. Cicchetti & M. Beeghly (Eds.), *The self in transi-*

tion: *Infancy to childhood* (pp. 165–182). Chicago: University of Chicago Press.

Bechara, A., Damasio, H., & Damasio, A. R. (2000). Emotion, decision making and the orbitofrontal cortex. *Cerebral Cortex, 10*(3), 295–307.

Beckmann, C. F., DeLuca, M., Devlin, J. T., & Smith, S. M. (2005). Investigations into resting-state connectivity using independent component analysis. *Philosophical Transactions of the Royal Society of London: Series B, Biological Sciences, 360*(1457), 1001–1013.

Berthoz, S., Armony, J. L., Blair, R. J. R., & Dolan, R. J. (2002). An fMRI study of intentional and unintentional (embarrassing) violations of social norms. *Brain, 125*(8), 1696–1708.

Bird, C. M., Castelli, F., Malik, O., Frith, U., & Husain, M. (2004). The impact of extensive medial frontal lobe damage on "Theory of Mind" and cognition. *Brain, 127*(Pt. 4), 914–928.

Blakemore, S. J. (2005). Recognizing the sensory consequences of one's own actions and delusions of control. In T. Feinberg & J. P. Keenan (Eds.), *The lost self: Pathologies of the brain and identity* (pp. 181–192). New York: Oxford University Press.

Blood, A. J., & Zatorre, R. J. (2001). Intensely pleasurable responses to music correlate with activity in brain regions implicated in reward and emotion. *Proceedings of the National Academy of Sciences of the United States of America, 98*(20), 11818–11823.

Broughton, J. (1978). Development of concepts of self, mind, reality, and knowledge. *New Directions for Child Development, 1*, 75–100.

Broughton, J. (1980). The divided self in adolescence. *Human Development, 24*, 13–32.

Brown, J. R., & Dunn, J. (1991). "You can cry, mum": The social and developmental implications of talk about internal states. *British Journal of Developmental Psychology, 9*, 237–256.

Butterworth, G. E. (1995). The self as an object of consciousness in infancy. In P. Rochat (Ed.), *The self in infancy: Theory and research* (pp. 35–51). Amsterdam: Elsevier.

Campos, J. J., & Stenberg, C. (1981). Perception, appraisal, and emotion: The onset of social referencing. In M. Lamb & L. Sherrod (Eds.), *Infant social cognition*. Hillsdale, NJ: Erlbaum.

Carmichael, S. T., & Price, J. L. (1996). Connectional networks within the orbital and medial prefrontal cortex of macaque monkeys. *Journal of Comparative Neurology, 371*(2), 179–207.

Carver, L. J., Bauer, P. J., & Nelson, C. A. (2000). Associations between infant brain activity and recall memory. *Developmental Science, 3*(2), 234–246.

Case, R. (1985). *Intellectual development: Birth to adulthood*. New York: Academic Press.

Case, R. (1992). *The mind's staircase*. Hillsdale, NJ: Erlbaum.

Cooley, C. H. (1902). *Human nature and the social order*. New York: Scribner.

Corbetta, M. (1998). Frontoparietal cortical networks for directing attention and the eye to visual locations: Identical, independent, or overlapping neural systems? *Proceedings of the National Academy of Sciences of the United States of America, 95*(3), 831–838.

Courage, M. L., & Howe, M. L. (2004). Advances in early memory development research: Insights about the dark side of the moon. *Developmental Review, 24*, 6–32.

Craig, A. D. (2002). How do you feel?: Interoception: The sense of the physiological condition of the body. *Nature Reviews: Neurosciences, 3*(8), 655–666.

Craig, A. D. (2003). Interoception: The sense of the physiological condition of the body. *Current Opinion in Neurobiology, 13*(4), 500–505.

Craig, A. D., Chen, K., Bandy, D., & Reiman, E. M. (2000). Thermosensory activation of insular cortex. *Nature Neuroscience, 3*(2), 184–190.

Craik, F. I. M., Moroz, T. M., Moscovitch, M., Stuss, D. T., Winocur, G., Tulving, E., et al. (1999). In search of the self: A positron emission tomography study. *Psychological Science, 10*(1), 26–34.

Critchley, H. D., Elliott, R., Mathias, C. J., & Dolan, R. J. (2000). Neural activity relating to generation and representation of galvanic skin conductance responses: A functional magnetic resonance imaging study. *Journal of Neuroscience, 20*(8), 3033–3040.

Critchley, H. D., Good, C. D., Ashburner, J., Frackowiak, R. S., Mathias, C. J., & Dolan, R. J. (2003). Changes in cerebral morphology consequent to peripheral autonomic denervation. *NeuroImage, 18*(4), 908–916.

Critchley, H. D., Mathias, C. J., & Dolan, R. J. (2001a). Neural activity in the human brain relating to uncertainty and arousal during anticipation. *Neuron, 29*(2), 537–545.

Critchley, H. D., Mathias, C. J., & Dolan, R. J. (2001b). Neuroanatomical basis for first- and second-order representations of bodily states. *Nature Neuroscience, 4*(2), 207–212.

Critchley, H. D., Mathias, C. J., Josephs, O., O'Doherty, J., Zanini, S., Dewar, B. K., et al. (2003). Human cingulate cortex and autonomic control: Converging neuroimaging and clinical evidence. *Brain, 126*(10), 2139–2152.

Critchley, H. D., Tang, J., Glaser, D., Butterworth, B., & Dolan, R. J. (2005). Anterior cingulate activity during error and autonomic response. *NeuroImage, 27*, 885–895.

Critchley, H. D., Wiens, S., Rotshtein, P., Ohman, A., & Dolan, R. J. (2004). Neural systems supporting interoceptive awareness. *Nature Neuroscience, 7*(2), 189–195.

Damasio, A. R. (1996). The somatic marker hypothesis and the possible functions of the prefrontal cortex. *Philosophical Transactions of the Royal Society of London: Series B, Biological Sciences, 351*(1346), 1413–1420.

Damasio, A. R. (1999). *The feeling of what happens:*

*Body and emotion in the making of consciousness.* Orlando, FL: Harcourt.

Damasio, A. R., Grahowski, T. J., Bechara, A., Damasio, H., Ponto, L. L., Parvizi, J., et al. (2000). Subcortical and cortical brain activity during the feeling of self-generated emotions. *Nature Neuroscience, 3*(10), 1049–1056.

Damon, W., & Hart, D. (1982). The development of self-understanding from infancy through adolescence. *Child Development, 53*(4), 841–864.

de Araujo, I. E., Kringelbach, M. L., Rolls, E. T., & McGlone, F. (2003). Human cortical responses to water in the mouth, and the effects of thirst. *Journal of Neurophysiology, 90*(3), 1865–1876.

de Veer, M. W., Gallup, G. G., Jr., Theall, L. A., van den Bos, R., & Povinelli, D. J. (2003). An 8-year longitudinal study of mirror self-recognition in chimpanzees (*Pan troglodytes*). *Neuropsychologia, 41*(2), 229–234.

Egan, G., Silk, T., Zamarripa, F., Williams, J., Federico, P., Cunnington, R., et al. (2003). Neural correlates of the emergence of consciousness of thirst. *Proceedings of the National Academy of Sciences of the United States of America, 100*(25), 15241–15246.

Eisenberger, N. I., & Lieberman, M. D. (2004). Why rejection hurts: A common neural alarm system for physical and social pain. *Trends in Cognitive Sciences, 8*(7), 294–300.

Eisenberger, N. I., Lieberman, M. D., & Williams, K. D. (2003). Does rejection hurt?: An FMRI study of social exclusion. *Science, 302*, 290–292.

Fay, W. H. (1979). Personal pronouns and the autistic child. *Journal of Autism and Developmental Disorders, 9*(3), 247–260.

Fink, G. R., Markowitsch, H. J., Reinkemeier, M., Bruckbauer, T., Kessler, J., & Heiss, W. D. (1996). Cerebral representation of one's own past: Neural networks involved in autobiographical memory. *Journal of Neuroscience, 16*(13), 4275–4282.

Fischer, K. W. (1980). A theory of cognitive development: The control and construction of hierarchies of skills. *Psychological Review, 87*, 477–531.

Fischer, K. W., Shaver, P., & Carnochan, P. (1990). How emotions develop and how they organize development. *Cognition and Emotion, 4*, 81–127.

Flavell, J. H., Green, F. L., & Flavell, E. R. (1993). Children's understanding of the stream of consciousness. *Child Development, 64*, 387–398.

Flavell, J. H., Green, F. L., & Flavell, E. R. (1995). Young children's knowledge of thinking. *Monographs of the Society for Research in Child Development, 60*(Serial No. 243).

Fossati, P., Hevenor, S. J., Lepage, M., Graham, S. J., Grady, C., Keightley, M. L., et al. (2004). Distributed self in episodic memory: Neural correlates of successful retrieval of self-encoded positive and negative personality traits. *NeuroImage, 22*, 1596–1604.

Frith, C. D., & Frith, U. (1999). Interacting minds—a biological basis. *Science, 286*, 1692–1695.

Frith, U., & Frith, C. D. (2003). Development and neurophysiology of mentalizing. In C. D. Frith & D. M. Wolpert (Eds.), *The neuroscience of social interaction* (pp. 45–76). New York: Oxford University Press.

Gallagher, H. L., Happe, F., Brunswick, N., Fletcher, P. C., Frith, U., & Frith, C. D. (2000). Reading the mind in cartoons and stories: An fMRI study of "theory of mind" in verbal and nonverbal tasks. *Neuropsychologia, 38*(1), 11–21.

Gallagher, I. I. (2000). Philosophical conceptions of the self: Implications for cognitive science. *Trends in Cognitive Sciences, 4*(1), 14–21.

Gallup, G. G., Jr. (1970). Chimpanzees: Self-recognition. *Science, 167*, 86–87.

Gallup, G. G., Jr. (1982). Self-awareness and the emergence of mind in primates. *American Journal of Primatology, 2*, 237–248.

Gallup, G. G., Jr. (1987). Toward a comparative psychology of self-awareness: Species limitations and cognitive consequences. In G. R. Goethals & J. Strauss (Eds.), *The self: An interdisciplinary approach* (pp. 121–135). New York: Springer.

Gallup, G. G., Jr. (1995). Mirrors, minds, and cetaceans. *Consciousness and Cognition, 4*(2), 226–228.

Gillihan, S. J., & Farah, M. J. (2005). The cognitive neuroscience of the self: insights from functional neuroimaging of the normal brain. In T. Feinberg & J. P. Keenan (Eds.), *The lost self: Pathologies of the brain and identity* (pp. 20–32). New York: Oxford University Press.

Greenberg, D. L., Rice, H. J., Cooper, J. J., Cabeza, R., Rubin, D. C., & Labar, K. S. (2005). Co-activation of the amygdala, hippocampus and inferior gyrus during autobiographical memory retrieval. *Neuropsychologia, 43*, 659–674.

Greicius, M. D., Krasnow, B., Reiss, A. L., & Menon, V. (2003). Functional connectivity in the resting brain: A network analysis of the default mode hypothesis. *Proceedings of the National Academy of Sciences of the United States of America, 100*(1), 253–258.

Griffin, N. (1992). Structural analysis of the development of their inner world: A neo-structural analysis of the development of intrapersonal intelligence. In R. Case (Ed.), *The mind's staircase* (pp. 189–206). Hillsdale, NJ: Erlbaum.

Gusnard, D. A., Akbudak, E., Shulman, G. L., & Raichle, M. E. (2001). Medial prefrontal cortex and self-referential mental activity: Relation to a default mode of brain function. *Proceedings of the National Academy of Sciences of the United States of America, 98*(7), 4259–4264.

Gusnard, D. A., Ollinger, J. M., Shulman, G. L., Cloninger, C. R., Price, J. L., & Van Essen, D. C. (2003). Persistence and brain circuitry. *Proceedings of the National Academy of Sciences of the United States of America, 100*(6), 3479–3484.

Gusnard, D. A., & Raichle, M. E. (2001). Searching for

a baseline: Functional imaging and the resting human brain. *Nature Reviews: Neuroscience, 2*(10), 685–694.

Hains, S. M. J., & Muir, D. W. (1996). Infant sensitivity to adult eye direction. *Infant Behavior and Development, 67*(5), 1940–1951.

Haith, M. M., Bergman, T., & Moore, M. J. (1977). Eye contact and face scanning in early infancy. *Science, 198*, 853–855.

Harris, P. L. (1991). The work of the imagination. In A. Whiten (Ed.), *Natural theories of mind* (pp. 283–304). Oxford, UK: Blackwell.

Harter, S. (1998). The development of self-representations. In W. S. E. Damon & N. V. E. Eisenberg (Eds.), *Handbook of child psychology: Vol. 3. Social, emotional, and personality development* (pp. 553–617). New York: Wiley.

Harter, S. (2003). Development of self-representations during childhood and adolescence. In M. R. Leary & J. P. Tangney (Eds.), *Handbook of self and identity* (pp. 610–642). New York: Guilford Press.

Hauser, M. D., Kralik, J., Botto-Mahan, C., Garrett, M., & Oser, J. (1995). Self-recognition in primates: Phylogeny and the salience of species-typical features. *Proceedings of the National Academy of Sciences of the United States of America, 92*(23), 10811–10814.

Heidbreder, E., Ziegler, A., Schafferhans, K., Heidland, A., & Gruninger, W. (1984). Psychomental stress in tetraplegic man: Dissociation in autonomic variables and emotional responsiveness. *Journal of Human Stress, 10*(4), 157–164.

Higgins, E. T. (1991). Development of self-regulatory and self-evaluative processes: Costs, benefits, and tradeoff. In M. R. Gunnar & L. A. Sroufe (Eds.), *The Minnesota Symposia on Child Development: Self-processes and development* (Vol. 23, pp. 125–166). Hillsdale, NJ: Erlbaum.

Howe, M. L. (2004). Early memory, early self, emergence of autobiographical memory. In D. R. Beike, J. M. Lampinen, & D. A. Behrend (Eds.), *The self and memory* (pp. 45–72). New York: Psychology Press.

Howe, M. L., & Courage, M. L. (1997). The emergence and early development of autobiographical memory. *Psychological Review, 104*, 499–523.

Howe, M. L., Courage, M. L., & Edison, S. C. (2003). When autobiographical memory begins. *Developmental Review, 23*, 471–494.

Ickes, W., Reidhead, S., & Patterson, M. (1986). Machiavellianism and self-monitoring: As different as "you" and "me." *Social Cognition, 4*(1), 58–74.

Ingvar, D. H. (1979). "Hyperfrontal" distribution of the cerebral grey matter flow in resting wakefulness: On the functional anatomy of the conscious state. *Acta Neurologica Scandinavica, 60*(1), 12–25.

Insel, T. R., & Young, L. J. (2001). The neurobiology of attachment. *Nature Reviews: Neuroscience, 2*(2), 129–136.

James, W. (1890). *Principles of psychology.* Boston: Harvard University Press.

Jasmin, L., Burkey, A. R., Granato, A., & Ohara, P. T. (2004). Rostral agranular insular cortex and pain areas of the central nervous system: A tract-tracing study in the rat. *Journal of Comparative Neurology, 468*(3), 425–440.

Joffe, T. H., & Dunbar, R. I. (1997). Visual and socio-cognitive information processing in primate brain evolution. *Proceedings of the Royal Society of London: Series B, Biological Sciences, 264*, 1303–1307.

Johnson, S. C., Baxter, L. C., Wilder, L. S., Pipe, J. G., Heiserman, J. E., & Prigatano, G. P. (2002). Neural correlates of self-reflection. *Brain 125*(8), 1808–1814.

Kagan, J. (1984). *The nature of the child.* New York: Basic Books.

Kagan, J. (1989). *Unstable ideas: Temperament, cognition, and self.* Cambridge, MA: Harvard University Press.

Kelley, W. M., Macrae, C. N., Wyland, C. L., Caglar, S., Inati, S., & Heatherton, T. E. (2002). Finding the self? An event-related fMRI study. *Journal of Cognitive Neuroscience, 14*(5), 785–794.

Kircher, T. T., Senior, C., Phillips, M. L., Benson, P. J., Bullmore, E. T., Brammer, M., et al. (2000). Towards a functional neuroanatomy of self processing: Effects of faces and words. *Cognitive Brain Research, 10*(1–2), 133–144.

Korner, A. F., & Kraemer, H. C. (1972). Individual differences in spontaneous oral behavior in neonates. In J. F. Bosma (Ed.), *Third Symposium on Oral Sensation and Perception* (pp. 335–346). Bethesda, MD: U.S. Department of Health Education and Welfare.

Lane, R. D., Fink, G. F., Chau, P. M.-L., & Dolan, R. J. (1997). Neural activation during selective attention to subjective emotional responses. *NeuroReport, 8*, 3969–3972.

Levine, B. (2004). Autobiographical memory and the self in time: Brain lesion effects, functional neuroanatomy, and lifespan development. *Brain Cognition, 55*(1), 54–68.

Levine, B., Black, S. E., Cabeza, R., Sinden, M., Mcintosh, A. R., Toth, J. P., et al. (1998). Episodic memory and the self in a case of isolated retrograde amnesia. *Brain, 121*(10), 1951–1973.

Levine, B., Turner, G. R., Tisserand, D., Hevenor, S. J., Graham, S. J., & Mcintosh, A. R. (2004). The functional neuroanatomy of episodic and semantic autobiographical remembering: A prospective functional MRI study. *Journal of Cognitive Neuroscience, 16*(9), 1633–1646.

Lewis, M., & Brooks-Gunn, J. (1985). Individual differences in early visual self-recognition. *Developmental Psychology, 21*, 1181–1187.

Lewis, M., Sullivan, M. W., Stanger, C., & Weiss, M. (1989). Self-development and self-conscious emotions. *Child Development, 60*, 146–156.

Lou, H. C., Luber, B., Crupain, M., Keenan, J. P.,

Nowak, M., Kjaer, T. W., et al. (2004). Parietal cortex and representation of the mental self. *Proceedings of the National Academy of Sciences of the United States of America, 101*(7), 6827–6832.

Maddock, R. J., Garrett, A. S., & Buonocore, M. H. (2001). Remembering familiar people: The posterior cingulate cortex and autobiographical memory retrieval. *Neuroscience, 104*(3), 667–676.

Maguire, E. A. (2001). Neuroimaging studies of autobiographical event memory. *Philosophical Transactions of the Royal Society of London, Series B, 356,* 1441–1451.

Maguire, E. A., & Mummery, C. J. (1999). Differential modulation of a common memory retrieval network revealed by positron emission tomography. *Hippocampus, 9*(1), 54–61.

Markus, H. (1977). Self-schemata and processing information about the self. *Journal of Personality and Social Psychology, 35*(2), 63–78.

Marten, K., & Psarakos, S. (1995). Using self-view television to distinguish between self-examination and social behavior in the bottlenose dolphin (*Tursiops truncatus*). *Consciousness and Cognition, 4*(2), 205–224.

Maurer, D. (1985). Infants' perception of faceness. In T. N. Field & N. Fox (Eds.), *Social perception in infants* (pp. 37–66). Hillsdale, NJ: Erlbaum.

McGuire, P. K., Paulesu, E., Frackowiak, R. S., & Frith, C. D. (1996). Brain activity during stimulus independent thought. *NeuroReport, 7*(13), 2095–2099.

Meltzoff, A. N. (1990). Towards a developmental cognitive science: The implications of cross-modal matching and imitation for the development of representation and memory in infancy. *Annals of the New York Academy of Sciences, 608,* 1–31.

Meltzoff, A. N., & Borton, R. W. (1979). Intermodal matching by human neonates. *Nature, 282,* 403–404.

Meltzoff, A. N., & Moore, M. K. (1983). Newborn infants imitate adult facial gestures. *Child Development, 54*(3), 702–709.

Meltzoff, A. N., & Moore, M. K. (1997). Explaining facial imitation: A theoretical model. *Early Development and Parenting, 63*(3–4), 179–192.

Mesulam, M. M. (1981). A cortical network for directed attention and unilateral neglect. *Annals of Neurology, 10*(4), 309–325.

Miller, B. L., Seeley, W. W., Mychack, P., Rosen, H. J., Mena, I., & Boone, K. (2001). Neuroanatomy of the self: Evidence from patients with frontotemporal dementia. *Neurology, 57*(5), 817–821.

Morton, J., & Johnson, M. H. (1991). CONSPEC and CONLEARN: A two-process theory of infant face recognition. *Psychological Review, 98*(2), 164–181.

Nauta, W. J. (1971). The problem of the frontal lobe: A reinterpretation. *Journal of Psychiatric Research, 8*(3), 167–187.

Neisser, U. (1988). Five kinds of self-knowledge. *Philosophical Psychology, 1,* 35–59.

Neisser, U. (1991). Two perceptually given aspects of self and their development. *Developmental Review, 11*(3), 197–209.

Neisser, U. (1993). *The perceived self.* New York: Cambridge University Press.

Nelson, C. A. (1987). The recognition of facial expressions in the first two years of life: Mechanisms of development. *Child Development, 58*(4), 889–909.

Nelson, F. (1993). The psychological and social origins of autobiographical memory. *Psychological Science, 4,* 7–14.

Nimchinsky, E. A., Gilissen, E., Allman, J. M., Perl, D. P., Erwin, J. M., & Hof, P. R. (1999). A neuronal morphologic type unique to humans and great apes. *Proceedings of the National Academy of Sciences of the United States of America, 96*(9), 5268–5273.

Nimchinsky, E. A., Vogt, B. A., Morrison, J. H., & Hof, P. R. (1995). Spindle neurons of the human anterior cingulate cortex. *Journal of Comparative Neurology, 355*(1), 27–37.

Nyberg, L., Forkstam, C., Peterson, K. M., Cabeza, R., & Ingvar, M. (2002). Brain imaging of human memory systems: Between-systems similarities and within-systems differences. *Cognitive Brain Research, 13,* 281–292.

Ochsner, K. N., Knierim, K., Ludlow, D. H., Hanelin, J., Ramachandran, T., Glover, G., et al. (2004). Reflecting upon feelings: An fMRI study of neural systems supporting the attribution of emotion to self and other. *Journal of Cognitive Neuroscience, 16*(10), 1746–1772.

Olausson, H., Lamarre, Y., Backlund, H., Morin, C., Wallin, B. G., Starck, G., et al. (2002). Unmyelinated tactile afferents signal touch and project to insular cortex. *Nature Neuroscience, 5*(9), 900–904.

Ongur, D., & Price, J. L. (2000). The organization of networks within the orbital and medial prefrontal cortex of rats, monkeys and humans. *Cerebral Cortex, 10*(3), 206–219.

Papousek, H., & Papousek, M. (1974). Mirror and image self-recognition in young human infants: Vol. 1. A new method of experimental analysis. *Developmental Psychobiology, 7*(2), 149–157.

Parker, S. T. (1997). A general model for the adaptive function of self-knowledge in animals and humans. *Consciousness and Cognition, 6*(1), 75–86.

Patterson, F. (1984). Self-recognition by gorilla (*Gorilla gorilla*). *Gorilla, 7,* 2–3.

Pezawas, L., Meyer-Lindenberg, A., Drabant, E. M., Verchinski, B. A., Munoz, K. E., Kolachana, B. S., et al. (2005). 5-HTTLPR polymorphism impacts human cingulate–amygdala interactions: A genetic susceptibility mechanism for depression. *Nature Neuroscience, 8*(6), 828–834.

Ploghaus, A., Tracey, I., Gati, J. S., Clare, S., Menon, R. S., Matthews, P. M., et al. (1999). Dissociating pain from its anticipation in the human brain. *Science, 284*(5422), 1979–1981.

Potts, R. (2004). Paleoenvironmental basis of cognitive evolution in great apes. *American Journal of Primatology, 62*(3), 209–228.

Povinelli, D. J. (1993). Reconstructing the evolution of mind. *American Psychologist, 48*(5), 493–509.

Povinelli, D. J., & Cant, J. G. (1995). Arboreal clambering and the evolution of self-conception. *Quarterly Review of Biology, 70*(4), 393–421.

Radke-Yarrow, M., Belmont, B., Nottelmann, E., & Bottomly, L. (1990). Young children's self-conceptions: Origins in the natural course of depressed and normal mothers and their children. In D. Cicchetti & M. Beeghly (Eds.), *The self in transition: Infancy to childhood* (pp. 345–362). Chicago: University of Chicago Press.

Raichle, M. E., MacLeod, A. M., Snyder, A. Z., Powers, W. J., & Gusnard, D. A. (2001a). A default mode of brain function. *Proceedings of the National Academy of Sciences of the United States of America, 98*(2), 676–682.

Raichle, M. E., MacLeod, A. M., Snyder, A. Z., Powers, W. J., Gusnard, D. A., & Shulman, G. L. (2001b). A default mode of brain function. *Proceedings of the National Academy of Sciences of the United States of America, 98*(2), 676–682.

Reiss, D., & Marino, L. (2001). Mirror self-recognition in the bottlenose dolphin: A case of cognitive convergence. *Proceedings of the National Academy of Sciences of the United States of America, 98*(10), 5937–5942.

Repacholi, B. M., & Gopnik, A. (1997). Early reasoning about desires: Evidence from 14- and 18-month-olds. *Developmental Psychobiology, 33*, 12–21.

Rochat, P. (1998). Self-perception and action in infancy. *Experimental Brain Research, 123*, 102–109.

Rochat, P. (2001). *The infant's world*. Cambridge, MA: Harvard University Press.

Rolls, E. T., O'Doherty, J., Kringelbach, M. L., Francis, S., Bowtell, R., & McGlone, F. (2003). Representations of pleasant and painful touch in the human orbitofrontal and cingulate cortices. *Cerebral Cortex, 13*(3), 308–317.

Rosenbaum, R. S., Kohler, S., Schacter, D. L., Moscovitch, M., Westmacott, R., Black, S. E., et al. (2005). The case of K.C.: Contributions of a memory-impaired person to memory theory. *Neuropsychologia, 43*(7), 989–1021.

Rovee-Collier, C. K. (1997). Dissociations in infant memory: Rethinking the development of implicit and explicit memory. *Psychological Review, 104*(2), 467–498.

Ryan, L., Nadel, L., Keil, K., Putnam, K., Schnyer, D., Trouard, T., et al. (2001). Hippocampal complex and retrieval of recent and very remote autobiographical memories: Evidence from functional magnetic resonance imaging in neurologically intact people. *Hippocampus, 11*, 707–714.

Schmitz, T. W., Kawahara-Baccus, T. N., & Johnson, S. C. (2004). Metacognitive evaluation, self-relevance, and the right prefrontal cortex. *NeuroImage, 22*(2), 941–947.

Schwartz, C. E., Wright, C. I., Shin, L. M., Kagan, J., & Rauch, S. L. (2003). Inhibited and uninhibited infants "grown up": Adult amygdalar response to novelty. *Science, 300*, 1952–1953.

Seeley, W., & Miller, B. (2005). Disorders of the self in dementia. In T. E. Feinberg & J. P. Keenan (Eds.), *The lost self: Pathologies of brain and identity* (pp. 147–165). New York: Oxford University Press.

Seeley, W. W., Lomen-Hoerth, C., & Miller, B. (2005). Pain without worry and suffering: Altered pain processing in frontotemporal lobar degeneration and Alzheimer's disease. *Neurology, 64*(6, Suppl. 1), A225.

Seger, C. A., Stone, M., & Keenan, J. P. (2004). Cortical activations during judgments about the self and an other person. *Neuropsychologia, 42*, 1168–1177.

Selman, R. (1980). *The growth of interpersonal understanding*. New York: Academic Press.

Sewards, T. V., & Sewards, M. A. (2000). The awareness of thirst: Proposed neural correlates. *Consciousness and Cognition, 9*(4), 463–487.

Shillito, D. J., Gallup, G. G., Jr., & Beck, B. B. (1999). Factors affecting mirror behaviour in western lowland gorillas, Gorilla gorilla. *Animal Behavior, 57*(5), 999–1004.

Siegel, D. J. (1999). *The developing mind: How relationships and the brain interact to shape who we are*. New York: Guilford Press.

Singer, T., Seymour, B., O'Doherty, J., Kaube, H., Dolan, R. J., & Frith, C. D. (2004). Empathy for pain involves the affective but not sensory components of pain. *Science, 303*, 1157–1162.

Smith, J. D., Shields, W. E., & Washburn, D. A. (2003). The comparative psychology of uncertainty monitoring and metacognition. *Behavioral and Brain Sciences, 26*(3), 317–339; discussion, 340–373.

Snow, K. (1990). Building memories: The ontogeny of autobiography. In D. Cicchetti & M. Beeghly (Eds.), *The self in transition: Infancy to childhood* (pp. 213–242). Chicago: University of Chicago Press.

Squire, L., Knowlton, B., & Musen, G. (1993). The structure and organization of memory. *Annual Review of Psychology, 44*, 453–495.

Takahashi, H., Yahata, N., Koeda, M., Matsuda, T., Asai, K., & Okubo, Y. (2004). Brain activation associated with evaluative processes of guilt and embarrassment: An fMRI study. *NeuroImage, 23*, 967–974.

Tangney, J. P. (1999). The self-conscious emotions: Shame, guilt, embarrassment, and pride. In T. Dalgleish & M. J. Power (Eds.), *Handbook of cognition and emotion* (pp. 541–568). New York: Wiley.

Teasdale, J. D., Dritschel, B. H., Taylor, M. J., Proctor, L., Lloyd, C. A., Nimmo-Smith, I., et al. (1995). Stimulus-independent thought depends on central executive resources. *Memory and Cognition, 23*(5), 551–559.

Tronick, E. Z. (1989). Emotions and emotional communication in infants. *American Psychologist, 44*(2), 112–119.

Vandenbergh, J., Dupont, P., Fischler, B., Bormans, G., Persoons, P., Janssens, J., et al. (2005). Regional brain activation during proximal stomach distention in humans: A positron emission tomography study. *Gastroenterology, 128*(3), 564–573.

Vogeley, K., Bussfeld, P., Newen, A., Herrmann, S., Happe, F., Falkai, P., et al. (2001). Mind reading: Neural mechanisms of Theory of Mind and self-perspective. *NeuroImage, 14*(1), 170–181.

Vogeley, K., & Fink, G. R. (2003). Neural correlates of the first-person-perspective. *Trends in Cognitive Sciences, 7*(1), 38–42.

Vogeley, K., May, M., Ritzl, A., Falkai, P., Zilles, K., & Fink, G. R. (2004). Neural correlates of first-person perspective as one constituent of human self-consciousness. *Journal of Cognitive Neuroscience, 16*(5), 817–827.

von Economo, C. (1926). Eine neue Art Spezialzellen des Lobus cinguli und Lobus insulae. *Zeitschrift für die Gesamte Neurologie Psychiatrie, 100,* 706–712.

Wellman, H. M., Cross, D., & Watson, J. (2001). Meta-analysis of theory-of-mind development: The truth about false belief. *Child Development, 72*(3), 655–684.

Wellman, H. M., & Estes, D. (1986). Early understanding of mental entities: A reexamination of childhood realism. *Child Development, 57,* 910–923.

Wheeler, M. A., Stuss, D. T., & Tulving, E. (1997). Toward a theory of episodic memory: The frontal lobes and autonoetic consciousness. *Psychological Bulletin, 121,* 331–354.

Zysset, S., Huber, O., Ferstl, E., & von Cramon, D. Y. (2002). The anterior frontomedian cortex and evaluative judgment: An fMRI study. *NeuroImage, 15*(4), 983–991.

# CHAPTER 22

# Frontal Dysfunction and Capacity to Consent to Treatment or Research

## CONCEPTUAL CONSIDERATIONS AND EMPIRICAL EVIDENCE

*Laura B. Dunn*
*Barton W. Palmer*
*Jason H. T. Karlawish*

Clinical research is necessary for the advancement of science and to improve clinical methods. Yet there is legitimate concern about the competence of persons with neuropathological disorders affecting frontal systems to provide informed consent to enter clinical research. Similar concerns occur in treatment settings, in particular the competency to refuse a prescribed treatment. Specifically, neuropathological disorders affecting frontal systems may impair a person's self-regulatory processes and self-awareness, which in turn may hinder cognitive processes that are core components of the competency to consent to treatment or research.

In this chapter, we review the influence of frontal systems and dysfunction in those systems on the ability to provide consent to treatment or research participation. First, we review the concepts of decision-making capacity and competency, and summarize when and how clinicians and researchers can most effectively screen or evaluate patients or potential research participants. Next, we consider the frontal–subcortical circuits, and the cognitive, behavioral, and affective functions they serve, that may be relevant to consent capacity. Then we consider empirical evidence regarding the influence of frontal neuropathology on decision-making skills. We conclude with a summary and tentative recommendations for clinicians and researchers working with patients who have frontal pathology, and point to areas needing additional empirical attention.

## COMPETENCY AND DECISION-MAKING CAPACITY

The concept of competency, one of three components of the modern-day model of informed consent, which we discuss in the context of consent for treatment- or research-related decisions, evolved from case law and consensus of experts in the field. The components are (1) disclosure of relevant information; (2) voluntariness of the decision (i.e., absence of coercion or undue influence); and (3) competency to make the decision (Faden, Beauchamp, & King, 1986; Grisso, 2003; Grisso & Appelbaum, 1998). The focus of this chapter is the third component: competency.

Competency has traditionally been viewed as a legal construct (i.e., a court or other legal proceeding leading to a finding of competency or incompetency). The bioethics principle of respect for persons (National Commission for the Protection of Human Subjects of Biomedical and Behavioral Research, 1978), as well as Western societies' general emphasis on treating individuals as autonomous agents, mean that our legal system generally views adults as competent to decide until proven otherwise. With certain exceptions, children, that is, persons under age 18, are generally presumed not to be competent. This is in part due to the presumed lack of full, reasoned judgment among non-adults; in this regard, it is noteworthy that the frontal lobes are among the last brain regions to complete neurodevelopment.

The proof that someone is not competent relies on an assessment of his or her decision-making capacity. In this chapter, we generally use the term "decision-making capacity" to maintain the distinction between competency as a legal concept versus capacity as a clinical construct. However, decision-making capacity is at the core of the contemporary concept of competency, because persons who lack capacity are not competent. A finding of the lack of capacity for *all* decisions in a given realm of functioning (e.g., finances, health care) requires a legal proceeding and the final determination is generally made by the courts, not clinicians or researchers, or policymakers/regulatory authorities.

A capacity assessment is required when there is concern about a person's ability to make a decision. When persons are found incompetent because they lack decision-making capacity, they forfeit their right to make their own decisions, *not* because we disagree with their reasons and their choice, but because they lack the requisite abilities to make that choice. However, in clinical practice, there may indeed be some functional bias to use either a person's reasons or choice as a prompt to assess his or her decision-making capacity. In particular, few physicians initiate a competency evaluation when patients accept their recommended treatment. Such evaluations commonly arise when patients refuse the clinician's recommended treatment (e.g., when a psychotic patient refuses hospitalization and/or treatment with antipsychotic medications).

The focus on the ability to make a decision has considerable conceptual and ethical advantages over concepts of competency that were common until the 1980s. Previously, competency was largely conceptualized on the basis of two things: a person's status and his or her choice. Competency was indicated by the choice of a reasonable adult in good mental health. In cases when a person's competency was called into question, a competency assessment typically focused on whether a person's choice conformed to notions of what constitutes a "reasonable choice." A judgment of incompetency was further supplemented by clinical information that described the severity of the person's mental illness to explain why the choice was judged "unreasonable." Such competency assessment largely relied on informal exchanges between an examiner and the person, rather than any structured or standardized evaluation, so the results were vulnerable to the idiosyncratic biases of the individual interviewer or court judge.

This model has substantial shortcomings. Chief among these is its failure to serve the ethical purpose of a competency assessment—that is, finding an appropriate balance between the ethical principles of respect for autonomy and beneficence (Faden et al., 1986). Placing the emphasis on the so-called "reasonableness" of the decision disregards the fact that individuals incorporate unique values and motivations into their decision making. "Reasonableness" is to a large degree in the eye of the beholder. Using this as the sole standard for competency is thus problematic. Instead, reasoning is best assessed by examining the logic behind individuals' choices, taking into account their personal values. A competent person has a personal claim relative to judging what is in his or her best interests.

The construct of decision-making capacity relies on an assessment of at least one of a person's decision-making abilities (Grisso & Appelbaum, 1998). There are four widely recognized decision-making abilities: understanding, appreciation, reasoning, and choice. Understanding is a core ability, because in some legal jurisdictions, it is the sole ability a person needs to demonstrate in order to be judged competent. It entails knowing the meaning of the information relevant to a decision. The second ability, appreciation, is distinct from understanding in that it describes the ability to recognize how information applies to the person. In the case of appreciation of a disorder, this ability is akin to the psychologist's construct of insight, or awareness. For example, in the context of treatment capacity, a person with adequate insight recognizes the nature and extent of his or her disorder. The ability to reason describes the presence of reasoning abilities (ability to manipulate information) and *not* the outcome of that reasoning process. For example, in the model put forth by Grisso and Appelbaum (1988), the "reasoning" component of decision-making capacity can be met by demonstrating the presence and application of comparative and consequential reasoning processes. The former describes explaining how one option is better than another, and the latter, explaining the potential consequences of following one course or another (e.g., the impact of likely consequences on one's daily life). The ability to express a choice is the simplest of the abilities, because it describes the ability to articulate a clear and consistent decision. The issue here is not individuals' explanation of their decision, but simply that they can make a choice.

"Decision-making capacity" is not the same kind of a person-centered trait as a cognitive ability. The construct of the abilities needed to make a choice is the product of an interaction between intrapersonal factors, the inherent complexity of the information or choice to be made, as well as the quality of the consent process (see Figure 22.1). Intrapersonal factors may include transitory or potentially modifiable factors (arousal, sleepiness, state anxiety, interest/motivation, etc.), stable but potentially modifiable factors (e.g., trait anxiety, vocabulary, familiarity with treatment or research concepts, and perhaps insight), and stable factors that are resistant to most forms of modification (e.g., cognitive functioning). The inherent complexity of the information is not readily modifiable, but the manner in which that information is communicated to the person may be, and the latter may be the most obvious target for "consent enhancement" (Carpenter et al., 2000; Dunn & Jeste, 2001; Dunn et al., 2002). For instance, Dunn and colleagues have shown that provision of research consent forms in a PowerPoint-based (bulleted text) format, as well as checking for misunderstood information with feedback, can improve understanding of relevant information regarding research among middle-age and older patients with schizophrenia.

## ASSESSING DECISION-MAKING CAPACITY

A capacity assessment is a decision-specific assessment. If a patient is being asked to make a decision about a surgical procedure, questioning needs to be directed to evaluating the patient's capacity to understand, appreciate, reason, and express a choice regarding this *specific* decision, rather than about general medical treatment or general decision making in the patient's life. Also, decision-making capacity assessments do not focus on whether people make ideal, logical decisions (which, if held as a rigid standard, few of us would meet) (Tversky & Kahneman, 1974). Instead, they focus on the ability to make a specific decision. In the clinical treatment context, a finding of incompetence means that it may be appropriate, *in a given situation at a specific time*, to disregard the person's choice and instead permit someone else to make the decision for that person (Grisso & Appelbaum, 1998).

### Capacity Instruments

Information about a person's decision-making capacity can be obtained through a structured interview that includes a decisional capacity instrument. A number of instruments specifically designed to assist clinicians and researchers in their evaluations of decision-making capacity have been developed (reviewed in Dunn, Nowrangi, Palmer, Jeste, & Saks, 2006; Grisso, 2003). Two of the most widely used and best validated are the MacArthur Competence Assessment Tools for Treatment (MacCAT-T) and for Clinical Research (MacCAT-CR).

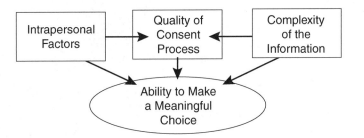

FIGURE 22.1. Decisional capacity as a social-cognitive construct.

The MacCAT-T and MacCAT-CR are semi-structured interviews that are adaptable to any treatment- or research-related decision. The content of disclosures must be modified for the specific decision facing the patient or participant (Appelbaum & Grisso, 2001; Grisso, Appelbaum, & Hill-Fotouhi, 1997). Each takes about 15–20 minutes to administer, and was derived from substantially lengthier instruments used in a large study of competency among psychiatric and medical patients, as well as healthy controls (Appelbaum & Grisso, 1995; Grisso & Appelbaum, 1995; Grisso, Appelbaum, Mulvey, & Fletcher, 1995). The MacCAT-T and MacCAT-CR have demonstrated good interrater reliability in trained raters. Training manuals and detailed scoring guidelines are available. Unfortunately, there are presently no data regarding the equivalency of such instruments across sites or versions; this is clearly an area needing further empirical attention (Dunn et al., 2006).

Neither the MacCAT-T, the MacCAT-CR, nor most similar instruments (reviewed in Dunn et al., 2006; Grisso, 2003) provide a final determination of whether a patient possesses or lacks decision-making capacity. The MacCAT-T and MacCAT-CR authors explicitly acknowledge the need to utilize a "sliding scale" concept of capacity: A lower threshold for capacity is desirable for decisions with minimal risks, whereas decisions that involve greater risk necessitate a greater level of capacity. This sliding scale raises unanswered questions regarding who gets to decide where to set the threshold of capacity–incapacity.

Another capacity assessment tool with sufficient validation in patients with dementia is the Competency to Consent to Treatment Inventory (CCTI) (Marson, Chatterjee, Ingram, & Harrell, 1996; Marson, Cody, Ingram, & Harrell, 1995; Marson, Ingram, Cody, & Harrell, 1995; Marson, Schmitt, Ingram, & Harrell, 1994). This tool utilizes two hypothetical treatment vignettes with standardized questions to evaluate competency under each of five legal standards (evidencing a choice; reasonableness of choice; appreciation of consequences; providing rational reasons for one's choice; and understanding the situation and choices). Given the contextual nature of the construct of capacity, assessment tools using hypothetical vignettes ideally should demonstrate correlation with actual decision-making performance.

The field of capacity assessment is relatively young, and research is ongoing into the best methods for assessing capacity in various contexts. It is virtually impossible to eliminate fully subjectivity in capacity assessment, but use of a structured instrument can at least improve the data collection process upon which the final judgment may ultimately be based.

## Cognitive Testing

Formal capacity assessments in the clinical context usually include a bedside interview, brief cognitive testing, and occasionally referral for more comprehensive/standardized (validated) neuropsychological evaluation, as well as reliance on collateral reports. All available sources of information are sought and integrated to develop a full and accurate picture of an individual's mental capacity for meaningful decision making. Although requests for competency evaluation are generally directed to psychiatrists (typically the consultation/liaison service), the input of other mental health professionals can be particularly relevant and helpful. For instance, neuropsychologists can provide a thorough standardized evaluation of patients' cognitive abilities within a range of specific cognitive domains relevant to decisional capacity, such as those identified in the Marson and Harrell (1999) tripartite cognitive model of consent capacity (discussed below). Neuropsychological evaluation is also helpful in placing apparent cognitive deficits within the broader context of personality, psychiatric, and motivational factors that may impinge upon apparent decision-making deficits.

Brief cognitive impairment/dementia screening measures, particularly the Folstein Mini-Mental State Examination (MMSE; Folstein, Folstein, & McHugh, 1975), can provide useful collateral information for decision-making capacity assessments. Although the MMSE has been shown in several studies to correlate with performance on measures of decision-making capacity (Dellasega, Frank, & Smyer, 1996; Karlawish, Casarett, & James, 2002; Kim & Caine, 2002; Kim, Caine, Currier, Leibovici, & Ryan, 2001; Lapid et al., 2003; Palmer et al., 2005; Raymont et al., 2004), it does not have adequate predictive validity to be used as a stand-alone or surrogate marker for decisional capacity impairment (Fitten, Lusky, & Hamann, 1990; Kim & Caine, 2002; Raymont et al., 2004). Also, the MMSE may be less sensitive to some of the higher-order executive deficits seen in patients with frontal-focused neuropathology (Malloy et al., 1997).

As noted earlier, comprehensive neuropsychological evaluations with standardized cognitive tests may be helpful in informing clinicians about patterns of cognitive strength and deficit, such as those highlighted in Marson and Harrell's tripartite cognitive model of decisional capacity (1999; discussed below), and there is considerable evidence that neuropsychological tests are strongly correlated with decision-making capacity skills (Carpenter et al., 2000; Casarett, Karlawish, & Hirschman, 2003; Marson et al., 1996; Moser et al., 2002; Palmer, Dunn, Appelbaum, & Jeste, 2004). Yet it is also important to keep in mind that although the cognitive abilities as measured by standard neuropsychological tests influence a person's ability to make a decision in a specific context, the abilities measured by such tests are not generally synonymous with decision-making capacity. For instance, a person with relatively low verbal skills may lack capacity to consent to a complex or high-risk research protocol or treatment, but may have sufficient ability to understand a procedurally simple study or treatment, particularly if the disclosure of the relevant information has been provided in an optimal format. Thus, the ultimate determination of decisional capacity should include evaluation of the person's specific capacity to understand, appreciate, and reason with regard to the information that is specifically relevant to the choice facing him or her. Decision-making capacity scales such as the MacCAT-T (Grisso & Appelbaum, 1998; Grisso et al., 1997) and MacCAT-CR (Appelbaum & Grisso, 2001) provide the latter sort of decision-specific information.

## RELATIONSHIPS BETWEEN DECISION-MAKING CAPACITY AND FRONTAL LOBE FUNCTIONING

Marson and Harrell (1999) proposed a tripartite cognitive conceptual model of loss of consent capacity in Alzheimer's disease (AD) that serves as a useful model for discussing the relationship of frontal lobe functions and decision-making capacity. Because the model integrates the various neurocognitive abilities necessary for the construct of capacity, it is relevant not only to AD patients but also to those with any cognitive disorder—although persons with predominant frontal lobe pathology present some additional challenges that we explore further below.

In the tripartite model, the first of the cognitive abilities necessary for consent capacity is comprehension of treatment-related information. This task is often impaired in early AD secondary to memory deficits. Although decrements in this aspect of consent capacity are not specific to frontal lobe functioning, impairments in working memory and conceptualization do contribute. The second ability, processing the information and forming a treatment decision by using logical decision making, relies on executive functioning in large degree. Intact executive functioning is needed for a patient to organize the information that has been encoded, to reason logically, and to shift set when necessary. The third component of the tripartite model engages the patient's ability to communicate a choice, involving some form of effective communication of that choice.

The second ability relies substantially on frontal lobe function. As Marson (2001) noted, "Conceptualization and executive function measures are important to consent capacity because of their relevance to organized processing of treatment information. Measures of judgment and reasoning are equally important as they make possible a patient's rational weighing of all this information, and his/her internal determination of a treatment choice" (p. 273). Studies that compare relationships between cognitive abilities and measures of decision-making abilities confirm that measures of executive functions, as well as those of verbal memory, are strongly correlated to clinical determinations of consent capacity (Marson, Hawkins, McInturff, & Harrell, 1997).

Separating out the skills subsumed under the terms "executive" and/or "frontal" functions further clarifies the role of deficits caused by frontotemporal dementia and other "frontal syndromes" relative to consent capacity. The term "executive functions" can be broadly defined as those cognitive processes involved in controlling the adaptive balance of initiation, maintenance, and shifting of responses to environmental demands permitting complex, goal-directed behavior rather than reflexive response to immediately salient stimuli (Loring, 1999; Palmer & Heaton, 2000; Royall et al., 2002). Historically, the terms "executive" and "frontal" were used interchangeably (e.g., "frontal–executive skills"), but it is clear that the frontal lobes also control more basic processes that are not "executive" in nature, and that some of the "executive functions" are also dependent on nonfrontal brain regions and systems. Also, though earlier neuropathological descriptions of "frontal–executive syndromes" tended to emphasize the frontal cortex (particularly the left prefrontal region), the last 20 years have witnessed increased emphasis and recognition of the role of frontal–subcortical connections in these functions (Cummings, 1993; Lichter & Cummings, 2001).

Presently, five frontal–subcortical circuits are generally recognized (Lichter & Cummings, 2001; Tekin & Cummings, 2002). Two, the motor and oculomotor circuits, serve primarily motor functions that may be of less direct relevance to decision-making capacity. However, the remaining circuits (dorsolateral prefrontal, orbitofrontal, and anterior cingulate circuits) together serve affective, behavioral, and cognitive functions that seem to have direct relevance to understanding, appreciation, and reasoning.

The dorsolateral prefrontal circuit is associated with abilities that are most prototypical of the concept of "executive functions." Such abilities include abstraction, problem solving, hypothesis generation, planning, goal selection, self-monitoring, sequencing, mental flexibility/maintenance, and appropriate shifting of response set in light of changing environmental contingencies, working memory, and motor programming (Lichter & Cummings, 2001; Royall et al., 2002; Tekin & Cummings, 2002). These abilities have obvious relevance to abilities of patients and research participants to monitor and envision present and future circumstances, and are thus clearly germane to the task of appreciation and reasoning during the informed consent process. Because damage to the dorsolateral prefrontal area or circuit is associated with concrete thinking, impairment in genuine understanding of disclosed information might also be anticipated. Royall and colleagues (2002) suggest that this circuit may also be involved in self-awareness and insight; if so, impairment in this circuit would also be clearly relevant to one's ability to appreciate the relevance of disclosed information for one's own condition or situation.

The anterior cingulate circuit is involved in affect regulation and motivation; patients with anterior cingulate lesions may manifest extreme apathy or emotional dysregulation (Lichter & Cummings, 2001; Royall et al., 2002; Tekin & Cummings, 2002). Impaired affect or inability to place appropriate valence on present and future possible outcomes could clearly hinder one's ability to fully appreciate and reason about risks and benefits of treatment alternatives or research participation. Tekin and Cummings also note that such patients may manifest reduced ability to understand new thoughts and to engage in creative thought processes, so, again, this region might be relevant to the abilities to understand and reason.

The orbitofrontal circuit is involved in the organization of information and impulse regulation (facilitation of socially appropriate responses and inhibition of socially inappropriate ones) (Lichter & Cummings, 2001; Royall et al., 2002; Tekin & Cummings, 2002). Impulse regulation may be particularly relevant to the reasoning component of decision-making capacity, in that patients with orbitofrontal impairments may not properly reflect on the long-term impact of their immediate choices (Bechara, Damasio, Damasio, & Anderson, 1994). Royall and colleagues (2002) also suggest that orbitofrontal function may be involved in risk assessment, and response to short- versus long-term goals and risks. Thus, those with orbitofrontal lesions might be unduly swayed by short-term benefits (e.g., such as payment for research participation), while not appropriately weighing costs in terms of potential long-term risks of a research protocol.

## EMPIRICAL EVIDENCE REGARDING DECISION-MAKING CAPACITY AND THE FRONTAL LOBES

Unfortunately, much of the aforementioned speculation about the relationship between the executive and frontal–subcortical circuit functions and capacity to consent to treatment or research remains precisely that, speculation. There is an enormous literature on decision processes from cognitive neuroscience involving primate and other animal lesion studies, case descriptions and clinical studies of people who have sustained discrete frontal injuries, as well as functional neuroimaging studies of patients and healthy controls evaluated while performing decision-making tasks (Bechara, 2004; Bechara et al., 1994; Rogers et al., 1999). Individuals with focal lesions show impairments ranging from indecision to poor planning, to problems weighing options rationally, to disregard for risk (Gomez-Beldarrain, Harries, Garcia-Monco, Ballus, & Grafman, 2004; Manes et al., 2002; Shuren & Grafman, 2002). Interested readers are referred to any of several excellent recent reviews of the literature on frontal systems in decision-making processes (e.g., Bechara, 2004; Clark, Cools, & Robbins, 2004; Krawczyk, 2002).

In terms of the focus of this chapter on consent capacity, a bridge remains to be built that would link the neuroscience and other decision-making literature to the empirical bioethics literature on decision-making capacity. For instance, there is strong evidence that the orbitofrontal region processes information regarding reward value of stimuli (reviewed in Krawcyzk, 2002). An impairment in ability to place appropriate valence on potential outcomes would seem to have at least a superficial relationship to the notions of "appreciation" and "reasoning" in the consent capacity literature, but what are the precise relationships? How precisely would the construct of reward value fit into a competency determination? Similarly, when do differences in risk preference (weighing of short- vs. long-term risks and benefits), another frontally mediated function, become an issue of pathology that explains incompetence versus acceptable variation in human preferences? The process of answering such questions will likely lead to refinement in our notions of consent capacity.

Recent years have witnessed a large body of empirical bioethics research on capacity issues among patients with various neuropsychiatric and medical conditions (Carpenter et al., 2000; Casarett et al., 2003; Dunn et al., 2002; Grisso & Appelbaum, 1995; Karlawish et al., 2002; Kim & Caine, 2002; Kim et al., 2001; Marson et al., 1996; Moser et al., 2002; Palmer et al., 2004, 2005; Roberts, 1998; Wirshing, Wirshing, Marder, Liberman, & Mintz, 1998), but there has been almost no research directly evaluating how specific brain regions influence consent capacity. One exception is a recent small functional magnetic resonance imaging (fMRI) study by Eyler and colleagues (paper presented at the annual meeting of the American Association of Geriatric Psychiatry, February 23, 2003, Baltimore, MD). These investigators studied 15 middle-age and older patients with schizophrenia. They found that MacCAT-CR Understanding scores (regarding participation in this fMRI study) were correlated with brain response to a verbal learning task in bilateral inferior frontal gyrus (as well as bilat-

eral hippocampus); no significant relationships were observed between brain response and MacCAT-CR Reasoning scores.

Although there are few studies of consent capacity among patients with focal frontal lesions, a number of studies of patient populations with more diffuse neurocognitive deficits have examined measures of executive functions as possible predictors of competency. For instance, several studies suggest that neuropsychological tests sensitive to impaired executive functions (plus tests of verbal learning/memory skills) tend to be among the best predictors of physician or other clinician determinations of decisional capacity (Holzer, Gansler, Moczynski, & Folstein, 1997; Marson et al., 1997; Royall, Mahurin, & Gray, 1992).

Tests sensitive to executive functions also tend to be among the best correlates of scores on decision-making capacity scales. For instance, using stepwise regression analysis to predict CCTI scores among AD patients, Marson, Cody, and colleagues (1995) found phonemic fluency to be the best cognitive predictor of appreciating consequences of a treatment choice, and Dementia Rating Scale (DRS) Initiation/Perseveration subscale scores were the best predictor of ability to provide rational reasons for a treatment choice.

Palmer and colleagues (2004) found that abstraction/cognitive flexibility scores (a composite of scores on the Wisconsin Card Sorting Test, Booklet Category Test, and Trail Making Test Part B) were significantly correlated with the capacity to consent to treatment among middle-age and older patients with schizophrenia, particularly the MacCAT-T Understanding, Reasoning, and Expression of a Choice subscales, although scores from other cognitive domains, particularly learning and recall, were also strong correlates of MacCAT-T scores.

Cassarett and colleagues (2003) provided another example of the relationship of executive tests to decisional capacity in their study of competence to consent to research among cancer patients. Using performance on the MacCAT-CR, patients were categorized as having or lacking decision-making capacity. Those lacking capacity had lower education and lower literacy scores, but also did worse on the Trail Making Test Part B (a task sensitive to mental flexibility, as well as psychomotor speed and efficiency of visual spatial scanning) and had lower scores on the MMSE backwards spelling item (i.e., "world," a task sensitive to working memory and spelling ability).

Studies from patients with disorders associated with nonfocal patterns of cognitive deficits have an interpretive limitation. It is difficult to identify definitive relationships between specific cognitive abilities and specific dimensions of decision-making capacity when the various cognitive constructs (and domains of decision-making capacity) may be assessed with measures of uncertain psychometric equivalence (Chapman & Chapman, 1973). Nonetheless, the overall picture that emerges from this growing empirical bioethics literature, as well as the larger neuroscience literature on decision-making processes, is one that strongly suggests the frontal–executive systems have a central role in ability to provide meaningful consent (Marson & Harrell, 1999).

## CONCLUSIONS

We venture several recommendations regarding consent for research. First, as is becoming more commonly required by institutional review boards (e.g., the University of California at San Diego), formal assessment of decisional capacity should be included in any greater than minimal risk study of patients with frontal disorders. Second, given the deficits associated with frontal dysfunction, researchers should be particularly alert to deficits in appreciation and reasoning, even when the basic ability to parrot superficially the details of a protocol appears intact. Third, the use of a structured instrument such as the MacCAT-CR (Appelbaum & Grisso, 2001) may facilitate that evaluation process. Fourth, it is important to consider the degree to which the particular person's lack of capacity may reflect transient and/or modifiable factors versus stable/unmodifiable ones (see Figure 22.1)—although empirical studies of means to improve appreciation and reasoning (to which patients with frontal dysfunction may be particularly vulnerable) have been less common than studies focused on the understanding component of consent capacity. Fifth, when patients lack decisional capacity, researchers need to consider local provisions for enrolling individuals via surrogate consent (consent provided by a legally authorized representative) in combination with participant assent, rather than simply limiting enrollment to those with capacity. Without the possibility of surrogate consent, research will be severely impeded on increasingly prevalent disorders (e.g., dementia) that by their very nature impair

decision-making capacity (Appelbaum, 2002). Finally, there is a need for legislation to promote both the use of advance directives for research, as well as to clarify the status of surrogate consent in most states (Appelbaum, 2002).

With regard to consent for treatment, our recommendation is to consider capacity evaluations not only when patients refuse treatment but also when they accept higher risk treatments. We also would recommend that clinicians consider including the MacCAT-T (Grisso et al., 1997; or other treatment capacity assessment instruments [Dunn et al., 2006]) as part of their capacity assessment procedure. Finally, addressing the need for advance directives for both treatment and research is an important piece of the clinical picture for all patients with frontal dysfunction.

Future research should build on the multiple lines of evidence that have established the centrality of the frontal lobes and systems subserving them in decision making (Damasio, 1995; Paulus et al., 2001; Shuren & Grafman, 2002; Stuss & Benson, 1986). Substantial empirical and conceptual work is needed to link data on cognitive and decision-making processes to data on the capacity to consent to research or treatment. This work will require integrating the perspectives of the neurosciences with law and bioethics, studying the decision-making capacity of patients with frontal lobe disorders, and employing emerging imaging and other technologies to link basic neuroscience findings with clinical and legal concepts of consent capacity. Important work is also required to develop further and refine methods and instruments for capacity assessment (Dunn et al., 2006; Grisso, 2003). These lines of research will help to elucidate the basic mechanisms underlying the frontal lobes' importance in meeting a critical requirement for patients to flourish as human beings: the ability to make a decision.

## REFERENCES

Appelbaum, P., & Grisso, T. (2001). *MacCAT-CR: MacArthur Competence Assessment Tool for Clinical Research.* Sarasota, FL: Professional Resource Press.

Appelbaum, P. S. (2002). Involving decisionally impaired subjects in research: The need for legislation. *American Journal of Geriatric Psychiatry, 10*(2), 120–124.

Appelbaum, P. S., & Grisso, T. (1995). The MacArthur Treatment Competence Study: I. Mental illness and competence to consent to treatment. *Law and Human Behavior, 19*(2), 105–126.

Bechara, A. (2004). The role of emotion in decision-making: Evidence from neurological patients with orbitofrontal damage. *Brain and Cognition, 55*(1), 30–40.

Bechara, A., Damasio, A. R., Damasio, H., & Anderson, S. W. (1994). Insensitivity to future consequences following damage to human prefrontal cortex. *Cognition, 50*(1–3), 7–15.

Carpenter, W. T., Jr., Gold, J. M., Lahti, A. C., Queern, C. A., Conley, R. R., Bartko, J. J., et al. (2000). Decisional capacity for informed consent in schizophrenia research. *Archives of General Psychiatry, 57*(6), 533–538.

Casarett, D. J., Karlawish, J. H., & Hirschman, K. B. (2003). Identifying ambulatory cancer patients at risk of impaired capacity to consent to research. *Journal of Pain and Symptom Management, 26*(1), 615–624.

Chapman, L. J., & Chapman, J. P. (1973). Problems in the measurement of cognitive deficit. *Psychological Bulletin, 79*(6), 380–385.

Clark, L., Cools, R., & Robbins, T. W. (2004). The neuropsychology of ventral prefrontal cortex: Decision-making and reversal learning. *Brain and Cognition, 55*(1), 41–53.

Cummings, J. L. (1993). Frontal–subcortical circuits and human behavior. *Archives of Neurology, 50*(8), 873–880.

Damasio, A. R. (1995). On some functions of the human prefrontal cortex. *Annals of the New York Academy of Sciences, 769,* 241–251.

Dellasega, C., Frank, L., & Smyer, M. (1996). Medical decision-making capacity in elderly hospitalized patients. *Journal of Ethics, Law, and Aging, 2*(2), 65–74.

Dunn, L. B., & Jeste, D. V. (2001). Enhancing informed consent for research and treatment. *Neuropsychopharmacology, 24*(6), 595–607.

Dunn, L. B., Lindamer, L. A., Palmer, B. W., Golshan, S., Schneiderman, L. J., & Jeste, D. V. (2002). Improving understanding of research consent in middle-aged and elderly patients with psychotic disorders. *American Journal of Geriatrics Psychiatry, 10*(2), 142–150.

Dunn, L. B., Nowrangi, M., Palmer, B. W., Jeste, D. V., & Saks, E. (2006). Assessing decisional capacity for clinical research or treatment: A review of instruments. *American Journal of Psychiatry, 163*(8), 1323–1334.

Faden, R., Beauchamp, T., & King, N. (1986). *A history and theory of informed consent.* New York: Oxford University Press.

Fitten, L. J., Lusky, R., & Hamann, C. (1990). Assessing treatment decision-making capacity in elderly nursing home residents. *Journal of the American Geriatric Society, 38*(10), 1097–1104.

Folstein, M. F., Folstein, S. E., & McHugh, P. R. (1975). "Mini-Mental State": A practical method for grading the cognitive state of patients for the clinician. *Journal of Psychiatric Research, 12*(3), 189–198.

Gomez-Beldarrain, M., Harries, C., Garcia-Monco, J. C., Ballus, E., & Grafman, J. (2004). Patients with right frontal lesions are unable to assess and use advice to make predictive judgments. *Journal of Cognitive Neuroscience, 16*(1), 74–89.

Grisso, T. (2003). *Evaluating competencies: Forensic assessments and instruments* (2nd ed.). New York: Kluwer Academic.

Grisso, T., & Appelbaum, P. S. (1995). The MacArthur Treatment Competence Study: III. Abilities of patients to consent to psychiatric and medical treatments. *Law and Human Behavior, 19*(2), 149–174.

Grisso, T., & Appelbaum, P. (1998). *Assessing competence to consent to treatment: A guide for physicians and other health professionals.* New York: Oxford University Press.

Grisso, T., Appelbaum, P. S., & Hill-Fotouhi, C. (1997). The MacCAT-T: A clinical tool to assess patients' capacities to make treatment decisions. *Psychiatric Services, 48*(11), 1415–1419.

Grisso, T., Appelbaum, P. S., Mulvey, E. P., & Fletcher, K. (1995). The MacArthur Treatment Competence Study: II. Measures of abilities related to competence to consent to treatment. *Law and Human Behavior, 19*(2), 127–148.

Holzer, J. C., Gansler, D. A., Moczynski, N. P., & Folstein, M. F. (1997). Cognitive functions in the informed consent evaluation process: A pilot study. *Journal of the American Academy of Psychiatry and the Law, 25*(4), 531–540.

Karlawish, J. H., Casarett, D. J., & James, B. D. (2002). Alzheimer's disease patients' and caregivers' capacity, competency, and reasons to enroll in an early-phase Alzheimer's disease clinical trial. *Journal of American Geriatric Society, 50*(12), 2019–2024.

Kim, S. Y., & Caine, E. D. (2002). Utility and limits of the Mini-Mental State Examination in evaluating consent capacity in Alzheimer's disease. *Psychiatric Services, 53*(10), 1322–1324.

Kim, S. Y., Caine, E. D., Currier, G. W., Leibovici, A., & Ryan, J. M. (2001). Assessing the competence of persons with Alzheimer's disease in providing informed consent for participation in research. *American Journal of Psychiatry, 158*(5), 712–717.

Krawczyk, D. C. (2002). Contributions of the prefrontal cortex to the neural basis of human decision making. *Neuroscience and Biobehavioral Reviews, 26*(6), 631–664.

Lapid, M. I., Rummans, T. A., Poole, K. L., Pankratz, V. S., Maurer, M. S., Rasmussen, K. G., et al. (2003). Decisional capacity of severely depressed patients requiring electroconvulsive therapy. *Journal of ECT, 19*(2), 67–72.

Lichter, D. G., & Cummings, J. L. (2001). Introduction and overview. In D. G. Lichter & J. L. Cummings (Eds.), *Frontal–subcortical circuits in psychiatric and neurological disorders* (pp. 1–43). New York: Guilford Press.

Loring, D. W. (Ed.). (1999). *INS dictionary of neuropsychology.* New York: Oxford University Press.

Malloy, P. F., Cummings, J. L., Coffey, C. E., Duffy, J., Fink, M., Lauterbach, E. C., et al. (1997). Cognitive screening instruments in neuropsychiatry: a report of the Committee on Research of the American Neuropsychiatric Association. *Journal of Neuropsychiatry and Clinical Neurosciences*, 9(2), 189–197.

Manes, F., Sahakian, B., Clark, L., Rogers, R., Antoun, N., Aitken, M., et al. (2002). Decision-making processes following damage to the prefrontal cortex. *Brain*, 125(3), 624–639.

Marson, D., Dymek, M., & Geyer, J. (2001). Informed consent, competency, and the neurologist. *Neurologist*, 7(6), 317–326.

Marson, D., & Harrell, L. (1999). Executive dysfunction and loss of capacity to consent to medical treatment in patients with Alzheimer's disease. *Seminars in Clinical Neuropsychiatry*, 4(1), 41–49.

Marson, D. C. (2001). Loss of competency in Alzheimer's disease: Conceptual and psychometric approaches. *International Journal of Law and Psychiatry*, 24, 267–283.

Marson, D. C., Chatterjee, A., Ingram, K. K., & Harrell, L. E. (1996). Toward a neurologic model of competency: Cognitive predictors of capacity to consent in Alzheimer's disease using three different legal standards. *Neurology*, 46(3), 666–672.

Marson, D. C., Cody, H. A., Ingram, K. K., & Harrell, L. E. (1995). Neuropsychologic predictors of competency in Alzheimer's disease using a rational reasons legal standard. *Archives of Neurology*, 52(10), 955–959.

Marson, D. C., Hawkins, L., McInturff, B., & Harrell, L. E. (1997). Cognitive models that predict physician judgments of capacity to consent in mild Alzheimer's disease. *Journal of the American Geriatrics Society*, 45(4), 458–464.

Marson, D. C., Ingram, K. K., Cody, H. A., & Harrell, L. E. (1995). Assessing the competency of patients with Alzheimer's disease under different legal standards: A prototype instrument. *Archives of Neurology*, 52(10), 949–954.

Marson, D. C., Schmitt, F. A., Ingram, K. K., & Harrell, L. E. (1994). Determining the competency of Alzheimer patients to consent to treatment and research. *Alzheimer Disease and Associated Disorders*, 8(Suppl. 4), 5–18.

Moser, D. J., Schultz, S. K., Arndt, S., Benjamin, M. L., Fleming, F. W., Brems, C. S., et al. (2002). Capacity to provide informed consent for participation in schizophrenia and HIV research. *American Journal of Psychiatry*, 159(7), 1201–1207.

National Commission for the Protection of Human Subjects of Biomedical and Behavioral Research. (1978). *The Belmont Report* (DHEW Publ. No. OS-78-0012). Washington, DC: U.S. Government Printing Office.

Palmer, B. W., Dunn, L. B., Appelbaum, P. S., & Jeste, D. V. (2004). Correlates of treatment-related decision-making capacity among middle-aged and older patients with schizophrenia. *Archives of General Psychiatry*, 61(3), 230–236.

Palmer, B. W., Dunn, L. B., Appelbaum, P. S., Mudaliar, S., Thal, L., Henry, R., et al. (2005). Assessment of capacity to consent to research among older persons with schizophrenia, Alzheimer disease or diabetes mellitus: Comparison of a three-item questionnaire with a comprehensive standardized capacity instrument. *Archives of General Psychiatry*, 62(7), 726–733.

Palmer, B. W., & Heaton, R. (2000). Executive dysfunction in schizophrenia. In T. Sharma & P. Harvey (Eds.), *Cognition in schizophrenia: Impairments, importance and treatment strategies* (pp. 52–72). New York: Oxford University Press.

Paulus, M. P., Hozack, N., Zauscher, B., McDowell, J. E., Frank, L., Brown, G. G., et al. (2001). Prefrontal, parietal, and temporal cortex networks underlie decision-making in the presence of uncertainty. *NeuroImage*, 13(1), 91–100.

Raymont, V., Bingley, W., Buchanan, A., David, A. S., Hayward, P., Wessely, S., et al. (2004). Prevalence of mental incapacity in medical inpatients and associated risk factors: Cross-sectional study. *Lancet*, 364, 1421–1427.

Roberts, L. W. (1998). The ethical basis of psychiatric research: Conceptual issues and empirical findings. *Comprehensive Psychiatry*, 39(3), 99–110.

Rogers, R. D., Owen, A. M., Middleton, H. C., Williams, E. J., Pickard, J. D., Sahakian, B. J., et al. (1999). Choosing between small, likely rewards and large, unlikely rewards activates inferior and orbital prefrontal cortex. *Journal of Neuroscience*, 19(20), 9029–9038.

Royall, D. R., Lauterback, E. C., Cummings, J. L., Reeve, A., Rummans, T. A., Kaufer, D. I., et al. (2002). Executive control function: A review of its promise and challenges for clinical research: A report from the Committee on Research of the American Neuropsychiatric Association. *Jounal of Neuropsychiatry and Clinical Neurosciences*, 14(4), 377–405.

Royall, D. R., Mahurin, R. K., & Gray, K. F. (1992). Bedside assessment of executive cognitive impairment: The executive interview. *Journal of the American Geriatrics Society*, 40(12), 1221–1226.

Shuren, J. E., & Grafman, J. (2002). The neurology of reasoning. *Archives of Neurology*, 59(6), 916–919.

Stuss, D. T., & Benson, D. F. (1986). *The frontal lobes.* New York: Raven.

Tekin, S., & Cummings, J. L. (2002). Frontal–subcortical neuronal circuits and clinical neuropsychiatry: an update. *Journal of Psychosomatic Research*, 53(2), 647–654.

Tversky, A., & Kahneman, D. (1974). Judgment under uncertainty: Heuristics and biases. *Science*, 185, 1124–1131.

Wirshing, D. A., Wirshing, W. C., Marder, S. R., Liberman, R. P., & Mintz, J. (1998). Informed consent: Assessment of comprehension. *American Journal of Psychiatry*, 155(11), 1508–1511.

# CHAPTER 23

# Social Cognition in Frontal Injury

*Katherine P. Rankin*

The goal of this chapter is to summarize recent evidence for the unique contributions of the frontal lobes to social functioning, with a particular emphasis on data from patients with brain injuries. In the past 5–10 years, tremendous advances in brain imaging have allowed more precise taxonomy of brain–behavior relationships, even for domains such as social behavior, which have traditionally been considered too abstract to have a specific neural substrate. Certainly, complex behaviors such as personality and social conduct are derived from multiple distributed networks of functional circuits. Because of this, it is impossible to discuss this topic without frequent reference to the substantial clarifications made by recent functional imaging work with normal controls. However, human lesion studies do provide unique supportive evidence to confirm or disprove the contribution of particular nodes in hypothesized functional networks and, as such, provide a rich body of work that can be used to inform and augment the functional imaging literature.

To delineate the frontal lobe contributions to social functioning, the constructs of "social behavior" and "personality" must be defined. To limit its scope, this chapter focuses only on cognitive processes that directly relate to interpersonal functioning. For instance, frontal contributions to emotion comprehension are examined in some detail, because understanding what someone else is feeling has direct relevance for social cognition and behavior; however, the aspects of emotion production that may directly affect social relationships are only

briefly addressed. The term "personality" has been used to describe many behavioral characteristics (e.g., apathy, irritability, or impulsivity), but decades of psychosocial research suggest that this term is more appropriately reserved for complex, psychometrically validated constructs such as those from the Big Five theory of personality, such as "extraversion," and "agreeableness."

Though the evidence for specific brain–behavior relationships in the area of social cognition is still being sifted and formed into more comprehensive theories, this chapter organizes the data into rough anatomical groups corresponding to the orbitofrontal cortex (OFC), the dorsomedial prefrontal cortex (DMPFC), and the dorsolateral prefrontal cortex (DLPFC).

## ORBITOFRONTAL CORTEX

For the purposes of this chapter, the OFC is defined as the portion of the frontal cortex that receives input from the magnocellular portions of the medial nucleus of the mediodorsal thalamus, in contrast to other frontal lobe structures that receive input from the lateral, parvocellular areas of the mediodorsal thalamus, corresponding to Brodmann's areas (BAs) 11, 12, 13, and 14 (Kringelbach & Rolls, 2004). BA 10 also receives magnocellular input from the thalamus, but for the purposes of this chapter, this region has been included in the section on the dorsomedial frontal lobe because of the functional links between the frontal pole and other paracingulate structures.

Studies of cognition and the OFC in both animal and human models suggest that its primary function is the analysis of rewards and punishments. More specifically, as the recipient of input from the "what is it?" pathways from all sensory modalities, the highly multimodal OFC is uniquely suited to evaluate rapidly the costs and benefits of specific behavioral responses to the environment, particularly in situations where those reinforcers must be inferred from minimal or complex input. In their excellent review of OFC functional neuroanatomy, Kringelbach and Rolls (2004) break the function of the OFC into four parts. First, the OFC (1) represents both concrete primary, unlearned reinforcers, such as touch and taste (processed in the posterior ventral OFC), and more abstract secondary, learned reinforcers emanating from visual, auditory, olfactory, and multimodal sources (processed in the anterior ventral OFC). The OFC then (2) detects changes in the value of those reinforcers, with the medial OFC involved in monitoring and decoding reward values, whereas the lateral OFC evaluates punishers and motivates behavior change. The OFC is then critical for (3) rapidly reprogramming the association between a stimulus and its reinforcement value, and finally, (4) facilitating rapid shifts in behavior as a result of these altered reward contingencies. In addition to evaluating rewards and punishments, there is evidence that the OFC may also perform dynamic filtering of emotional stimuli, in effect dampening arousal related to irrelevant emotional input while maintaining neural activations that are task-relevant (Rule, Shimamura, & Knight, 2002). A third hypothesis about the OFC function, the "somatic marker hypothesis," agrees that the OFC is involved in rapid attribution of valence to potential reinforcers. However, it suggests that rather than being encoded in the OFC, valence comes from the peripheral nervous system (or an "as if" representation of the peripheral nervous system) in the form of an emotional "marker" that is used by the OFC to guide behavior (Damasio, 1994).

The "reinforcer value" framework for understanding the function of the OFC quickly makes clear the reasons why OFC damage is likely to result in abnormal social behavior. In an individual who can neither recognize the reward value of interpersonal stimuli nor sense how his or her behavior might be viewed negatively by others and thus be socially punished, and who cannot rapidly mobilize appropriate behaviors to acquire interpersonal rewards or avoid punishments, appropriate social behavior would quickly disintegrate. Studies of populations with brain injuries have provided evidence for specific deficits in both the detection and the evaluation of social information, and have delineated a broad array of behavior deficits that result from OFC damage.

## Emotion Recognition

While there is certainly evidence that emotion comprehension and expression are primarily mediated by structures outside of the frontal lobes, particularly the temporal, insular, and somatosensory cortex (Adolphs, Damasio, Tranel, Cooper, & Damasio, 2000), a number of studies have suggested that patients with OFC lesions show deficits in emotion recognition, both in facial and vocal modalities. Hornak, Rolls, and Wade (1996) found that patients with diverse ventral frontal damage were significantly impaired on a facial emotion recognition tests, though they later showed that patients with more discrete lesions in only the lateral portions of the OFC could perform facial emotion recognition normally (Hornak et al., 2003). However, OFC patients in both studies had deficits in identifying non-verbal vocal expressions of emotion. Beer, Heerey, Keltner, Scabini, and Knight (2003) found that a group of five patients with focal bilateral OFC damage were significantly worse than normal controls at identifying self-conscious emotions (embarrassment, shame), but not other emotions (anger, disgust, fear, happiness, sadness, contempt, surprise, or amusement). Blair and Cipolotti (2000) showed that a patient with a unilateral right OFC lesion was not only impaired in recognizing angry and disgusted facial expressions but also had a lower autonomic response to these expressions than did controls. Mah, Arnold, and Grafman (2005) grouped together patients with both unilateral and bilateral OFC lesions, but showed they had poorer matching of emotion expressions (facial expressions, hand gestures, and body postures) than either healthy controls or patients with dorsolateral frontal injury.

Additional information can be gained from studies that lack anatomical specificity but that analyze patient groups based on hemispheric laterality. Certainly, there is strong, consistent evidence for dominance of the right hemisphere for emotion perception (facial expression and voice prosody) and emotion expression in studies of normal functioning (Borod, 2000). Among patients with lateralized lesions, those with right-hemisphere damage perform more poorly at recognizing facial emotions (Adolphs et al., 2000; Mandal et al., 1999) and voice prosody (Kucharska-Pietura, Phillips, Gernand, & David, 2003).

Though studies of patients with generalized traumatic brain injury (TBI) often do not provide direct imaging evidence of OFC dysfunction, they consistently suggest that emotion recognition deficits are common sequelae to head injury. Given the considerable evidence that TBI results in OFC disconnection via axonal shearing (Abdel-Dayem et al., 1998; Abu-Judeh et al., 1999; Tomaiuolo et al., 2005; Wallesch et al., 2001), these studies may be taken as indirect support for the role of the OFC in emotion detection. In one of the first studies to investigate specifically perception of facial affect in TBI patients, Prigatano and Pribram (1982) found that patients with closed head injuries performed more poorly than patients with strokes or tumors. Jackson and Moffat (1987) later broadened this finding by showing that patients with TBI had difficulty identifying not only emotional faces but also emotional postures. Green, Turner, and Thompson (2004) found that these facial emotion recognition deficits in TBI were accompanied by impaired lexical naming of emotions. Hopkins, Dywan, and Segalowitz (2002) went on to demonstrate that they have abnormal electrodermal activity in response to faces showing negative emotions. Spell and Frank (2000) added that patients with TBI have difficulty interpreting nonverbal vocal emotions as well.

Patients with frontotemporal lobar degeneration (FTLD), a neurodegenerative disease causing significant damage to the orbitofrontal cortex (Rosen et al., 2002), perform worse on tests of emotion perception than dementia control groups without OFC damage. Studies of these patients have consistently found that comprehension of negative facial affect is impaired (Keane, Calder, Hodges, & Young, 2002; Lavenu & Pasquier, 2005; Lavenu, Pasquier, Lebert, Petit, & Van der Linden, 1999; Rosen et al., 2004), although there is some evidence that recognition of positive emotions such as happiness may be initially preserved, but may decline with disease sever-

ity (Lavenu & Pasquier, 2005; Rosen et al., 2002). This effect might be explained in part by the evidence that happiness is easier to identify than any of the negative emotions (Hager & Ekman, 1979).

Given the preponderance of evidence that emotion processing occurs primarily in the temporal lobes and insula, it has not yet been ruled out that the emotion comprehension deficits seen in OFC lesion patients result from disconnection between the OFC and temporal lobe structures, including the amygdala. However, other mechanisms consistent with known OFC functioning, such as inaccurate evaluation of the reinforcer value of emotional expressions, might also be responsible. Additional evidence is needed to delineate the precise neuroanatomical etiology of these observed emotion detection deficits after right OFC lesions.

## Evaluation of Social Information

Another important role of the OFC in social behavior is to evaluate and quickly recognize alterations in feedback both from external (social) and internal (subjective emotional) sources. OFC injury can interfere with this evaluation process on multiple levels.

### Subjective Emotional Experience

Hornak and colleagues (2003) found that patients with circumscribed bilateral OFC lesions reported large changes in their subjective experience of emotions, an effect that was present, though diminished, in patients with unilateral OFC lesions. In a previous study (Hornak et al., 1996), patients with more extensive OFC damage showed significantly greater change in subjective emotional experience than patients with frontal lobe damage outside of the OFC. Eight out of 10 patients with OFC lesions reported sizable reductions in their capacity to experience fear, whereas on the other emotions they showed high intra- and interindividual variability, with sizable increases or decreases in intensity or frequency of experienced emotions. These subjective reports are confirmed by evidence that patients with OFC lesions have decreased autonomic arousal to stimuli designed to elicit reliably an emotional response in healthy normals. Two case reports involving patients with predominantly right-sided orbitofrontal damage indicated that they had abnormally low skin conductance responses to both negative stimuli (threatening objects and scenes, e.g., pointed weapons, war scenes, blood/injuries) and positive stimuli (happy people, sports scenes) despite otherwise normal autonomic functioning (Angrilli, Palomba, Cantagallo, Maietti, & Stegagno, 1999; Blair & Cipolotti, 2000). One caveat to these studies is that at least some of the patients appeared to have lesions extending to the anterior cingulate cortex (ACC), an area that has also been demonstrated to mediate subjective emotional experience (see below). In support of the hypothesis that OFC damage can cause lability of subjective emotion, Beer and colleagues (2003) showed that patients with localized OFC lesions tended to become more embarrassed and self-conscious than controls during a task in which they received exaggerated praise.

### Contingency-Based Learning and Social Norms

The capacity for contingency-based learning can be conceptualized as the ability to evaluate possible behaviors based on either explicit or implicit feedback about potential outcomes. This skill is central to interpersonal functioning, particularly in situations in which a social behavior that was once rewarding becomes inappropriate (e.g., a joke that was funny in the lunchroom may not be well received at a funeral). It also underpins our ability to recognize that certain of our impulses would violate implicit social norms for our cultural group and might result in censure or outright punishment. A number of studies suggest that patients with OFC lesions have difficulty assigning an appropriate valence to stimuli that have an ambiguous potential for reward or punishment, which has widespread ramifications for behavior.

Bechara and colleagues (Bechara, Damasio, Damasio, & Anderson, 1994) designed a computerized gambling task (GT) to simulate real-life decision-making behavior in subjects. Subjects choose from decks of cards that have a mixed probability of reward or punishment. Healthy control subjects learn, over the course of 40–60 trials, that two of the decks have a net worth that is advantageous despite smaller increments of reward, whereas the two other decks are disadvantageous overall, despite providing an occasional large reward. Patients with OFC damage continue to lose money over the course of the learning trials because they

gravitate to the decks with larger rewards, failing to consider that these decks also have larger punishments and are thus disadvantageous overall (Bechara et al., 1994; Bechara, Tranel, Damasio, & Damasio, 1996; Bar-On, Tranel, Denberg, & Bechara, 2003). Unlike healthy controls, patients with OFC damage fail to generate skin conductance responses (SCRs) before choosing a risky deck, though they show a normal SCR pattern after receiving either rewards or punishments (Bechara, Damasio, Damasio, & Lee, 1999). This pattern occurs even when the punishment versus reward disparity is heightened and the delay before rewards or punishments is changed (Bechara, Damasio, & Damasio, 2000). A pair of complementary studies using the GT with patients with unilateral OFC damage have suggested that while patients with right OFC damage show a typically impaired pattern, patients with left OFC damage perform at near-normal levels and do show anticipatory SCRs (Manes et al., 2002; Tranel, Bechara, & Denburg, 2002).

The relevance of these studies to understanding the role of the OFC in inappropriate behavior, according to the authors of the test, is that patients with OFC damage make poor decisions because they are insensitive to future consequences and respond only to the immediate prospect of gratification or punishment (Bechara et al., 2000). It is important to note that such patients appear to experience the reward or punishment normally after it has occurred; their deficit is in imagining the reinforcer ahead of time. Applying the Kringelbach and Rolls (2004) theory, these patients show impairment in three of the four major functions of the OFC: (1) monitoring and decoding reward values, (2) rapidly reprogramming the reward value of a stimulus based on feedback, and (3) rapidly shifting behavior based on this new evaluation of the stimulus. The gambling task performance of patients with OFC damage is one of the best sources of support for the hypothesis that they cannot accurately evaluate social input to intuit rapidly the best course of action, or to inhibit an inappropriate one. Perhaps the most direct application of this failure of contingency-based learning to social behavior is seen in the violation of social norms. The medial OFC has repeatedly been demonstrated to be part of the circuit involved with moral reasoning (Moll, Oliveira-Souza, & Eslinger, 2003), ostensibly because it links potential violations of social norms with the possibility of punishment, thereby curbing bad behavior. Combined with the emotion detection deficits described earlier, individuals with OFC damage are likely to fail to recognize the often subtle signals for social disapproval, and do not realize that others' frowns are intended as a punishment in themselves. They are unlikely to recognize that they have crossed a line until a direct, concrete punishment occurs, such as being arrested or perhaps slapped by an indignant acquaintance. Individuals who sustain damage to the OFC from childhood never do develop a body of knowledge about moral and social norms, ostensibly because they were never able to process the personal rewards and punishments derived from following or breaking such rules (Anderson, Bechara, Damasio, Tranel, & Damasio, 1999).

### Attitudes and Stereotypes

Because the OFC functions as the brain's repository for information about the valence of reinforcers and is designed to yield this information rapidly to aid in the types of instantaneous decisions we must often make, researchers have hypothesized that our implicit social stereotypes and attitudes are generated by the OFC. Healthy controls respond more quickly when testing material is designed to match traditional gender stereotypes, ostensibly because stereotypes provide a cognitive "shorthand" for instantaneously decoding social situations in order to allow rapid behavioral responses. Using a task designed to test subjects' biases about women, Milne and Grafman (2001) showed that male patients with OFC damage did not show the expected shorter response time for social stereotypes, despite the fact that on explicit questionnaires they espoused the same gender stereotypes as control subjects. In a related study, the same group found that both normal controls and patients with right frontal lobe lesions found it easier to perform logical reasoning about social situations than about abstract relationships (Goel, Shuren, Sheesley, & Grafman, 2004). However, patients with left frontal lobe lesions did not show this normal facilitation, taking equally long with social rules (e.g., "If a person is to drink alcohol, he or she must be at least 21 years old") and abstract rules (e.g., "If a card has an A on one side, it will have a four on the other side"). Taken together, these studies converge to suggest that OFC damage interferes with the rapid

evaluation of complex social information based on previously learned associations.

### Behavioral Control

One of the major results of the Kringelbach and Rolls (2004) meta-analysis of OFC function was that they found a medial–lateral gradient in which the medial sections of the OFC were involved in decoding and monitoring the reward value of reinforcers, whereas the more lateral areas were more involved in evaluating a reinforcer's potential for punishment, facilitating a change in behavior based on this evaluation. Thus, deficits in social behavior may result from dysfunction at any level of processing by the OFC: inadequate social information detection or inaccurate evaluation/reevaluation of that information, as presented in the previous section, or as a direct result of an inability to rapidly facilitate shifts in behavior, even in cases where social rewards and punishments have been adequately perceived and evaluated. It is clear that the specific mechanisms for behavioral dysfunction in clinical populations with OFC damage may be multifactorial, and upon more precise study may in fact diverge, depending on which areas of the OFC are damaged. However, whatever the precise neuroanatomical etiologies, the fact that OFC injury alters interpersonal behavior has been confirmed by more than a century of literature that bears mentioning here.

A few caveats to the following summary are necessary. Studies examining patients with lesions in the frontal lobe outside of the OFC consistently fail to reveal the same magnitude of generalized behavior and personality disturbances, providing strong support for the hypothesis that OFC damage or disconnection is primarily responsible. Based on this assumption of OFC predominance in behavioral disturbance, this section includes some studies of behavior dyscontrol after frontal injury that do not clearly localize lesions to the OFC. Another issue is that historically, attempts to derive a clear, consistent taxonomy of these behavior and personality changes have been hampered by the use of a wide variety of different terminologies and assessment tools. For instance, in this context, the term "personality" has been applied to everything from specific behavior symptoms such as "impulsivity" or "apathy" to clinical psychopathology such as is measured by the Minnesota Multiphasic Personality Inventory, to traits from psychometrically derived theories of interpersonal and intrapersonal behavior, such as the Five Factor Theory. For the purposes of this chapter, the term "personality" will be reserved only for this last category. In this section OFC-related alterations are described as "behavior changes," and inferences are not made about the OFC's contributions to the larger, more complex construct of personality. With that caveat, some consistent patterns of OFC-related behavior deficits do emerge from a review of the clinical literature across multiple patient populations.

### Frontal Lobe Lesion or Trauma

Patients with lesions to the frontal cortex have often been described as having alterations in personality and social behavior (Bar-On et al., 2003; Bechara et al., 1994, 2000; Beer et al., 2003; Damasio, 1994; Grafman et al., 1996; Hornak et al., 1996). One very useful attempt to provide an exhaustive overview of these symptoms was performed by Barrash, Tranel, and Anderson (2000). For this study, they used an instrument called the Iowa Rating Scales of Personality Change to demonstrate an OFC-specific behavior syndrome that can be distinguished from that which results from non-OFC frontal lobe damage. They organized this syndrome into five components, including (1) a general dampening of emotional experience, (2) poorly modulated emotional reactions (including poor frustration tolerance, lability, and irritability), (3) disturbances in (particularly social) decision making (including indecisiveness, poor judgment, inflexibility, social inappropriateness, and lack of empathy/sensitivity), (4) disturbances in goal-directed behavior, and (5) lack of insight into these personality disturbances. Later, this same group demonstrated that only right-sided OFC damage produces this syndrome; the scores of patients with unilateral left OFC lesions on the Iowa Rating Scales of Personality were indistinguishable from those of healthy controls (Tranel et al., 2002).

### Neurodegenerative Disease

Although patients with specific neurodegenerative diseases demonstrate interindividual variability in the location of their brain injury, there are consistent patterns within disease groups that can provide useful information about brain–behavior relationships. Frontotemporal dementia (FTD), also known as the frontal variant of FTLD, causes severe injury throughout the frontal lobes, including the medial OFC, with relative sparing of posterior structures (Rosen et al., 2002). Clinical diagnosis of the disease is based primarily on the dramatic social and personality changes that are the hallmark of the disease, including (1) early decline in social interpersonal conduct, (2) early impairment in regulation of personal conduct, (3) early emotional blunting, and (4) early loss of insight (Neary et al., 1998). Compared to AD patients, FTD patients have significantly more disinhibition, euphoria, apathy, and aberrant motor behavior (Levy, Miller, Cummings, Fairbanks, & Craig, 1996). With regard to their social and emotional behavior, Bathgate, Snowden, Varma, Blackshaw, and Neary (2001) found that patients with FTD were significantly more likely than patients with AD or vascular dementia to have decreased emotional expression, decreased embarrassment, loss of hygiene, loss of interest in others, and increased selfishness and social disinhibition. They are more socially submissive (Rankin, Kramer, Mychack, & Miller, 2003), and show less empathy (Rankin, Kramer, & Miller, 2005). In one study directly linking behavior change of patients with FTD to orbitofrontal damage, Rankin, Rosen, and colleagues (2004) found a dissociation between the functions of the right and left OFC, showing that patients' right medial OFC damage positively correlated with decreased attentiveness to the needs of others in social interactions.

### Head Injury

Much of the literature examining behavior and personality changes following closed head injury does not attempt to describe differences among patients based on estimated location of brain damage. However, given the established connection between TBI and OFC disconnection via axonal shearing, OFC dysfunction is suspected to play a part in many posttraumatic behavioral sequelae (Abdel-Dayem et al., 1998; Abu-Judeh et al., 1999; Tomaiuolo et al., 2005; Wallesch et al., 2001). In a review of studies examining emotional and social disturbances in patients with head injuries, Prigatano (1999) demonstrated that a number of symptom clusters appear repeatedly: emotional lability, self-centered and socially insensitive responses, interpersonal irritability and belligerence, paranoia, and loss of interest and initiative. Given the high rates at which aggression and disinhibition appear after mild to moderate TBI, it can be difficult to determine whether a particular patient's inappropriate social choices result from acquired deficits in social cue processing or merely a failure to attend to others in the heat of the moment. In fact, when Lanoo, de Deyne, Colardyn, de Soete, and Jannes (1997) measured higher-level personality changes in psychometrically robust domains such as Agreeableness, Extraversion, Neuroticism, Openness, and Conscientiousness (the Big Five personality factors) in both patients with TBI ($N = 63$) and controls with traumatic injuries to parts of the body other than the head ($N = 28$), there were no differences, suggesting that many postconcussive personality changes may originate in psychosocial rather than neurological factors. However, after recovery from more severe forms of head injury, patients' interpersonal behaviors do show a general impoverishment and lack of spontaneity that are unrelated to decreased information-processing speed (Godfrey, Knight, Marsh, Moroney, & Bishara, 1989). Further research is needed, ideally using technologies such as diffusion tensor imaging, to more precisely quantify axonal disconnection syndromes to determine which behavior changes have a specific frontal etiology in this patient group.

### Psychiatric Disorders

Imaging studies of patients with psychiatric disorders also show a relationship between the OFC and behavioral dyscontrol. For instance, in examining patients with schizophrenia, Chemerinski, Noupoulos, Crespo-Facorro, Andreasen, and Magnotta (2002) demonstrated an inverse relationship between OFC volumes and changes in social functioning using the Scale for Assessing Negative Symptoms. The behaviors significantly related to the OFC were affective nonresponsivity, poor grooming and hygiene, decreased recreational interests and activities, decreased ability to feel intimacy, poorer relationships with friends and peers, and social inattentiveness. In a recent volumetric study of patients with obsessive–compulsive disorder (OCD), Pujol and colleagues (2004) demonstrated reduced medial OFC gray matter volume. Additional studies implicate reduced left OFC volumes in poor planning, reasoning, and organization in OCD (Choi et al., 2004). This may be further supported by functional imaging studies that demonstrate increased OFC activation in patients with OCD. Several authors suggest that in OCD, the hyperactivation of the orbitostriatal system reflects a dysregulation that requires constant effort to inhibit behavioral patterns that fail to terminate normally (Evans, Lewis, & Iobst, 2004).

Whereas there has been some evidence to suggest that patients with social phobia show reduced orbitofrontal and increased amygdala activation in response to social stress (Tillfors et al., 2001), many other studies associate social anxiety with enhanced perfusion of the OFC (Bell, Malizia, & Nutt, 1999; Malizia, 1997). When patients with social phobia were tested on an anxiogenic script-guided imagery paradigm, a network of frontal areas including the OFC, right medial frontal cortex, left precentral and postcentral gyrus, and insula had increased cerebral blood flow (CBF) (Marcin & Nemeroff, 2003). Some researchers have suggested that this decrease in OFC function may result when patients down-regulate their anxiety through visual avoidance in response to a social stressor (Van Ameringen et al., 2004).

### Summary

Despite the diverse etiologies for the frontal injuries described in the aforementioned populations, a cohesive pattern of behavioral dyscontrol can be seen to emerge. The symptoms of behavior and personality change that emerge repeatedly as a result of OFC damage are (1) altered emotional experience, including either emotional blunting and emotional lability, which may include an insensitivity to others emotions; (2) deficient decision making, including poor social and nonsocial judgment, lack of self-monitoring, and/or inflexibility; and (3) deficient goal-directed behavior, including apathy, disinhibition, task impersistence, and general disorganization. Additional studies are needed to determine more precisely the functional anatomy of these behavior deficits, particularly in light of recent advances in the precision of our understanding of nonsocial

OFC functions. Care will also need to be taken to distinguish OFC-related behavior changes from changes caused by damage to more dorsal structures in the frontal lobes.

## DORSOMEDIAL FRONTAL CORTEX

The dorsomedial aspect of the prefrontal cortex (DMPFC; BA medial 8 and 9, 10, 24 and 25, 32 and 33, including the ACC), plays a role in affective processing and self-evaluation. With respect to social behavior and personality, its primary function appears to be regulation of the interaction between self-awareness and the awareness of others to improve social sensitivity. Seeley and Sturm, Chapter 21, this volume, have examined the DMPFC's role in self-awareness in detail, so I only briefly touch on this topic by addressing the DMPFC contribution to the subjective experience of emotions. However, evidence is growing that the anterior frontomedial cortex, roughly corresponding to the superior frontal gyrus and BAs 9/10, is associated with important social functions, most importantly the capacity to take another person's perspective. Although, based on its cytoarchitectonics and the fact that it too receives inputs from the magnocellular portion of the mediodorsal thalamus, BA 10 of the frontal pole might be considered to be part of the OFC in some taxonomies (Kringelbach & Rolls, 2004), I have categorized it with the other dorsomedial frontal structures, because their functions are more closely related.

### Subjective Experience of Emotions

Although the ability to gauge one's own emotional state appears to be partly mediated by the OFC (discussed previously), lesions to the DMPFC appear to cause more profound deficits in this function. Hornak and colleagues (2003) found in their study of patients with frontal injury that those reporting drastic changes to their subjective experience of emotion all had damage to a key region involving medial BA 9 and/or the ACC, whereas patients with damage outside of these areas reported little or no change. The damage to this key medial region could be unilateral on either side of the brain but still resulted in profound alterations in experience of both positive and negative emotions consistent with greater lability

and hypersensitivity. Importantly, this study reinforced the link between subjective awareness of emotions and social behavior by finding that patients with greater changes in subjective emotion were rated by family informants as having poorer social adjustment. The findings of this lesion study are consistent with functional neuroimaging of normals, which has shown activation of medial BA 9 and the ACC during the experience of emotion (Lane, Reiman, Ahern, Schwartz, & Davidson, 1977; Lane et al., 1998). Given the degree to which the "affective" or subgenual portion of the ACC is interconnected with the hypothalamus and insula, these authors suggest that parts of the DMPFC may function to interpret autonomic emotional input. In a study of a patient with orbitofrontal damage who also had extensive damage to the DMPFC (BA 8, 9, 32, and anterior 24), Angrilli and colleagues (1999) demonstrated that the patient failed to produce a heightened autonomic response to emotionally arousing (positive and negative) stimuli.

There is considerable clinical evidence of decreased emotional insight in other populations with DMPFC damage such as patients with TBI or with neurodegenerative disease (Bathgate et al., 2001; Rankin, Baldwin, Pace-Savitsky, Kramer, & Miller, 2004). Recently, emerging studies have directly linked this loss of self-awareness with a specific neuroanatomy in patients with neurodegenerative disease. Rankin and colleagues (2006) examined questionnaire data by caregivers describing the ability of patients with FTLD, AD, corticobasal degeneration, and progressive supranuclear palsy to recognize implicit feedback from others about their own social behavior. Using voxel-based morphometry of the patients' structural MRI scans, she showed strong correlations between poor social self-monitoring and decreased volume in the right superior frontal gyrus, the right superior middle frontal gyrus, and the right OFC.

### Perspective Taking

During the past decade of research, "perspective taking" has frequently been connected with constructs such as theory of mind (ToM), mentalizing, mind-blindness, sympathy, and empathy. The concept of ToM arose primarily out of the autism literature, and suggests that humans do not merely respond to others' overt behavior, but to a belief that others have an invisible "mind," the workings of which can be partly predicted based on comparison with one's own mind. A strict definition of ToM delineates a conceptual hierarchy in which a "first-order" ToM task is to infer what person X is thinking, while a "second-order" task is to infer what person Y believes person X is thinking, or "belief about belief." Studies often employ tests of *faux pas* detection as an extension of ToM testing, since they require additional inferences about a person's feelings [e.g., Sam unwittingly tells George he dislikes a picture that turns out to have been painted by George's wife. Recognition that this is a faux pas requires two inferences: (1) that because Sam did not know the painter was George's spouse, he did not intend to insult George, and (2) that George would be hurt by Sam's comment]. Irony recognition is assumed to require some degree of perspective taking, because one must understand the speaker's intention to recognize that it does not match his or her words. Depending upon the modality in which it is delivered, sarcasm, on the other hand, usually requires that one recognize that the speaker's exaggerated or atypical nonverbal signals (voice prosody, facial expressions) are a cue to disregard his or her mismatched words, making sarcasm more of an emotion detection task than a ToM task. The exception is in certain cases of sarcasm, such as in written texts, where no nonverbal signals are provided, and one must recognize sarcasm based upon an inference about the true intention of the speaker.

Empathy is often considered to be a construct related to ToM. It is generally argued to have multiple components, roughly corresponding to an implicit or automatic awareness of another's emotional state, and a less automatic cognitive component that can involve making inferences about others' thoughts or feelings. In his review of empathy, Decety and Jackson (2004) suggest that the cognitive element of the empathic response is probably under voluntary control, and argue that healthy, socially normal individuals often do not choose to take another's perspective despite having the capacity to do so. Thus far, there is controversy in the field over whether sympathy and empathy differ, and what their respective definitions should be. Some consider sympathy to be synonymous with the cognitive perspective taking, nonemotional elements of empathy

(Dolan, 2004), whereas others define it as a feeling of affinity based on a sense of emotional identification with and similarity to the other (Decety & Chaminade, 2003).

In response to the complexity and confusion of ToM-related tasks in the social cognition literature, attempts have been made to break this construct down into its simplest component parts, the most fundamental of which appears to be perspective taking. In its simplest incarnation, perspective taking occurs when one individual infers another's knowledge based on information about other's physical location and visual point of view, also called "visual perspective taking" (Stuss, Gallup, & Alexander, 2001). Visual perspective-taking tasks intentionally avoid complex abstract reasoning, because they deal straightforwardly with objects in a room and require decisions only about what someone knows based on what he or she has physically seen. They also do not have an emotional element, so emotion processing deficits should not affect visual perspective-taking performance. However, the term "perspective taking" is also often used more generally to refer to the capacity to infer another's mental or emotional state, and perspective taking can be performed based on complex constellations of information from multiple situational and emotional modalities. Thus, perspective taking is a necessary component of accurate ToM inferences, though additional factors such as emotion detection may be required to perform ToM tasks such as detection of *faux pas*, recognition of irony, and cognitive empathy.

In a review of evidence from clinical and neuroimaging studies, Decety and Jackson (2004) suggest that there is significant convergent evidence that perspective taking is mediated by the DMPFC. They suggest that these brain areas may facilitate perspective taking by inhibiting or "toning down" the default self-perspective, in order to temporarily attend to and make inferences about the other's point of view. Importantly, functional imaging demonstrates that these areas also show significant activations, after subtracting out activations related to emotions, when normal individuals are asked to judge another's behavior as "right" or "wrong," suggesting that taking another's perspective may be involved in complex moral judgments (Moll, Eslinger, & Olivera-Souza, 2001). Studies comparing brain injured patients to normals have documented worse perspective taking in patients with lesions to the dorsomedial and frontopolar areas, including BA 10. One of the first studies suggesting an anatomic specificity to perspective taking showed that 5 patients with OFC damage performed worse than controls on a faux pas detection task despite normal 1° and 2° ToM performance; notably, 4 of the 5 patients had damage to BA 10 (Stone, Baron-Cohen, & Knight, 1998). Shamay-Tsoory, Tomer, Berger, and Aharon-Peretz (2003) conducted a series of studies of perspective taking in patients with OFC lesions. In the first, they showed that among patients with diverse frontal lobe injury, those with damage to the right frontal pole had the lowest levels of self-reported empathic perspective taking. They then showed that the only patients with frontal lobe injury who had significant deficits in both affective and cognitive components of empathy were the groups that included patients with BA 10 lesions, regardless of hemispheric laterality (Shamay-Tsoory, Tomer, Goldsher, & Aharon-Peretz, 2004). Third, they performed a study that confirmed Stone and colleagues' finding (1998) that patients with OFC lesions (N = 12) performed normally on first- and second-order ToM tasks but were impaired on *faux pas* recognition (Shamay-Tsoory, Tomer, Berger, Goldsher, & Aharon-Peretz, 2005). In addition, Shamay-Tsoory and colleagues showed that the deficits in irony and *faux pas* detection were most likely to occur in patients with damage to the right frontal pole, a finding seen earlier in less anatomically specific studies comparing the impact of right- versus left-hemisphere lesions on ToM (Rowe, Bullock, Polkey, & Morris, 2001; Surian & Siegal, 2001; Winner, Brownell, Happe, Blum, & Pincus, 1998), as well as perspective taking and deception (Stuss et al., 2001). Shamay-Tsoory and colleagues' most recent study (2005) also demonstrated that patients with poor irony and *faux pas* detection also had lower cognitive perspective-taking scores on an empathy measure, but that these deficits were dissociated from their performance on facial and vocal emotion recognition tasks. This supports the hypothesis that although the ventral OFC appears to be at least peripherally involved in emotion processing, it is not necessary for perspective taking, and that perspective-taking deficits are not explained by poor emotion recognition.

Perspective-taking deficits have also been correlated with frontal damage in other patient populations. Happe, Malhi, and Checkley (2001) found a new-onset impairment in perspective taking in a patient after he underwent an anterior capsulotomy that severed connections from the thalamus to the OFC (and other portions of the frontal lobe). In a review of ToM performance after TBI, which can also cause frontal–subcortical disconnection, Bibby and McDonald (2005) concluded that there is adequate evidence that this group also demonstrates weak inferential reasoning in general, as well as deficits in performing second-order ToM tasks. Gregory and colleagues (2002) showed that impaired ToM correlates directly to degree of frontal lobe atrophy in patients with FTD, though they divided their patients into DLPFC or OFC groups without specifically examining the contribution of the dorsomedial areas. Autistic individuals have long been demonstrated to have deficits in ToM, though the degree to which these deficits are due to inadequate perspective taking or failure to comprehend emotions depends somewhat on the severity of the autism. Morphometric analysis of the brains of autistic subjects found decreased volume in the right paracingulate gyrus and the left inferior frontal gyrus compared to controls, in addition to volume loss in the periamygdalar areas (Abell et al., 1999). In a recent case study arguing against the necessity of the dorsomedial frontal cortex in perspective taking, Bird, Castelli, Malik, Frith, and Husain (2004) showed that a patient with isolated but extensive bilateral damage to the medial surface of the frontal lobes performed normally on many ToM tasks. However, all of their ToM tasks were complicated by additional emotional or inferential reasoning requirements, and no simple visual perspective-taking tasks were included in the battery. This case reiterates the need for more detailed study to clarify the precise role of the DMPFC in perspective taking.

Though these studies of patients with brain damage converge with neuroimaging research (Gallagher & Frith, 2003) to implicate the frontal pole in the capacity for taking another person's perspective, the mechanism for this function has yet to be clarified. If the superior frontal gyrus and paracingulate gyrus can be assumed to function in a manner related to the affective division of the anterior cingulate, these dorsolateral areas may perform complex, dynamic evaluations of others' mental states in a manner that allows them to be represented separately from, and compared to, both one's own mental state and reality (Gallagher & Frith, 2003; Zysset, Huber, Ferstl, & von Cramon, 2002).

## DORSOLATERAL FRONTAL CORTEX

The evidence suggests that the dorsolateral regions of the frontal lobes probably make the least direct contribution to social functioning and personality; however, the dorsolateral prefrontal cortex (DLPFC; BAs 46, 47, and 6; lateral 8 and 9) does appear to lend clarity and organization to social cognition. The DLPFC is known to be involved in classical executive functions, including working memory, set shifting, sequencing, planning, inhibition, and abstract reasoning. Along these lines, the main contribution of the DLPFC to social functioning appears to be the application of these executive processes to social contexts by facilitating complex social reasoning and logical, deliberate regulation of social behavior. Recent experimental research suggests that the DLPFC may also be involved in the development and storage of complex social behavior schemas that provide a shorthand guide when conducting familiar social exchanges.

### Complex Deliberation, Planning, and Control in Social Contexts

Given the complexity of social contexts and their demands on our behavior, it is not surprising that better executive functioning (inhibition, planning, working memory, etc.) improves social comprehension and performance. Studies have indicated that patients with DLPFC damage have preserved emotion comprehension (Mah et al., 2005), normal "emotional intelligence" (Bar-On et al., 2003), and are no more likely than healthy controls to show increased aggression and violent behavior (Grafman et al., 1996). Unlike childhood injury to other areas of the frontal lobes, early, isolated DLPFC damage can yield normal personality and social behavior in adulthood (Eslinger, Flaherty-Craig, & Benton, 2004). Studies that have found social testing deficits in patients with DLPFC damage have frequently linked these deficits with abnormal executive functioning. For instance, poorer performance

by patients with DLPFC damage on ToM tasks (Stone et al., 1998), and risky decision-making tasks (Manes et al., 2002) have been directly associated with working memory impairments. Impaired performance on social reasoning tasks in these patients has been correlated with deficits in logical sequencing (Mah et al., 2005) and other executive functions (Channon & Crawford, 2000). Deficits in empathy correlate with poorer set shifting and generation in patients with DLPFC damage but not in patients with lesions outside the DLPFC (Shamay-Tsoory et al., 2003). Functional imaging studies suggest that the lateral DLPFC is involved in voluntarily suppressing negative emotions, a function that could have direct relevance for personality and social behavior (Levesque et al., 2003; Ochser, Bunge, Gross, & Gabrieli, 2002), though no lesion studies have provided direct evidence for this phenomenon yet.

Despite the fact that these studies suggest that the DLPFC does not make a unique contribution to social cognition, they do make clear that the executive dysfunction caused by damage to this area does result in real social cognition deficits. Mah, Arnold, and Grafman (2004) found that on a complex measure of realistic interpersonal inference making, patients with DLPFC damage were as impaired as patients with OFC damage, particularly on tests of lie detection and awareness of their own deficits. Also, though studies using the GT have provided variable evidence regarding patients with DLPFC damage, right DLPFC damage may correlate with poorer decision making in this complex, inferential task (Clark, Manes, Antoun, Sahakian, & Robbins, 2003). The executive demands of real tasks in the social realm can be enormously complex, and executive skills are probably necessary to perform the kind of slow, deliberative logical processing necessary to synthesize implicit, multimodal, often conflicting social information from multiple sources and plan behavior accordingly. The relative contributions of right versus left DLPFC to the executive processing of social and emotional material remain an open question that requires additional, focused investigation.

### Structured Event Complexes

One group of investigators has suggested that the DLPFC performs an additional function that is specific to social functioning. According to Grafman (2002), as we realize that certain social events and interactions have a similar internal event structure (e.g., "going out to dinner" or "putting a child to bed"), we develop a coherent schema of expected elements and goals (tell the child it's time for bed, put on her nightclothes, put the child in bed, read a story, etc.). Probably stored in the DLPFC, these social "structured event complexes" (SECs) function as a recipe for these complex series of behaviors and may control our behavior via a slower, more deliberate route than the kind of rapidly accessed stimulus–behavior associations that typify OFC function and are characteristic of the stereotypes discussed earlier (Wood, Knutson, & Grafman, 2004). According to this theory, we may conduct our social behavior via these SECs over long periods of time to achieve long-term goals (e.g., maintain a healthy marriage), which requires that more short-term impulses be overridden (e.g., not flirting with the flight attendant in front of one's spouse). Wood and colleagues (2004) speculate that these SECs may be involved in learned aggressive behaviors, as well as non-aggressive conflict resolution, and may provide models for our inferential reasoning about others' mental states based on situational cues. They suggest that SECs may also be involved in "relationship-specific repertoires of behavior," that is, interpersonal routines that are situation- or group-specific (e.g., telling personal stories at a dinner party with friends but not at a dinner with clients). Hypothetically, these stored behavioral repertoires may even be involved in enduring personality styles, though further research is needed to investigate this connection.

## SUMMARY AND CONCLUSIONS

This chapter has summarized the current evidence from patients with brain injuries for specifically frontal lobe contributions to social cognition. Though the behavioral outcome of injury to the OFC has been well described for more than a century, research during the past decade has allowed more precise explanations of how the OFC functions, resulting in clarification of the mechanisms by which OFC damage can result in disordered social and emotional behavior. Disruptions in the OFC's capacity to assign stimulus–reinforcer associations rapidly can result in emotion perception

deficits. Inaccurate evaluation of the reward or punishment value of social information is probably the mechanism by which some patients with frontal lobe injury fail to adhere to social norms. The failure to translate social information rapidly into altered behavior may also be responsible for some OFC-related social deficits. Recent studies suggest that our attitudes and stereotypes are also mediated by the OFC, which is uniquely suited to encode flexible assumptions about our social environment for instantaneous retrieval in circumstances where slow, deliberative evaluation would hinder effective social responses. In behavioral terms, patients with damage to the OFC, particularly in the right hemisphere, show a pattern of behavioral dyscontrol that may involve (1) either emotional blunting or emotional lability, including an insensitivity to others emotions; (2) deficient decision making, including poor social and nonsocial judgment, lack of self-monitoring, and/or inflexibility; and (3) deficient goal-directed behavior, including apathy, disinhibition, task impersistence, and general disorganization.

The more precise account that neuroscience has provided to describe the roles of the OFC in social functioning has also helped clarify which social functions are *not* performed by the ventral OFC. The dorsomedial portions of the frontal lobes, including the anterior cingulate, paracingulate, superior frontal gyrus, and frontal pole (BAs 9/10) appear to be involved in higher-level social cognition. There is increasing evidence that the complex processes of self-monitoring and taking the perspective of others are highly interdependent, and both are mediated by these dorsomedial frontal structures.

Unlike the OFC and DMPFC, there is little evidence as yet that systems in the DLPFC areas are uniquely dedicated to specific social functions. However, many studies have highlighted the fact that conventional executive skills mediated by lateral frontal lobe areas, such as planning, sequencing, inhibition, generation, working memory, and abstract reasoning, directly impact our ability to perform complex reasoning about social information. Our ability intentionally to regulate, organize, and plan our own behavior, as well as to deliberate about the behaviors of others, is dependent on the "cold cognition" systems in the lateral frontal lobes. There is evidence that we even guide our social behavior based on previously learned sequences of expected events and behaviors that we can select from a dorsolaterally mediated "social library" to fit the needs of a particular situation.

Cognitive neuroscience has made it increasingly clear that all social functioning is dependent on multiple functional circuits throughout not only the frontal lobes but also the rest of the cortex and subcortex. However, the explicitly frontal contributions to our social selves can be delineated, and the next decade holds extraordinary promise for continued discovery and illumination of this fascinating relationship.

## REFERENCES

Abdel-Dayem, H. M., Abu-Judeh, H., Kumar, M., Atay, S., Naddaf, S., El-Zeftawy, H., et al. (1998). SPECT brain perfusion abnormalities in mild or moderate traumatic brain injury. *Clinical Nuclear Medicine*, 23(5), 309–317.

Abell, F., Krams, M., Ashburner, J., Passingham, R., Friston, K., Frackowiak, R., et al. (1999). The neuroanatomy of autism: A voxel-based whole brain analysis of structural scans. *NeuroReport*, 10(8), 1647–1651.

Abu-Judeh, H., Parker, R., Singh, M., El-Zeftawy, H., Atay, S., Kumar, M., et al. (1999). SPECT brain perfusion imaging in mild traumatic brain injury without loss of consciousness and normal computed tomography. *Nuclear Medicine Communications*, 20(6), 505–510.

Adolphs, R., Damasio, H., Tranel, D., Cooper, G., & Damasio, A. R. (2000). A role for somatosensory cortices in the visual recognition of emotion as revealed by three-dimensional lesion mapping. *Journal of Neuroscience*, 20(7), 2683–2690.

Anderson, S. W., Bechara, A., Damasio, H., Tranel, D., & Damasio, A. R. (1999). Impairment of social and moral behavior related to early damage in human prefrontal cortex. *Nature Neuroscience*, 2, 1032–1037.

Angrilli, A., Palomba, D., Cantagallo, A., Maietti, A., & Stegagno, L. (1999). Emotional impairment after right orbitofrontal lesion in a patient without cognitive deficits. *NeuroReport*, 10(8), 1741–1746.

Bar-On, R., Tranel, D., Denberg, N. L., & Bechara, A. (2003). Exploring the neurological substrate of emotional and social intelligence. *Brain*, 126, 1790–1800.

Barrash, J., Tranel, D., & Anderson, S. W. (2000). Acquired personality disturbances associated with bilateral damage to the ventromedial prefrontal region. *Developmental Neuropsychology*, 18(3), 355–381.

Bathgate, D., Snowden, J. S., Varma, A., Blackshaw, A., & Neary, D. (2001). Behaviour in frontotemporal dementia, Alzheimer's disease and vascular dementia. *Acta Neurologica Scandinavica*, 103(6), 367–378.

Bechara, A., Damasio, A. R., Damaso, H., & Anderson, S. (1994). Insensitivity to future consequences following damage to human prefrontal cortex. *Cognition*, 50, 7–12.

Bechara, A., Damasio, H., Damasio, A. R., & Lee, G. P. (1999). Different contributions of the human amygdala and ventromedial prefrontal cortex to decision-making. *Journal of Neuroscience*, 19(13), 5473–5481.

Bechara, A., Damasio, H., & Damasio, A. R. (2000). Emotion, decision making and the orbitofrontal cortex. *Cerebral Cortex*, 10(3), 295–307.

Bechara, A., Tranel, D., Damasio, H., & Damasio, A. R. (1996). Failure to respond autonomically to anticipated future outcomes following damage to prefrontal cortex. *Cerebral Cortex*, 6(2), 215–225.

Beer, J. S., Heerey, E., Keltner, D., Scabini, D., & Knight, R. (2003). The regulatory function of self-conscious emotion: Insights from patients with orbitofrontal damage. *Journal of Personality and Social Psychology*, 85(4), 589–593.

Bell, C. J., Malizia, A. L., & Nutt, D. J. (1999). The neurobiology of social phobia. *European Archives of Psychiatry and Clinical Neuroscience*, 249(Suppl. 1), S11–S18.

Bibby, H., & McDonald, S. (2005). Theory of mind after traumatic brain injury. *Neuropsychologia*, 43(1), 99–114.

Bird, C. M., Castelli, F., Malik, O., Frith, U., & Husain, M. (2004). The impact of extensive medial frontal lobe damage on "theory of mind" and cognition. *Brain*, 127, 914–928.

Blair, R. J., & Cipolotti, L. (2000). Impaired social response reversal: A case of "acquired sociopathy." *Brain*, 123(6), 1122–1141.

Borod, J. C. (Ed.). (2000). *The neuropsychology of emotion*. New York: Oxford University Press.

Channon, S., & Crawford, S. (2000). The effects of anterior lesions on performance on a story comprehension test: Left anterior impairment on a theory of mind-type task. *Neuropsychologia*, 38(7), 1006–1017.

Chemerinski, E., Nopoulos, P. C., Crespo-Facorro, B., Andreasen, N. C., & Magnotta, V. (2002). Morphology of the ventral frontal cortex in schizophrenia: Relationship with social dysfunction. *Biological Psychiatry*, 52(1), 1–8.

Choi, J. S., Kang, D. H., Kim, J. J., Ha, T. H., Lee, J. M., Youn, T., et al. (2004). Left anterior subregion of orbitofrontal cortex volume reduction and impaired organizational strategies in obsessive–compulsive disorder. *Journal of Psychiatric Research*, 38(2), 193–199.

Clark, L., Manes, F., Antoun, N., Sahakian, B. J., & Robbins, T. W. (2003). The contributions of lesion laterality and lesion volume to decision-making impairment following frontal lobe damage. *Neuropsychologia*, 41(11), 1474–1483.

Damasio, A. R. (1994). *Descartes' error: Emotion, reason and the human brain*. New York: Grosset/Putnam.

Decety, J., & Chaminade, T. (2003). Neural correlates of feeling sympathy. *Neuropsychologia, 41,* 127–138.

Decety, J., & Jackson, P. L. (2004). The functional architecture of human empathy. *Behavioral and Cognitive Neuroscience Reviews, 3*(2), 71–100.

Dolan, R. J. (2004). *The brain, emotion, and aesthetic judgments.* Paper presented at the 3rd Annual International Conference on Neuroesthetics, Berkeley, CA.

Eslinger, P. J., Flaherty-Craig, C. V., & Benton, A. L. Developmental outcomes after early prefrontal cortex damage. *Brain and Cognition, 55*(1), 84–103.

Evans, D. W., Lewis, M. D., & Iobst, E. (2004). The role of the orbitofrontal cortex in normally developing compulsive-like behaviors and obsessive–compulsive disorder. *Brain and Cognition, 55*(1), 220–234.

Gallagher, H. L., & Frith, C. D. (2003). Functional imaging of "theory of mind." *Trends in Cognitive Science, 7*(2), 77–83.

Godfrey, H. P., Knight, R. G., Marsh, N. V., Moroney, B., & Bishara, S. N. (1989). Social interaction and speed of information processing following very severe head-injury. *Psychological Medicine, 19*(1), 175–182.

Goel, V., Shuren, J., Sheesley, L., & Grafman, J. (2004). Asymmetrical involvement of frontal lobes in social reasoning. *Brain, 127*(4), 783–790.

Grafman, J. (2002). The human prefrontal cortex has evolved to represent components of structured event complexes. In *Handbook of neuropsychology* (pp. 157–174). Amsterdam: Elsevier.

Grafman, J., Schwab, K., Warden, D., Pridgen, A., Brown, H. R., & Salazar, A. M. (1996). Frontal lobe injuries, violence, and aggression: A report of the Vietnam Head Injury Study. *Neurology, 46*(5), 1231–1238.

Green, R. E., Turner, G. R., & Thompson, W. F. (2004). Deficits in facial emotion perception in adults with recent traumatic brain injury. *Neuropsychologia, 42*(2), 133–141.

Gregory, C., Lough, S., Stone, V., Erzinclioglu, S., Martin, L., Baron-Cohen, S., et al. (2002). Theory of mind in patients with frontal variant frontotemporal dementia and Alzheimer's disease: Theoretical and practical implications. *Brain, 125*(4), 752–764.

Hager, J. C., & Ekman, P. (1979). Long-distance transmission of facial affect signals. *Ethology and Sociobiology, 1,* 77–92.

Happe, F., Malhi, G. S., & Checkley, S. (2001). Acquired mind-blindness following frontal lobe surgery?: A single case study of impaired "theory of mind" in a patient treated with stereotactic anterior capsulotomy. *Neuropsychologia, 39*(1), 83–90.

Hopkins, M. J., Dywan, J. , & Segalowitz, S. J. (2002). Altered electrodermal response to facial expression after closed head injury. *Brain Injury, 16*(3), 245–257.

Hornak, J., Bramham, J., Rolls, E. T., Morris, R. G., O'Doherty, J., Bullock, P. R., et al. (2003). Changes in emotion after circumscribed surgical lesions of the orbitofrontal and cingulate cortices. *Brain, 126*(7), 1691–1712.

Hornak, J., Rolls, E. T., & Wade, D. (1996). Face and voice expression identification in patients with emotional and behavioural changes following ventral frontal lobe damage. *Neuropsychologia, 34*(4), 247–261.

Jackson, H. F., & Moffat, N. J. (1987). Impaired emotional recognition following severe head injury. *Cortex, 23*(2), 293–300.

Keane, J., Calder, A. J., Hodges, J. R., & Young, A. W. (2002). Face and emotion processing in frontal variant frontotemporal dementia. *Neuropsychologia, 40*(6), 655–665.

Kringelbach, M. L., & Rolls, E. T. (2004). The functional neuroanatomy of the human orbitofrontal cortex: Evidence from neuroimaging and neuropsychology. *Progress in Neurobiology, 72*(5), 341–372.

Kucharska-Pietura, K., Phillips, M. L., Gernand, W., & David, A. S. (2003). Perception of emotions from faces and voices following unilateral brain damage. *Neuropsychologia, 41,* 1082–1090.

Lane, R. D., Reiman, E. M., Ahern, G. L., Schwartz, G. E., & Davidson, R. J. (1997). Neuroanatomical correlates of happiness, sadness, and disgust. *American Journal of Psychiatry, 154*(7), 926–933.

Lane, R. D., Reiman, E. M., Axelrod, B., Yun, L.-S., Holmes, A. H., & Schwartz, G. E. (1998). Neural correlates of levels of emotional awareness: Evidence of an interaction between emotion and attention in the anterior cingulate cortex. *Journal of Cognitive Neuroscience, 10,* 525–535.

Lannoo, E., de Deyne, C., Colardyn, F., de Soete, G., & Jannes, C. (1997). Personality change following head injury: Assessment with the NEO Five-Factor Inventory. *Journal of Psychosomatic Research, 43*(5), 505–511.

Lavenu, I., Pasquier, F., Lebert, F., Petit, H., & Van der Linden, M. (1999). Perception of emotion in frontotemporal dementia and Alzheimer disease. *Alzheimer Disease and Associated Disorders, 13*(2), 96–101.

Lavenu, I., & Pasquier, F. (2005). Perception of emotion on faces in frontotemporal dementia and Alzheimer's disease: A longitudinal study. *Dementia and Geriatric Cognitive Disorders, 19*(1), 37–41.

Levesque, J., Eugene, F., Joanette, Y., Paquette, V., Mensour, B., Beaudoin, G., et al. (2003). Neural circuitry underlying voluntary suppression of sadness. *Biological Psychiatry, 53*(6), 502–510.

Levy, M. L., Miller, B. L., Cummings, J. L., Fairbanks, L. A., & Craig, A. (1996). Alzheimer disease and Frontotemporal dementias: Behavioural distinctions. *Archives of Neurology, 53,* 687–690.

Mah, L., Arnold, M. C., & Grafman, J. (2004). Impairment of social perception associated with lesions of the prefrontal cortex. *American Journal of Psychiatry, 161*(7), 1247–1255.

Mah, L., Arnold, M. C., & Grafman, J. (2005). Deficits

in social knowledge following damage to ventromedial prefrontal cortex. *Journal of Neuropsychiatry and Clinical Neurosciences, 17*(1), 66–74.

Malizia, A. L. (1997). The frontal lobes and neurosurgery for psychiatric disorders. *Journal of Psychopharmacology, 11*(2), 179–187.

Mandal, M. K., Borod, J. C., Asthana, H. S., Mohanty, A., Mohanty, S., & Koff E. (1999). Effects of lesion variables and emotion type on the perception of facial emotion. *Journal of Nervous and Mental Disease, 187*(10), 603–609.

Manes, F., Sahakian, B., Clark, L., Rogers, R., Antoun, N., Aitken, M., et al. (2002). Decision-making processes following damage to the prefrontal cortex. *Brain, 125*(3), 624–639.

Marcin, M. S., & Nemeroff, C. B. (2003). The neurobiology of social anxiety disorder: The relevance of fear and anxiety. *Acta Psychiatrica Scandinavica, 417*(Suppl.), 51–64.

Milne, E., & Grafman, J. (2001). Ventromedial prefrontal cortex lesions in humans eliminate implicit gender stereotyping. *Journal of Neuroscience, 21*(12), RC150.

Moll, J., Eslinger, P. J., & Oliveira-Souza, R. (2001). Frontopolar and anterior temporal cortex activation in a moral judgment task: Preliminary functional MRI results in normal subjects. *Arquivos de Neuro-Psiquiatria, 59*(3–B), 657–664.

Moll, J., Oliveira-Souza, R., & Eslinger, P. J. (2003). Morals and the human brain: A working model. *NeuroReport, 14*, 299–305.

Neary, D., Snowden, J. S., Gustafson, L., Passant, U., Stuss, D., Black, S., et al. (1998). Frontotemporal lobar degeneration: A consensus on clinical diagnostic criteria. *Neurology, 51*(6), 1546–1554.

Ochsner, K. N., Bunge, S. A., Gross, J. J., & Gabrieli, J. D. E. (2002). Rethinking feelings: An fMRI study of the cognitive regulation of emotion. *Journal of Cognitive Neuroscience, 14*(8), 1215–1229.

Prigatano, G. P. (1999). Personality disturbances and brain damage: Theoretical perspectives. In G. P. Prigatano, *Principles of neuropsychological rehabilitation* (pp. 117–147). New York: Oxford University Press.

Prigatano, G. P., & Pribram K. H. (1982). Perception and memory of facial affect following brain injury. *Perceptual and Motor Skills, 54*(3), 859–869.

Pujol, J., Soriano-Mas, C., Alonso, P., Cardoner, N., Menchon, J. M., Deus, J., et al. (2004). Mapping structural brain alterations in obsessive–compulsive disorder. *Archives of General Psychiatry, 61*(7), 720–730.

Rankin, K. P., Baldwin, E., Pace-Savitsky, C., Kramer, J. H., & Miller, B. L. (2004). Self awareness and personality change in dementia. *Journal of Neurology, Neurosurgery and Psychiatry, 76*, 632–639.

Rankin, K. P., Glenn, S., Stanley, C. M., Allison, S., Kramer, J. H., & Miller, B. L. (2006). Right frontal correlates of utilizing social feedback in self-monitoring. *Neurology, 66*(Suppl. 12), A122–123.

Rankin, K. P., Kramer, J. H., & Miller, B. (2005). Patterns of cognitive and emotional empathy in frontotemporal dementia. *Cognitive and Behavioral Neurology, 18*(1), 28–36.

Rankin, K. P., Kramer, J. H., Mychack, P., & Miller, B. L. (2003). Double dissociation of social functioning in frontotemporal dementia. *Neurology, 60*(2), 266–271.

Rankin, K. P., Rosen, H. J., Kramer, J. H., Schauer, G. F., Weiner, M. W., Schuff, N., et al. (2004). Right and left medial orbitofrontal volumes show an opposite relationship to agreeableness in FTD. *Dementia and Geriatric Cognitive Disorders, 17*(4), 328–332.

Rosen, H. J., Gorno-Tempini, M. L., Goldman, W. P., Perry, R. J., Schuff, N., Weiner, M., et al. (2002). Patterns of brain atrophy in frontotemporal dementia and semantic dementia. *Neurology, 58*(2), 198–208.

Rosen, H. J., Pace-Savitsky, C., Perry, R. J., Kramer, J. H., Miller, B., & Levinson, R. W. (2004). Recognition of emotion in the frontal and temporal variants of frontotemporal dementia. *Dementia and Geriatric Cognitive Disorders, 17*(4), 277–281.

Rosen, H. J., Perry, R. J., Murphy, J., Kramer, J. H., Mychack, P., Schuff, N., et al. (2002). Emotion comprehension in the temporal variant of frontotemporal dementia. *Brain, 125*, 2286–2295.

Rowe, A. D., Bullock, P. R., Polkey, C. E., & Morris, R. G. (2001). "Theory of mind" impairments and their relationship to executive functioning following frontal lobe excisions. *Brain, 124*(3), 600–616.

Rule, R. R., Shimamura, A. P., & Knight, R. T. (2002). Orbitofrontal cortex and dynamic filtering of emotional stimuli. *Cognitive, Affective and Behavioral Neuroscience, 2*(3), 264–270.

Shamay-Tsoory, S. G., Tomer, R., Berger, B. D., & Aharon-Peretz, J. (2003). Characterization of empathy deficits following prefrontal brain damage: The role of the right ventromedial prefrontal cortex. *Journal of Cognitive Neuroscience, 15*(3), 324–337.

Shamay-Tsoory, S. G., Tomer, R., Berger, B. D., Goldsher, D., & Aharon-Peretz, J. (2005). Impaired "affective theory of mind" is associated with right ventromedial prefrontal damage. *Cognitive and Behavioral Neurology, 18*(1), 55–67.

Shamay-Tsoory, S. G., Tomer, R., Goldsher, D., Berger, B. D., & Aharon-Peretz, J. (2004). Impairment in cognitive and affective empathy in patients with brain lesions: Anatomical and cognitive correlates. *Journal of Clinical and Experimental Neuropsychology, 26*(8), 1113–1127.

Spell, L., & Frank, E. (2000). Recognition of nonverbal communication of affect following traumatic brain injury. *Journal of Nonverbal Behavior, 24*(4), 285–300.

Stone, V. E., Baron-Cohen, S., & Knight, R. T. (1998). Frontal lobe contributions to theory of mind. *Journal of Cognitive Neuroscience, 10*(5), 640–656.

Stuss, D., Gallup, G. G., & Alexander, M. P. (2001). The frontal lobes are necessary for "theory of mind." *Brain, 124*, 279–286.

Surian, L., & Siegal, M. (2001). Sources of performance on theory of mind tasks in right hemisphere–damaged patients. *Brain and Language*, 78(2), 224–232.

Tillfors, M., Furmark, T., Marteinsdottir, I., Fischer, H., Pissiota, A., Langstrom, B., et al. (2001). Cerebral blood flow in subjects with social phobia during stressful speaking tasks: A PET study. *American Journal of Psychiatry*, 158(8), 1220–1226.

Tomaiuolo, F., Worsley, K., Lerch, J., Di Paola, M., Carlesimo, G. A., Bonanni, R., et al. (2005). Changes in white matter in long-term survivors of severe non-missile traumatic brain injury: A computational analysis of magnetic resonance images. *Journal of Neurotrauma*, 22(1), 76–82.

Tranel, D., Bechara, A., & Denburg, N. L. (2003). Asymmetric functional roles of right and left ventromedial prefrontal cortices in social conduct, decision-making, and emotional processing. *Cortex*, 38(4), 589–612.

Van Ameringen, M., Mancini, C., Szechtman, H., Nahmias, C., Oakman, J. M., Hall, G. B., et al. (2004). A PET provocation study of generalized phobia. *Psychiatry Research*, 132(1), 13–18.

Wallesch, C. W., Curio, N., Kutz, S., Jost, S., Bartels, C., & Synowitz, H. (2001). Outcome after mild-to-moderate blunt head injury: Effects of focal lesions and diffuse axonal injury. *Brain Injury*, 15(5), 401–412.

Winner, E., Brownell, H., Happe, F., Blum, A., & Pincus, D. (1998). Distinguishing lies from jokes: Theory of mind deficits and discourse interpretation in right hemisphere brain-damaged patients. *Brain and Language*, 62(1), 89–106.

Wood, J. N., Knutson, K. M., & Grafman J. (2004). Psychological structure and neural correlates of event knowledge. *Cerebral Cortex*, 15, 1155–1161.

Zysset, S., Huber, O., Ferstl, E., & von Cramon, D. Y. (2002). The anterior frontomedian cortex and evaluative judgment: An fMRI study. *NeuroImage*, 15(4), 983–991.

# PART VI

## NEUROLOGICAL DISEASES

# SECTION A

# Frontotemporal Dementia and Related Disorders

# CHAPTER 24

# Clinical Aspects of Frontotemporal Dementia

*Pei-Ning Wang*
*Bruce L. Miller*

Frontotemporal lobar degeneration (FTLD) is a neurodegenerative disease that selectively attacks the frontal and anterior temporal regions. In 1892 Arnold Pick described a 71-year-old patient with progressive language loss and cognitive decline. Pick commented upon the focal nature of this patient's neurodegenerative condition and described the unique language deficits of his patient. Autopsy revealed prominent left anterior temporal atrophy. Today, this patient would be considered to suffer from the FTLD subtype semantic dementia (SD). Sadly, even more than 100 years after the first description of this fascinating disorder, diagnostic accuracy remains flawed, and FTLD and related disorders are still greatly underdiagnosed (Baldwin & Forstl, 1993; Kertesz & Munoz, 2002).

## EPIDEMIOLOGY AND DEMOGRAPHICS

FTLD occurs in 5–15% of patients with dementia (Hokoishi et al., 2001; Ikeda, Ishikawa, & Tanabe, 2004; Kertesz, 1997; Ratnavalli et al., 2002) and it is the third most common degenerative dementia, following only Alzheimer's disease (AD) and dementia with Lewy bodies (Harvey, Skelton-Robinson, & Rossor, 2003; Ikeda et al., 2004; Pasquier & Delacourte, 1998). Typical age of onset is between 50 and 60 years, although FTLD can occur as early as the 20s and has been reported in the ninth decade (Knopman, Petersen, Edland,

Cha, & Rocca, 2004; Ratnavalli, Brayne, Dawson, & Hodges, 2002; Rosso et al., 2003).

Community-based studies on the incidence and overall prevalence of FTLD are lacking (Lund and Manchester Groups, 1994; Ratnavalli et al., 2002). Recent work suggests that in patients with dementia ages 45–70 years, the prevalence of FTLD approaches that of AD, whereas in patients below age 50 years, FTLD is probably more common than AD. The first studies to address this issue revealed that the prevalence of FTLD between the ages of 45 and 64 years varied from 4 to 15 per 100,000 (Harvey et al., 2003; Ratnavalli et al., 2002; Rosso et al., 2003). In a recent study, the incidence rate of FTLD was 2.2 per 100,000 between ages 40 and 49, 3.3 per 100,000 between ages 50 and 59 years, and 8.9 per 100,000 between ages 60 and 69 years (Knopman et al., 2004). FTLD has been reported more frequently in Western compared to Asian populations (Ikeda et al., 2004). Genetic factors may contribute to this discrepancy, and approximately one-third of patients with FTLD in the United States and Europe have a positive family history (Chow, Miller, Hayashi, & Geschwind, 1999; Stevens et al., 1998), whereas most Japanese FTLD cases have been sporadic (Ikeda, 2000). However, diminished recognition of FTLD and related disorders is likely to be a major factor for the low prevalence reported in Asian countries.

With the development of new research criteria for FTLD, the demographics and relative age and sex distribution of the various FTLD patient populations are now being explored. There are important demographic differences between the three subtypes originally defined by Neary and colleagues (1998). In work from Cambridge, United Kingdom, and in a separate three-site study from the University of California at San Francisco (UCSF), the University of California at Los Angeles (UCLA), and Munich, Germany, the frontotemporal dementia (FTD) subtype of FTLD has shown a strong male predominance. The relative sex distribution for the other FTLD subtypes, SD, and nonfluent progressive aphasia (NFPA) is still unknown, although our preliminary work suggests that SD is more common in males and NFPA is more common in females. There is a strong link between FTD and motor neuron disease, and atypical Parkinsonian syndromes, including corticobasal degeneration (CBD) and progressive supranuclear palsy (PSP) (Kertesz,

Hillis, & Munoz, 2003; Spillantini, Bird, & Ghetti, 1998; Talbot, 1996). The appearance of motor neuron disease or parkinsonism strongly influences survival in FTD (Grasbeck, Englund, Horstmann, Passant, & Gustafson, 2003; Hodges, Davies, Xuereb, Kril, & Halliday, 2003). FTD tends to occur at a slightly younger age and has the shortest life expectancy from time of presentation.

Genetics remain the only known risk factor for FTLD. The majority of cases are sporadic, but approximately 10% of cases seem to follow an autosomal dominant pattern of inheritance (Chow et al., 1999; Stevens et al., 1998). Mutations in tau introns and exons represent the most common known cause for these dominant forms of FTLD (Foster et al., 1997; Spillantini & Goedert, 2001; Yoshiyama, Lee, & Trojanowski, 2001), although many genes remain to be discovered, even in autosomal dominant families (Bird, 2001; Goldman et al.,

**TABLE 24.1. Features of Patients with Different FTLD Subtypes**

| Diagnosis | FTLD subtype | | |
| --- | --- | --- | --- |
| | FTD | SD | NFPA |
| Sex distribution | Male > female | Male > female | Female > male |
| Age at onset | Mid-50s | Late 50s | Early 60s |
| Genetics | Strongly familial | Rarely familial | Intermediate |
| Motor neuron disease | Common | Unusual | Unusual |
| Survival from time of diagnosis | 3.1 years | 5.3 years | 4.2 years |
| Behavior | Overeating, apathy, disinhibition, personality change, repetitive behaviors | Similar to FTD in right-sided cases; FTD-type behaviors emerge after a few years in left-sided cases | Tends to remain normal; depression is common |
| Neuropsychology | Poor generation, set-shifting, inhibition; good drawing, naming | Poor naming, verbal memory; good drawing, working memory | Nonfluent, verbal apraxia; good comprehension |
| Neurology | Look for ALS, Parkinsonian features | Look for ALS, often normal | Overlap with PSP and CBD |
| Neuroimaging | Bilateral (right > left) frontal–ventral–insular and cingulated atrophy/ hypometabolism (left > right) anterior temporal, amygdala and insular atrophy/hypometabolism | Bilateral | Bilateral (left > right) fronto-insular atrophy/ hypometabolism |
| Neuropathology | Most common: FTD-ubiquitin inclusions; less common: no inclusions or tau inclusions | Most common pathology is FTD-ubiquitin inclusions | Most common pathology is FTD-tau; often overlaps with CBD or PSP |

2004; Tolnay & Probst, 2002; Wilhelmsen, 1998). FTD and FTD with amyotrophic lateral sclerosis (ALS) are the most genetic forms of FTLD, whereas SD is the least familial (Chow et al., 1999). Table 24.1 describes the demographic features of patients with the different FTLD subtypes.

## CLINICAL MANIFESTATIONS

The clinical presentation of FTLD is heterogeneous, driven by the variable involvement of the left or right frontal or temporal regions. Additionally, the basal ganglia, motor neurons, and spinal cord are vulnerable in FTLD (Brun, 1987; Mann, South, Snowden, & Neary, 1993; Tolnay & Probst, 2001). In some instances,

motor involvement precedes cortical disease; in others, it follows cortical deficits, and in still others, it develops concurrently with the cortical presentations (Brun & Passant, 1996). FTLD is divided into three clinical subtypes, FTD, NFPA, and SD (Neary et al., 1998). Each subtype presents distinctive clinical manifestations driven by the different brain areas that are predominantly involved. With FTD, the disorder is frontally predominant and involves the right hemisphere more than the left. NFPA involves the left frontal region, whereas SD is a temporally predominant syndrome that tends to affect the anterior temporal regions (see Figure 24.1).

In this chapter we review the symptoms of FTLD, delineate the different FTLD subtypes, describe the motor disorders strongly linked

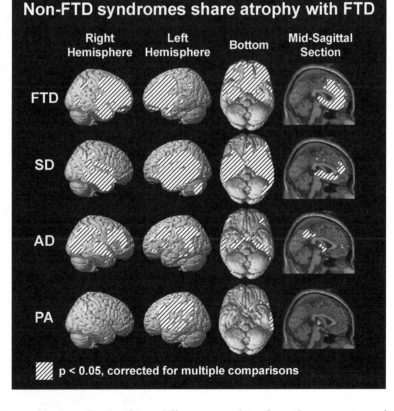

FIGURE 24.1. Maps of statistically significant differences resulting from the comparison of structural images in different dementia syndromes with control images. Patterns of frontal involvement differ according to the clinical syndrome, with FTD particularly affecting medial and lateral frontal regions, AD affecting the lateral frontal regions and parietal, and PA affecting mainly the left lateral frontoparietal (perisylvian) region. FTD, frontotemporal dementia; SD, semantic dementia; AD, Alzheimer's disease; PA, progressive nonfluent aphasia.

with FTLD, including CBD, PSP, and motor neuron disease, and outline the neuropsychological features of FTLD.

## Early Symptoms

First symptoms often help with the differentiation of FTLD from other dementias and facilitate accurate classification of the three clinical subtypes. In contrast to AD, in which memory loss is usually the first symptom, the initial symptoms of FTLD often involve changes in personality, behavior, affective symptoms, and language function (Hodges, 2001; Lindau et al., 2000). These early behavioral symptoms are easily misdiagnosed as the manifestation of a primary psychiatric disorder, and many FTLD patients are initially seen by psychiatrists.

Behavior change is the most common first symptom in FTD (62%), whereas speech and language problems are most common in NFPA (100%) and SD (58%). About 10% of patients with FTD present with memory problems as a first symptom. Common behavioral symptoms in FTD include apathy (32%) and disinhibition (16%). Also strongly distinguishing NFPA from FTD is the fact that insight is often exquisitely preserved in NFPA (Liu et al., 2004). Most patients with SD begin with language (left-sided cases) or emotional (right-sided cases) changes (Seeley et al., 2005). The lack of insight seen in FTD, and sometimes in SD, leads patients to ignore or deny their deficits, often delaying diagnosis.

Nomenclature issues are greatly confounded by the overlap among FTLD, CBD, PSP, and ALS (Hou, Carlin, & Miller, 2004; Kertesz, 2003). Fluid changes between these different syndromes and FTLD are common. For example, patients can begin with NFPA and then develop asymmetric parkinsonism with alien limb, suggesting CBD. Conversely, asymmetric parkinsonism as a first symptom may suggest CBD, but many such patients then go on to an FTD or NFPA cortical syndrome. Hence, first symptoms often define the initial diagnosis, but diagnosis may change as the illness progresses. Distinguishing FTLD from AD during life is relatively straightforward, with 80–90% of cases correctly separated in several studies (Diehl et al., 2005; Knopman et al., 2005; Kramer et al., 2003; Rosen, Hartikainen, et al., 2002). In contrast, predicting whether a patient

will show CBD, FTD with tau, FTD with ubiquitin, or FTD without inclusions (so-called dementia lacking distinctive histology) is currently impossible. Classical silver-staining, tau-positive cellular inclusions, so-called Pick bodies, account for < 20% of cases.

## FTLD Subtypes

### Frontotemporal Dementia

The core features of FTD as defined by the Neary criteria (Neary et al., 1998) are early decline in social and personal conduct, emotional blunting, and loss of insight. Selective brain degeneration is seen in the dorsolateral, orbital, and medial frontal cortex (Frisoni et al., 1996; Larsson et al., 2000; Rosen, Gorno-Tempini, et al., 2002). The insular cortex is also severely atrophic (Rosen, Gorno-Tempini, et al., 2002). The anterior temporal lobes are variably involved, but the parietal regions are relatively spared, and occipital cortex is often normal. The degeneration associated with FTD involves the right hemisphere more severely than the left (Gee et al., 2003; Miller, Chang, Mena, Boone, & Lesser, 1993; Rosen, Gorno-Tempini, et al., 2002). Personality change, disinhibition, and apathy are prominent and frequently noted by informants. Personality shifts in the direction of submissiveness are typical of FTD, although extraversion can emerge in previously introverted individuals (Rankin, Kramer, Mychack, & Miller, 2003). There is a shift from warmth to coldness on personality scales. Changes in established religious or political beliefs and patterns of dress suggesting changes in the sense of self are common (Miller et al., 2001). Respect for personal boundaries disappears, and some patients stare or become overfriendly, talking openly to strangers (including children) (Miller et al., 2001). Increased trust for others makes these patients vulnerable to financial scams or sexual exploitation. One patient accepted repeated telephone calls from a fraudulent land company and spent many thousands of dollars over the phone buying nonexistent land, despite repeated warnings from relatives and lawyers.

Indiscretion causes embarrassment to the family, and disinhibited verbal outbursts or socially inappropriate behaviors are common (Mendez, Perryman, Miller, Swartz, & Cummings, 1997; Mendez, Solwood, Mastri,

& Frey, 1993). Antisocial behaviors, including crimes, develop de novo, and often reflect poor judgment and impaired impulse control (Miller et al., 1997). Shoplifting, sexual exhibitionism, speeding, and running stop signs are common, but highly organized and well-planned criminal activities are rare in these patients. Verbal discussion of sexual matters, is seen but hyposexuality is far more common than hypersexuality (Cummings & Duchen, 1981; Miller, Darby, Swartz, Yener, & Mena, 1995). Impairment in personal conduct is a core feature. Some patients are overactive, with increased verbal and motor activities, whereas others become inactive and withdrawn. Some patients fluctuate between overactivity and apathy. Decreased concern regarding personal grooming and appearance are also common.

Loss of concern for others and prominent emotional blunting tend to isolate the patient with FDT (Gregory & Hodges, 1996; Keane, Calder, Hodges, & Young, 2002; Rosen et al., 2004). A constellation of cognitive and emotional changes contribute to this emotional blunting. For example, comprehension and expression of emotion are deficient, and the inability to comprehend the emotions that others are feeling, particularly negative emotions, contributes to the feeling that the patient is no longer concerned about his or her loved ones. In addition, patients become self-centered and tend to focus on their own particular needs and desires. In a medical crisis setting, patients may respond with inappropriate lack of concern, sometimes in a bizarre manner. One patient flew back home the day that his wife was to undergo a bone marrow transplantation, in order to complete his tax returns, whereas another drove slowly to the hospital so as not to get a ticket when his father was bleeding to death.

Depression occurs and many patients with FTD are diagnosed with depressive disorders before dementia is evident (Chow, Miller, Boone, Mishkin, & Cummings, 2002; Miller et al., 1991). Often, the depression has atypical features that are a clue to the real diagnosis. Loss of insight regarding behavioral changes, diminished empathy for others, denial of depression, apathy, and blunted affect are present in many patients with FTD and depressive features. Psychotic features, such as delusions and hallucinations, occur but are infrequent. In one study 13% of patients had hallucinations and 22% showed delusions (Liu et al., 2004). Delu-

sions differ from those in patients with AD and are typically grandiose or bizarre. One patient insisted that she had won the lottery and spent $100,000 on clothes; another ritualistically lined up dead cockroaches in a closet.

Perseverative and stereotyped behaviors emerge in the middle stages of FTD (Ames, Cummings, Wirshing, Quinn, & Mahler, 1994; Mendez et al., 1997; Mendez, Shapira, & Miller, 2005; Miller et al., 1995; Swartz, Miller, Lesser, & Darby, 1997). Simple repetitive motor or verbal acts such as lip smacking, hand rubbing, or humming are common (Snowden et al., 2001). More complex behaviors, such as collecting (garbage, rocks, stamps, plastic figures, etc.), wandering a fixed route, or counting money, evolve in many patients. Also, eating change and hyperorality are common (Bozeat, Gregory, Ralph, & Hodges, 2000; Miller et al., 1995). Hyperorality manifests in overeating, change in food preference to a certain type of food, or even the consumption of inedible objects (Swartz, Miller, Lesser, & Darby, 1997). Excessive smoking and alcohol or drug abuse can lead to the misdiagnosis of alcohol or drug addiction. Patients with FTD tend to overeat in a gluttonous manner, whereas patients with SD may compulsively eat one or several items without gaining weight (Snowden et al., 2001).

Loss of executive functions leads to impaired multitasking, shifting, abstracting, making sound judgments, planning, and problem solving (Johanson & Hagberg, 1989; Kramer et al., 2003). These executive problems can be the first manifestation of FTD, preceding behavioral deficits (Lindau et al., 2000). Poor performance at jobs leads these patients to get fired, and they tend to work at progressively simpler occupations. Similarly, catastrophic financial loss due to poor decision making is common prior to presentation at the physician's office. Deficits in working memory, set shifting, and generation are evident on bedside testing. Episodic memory deficits can be prominent, leading to a misdiagnosis of AD.

### Nonfluent Progressive Aphasia

NFPA is defined by the Neary criteria as an expressive language disorder with nonfluent spontaneous speech, agrammatism, phonemic paraphasias, and anomia. According to this relatively vague definition, many patients diagnosed with NFPA will have a degenerative disorder that begins in the left frontal insular region. However, others meeting the Neary criteria for NFPA have a degenerative disorder that begins in the left angular gyrus or posterior temporal region. We suspect that the majority of patients with the posterior anatomical variant of NFPA suffer from an asymmetrical cortical variation of AD (Gorno-Tempini, Dronkers, et al., 2004).

Speech or language problems are almost always the earliest symptoms associated with NFPA. Patients have effortful, hesitant and broken speech, and the number of words and phrases diminishes. Phonemic paraphasias, particularly during repetition, become evident. Deficits in working memory are common due to involvement of the frontal and sometimes parietal regions. Reading, writing, and confrontation naming are also impaired. Comprehension is relatively preserved, especially comprehension for simple sentences and single words. When abnormalities in sentence comprehension are present early in the illness, posterior progressive aphasia due to AD should be considered. Expressive speech difficulty may affect the performance on verbal memory tasks, but visual memory is relatively preserved in NFPA.

As the disease advances, the speech of patients with NFPA becomes less fluent, and naming and repetition decline. Comprehension of single words eventually fails as NFPA spreads posteriorly. Ultimately patients with NFPA become mute. Comprehension of verbs is more impaired than is comprehension for nouns (Bak, O'Donovan, Xuereb, Boniface, & Hodges, 2001; Rhee, Antiquena, & Grossman, 2001). Apraxia of speech, articulatory groping, and impaired sequencing of phonemesis common. The anatomical correlate of these findings is atrophy in the left inferior frontal gyrus, premotor cortex, and anterior insula (Gorno-Tempini, Dronkers, et al., 2004; Kertesz, Hillis, & Munoz, 2003; Radanovic et al., 2001), brain regions that participate in motor speech and syntax processing.

In some patients, speech abnormalities are the presenting feature of NFPA. Typically these patients become mute relatively early in the illness. In many instances, patients with NFPA patient are better able to communicate by writing. Sometimes a full-blown CBD syndrome with an alien hand, focal dystonia, and asym-

metric parkinsonism emerge. We suspect that many patients that begin with speech abnormalities will go on to demonstrate CBD neuropathology (Gorno-Tempini, Dronkers, et al., 2004; Graham, Bak, & Hodges, 2003). Although apathy, depression, and social withdrawal are common, other behavioral abnormalities seen in FTD are not typically found in the early stages of NFPA. As the disease progress, similar behavior problems may develop when the degeneration spreads to the right side of brain.

## Semantic Dementia

Patients with SD show impairment of word meaning and object identity, and exhibit fluent empty, spontaneous speech (Hodges, Patterson, Oxbury, & Funnell, 1992; Snowden, 1999). Language output is grammatical but empty because of loss of knowledge regarding words and word meanings. Comprehension of single words is impaired. Prosody, phonology, and speech syntax are relatively preserved. Repetition is usually good, and it is common to see patients with SD repeat or write a word that they do not know. In reading and writing, patients perform well with phonetically and orthographically regular words but are impaired with irregular words (Hodges et al., 1992; Noble, Glosser, & Grossman, 2000; Patterson, Lambon Ralph, Hodges, & McClelland, 2001). Words such as "yacht," "knight," "gnat," or "choir" are semantically irregular words that are difficult for patients to read or spell. Hence, "yacht" is pronounced "yached," whereas a patient given the word "yacht" might spell it "YOT," while "gnat is read "gunat" and spelled "NAT." SD is not simply a language deficit but represents a fundamental loss of semantic memory and knowledge: long-term memories that contain knowledge about items in the world, as well as an understanding of their relationship (Murre, Graham, & Hodges, 2001). Facts, concepts, and words disappear, as do autobiographical items (Westmacott, Leach, Freedman, & Moscovitch, 2001).

As the knowledge surrounding a word is lost, patients with SD use general rather than precise terms to describe objects, facts, people, or faces. Their deficits reflect loss of specific knowledge regarding a category of animals, vehicles, tools, and so forth. For example, a "golden eagle" becomes an "eagle," then a "bird," then an "animal," and finally a "thing." Semantic, but not phonemic, paraphasias are present, and patients replace the correct word with semantically related ones, such as substituting "dog" with "cat." Unlike a visual or auditory agnosia in which perception is disassociated from meaning in a single modality, the abnormalities in SD involve multiple modalities. The deficits in recognition are multimodal and are not improved by pictures, sound, touch, or smell (Snowden, 1999). Until the latest stages, patients with SD perform normally in perceptual matching task to identify which two objects are identical.

The Pyramid and Palm Trees test allows comparison of semantic knowledge for words and pictures. Most patients with SD perform poorly on this test. A poorer performance in the word than in the picture version suggests greater left temporal involvement, whereas poorer performance on the picture version shows more right temporal disease. In contrast to AD, often orientation and day-to-day memory remains intact. Quantitative assessments show that patients with SD are more impaired in the recall of distant life events than recent ones (Graham, Becker, & Hodges, 1997; Hodges & Graham, 1998). This pattern of memory loss contrasts dramatically with that in AD, in which more remote events tend to be relatively spared.

Behavioral and emotional disorders also are noted in SD, but differ qualitatively from those in FTD (Rosen, Gorno-Tempini, et al., 2002; Rosen et al., 2004; Snowden et al., 2001). These behavioral and emotional changes strongly correlate with degeneration of the orbitofrontal cortex and right anterior temporal lobe. The ratio of patients with predominantly left-sided temporal degeneration compared to right-sided temporal degeneration is around five to one in our clinic. In contrast to left-sided patients, in whom language syndromes are dominant, patients with asymmetric right-sided disease tend to present with behavioral rather than language deficits (Seeley et al., 2005). Depression, loss of empathy, fatigue, and intensification of beliefs are common first symptoms in these patients with right-sided damage. Hence, these patients with right temporal lobe degeneration are easily misdiagnosed as having disorders that are psychiatric in origin.

As the right temporal lobe progressively degenerates, deficits in the recognition of negative emotions commonly contribute to loss of empathy. Snowden and his colleagues (2001) found that patients with SD had a diminished fear response, and Rosen, Perry, and colleagues (2002) reported that temporal variant patients with FTLD had greater impairment in emotion with a negative valence, including sadness, anger, and fear. Seeley and colleagues (2005) suggest that the disease spreads from one temporal lobe to the other and then involves the orbitofrontal cortex. As either the left-sided or right-sided damage progresses, patients' compulsive attraction for words or symbols becomes evident. The aberrant motor behaviors seen in FTD are often simple repetitive stereotypes, such as hand rubbing or foot tapping, but rarely involve more creative outputs such as painting or music. By contrast, complex repetitive behaviors occur more often in SD (Snowden et al., 2001). As these patients show a narrowing of interest, they may become obsessed with a single activity, such as completing jigsaw puzzles, singing the same song, or painting or playing solitaire over and over again. Eating behavior change in patients with SD becomes increasingly selective, and patients may focus on eating a single food or a series of food items. This contrasts the overeating and indiscriminate eating seen in FTD (Snowden et al., 2001).

SD represents a temporal variant of FTLD. The language deficits in SD are largely driven by left anterior temporal degeneration, and the depressive features, loss of empathy, and emotional blunting come from right temporal lobe disease (Edwards-Lee et al., 1997; Hodges et al., 1992; Seeley et al., 2005). These findings usually precede disinhibition, which is driven by the orbitofrontal injury. Most patients with SD reveal bilateral anterior temporal lobe atrophy, with inferior and middle temporal gyri being more predominantly affected (Chan et al., 2001; Gorno-Tempini, Dronkers, et al., 2004; Mummery et al., 2000). The left anterior temporal pole is the most consistently affected region, but there is also extensive tissue loss in the orbitofrontal and insular cortex (Galton et al., 2001; Gorno-Tempini, Dronkers, et al., 2004; Mummery et al., 2000; Rosen, Gorno-Tempini, et al., 2002). The amygdala is severely involved in nearly all cases of SD and appears to be the site where the illness begins (Galton et al., 2001; Rosen, Perry, et al., 2002).

*FTD–Motor Neuron Disease*

There is great overlap between FTD and ALS both clinically and pathologically (Bigio, Lipton, White, Dickson, & Hirano, 2003; Neary et al., 1990). FTD is associated with both familial and sporadic ALS, although recent work from the UCSF suggests that FTD with ALS may be the most strongly genetic of all FTLD subtypes (Hosler et al., 2000). To date, no one has found a gene, or group of genes, that causes the combination of FTD and ALS.

The symptoms of motor weakness with FTLD-ALS can appear before, after, or concomitant with the symptoms of dementia. In a UCSF FTLD cohort, ALS findings eventually arose in approximately 15% of all patients. Similarly, nearly one-half of ALS patients develop frontal executive or behavioral deficits, and some of these individuals go on to develop a full-blown FTLD syndrome (Lomen-Hoerth, 2004). ALS features associated with FTLD typically suggest lower motor neuron dysfunction, particularly in the bulbar region, and many patients do not show pyramidal tract abnormalities (Lomen-Hoerth, 2004; Nakano, 2000; Neary, Snowden, & Mann, 2000).

The FTLD clinical picture is usually the FTD subtype, although NFPA and SD presentations do occur with ALS (Catani et al., 2004; Garraux, Salmon, Degueldre, Lemaire, & Franck, 1999; Gentileschi, Muggia, Poloni, & Spinnler, 1999; Lopez, Becker, & DeKosky, 1994; Talbot, 1996). The cognitive and behavioral abnormalities seen in patients with ALS are quite broad, and deficits can range from subtle deficits in frontal executive function to a full-blown frontal dementia syndrome (Bak & Hodges, 1999; Gentileschi et al., 1999; Lomen-Hoerth, 2004; Neary et al., 2000).

Whether FTLD and ALS represent two ends of a continuum or separate disorders is debated. The illness begins with changes in personality or behavior, impaired insight, apathy, euphoria, and disinhibition or irritability. Some of the classical behavioral alterations of FTD, such as pacing, collecting, or overeating, can be masked by the motor neuron disorder. There has been a tendency to excuse the behavioral or cognitive syndrome of FTD as a natural reaction to the ALS. FTD that occurs with ALS adds a unique burden to caregiving. Beyond the behavioral and cognitive deficits that emerge, the patient has difficulty participating in the consent process related to advanced directives, feeding tubes, and ventilation. These issues need to be addressed carefully in each individual patient.

*CBD and PSP*

As with ALS, the overlap with these two parkinsonian syndromes and FTLD is extensive (Kertesz, 2003; Kertesz, Hillis, & Munoz, 2003; Kertesz & Munoz, 2004). It is common to see patients with FTD develop diminished vertical or horizontal gaze, axial rigidity, and frequent falling or asymmetric parkinsonism with dystonia, myoclonus, or alien hand. Conversely, many patients with PSP and CBD develop cognitive and behavioral disorders that suggest FTD or NFPA. In the setting of an FTD or NFPA syndrome, when parkinsonian changes occur early, particularly axial rigidity, falls, and supranuclear horizontal or vertical opthalmoplegia, the likelihood that CBD or PSP pathology will be demonstrated at autopsy greatly increases (Feany, Mattiace, & Dickson, 1996; Jendroska, Rossor, Mathias, & Daniel, 1995; Kertesz, Davidson, & Munoz, 1999; Lang, Bergeron, Pollanen, & Ashby, 1994). The clinical, genetic, and pathological overlap among CBD, PSP, and FTD is so extensive that some researchers have suggested that they represent different presentations of the same disease.

## Neuropsychological Assessments

The Mini-Mental State Examination (MMSE) has limited value for diagnosing FTLD spectrum disorders, lacking both sensitivity and specificity. Patients with FTD may achieve a normal score or only a slightly lowered MMSE, despite the presence of profound behavioral and cognitive deficits (Gregory, Serra-Mestres, & Hodges, 1999; Neary et al., 1986; Pachana, Boone, Miller, Cummings, & Berman, 1996). Only a minority of patients show severe memory deficits, although poor effort can lead to global deficits in testing. The profile is characterized by impairment in executive control and attention disproportionate to memory loss (Hodges & Miller, 2001; Neary, 1995; Turner, Kenyon, Trojanowski, Gonatas, & Grossman, 1996). Impaired executive functions include difficulty with set shifting, concept formation, abstraction and reasoning, inhibition of overlearned responses, response generation, organization, planning, and self-monitoring. Frontal lobe tasks such as the Wisconsin Card Sorting Test, Trail Making Test, Stroop Category Test, and verbal or visual fluency tests often reveal impairment.

Memory performance usually falls below the normal range, but the pattern differs from that seen in AD (Glosser, Gallo, Clark, & Grossman, 2002; Pasquier, Grymonprez, Lebert, & Van der Linden, 2001; Thomas-Anterion, Jacquin, & Laurent, 2000). Clinicians need to consider the pattern of memory deficit on the specific task. Factors that disproportionately influence memory performance in FTD include poor effort, abnormal attention, diminished working memory, and deficient retrieval. When effort is sustained, many patients are able to encode a list of words. Therefore, even though the patient with FTD may fail on spontaneous recall on a verbal or visual memory task, the performance typically improves when the examiner offers the patient choices. Other tasks that are spared in FTD include copying and naming (Hodges et al., 1999; Perry & Hodges, 2000).

Beyond the deficits in speech and fluency, the greatest cognitive deficits of patients with NFPA fall in the area of working memory, letter fluency, verbal abstraction, and repetition (Graham, Patterson, & Hodges, 2004; Grossman, 2002). Visuospatial skills are spared, and patients often are able to draw the intersecting pentagons when their MMSE score is less than 10. Similarly, visual memory is usually normal (Mesulam, 2001). Profound deficits in arithmetic, reading, and visual memory should raise concerns that the patient with NFPA has AD, not FTLD.

With SD, the greatest deficits appear on naming, general information, and comprehension tasks that require an understanding of low-frequency words and remote memory of facts or faces. The Neary criteria emphasize the inability of the patient with SD to recognize familiar faces (prosopagnosia) or objects (visual agnosia) in order to capture patients' right temporal–predominant dysfunction, although these deficits occur much later in the illness. In the earlier stages of the right temporal variant of SD, patients' subtle changes in social cognition include deficits in encoding emotion perception and loss of empathy (Seeley et al., 2005).

The results of neuropsychological assessments in patients with FTLD tend to be some-what variable, and the neuropsychological results cannot be considered in isolation. Every patient comes to the assessment with different premorbid abilities and slightly different brain degeneration. Also, the behavioral problems associated with FTD also influence the test results. Therefore, it is not possible to have a simple neuropsychological formula that will diagnose every patient. Each patient needs to be assessed in a manner that takes into account his or her behavior presentations and neuroimaging data.

## Neurological Examination

Neurological examinations in patients with FTLD are usually normal early in the illness, but in some patients, subtle parkinsonism is present at diagnosis. Swallowing difficulty, with poor gag reflex, is common (Hodges et al., 2003). Nearly 80% of patients with FTLD show basal ganglia and midbrain degeneration by the time of death, which explains why so many patients eventually exhibit parkinsonian features (Kersaitis, Halliday, & Kril, 2004; Tolnay & Probst, 2001). Some patients show stimulus-bound behavior such as echolalia or utilization behavior. Approximately 10–15% of patients go on to develop findings suggestive of motor neuron disease, including fasciculations, dysarthria, dysphagia, muscle wasting, and weakness.

## Clinical Course

The clinical onset is insidious, with a slow gradual progression. Although the neuropsychiatric profile for patients with FTLD varies between the three clinical subtypes, behavior problems such as overeating, repetitive compulsive behaviors, apathy, and agitation and disinhibition, develop in the majority of these patients as the disease progresses (Chow et al., 2002; Marczinski, Davidson, & Kertesz, 2004). Patients with FTD also go on to develop speech and language problems during the evolution of disease (Neary et al., 1998; Pasquier, Lebert, Lavenu, & Guillaume, 1999).

Because the initial symptoms usually present as affective problems or personality change, the age at onset and, consequently, the duration of the disease are difficult to precisely localize. The mean age of onset is around the 50s, and the estimated duration of the illness is around 6–10 years (Mendez et al., 1993; Pasquier et al., 1999; Pasquier, Richard, & Lebert, 2004). Patients with FTD have the shortest lifespan, with a mean survival of 3.4 years from the time of diagnosis (Grasbeck et al., 2003; Hodges et al., 2003; Pasquier et al., 2004). Patients with NFPA live closer to 4.5 years, whereas patients with SD have the longest survival. The presence of ALS or parkinsonian features greatly shortens survival (Grasbeck et al., 2003). Other factors linked to a shorter survival are mutism, dysphagia, neurological abnormalities (e.g., parkinsonism, primitive reflexes, incontinence, and seizures) (Hodges et al., 2003). Underlying pathology also may play a role in the survival of patients with FTLD. Those with tau-positive pathology seem to have a slower progression than patients with ubiquitin inclusions or no inclusions (Hodges et al., 2003; Roberson et al., 2005).

### Differential Diagnosis

In clinical practice, because many physicians are unfamiliar with its specific features, FTLD is commonly misdiagnosed as AD. In early AD, memory impairment usually is the most prominent problem, with preserved social skills and personality propriety. Conversely, decline in social and personal conduct, emotional blunting, loss of insight, and progressive speech disorder develop early in FTLD (Barber, Snowden, & Craufurd, 1995; Lindau et al., 2000; Mendez et al., 1993). Patients with FTLD usually perform better on visuospatial tasks, calculation, praxis, and episodic memory tests, due to a relative sparing of posterior temporal and parietal lobe involvement in the early stage (Hodges et al., 1999; Mendez, Doss, & Cherrier, 1998). Patients with FTLD can be separated from those with AD with approximately 90% accuracy, but it is not possible to separate the various types of FTLD-related pathologies based upon clinical or imaging features (Knopman et al., 2005). As a rule of thumb, the presence of early parkinsonism suggests tau-related pathology (Baba et al., 2005; van Swieten et al., 2004; Verpillat et al., 2002), whereas motor neuron disease in FTLD is usually associated with FTD with ubiquitin inclusions (Hodges et al., 2004; Tan et al., 2003; Yoshida, 2004).

Other neurodegenerative diseases that present with frontal or anterior temporal lobe dysfunction include Kreutzfeldt–Jakob disease, subcortical ischemic disease, Huntington's disease, and a frontal variant of AD. Usually these

patients can be separated from those with FTD based upon the clinical course or the neuroimaging findings. Patients with Kreutzfeldt–Jakob disease show cortical ribboning and basal ganglia changes with fluid-attenuated inversion recovery (FLAIR) and diffusion-weighted imaging, and have a much more rapid disease course (Meissner et al., 2004; Shiga et al., 2004; Ukisu et al., 2005). Frontal lobe vascular syndromes are associated with extensive white matter disease and lacunar or frontal infarctions. Chorea is extremely unusual in FTLD, even in autosomal dominant forms of FTLD, easily separating this from Huntington's disease (Haddad & Cummings, 1997; McCusker, Richards, Sillence, Wilson, & Trent, 2000).

### Treatments

The development of pharmacological therapies in FTLD has lagged far behind that in AD. In one open-label and one placebo-controlled study, serotonin reuptake inhibitors improved a variety of psychiatric symptoms, including irritability, depression, repetitive behaviors, and hyperorality (Swartz, Miller, Lesser, Booth, et al., 1997). In some studies, acetylcholinesterase compounds showed efficacy in both behavioral and cognitive symptomatic treatments of AD (Mega, Masterman, O'Connor, Barclay, & Cummings, 1999; Morris et al., 1998; Raskind, Sadowsky, Sigmund, Beitler, & Auster, 1997; Tariot et al., 2000; Trinh, Hoblyn, Mohanty, & Yaffe, 2003). However, there is no evidence for a cholinergic deficit associated with any subtypes FTLD, and in our experience, cholinesterase inhibitors can precipitate worsening of behavior. Therefore, we do not recommend these compounds for either the cognitive or behavioral disorder associated with FTLD.

There is a profound loss of glutamatergic neurons in frontal cortex in FTLD (Ernst, Chang, Melchor, & Mehringer, 1997), but no data suggest that the mechanism for this loss is via excessive excitotoxic activity at the level of N-methyl-D-aspartate (NMDA) receptors. Despite the absence of a strong scientific rationale for NMDA-blockers, the recent successes with these compounds in slowing progression of AD (Reisberg et al., 2003; Tariot et al., 2004) have encouraged an interest in their use for FTLD. Several treatment studies with the new NMDA receptor blocker, memantine, are under way. Whether this compound will have either symptomatic benefits or slow the progression of any of the FTLD subtypes remains unknown.

Typical and atypical antipsychotics have been used for controlling aggressive and psychotic symptoms. However, considering the possible adverse response with deteriorating motor symptoms and dysphagia, antipsychotics should only be used as a last resort. Anticonvulsants, such as valproic acid and carbamazepine, have not been studied in FTLD but may play a minor role in the treatment of FTLD-related agitation or aggression.

There have been a variety of creative approaches to the treatment of FTLD based on the finding that tau mutations cause this disorder (Benitez-King, Ramirez-Rodriguez, Ortiz, & Meza, 2004; Iqbal et al., 2000; Iqbal & Grundke-Iqbal, 2004). Either overexpression of animal tau, or expression of human tau in transgenic mice cause degenerative disorders with features of FTLD (Ho et al., 2001; Lambourne et al., 2005; Lewis et al., 2000; Lim et al., 2001; Rademakers, Cruts, & van Broeckhoven, 2004; Tanemura et al., 2002). Treatments that will stabilize tau are being explored in these animal models and, if successful, could lead to more rational and better therapies for FTLD.

## Caregiver Strategies

Many aspects of this disorder make it particularly troublesome for caregivers (Merrilees & Miller, 2003; Mourik et al., 2004; Perry & Miller, 2001), including the loss of empathy for others, apathy, diminished insight, and inappropriate social behaviors that characterize these patients. FTLD strikes at a relatively young age, so the disease often causes dramatic economic and social consequences before the patient arrives in clinic. Patients lose their intellectual and emotional rapport as an adult partner, and caregivers are forced to perform the role of a parent. Generally, the caregivers' burden in FTLD is much more arduous than that with AD. Caregivers require comprehensive information for this disease and group support. FTD–motor neuron disease is significant because of the early death of patients due to inability to swallow and respiratory system problems. So it is important to assess muscle strength, swallowing ability, and balance with gait to optimize functional abilities throughout the disease course. Educating the patient and family about the prognosis and planning ahead

regarding subsequent treatment of swallowing problems and infections before feeding tube placement is important.

## REFERENCES

Ames, D., Cummings, J. L., Wirshing, W. C., Quinn, B., & Mahler, M. (1994). Repetitive and compulsive behavior in frontal lobe degenerations. *Journal of Neuropsychiatry and Clinical Neuroscience*, 6(2), 100–113.

Baba, Y., Tsuboi, Y., Baker, M. C., Uitti, R. J., Hutton, M. L., Dickson, D. W., et al. (2005). The effect of tau genotype on clinical features in FTDP-17. *Parkinsonism and Related Disorders*, 11(4), 205–208.

Bak, T. H., & Hodges, J. R. (1999). Cognition, language and behaviour in motor neurone disease: Evidence of frontotemporal dysfunction. *Dementia and Geriatric Cognitive Disorders*, 10(Suppl. 1), 29–32.

Bak, T. H., O'Donovan, D. G., Xuereb, J. H., Boniface, S., & Hodges, J. R. (2001). Selective impairment of verb processing associated with pathological changes in Brodmann areas 44 and 45 in the motor neurone disease–dementia–aphasia syndrome. *Brain*, 124(1), 103–120.

Baldwin, B., & Forstl, H. (1993). "Pick's disease"—101 years on still there, but in need of reform. *British Journal of Psychiatry*, 163, 100–104.

Barber, R., Snowden, J. S., & Craufurd, D. (1995). Frontotemporal dementia and Alzheimer's disease: Retrospective differentiation using information from informants. *Journal of Neurology, Neurosurgery, and Psychiatry*, 59(1), 61–70.

Benitez-King, G., Ramirez-Rodriguez, G., Ortiz, L., & Meza, I. (2004). The neuronal cytoskeleton as a potential therapeutical target in neurodegenerative diseases and schizophrenia. *Current Drug Targets: CNS and Neurological Disorders*, 3(6), 515–533.

Bigio, E. H., Lipton, A. M., White, C. L., III, Dickson, D. W., & Hirano, A. (2003). Frontotemporal and motor neurone degeneration with neurofilament inclusion bodies: Additional evidence for overlap between FTD and ALS. *Neuropathology and Applied Neurobiology*, 29(3), 239–253.

Bird, T. D. (2001). Frontotemporal dementia: Genotypes, phenotypes and more problems to be solved. *Neurobiology of Aging*, 22(1), 113–114.

Bozeat, S., Gregory, C. A., Ralph, M. A., & Hodges, J. R. (2000). Which neuropsychiatric and behavioural features distinguish frontal and temporal variants of frontotemporal dementia from Alzheimer's disease? *Journal of Neurology, Neurosurgery, and Psychiatry*, 69(2), 178–186.

Brun, A. (1987). Frontal lobe degeneration of non-Alzheimer type: I. Neuropathology. *Archives of Gerontology and Geriatrics*, 6(3), 193–208.

Brun, A., & Passant, U. (1996). Frontal lobe degeneration of non-Alzheimer type: Structural characteristics, diagnostic criteria and relation to other frontotemporal dementias. *Acta Neurologica Scandavica Supplement*, 168, 28–30.

Catani, M., Piccirilli, M., Geloso, M. C., Cherubini, A., Finali, G., Pelliccioli, G., et al. (2004). Rapidly progressive aphasic dementia with motor neuron disease: A distinctive clinical entity. *Dementia and Geriatric Cognitive Disorders*, 17(1–2), 21–28.

Chan, D., Fox, N. C., Scahill, R. I., Crum, W. R., Whitwell, J. L., Leschziner, G., et al. (2001). Patterns of temporal lobe atrophy in semantic dementia and Alzheimer's disease. *Annals of Neurology*, 49(4), 433–442.

Chow, T. W., Miller, B. L., Boone, K., Mishkin, F., & Cummings, J. L. (2002). Frontotemporal dementia classification and neuropsychiatry. *Neurologist*, 8(4), 263–269.

Chow, T. W., Miller, B. L., Hayashi, V. N., & Geschwind, D. H. (1999). Inheritance of frontotemporal dementia. *Archives of Neurology*, 56(7), 817–822.

Cummings, J. L., & Duchen, L. W. (1981). Kluver–Bucy syndrome in Pick disease: Clinical and pathologic correlations. *Neurology*, 31(11), 1415–1422.

Diehl, J., Monsch, A. U., Aebi, C., Wagenpfeil, S., Krapp, S., Grimmer, T., et al. (2005). Frontotemporal dementia, semantic dementia, and Alzheimer's disease: The contribution of standard neuropsychological tests to differential diagnosis. *Journal of Geriatric Psychiatry and Neurology*, 18(1), 39–44.

Edwards-Lee, T., Miller, B. L., Benson, D. F., Cummings, J. L., Russell, G. L., Boone, K., et al. (1997). The temporal variant of frontotemporal dementia. *Brain*, 120(6), 1027–1040.

Ernst, T., Chang, L., Melchor, R., & Mehringer, C. M. (1997). Frontotemporal dementia and early Alzheimer disease: Differentiation with frontal lobe H-1 MR spectroscopy. *Radiology*, 203(3), 829–836.

Feany, M. B., Mattiace, L. A., & Dickson, D. W. (1996). Neuropathologic overlap of progressive supranuclear palsy, Pick's disease and corticobasal degeneration. *Journal of Neuropathology and Experimental Neurology*, 55(1), 53–67.

Foster, N. L., Wilhelmsen, K., Sima, A. A., Jones, M. Z., D'Amato, C. J., & Gilman, S. (1997). Frontotemporal dementia and parkinsonism linked to chromosome 17: A consensus conference. *Annals of Neurology*, 41(6), 706–715.

Frisoni, G. B., Beltramello, A., Geroldi, C., Weiss, C., Bianchetti, A., & Trabucchi, M. (1996). Brain atrophy in frontotemporal dementia. *Journal of Neurology, Neurosurgery, and Psychiatry*, 61(2), 157–165.

Galton, C. J., Patterson, K., Graham, K., Lambon Ralph, M. A., Williams, G., Antoun, N., et al. (2001). Differing patterns of temporal atrophy in Alzheimer's disease and semantic dementia. *Neurology*, 57(2), 216–225.

Garraux, G., Salmon, E., Degueldre, C., Lemaire, C., & Franck, G. (1999). Medial temporal lobe metabolic impairment in dementia associated with motor neuron disease. *Journal of Neurological Sciences*, 168(2), 145–150.

Gee, J., Ding, L., Xie, Z., Lin, M., DeVita, C., & Grossman, M. (2003). Alzheimer's disease and frontotemporal dementia exhibit distinct atrophy-behavior correlates: A computer-assisted imaging study. *Academic Radiology*, 10(12), 1392–1401.

Gentileschi, V., Muggia, S., Poloni, M., & Spinnler, H. (1999). Fronto-temporal dementia and motor neuron disease: A neuropsychological study. *Acta Neurologica Scandinavica*, 100(5), 341–349.

Glosser, G., Gallo, J. L., Clark, C. M., & Grossman, M. (2002). Memory encoding and retrieval in frontotemporal dementia and Alzheimer's disease. *Neuropsychology*, 16(2), 190–196.

Goldman, J. S., Farmer, J. M., Van Deerlin, V. M., Wilhelmsen, K. C., Miller, B. L., & Grossman, M. (2004). Frontotemporal dementia: Genetics and genetic counseling dilemmas. *Neurologist*, 10(5), 227–234.

Gorno-Tempini, M. L., Dronkers, N. F., Rankin, K. P., Ogar, J. M., Phengrasamy, L., Rosen, H. J., et al. (2004). Cognition and anatomy in three variants of primary progressive aphasia. *Annals of Neurology*, 55(3), 335–346.

Gorno-Tempini, M. L., Murray, R. C., Rankin, K. P., Weiner, M. W., & Miller, B. L. (2004). Clinical, cognitive and anatomical evolution from nonfluent progressive aphasia to corticobasal syndrome: A case report. *Neurocase*, 10(6), 426–436.

Graham, K. S., Becker, J. T., & Hodges, J. R. (1997). On the relationship between knowledge and memory for pictures: Evidence from the study of patients with semantic dementia and Alzheimer's disease. *Journal of the International Neuropsychological Society*, 3(6), 534–544.

Graham, N. L., Bak, T. H., & Hodges, J. R. (2003). Corticobasal degeneration as a cognitive disorder. *Movement Disorders*, 18(11), 1224–1232.

Graham, N. L., Patterson, K., & Hodges, J. R. (2004). When more yields less: Speaking and writing deficits in nonfluent progressive aphasia. *Neurocase*, 10(2), 141–155.

Grasbeck, A., Englund, E., Horstmann, V., Passant, U., & Gustafson, L. (2003). Predictors of mortality in frontotemporal dementia: A retrospective study of the prognostic influence of pre-diagnostic features. *International Journal of Geriatric Psychiatry*, 18(7), 594–601.

Gregory, C. A., & Hodges, J. R. (1996). Clinical features of frontal lobe dementia in comparison to Alzheimer's disease. *Journal of Neural Transmission: Supplementum*, 47, 103–123.

Gregory, C. A., Serra-Mestres, J., & Hodges, J. R. (1999). Early diagnosis of the frontal variant of frontotemporal dementia: How sensitive are standard neuroimaging and neuropsychologic tests? *Neuropsychiatry, Neuropsychology and Behavioral Neurology*, 12(2), 128–135.

Grossman, M. (2002). Progressive aphasic syndromes: Clinical and theoretical advances. *Current Opinion in Neurology, 15*(4), 409–413.

Haddad, M. S., & Cummings, J. L. (1997). Huntington's disease. *Psychiatric Clinics of North America, 20*(4), 791–807.

Harvey, R. J., Skelton-Robinson, M., & Rossor, M. N. (2003). The prevalence and causes of dementia in people under the age of 65 years. *Journal of Neurology, Neurosurgery, and Psychiatry, 74*(9), 1206–1209.

Ho, L., Xiang, Z., Mukherjee, P., Zhang, W., De Jesus, N., Mirjany, M., et al. (2001). Gene expression profiling of the tau mutant (P301L) transgenic mouse brain. *Neuroscience Letters, 310*(1), 1–4.

Hodges, J. R. (2001). Frontotemporal dementia (Pick's disease): Clinical features and assessment. *Neurology, 56*(11, Suppl. 4), S6–S10.

Hodges, J. R., Davies, R. R., Xuereb, J. H., Casey, B., Broe, M., Bak, T. H., et al. (2004). Clinicopathological correlates in frontotemporal dementia. *Annals of Neurology, 56*(3), 399–406.

Hodges, J. R., Davies, R., Xuereb, J., Kril, J., & Halliday, G. (2003). Survival in frontotemporal dementia. *Neurology, 61*(3), 349–354.

Hodges, J. R., & Graham, K. S. (1998). A reversal of the temporal gradient for famous person knowledge in semantic dementia: Implications for the neural organisation of long-term memory. *Neuropsychologia, 36*(8), 803–825.

Hodges, J. R., & Miller, B. (2001). The neuropsychology of frontal variant frontotemporal dementia and semantic dementia: Introduction to the special topic papers: Part II. *Neurocase, 7*(2), 113–121.

Hodges, J. R., Patterson, K., Oxbury, S., & Funnell, E. (1992). Semantic dementia: Progressive fluent aphasia with temporal lobe atrophy. *Brain, 115*(6), 1783–1806.

Hodges, J. R., Patterson, K., Ward, R., Garrard, P., Bak, T., Perry, R., et al. (1999). The differentiation of semantic dementia and frontal lobe dementia (temporal and frontal variants of frontotemporal dementia) from early Alzheimer's disease: A comparative neuropsychological study. *Neuropsychology, 13*(1), 31–40.

Hokoishi, K., Ikeda, M., Maki, N., Nebu, A., Shigenobu, K., Fukuhara, R., et al. (2001). Frontotemporal lobar degeneration: A study in Japan. *Dementia and Geriatric Cognitive Disorders, 12*(6), 393–399.

Hosler, B. A., Siddique, T., Sapp, P. C., Sailor, W., Huang, M. C., Hossain, A., et al. (2000). Linkage of familial amyotrophic lateral sclerosis with frontotemporal dementia to chromosome 9q21-q22. *Journal of the American Medical Association, 284*(13), 1664–1669.

Hou, C. E., Carlin, D., & Miller, B. L. (2004). Non-Alzheimer's disease dementias: Anatomic, clinical, and molecular correlates. *Canadian Journal of Psychiatry, 49*(3), 164–171.

Ikeda, K. (2000). Neuropathological discrepancy between Japanese Pick's disease without Pick bodies and frontal lobe degeneration type of frontotemporal dementia proposed by Lund and Manchester Group. *Neuropathology, 20*(1), 76–82.

Ikeda, M., Ishikawa, T., & Tanabe, H. (2004). Epidemiology of frontotemporal lobar degeneration. *Dementia and Geriatric Cognitive Disorders, 17*(4), 265–268.

Iqbal, K., Alonso, A. D., Gondal, J. A., Gong, C. X., Haque, N., Khatoon, S., et al. (2000). Mechanism of neurofibrillary degeneration and pharmacologic therapeutic approach. *Journal of Neural Transmission: Supplementum, 59*, 213–222.

Iqbal, K., & Grundke-Iqbal, I. (2004). Inhibition of neurofibrillary degeneration: A promising approach to Alzheimer's disease and other tauopathies. *Current Drug Targets, 5*(6), 495–502.

Jendroska, K., Rossor, M. N., Mathias, C. J., & Daniel, S. E. (1995). Morphological overlap between corticobasal degeneration and Pick's disease: A clinicopathological report. *Movement Disorders, 10*(1), 111–114.

Johanson, A., & Hagberg, B. (1989). Psychometric characteristics in patients with frontal lobe degeneration of non-Alzheimer type. *Archives of Gerontology and Geriatrics, 8*(2), 129–137.

Keane, J., Calder, A. J., Hodges, J. R., & Young, A. W. (2002). Face and emotion processing in frontal variant frontotemporal dementia. *Neuropsychologia, 40*(6), 655–665.

Kersaitis, C., Halliday, G. M., & Kril, J. J. (2004). Regional and cellular pathology in frontotemporal dementia: Relationship to stage of disease in cases with and without Pick bodies. *Acta Neuropathologica (Berlin), 108*, 515–523.

Kertesz, A. (1997). Frontotemporal dementia, Pick disease, and corticobasal degeneration: One entity or 3? 1. *Archives of Neurology, 54*(11), 1427–1429.

Kertesz, A. (2003). Pick complex: an integrative approach to frontotemporal dementia: primary progressive aphasia, corticobasal degeneration, and progressive supranuclear palsy. *Neurologist, 9*(6), 311–317.

Kertesz, A., Davidson, W., McCabe, P., Takagi, K., & Munoz, D. (2003). Primary progressive aphasia: Diagnosis, varieties, evolution. *Journal of the International Neuropsychological Society, 9*(5), 710–719.

Kertesz, A., Davidson, W., & Munoz, D. G. (1999). Clinical and pathological overlap between frontotemporal dementia, primary progressive aphasia and corticobasal degeneration: The Pick complex. *Dementia and Geriatric Cognitive Disorders, 10*(Suppl. 1), 46–49.

Kertesz, A., Hillis, A., & Munoz, D. G. (2003). Frontotemporal degeneration, Pick's disease, Pick complex, and Ravel. *Annals of Neurology, 54*(Suppl. 5), S1–S2.

Kertesz, A., & Munoz, D. (2004). Relationship between

frontotemporal dementia and corticobasal degeneration/progressive supranuclear palsy. *Dementia and Geriatric Cognitive Disorders, 17*(4), 282–286.

Kertesz, A., & Munoz, D. G. (2002). Frontotemporal dementia. *Medical Clinics of North America, 86*(3), 501–518, vi.

Knopman, D. S., Boeve, B. F., Parisi, J. E., Dickson, D. W., Smith, G. E., Ivnik, R. J., et al. (2005). Antemortem diagnosis of frontotemporal lobar degeneration. *Annals of Neurology, 57*(4), 480–488.

Knopman, D. S., Petersen, R. C., Edland, S. D., Cha, R. H., & Rocca, W. A. (2004). The incidence of frontotemporal lobar degeneration in Rochester, Minnesota, 1990 through 1994. *Neurology, 62*(3), 506–508.

Kramer, J. H., Jurik, J., Sha, S. J., Rankin, K. P., Rosen, H. J., Johnson, J. K., et al. (2003). Distinctive neuropsychological patterns in frontotemporal dementia, semantic dementia, and Alzheimer disease. *Cognitive and Behavioral Neurology, 16*(4), 211–218.

Lambourne, S. L., Sellers, L. A., Bush, T. G., Choudhury, S. K., Emson, P. C., Suh, Y. H., et al. (2005). Increased tau phosphorylation on mitogen-activated protein kinase consensus sites and cognitive decline in transgenic models for Alzheimer's disease and FTDP-17: Evidence for distinct molecular processes underlying tau abnormalities. *Molecular and Cellular Biology, 25*(1), 278–293.

Lang, A. E., Bergeron, C., Pollanen, M. S., & Ashby, P. (1994). Parietal Pick's disease mimicking cortical-basal ganglionic degeneration. *Neurology, 44*(8), 1436–1440.

Larsson, E., Passant, U., Sundgren, P. C., Englund, E., Brun, A., Lindgren, A., et al. (2000). "Magnetic resonance imaging and histopathology in dementia, clinically of frontotemporal type. *Dementia and Geriatric Cognitive Disorders, 11*(3), 123–134.

Lewis, J., McGowan, E., Rockwood, J., Melrose, H., Nacharaju, P., Van Slegtenhorst, M., et al. (2000). Neurofibrillary tangles, amyotrophy and progressive motor disturbance in mice expressing mutant (P301L) tau protein. *Nature Genetics, 25*(4), 402–405.

Lim, F., Hernandez, F., Lucas, J. J., Gomez-Ramos, P., Moran, M. A., & Avila, J. (2001). FTDP-17 mutations in tau transgenic mice provoke lysosomal abnormalities and Tau filaments in forebrain. *Molecular and Cellular Neuroscience, 18*(6), 702–714.

Lindau, M., Almkvist, O., Kushi, J., Boone, K., Johansson, S. E., Wahlund, L. O., et al. (2000). First symptoms—frontotemporal dementia versus Alzheimer's disease. *Dementia and Geriatric Cognitive Disorders, 11*(5), 286–293.

Liu, W., Miller, B. L., Kramer, J. H., Rankin, K., Wyss-Coray, C., Gearhart, R., et al. (2004). Behavioral disorders in the frontal and temporal variants of frontotemporal dementia. *Neurology, 62*(5), 742–748.

Lomen-Hoerth, C. (2004). Characterization of amyotrophic lateral sclerosis and frontotemporal dementia. *Dementia and Geriatric Cognitive Disorders, 17*(4), 337–341.

Lopez, O. L., Becker, J. T., & DeKosky, S. T. (1994). Dementia accompanying motor neuron disease. *Dementia, 5*(1), 42–47.

Mann, D. M., South, P. W., Snowden, J. S., & Neary, D. (1993). Dementia of frontal lobe type: neuropathology and immunohistochemistry. *Journal of Neurology, Neurosurgery, and Psychiatry, 56*(6), 605–614.

Marczinski, C. A., Davidson, W., & Kertesz, A. (2004). A longitudinal study of behavior in frontotemporal dementia and primary progressive aphasia. *Cognitive and Behavioral Neurology, 17*(4), 185–190.

McCusker, E., Richards, F., Sillence, D., Wilson, M., & Trent, R. J. (2000). Huntington's disease: Neurological assessment of potential gene carriers presenting for predictive DNA testing. *Journal of Clinical Neuroscience, 7*(1), 38–41.

Mega, M. S., Masterman, D. M., O'Connor, S. M., Barclay, T. R., & Cummings, J. L. (1999). The spectrum of behavioral responses to cholinesterase inhibitor therapy in Alzheimer disease. *Archives of Neurology, 56*(11), 1388–1393.

Meissner, B., Kortner, K., Bartl, M., Jastrow, U., Mollenhauer, B., Schroter, A., et al. (2004). Sporadic Creutzfeldt–Jakob disease: Magnetic resonance imaging and clinical findings. *Neurology, 63*(3), 450–456.

Mendez, M. F., Doss, R. C., & Cherrier, M. M. (1998). Use of the cognitive estimations test to discriminate frontotemporal dementia from Alzheimer's disease. *Journal of Geriatric Psychiatry and Neurology, 11*(1), 2–6.

Mendez, M. F., Perryman, K. M., Miller, B. L., Swartz, J. R., & Cummings, J. L. (1997). Compulsive behaviors as presenting symptoms of frontotemporal dementia. *Journal of Geriatric Psychiatry and Neurology, 10*(4), 154–157.

Mendez, M. F., Selwood, A., Mastri, A. R., & Frey, W. H., II. (1993). Pick's disease versus Alzheimer's disease: A comparison of clinical characteristics. *Neurology, 43*(2), 289–292.

Mendez, M. F., Shapira, J. S., & Miller, B. L. (2005). Stereotypical movements and frontotemporal dementia. *Movement Disorders, 20*(6), 742–745.

Merrilees, J. J., & Miller, B. L. (2003). Long-term care of patients with frontotemporal dementia. *Journal of the American Medical Directors Association, 4*(Suppl. 6), S162–S164.

Mesulam, M. M. (2001). Primary progressive aphasia. *Annals of Neurology, 49*(4), 425–432.

Miller, B. L., Chang, L., Mena, I., Boone, K., & Lesser, I. M. (1993). Progressive right frontotemporal degeneration: Clinical, neuropsychological and SPECT characteristics. *Dementia, 4*(3–4), 204–213.

Miller, B. L., Cummings, J. L., Villanueva-Meyer, J., Boone, K., Mehringer, C. M., Lesser, I. M., et al. (1991). Frontal lobe degeneration: Clinical, neuropsychological, and SPECT characteristics. *Neurology, 41*(9), 1374–1382.

Miller, B. L., Darby, A., Benson, D. F., Cummings, J. L., & Miller, M. H. (1997). Aggressive, socially disruptive and antisocial behaviour associated with frontotemporal dementia. *British Journal of Psychiatry, 170,* 150–154.

Miller, B. L., Darby, A. L., Swartz, J. R., Yener, G. G., & Mena, I. (1995). Dietary changes, compulsions and sexual behavior in frontotemporal degeneration. *Dementia, 6*(4), 195–199.

Miller, B. L., Seeley, W. W., Mychack, P., Rosen, H. J., Mena, I., & Boone, K. (2001). Neuroanatomy of the self: Evidence from patients with frontotemporal dementia. *Neurology, 57*(5), 817–821.

Morris, J. C., Cyrus, P. A., Orazem, J., Mas, J., Bieber, F., Ruzicka, B. B., et al. (1998). Metrifonate benefits cognitive, behavioral, and global function in patients with Alzheimer's disease. *Neurology, 50*(5), 1222–1230.

Mourik, J. C., Rosso, S. M., Niermeijer, M. F., Duivenvoorden, H. J., Van Swieten, J. C., & Tibben, A. (2004). Frontotemporal dementia: Behavioral symptoms and caregiver distress. *Dementia and Geriatric Cognitive Disorders, 18*(3–4), 299–306.

Mummery, C. J., Patterson, K., Price, C. J., Ashburner, J., Frackowiak, R. S., & Hodges, J. R. (2000). A voxel-based morphometry study of semantic dementia: Relationship between temporal lobe atrophy and semantic memory. *Annals of Neurology, 47*(1), 36–45.

Murre, J. M., Graham, K. S., & Hodges, J. R. (2001). Semantic dementia: Relevance to connectionist models of long-term memory. *Brain, 124*(4), 647–675.

Nakano, I. (2000). Frontotemporal dementia with motor neuron disease (amyotrophic lateral sclerosis with dementia). *Neuropathology, 20*(1), 68–75.

Neary, D. (1995). Neuropsychological aspects of frontotemporal degeneration. *Annals of the New York Academy of Sciences, 769,* 15–22.

Neary, D., Snowden, J. S., Bowen, D. M., Sims, N. R., Mann, D. M., Benton, J. S., et al. (1986). Neuropsychological syndromes in presenile dementia due to cerebral atrophy. *Journal of Neurology, Neurosurgery, and Psychiatry, 49*(2), 163–174.

Neary, D., Snowden, J. S., Gustafson, L., Passant, U., Stuss, D., Black, S., et al. (1998). Frontotemporal lobar degeneration: A consensus on clinical diagnostic criteria. *Neurology, 51*(6), 1546–1554.

Neary, D., Snowden, J. S., & Mann, D. M. (2000). Cognitive change in motor neurone disease/amyotrophic lateral sclerosis (MND/ALS). *Journal of Neurological Sciences, 180*(1–2), 15–20.

Neary, D., Snowden, J. S., Mann, D. M., Northen, B., Goulding, P. J., & Macdermott, N. (1990). Frontal lobe dementia and motor neuron disease. *Journal of Neurology, Neurosurgery, and Psychiatry, 53*(1), 23–32.

Noble, K., Glosser, G., & Grossman, M. (2000). Oral reading in dementia. *Brain and Language, 74*(1), 48–69.

Pachana, N. A., Boone, K. B., Miller, B. L., Cummings, J. L., & Berman, N. (1996). Comparison of neuropsychological functioning in Alzheimer's disease and frontotemporal dementia. *Journal of the International Neuropsychological Society, 2*(6), 505–510.

Pasquier, F., & Delacourte, A. (1998). Non-Alzheimer degenerative dementias. *Current Opinion in Neurology, 11*(5), 417–427.

Pasquier, F., Grymonprez, L., Lebert, F., & Van der Linden, M. (2001). Memory impairment differs in frontotemporal dementia and Alzheimer's disease. *Neurocase, 7*(2), 161–171.

Pasquier, F., Lebert, F., Lavenu, I., & Guillaume, B. (1999). The clinical picture of frontotemporal dementia: diagnosis and follow-up. *Dementia and Geriatric Cognitive Disorders, 10*(Suppl. 1), 10–14.

Pasquier, F., Richard, F., & Lebert, F. (2004). Natural history of frontotemporal dementia: Comparison with Alzheimer's disease. *Dementia and Geriatric Cognitive Disorders, 17*(4), 253–257.

Patterson, K., Lambon Ralph, M. A., Hodges, J. R., & McClelland, J. L. (2001). Deficits in irregular past-tense verb morphology associated with degraded semantic knowledge. *Neuropsychologia, 39*(7), 709–724.

Perry, R. J., & Hodges, J. R. (2000). Differentiating frontal and temporal variant frontotemporal dementia from Alzheimer's disease. *Neurology, 54*(12), 2277–2284.

Perry, R. J., & Miller, B. L. (2001). Behavior and treatment in frontotemporal dementia. *Neurology, 56*(11, Suppl. 4), S46–S51.

Pick, A. (1892). Uber die Beziehungen der senilen Hirnatrophie zur Aphasie. *Prager Medizinische Wochenschrift, 17,* 165–167.

Radanovic, M., Senaha, M. L., Mansur, L. L., Nitrini, R., Bahia, V. S., Carthery, M. T., et al. (2001). Primary progressive aphasia: Analysis of 16 cases. *Arquivos de Neuropsiquiatria, 59*(3-A), 512–520.

Rademakers, R., Cruts, M., & van Broeckhoven, C. (2004). The role of tau (MAPT) in frontotemporal dementia and related tauopathies. *Human Mutation, 24*(4), 277–295.

Rankin, K. P., Kramer, J. H., Mychack, P., & Miller, B. L. (2003). Double dissociation of social functioning in frontotemporal dementia. *Neurology, 60*(2), 266–271.

Raskind, M. A., Sadowsky, C. H., Sigmund, W. R., Beitler, P. J., & Auster, S. B. (1997). Effect of tacrine on language, praxis, and noncognitive behavioral problems in Alzheimer disease. *Archives of Neurology, 54*(7), 836–840.

Ratnavalli, E., Brayne, C., Dawson, K., & Hodges, J. R. (2002). The prevalence of frontotemporal dementia. *Neurology, 58*(11), 1615–1621.

Reisberg, B., Doody, R., Stoffler, A., Schmitt, F., Ferris, S., & Mobius, H. J. (2003). Memantine in moderate-to-severe Alzheimer's disease. *New England Journal of Medicine, 348*(14), 1333–1341.

Rhee, J., Antiquena, P., & Grossman, M. (2001). Verb comprehension in frontotemporal degeneration: The role of grammatical, semantic and executive components. *Neurocase, 7*(2), 173–184.

Roberson, E. D., Hesse, J. H., Rose, K. D., Slama, H., Johnson, J. K., Yaffe, K., et al. (2005). Frontotemporal dementia progresses to death faster than Alzheimer disease. *Neurology, 65,* 719–725.

Rosen, H. J., Gorno-Tempini, M. L., Goldman, W. P., Perry, R. J., Schuff, N., Weiner, M., et al. (2002). Patterns of brain atrophy in frontotemporal dementia and semantic dementia. *Neurology, 58*(2), 198–208.

Rosen, H. J., Hartikainen, K. M., Jagust, W., Kramer, J. H., Reed, B. R., Cummings, J. L., et al. (2002). Utility of clinical criteria in differentiating frontotemporal lobar degeneration (FTLD) from AD. *Neurology, 58*(11), 1608–1615.

Rosen, H. J., Kramer, J. H., Gorno-Tempini, M. L., Schuff, N., Weiner, M., & Miller, B. L. (2002). Patterns of cerebral atrophy in primary progressive aphasia. *American Journal of Geriatric Psychiatry, 10*(1), 89–97.

Rosen, H. J., Pace-Savitsky, K., Perry, R. J., Kramer, J. H., Miller, B. L., & Levenson, R. W. (2004). Recognition of emotion in the frontal and temporal variants of frontotemporal dementia. *Dementia and Geriatric Cognitive Disorders, 17*(4), 277–281.

Rosen, H. J., Perry, R. J., Murphy, J., Kramer, J. H., Mychack, P., Schuff, N., et al. (2002). Emotion comprehension in the temporal variant of frontotemporal dementia. *Brain, 125*(10), 2286–2295.

Rosso, S. M., Donker Kaat, L., Baks, T., Joosse, M., de Koning, I., Pijnenburg, Y., et al. (2003). Frontotemporal dementia in The Netherlands: Patient characteristics and prevalence estimates from a population-based study. *Brain, 126*(9), 2016–2022.

Rozzini, L., Lussignoli, G., Padovani, A., Bianchetti, A., & Trabucchi, M. (1997). Alzheimer disease and frontotemporal dementia. *Archives of Neurology, 54*(4), 350.

Seeley, W. W., Bauer, A. M., Miller, B. L., Gorno-Tempini, M. L., Kramer, J. H., Weiner, M., et al. (2005). The natural history of temporal variant frontotemporal dementia. *Neurology, 64*(8), 1384–1390.

Shiga, Y., Miyazawa, K., Sato, S., Fukushima, R., Shibuya, S., Sato, Y., et al. (2004). Diffusion-weighted MRI abnormalities as an early diagnostic marker for Creutzfeldt–Jakob disease. *Neurology, 63*(3), 443–449.

Snowden, J. S. (1999). Semantic dysfunction in frontotemporal lobar degeneration. *Dementia and Geriatric Cognitive Disorders, 10*(Suppl. 1), 33–36.

Snowden, J. S., Bathgate, D., Varma, A., Blackshaw, A., Gibbons, Z., C. & Neary, D. (2001). Distinct behavioural profiles in frontotemporal dementia and semantic dementia. *Journal of Neurology, Neurosurgery, and Psychiatry, 70*(3), 323–332.

Spillantini, M. G., Bird, T. D., & Ghetti, B. (1998). Frontotemporal dementia and Parkinsonism linked to chromosome 17: A new group of tauopathies. *Brain Pathology, 8*(2), 387–402.

Spillantini, M. G., & Goedert, M. (2001). Tau gene mutations and tau pathology in frontotemporal dementia and parkinsonism linked to chromosome 17. *Advances in Experimental Medicine and Biology, 487,* 21–37.

Stevens, M., van Duijn, C. M., Kamphorst, W., de Knijff, P., Heutink, P., van Gool, W. A., et al. (1998). Familial aggregation in frontotemporal dementia. *Neurology, 50*(6), 1541–1545.

Swartz, J. R., Miller, B. L., Lesser, I. M., Booth, R., Darby, A., Wohl, M., et al. (1997). Behavioral phenomenology in Alzheimer's disease, frontotemporal dementia, and late-life depression: A retrospective analysis. *Journal of Geriatric Psychiatry and Neurology, 10*(2), 67–74.

Swartz, J. R., Miller, B. L., Lesser, I. M., & Darby, A. L. (1997). Frontotemporal dementia: Treatment response to serotonin selective reuptake inhibitors. *Journal of Clinical Psychiatry, 58*(5), 212–216.

Talbot, P. R. (1996). Frontal lobe dementia and motor neuron disease. *Journal of Neural Transmission: Supplementum, 47,* 125–132.

Tan, C. F., Kakita, A., Piao, Y. S., Kikugawa, K., Endo, K., Tanaka, M., et al. (2003). Primary lateral sclerosis: A rare upper-motor-predominant form of amyotrophic lateral sclerosis often accompanied by frontotemporal lobar degeneration with ubiquitinated neuronal inclusions?: Report of an autopsy case and a review of the literature. *Acta Neuropathologica (Berlin), 105*(6), 615–620.

Tanemura, K., Murayama, M., Akagi, T., Hashikawa, T., Tominaga, T., Ichikawa, M., et al. (2002). Neurodegeneration with tau accumulation in a transgenic mouse expressing V337M human tau. *Journal of Neuroscience, 22*(1), 133–141.

Tariot, P. N., Farlow, M. R., Grossberg, G. T., Graham, S. M., McDonald, S., & Gergel, I. (2004). Memantine treatment in patients with moderate to severe Alzheimer disease already receiving donepezil: A randomized controlled trial. *Journal of the American Medical Association, 291*(3), 317–324.

Tariot, P. N., Solomon, P. R., Morris, J. C., Kershaw, P., Lilienfeld, S., & Ding, C. (2000). A 5-month, randomized, placebo-controlled trial of galantamine in AD: The Galantamine USA-10 Study Group. *Neurology, 54*(12), 2269–2276.

Lund and Manchester Groups. (1994). Clinical and neuropathological criteria for frontotemporal dementia: The Lund and Manchester Groups. *Journal of Neurology, Neurosurgery, and Psychiatry, 57*(4), 416–418.

Thomas-Anterion, C., Jacquin, K., & Laurent, B. (2000). Differential mechanisms of impairment of remote memory in Alzheimer's and frontotemporal dementia. *Dementia and Geriatric Cognitive Disorders, 11*(2), 100–106.

Tolnay, M., & Probst, A. (2001). Frontotemporal lobar degeneration: An update on clinical, pathological and genetic findings. *Gerontology, 47*(1), 1–8.

Tolnay, M., & Probst, A. (2002). Frontotemporal lobar

degeneration—tau as a pied piper? *Neurogenetics*, *4*(2), 63–75.

Trinh, N. H., Hoblyn, J., Mohanty, S., & Yaffe, K. (2003). Efficacy of cholinesterase inhibitors in the treatment of neuropsychiatric symptoms and functional impairment in Alzheimer disease: A meta-analysis. *Journal of the American Medical Association*, *289*(2), 210–216.

Turner, R. S., Kenyon, L. C., Trojanowski, J. Q., Gonatas, N., & Grossman, M. (1996). Clinical, neuroimaging, and pathologic features of progressive nonfluent aphasia. *Annals of Neurology*, *39*(2), 166–173.

Ukisu, R., Kushihashi, T., Kitanosono, T., Fujisawa, H., Takenaka, H., Ohgiya, Y., et al. (2005). Serial diffusion-weighted MRI of Creutzfeldt–Jakob disease. *AJR: American Journal of Roentgenology*, *184*(2), 560–566.

van Swieten, J. C., Rosso, S. M., van Herpen, E., Kamphorst, W., Ravid, R., & Heutink, P. (2004). Phenotypic variation in frontotemporal dementia and parkinsonism linked to chromosome 17. *Dementia and Geriatric Cognitive Disorders*, *17*(4), 261–264.

Verpillat, P., Camuzat, A., Hannequin, D., Thomas-Anterion, C., Puel, M., Belliard, S., et al. (2002). Association between the extended tau haplotype and frontotemporal dementia. *Archives of Neurology*, *59*(6), 935–939.

Westmacott, R., Leach, L., Freedman, M., & Moscovitch, M. (2001). Different patterns of autobiographical memory loss in semantic dementia and medial temporal lobe amnesia: A challenge to consolidation theory. *Neurocase*, *7*(1), 37–55.

Wilhelmsen, K. C. (1998). Frontotemporal dementia genetics. *Journal of Geriatric Psychiatry and Neurology*, *11*(2), 55–60.

Yoshida, M. (2004). Amyotrophic lateral sclerosis with dementia: The clinicopathological spectrum. *Neuropathology*, *24*(1), 87–102.

Yoshiyama, Y., Lee, V. M., & Trojanowski, J. Q. (2001). Frontotemporal dementia and tauopathy. *Current Neurology and Neuroscience Reports*, *1*(5), 413–421.

# CHAPTER 25

# Genetics and Neuropathology of Frontotemporal Dementia

*Nigel J. Cairns*
*Virginia M.-Y. Lee*
*John Q. Trojanowski*

Frontotemporal dementia (FTD) is a clinical syndrome associated with several neurodegenerative diseases characterized by frontotemporal lobar degeneration (FTLD) (Brun et al., 1994; McKhann et al., 2001; Trojanowski & Dickson, 2001). After Alzheimer's disease (AD) and dementia with Lewy bodies (DLB), FTLD is the most common early-onset neurodegenerative disorder. Men and women are both affected, and the disorder has a worldwide distribution. Many cases of FTD have a family history of a similar dementing disorder (Chow, Miller, Hayashi, & Geschwind, 1999; Knopman, Mastri, Frey, Sung, & Rustan, 1990). Rapid progress is being made in the molecular classification of these diseases that are both clinically and neuropathologically heterogeneous. Most of these diseases are characterized by the pathological aggregation of misfolded proteins, either in neurons or glial cells, or both. A minority of cases have abnormal intracellular cytoplasmic accumulations of the microtubule-associated protein (MAP) tau. The term "tauopathies" has been applied to this apparently unrelated group of diseases that includes Pick's disease (PiD), corticobasal degeneration (CBD), progressive supranuclear palsy (PSP), and FTD with parkinsonism linked to chromosome 17 (FTDP-17).

A second group of patients with FTLD lacks filamentous tau inclusions. The molecular classification of this group is evolving and includes FTLD (Neary et al., 1998; Trojanowski & Dickson, 2001), also called dementia lacking distinctive histopathology (DLDH) (Knopman et al., 1990) or frontal lobe degeneration of non-Alzheimer type (Brun & Passant 1996); FTLD with motor neuron disease–type inclusions (FTLD-MND) (Trojanowski & Dickson, 2001), also called motor neuron disease–inclusion dementia (Jackson, Lennox, & Lowe, 1996); neuronal intermediate filament inclusion disease (NIFID) (Cairns et al., 2004), basophilic inclusion body disease (BIBD) (Munoz-Garcia & Ludwin, 1984); and inclusion body myopathy associated with Paget's disease of bone and early-onset frontotemporal dementia (IBMPFD) (Watts et al., 2004). The practicing neuropathologist should also be aware that sporadic and familial cases of FTD may be associated with AD and other neurodegenerative diseases, including DLB (Bonner et al., 2003).

## TAUOPATHIES

Several sporadic and familial neurodegenerative diseases are characterized by the formation of argyrophilic, filamentous deposits of abnormal brain proteins. Thus, a heterogeneous group of FTLDs is linked by the presence of pathological intracellular glial and neuronal inclusions of tau (Table 25.1). Despite the diverse phenotypic expression, brain dysfunction and neurodegeneration are linked to the progressive accumulation of abnormal filamentous protein, and this, together with the absence of other disease-specific neuropathological abnormalities, provides evidence implicating tau in disease onset and progression. The discovery of multiple mutations in the *tau* gene in FTD with parkinsonism linked to chromosome 17 (FTDP-17) has led to the unequivocal evidence that tau abnormalities alone are sufficient to cause neurodegenerative disease. These discoveries have opened up new avenues of research into the role of tau in mechanisms of brain dysfunction and neurodegeneration.

Tau proteins are low-molecular-weight MAPs that are abundant in the central nervous system (CNS), where they are expressed predominantly in axons, and at low levels in astrocytes and oligodendrocytes. Human tau proteins are encoded by a single-copy gene on chromosome 17q21 of 16 exons with CNS isoforms generated by alternative messenger RNA (mRNA) splicing of 11 of these exons (Figure 25.1). In the adult human brain, alternative splicing of exons 2, 3, and 10 generates 6 tau isoforms ranging from 352 to 441 amino acids in length, which differ by the presence of either 3 or 4 microtubule (MT) binding repeats (3R tau or 4R tau, respectively) consisting of repeat sequences of 31 or 32 amino acids each that are encoded by exons 9 to 12. Additionally, alternative splicing of exons 2 and 3 leads to the absence (0N) or presence of inserted sequences of

**TABLE 25.1. Molecular Classification of Inclusion Bodies in FTLDs**

| Disease | Protein aggregate | Chromosomal linkage, *gene defect/haplotype* | Isoform |
|---|---|---|---|
| | | Tauopathies | |
| PiD sporadic | Tau | Unknown1 | 3R |
| PiD familial | Tau | *Presenilin 1 (PS1 G183V)* | — |
| CBD sporadic | Tau | *Tau H1 haplotype* | 4R |
| PSP sporadic | Tau | *Tau H1 haplotype* | 4R; 4R > 3R |
| FTDP-17 familial | Tau | Chromosome 17, *Tau[b]* | 4R; 4R and 3R; 4R > 3R |
| | | FTLDs without tau-positive inclusions | |
| FTLD sporadic | ND | Unknown | — |
| FTLD familial | ND | Chromosome 3, *CHMP2B* | — |
| FTLD familial | ND | Chromosome 17 *Tau intron 10 + 19, + 29[b]* | 3R |
| FTLD-MND sporadic | Ubiquitin[a] | Unknown | — |
| FTLD-MND familial | Ubiquitin[a] | Chromosome 9 | — |
| FTLD-MND familial | Ubiquitin[a] | Chromosome 17, *PRGN* | — |
| NIFID sporadic | Ubiquitin[a] + Neuronal intermediate filaments | Unknown | — |
| BIBD sporadic | Ubiquitin[a] | Unknown | — |
| IBMPFD familial | Ubiquitin[a] + Valosin-containing protein | Chromosome 9, *Valosin-containing protein* | — |

*Note.* FTLD, frontotemporal lobar degeneration; FTLD-MND, frontotemporal lobar degeneration with motor neuron–type inclusions; NIFID, neuronal intermediate filament inclusion disease; BIBD, basophilic inclusion body disease; IBMPFD, inclusion body myopathy associated with Paget's disease of bone and frontotemporal dementia; PiD, Pick's disease; CBD, corticobasal degeneration; PSP, progressive supranuclear palsy; FTDP-17, frontotemporal dementia with parkinsonism linked to chromosome 17; 3R, the predominant number of tau isoforms with three microtubule-binding domains: *CHMP2B*, charged multivesicular body protein 2B; PRGN, progranulin.
[a] Inclusions in these diseases contain ubiquitin, but other proteins have not yet been identified.
[b] Mutations in *tau* are described in Table 25.2.

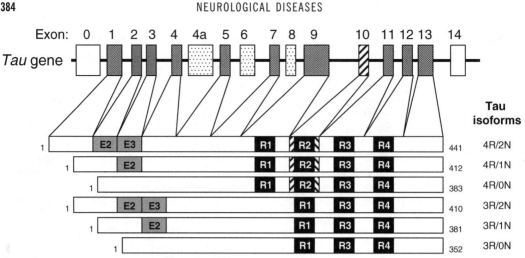

FIGURE 25.1. Schematic representation of the human *tau* gene and six human CNS tau isoforms generated by alternative splicing. Exons 1, 4, 5, 7, 9, and 11–13 are constitutively expressed. Alternative splicing of exons 2 (E2), 3 (E3), and 10 produces the six alternative tau isoforms. The black bars depict the 18–amino acid microtubule-binding repeats and are designated R1 to R4. The relative sizes of the exons and introns are not drawn to scale.

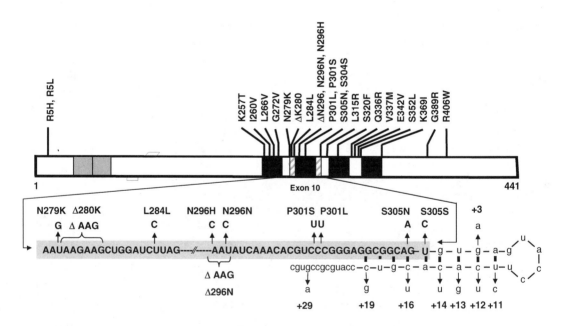

FIGURE 25.2. Schematic representation of mutations in the *tau* gene in FTDP-17. The structure of the largest tau isoform is shown, with known coding region mutations indicated above. The gray boxes near the amino terminus represent the alternatively spliced inserts encoded for by exons 2 and 3, whereas the black boxes represent each of the four microtubule (MT)-binding repeats (not drawn to scale). The second MT-binding repeat is encoded by exon 10. Part of the mRNA sequence encoding exon 10 and the intron following exon 10 is enlarged to visualize the 5' splice site, as well as the mutations in both exon 10 and within the 5' splice site. Nucleotides of intron 10 are shown in lowercase letters.

29 (1N) or 58 (2N) amino acids in the amino-terminal third of the molecule. In the adult human brain, the ratio of 3R:4R tau isoforms is approximately 1:1.

Tau binds to and stabilizes MTs and promotes MT polymerization. The MT-binding domains of tau are localized within the four MT-binding motifs (Figures 25.1 and 25.2). These motifs are composed of highly conserved binding elements. The function of tau as an MT-binding protein is regulated by phosphorylation. Several protein kinases and protein phosphatases have been implicated in regulating the phosphorylation state and thus the

function of tau. The phosphorylation sites are clustered in regions flanking the MT-binding repeats, and increasing tau phosphorylation at multiple sites regulates MT binding (Bramblett et al., 1993). However, in both sporadic and familial tauopathies, tau is hyperphosphorylated, and it is this "abnormal" tau that is the principle component of the filamentous aggregates in neurons and glia that are the pathological hallmarks of these disorders. The tauopathies may be broadly grouped according to the pattern of tau immunostaining and tau isoform ratios as demonstrated by Western blotting (Figure 25.3).

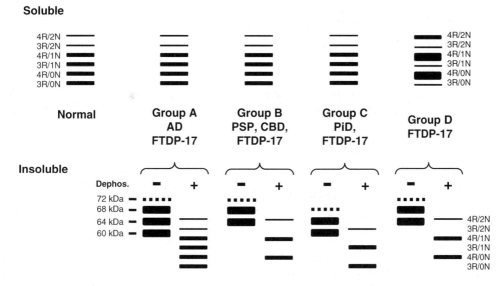

FIGURE 25.3. Cartoon representing Western blot banding patterns of soluble and insoluble tau from different tauopathies. The figure depicts the typical banding pattern of soluble tau (top panels) and insoluble and filamentous tau (bottom panels) from the brains of patients with FTDP-17, as well as sporadic tauopathies resolved by electrophoresis and demonstrated by immunoblotting with antitau antibodies. The FTDP-17 mutations show several different Western blot banding patterns of soluble and insoluble tau protein that are depicted as groups A to D. The soluble fraction from the brains of unaffected (normal) individuals, sporadic tauopathies, and FTDP-17, with mutations that do not affect tau splicing (Groups A, B, and C), show expression of all six tau isoforms. Insoluble tau from the brain of patients with FTDP-17, group A (S320F, V337M, K369I, G389R, and R406W), resolve as three major 68-, 64-, and 60-kDa proteins, and a minor band of 72 kDa similar to that observed in AD. When dephosphorylated, they resolve into six proteins that correspond to all six tau isoforms similar to the soluble fraction. In FTDP-17 group B (R5H, P301L, and G342V), two prominent 68 and 64 kDa protein bands are detected (the 72 kDa minor band is variably detected) that align with 4R tau following dephosphorylation similar to that observed in PSP and CBD, indicating the selective aggregation of 4R tau. In FTDP-17 group C (K257T) and PiD, the 64- and 60-kDa insoluble tau protein isoforms predominate and align with 3R tau isoforms following dephosphorylation, indicating selective aggregation of 3R tau. In contrast, in FTDP-17 mutations that affect mRNA splicing (Group D: N279K, L284L, N296N, N296H, S305S, S305N, and intron 10 mutations), there is expression of predominantly 4R tau throughout the entire brain, which is reflected in the insoluble tau aggregates.

## Pick's Disease

### Genetics

Arnold Pick first reported a form of presenile dementia with circumscribed lobar atrophy in 1892. However, it was Alois Alzheimer who first described in 1911 the histological lesions that are characteristic of the disease: intraneuronal, argyrophilic, and globular inclusions. Classical cases of PiD may be readily distinguished from AD on clinical grounds but many patients with PiD have symptoms that are indistinguishable from those found in AD. In contrast, it is easier to distinguish PiD from AD pathologically. PiD is an uncommon cause of dementia and accounts for less than 5% of cases (Boller, Lopez, & Moossey, 1989). The age at onset varies between 45 and 65 years, and rarely beyond 75 years. Thus, unlike most patients with AD, patients with PiD typically have an early-onset dementia. The duration of the disease is on average 5 to 10 years. Women appear to be slightly more affected than men and the disease has a worldwide distribution. It is largely a sporadic disease, and because familial cases have come under greater scrutiny, the original diagnosis in some has been revised to take into account advances in immunohistochemistry and molecular genetics. Most familial cases have now been reassigned to FTDP-17 (see below). However, in one family with tau-positive inclusions, a novel *presenilin 1* mutation was reported (Dermaut et al., 2004) demonstrating that PiD, like AD, is genetically heterogeneous. Two extended haplotypes cover the human *tau* gene, and there is complete disequilibrium between polymorphisms that span the gene (which covers approximately 100 kb

of DNA). This suggests that the establishment of the two haplotypes was an ancient event, and that either recombination is suppressed in this region, or recombinant genes are selected against. The more common haplotype (H1) is significantly overrepresented in patients with progressive supranuclear palsy (PSP) (Baker et al., 1999), but there is no difference between the tau H2 haplotype or H2/H2 genotype frequency in PiD cases when compared with control subjects, and no *tau* mutations have been found in pathologically typical cases of PiD (Morris, Baker, et al., 2002).

### Neuropathology

The appearance of the PiD brain is one of the most dramatic in all neuropathology (Figure 25.4). What is striking is the severity of atrophy and its localization to the frontal or temporal lobe, or both, and less commonly to the parietal lobe. The loss of tissue can be so severe as to give the appearance of a shrivelled walnut. In classical cases the temporal pole may be particularly affected, with relative sparing of the posterior part of the superior temporal gyrus. In the frontal lobes, the inferior aspect including the orbitofrontal region is often severely shrunken. The loss of brain substance may lead to a brain weight below 1,000 g.

Coronal slicing of the cerebral hemispheres reveals narrowing of the gyri and widening of sulci in the frontal and temporal lobes. The amygdala and hippocampus are often severely affected, and the caudate nucleus may be so atrophied as to give the appearance of that seen in Huntington's disease. Associated with this devastation, the lateral ventricles may be

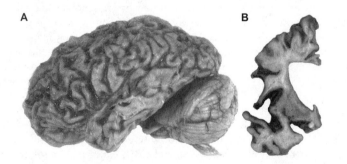

A                          B

FIGURE 25.4. A Pick's disease brain. (A) There is striking atrophy of the frontal and temporal lobes, and the parietal lobe is also affected. The gyri are markedly thinned and the sulci are widened. (B) A coronal slice of the hemibrain of A. The lateral ventricle is severely dilated; the lateral fissure is enlarged, gyri are narrowed, and the cortical ribbon is thinned.

grossly dilated. These changes can be contrasted with the relatively well-preserved remainder of the brain. Although these changes are typical of PD, they may not be present in all cases. The patient may die at an early stage of the disease, and the atrophy may not be particularly extensive. In those patients who have the longest clinical history, the brain may be the most atrophied.

The diagnostic histological feature of PiD is the Pick body (Figure 25.5). Pick bodies are well-circumscribed, spherical, argyrophilic, tau-immunoreactive neuronal intracytoplasmic inclusions. In addition, there are swollen achromatic so-called "ballooned" neurons or Pick cells, neuronal loss, and astrocytosis. Granulovacuolar degeneration may be seen in the hippocampus. These additional changes are not specific to PiD, because they are also found in other neurodegenerative disorders. Pick bodies are found most abundantly in the granule cells of the dentate gyrus. The predilection for the cells of the dentate gyrus distinguishes PiD from AD, in which neurofibrillary tangles (NFTs) are rarely found in the granule cells. Pick bodies are found at lower densities in the pyramidal neurons of the frontal and temporal neocortex. The distribution of Pick bodies may be uni- or bilaminar, and this difference may reflect the stage of progression of the disease. A prominent band may be seen in layer II and upper layer III, and a band in layer IV (Figure 25.5A). These neurons can be contrasted with those in AD, in which NFTs are found predominantly in the large pyramidal neurons of layers III and V, the major corticocortical projecting neurons. Spatial pattern analysis has shown that Pick bodies appear in regular clusters throughout affected cortical areas (Armstrong, Cairns, & Lantos, 1998). The size of Pick bodies depends on the size of the neuron in which they are found: Pick bodies in the pyramidal cells of the hippocampus are larger than those found in dentate granule cells. They may be found outside the hippocampus, temporal and frontal neocortex, including the amygdala, striatum, thalamus, hypothalamus, brainstem nuclei, and the spinal cord.

Ultrastructurally, Pick bodies consist mainly of bundles of disorganized straight fibrils that are labeled by antitau antibodies. Although Pick bodies are well demarcated by light microscopy, ultrastructurally, they do not appear to have a limiting membrane (Figure 25.5D). Immunohistochemically, Pick bodies are labeled most intensely by antiubiquitin and antitau antibodies. They have a similar staining pattern to NFTs, but the immunohistochemical and biochemical profile of tau in PiD is different from that in AD: In PiD, 3R tau isoforms are predominant (Bell, Cairns, Lantos, & Rossor, 2000; Delacourte, 1999; Delacourte et al., 1996).

Swollen achromatic neurons are readily seen in hematoxylin and eosin-stained sections. The nucleus is usually in an eccentric position in relation to the cytoplasm. They are typically present in the deep layers of the cortex. They are not present in all cases and are usually absent from the most severely affected regions of the cortex. Electron microscopic studies reveal filaments similar to those seen in Pick bodies,

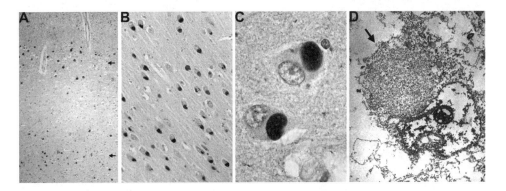

FIGURE 25.5. Pick bodies in Pick's disease. (A) Bilaminar distribution of Pick bodies in superficial (*upper arrow*) and deep laminae (*lower arrow*) of the temporal lobe. (B) Numerous neuronal cytoplasmic Pick bodies in the subiculum. Tau immunohistochemistry. (C) Pick bodies. Ubiquitin immunohistochemistry. (D) An electron micrograph revealing the filaments of a non-membrane-bound Pick body (*arrow*).

together with granular material and some degenerate organelles. Ballooned neurons have a slightly different immunohistochemical profile than that of Pick bodies. Like Pick bodies, the swollen neurons are labeled by antiubiquitin and antitau antibodies, but the intensity of staining is usually less, and variable within the cytoplasm of ballooned neurons. They are also labeled by the heat-shock protein anti-αB-crystallin antibodies (Figure 25.6) (Cooper, Jackson, Lennor, Lowe, & Mann, 1995). The significance of ballooned neurons in the pathogenesis of PiD is unclear.

## Corticobasal Degeneration

### Genetics

The clinicopathological description of corticodentatonigral degeneration with neuronal achromasia was first made by Rebeiz, Kolody, and Richardson in 1967 and 1968, but it was Gibb, Luthert, and Marsden who coined the term "corticobasal degeneration" (CBD) in 1989. Males and females are equally affected, and the age at onset of sporadic cases is the sixth to eighth decades. In the rare familial cases that have been reported, there is an earlier age at onset. Duration of illness ranges from 7 to 10 years. The neuronal and glial inclusions of CBD may be compared with those of PiD and PSP. The presence of swollen neurons, particularly when demonstrated by immunohistochemistry, is the most striking feature of this disease. As with familial cases of PiD, the discovery of mutations in the *tau* gene in familial cases of CBD has resulted in these cases being reassigned to FTDP-17 (see below). In sporadic cases, genetic analysis of the *tau*

gene has resulted in two major forms, or haplotypes, called H1 and H2 (Baker et al., 1999). The frequency of the H1 haplotype is increased in CBD and several cases are H1/H1 homozygous (Houlden et al., 2001).

### Neuropathology

Characteristically, the brain is atrophied asymmetrically in the posterior frontal and parietal lobes; both the pre- and postcentral gyri are affected. Cortical atrophy is not usually as pronounced as in PiD. There is dilatation of the lateral ventricles and the striatum may be shrunken. The corticospinal tracts and corpus callosum may appear thinned. The substantia nigra appears pale in the majority of cases, but there is not the brainstem atrophy typically found in patients with progressive supranuclear palsy.

The loss of neurons may be more severe in the outer cortical laminae and generate status spongiosus. The white matter underlying the affected areas of cortex may be rarefied and display a reactive astrocytosis. Ballooned neurons are readily seen. They are found most frequently in the deeper cortical laminae (III, V, and VI) and occasionally in subcortical areas, but may be absent in the most severely affected cortical areas. As in PiD, swollen neurons are variably labeled by ubiquitin, neurofilament, and tau antibodies; they are best demonstrated by αB-crystallin immunohistochemistry (Lowe et al., 1992). Ultrastructurally, swollen neurons contain 10–15 nm filaments and a smaller number of thicker 25–30 nm filaments, granular material, and lipofuscin (Wakabayashi et al., 1994). The swollen neurons of corticobasal degeneration may be distinguished from Pick cells of PiD by epitope-specific antitau antibodies (Bell, Cairns, Lantos, & Rossor, 2000).

There is usually severe neuronal loss and accompanying astrocytosis in the substantia nigra. A characteristic feature is the intraneuronal basophilic inclusion. These "corticobasal inclusions" are argyrophilic and fibrillar, and are labeled by antiubiquitin and antitau antibodies (Figure 25.7). Histologically, they resemble the neurofibrillary tangles of PSP. Ultrastructurally, the filaments of the inclusions are mainly straight, with a diameter of 15 nm (Wakabayashi et al., 1994). Similar inclusions may be found in the locus coeruleus and other brainstem nuclei. In addition to these corticobasal inclusions, small neuronal tau-

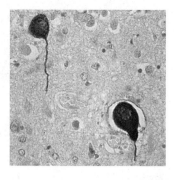

FIGURE 25.6. Swollen achromatic neurons, so-called "ballooned" or Pick cells, in the frontal lobe in PiD. αB-crystallin immunohistochemistry.

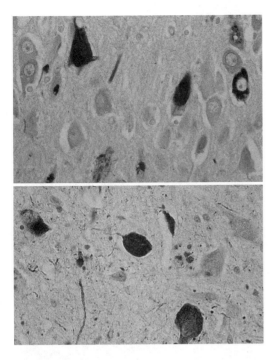

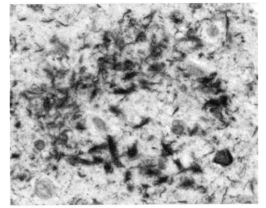

FIGURE 25.8. CBD. An astrocytic plaque in the superior temporal gyrus. Tau immunohistochemistry.

FIGURE 25.7. CBD. Neurofibrillary tangles in the CA1 subfield of the hippocampus (upper panel) and subthalamic nucleus (lower panel). Tau immunohistochemistry.

positive inclusions and neuropil threads can be found in the superficial layers of the cortex.

A striking feature of CBD is glial pathology in the affected areas. Filamentous argyrophilic structures are seen most commonly in astrocytes and less frequently in oligodendrocytes. Clusters of astrocytic tangles may form astrocytic plaques (Figure 25.8). The inclusions in oligodendrocytes are argyrophilic fibrillar structures. Both the astrocytic and oligodendroglial inclusions in CBD are labeled by anti-ubiquitin and antitau antibodies. They are not recognized by anti-α-synuclein antibodies, the major component of the glial cytoplasmic inclusions (GCIs) of multiple system atrophy (MSA) (Spillantini, Crowther, et al. 1998a; Tu et al., 1998). Although it has been suggested that the GCIs are not specific to MSA and are also found in CBD and PSP, the oligodendroglial inclusions of CBD are morphologically and immunohistochemically different from the GCIs of MSA. The tau protein in CBD is predominantly 4R tau, which is different from that of both AD and PiD.

## Progressive Supranuclear Palsy

### Genetics

Progressive supranuclear palsy (PSP) was first defined as a clinical and neuropathological entity in 1964 by Steele, Richardson, and Olszewski. Approximately 4% of parkinsonian patients have PSP, or four cases per million per year. The age at onset is around 60 years, with an average duration of 6 years and a slight male preponderance; the male-to-female ratio is 60% to 40%. The clinical features include parkinsonism, vertical supranuclear gaze palsy, cognitive impairment consistent with FTD, dysarthria, and dysphasia. Frontal lobe signs may be prominent (Golbe, Davis, Schoenberg, & Duvoisin, 1988). The parkinsonian symptoms include bradykinesia, rigidity, gait disorder, masked fascies, neck dystonia, and falls, but there is no tremor and the patient does not respond to levodopa. The disease is sporadic, although rare autosomal dominant familial cases have been reported. Some familial cases with a PSP-phenotype have *tau* mutations, and these have been reassigned to FTDP-17 (see below); however, some familial cases of PSP fail to show mutations in *tau* (Morris, Katzenschlager, et al., 2002b). Two extended haplotypes cover the human *tau* gene, and there is complete disequilibrium between polymorphisms that span the gene. The more common haplotype (H1) is significantly overrepresented in patients with PSP, extending earlier reports of an association between an intronic dinucleotide polymorphism and PSP (Baker et al., 1999).

## Neuropathology

Macroscopically, the brain may appear normal or atrophied. The atrophy may include the globus pallidus, thalamus, subthalamic nucleus, and occasionally the brainstem and cerebellum (Figure 25.9). The substantia nigra and locus coeruleus often appear pale. Histology reveals NFTs, neuropil threads, glial inclusions, neuronal loss, and astrocytosis (Bergeron, Davis, & Lang, 1998). The predominant hallmark of PSP is the NFT (Figure 25.10). They are found in the substantia nigra, globus pallidus, subthalamic nucleus, nucleus basalis of Meynert, pretectal area, tegmentum of the midbrain and pons, locus coeruleus, raphe nuclei, and the nuclei of various cranial nerves. The tangles are readily seen by silver impregnation methods but are best visualized by tau immunohistochemistry. Electron microscopy demonstrates that the tangles contain straight filaments of 12–15 nm (Tellez-Nagel & Wisniewski, 1973), which in turn are com-

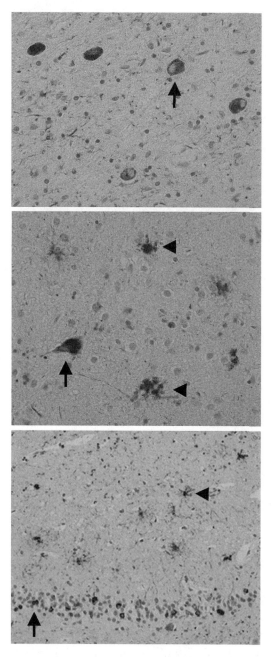

FIGURE 25.10. PSP. Neurofibrillary tangle (*arrow*) in the subthalamic nucleus (upper panel), a neurofibrillary tangle (*arrow*) and thorny astrocytes (*arrowheads*) in the globus pallidus (middle panel), and hippocampus (lower panel). Tau immunohistochemistry.

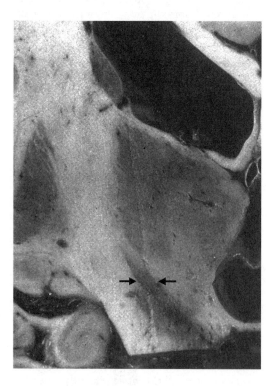

FIGURE 25.9. Atrophy of the subthalamic nucleus (*between arrow*s) in PSP.

posed of six or more protofilaments of 2–5 nm (Montpetit, Clapin, & Guberman, 1985). Paired helical filaments (PHFs) and intermediate forms may be seen. Many astrocytes show inclusions, so-called "astrocytic tangles," and tuft-shaped or thorn-shaped astrocytes have also been observed. Oligodendrocytes may also contain tau-positive inclusions called coiled bodies, which are different from the GCIs of MSA. Predominantly 4R tau isoforms are present in PSP (Delacourte, 1999).

The diagnosis is based on a semiquantitative assessment of the distribution of neurofibrillary tangles. The criteria also take into account the presence of neuropil threads and tau-positive astrocytes. Based on neuropathological criteria, three types of PSP can be distinguished: typical, atypical, and combined (Hauw et al., 1994). Typical cases show the pathological features as originally described, whereas atypical cases are variants of the histological changes characteristic of PSP. In combined cases, in addition to PSP, there is another disease process such as AD or vascular disease.

## FTD with Parkinsonism Linked to Chromosome 17

### Genetics

In recent years, a number of families with FTD, with and without movement disorder, have been identified with mutations in the *tau* gene on chromosome 17. Although this group of disorders has been referred to as frontotemporal dementia and parkinsonism linked to chromosome 17 (FTDP-17) not all cases have parkinsonism. *Tau* gene mutations cause tau dysfunction by several mechanisms. Intronic and some exonic mutations affect the alternative splicing of exon 10 and consequently alter the relative proportions of 3R and 4R tau. Other exonic mutations impair the ability of tau to bind MTs and to promote MT assembly. Some mutations also promote the assembly of tau into pathological amyloid filaments. Intronic mutations clustered around the 5′ splice site of exon 10, as well as several mutations within exon 10, increase the ratio of 4R:3R tau by altering exon splicing (D'Souza et al., 1999; D'Souza & Schellenberg, 2000; Grover et al., 1999; Hutton et al., 1998). As a result of these mutations there is a relative increase in mRNA containing exon 10. Biochemical analysis of insoluble tau extracted from FTDP-17 brain tissue reveals predominantly 4R tau isoforms (Figure 25.3). Furthermore, 4R tau protein levels are increased in both affected and unaffected regions of FTDP-17 brains (Goedert, Spillantini, et al., 1999; Hong et al., 1998; Spillantini, Murrell, et al., 1998).

Mutations alter exon 10 splicing of *tau* by affecting several of the regulatory elements described above. For example, the intronic mutations, as well as the exonic mutations at codon 305 (S305N and S305S), may destabilize the inhibitory stem–loop structure and alter the ratio of 3R:4R tau (D'Souza et al., 1999; Hutton et al., 1998). The mechanisms by which changes in the ratio of 3R:4R tau lead to neuronal and glial dysfunction and cell death remain unclear. However, 3R and 4R tau may bind to distinct sites on MTs (Goode & Feinstein, 1994), and it is possible that a specific ratio of tau isoforms is necessary for normal MT function (Goode et al., 1997). Thus, the altered ratio of 3R:4R tau may directly affect MT function. In addition, overproduction of 4R tau isoforms may lead to an excess of free tau in the cytoplasm that is prone to aggregate and polymerize into filaments over time. Conversely, overproduction of 3R tau may have the opposite effect: an absence of tau inclusions and the phenotype of FTLD (Stanford et al., 2003).

Another subset of the mutations has no effect on splicing, but instead alters the ability of tau to interact with MTs: missense mutations K257T, G272V, ΔK280, ΔN296, P301L, P301S, V337M, G389R, and R406W reduce the binding of tau to MTs and decrease its ability to promote MT stability and assembly *in vitro* (Hasegawa, Smith, & Goedert, 1998; Rizzini et al., 2000; Rizzu et al., 1999). In contrast to mutations that affect the splicing of *tau*, these mutations do not alter the expression pattern of 3R and 4R tau (Hong et al., 1998). A moderate decrease in soluble 4R tau with the *P301L* mutation is caused by the selective aggregation of mutant 4R tau isoforms (Hong et al., 1998; Miyasaka et al., 2001; Rizzu et al., 2000). These mutations generate a variety of biochemical patterns of insoluble tau extracted from brain tissue of patients.

Tau aggregation in FTDP-17 may be caused, in part, by a subset of missense *tau* mutations. *In vitro* studies demonstrate that mutations, including K257T, G272V, ΔK280, ΔN296, P301L, P301S, V337M, and R406W, promote heparin- or arachidonic acid–induced tau filament formation relative to wild-type tau (Gamblin et al., 2000; Miyasaka et al., 2001). Tau function may also be altered by *tau* mutations by altering its phosphorylation state, and several mutations decrease the binding affinity of tau for phosphatase 2A, a phosphatase implicated in the regulation of the MT-binding activity of tau (Goedert et al., 2000).

### Neuropathology

These familial cases typically have atrophy of the frontal and temporal lobes (Figure 25.11). Microscopically, neuronal loss, astrocytosis, microvacuolation, and swollen neurons are found in affected areas, together with a spectrum of tau pathology, including intraneuronal neurofibrillary tangle-like inclusions, neuronal globose tangle-like inclusions, intraneuronal Pick body–like inclusions, astrocytic tangle-like inclusions, and oligodendroglial inclusions resembling coiled bodies and dystrophic neurites (Figure 25.12). In a subset of cases with *tau* mutations, there may be sufficient NFTs and β-amyloid plaques to fulfill the neuropathological criteria for AD, but these cases, in addition to the *tau* mutation, may also have an apolipoprotein E ε4 allele (Lantos et al., 2002). Mutations in the *tau* gene generate a heterogeneous biochemical phenotype: Mutations may generate predominantly either 3R or 4R tau, or a combination of the two (see Table 25.2). Thus, an extraordinarily wide-range of tau pathology has been observed in these familial cases.

Although there is clinical and neuropathological overlap between the neurodegenerative tauopathies, each can be distinguished with variable probability by the distribution, severity, and morphology of tau-positive inclusions. In cases with a *tau* gene mutation, in addition to extensive neuronal loss and astrocytosis, tau-positive neuronal and glial inclusions may resemble those seen in AD, PSP, CBD, and PiD. This neuropathological heterogeneity is a striking feature of FTDP-17, and it is complemented by biochemical heterogeneity in which there is variation in the proportions of tau isoforms, not only with different mutations but also within the same brain. Nevertheless, cases with *tau* gene mutations may be broadly grouped according to the pattern of tau immunostaining and tau isoform ratios, as demonstrated by Western blotting (Figure 25.3).

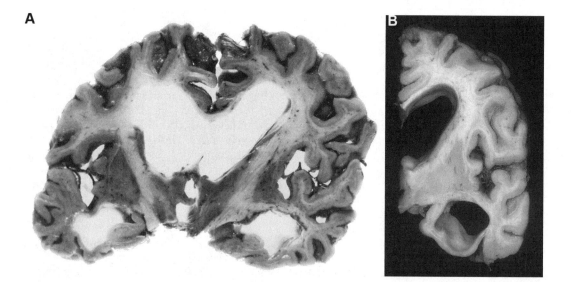

FIGURE 25.11. FTDP-17. Atrophy of the frontal and temporal lobes at the level of the red nucleus in a case with intron *tau* 10[+16] mutation (A) and atrophy of the right hemibrain of a case of *tau* mutation G389R at the level of the globus pallidus (B). In each hemisphere there is narrowing of gyri, widening of the sylvian fissure, severe dilatation of the lateral ventricle and its inferior horn, and atrophy of the hippocampus (A) and amygdala (B).

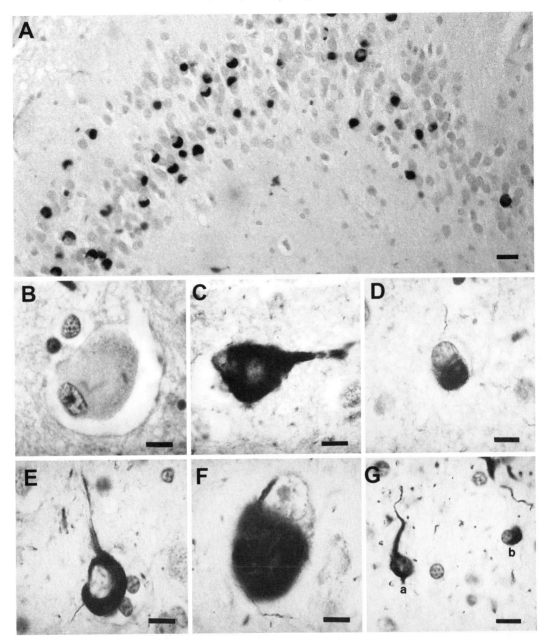

FIGURE 25.12. Spectrum of neuronal and glial tau inclusions in FTDP-17. Inclusions in *tau* G389R mutation (A) and intron *tau* 10+16 mutation (B–G). (A) Numerous Pick body–like inclusions in the granule neurons of the dentate fascia. (B) A swollen achromatic neuron (hematoxylin and eosin). (C) A swollen neuron with a central area of pale antitau immunoreactivity surrounded by more intense staining. (D) An intraneuronal inclusion resembling a Pick body in the frontal lobe. (E) A NFT-like inclusion in a pyramidal neuron of the frontal lobe. (F) A globose NFT-like inclusion in the dorsal raphe nucleus. (G) An astrocytic fibrillary inclusion (a) and a coiled body (b) in an oligodendrocyte in the white matter of the frontal lobe. (A, C–G) Tau immunohistochemistry. Scale bars = 10 μm.

**TABLE 25.2.** *Tau* Mutations in FTDP-17

| Protein Mutation[a] | Region | Effect on exon 10 splicing | Effect on MT assembly | Pathological phenotype | Reference |
|---|---|---|---|---|---|
| R5H | Exon 1 | No | Yes | FTDP-17 | Hayashi et al. (2002) |
| R5L | Exon 1 | No | Yes | PSP-like | Poorkaj et al. (2002) |
| K257T | Exon 9 | ND | Yes | PiD-like | Pickering-Brown et al. (2000); Rizzini et al. (2000) |
| I260V | Exon 9 | No | Yes | FTDP-17 | Grover et al. (2003) |
| L266V | Exon 9 | 4R ↑ | Yes | PiD-like | Kobayashi et al. (2003) |
| G272V | Exon 9 | ND | Yes | FTDP-17 | Hutton et al. (1998) |
| E9+33 | Intron 9 | ND | ND | ND | Rizzu et al. (1999) |
| N279K | Exon 10 | 4R ↑ | No | PSP-like | Clark et al. (1998) |
| Δ280 | Exon 10 | 3R ↑ | Yes | FTDP-17 | Rizzu et al. (1999) |
| L284L | Exon 10 | 4R ↑ | No | AD-like | D'Souza et al. (1999) |
| N296N | Exon 10 | 4R ↑ | Yes | CBD-like | Spillantini et al. (2000) |
| N296H | Exon 10 | 4R ↑ | Yes | FTDP-17 | Iseki et al. (2001) |
| ΔN296 | Exon 10 | 4R ↑ | No | PSP-like | Pastor et al. (2001) |
| P301L | Exon 10 | No | Yes | FTDP-17 | Hutton et al. (1998) |
| P301S | Exon 10 | No | Yes | CBD-like, FTDP-17 | Bugiani et al. (1999); Sperfeld et al. (1999) |
| S305N | Exon 10 | 4R ↑ | Yes | CBD-like | Hasegawa et al. (1999); Iijima et al. (1999) |
| S305S | Exon 10 | 4R ↑ | No | PSP-like | Stanford et al. (2000) |
| E10+3 | Intron 10 | 4R ↑ | No | FTDP-17 | Spillantini, Bird, & Ghetti (1998) |
| E10+11 | Intron 10 | 4R ↑ | No | FTDP-17 | Miyamoto et al. (2001) |
| E10+12 | Intron 10 | 4R ↑ | No | FTDP-17 | Yasuda et al. (2000) |
| E10+13 | Intron 10 | 4R ↑ | No | NA | Hutton et al. (1998) |
| E10+14 | Intron 10 | 4R ↑ | No | PSP-like, FTDP-17 | Hutton et al. (1998) |
| E10+16 | Intron 10 | 4R ↑ | No | AD-, PiD-, PSP-, and CBD-like, FTDP-17 | Hutton et al. (1998) |
| E10+19 | Intron 10 | 3R ↑ | No | FTLD | Stanford et al. (2003) |
| E10+29 | Intron 10 | 3R ↑ | No | FTLD | Stanford et al. (2003) |
| L315R | Exon 11 | ND | Yes | PiD-like | van Herpen et al. (2003) |
| S320F | Exon 11 | ND | Yes | PiD-like | Rosso et al. (2002) |
| Q336R | Exon 12 | ND | Yes | PiD-like | Pickering-Brown et al. (2004) |
| V337M | Exon 12 | ND | Yes | FTDP-17 | Poorkaj et al. (1998) |
| E342V | Exon 12 | 4R ↑ | ND | FTDP-17 | Lippa et al. (2000) |
| S352L | Exon 12 | ND | Yes | Atypical | Nicholl et al. (2003) |
| K369I | Exon 12 | ND | Yes | PiD-like | Neumann et al. (2001) |
| G389R c2170G>C | Exon 13 | ND | Yes | PiD-like | Murrell (1999) |
| G389R c2170G>A | Exon 13 | No | Yes | PiD-like | Pickering-Brown et al. (2000) |
| R406W | Exon 13 | ND | Yes | PSP-like | Hutton et al. (1998) |

*Note.* MT, microtubule; Δ, deletion; 4R ↑, increase in the ratio of 4R:3R tau isoforms; ND, not determined.
[a] Protein mutation name relative to the longest, four microtubule binding repeats (4R) and two inserts (2N), human adult tau isoform.

## Transgenic Models of Tauopathies

To simulate the pathogenesis of tau inclusion bodies, transgenic (TG) models have been generated by overexpressing human tau proteins in mice (Götz, 2001; Götz, Chen, Barmettler, & Nitsch, 2001). However, these mice are either asymptomatic or develop pathology that is localized to the spinal cord, or that lacks many of the pathological changes of tau-based disorders. In contrast, the introduction of the *P301L* mutation led to the development of TG mice that develop age- and gene dose-dependent accumulation of tau tangles in the brain and spinal cord, with associated nerve cell loss and gliosis, as well as behavioral abnormalities (Götz et al., 2001). The tau inclusions were composed of only mutant human *tau* thus implicating the *P301L* mutation in the aggregation of mutant *tau*. Various aspects of human tauopathies have been modeled, including a TG mouse overexpressing the shortest human tau isoform, which acquired age-dependent tau pathology similar to that seen in FTDP-17 and amyotrophic lateral sclerosis–parkinsoniam dementia complex (ALS/PDC) (Ishihara et al., 1999). The fruit fly, *Drosophila melanogaster*, has been used to overexpress either wild-type or mutant *tau* (*R406W* and *V337M*) and shows features of tauopathy, including adult-onset progressive neurodegeneration with accumulation of abnormal tau (Wittmann et al., 2001), but the neurodegeneration occurs in the absence of NFT formation. NFT-like pathology has been generated in another fly model when tau was coexpressed with shaggy, a homologue of glycogen synthase 3-kinase, an enzyme implicated in tau phosphorylation (Jackson et al., 2002). A tau TG *Caenorhabditis elegans* model has been used to demonstrate neurodegeneration and defective neurotransmission. In this model, pan-neuronal expression of normal and mutant tau resulted in altered behavior, accumulation of insoluble phosphorylated tau, age-dependent loss of axons and neurons, and structural damage to axonal tracts (Kraemer et al., 2003). Thus, a spectrum of models is being developed that recapitulates various features of tau pathology, and these models will facilitate understanding of the molecular mechanisms underlying neurodegeneration in the tauopathies.

## FTLDs WITHOUT TAU-POSITIVE INCLUSIONS

### Frontotemporal Lobar Degeneration

#### Genetics

Among the neurodegenerative diseases, the FTLDs are neuropathologically strikingly heterogeneous. This pathological heterogeneity may be explained by different genetic loci in familial FTLDs. In addition to the over 30 mutations in the *tau* gene that have been identified in cases of FTDP-17 (Table 25.2), extensive sequencing of *tau* in familial FTD cases, with and without abnormal tau inclusions, excludes *tau* as the genetic locus in those cases. Molecular genetics studies have linked familial FTLDs to loci on chromosomes 3, 9, and 17 (Table 25.1). FTLD in a Danish family has been linked to a 12-cM (centimorgan) region of the centromeric area of chromosome 3 (Brown et al., 1995) and mutations have been reported in the charged multi-vesicular body protein 2B gene (*CHMP2B*) (Skibinski et al., 2005). Initially, this FTLD family was described as having no inclusions, but one report has shown that in three brains, tau inclusions were present in neurons and some glial cells in the absence of β-amyloid deposits. The presence of filamentous tau protein in the frontal cortex of these patients suggests a possible link between *tau* and the genetic defect present on chromosome 3 and associated with FTLD, although the limited amount of tau deposits in relation to the severe neuronal loss indicate that these cases are unlikely to be a tauopathy (Yancopoulou et al., 2003). Conversely, the absence of any tau inclusions in familial FTLD may be associated with *tau* mutation. In one family with FTLD lacking tau- and ubiquitin-positive inclusions, sequence analysis revealed intronic *tau* 10+19 and +29 mutations that were associated with increased 3R isoforms of tau (Stanford et al., 2003). Thus, FTLD, like FTDP-17 (see below), is genetically heterogeneous. Biochemically, patients with FTLD without distinctive tau pathology have been shown to have decreased soluble tau, but tau mRNA levels were unaltered (Zhukareva et al., 2001, 2003). However, in a study of 33 patients with FTLD without tau inclusions, the loss of soluble tau was associated with the loss of another neuronal protein, NeuN, indicating that loss of tau may reflect a general neurodegenerative response in these cases (Taniguchi et al., 2004).

*Neuropathology*

FTLD is characterized by stereotypical features: atrophy of the frontal and temporal lobes, neuronal loss, microvacuolation, and astrocytosis (Figure 25.13) (McKhann et al., 2001; Trojanowski & Dickson, 2001). This disease is distinguished by the absence of any hallmark inclusion. Previously, this nosological entity combined clinical syndromes with pathological substrates and was referred to variously as PiD Group C in the classification scheme of Constantinidis, Richard, and Tissot (1974), frontal lobe degeneration of non-Alzheimer type (Brun, 1987), dementia of frontal type, FTD, and DLDH (Knopman et al., 1990). As new techniques are developed, such as ubiquitin immunohistochemistry, inclusions have been identified in cases previously considered to be FTLD, resulting in this diagnostic entity being assigned to a dwindling number of cases.

Atrophy in FTLD is variable. It may be limited to the frontal lobe or may be more pronounced in the anterior temporal lobe. The parietal lobes are typically relatively well preserved, and most cases show symmetrical cerebral atrophy, although a few cases show asymmetrical atrophy. In addition to neocortical thinning, there may also be atrophy of nuclei of the limbic system, particularly the amygdala and hippocampus. The striatum is often affected, and there may be pallor of the pigmented nuclei of the brainstem. These cases often show extrapyramidal signs and the combination of neocortical, limbic, and nigral involvement has been referred to as "mesolimbocortical dementia" (Torack & Morris, 1986). Microscopy typically reveals neuronal loss in superficial cortical laminae (II and III), which is often associated with microvacuolation, and in the most severe cases this extends to the full thickness of the cortex. As status spongiosus is often the only dramatic feature of the histology, the possibility of prion disease arises. However, prion protein immunohistochemistry (Caselli et al., 1993) and Western blotting (Pollanen, Bergeron, & Weyer, 1993) exclude prion disease from the differential diagnosis. The distribution of neuronal loss is accompanied by gliosis, and swollen achromatic neurons are seen in most cases. The complete absence of argyrophilic inclusions by silver impregnation methods and the absence of abnormal protein aggregates by immunohistochemistry for ubiquitin, tau, α-synuclein, prion, polyglutamine, valosin-containing protein, and neuronal intermediate filaments lead to FTLD

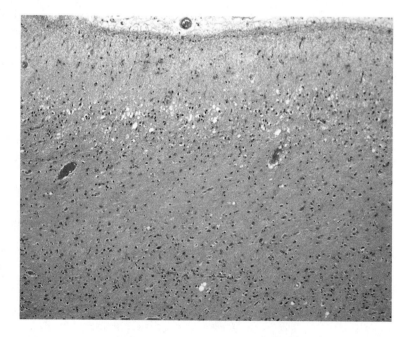

FIGURE 25.13. FTLD. There is neuronal loss and microvacuolation in the superficial cortical layers. In the most severely affected areas, neuronal loss and vacuolation may extend to the full thickness of the cortex.

being a neuropathological diagnosis of exclusion.

## FTLD with Motor Neuron Disease–Type Inclusions

### Genetics

The association between motor neuron disease (MND) and dementia has been recognized in several studies (Mitsuyama & Takamiya, 1979; Neary et al., 1990), and in a number of patients, dementia may be present without the pathological changes seen in the spinal cord in MND (Jackson et al., 1996). Among patients with FTD, FTLD-MND-type, also called motor neuron disease–type inclusion dementia, is one of the more common neuropathological diagnoses. FTLD-MND-type, with or without the clinical and pathological features of classical MND, presents with cognitive impairment and in some, but not all patients, an amyotrophic picture develops (weakness and wasting of limb muscles and bulbar palsy leading to dysarthria, dysphagia, and wasting of the tongue). The disease often starts in the sixth decade of life and has an average duration of 2–3 years, considerably shorter than that of AD. More men are affected than women, with a ratio of 2:1. Although mainly a sporadic disorder, familial occurrence may account for 15–20% of cases. The sex ratio, age at onset, and disease duration do not vary between familial and sporadic forms (Mann, 1998). A number of families with FTLD-MND have been linked to chromosome 9q21-q22 (Hosler et al., 2000; Savioz et al., 2000, 2003) and chromosome 17q21 (Froelich, Axelman, Almkvist, Basun, & Lannfelt, 2003; Kertesz et al., 2000; Rademakers et al., 2002; Rosso et al., 2001). Recently, mutations in the progranulin gene in familiar FTLD-MND-type linked to chromosome 17 were discovered (Baker et al., in press).

### Neuropathology

Macroscopically, there is mild to moderate atrophy of the frontal, anterior temporal, and parietal lobes (Figure 25.14). The atrophy is often less dramatic than that seen in PD. Coronal slices often have dilated lateral ventricles with rounding of the angles, and the corpus callosum is thin. There may be loss of pigment from the substantia nigra. Microscopy shows neuronal loss, microvacuolation, astrocyto-

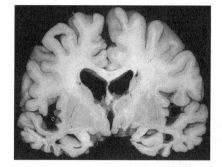

FIGURE 25.14. FTLD-MND-type. There is dilatation of the lateral ventricles, increased space in the lateral fissure, and pronounced atrophy of the temporal lobes.

sis in the superficial layers of the cortex, and intraneuronal nonargyrophilic, ubiquitin-positive, tau-negative dystrophic neurites and inclusions both in the cortex and in the granule cells of the dentate gyrus (Figure 25.15). Neuronal inclusions are also seen in the amygdala (Anderson, Cairns, & Leigh, 1995), but the highest densities are observed in the dentate fascia. Ubiquitin-positive neuronal in-

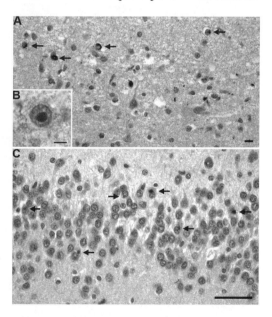

FIGURE 25.15. FTLD-MND-type. Ubiquitin-positive, tau-negative inclusions (*arrows*) in the middle frontal gyrus (A), a neuronal intranuclear inclusion in an adjacent field (B), and cytoplasmic inclusions in granule neurons of the dentate gyrus (C). Scale bars: A = 10 µm, B = 10 µm, C = 50 µm. Ubiquitin immunohistochemistry.

clusions have been reported in familial cases of FTLD-MND (Cairns, Brännström, Khan, Rossor, & Lantos, 2003; Mackenzie & Feldman, 2003) and more recently in sporadic cases (Bigio et al., 2004). In the most severely affected areas neuronal loss may extend across all cortical laminae, with widespread astrocytosis and microglial activation. There is usually severe neuronal loss in the substantia nigra. The pathological changes found in MND may also be present (FTLD-MND with clinical and pathological MND), including neuron loss in the anterior horns of the spinal cord, motor nuclei of the brainstem, and motor cortex. Surviving neurons contain ubiquitin-positive, skein-like, and other inclusions of MND. In addition to the clinical phenotypes of FTD and MND, the pathological changes of FTLD-MND may also be present in cases of semantic dementia (Rossor, Revesz, Lantos, & Warrington, 2000). The occurrence of FTD, semantic dementia, and MND with similar pathological changes may relate to neuronal loss, vacuolation, and dendritic and synaptic loss in neocortex, limbic, and subcortical nuclei. Thus, the presence of ubiquitin inclusions links FTLD-MND-type with FTLD-MND and MND.

## Neuronal Intermediate Filament Inclusion Disease

### Genetics

Neuronal intermediate filament (IF) inclusion disease (NIFID) is a novel neurological disease with a clinically heterogeneous phenotype including atypical dementia, and pyramidal and extrapyramidal signs presenting at a young age (Bigio, Lipton, White, Dickson, & Hirano, 2003; Cairns et al., 2004; Josephs et al., 2003). In a series of 10 cases, the mean age at onset was 40 (range 23 to 56) years, the mean duration of disease was 4.5 (range 2.7 to 13.0) years, and the mean age at death was 45 (range 28 to 61) years (Cairns et al., 2004). Both sexes are affected; the ratio of men to women is 2:3. NIFID is largely a sporadic disorder, and only one case has been reported in which the father had parkinsonism and dementia indicating evidence of heredity (Josephs, Tsuboi, Cookson, Watt, & Dickson, 2004). Presenting symptoms include personality change, apathy, blunted affect, and disinhibition. There may also be memory loss, cognitive impairment, and language deficits, as seen in half of the cases. Motor weakness may be evident at pre-

sentation in a minority of patients. Extrapyramidal features are present in most cases, and less frequently, buccofacial apraxia and supranuclear ophthalmoplegia. Personality and behavioral changes, and memory and language deficits are seen in the majority of patients. Hyperreflexia is a common finding, and most patients became mute with advanced disease. Structural brain imaging typically shows atrophy of the frontal and temporal lobe, and the caudate nucleus may be atrophied. Atrophy of the caudate may raise the possibility of Huntington's disease, but no expansion in the *huntingtin* gene has been reported.

### Neuropathology

The brain often shows severe atrophy of the frontal and temporal lobes, with mild parietal

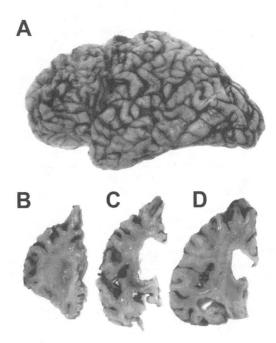

FIGURE 25.16. The lateral aspect of the left hemibrain of 27-year-old woman with NIFID. There is pronounced atrophy of the frontal and anterior temporal lobes. Coronal slices of the left hemisphere reveal enlargement of the lateral ventricle and marked atrophy of the anterior frontal lobe (B) and striatum (C). The sylvian fissure is widened; the caudate nucleus is reduced to a narrow band (C); and the hippocampus (D) is small. The parietal and occipital lobes are only mildly affected.

atrophy (Figure 25.16). The loss of brain substance may lead to a brain weight below 1,000 g. The caudate nucleus is markedly atrophied in most cases. Although the severity and pattern of atrophy varies from case to case, the frontal and temporal poles and caudate nucleus are often the most severely affected. In all cases, there is variable atrophy of subcortical nuclei, including the basal ganglia, amygdala, and thalamus. The brainstem, cerebellum, and spinal cord appear unremarkable. Coronal slices further confirm frontotemporal atrophy: The gyri are narrowed and the intervening sulci are widened, with enlargement of the lateral ventricles. In more severely affected cases the cortical ribbon is thinned. In some cases there is striking atrophy of the amygdala and hippocampus. The histological changes included the stereotypical lesions of FTLDs: neuronal loss, status spongiosus, and astrocytosis in temporal

and frontal isocortex. Swollen achromatic neurons are also seen. However, the most striking feature is the presence of inclusions containing neuronal IF proteins (i.e., the neurofilament [NF] triplet proteins and α-internexin [Figure 25.17]). The severity of each of these histological abnormalities varies from case to case.

Microscopy reveals extensive neuronal loss and reactive astrocytosis in the frontal, medial temporal, and parietal lobes, and varying degrees of loss in subcortical nuclei, including the caudate nucleus, putamen, globus pallidus, amygdala, substantia nigra, and locus coeruleus. A variable degree of neuronal loss and axonal swellings may be present in the cerebellum. Occasional swollen achromatic neurons are observed in affected areas. In areas of neuronal loss, faintly eosinophilic, intraneuronal, cytoplasmic inclusions are present. In both hematoxylin and eosin and cresyl violet-

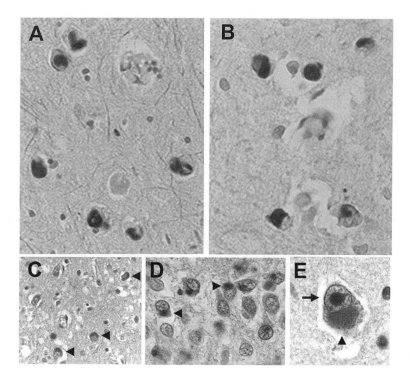

FIGURE 25.17. Neuronal inclusions in NIFID are pleomorphic and may be seen in the same section with normal axons that also contain neuronal IFs. Pick body–like inclusions are the most common morphological type. Inclusions are present throughout the neuraxis: inclusions in the subiculum (A) and thalamus (B). α-Internexin immunohistochemistry. Neuronal inclusions in NIFID are variably ubiquitinated: inclusions (*arrowheads*) in the frontal lobe (C) and granule cells of the dentate gyrus (D). A neuronal cytoplasmic (*arrowhead*) and intranuclear inclusion (*arrow*) are present in the same neuron (E). Intranuclear inclusions appear as round or elongated structures, either as a single inclusion or as multiple forms (C–E). Ubiquitin immunohistochemistry.

stained sections, hyaline aggregates of neuronal IFs are observed. The inclusions are variably argyrophilic, with modified Bielschowsky and Bodian silver impregnations, and superficially resemble the Pick bodies of PiD. Immuno-histochemistry demonstrates the presence within the inclusions of all class IV IF proteins (NF-H, NF-M, NF-L, and α-internexin). The morphology of the inclusions is extremely variable throughout the neuraxis. Axonal swellings, similar to those found in MND and normal aging, but which are not specific to any neurodegenerative disease, are also seen in affected areas and in underlying white matter, corticospinal tracts, and other white matter tracts. In cases with pyramidal signs, there may be evidence of corticospinal tract degeneration in the spinal cord. However, motor neurons in the anterior horns are relatively spared, and the number of pyknotic neurons is much lower than that typically seen in classical MND.

The cytoplasmic inclusions of NIFID are variably ubiquitinated, as demonstrated by immunohistochemistry. Ubiquitinated and neuronal IF-positive inclusions are most numerous in the youngest cases (Cairns et al., 2004). Ubiquitinated inclusions are found in cortex and subcortical nuclei, and in the neurons of the dentate gyrus in all cases, and resemble those seen in FTLD-MND-type. Rare single (Figure 25.17E) and multiple round and elongated intranuclear inclusions may also be observed in neurons containing cytoplasmic inclusions. The intranuclear inclusions in NIFID are not labeled by antineuronal IF antibodies.

Ultrastructural study of the neuronal cytoplasmic inclusions in NIFID, like those of other inclusions in FTLDs, reveal aggregates of granular filamentous material with no apparent limiting membrane. The granular material resembles the morphology of ribosomes, and the filaments have an apparent diameter of 10–25 nm. Immunoelectron microscopy demonstrates that the filaments of the cytoplasmic inclusions contain epitopes of neuronal IF proteins (Cairns et al., 2004).

## Basophilic Inclusion Body Disease

### Genetics

Rare cases of BIBD may present as juvenile (Matsumoto et al., 1992; Nelson & Prensky, 1972) or adult-onset MND (Kusaka, Matsumoto, & Imai, 1990, 1993), FTD (Munoz-Garcia &

Ludwin, 1984), or a combination of both (Hamada et al., 1995). Typically, patients are younger when symptoms develop (29–30 years [Munoz-Garcia & Ludwin, 1984] and 52–58 years [Ito, Kusaka, Matsumoto, & Imai, 1995]) than those with PiD. Features of MND and FTD are comparable to the heterogeneous phenotype of NIFID. The early age at onset of this widespread but rare disease hints at a genetic cause, but none has been identified.

### Neuropathology

Cases typically show pronounced atrophy of the frontal and temporal lobes, with less involvement of the parietal lobe. Coronal slices reveal marked atrophy of the striatum, often with a thinned caudate nucleus, thalamus, and amygdala. The substantia nigra is also depigmented. Microscopy shows the stereotypical features of FTLDs: severe neuronal loss, superficial microvacuolation, and reactive astrocytosis. The histological hallmark of this disease is the presence of basophilic inclusion bodies (Munoz-Garcia & Ludwin, 1984) that contain neither tau nor α-synuclein nor neuronal IF proteins (Figure 25.18). Basophilic inclusion bodies are found in affected neocortex, preferentially affecting the superficial laminae similar to the distribution in PD (Armstrong, Cairns, & Lantos, 1999). Unlike Pick bodies in PiD, basophilic inclusion bodies are not usually found in the hippocampus and dentate gyrus. However, inclusions are found in subcortical nuclei including the putamen, caudate nucleus, globus pallidus, nucleus basalis of Meynert, red nucleus, subthalamic nucleus, periaqueductal gray, and in the anterior horns of the spinal cord. Unlike in MND, no Bunina bodies and

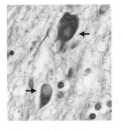

FIGURE 25.18. Neuronal cytoplasmic inclusions in the pons of BIBD. The inclusions (*arrows*) are outlined, but not labeled, by antineuronal IF protein antibodies. α-Internexin immunohistochemistry.

no ubiquitin-positive, skein-like inclusions are seen in cases of BIBD. The inclusions are variably basophilic, and occasionally eosinophilic, in hematoxylin- and eosin-stained sections. The inclusions are variably ubiquitinated and contain variable amounts of RNA, as shown by acridine orange staining. Misfolded proteins seen in tauopathies and synucleinopathies and neuronal IF proteins are absent from these inclusions. Electron microscopy shows that the inclusions are not membrane bound and contain fibrils with a diameter between 13 and 25 nm and variably granular in appearance (Munoz-Garcia & Ludwin, 1984). Swollen axons and axonal spheroids are also present, but these are not specific to BIBD, because they are commonly seen in other neurodegenerative diseases and normal aging.

## Inclusion Body Myopathy with Paget's Disease of Bone and FTD

### Genetics

Hereditary inclusion body myopathy (IBM) associated with Paget's disease of bone (PDB) and early-onset FTD is a rare, lethal, autosomal dominant progressive disease linked to chromosome 9p13.3-p12 (Kovach et al., 2001). The disease features adult-onset proximal and distal muscle weakness, early-onset PDB and, in most cases, FTD. The phenotypic variation in this disease is remarkable in that death may precede overt clinical symptoms in one or more of the affected tissues. Thus, in 13 families in which mutations in *valosin-containing protein* (*VCP*) gene were reported, 82% had myopathy, 49% had PDB, and 30% had early-onset FTD (Watts et al., 2004). The mean age at presentation was 42 years for both IBM and PDB, whereas FTD typically developed somewhat later at age 53, possibly indicating greater functional reserve in brain tissue. In IBMPFD myopathic muscle and PDB osteoclasts, similar inclusions are seen, indicating common pathogenetic mechanisms. Six missense mutations in *VCP* have been reported, resulting in the amino acid substitutions R95G, R191Q, R155H, R155C, R155P, and A232E (Watts et al., 2004). Human VCP (also called p97, ter94, or CDC48) is a 644–amino acid protein encoded by a gene with 17 exons that maps to chromosome 9p13-p12. It is a member of the AAA-ATPase (ATPases [adenosine triphosphatase] Associated with various cellular Activities)

superfamily involved in vesicle transport and fusion, 26S proteasome function, and assembly of peroxisomes. VCP is a structural protein associated with the assembly of clathrin and the heat-shock protein HSP70. VCP has been implicated in a number of cellular events regulated during mitosis, including homotypic membrane fusion, spindle pole body function, and ubiquitin-dependent protein degradation. Ten of the 13 families with IBMPFD had an amino acid substitution at codon 155 in VCP, and all were present within the N-terminal CDC48 domain, which is involved in ubiquitin binding (Dai & Li, 2001), indicating that mutations in this region may compromise the normal ubiquitin protein degradation pathway.

### Neuropathology

To date, few brains of patients with IBMPFD have been examined. Of those patients with FTD, the characteristic features of FTLD have been observed: atrophy of the frontal lobe, neuronal loss, status spongiosus, and reactive astrocytosis. The atrophy is less pronounced than in other FTLDs. The disease is characterized microscopically by ubiquitin-positive neuronal intranuclear inclusions and dystrophic neurites and sparse cytoplasmic inclusions; a variable proportion of the inclusions are visualized by anti-VCP antibodies (Figure 25.19). Large focal inclusions and smaller foci containing VCP are present in muscle fibers of patients with IBMPFD. This pattern of staining is not specific to IBMPFD, because VCP aggregates are also seen in muscle fibers in sporadic IBM. In brain of affected patients, ubiquitin-positive, VCP-positive neuronal inclusions are seen, and this immunoractive profile of the in-

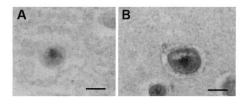

FIGURE 25.19. Neuronal intranuclear inclusions in the frontal lobe of a case of IBMPFD. An inclusion in layer III of the parietal cortex (A) and layer III of the parahippocampal gyrus (B). (A and B) Valosin-containing protein and ubiquitin immunohistochemistry, respectively. Scale bars = 10 μm.

clusion bodies is not unique to IBMPFD, because VCP has also been shown to be a component of a subset of inclusions in other neurodegenerative diseases, including expanded polyglutamine protein aggregates, dystrophic neurites of AD, α-synuclein aggregates in dementia with Lewy bodies (DLB), Parkinson's disease and MSA, and ubiquitinated inclusions in MND (Ishigaki et al., 2004; Mizuno, Hori, Kakizuka, & Okamoto, 2003). Thus, the presence of VCP in the inclusions of IMBPFD implicates this protein in the pathogenesis of several protein-folding diseases.

## CONCLUSIONS

The accumulation of misfolded proteins in inclusion bodies is a common feature of a wide variety of sporadic and familial neurodegenerative disorders that present clinically with FTD. These diseases are distinguished by the distinct topographic and cell type–specific distribution of inclusions. The biochemical and ultrastructural characteristics of the inclusions also reveal a significant phenotypic overlap. The discovery of multiple mutations in the *tau* gene, leading to abnormal filamentous inclusions, demonstrates that tau dysfunction is sufficient to produce neurodegenerative disease. Experimental evidence indicates that mutations lead to specific alterations in expression, function, and biochemistry of tau proteins. Similarly, mutations in *VCP* result in protein aggregation, inclusion formation, and neurodegeneration in a subset of cases with IBMPFD. The identification of additional gene mutations in the FTLDs or polymorphisms at distinct genetic loci that either cause or are risk factors for disease will provide additional insights into disease pathogenesis, as well the development of novel strategies for treatment and prevention.

## ACKNOWLEDGMENTS

Support for this work was provided by grants from the National Institute on Aging of the National Institutes of Health (Nos. AG-03991 and AG-05681 to NJC; Nos. AG-09215, AG-10124, and AG-17586 to VM-YL and JQT), and from the Wellcome Trust, United Kingdom (No. GR066166AIA to NJC). We would also like to thank the members of the Alzheimer's Disease Research Center, Washington University, St. Louis, and the Center for Neurodegenerative Disease Research, University of Pennsylvania, who contributed to the work, and the many patients studied and their families, for making the research reviewed here possible.

## REFERENCES

Alzheimer, A. (1911). Über eigenartige Krankheitsfälle des späteren Alters [On certain peculiar disease of old age]. *Zeitschrift für die Gesamte Neurologie und Psychiatrie, 4,* 356–385.

Anderson, V. E., Cairns, N. J., & Leigh, P. N. (1995). Involvement of the amygdala, dentate and hippocampus in motor neuron disease. *Journal of the Neurological Sciences, 129*(Suppl.), 75–78.

Armstrong, R. A., Cairns, N. J., & Lantos, P. L. (1998). Clustering of Pick bodies in patients with Pick's disease. *Neuroscience Letters, 242,* 81–84.

Armstrong, R. A., Cairns, N. J., & Lantos, P. L. (1999). Laminar distribution of Pick bodies, pick cells and Alzheimer disease pathology in the frontal and temporal cortex in Pick's disease. *Neuropathology and Applied Neurobiology, 25,* 266–271.

Baker, M., Litvan, I., Houlden, H., Adamson, J. Dickson, D., Perez-Tur, J., et al. (1999). Association of an extended haplotype in the *tau* gene with progressive supranuclear palsy. *Human Molecular Genetics, 8,* 711–715.

Baker, M., MacKenzie, I. R., Pickering-Brown, S. M., Gass, J., Rademakers, R., Lindholm, C., et al. (in press). Mutations in progranulin cause tau-negative frontotemporal dementia linked to chromosome 17. *Nature.*

Bell, K., Cairns, N. J., Lantos, P. L., & Rossor, M. N. (2000). Immunohistochemistry distinguishes between Pick's disease and corticobasal degeneration. *Journal of Neurology, Neurosurgery, and Psychiatry, 69,* 835–836.

Bergeron, C., Davis, A., & Lang, A. E. (1998). Corticobasal ganglionic degeneration and progressive supranuclear palsy presenting with cognitive decline. *Brain Pathology, 8,* 355–365.

Bigio, E. H., Johnson, N. A., Rademaker, A. W., Fung, B. B., Mesulam, M. M., Siddique, N., et al. (2004). Neuronal ubiquitinated intranuclear inclusions in familial and non-familial frontotemporal dementia of the motor neuron disease type associated with amyotrophic lateral sclerosis. *Journal of Neuropathology and Experimental Neurology, 63,* 801–811.

Bigio, E. H., Lipton, A. M., White, C. L., III, Dickson, D. W., & Hirano, A. (2003). Frontotemporal and motor neurone degeneration with neurofilament inclusion bodies: Additional evidence for overlap between FTD and ALS. *Neuropathology and Applied Neurobiology, 29,* 239–253.

Boller, F., Lopez, O. L., & Moossy, J. (1989). Diagnosis of dementia: Clinicopathologic correlations. *Neurology, 39,* 76–79.

Bonner, L. T., Tsuang, D. W., Cherrier, M. M., Eugenio,

C. J., Du Jennifer, Q., Steinbart, E. J., et al. (2003). Familial dementia with Lewy bodies with an atypical clinical presentation. *Journal of Geriatric Psychiatry and Neurology, 16*, 59–64.

Bramblett, G. T., Goedert, M., Jakes, R., Merrick, S. E., Trojanowski, J. Q., & Lee, V.-M. (1993). Abnormal tau phosphorylation at Ser396 in Alzheimer's disease recapitulates development and contributes to reduced microtubule binding. *Neuron, 10*, 1089–1099.

Brown, J., Ashworth, A., Gydesen, S., Sorensen, A., Rossor, M., Hardy, J., et al. (1995). Familial nonspecific dementia maps to chromosome 3. *Human Molecular Genetics, 4*, 1625–1628.

Brun, A. (1987). Frontal lobe degeneration of non-Alzheimer type: I. Neuropathology. *Archives of Gerontology and Geriatrics, 6*, 193–208.

Brun, A., Englund, B., Gustafson, L., Passant, U., Mann, D. M. A., Neary, D., et al. (1994). Clinical and neuropathological criteria for frontotemporal dementia. *Journal of Neurology, Neurosurgery, and Psychiatry, 57*, 416–418.

Brun, A., & Passant, U. (1996). Frontal lobe degeneration of non-Alzheimer type: Structural characteristics, diagnostic criteria and relation to other frontotemporal dementias. *Acta Neurologica Scandinavica Supplement, 168*, 28–30.

Bugiani, O., Murrell, J. R., Giaccone, G., Hasegawa, M., Ghigo, G., Tabaton, M., et al. (1999). Frontotemporal dementia and corticobasal degeneration in a family with a P301S mutation in tau. *Journal of Neuropathology and Experimental Neurology, 58*, 667–677.

Cairns, N. J., Brännström, T., Khan, M. N., Rossor, M. N., & Lantos, P. L. (2003). Neuronal loss in familial frontotemporal dementia with ubiquitin-positive, tau-negative inclusions. *Experimental Neurology, 181*, 319–326.

Cairns, N. J., Grossman, M., Arnold, S. E., Burn, D. J., Jaros, E., Perry, R. H., et al. (2004). Clinical and neuropathologic variation in neuronal intermediate filament inclusion disease. *Neurology, 63*, 1376–1384.

Caselli, R. J., Windebank, A. J., Petersen, R. C., Komori, T., Parisi, J. E., Okazaki, H., et al. (1993). Rapidly progressive aphasic dementia and motor neuron disease. *Annals of Neurology, 33*, 200–207.

Chow, T. W., Miller, B. L., Hayashi, V. N., & Geschwind, D. H. (1999). Inheritance of frontotemporal dementia. *Archives of Neurology, 56*, 817–822.

Clark, L. N., Poorkaj, P., Wszolek, Z., Geschwind, D. H., Nasreddine, Z. S., Miller, B., et al. (1998). Pathogenic implications of mutations in the tau gene in pallido-ponto-nigral degeneration and related neurodegenerative disorders linked to chromosome 17. *Proceedings of the National Academy of Sciences of the United States of America, 95*, 13103–13107.

Constantinidis, J., Richard, J., & Tissot, R. (1974). Pick's disease: Histological and clinical correlations. *European Neurology, 11*, 208–217.

Cooper, P. N., Jackson, M., Lennox, G., Lowe, J., & Mann, D. M. (1995). Tau, ubiquitin, and alpha B-crystallin immunohistochemistry define the principal causes of degenerative frontotemporal dementia. *Archives of Neurology, 52*, 1011–1015.

Dai, R. M., & Li, C. C. (2001). Valosin-containing protein is a multi-ubiquitin chain-targeting factor required in ubiquitin–proteasome degradation. *Nature Cell Biology, 3*, 740–744.

Delacourte, A. (1999). Biochemical and molecular characterization of neurofibrillary degeneration in frontotemporal dementias. *Dementia and Geriatric Cognitive Disorders, 10*(Suppl. 1), 75–79.

Delacourte, A., Robitaille, Y., Sergeant, N., Buee, L., Hof, P. R., Wattez, A., et al. (1996). Specific pathological *tau* protein variants characterize Pick's disease. *Journal of Neuropathology and Experimental Neurology, 55*, 159–168.

Dermaut, B., Kumar-Singh, S., Engelborghs, S., Theuns, J., Rademakers, R., Saerens, J., et al. (2004). A novel presenilin 1 mutation associated with Pick's disease but not beta-amyloid plaques. *Annals of Neurology, 55*, 617–626.

D'Souza, I., Poorkaj, P., Hong, M., Nochlin, D., Lee, V.-M., Bird, T. D., et al. (1999). Missense and silent *tau* gene mutations cause frontotemporal dementia with parkinsonism-chromosome 17 type, by affecting multiple alternative RNA splicing regulatory elements. *Proceedings of the National Academy of Sciences of the United States of America, 96*, 5598–5603.

D'Souza, I., & Schellenberg, G.D. (2000). Determinants of 4-repeat tau expression: Coordination between enhancing and inhibitory splicing sequences for exon 10 inclusion. *Journal of Biological Chemistry, 275*, 17700–17709.

Froelich, F. S., Axelman, P., Almkvist, A., Basun, H., & Lannfelt, L. (2003). Extended investigation of *tau* and mutation screening of other candidate genes on chromosome 17q21 in a Swedish FTDP-17 family. *American Journal of Medical Genetics, 121B*, 112–118.

Gamblin, T. C., King, M. E., Dawson, H., Vitek, M. P., Kuret, J., Berry, R. W., et al. (2000). In vitro polymerization of tau protein monitored by laser light scattering: Method and application to the study of FTDP-17 mutants. *Biochemistry, 39*, 6136–6144.

Gibb, W. R., Luthert, P. J., & Marsden, C. D. (1989). Corticobasal degeneration. *Brain, 112*, 1171–1192.

Goedert, M., Jakes, R., & Crowther, R. A. (1999). Effects of frontotemporal dementia FTDP-17 mutations on heparin-induced assembly of tau filaments. *FEBS Letters, 450*, 306–311.

Goedert, M., Satumtira, S., Jakes, R., Smith, M. J., Kamibayashi, C., White, C. L., III, et al. (2000). Reduced binding of protein phosphatase 2A to *tau* protein with frontotemporal dementia and parkinsonism linked to chromosome 17 mutations. *Journal of Neurochemistry, 75*, 2155–2162.

Goedert, M., Spillantini, M. G., Crowther, R. A., Chen,

S. G., Parchi, P., Tabaton, M., et al. (1999). Tau gene mutation in familial progressive subcortical gliosis. *Nature Medicine, 5,* 454–457.

Golbe, L. I., Davis, P. H., Schoenberg, B. S., & Duvoisin, R. C. (1988). Prevalence and natural history of progressive supranuclear palsy. *Neurology, 38,* 1031–1034.

Goode, B. L., Denis, P. E., Panda, D., Radeke, M. J., Miller, H. P., Wilson, L., et al. (1997). Functional interactions between the proline-rich and repeat regions of tau enhance microtubule binding and assembly. *Molecular Biology of the Cell, 8,* 353–365.

Goode, B. L., & Feinstein, S. C. (1994). Identification of a novel microtubule binding and assembly domain in the developmentally regulated inter-repeat region of tau. *Journal of Cell Biology, 124,* 769–782.

Götz, J. (2001). Tau and transgenic animal models. *Brain Research: Brain Research Reviews, 35,* 266–286.

Götz, J., Chen, F., Barmettler, R., & Nitsch, R. M. (2001). Tau filament formation in transgenic mice expressing P301L tau. *Journal of Biological Chemistry, 276,* 529–534.

Grover, A., England, E., Baker, M., Sahara, N., Adamson, J., Granger, B., et al. (2003). A novel tau mutation in exon 9 (I260V) causes a four-repeat tauopathy. *Experimental Neurology, 184,* 131–140.

Grover, A., Houlden, H., Baker, M., Adamson, J., Lewis, J., Prihar, G., et al. (1999). 5' Splice site mutations in tau associated with the inherited dementia FTDP-17 affect a stem-loop structure that regulates alternative splicing of exon 10. *Journal of Biological Chemistry, 274,* 15134–15143.

Hamada, K., Fukazawa, T., Yanagihara, T., Yoshida, K., Hamada, T., Yoshimura, N., et al. (1995). Dementia with ALS features and diffuse Pick body–like inclusions (atypical Pick's disease?). *Clinical Neuropathology, 14,* 1–6.

Hasegawa, M., Smith, M. J., & Goedert, M. (1998). Tau proteins with FTDP-17 mutations have a reduced ability to promote microtubule assembly. *FEBS Letters, 437,* 207–210.

Hasegawa, M., Smith, M. J., Iijima, M., Tabira, T., & Goedert, M. (1999). FTDP-17 mutations N279K and S305N in tau produce increased splicing of exon 10. *FEBS Letters, 443,* 93–96.

Hauw, J.-J., Daniel, S. E., Dickson, D., Horoupian, D. S., Jellinger, K., Lantos, P. L., et al. (1994). Preliminary NINDS neuropathologic criteria for Steele–Richardson–Olszewski syndrome (progressive supranuclear palsy). *Neurology, 44,* 2015–2019.

Hayashi, S., Toyoshima, Y., Hasegawa, M., Umeda, Y., Wakabayashi, K., Tokiguchi, S., et al. (2002). Late-onset frontotemporal dementia with a novel exon 1 (Arg5His) tau gene mutation. *Annals of Neurology, 51,* 525–530.

Hong, M., Zhukareva, V., Vogelsberg-Ragaglia, V., Wszolek, Z., Reed, L., Miller, B. I., et al. (1998). Mutation-specific functional impairments in distinct tau isoforms of hereditary FTDP-17. *Science, 282,* 1914–1917.

Hosler, B. A., Siddique, T., Sapp, P. C., Sailor, W., Huang, M. C., Hossain, A., et al. (2000). Linkage of familial amyotrophic lateral sclerosis with frontotemporal dementia to chromosome 9q21-q22. *Journal of the American Medical Association, 284,* 1664–1669.

Houlden, H., Baker, M., Morris, H. R., MacDonald, N., Pickering-Brown, S., Adamson, J., et al. (2001). Corticobasal degeneration and progressive supranuclear palsy share a common tau haplotype. *Neurology, 56,* 1702–1706.

Hutton, M., Lendon, C. L., Rizzu, P., Baker, M., Froelich, S., Houlden, H., et al. (1998). Association of missense and 5'-splice-site mutations in tau with the inherited dementia FTDP-17. *Nature, 393,* 702–705.

Iijima, M., Tabira, T., Poorkaj, P., Schellenberg, G. D., Trojanowski, J. Q., Lee, V. M., et al. (1999). A distinct familial presenile dementia with a novel missense mutation in the tau gene. *NeuroReport, 10,* 497–501.

Iseki, E., Matsumura, T., Marui, W., Hino, H., Odawara, T., Sugiyama, N., et al. (2001). Familial frontotemporal dementia and parkinsonism with a novel N296H mutation in exon 10 of the tau gene and a widespread tau accumulation in the glial cells. *Acta Neuropathologica, 102,* 285–292.

Ishigaki, S., Hishikawa, N., Niwa, J. I., Iemura, S. I., Natsume, T., Hori, S., et al. (2004). Physical and functional interaction between dorfin and valosin-containing protein that are colocalized in ubiquitylated inclusions in neurodegenerative disorders. *Journal of Biological Chemistry, 279,* 51376–51385.

Ishihara, T., Hong, M., Zhang, B., Nakagawa, Y., Lee, M. K., Trojanowski, J. Q., et al. (1999). Age-dependent emergence and progression of a tauopathy in transgenic mice overexpressing the shortest human tau isoform. *Neuron, 24,* 751–762.

Ito, H., Kusaka, H., Matsumoto, S., & Imai, T. (1995). Topographic involvement of the striatal efferents in basal ganglia of patients with adult-onset motor neuron disease with basophilic inclusions. *Acta Neuropathologica, 89,* 513–518.

Jackson, G. R., Wiedau-Pazos, M., Sang, T. K., Wagle, N., Brown, C. A., Massachi, S., et al. (2002). Human wild-type tau interacts with wingless pathway components and produces neurofibrillary pathology in *Drosophila. Neuron, 34,* 509–519.

Jackson, M., Lennox, G., & Lowe. J. (1996). Motor neurone disease–inclusion dementia. *Neurodegeneration, 5,* 339–350.

Josephs, K. A., Holton, J. L., Rossor, M. N., Braendgaard, H., Ozawa, T., Fox, N. C., et al. (2003). Neurofilament inclusion body disease: A new proteinopathy? *Brain, 126,* 2291–2303.

Josephs, K. A., Tsuboi, Y., Cookson, N., Watt, H., & Dickson, D. W. (2004). Apolipoprotein E epsilon 4 is a determinant for Alzheimer-type pathologic features in tauopathies, synucleinopathies, and frontotemporal degeneration. *Archives of Neurology, 61,* 1579–1584.

Kertesz, A., Kawarai, T., Rogaeva, E., George-Hyslop, P., Poorkaj, P., Bird, T. D., et al. (2000). Familial frontotemporal dementia with ubiquitin-positive, tau-negative inclusions. *Neurology, 54,* 818–827.

Knopman, D. S., Mastri, A. R., Frey, W. H., Sung, J. H., & Rustan, T. (1990). Dementia lacking distinctive histologic features: A common non-Alzheimer degenerative dementia. *Neurology, 40,* 251–256.

Kobayashi, T., Ota, S., Tanaka, K., Ito, Y., Hasegawa, M., Umeda, Y., et al. (2003). A novel L266V mutation of the tau gene causes frontotemporal dementia with a unique tau pathology. *Annals of Neurology, 53,* 133–137.

Kovach, M. J., Waggoner, B., Leal, S. M., Gelber, D., Khardori, R., Levenstien, M. A., et al. (2001). Clinical delineation and localization to chromosome 9p13.3-p12 of a unique dominant disorder in four families: Hereditary inclusion body myopathy, Paget disease of bone, and frontotemporal dementia. *Molecular Genetics and Metabolism, 74,* 458–475.

Kraemer, B. C., Zhang, B., Leverenz, J. B., Thomas, J. H., Trojanowski, J. Q., & Schellenberg, G. D. (2003). Neurodegeneration and defective neurotransmission in a *Caenorhabditis elegans* model of tauopathy. *Proceedings of the National Academy of Sciences of the United States of America, 100,* 9980–9985.

Kusaka, H., Matsumoto, S., & Imai, T. (1990). An adult-onset case of sporadic motor neuron disease with basophilic inclusions. *Acta Neuropathologica, 80,* 660–665.

Kusaka, H., Matsumoto, S., & Imai, T. (1993). Adult-onset motor neuron disease with basophilic intraneuronal inclusion bodies. *Clinical Neuropathology, 12,* 215–218.

Lantos, P. L., Cairns, N. J., Khan, M. N., King, A., Revesz, T., Janssen, J. C., et al. (2002). Neuropathologic variation in frontotemporal dementia due to the intronic *tau* 10$^{+16}$ mutation. *Neurology, 58,* 1169–1175.

Lippa, C. F., Zhukareva, V., Kawarai, T., Uryu, K., Shafiq, M., Nee, L. E., et al. (2000). Frontotemporal dementia with novel tau pathology and a Glu342Val tau mutation. *Annals of Neurology, 48,* 850–858.

Lowe, J., Errington, D. R., Lennox, G., Pike, I., Spendlove, I., Landon, M., et al. (1992). Ballooned neurons in several neurodegenerative diseases and stroke contain alpha B crystallin. *Neuropathology and Applied Neurobiology, 18,* 341–350.

Mackenzie, I. R., & Feldman H. (2003). Neuronal intranuclear inclusions distinguish familial FTD-MND type from sporadic cases. *Acta Neuropathologica, 105,* 543–548.

Mann, D. M. (1998). Dementia of frontal type and dementias with subcortical gliosis. *Brain Pathology, 8,* 325–338.

Matsumoto, S., Kusaka, H., Murakami, N., Hashizume, Y., Okazaki, H., & Hirano, A. (1992). Basophilic inclusions in sporadic juvenile amyotrophic lateral sclerosis: An immunocytochemical and ultrastructural study. *Acta Neuropathologica, 83,* 579–583.

McKhann, G. M., Albert, M. S., Grossman, M., Miller, B., Dickson, D., & Trojanowski, J. Q. (2001). Clinical and pathological diagnosis of frontotemporal dementia: Report of the Work Group on Frontotemporal Dementia and Pick's Disease. *Archives of Neurology, 58,* 1803–1809.

Mitsuyama, Y., & Takamiya, S. (1979). Presenile dementia with motor neuron disease in Japan: A new entity? *Archives of Neurology, 36,* 592–593.

Miyamoto, K., Kowalska, A., Hasegawa, M., Tabira, T., Takahashi, K., Araki, W., et al. (2001). Familial frontotemporal dementia and parkinsonism with a novel mutation at an intron 10+11-splice site in the tau gene. *Annals of Neurology, 50,* 117–120.

Miyasaka, T., Morishima-Kawashima, M., Ravid, R., Kamphorst, W., Nagashima, K., & Ihara, Y. (2001). Selective deposition of mutant *tau* in the FTDP-17 brain affected by the *P301L* mutation. *Journal of Neuropathology and Experimental Neurology, 60,* 872–884.

Mizuno, Y., Hori, S., Kakizuka, A., & Okamoto, K. (2003). Vacuole-creating protein in neurodegenerative diseases in humans. *Neuroscience Letters, 343,* 77–80.

Montpetit, V., Clapin, D. F., & Guberman, A. (1985). Substructure of 20 nm filaments of progressive supranuclear palsy. *Acta Neuropathologica, 68,* 311–318.

Morris, H. R., Baker, M., Yasojima, K., Houlden, H., Khan, M. N., Wood, N. W., et al. (2002). Analysis of tau haplotypes in Pick's disease. *Neurology, 59,* 443–445.

Morris, H. R., Katzenschlager, R., Janssen, J. C., Brown, J. M., Ozansoy, M., Quinn, N., et al. (2002). Sequence analysis of tau in familial and sporadic progressive supranuclear palsy. *Journal of Neurology, Neurosurgery, and Psychiatry, 72,* 388–390.

Munoz-Garcia, D., & Ludwin, S. K. (1984). Classic and generalized variants of Pick's disease: A clinicopathological, ultrastructural, and immunocytochemical comparative study. *Annals of Neurology, 16,* 467–480.

Murrell, J. R., Spillantini, M. G., Zolo, P., Guazzelli, M., Smith, M. J., Hasegawa, M., et al. (1999). Tau gene mutation G389R causes a tauopathy with abundant pick body-like inclusions and axonal deposits. *Journal of Neuropathology and Experimental Neurology, 58,* 1207–1226.

Neary, D., Snowden, J. S., Gustafson, L., Passant, U., Stuss, D., Black, S., et al. (1998). Frontotemporal lobar degeneration: A consensus on clinical diagnostic criteria. *Neurology, 51,* 1546–1554.

Neary, D., Snowden, J. S., Mann, D. M., Northen, B., Goulding, P. J., & Macdermott, N. (1990). Frontal lobe dementia and motor neuron disease. *Journal of Neurology, Neurosurgery, and Psychiatry, 53,* 23–32.

Nelson, J. S., & Prensky, A. L. (1972). Sporadic juvenile amyotrophic lateral sclerosis: A clinicopathological study of a case with neuronal cytoplasmic inclusions containing RNA. *Archives of Neurology, 27,* 300–306.

Neumann, M., Schulz-Schaeffer, W., Crowther, R. A., Smith, M. J., Spillantini, M. G., Goedert, M., et al. (2001). Pick's disease associated with the novel Tau gene mutation K369I. *Annals of Neurology, 50,* 503–513.

Nicholl, D. J., Greenstone, M. A., Clarke, C. E., Rizzu, P., Crooks, D., Crowe, A., et al. (2003). An English kindred with a novel recessive tauopathy and respiratory failure. *Annals of Neurology, 54,* 682–686.

Pastor, P., Pastor, E., Carnero, C., Vela, R., Garcia, T., Amer, G., et al. (2001). Familial atypical progressive supranuclear palsy associated with homozygosity for the delN296 mutation in the tau gene. *Annals of Neurology, 49,* 263–267.

Pick, A. (1892). Über die Beziehungen der senilen Hirnatrophie zur Aphasie [Pertaining to senile brain-atrophy and aphasia]. *Prager Medizinische Wochenschrisft, 17,* 165–167.

Pickering-Brown, S. M., Baker, M., Nonaka, T., Ikeda, K., Sharma, S., Mackenzie, J., et al. (2004). Frontotemporal dementia with Pick-type histology associated with Q336R mutation in the tau gene. *Brain, 127,* 1415–1426.

Pickering-Brown, S., Baker, M., Yen, S. H., Liu, W. K., Hasegawa, M., Cairns, N., et al. (2000). Pick's disease is associated with mutations in the tau gene. *Annals of Neurology, 48,* 859–867.

Pollanen, M. S., Bergeron, C., & Weyer, L. (1993). Absence of protease-resistant prion protein in dementia characterized by neuronal loss and status spongiosus. *Acta Neuropathologica, 86,* 515–517.

Poorkaj, P., Bird, T. D., Wijsman, E., Nemens, E., Garruto, R. M., Anderson, L., et al. (1998). Tau is a candidate gene for chromosome 17 frontotemporal dementia. *Annals of Neurology, 43,* 815–825.

Poorkaj, P., Muma, N. A., Zhukareva, V., Cochran, E. J., Shannon, K. M., Hurtig, H., et al. (2002). An R5L tau mutation in a subject with a progressive supranuclear palsy phenotype. *Annals of Neurology, 52,* 511–516.

Rademakers, R., Cruts, M., Dermaut, B., Sleegers, K., Rosso, S. M., van den Broeck, M., et al. (2002). Tau negative frontal lobe dementia at 17q21: Significant finemapping of the candidate region to a 4.8 cM interval. *Molecular Psychiatry, 7,* 1064–1074.

Rebeiz, J. J., Kolodny, E. H., & Richardson, E. P., Jr. (1967). Corticodentatonigral degeneration with neuronal achromasia: A progressive disorder of late adult life. *Transactions of the American Neurological Association, 92,* 23–26.

Rebeiz, J. J., Kolodny, E. H., & Richardson, E. P., Jr.

(1968). Corticodentatonigral degeneration with neuronal achromasia. *Archives of Neurology, 18,* 20–33.

Rizzini, C., Goedert, M.. Hodges, J. R., Smith, M. J., Jakes, R., Hills, R., et al. (2000). Tau gene mutation K257T causes a tauopathy similar to Pick's disease. *Journal of Neuropathology and Experimental Neurology, 59,* 990–1001.

Rizzu, P., Joosse, M., Ravid, R., Hoogeveen, A., Kamphorst, W., van Swieten, J. C., et al. (2000). Mutation-dependent aggregation of tau protein and its selective depletion from the soluble fraction in brain of P301L FTDP-17 patients. *Human Molecular Genetics, 9,* 3075–3082.

Rizzu, P., van Swieten, J. C., Joosse, M., Hasegawa, M., Stevens, M., Tibben, A., et al. (1999). High prevalence of mutations in the microtubule-associated protein tau in a population study of frontotemporal dementia in the Netherlands. *American Journal of Human Genetics, 64,* 414–421.

Rosso, S. M., Kamphorst, W., de Graaf, B., Willemsen, R., Ravid, R., Niermeijer, M. F., et al. (2001). Familial frontotemporal dementia with ubiquitin-positive inclusions is linked to chromosome 17q21-22. *Brain, 124,* 1948–1957.

Rosso, S. M., van Herpen, E., Deelen, W., Kamphorst, W., Severijnen, L. A., Willemsen, R., et al. (2002). A novel tau mutation, S320F, causes a tauopathy with inclusions similar to those in Pick's disease. *Annals of Neurology, 51,* 373–376.

Rossor, M. N., Revesz, T., Lantos, P. L., & Warrington, E. K. (2000). Semantic dementia with ubiquitin-positive tau-negative inclusion bodies. *Brain, 123,* 267–276.

Savioz, A., Kovari, E., Anastasiu, R., Rossier, C., Saini, K., Bouras, C., et al. (2000). Search for a mutation in the *tau* gene in a Swiss family with frontotemporal dementia. *Experimental Neurology, 161,* 330–335.

Savioz, A., Riederer, B. M., Heutink, P., Rizzu, P., Tolnay, M., Kovari, E., et al. (2003). Tau and neurofilaments in a family with frontotemporal dementia unlinked to chromosome 17q21-22. *Neurobiology of Disease, 12,* 46–55.

Skibinski, G., Parkinson, N. J., Brown, J. M., Chakrabarti, L., Lloyd, S. L., Hummerich, H., et al. (2005). Mutations in the endosomal ESCRTIII complex subunit CHMP2B in frontotemporal dementia. *Nature Genetics, 37,* 806–808.

Sperfeld, A. D., Collatz, M. B., Baier, H., Palmbach, M., Storch, A., Schwarz, J., et al. (1999). FTDP-17: An early-onset phenotype with parkinsonism and epileptic seizures caused by a novel mutation. *Annals of Neurology, 46,* 708–715.

Spillantini, M. G., Bird, T. D., & Ghetti, B. (1998). Frontotemporal dementia and parkinsonism linked to chromosome 17: A new group of tauopathies. *Brain Pathology, 8,* 387–402.

Spillantini, M. G., Crowther, R. A., Jakes, R., Cairns, N. J., Lantos, P. L., & Goedert, M. (1998). Filamentous alpha-synuclein inclusions link multiple system atrophy with Parkinson's disease and dementia with Lewy bodies. *Neuroscience Letters, 251*, 205–208.

Spillantini, M. G., Murrell, J. R., Goedert, M., Farlow, M. R., Klug, A., & Ghetti, B. (1998). Mutation in the *tau* gene in familial multiple system tauopathy with presenile dementia. *Proceedings of the National Academy of Sciences of the United States of America, 95*, 7737–7741.

Spillantini, M. G., Yoshida, H., Rizzini, C., Lantos, P. L., Khan, N., Rossor, M. N., et al. (2000). A novel tau mutation (N296N) in familial dementia with swollen achromatic neurons and corticobasal inclusion bodies. *Annals of Neurology, 48*, 939–943.

Stanford, P. M., Halliday, G. M., Brooks, W. S., Kwok, J. B., Storey, C. E., Creasey, H., et al. (2000). Progressive supranuclear palsy pathology caused by a novel silent mutation in exon 10 of the tau gene: Expansion of the disease phenotype caused by tau gene mutations. *Brain, 123*, 880–893.

Stanford, P. M., Shepherd, C. E., Halliday, G. M., Brooks, W. S., Schofield, P. W., Brodaty, H., et al. (2003). Mutations in the *tau* gene that cause an increase in three repeat tau and frontotemporal dementia. *Brain, 126*, 814–826.

Steele, J. C., Richardson, J. C., & Olszewski, J. (1964). Progressive supranuclear palsy: A heterogeneous degeneration involving the brain stem, basal ganglia and cerebellum with vertical gaze pseudobulbar palsy, nuchal dystonia and dementia. *Archives of Neurology, 10*, 333–359.

Taniguchi, S., McDonagh, A. M., Pickering-Brown, S. M., Umeda, Y., Iwatsubo, T., Hasegawa, M., et al. (2004). The neuropathology of frontotemporal lobar degeneration with respect to the cytological and biochemical characteristics of tau protein. *Neuropathology and Applied Neurobiology, 30*, 1–18.

Tellez-Nagel, I., & Wisniewski, H. M. (1973). Ultrastructure of neurofibrillary tangles in Steele–Richardson–Olszewski syndrome. *Archives of Neurology, 29*, 324–327.

Torack, R. M., & Morris, J. C. (1986). Mesolimbocortical dementia: A clinicopathologic case study of a putative disorder. *Archives of Neurology, 43*, 1074–1078.

Trojanowski, J. Q., & Dickson, D. (2001). Update on the neuropathological diagnosis of frontotemporal dementias. *Journal of Neuropathology and Experimental Neurology, 60*, 1123–1126.

Tu, P. H., Galvin, J. E., Baba, M., Giasson, B., Tomita, T., Leight, S., et al. (1998). Glial cytoplasmic inclusions in white matter oligodendrocytes of multiple system atrophy brains contain insoluble alpha-synuclein. *Annals of Neurology, 44*, 415–422.

van Herpen, E., Rosso, S. M., Serverijnen, L. A., Yoshida, H., Breedveld, G., van der Graaf, R., et al. (2003). Variable phenotypic expression and extensive tau pathology in two families with the novel tau mutation L315R. *Annals of Neurology 54*, 573–581.

Wakabayashi, K., Oyanagi, K., Makifuchi, T., Ikuta, F., Homma, A., Homma, Y., et al. (1994). Corticobasal degeneration: Etiopathological significance of the cytoskeletal alterations. *Acta Neuropathologica, 87*, 545–553.

Watts, G. D., Wymer, J., Kovach, M. J., Mehta, S. G., Mumm, S., Darvish, D., et al. (2004). Inclusion body myopathy associated with Paget disease of bone and frontotemporal dementia is caused by mutant valosin-containing protein. *Nature Genetics, 36*, 377–381.

Wittmann, C. W., Wszolek, M. F., Shulman, J. M., Salvaterra, P. M., Lewis, J., Hutton, M., et al. (2001). Tauopathy in *Drosophila*: Neurodegeneration without neurofibrillary tangles. *Science, 293*, 711–714.

Yancopouloù, D., Crowther, R. A., Chakrabarti, L., Gydesen, S., Brown, J. M., & Spillantini, M. G. (2003). Tau protein in frontotemporal dementia linked to chromosome 3 (FTD-3). *Journal of Neuropathology and Experimental Neurology, 62*, 878–882.

Yasuda, M., Takamatsu, J., D'Souza, I., Crowther, R. A., Kawamata, T., Hasegawa, M., et al. (2000). A novel mutation at position +12 in the intron following exon 10 of the tau gene in familial frontotemporal dementia (FTD-Kumamoto). *Annals of Neurology, 47*, 422–429.

Zhukareva, V., Sundarraj, S., Mann, D., Sjogren, M., Blenow, K., Clark, C. M., et al. (2003). Selective reduction of soluble tau proteins in sporadic and familial frontotemporal dementias: An international follow-up study. *Acta Neuropathologica, 105*, 469–476.

Zhukareva, V., Vogelsberg-Ragaglia, V., Van Deerlin, V. M., Bruce, J., Shuck, T., Grossman, M., et al. (2001). Loss of brain tau defines novel sporadic and familial tauopathies with frontotemporal dementia. *Annals of Neurology, 49*, 165–175.

# CHAPTER 26

# Imaging in Frontotemporal Dementia

## *Murray Grossman*

Frontotemporal dementia (FTD) is a neuro-degenerative condition with a relatively young age of onset, and a prevalence rate that is as common as Alzheimer's disease (AD) in individuals younger than 65 years of age (Knopman, Petersen, Edland, Cha, & Rocca, 2004; Rosso et al., 2003). The major clinical features of FTD are a progressive form of apha-sia and a disorder of social comportment and personality (Grossman, 2002; Grossman & Ash, 2004; Neary et al., 1998; Snowden, Neary, & Mann, 1996). It is obviously impor-tant to provide a correct diagnosis to the pa-tient and his or her family. Diagnosis plays a major determining role in prognosis and the fu-ture course of the disease (e.g., factors that are important for family planning). It is also cru-cial to distinguish between FTD and other pro-gressive neurodegenerative conditions such as AD, because of the imminent development of etiologically specific treatments.

Unfortunately, the accurate clinical diagnosis of FTD is not trivial (Litvan et al., 1997), due in part to the fact that neurodegenerative con-ditions such as FTD and AD are both associ-ated with impairments in domains such as naming and executive functioning (Elfgren et al., 1994; Frisoni et al., 1995; Jagust, Reed, Seab, Kramer, & Budinger, 1989; Knopman, Christiansen, & Schut, 1989; Mendez et al., 1996; Pachana, Boone, Miller, Cummings, & Berman, 1996). Whereas one report associates the nonfluent form of progressive aphasia with histopathological features of Pick's disease (Hodges et al., 2004), others have not con-firmed this observation (Forman et al., 2006).

Autopsy-proven cases of AD can present with a clinical pattern known as a "frontal variant," or a progressive form of aphasia that mimics FTD (Galton, Patterson, Xuereb, & Hodges, 2000; Johnson, Head, Kim, Starr, & Cotman, 1999). Conversely, patients with FTD may have disease at autopsy that involves the hippo-campus, resulting in a clinical profile of mem-ory difficulty resembling AD (Arnold, Trojanowski, Clark, Grossman, & Han, 2000; Graham et al., 2005).

Because of the apparent difficulty diagnosing FTD based solely on clinical characteristics, it is important to develop biomarkers than can supplement clinical observations and help dis-tinguish between overlapping neurodegenera-tive conditions such as FTD and AD. Neuroim-aging is one such modality. In this chapter, I review the results of various imaging modali-ties that have been used to help identify pa-tients with FTD, and to distinguish between these patients and individuals suffering from other neurodegenerative conditions such as AD.

## EARLY IMAGING WORK IN FTD

Early researchers used a variety of techniques to characterize neuroimaging changes in pa-tients clinically diagnosed with FTD. These early studies often used structural imaging with computed tomography (CT) scan to show changes. Progressive aphasics and patients with semantic dementia were generally shown to have left hemisphere atrophy (Mesulam, 1982;

Warrington, 1975). These seminal studies, while difficult to assert their findings with confidence because of the limited spatial resolution and hardening artifact associated with CT, foreshadowed work for the next three decades. The first quantitative imaging study of FTD was a positron emission tomography (PET) study of a patient with primary progressive aphasia (Chawluk et al., 1986). This patient had reduced left-hemisphere glucose metabolism. In subsequent studies, carefully selected patients with FTD were found to have hypoperfusion in the frontal lobe using single-photon emission computed tomography (SPECT) (Jagust et al., 1989; Miller, Cummings, & Villanueva-Meyer, 1991; Neary, Snowden, Shields, & Burjan, 1987; Risberg, 1987).

These seminal observations fostered comparative studies of FTD and AD. The goal of these comparisons was to reveal distinct distributions of abnormality that would improve diagnostic accuracy and lend validity to imaging observations in FTD. For example, a visually based clinical rating of magnetic resonance imaging (MRI) scans showed temporal atrophy in a partially distinct distribution in FTD compared to AD, that is, equal involvement of the hippocampus but more prominent atrophy of anterior and ventral temporal cortex in FTD than in AD (Galton, Gomez-Anson, et al., 2001; Frisoni et al., 1999). Visual inspection of SPECT associated a bilateral anterior perfusion defect with the clinical diagnosis of FTD compared to AD, Lewy Body disease, and vascular dementia (Talbot, Lloyd, Snowden, Neary, & Testa, 1998). More detailed examination of these observations revealed several patterns of hypoperfusion that distinguished between clinically diagnosed patients with progressive aphasia ($n = 22$) or a nonaphasic social disorder ($n = 58$) and patients with AD. Patients with progressive aphasia were thus found to have significantly reduced unilateral posterior, bilateral anterior, or bilateral anterior plus unilateral posterior patterns of hypoperfusion relative to AD patients, whereas FTD patients with a social disorder showed significantly reduced bilateral anterior and bilateral anterior plus unilateral posterior hypoperfusion, as well as significantly increased bilateral posterior perfusion relative to patients with AD. Patients with progressive aphasia were more likely to have a pattern of unilateral posterior hypoperfusion relative to patients with nonaphasic

FTD. This was confirmed by a novel MRI technique that quantifies cerebral blood flow with an arterial spin-labeling technique (Alsop, Detre, & Grossman, 2000). A significant perfusion defect was seen in a frontal distribution in FTD, and this differed from the distribution of hypoperfusion in AD.

Semiquantitative data have used a region-of-interest (ROI) approach to compare FTD and AD more directly. One ROI evaluation of the corpus callosum on the midsagittal plane of MRIs revealed significant atrophy in an anterior distribution in 16 patients with FTD relative to patients with AD, for example, presumably reflecting reduced interhemispheric projections from atrophied frontal and anterior temporal cortical regions (Kaufer et al., 1997). An ROI analysis of the temporal lobe revealed predominantly anterior hippocampal atrophy in 13 patients with FTD relative to patients with AD, although posterior hippocampal and entorhinal cortex atrophy was equivalent across these groups (Laakso et al., 2000). A ROI analysis of SPECT imaging in 20 patients with the clinical diagnosis of FTD demonstrated reduced frontal perfusion relative to patients with AD (Charpentier et al., 2000). The perfusion defect was most prominent in right median frontal and left lateral frontal ROIs. A ROI analysis of PET in 21 patients with the clinical diagnosis of FTD showed reduced glucose metabolism relative to patients with AD in orbital, middle and superior frontal, anterior temporal, anterior cingulate, and hippocampal regions bilaterally, as well as in left inferior frontal cortex (Ishii et al., 1998).

Another way to improve the validity of imaging in FTD is through longitudinal studies. The clinical diagnosis in patients followed longitudinally is more assured when followed over time. Moreover, given the great variability of cortical volume loss in older populations, longitudinal change provides a more valid picture of the specific brain regions that are becoming systematically atrophic more rapidly than would be expected in healthy aging. In the first longitudinal study, 30 patients with FTD showed much greater cortical atrophy (average annual atrophy of 3.2%) compared to individuals with AD (Chan, Fox, Jenkins, et al., 2001). Patients with FTD who have a social disorder showed more rapid longitudinal change in anterior ROIs bilaterally, whereas patients with semantic dementia showed progressive atrophy in a unilateral anterior ROI. More recent work has examined longitudinal imaging changes quantitatively. In a study of 46 patients with FTD, serial MRIs were registered in a user-independent manner and voxel-level analyses were performed (Whitwell, Anderson, Scahill, Rossor, & Fox, 2004). This work showed significant changes in frontal, temporal, and parietal regions, with patterns of longitudinal change differing across subgroups of patients with FTD. Similarly, automated registration, segmentation, and voxel-based analyses were performed on pairs of images in 8 patients with FTD (Avants, Grossman, & Gee, 2005). This analysis showed progressive annualized cortical atrophy that was most prominent in frontal, temporal, and parietal regions bilaterally. Correspondingly, loss of white matter volume was most evident in bilateral frontal and anterior temporal regions, accompanied by expanded cerebrospinal fluid (CSF) spaces anteriorly. Longitudinal atrophy was associated with longitudinal changes on language measures, and these analyses revealed prominent correlations in the left hemisphere: Confrontation naming showed the greatest correlation with inferolateral and ventral portions of left temporal cortex; semantic category membership judgments correlated most significantly with left lateral temporal and bilateral dorsolateral prefrontal cortex; and category naming fluency for a semantic category ("animals") correlated extensively with temporal and frontal cortices.

The consensus emerging from this work appears to suggest that atrophy in a frontal and anterior temporal distribution signals a diagnosis compatible with FTD. More recent work emphasizes some caution in this conclusion, based on direct, quantitative comparisons of images in FTD and AD. Using fully automated registration, normalization, and segmentation procedures, and an analysis at a fine-grained voxel level, this work revealed relatively subtle differences in the anatomic distribution of cortical atrophy in FTD ($n = 29$) compared to AD (Grossman, McMillan, et al., 2004). Significantly greater atrophy was seen in left medial frontal and right dorsolateral and superior prefrontal cortex in FTD compared to AD, whereas FTD also showed significantly less atrophy in left hippocampus, bilateral temporal–parietal cortex, and bilateral occipital association cortex.

Perhaps the most important validation of imaging studies in FTD comes from comparisons with other biomarkers of disease. In one such study, a significant correlation was found between cortical atrophy demonstrated at a voxel level in right frontal and left temporal regions and the level of tau in the CSF of patients with FTD (Grossman et al., 2005). The gold standard for validating imaging studies is a histopathological diagnosis of FTD in the imaged patients. However, there have been remarkably few quantitative imaging studies in autopsy-proven cases of FTD (Lieberman et al., 1998; Turner, Kenyon, Trojanowski, Gonatas, & Grossman, 1996). Carefully examined series of cases such as these, while small, have shown imaging defects in a frontal and anterior temporal distribution. However, imaging studies alone do not appear to distinguish between histopathologically distinct subgroups of patients with FTD. Imaging in autopsy-proven cases of FTD with tau-positive pathology thus does not differ substantially from cases with tau-negative pathology, for example (Whitwell et al., 2004).

In summary, there are important suggestions that imaging can play a role in the differential diagnosis of FTD. Imaging observations such as these contribute to the evaluation of criteria for the clinical diagnosis of FTD (e.g., Miller et al., 1997). Many studies have thus shown imaging defects in a frontal and anterior temporal distribution in FTD. However, caution is advised on the basis of studies that directly compare FTD with other neurodegenerative conditions, such as AD, that evaluate imaging against other biomarkers of disease, and that assess imaging quantitatively in autopsy-proven cases of FTD. These observations suggest that imaging studies alone are unlikely to be sufficient on their own to provide a diagnosis of FTD.

An important proviso in the work just described is that the highly variable clinical presentation of FTD makes it difficult to interpret the results of imaging in a group composed of such heterogeneous phenotypes. One potential way to improve the yield of imaging studies is to consider more closely the relationship between phenotype and the anatomical distribution of disease. It is thus possible that evaluations of imaging in less heterogeneous subgroups of patients with FTD will prove more informative in the diagnosis of this condition. Moreover, these studies are likely to contribute to our understanding of the neural basis for language and social functioning that is disturbed in these patients. I turn below to imaging studies that targeted clinically defined subgroups of patients with FTD.

## IMAGING STUDIES OF FTD PATIENT SUBGROUPS

A more critical eye toward the careful definition of the patient population has resulted in improved clinical diagnoses. Because of the great variability in clinical presentation across the entire population of patients with FTD, investigators have examined more narrowly defined subgroups of these individuals in an attempt to improve the informativeness of imaging studies. These profiles focus on patients with a particular form of progressive aphasia or a specific kind of social disorder. Through the use of a variety of imaging modalities in these well-defined groups, this body of work has led to important advances in our understanding of patients with FTD and the cognitive deficits that characterize these individuals.

### Progressive Nonfluent Aphasia

Primary progressive aphasia is generally thought to present in two major forms (Mesulam, Grossman, Hillis, Kertesz, & Weintraub, 2003), although recent observations raise the possibility of a third form (Gorno-Tempini et al., 2004; Grossman & Ash, 2004). Effortful, agrammatic, and dysarthric speech with frequent phonemic paraphasic errors are the hallmarks of progressive nonfluent aphasia (PNFA) (Grossman et al., 1996; Thompson, Ballard, Tait, Weintraub, & Mesulam, 1997). These patients also may have impaired sentence comprehension (Grossman, Rhee, & Antiquena, 2005; Hodges & Patterson, 1996). Several functional neuroimaging studies with PET or SPECT have assessed single cases or brief case series of carefully described patients with PNFA. A PET scan of the Kempler and colleagues patient with PNFA (Case 2) revealed hypometabolism in left frontal regions that extended into adjacent superior temporal and inferior parietal regions. The PET scans of the Tyrrell, Warrington, Frackowiak, and Rossor (1990) patients with PNFA showed defects in the frontal and superior temporal regions of the left hemisphere. In the three patients with PNFA described by Caselli, Jack, Petersen,

Walmer, and Yanagihara (1992), left frontal atrophy was seen on MRI, and SPECT scans demonstrated hypoperfusion centered in the left frontal region. SPECT imaging in the PNFA patient studied by Delecluse and her coworkers (1990) showed reduced frontal and temporal perfusion that was more prominent on the left than on the right. Grossman and colleagues (1996) associated the pattern of nonfluent language impairment seen longitudinally in four patients with PNFA with a PET defect in middle frontal, inferior frontal, and superior temporal regions of the left hemisphere. A ROI analysis of SPECT images in PNFA showed reduced perfusion in dorsolateral prefrontal and subcortical gray matter regions (Newberg, Mozley, Sadek, Grossman, & Alavi, 2000). Voxel-based morphometry (VBM) analysis of a PNFA case revealed predominantly frontal cortical atrophy that increased in the same region over the course of a year (Rosen, Kramer, et al., 2002).

Recently, the regional anatomical distribution of disease in PNFA has been studied in larger numbers of patients, and with more powerful, quantitative imaging techniques. VBM analyses of volumetric MRI and quantitative assessments of PET have shown statistically significant changes in PNFA that appear to be centered in left inferior frontal cortex and adjacent regions, such as the frontal operculum and anterior insula. For example, one VBM study of 11 patients with PNFA showed significant cortical atrophy in inferior frontal, middle frontal, precentral, anterior insula, and caudate regions of the left hemisphere (Gorno-Tempini et al., 2004).

There are several ways to improve confidence in the validity of imaging observations such as these. One way involves a direct comparison between patients with PNFA and those with other neurodegenerative diseases. One comparison with AD showed reduced PET glucose metabolic activity in the left anterior insula of patients with PNFA (Nestor et al., 2003). Another comparative study used VBM analyses of volumetric MRI to show significant cortical atrophy in PNFA involving left inferior, dorsolateral, premotor, and anterior insula regions of the left frontal lobe, as well as left anterior temporal cortex (Grossman, McMillan, et al., 2004). Relative to other patients with FTD, cortical atrophy was seen in an anatomical distribution involving left temporal cortex (relative to nonaphasic patients with FTD) and right frontal cortex (relative to patients with semantic dementia [SD]).

Another approach to validate the crucial contribution of left frontal disease to the syndrome of PNFA involves correlating a neuroimaging characteristic with a clinical feature of FTD, such as linguistic or cognitive functioning. One critical characteristic of patients with PNFA is their disorder of grammatical processing. A direct correlation between cognitive performance and SPECT imaging showed a significant relationship between impaired grammatical comprehension and reduced dorsolateral and inferior frontal perfusion in the left hemisphere (Grossman et al., 1998). More recently, we observed a significant correlation in PNFA between patients' comprehension of grammatically complex sentences and cortical volume in inferior frontal, frontal opercular, insula, dorsolateral frontal, and anterior temporal regions of the left hemisphere (Grossman, Work, Gee, McMillan, & Moore, submitted). These areas also had significant cortical atrophy, allowing us to infer that the correlations between grammatical comprehension and these regions are likely to represent significant interruptions of a large-scale neural network important for sentence comprehension in PNFA.

A related way to improve confidence in the meaningfulness of an imaging defect is to assess the distribution of reduced cortical recruitment during a cognitive challenge. For example, many functional MRI (fMRI) studies of healthy adults have shown activation of left inferior frontal cortex during performance of a sentence comprehension task. We might expect limited recruitment of left inferior frontal cortex in PNFA, based on the cognitive profile of poor sentence comprehension in patients with PNFA, the left frontal defect seen in these patients, and the correlations between impaired sentence processing and the frontal–cortical atrophy in PNFA mentioned earlier. In an fMRI study of sentence comprehension, patients with PNFA who also have limited grammatical comprehension in fact showed poor activation of the ventral portion of left inferior frontal cortex during attempts to understand a sentence (Cooke et al., 2003). By comparison, nonaphasic patients with limited working memory showed good activation of this portion of left inferior frontal cortex. Another study of sentence comprehension directly compared activation in patients with PNFA compared to patients with SD and patients with nonaphasic FTD who have social and executive deficits. Patients with PNFA showed reduced activation of dorsolateral prefrontal cortex in comparison to both patients with SD and those with a nonaphasic form of FTD (Grossman, Cooke, et al., 2004).

A final way to improve the validity and reliability of imaging studies is to examine imaging in patients with pathologically proven disease. In one study, a patient with PNFA due to Pick's disease showed reduced PET glucose metabolism in left inferior frontal cortex, as well as left superior frontal cortex (Lieberman et al., 1998). Another series of four patients with PNFA due to dementia lacking distinctive histopathology showed reduced left inferior frontal and anterior superior temporal glucose metabolism on PET (Turner et al., 1996).

Imaging studies of PNFA thus appear to suggest that left inferior frontal cortex and adjacent brain regions are compromised in PNFA. Furthermore, a specific imaging profile may imply a particular histopathological abnormality, because one study has reported that Pick's disease is a major cause of PNFA (Hodges et al., 2004). However, other work advises caution in making this kind of inference (Forman et al., 2006; Whitwell, Warren, et al., 2004). Even though the clinical phenotype by itself may not be able to determine the underlying pathology, future work may be able to use these imaging studies as part of a panel of biomarkers that can identify a specific subgroup of patients with FTD.

## Semantic Dementia

Semantic dementia (SD) is often considered another form of primary progressive aphasia. Patients with SD present with a fluent language disorder that involves impaired naming and single-word comprehension difficulty (Hodges, Patterson, Oxbury, & Funnell, 1992; Snowden, Goulding, & Neary, 1989). Over time, this evolves to include an impairment in understanding object appearance and object use (Bozeat, Lambon Ralph, Patterson, Garrard, & Hodges, 2000; Bozeat, Lambon Ralph, Patterson, & Hodges, 2002; Hodges, Bozeat, Lambon Ralph, Patterson, & Spatt, 2000; Lambon Ralph, McClelland, Patterson, Galton, & Hodges, 2001).

Early CT imaging studies of patients with semantic impairment (Warrington, 1975) revealed some nonspecific atrophy that was greater in the left hemisphere than in the right hemisphere. Unfortunately, CT imaging provides only limited structural detail due to poor spatial resolution and significant hardening artifact that prevents adequate imaging of the temporal lobe. One of Warrington's patients was reimaged with MRI. This revealed left-sided perisylvian and temporal atrophy (Tyrrell et al., 1990).

Functional neuroimaging studies obtained at rest have attempted to confirm the critical role of left temporal lobe functioning in this syndrome. A PET study of one of Warrington's (1975) patients with semantic impairment and three additional patients with SD revealed significantly reduced oxygen utilization in left temporal and perisylvian regions (Tyrrell et al., 1990). SPECT imaging in a patient with progressive fluent aphasia revealed left-hemisphere hypoperfusion that appeared to be most evident in the temporal region (Poeck & Luzzatti, 1988). In the Snowden and colleagues (1992) series, six patients with progressive fluent aphasia studied with SPECT imaging revealed hypoperfusion anteriorly that involved the left hemisphere in two patients and that was bilateral in four patients. The PET scans of two patients with progressive fluent aphasia showed glucose hypometabolism that was most prominent in the posterior temporal and inferior parietal regions of the left hemisphere (Kempler et al., 1990). Five well characterized patients with SD showed marked temporal lobe atrophy and a corresponding functional imaging defect on SPECT or PET (Hodges et al., 1992).

More recently, the distribution of atrophy in patients with SD has been defined in greater detail with semiquantitative MRI. This work has emphasized the role of left temporal cortex in SD. An anterior–posterior gradient of asymmetric atrophy of the left temporal lobe was observed in a series of 10 patients with SD, based on experimenter-implemented ROI analyses of high-resolution MRI (Chan, Fox, & Scahill, 2001). Areas of atrophy included entorhinal cortex; parahippocampal gyrus; fusiform gyrus; superior, middle, and inferior temporal gyri; and medial temporal structures, such as the amygdala and the hippocampus. Several investigators, focusing on medial temporal structures, confirmed hippocampal atrophy in SD that is more prominent in the left hemisphere (Frisoni et al., 1999; Laakso et al., 2000). This work also emphasized the rela-

tively anterior distribution of hippocampal atrophy in these patients. A study of 18 patients with SD used experimenter-drawn ROIs to show a pattern of atrophy affecting primarily anterior and inferior portions of the left temporal lobe (Galton, Patterson, et al., 2001).

Using a fully quantitative approach, the Mummery, Patterson, Price, and Hodges (2000) examined six clinically defined patients with SD with a VBM analysis of high resolution structural MRI. This showed cortical atrophy in the temporal pole bilaterally, in middle, inferior, and anterior fusiform gyri of the left temporal lobe, and in the ventromedial portion of the left frontal lobe. VBM and ROI analyses were performed on MRIs in 10 subjects with SD (Good et al., 2002). This revealed an anterior–posterior gradient of cortical atrophy that was most prominent in the left temporal lobe using either technique, affecting the amygdala, inferior and middle temporal gyri, and entorhinal cortex. There was also a reduction of white matter volume in the left temporal lobe and the corpus callosum. A fully automated normalization and segmentation procedure, with VBM analysis of high-dimensional imaging, showed gray matter atrophy in eight patients with SD that was most prominent in left inferior and middle temporal gyri, left fusiform gyrus, and the left temporal pole (Grossman, McMillan, et al., 2004). Another VBM study of 10 patients with SD showed significant cortical atrophy in polar, anterior fusiform, and lateral temporal regions of the left hemisphere, extending into posterior insula, ventromedial frontal, and deep gray structures (Gorno-Tempini et al., 2004). In a recent study, Studholme and colleagues (2004) used diffusion tensor imaging to show compromised white matter tracts in the left temporal lobe of patients with SD.

One way to validate the contribution of left temporal cortex to the clinical syndrome of SD is through longitudinal studies. In a longitudinal study that analyzed volumetric change of anterior and posterior halves of the left hemisphere and the right hemisphere (Chan, Fox, Jenkins, et al., 2001), the annualized rate of atrophy in the left anterior quadrant of patients with SD was 3.6%, greater than the annualized atrophy rate in the right anterior quadrant (2.6%). Atrophy in these anterior quadrants proceeded at a faster rate than that in the posterior quadrants of the left hemisphere (2.1%) or the right hemisphere (1.5%).

Another way to validate the left temporal locus of disease on imaging studies in patients with SD is by correlating patients' regional atrophy with their cognitive difficulties. These findings emphasize left temporal lobe atrophy in SD, and appear to correlate this distribution of atrophy with impairments of naming and semantic memory that are the hallmarks of this syndrome. In one study, poor performance on a measure of semantic memory correlated with atrophy of the left temporal pole, but not with left ventromedial frontal cortex (Mummery et al., 2000). In an ROI follow-up study (Galton, Patterson, et al., 2001), performance on a measure of semantic memory correlated with atrophy of the left fusiform gyrus, whereas naming difficulty correlated with atrophy of polar, middle, and inferior temporal regions of the left hemisphere. In a pair of VBM studies, difficulty on a measure of semantic memory correlated with inferolateral portions of left temporal cortex, whereas difficulty with confrontation naming correlated with left anterolateral temporal cortical atrophy (Grossman, McMillan, et al., 2004).

Another way to validate the contribution of left temporal cortex to the clinical syndrome of SD is through activation studies. This work has shown limited left temporal activation during cognitive challenges in SD. A variety of language-mediated measures activate the left temporal lobe during probes of word or sentence meaning. The posterolateral temporal area has been associated with semantic memory for single words in healthy subjects studied with fMRI (Joseph, 2001), for example, and in correlation and activation neuroimaging studies of AD (Desgranges et al., 1998; Grossman et al., 1997, 2003). A SPECT activation study revealed reduced left temporal activation during semantic decisions in SD (Cardebat, Demonet, Celsis, & Puel, 1996). A PET activation study of four patients with SD assessed cortical recruitment associated with a semantic decision about pictures, and showed reduced left lateral temporal activation (Mummery et al., 1999). However, a more recent study of patients with primary progressive aphasia with left lateral temporal atrophy showed essentially normal activation of this region (Sonty et al., 2003). Temporal regions are also recruited during activation studies of sentence comprehension (Ben-Shachar, Palti, & Grodzinsky, 2004; Cooke et al., 2002; Grossman et al., 2002; Just, Carpenter, Keller, Eddy, & Thulborn, 1996). In

a study of sentence comprehension, patients with SD showed limited activation of left temporal, left parietal, and left frontal regions compared to nonaphasic patients with FTD (Grossman, Cooke, et al., 2004).

These findings suggest that the left temporal lobe plays a crucial role in the semantic impairment of patients with SD, although several left temporal regions appear to be implicated by the work just described. This includes the left temporal pole, left ventral temporal cortex, and left lateral temporal cortex. Some of this ambiguity may be due in part to the observation of a fluent form of progressive aphasia, in which the dominant clinical feature is anomia, but there is less multimodal semantic memory impairment in these patients (Gorno-Tempini et al., 2004; Graham, Patterson, & Hodges, 1995). This appears to be associated with a posterolateral distribution of cortical atrophy on MRI. Additional work is needed to distinguish the clinical and imaging features of these progressive fluent aphasic syndromes, and to determine more precisely the role that these various temporal regions play in SD. Some work thus appears to associate the semantic memory impairment of SD with a modality-neutral deficit for object knowledge due to left inferolateral and/or anterior temporal disease, but other studies cannot rule out the potential contribution of a modality-specific impairment for visual–perceptual features in visual association regions of inferior temporal cortex or lexical phonological representations in auditory association regions of left lateral temporal cortex. Regardless of these emerging issues in the study of single-word meaning, there appears to be little conflict surrounding the distinction between the clinical and imaging features of fluent form(s) of progressive aphasia compared to PNFA. Direct comparison of these syndromes with clinical and imaging studies provide reasonably strong evidence that progressive aphasia is not an undifferentiated disorder, but instead underline distinct fluent and nonfluent forms of progressive aphasia.

## Nonaphasic Patients with a Disorder of Social Comportment and Executive Functioning

The most prominent feature of patients with FTD who do not have an aphasia is their disorder of social comportment and personality. Advances in our understanding of the nosology of these difficulties are continuing (Gregory et al., 2002; Liu et al., 2004; Rankin, Kramer, Mychack, & Miller, 2003; Snowden et al., 2003), although the precise characteristics of these impairments remain to be elucidated. Many of these individuals also have difficulty with executive functioning in cognitive domains, such as poor inhibitory control, limited working memory, and impaired planning and mental organization (Boone et al., 1999; Bozeat, Gregory, Lambon Ralph, & Hodges, 2000; Lough, Gregory, & Hodges, 2001; Rahman, Sahakian, Hodges, Rogers, & Robbins, 1999; Razani, Boone, Miller, Lee, & Sherman, 2001).

In this context, early work examined the distribution of clinically identified patients diagnosed by experts. These studies emphasize involvement of frontal and temporal regions of the right hemisphere. An early study of eight patients with behavioral disinhibition, social withdrawal, and neuropsychological evidence of executive limitations used an ROI analysis to show reduced right frontal and temporal perfusion with SPECT (Miller et al., 1991). Among seven patients with FTD who have a significant change of "self," as defined by changed political, social, and religious values, six patients had MRI or SPECT evidence for right frontal disease (Miller et al., 2003). A PET study of 29 nonaphasic patients with FTD showed reduced glucose metabolism predominantly in prefrontal regions but also in cingulate, anterior temporal, inferior parietal, insula, and deep gray structures (Jeong et al., 2005). In eight patients with this social and executive syndrome, a VBM analysis showed cortical atrophy in right dorsolateral prefrontal and left motor cortex, as well as in orbital frontal and anterior cingulate cortex (Rosen, Gorno-Tempini, et al., 2002). In a comparative study based on VBM analyses of cortical atrophy, a cohort of 14 patients with FTD and a social and executive disorder showed significant right dorsolateral frontal, right anterior cingulate, and right anterior insula cortical atrophy in a direct comparison with patients with SD, and significant right posterolateral temporal cortical atrophy was seen relative to patients with PNFA (Grossman, McMillan, et al., 2004).

Several studies have demonstrated social and cognitive deficits in groups of patients with FTD, defined by the presence of a right-hemisphere imaging defect, and distinct patterns of social and personality impairment appear to emerge depending on the right frontal or right temporal distribution of the imaging defect. Undesirable social behaviors such as criminality, aggression, financial recklessness, sexually deviant behavior, alienation from friends, and abnormal response to spousal crisis were associated with right-sided perfusion defects upon visual inspection of SPECT in 12 patients with FTD compared to 19 patients with left-sided defects (Mychack, Kramer, Boone, & Miller, 2001). An examination of personality revealed submissiveness in 16 patients with a so-called "frontal variant" of FTD (fvFTD), defined on the basis of visual inspection of MRI, whereas 10 patients with visually apparent temporal atrophy showed coldheartedness (Rankin et al., 2003). Five of 47 patients with FTD were examined in detail because of the presence of right temporal lobe hypoperfusion on SPECT imaging (Edwards-Lee et al., 1997). These patients showed irritability, impulsiveness, mental rigidity, decreased facial expression, increased visual alertness, and bizarre behaviors. Patients with predominantly right temporal atrophy ($n = 11$) on visual inspection of CT or MRI showed a behavioral disorder consisting of food fads, irritability, loss of insight, and social awkwardness (Thompson, Patterson, & Hodges, 2003).

Semiquantitative image analyses have been used to supplement these informal visual observations. A ROI analysis of frontal and temporal structures in nine patients with the so-called "temporal variant" of FTD (tvFTD) showed a significant correlation between poor comprehension of emotional faces, particularly those with negative valence, and atrophy in right amygdala and right orbitofrontal cortex (Rosen, Perry, et al., 2002). A ROI analysis of MRI in 51 patients found significantly greater atrophy bilaterally in temporal and amygdala regions in patients with tvFTD relative to patients with AD whereas significantly greater frontal atrophy was found bilaterally in patients with fvFTD relative to patients with AD. Both patients with fvFTD and tvFTD showed significantly greater atrophy in ventromedial frontal cortex bilaterally relative to patients with AD. An analysis of behavior in these FTD subgroups showed more apathy, anxiety, and eating disorders in patients with fvFTD than in patients with AD, and more apathy than in patients with tvFTD; a higher prevalence of sleeping disorders was seen in patients with tvFTD relative to patients with AD and fvFTD; and both fvFTD and tvFTD groups showed higher proportions of euphoria, disinhibition, and aberrant motor behavior than did patients with AD. An eating disorder was associated with atrophy in dorsolateral and ventromedial portions of right frontal cortex; disinhibition was associated with reduced volume in the amygdala, ventromedial frontal and anterior temporal ROIs of the right hemisphere; and depression was associated with right amygdala and right anterior temporal atrophy.

Several cognitive domains share many features with these social domains. Theory of mind judgments were assessed in 19 patients with personality and behavioral changes due to FTD without aphasia (Gregory et al., 2002). All aspects of theory of mind were impaired in these patients. A visual rating scale assessed the severity of frontal atrophy on MRI, and there was good concordance between the severity of theory of mind impairment and ventromedial frontal atrophy. Visual inspection of MRI identified 10 patients with FTD who have predominantly frontal atrophy and deficits in executive functioning, and this cognitive deficit distinguished these patients from patients with FTD who have temporal atrophy associated with impaired semantic memory, and from patients with AD who have significant episodic memory difficulty (Perry & Hodges, 2000).

There have been few direct correlations of social and executive functioning with cortical atrophy in these patients. One study examined the neural basis for category-naming fluency in patients with FTD and a disorder of social and executive functioning, and in patients with SD (Work, Gee, McMillan, Moore, & Grossman, 2004). Using VBM-determined MRI cortical atrophy, patients with a social and executive disorder demonstrated a correlation with left inferior frontal atrophy for both semantically guided ("animals") and letter-guided ("F-A-S") category naming. By comparison, patients with SD showed a correlation for letter-guided category naming with atrophy in left temporal–parietal cortex, and for semantically guided naming in left ventral temporal cortex, but no correlation with left inferior frontal atrophy. This emphasizes the importance of left inferior frontal cortex for tasks requiring selection during a mental search, regardless of the material being processed (Thompson-Schill, D'Esposito, Aguirre, & Farah, 1997; Wagner, Pare-Blagoev, Clark, & Poldrack, 2001).

Other studies have demonstrated reduced cortical activation during the performance of cognitive measures. One early study associated reduced frontal PET activation during a category-naming fluency task (Warkentin & Passant, 1997). Seven patients with FTD showed reduced activation during an fMRI study of working memory, and the linear increase in activation with increased working memory load was less in FTD than in AD (Rombouts et al., 2003). Another study showed limited activation of the dorsal portion of left inferior frontal cortex during attempts to understand sentences that stress working memory demands in patients with a disorder of social and executive functioning (Cooke et al., 2003).

Taken together, these findings emphasize the association between the disorder of social functioning that is so prominent in FTD and disease in right frontal and temporal cortical regions. Additional empirical work is needed to confirm the distribution of an imaging defect in patients with a social disorder who have not been preselected because of the presence of right-hemispheric changes on an imaging study.

## CONCLUSION

Imaging is an important biomarker that is part of the armamentarium of clinicians faced with the difficult task of diagnosing FTD. Imaging studies appear to suggest some features that distinguish FTD from AD. The reliability of these features is underlined by converging evidence from multiple studies using many different imaging modalities and statistical approaches. The validity of these features, however, remains limited by the rare report of quantitative imaging in well-studied patients with other biomarkers of FTD, or with autopsy-proven FTD. Perhaps the most common imaging findings in FTD reflect disease in anterior temporal cortex of the left hemisphere and dorsolateral frontal cortex of the right hemisphere. Of course, other regions related to these are frequently compromised as well. These areas are most compromised statistically in patients with FTD compared to healthy seniors, the most common comparative group. These areas also differ statistically when direct comparisons are made between patients with FTD and AD. Correlations between clinical features and imaging changes implicate these anatomical areas most closely in the symptomatology of FTD. This offers some reassurance that the observed imaging defects are valid. The few quantitative imaging studies in autopsy-proven patients with FTD are consistent with these views.

Because of the noninvasive nature of this diagnostic modality, it is likely that imaging will contribute importantly to criteria for entering a clinical trial, and to the endpoints that reflect efficacy following participation in a treatment trial. It is important to emphasize, however, that imaging data such as these do not provide pathognomonic evidence supporting the diagnosis of FTD. Together with other clinical and biomarker observations, it is likely that imaging data will enhance our ability to make an accurate diagnosis of FTD during life.

An important subsidiary issue addressed by these brain–behavior relationships is the neural basis for the linguistic and social disorders that are so prominent in FTD. Work with well-defined patients with FTD can improve our understanding of the neural basis for language and social functioning. Important advances are being made in the areas of word and sentence comprehension through the examination of patients with progressive aphasia, and novel approaches to the study of social functioning are being demonstrated through inventive examinations of patients with FTD and a disorder of personality and social comportment.

## ACKNOWLEDGMENTS

This work was supported in part by the U.S. Public Health Service (Grant Nos. AG17586, AG15116, and NS44266) and the Dana Foundation. I wish to express my appreciation to an outstanding group of collaborators (Sherry Ash, John Detre, Jennifer Farmer, Mark Forman, Jim Gee, Phyllis Koenig, Virginia M.-Y. Lee, and John Q. Trojanowski), and to the enthusiastic patients and families who live with frontotemporal dementia in their daily lives.

## REFERENCES

Alsop, D., Detre, J., & Grossman, M. (2000). Arterial spin labelling perfusion MRI in frontotemporal dementia and Alzheimer's disease: Correlation with language functions. *Annals of Neurology, 47,* 93–100.

Arnold, S. E., Trojanowski, J. Q., Clark, C. M., Grossman, M., & Han, L.-Y. (2000). Quantitative neurohistological features of frontotemporal degeneration. *Neurobiology of Aging, 21,* 913–939.

Avants, B., Grossman, M., & Gee, J. C. (2005). Frontotemporal dementia induced annualized gray matter loss using diffeomorphic morphometry. *Alzheimer's Disease and Associated Disorders, 19,* 525–528.

Ben-Shachar, M., Palti, D., & Grodzinsky, Y. (2004). Neural correlates of syntactic movement: Converging evidence from two fMRI experiments. *NeuroImage, 21,* 1320–1326.

Boone, K., Miller, B. L., Lee, A., Berman, N., Sherman, D., & Stuss, D. (1999). Neuropsychological patterns in right versus left frontotemporal dementia. *Journal of the International Neuropsychological Society, 5,* 616–622.

Bozeat, S., Gregory, C. A., Lambon Ralph, M. A., & Hodges, J. R. (2000). Which neuropsychiatric and behavioural features distinguish frontal and temporal variants of frontotemporal dementia from Alzheimer's disease? *Journal of Neurology, Neurosurgery, and Psychiatry, 69,* 178–186.

Bozeat, S., Lambon Ralph, M. A., Patterson, K., Garrard, P., & Hodges, J. R. (2000). Non-verbal semantic impairment in semantic dementia. *Neuropsychologia, 38,* 1207–1215.

Bozeat, S., Lambon Ralph, M. A., Patterson, K., & Hodges, J. R. (2002). When objects lose their meaning: What happens to their use? *Cognitive, Affective, and Behavioral Neuroscience, 2,* 236–251.

Cardebat, D., Demonet, J.-F., Celsis, P., & Puel, M. (1996). Living/nonliving dissociation in a case of semantic dementia: SPECT activation study. *Neuropsychologia, 34,* 1175–1179.

Caselli, R. J., Jack, C. R., Petersen, R. C., Walmer, H. W., & Yanagihara, T. (1992). Asymmetric cortical degenerative syndromes: Clinical and radiological correlations. *Neurology, 42,* 1462–1468.

Chan, D., Fox, N. C., Jenkins, R., Scahill, R. I., Crum, W. R., & Rossor, M. N. (2001). Rates of global and regional cerebral atrophy in AD and frontotemporal dementia. *Neurology, 57,* 1756–1763.

Chan, D., Fox, N. C., & Scahill, R. I. (2001). Patterns of temporal lobe atrophy in semantic dementia and Alzheimer's disease. *Annals of Neurology, 49,* 433–442.

Charpentier, P., Lavenu, I., Defebvre, L., Duhamel, A., Lecouffe, P., Pasquier, F., et al. (2000). Alzheimer's disease and frontotemporal dementia are differentiated by discriminant analysis applied to $^{99m}Tc$ HmPAO SPECT data. *Journal of Neurology, Neurosurgery, and Psychiatry, 69,* 661–663.

Chawluk, J., Mesulam, M.-M., Hurtig, H. I., Kushner, M., Weintraub, S., Saykin, A. J., et al. (1986). Slowly progressive aphasia without dementia: Studies with positron emission tomography. *Annals of Neurology, 19,* 68–74.

Cooke, A., DeVita, C., Gee, J. C., Alsop, D., Detre, J., Chen, W., et al. (2003). Neural basis for sentence comprehension deficits in frontotemporal dementia. *Brain and Language, 85,* 211–221.

Cooke, A., Zurif, E. B., DeVita, C., Alsop, D., Koenig, P., Detre, J., et al. (2002). The neural basis for sentence comprehension: Grammatical and short-term memory components. *Human Brain Mapping*, *15*, 80–94.

Delecluse, F., Andersen, A. R., Waldemar, G., Thomsen, A.-M., Kjaer, L., Lassen, N. A., et al. (1990). Cerebral blood flow in progressive aphasia without dementia. *Brain*, *113*, 1395–1404.

Desgranges, B., Baron, J.-C., de la Sayette, V., Petit-Taboue, M. C., Benali, K., Landeau, B., et al. (1998). The neural substrates of memory systems impairment in Alzheimer's disease: A PET study of resting brain glucose utilization. *Brain*, *121*, 611–631.

Edwards-Lee, T., Miller, B. L., Benson, D. F., Cummings, J. L., Russell, G. L., Boone, K., et al. (1997). The temporal variant of frontotemporal dementia. *Brain*, *120*, 1027–1040.

Elfgren, C., Brun, A., Gustafson, L., Johansen, A., Minthon, L., Passant, U., et al. (1994). Neuropsychological tests as discriminators between dementia of Alzheimer type and frontotemporal dementia. *International Journal of Geriatric Psychiatry*, *9*, 635–642.

Forman, M. S., Farmer, J., Johnson, J. K., Clark, C. M., Arold, S. G., Coslett, H. B., et al. (2006). Frontotemporal dementia: Clinicopathological correlations. *Annals of Neurology*, *59*, 952–962.

Frisoni, G. B., Laakso, M. P., Beltramello, A., Geroldi, C., Bianchetti, A., Soininen, H., et al. (1999). Hippocampal atrophy and entorhinal cortex atrophy in frontotemporal dementia and Alzheimer's disease. *Neurology*, *52*, 91–100.

Frisoni, G. B., Pizzolato, G., Geroldi, C., Rossato, A., Bianchetti, A., & Trabucchi, M. (1995). Dementia of the frontal lobe type: Neuropsychological and [$^{99}$Tc]-HM-PAO SPECT features. *Journal of Geriatric Psychiatry and Neurology*, *8*, 42–48.

Galton, C. J., Gomez-Anson, B., Antoun, N., Scheltens, P., Patterson, K., Graves, M., et al. (2001). Temporal lobe rating scale: Application to Alzheimer's disease and frontotemporal dementia. *Journal of Neurology, Neurosurgery, and Psychiatry*, *70*, 165–173.

Galton, C. J., Patterson, K., Graham, K. S., Lambon Ralph, M. A., Williams, G., Antoun, N., et al. (2001). Differing patterns of temporal atrophy in Alzheimer's disease and semantic dementia. *Neurology*, *57*, 216–225.

Galton, C. J., Patterson, K., Xuereb, J., & Hodges, J. R. (2000). Atypical and typical presentations of Alzheimer's disease: A clinical, neuropsychological, neuroimaging, and pathological study of 13 cases. *Brain*, *123*, 484–498.

Good, C. D., Scahill, R. I., Fox, N. C., Ashburner, J., Friston, K., Chan, D., et al. (2002). Automated differentiation of anatomical patterns in the human brain: Validation with studies of degenerative dementias. *NeuroImage*, *17*, 29–46.

Gorno-Tempini, M., Dronkers, N. F., Rankin, K. P., Ogar, J. M., Phengrasamy, L., Rosen, H. J., et al. (2004). Cognition and anatomy in three variants of primary progressive aphasia. *Annals of Neurology*, *55*, 335–346.

Graham, A., Davies, R., Xuereb, J., Halliday, G. M.,

Kril, J. J., Creasey, H., et al. (2005). Pathologically proven frontotemporal dementia presenting with severe amnesia. *Brain*, *128*, 597–605.

Graham, K. S., Patterson, K., & Hodges, J. R. (1995). Progressive pure anomia: Insufficient activation of phonology by meaning. *Neurocase*, *1*, 25–38.

Gregory, C. A., Lough, S., Stone, V., Erzinclioglu, S., Martin, L., Baron-Cohen, S., et al. (2002). Theory of mind in patients with frontal variant frontotemporal dementia and Alzheimer's disease: Theoretical and practical implications. *Brain*, *125*, 752–764.

Grossman, M. (2002). Frontotemporal dementia: A review. *Journal of the International Neuropsychological Society*, *8*, 564–583.

Grossman, M., & Ash, S. (2004). Primary progressive aphasia: A review. *Neurocase*, *10*, 3–18.

Grossman, M., Cooke, A., DeVita, C., Alsop, D., Detre, J., & Gee, J. C. (2002). Age-related changes in working memory during sentence comprehension: An fMRI study. *NeuroImage*, *15*, 302–317.

Grossman, M., Cooke, A., McMillan, C., Moore, P., Gee, J. C., & Work, M. (2004b). Sentence comprehension in progressive aphasia and frontotemporal dementia: An fMRI study. *Brain and Language*, *91*, 134–135.

Grossman, M., Farmer, J., Leight, S., Work, M., Moore, P., Van Deerlin, V. M. D., et al. (2005). Cerebrospinal fluid profile distinguishes frontotemporal dementia from Alzheimer's disease. *Annals of Neurology*, *57*, 721–729.

Grossman, M., Koenig, P., Glosser, G., DeVita, C., Moore, P., Rhee, J., et al. (2003). Neural basis for semantic memory difficulty in Alzheimer's disease: An fMRI study. *Brain*, *126*, 292–311.

Grossman, M., McMillan, C., Moore, P., Ding, L., Glosser, G., Work, M., et al. (2004c). What's in a name?: Voxel-based morphometric analyses of MRI and naming difficulty in Alzheimer's disease, frontotemporal dementia, and corticobasal degeneration. *Brain*, *127*, 628–649.

Grossman, M., Mickanin, J., Onishi, K., Hughes, E., D'Esposito, M., Ding, X.-S., et al. (1996). Progressive non-fluent aphasia: Language, cognitive and PET measures contrasted with probable Alzheimer's disease. *Journal of Cognitive Neuroscience*, *8*, 135–154.

Grossman, M., Moore, P., Work, M., Gee, J. C., Glosser, G., Koenig, P., et al. (submitted). *Semantic knowledge and categorization difficulty: A comparative study of neurodegenerative diseases*.

Grossman, M., Payer, F., Onishi, K., D'Esposito, M., Morrison, D., Sadek, A., et al. (1998). Language comprehension and regional cerebral defects in frontotemporal degeneration and Alzheimer's disease. *Neurology*, *50*, 157–163.

Grossman, M., Rhee, J., & Antiquena, P. (2005). Sentence processing in frontotemporal dementia. *Cortex*, *41*, 764–777.

Grossman, M., White-Devine, T., Payer, F., Onishi, K., D'Esposito, M., Robinson, K. M., et al. (1997). Constraints on the cerebral basis for semantic processing from neuroimaging studies of Alzheimer's disease. *Journal of Neurology, Neurosurgery, and Psychiatry*, *63*, 152–158.

Grossman, M., Work, M., Gee, J. C., McMillan, C., & Moore, P. (submitted). *Sentence comprehension difficulty in progressive non-fluent aphasia: A voxel-based morphometric analysis.*

Hodges, J. R., Bozeat, S., Lambon Ralph, M. A., Patterson, K., & Spatt, J. (2000). The role of conceptual knowledge in object use: Evidence from semantic dementia. *Brain*, *123*, 1913–1925.

Hodges, J. R., Davies, R. R., Xuereb, J., Casey, B. J., Broe, M., Bak, T., et al. (2004). Clinicopathological correlates in frontotemporal dementia. *Annals of Neurology*, *56*, 399–406.

Hodges, J. R., & Patterson, K. (1996). Nonfluent progressive aphasia and semantic dementia: A comparative neuropsychological study. *Journal of the International Neuropsychological Society*, *2*, 511–524.

Hodges, J. R., Patterson, K., Oxbury, S., & Funnell, E. (1992). Semantic dementia: Progressive fluent aphasia with temporal lobe atrophy. *Brain*, *115*, 1783–1806.

Ishii, K., Sakamoto, S., Sasaki, M., Kitagaki, H., Yamaji, S., Hashimoto, M., et al. (1998). Cerebral glucose metabolism in patients with frontotemporal dementia. *Journal of Nuclear Medicine*, *39*, 1875–1878.

Jagust, W. J., Reed, B. R., Seab, J. P., Kramer, J. H., & Budinger, T. F. (1989). Clinical–physiologic correlates of Alzheimer's disease and frontal lobe dementia. *American Journal of Physiological Imaging*, *4*, 89–96.

Jeong, Y., Cho, S. S., Park, J. M., Kang, S. J., Lee, J. S., Kang, E., et al. (2005). $^{18}$F-FDG PET findings in frontotemporal dementia: An SPM analysis of 29 patients. *Journal of Nuclear Medicine*, *46*, 233–239.

Johnson, J. K., Head, E., Kim, R., Starr, A., & Cotman, C. W. (1999). Clinical and pathological evidence for a frontal variant of Alzheimer disease. *Archives of Neurology*, *56*, 1233–1239.

Joseph, J. E. (2001). Functional neuroimaging studies of category specificity in object recognition: A critical review and meta-analysis. *Cognitive, Affective and Behavioral Neuroscience*, *1*, 119–136.

Just, M. A., Carpenter, P. A., Keller, T. A., Eddy, W. F., & Thulborn, K. R. (1996). Brain activation modulated by sentence comprehension. *Science*, *274*, 114–116.

Kaufer, D. I., Miller, B. L., Itti, L., Fairbanks, L., Li, J., Fishman, J., et al. (1997). Midline cerebral morphometry distinguishes frontotemporal dementia and Alzheimer's disease. *Neurology*, *48*, 978–985.

Kempler, D., Metter, E. J., Riege, W. H., Jackson, C., Benson, D. F., & Hanson, W. R. (1990). Slowly progressive aphasia: Three cases with language, memory, CT, and PET data. *Journal of Neurology, Neurosurgery, and Psychiatry*, *53*, 987–993.

Knopman, D. S., Christiansen, K. J., & Schut, L. J. (1989). The spectrum of imaging and neuropsycho-

logical findings in Pick's disease. *Neurology*, *39*, 362–368.

Knopman, D. S., Petersen, R. C., Edland, S. D., Cha, R. H., & Rocca, W. A. (2004). The incidence of frontotemporal lobar degeneration in Rochester, Minnesota, 1990 through 1994. *Neurology*, *62*, 506–508.

Laakso, M., Frisoni, G. B., Kononen, M., Mikkonen, M., Beltramello, A., Geroldi, C., et al. (2000). Hippocampal and entorhinal cortex in frontotemporal dementia and Alzheimer's disease: A morphometric MRI study. *Biological Psychiatry*, *47*, 1056–1063.

Lambon Ralph, M. A., McClelland, J. L., Patterson, K., Galton, C. J., & Hodges, J. R. (2001). No right to speak?: The relationship between object naming and semantic impairment: Neuropsychological evidence and a computational model. *Journal of Cognitive Neuroscience*, *13*, 341–356.

Lieberman, A. P., Trojanowski, J. Q., Lee, V. M. Y., Balin, B., Ding, X.-S., Greenberg, J., et al. (1998). Cognitive, neuroimaging, and pathologic studies in a patient with Pick's disease. *Annals of Neurology*, *43*, 259–264.

Litvan, I., Agid, Y., Sastrj, N., Jankovic, J., Wenning, G. K., Goetz, C. G., et al. (1997). What are the obstacles for an accurate clinical diagnosis of Pick's disease?: A clinicopathologic study. *Neurology*, *49*, 62–69.

Liu, W., Miller, B. L., Kramer, J. H., Rankin, K., Wyss-Coray, C., Gearhart, R., et al. (2004). Behavioral disorders in the frontal and temporal variants of frontotemporal dementia. *Neurology*, *62*, 742–748.

Lough, S., Gregory, C. A., & Hodges, J. R. (2001). Dissociation of social cognition and executive function in frontal variant fronto-temporal dementia. *Neurocase*, *7*, 123–130.

Mendez, M. F., Cherrier, M., Perryman, K. M., Pachana, N., Miller, B. L., & Cummings, J. L. (1996). Frontotemporal dementia versus Alzheimer's disease: Differential cognitive features. *Neurology*, *47*, 1189–1194.

Mesulam, M.-M. (1982). Slowly progressive aphasia without generalized dementia. *Annals of Neurology*, *11*, 592–598.

Mesulam, M.-M., Grossman, M., Hillis, A. E., Kertesz, A., & Weintraub, S. (2003). The core and halo of primary progressive aphasia and semantic dementia. *Annals of Neurology*, *54*, S11–S14.

Miller, B. L., Cummings, J. L., & Villanueva-Meyer, J. (1991). Frontal lobe degeneration: Clinical, neuropsychological, and SPECT characteristics. *Neurology*, *41*, 1374–1382.

Miller, B. L., Ikonte, C., Ponton, M., Levy, M., Boone, K., Darby, A., et al. (1997). A study of the Lund–Manchester research criteria for frontotemporal dementia: Clinical and single photon emission CT correlations. *Neurology*, *48*, 937–942.

Miller, B. L., Seeley, W. W., Mychack, P., Rosen, H. J., Mena, I., & Boone, K. (2003). Neuroanatomy of the self: Evidence from patients with frontotemporal dementia. *Neurology*, *57*, 817–821.

Mummery, C. J., Patterson, K., Price, C. J., & Hodges,

J. R. (2000). A voxel-based morphometry study of semantic dementia: Relationship between temporal lobe atrophy and semantic memory. *Annals of Neurology*, 47, 36–45.

Mummery, C. J., Patterson, K., Wise, R. J. S., Vandenbergh, R., Price, C. J., & Hodges, J. R. (1999). Disrupted temporal lobe connections in semantic dementia. *Brain*, 122, 61–73.

Mychack, P., Kramer, J. H., Boone, K. B., & Miller, B. L. (2001). The influence of right frontotemporal dysfunction on social behavior in frontotemporal dementia. *Neurology*, 56, 11–15.

Neary, D., Snowden, J. S., Gustafson, L., Passant, U., Stuss, D., Black, S., et al. (1998). Frontotemporal lobar degeneration: A consensus on clinical diagnostic criteria. *Neurology*, 51, 1546–1554.

Neary, D., Snowden, J. S., Shields, R. A., & Burjan, A. W. (1987). Single photon emission tomographic imaging of the brain using $^{99m}$Tc-HM-PAO in the investigation of dementia. *Journal of Neurology, Neurosurgery, and Psychiatry*, 50, 1101–1109.

Nestor, P. J., Graham, N. L., Fryer, T. D., Williams, G. B., Patterson, K., & Hodges, J. R. (2003). Progressive non-fluent aphasia is associated with hypometabolism centred on the left anterior insula. *Brain*, 126, 2406–2418.

Newberg, A., Mozley, P. D., Sadek, A., Grossman, M., & Alavi, A. (2000). The regional cerebral distribution of [$^{99m}$Tc]HMPAO in patients with progressive aphasia. *Journal of Neuroimaging*, 10, 162–168.

Pachana, N., Boone, K., Miller, B. L., Cummings, J. L., & Berman, N. (1996). Comparison of neuropsychological functioning in Alzheimer's disease and frontotemporal dementia. *Journal of the International Neuropsychological Society*, 2, 505–510.

Perry, R. J., & Hodges, J. R. (2000). Differentiating frontal and temporal variant frontotemporal dementia from Alzheimer's disease. *Neurology*, 54, 2277–2284.

Poeck, K., & Luzzatti, C. (1988). Slowly progressive aphasia in three patients. *Brain*, 111, 151–168.

Rahman, S., Sahakian, B. J., Hodges, J. R., Rogers, R. D., & Robbins, T. W. (1999). Specific cognitive deficits in mild frontal variant frontotemporal dementia. *Brain*, 122, 1469–1493.

Rankin, K. P., Kramer, J. H., Mychack, P., & Miller, B. L. (2003). Double dissociation of social functioning in frontotemporal dementia. *Neurology*, 60, 266–271.

Razani, J., Boone, K. B., Miller, B. L., Lee, A., & Sherman, D. (2001). Neuropsychological performance of right- and left-frontotemporal dementia compared to Alzheimer's disease. *Journal of the International Neuropsychological Society*, 7, 468–480.

Risberg, J. (1987). Frontal lobe degeneration of non-Alzheimer type: III. Regional cerebral blood flow. *Archives of Gerontology and Geriatrics*, 6, 225–233.

Rombouts, S. A., van Swieten, J. C., Pijnenburg, Y. A. L., Goekoop, R., Barkhof, F., & Scheltens, P. (2003). Loss of frontal fMRI activation in early frontotemporal dementia compared to early AD. *Neurology*, 60, 1904–1908.

Rosen, H. J., Gorno-Tempini, M. L., Goldman, W. P., Perry, R. J., Schuff, N., Weiner, M., et al. (2002). Patterns of brain atrophy in frontotemporal dementia and semantic dementia. *Neurology*, 58, 198–208.

Rosen, H. J., Kramer, J. H., Gorno-Tempini, M., Schuff, N., Weiner, M., & Miller, B. L. (2002). Patterns of cerebral atrophy in primary progressive aphasia. *American Journal of Geriatric Psychiatry*, 10, 89–97.

Rosen, H. J., Perry, R. J., Murphy, J., Kramer, J. H., Mychack, P., Schuff, N., et al. (2002). Emotion comprehension in the temporal variant of frontotemporal dementia. *Brain*, 125, 2286–2295.

Rosso, S. M., Kaat, L. D., Baks, T., Joosse, M., de Koning, I., Pijnenburg, Y. A. L., et al. (2003). Frontotemporal dementia in The Netherlands: Patient characteristics and prevalence estimates from a population-based study. *Brain*, 126, 2016–2022.

Snowden, J. S., Gibbons, Z. C., Blackshaw, A., Doubleday, E., Thompson, J., Craufurd, D., et al. (2003). Social cognition in frontotemporal dementia and Huntington's disease. *Neuropsychologia*, 41, 688–701.

Snowden, J. S., Goulding, P. J., & Neary, D. (1989). Semantic dementia: A form of circumscribed cerebral atrophy. *Behavioral Neurology*, 2, 167–182.

Snowden, J. S., Neary, D., & Mann, D. M. (1996). *Fronto-temporal lobar degeneration: Fronto-temporal dementia, progressive aphasia, semantic dementia*. New York: Churchill Livingstone.

Snowden, J. S., Neary, D., Mann, D. M. A., Goulding, P. J., & Testa, H. J. (1992). Progressive language disorder due to lobar atrophy. *Annals of Neurology*, 31, 174–183.

Sonty, S. P., Mesulam, M.-M., Thompson, C. K., Johnson, N., Weintraub, S., Parrish, T. B., et al. (2003). Primary progressive aphasia: PPA and the language network. *Annals of Neurology*, 53, 35–49.

Studholme, C., Cardenas, V., Blumenfeld, R., Schuff, N., Rosen, H. J., Miller, B. L., et al. (2004). Deformation tensor morphometry of semantic dementia with quantitative validation. *NeuroImage*, 21, 1387–1398.

Talbot, P. R., Lloyd, J. J., Snowden, J. S., Neary, D., & Testa, H. J. (1998). A clinical role for $^{99m}$Tc-HMPAO SPECT in the investigation of dementia? *Journal of Neurology, Neurosurgery, and Psychiatry*, 64, 306–313.

Thompson, C. K., Ballard, K. J., Tait, M. E., Weintraub, S., & Mesulam, M. (1997). Patterns of language decline in non-fluent primary progressive aphasia. *Aphasiology*, 11, 297–331.

Thompson, S. A., Patterson, K., & Hodges, J. R. (2003). Left/right asymmetry of atrophy in semantic dementia: Behavioral-cognitive implications. *Neurology*, 61, 1196–1203.

Thompson-Schill, S. L., D'Esposito, M., Aguirre, G., & Farah, M. J. (1997). Role of left inferior prefrontal cortex in retrieval of semantic knowledge: A reevaluation. *Proceedings of the National Academy of Sciences of the United States of America, 94,* 14792–14797.

Turner, R. S., Kenyon, L. C., Trojanowski, J. Q., Gonatas, N., & Grossman, M. (1996). Clinical, neuroimaging, and pathologic features of progressive non-fluent aphasia. *Annals of Neurology, 39,* 166–173.

Tyrrell, P. J., Warrington, E. K., Frackowiak, R. S. J., & Rossor, M. N. (1990). Heterogeneity in progressive aphasia due to focal cortical atrophy: A clinical and PET scan study. *Brain, 113,* 1321–1326.

Wagner, A. D., Pare-Blagoev, E. J., Clark, J., & Poldrack, R. A. (2001). Recovering meaning: Left prefrontal cortex guides controlled semantic retrieval. *Neuron, 31,* 329–336.

Warkentin, S., & Passant, U. (1997). Functional imaging of the frontal lobes in organic dementia: Regional cerebral blood flow findings in normals, in patients with frontotemporal dementia and in patients with Alzheimer's disease, performing a word fluency test. *Dementia and Geriatric Cognitive Disorders, 8,* 105–109.

Warrington, E. K. (1975). The selective impairment of semantic memory. *Quarterly Journal of Experimental Psychology, 27,* 635–657.

Whitwell, J. L., Anderson, V. M., Scahill, R. I., Rossor, M. N., & Fox, N. C. (2004). Longitudinal patterns of regional change on volumetric MRI in frontotemporal lobar degeneration. *Dementia and Geriatric Cognitive Disorders, 17,* 307–310.

Whitwell, J. L., Warren, J. D., Josephs, K. A., Godbolt, A., Revesz, T., Fox, N. C., et al. (2004). Voxel-based morphometry in tau-positive and tau-negative frontotemporal lobar degenerations. *Neurodegenerative Diseases, 1,* 225–230.

Work, M., Gee, J. C., McMillan, C., Moore, P., & Grossman, M. (2004). Voxel-based morphometric analysis of verbal fluency: Executive function vs. lexical content. *Neurology, 62,* A165–A166.

# CHAPTER 27

# Progressive Supranuclear Palsy, Corticobasal Degeneration, and the Frontal Cortex

*Irene van Balken*
*Irene Litvan*

Progressive supranuclear palsy (PSP) and corticobasal degeneration (CBD) are closely related, atypical, parkinsonian neurodegenerative disorders with prominent involvement of the frontal cortex. Since there are no biological markers for their clinical diagnosis, PSP and CBD are occasionally confused with each other and are frequently underdiagnosed (Boeve, Lang, & Litvan, 2003).

In this chapter we discuss the frontal cortical involvement in PSP and CBD, based upon current knowledge and understanding of the frontal subcortical circuits. We also focus on typical and atypical features of PSP and CBD, and their underlying neuropathological findings.

## PSP AND CBD

PSP and CBD present usually around 60 years of age, with an average disease survival of approximately 5–6 years. Both are considered 4-repeat tauopathies, because this protein aggregates in neurons and glia in affected brain areas (Dickson et al., 2002; Goedert, 2004). However, the exact underlying pathogenesis of these disorders is still unknown (Litvan, 2004).

PSP, also known as Steele–Richardson–Olszewski syndrome, and lately as the Richardson syndrome (Williams et al., 2005), is characterized by early postural instability and falls, bilateral parkinsonian involvement with tran-

sient or no benefit from levodopa therapy, oculomotor signs, and rapid disease progression (Litvan, 1998, 2004). CBD, on the other hand, can present in two ways: as an asymmetrical motor and cognitive lateralized syndrome (corticobasal syndrome) or as a bilateral frontal cognitive and parkinsonian syndrome (dementia corticobasal syndrome). The former phenotype, the corticobasal syndrome, is likely to present with a progressive unilateral parkinsonism, dystonia, myoclonus, and ideomotor or limb kinetic apraxia that spreads to the other limbs, eventually leading to severe generalized disability several years later (Boeve et al., 1999, 2003; Litvan et al., 1997). Little is known about the dementia corticobasal syndrome, for this phenotype is usually diagnosed postmortem (Grimes, Lang, & Bergeron, 1999). In this chapter, the term "corticobasal degeneration" is reserved for the pathologically confirmed disease.

## FRONTAL–SUBCORTICAL CIRCUIT INVOLVEMENT

PSP and CBD both exhibit a broad spectrum of clinical symptoms that can be related to the frontal cortex. The differences in symptomatology in PSP and CBD may in part be explained by differences in the frontosubcortical circuit involvement. The five main frontal subcortical circuits are involved in executive functions; social behavior; motivation; motor functioning and saccadic eye movements, and they affect, respectively, the dorsolateral prefrontal; orbitofrontal; medial frontal; motor and oculomotor circuits, and are discussed in this chapter.

## Dorsolateral Prefrontal Circuit

Executive dysfunction, including mechanistic planning, verbal reasoning and problem solving, is thought to be a manifestation of activity of the dorsolateral prefrontal circuit (Grafman & Litvan, 1999). This is supported by functional imaging studies (Berman et al., 1995; McIntosh, 2000; Nagahama et al., 1996), as well as neuropathological studies (Hattori et al., 2003).

In PSP, slowed information processing, poor information retrieval, concreteness in thinking, lack of insight, impaired reasoning, impaired control over attention or execution of sequential actions, and problems in shifting tasks are usually observed at early stages but become more frequent and severe with disease progression (Table 27.1) (Dubois et al., 2005; Grafman, Litvan, Gomez, & Chase, 1990; Grafman, Litvan, & Stark, 1995; Litvan, 1994; Litvan, Grafman, Gomez, & Chase, 1989; Litvan, Mega, Cummings, & Fairbanks, 1996; Pillar et al., 1994; Pillon, Dubois, Lhermitte, & Agid, 1986; Pillon, Dubois, Ploska, & Agid, 1991). With progression, patients with PSP may exhibit a dynamic aphasia, but they do not usually exhibit Broca's or Wernicke's type of aphasia. In PSP, lesions found in all regions involved in the dorsolateral prefrontal circuit (Hattori et al., 2003),[14] but mostly in the caudate, likely explain the slow information

processing and the broad spectrum of other cognitive dysfunctions.

Patients with corticobasal syndrome have varying cognitive symptoms that seem to relate to underlying pathology of cortical more than subcortical structures. In these patients the dorsolateral prefrontal cortex is usually affected; however, there is a wide interpatient variety in the severity of these lesions (Frasson et al., 1998; Litvan et al., 1997; Pillon & Dubois, 2000; Pillon et al., 1995). The degree of cognitive symptoms in an individual relates to the underlying pathology. The dysexecutive syndrome is eventually similar to that of patients with PSP. Aphasia, usually nonfluent, is observed in a significant number of patients with CBD (Frattali, Grafman, Patronas, Makhlouf, & Litvan, 2000; Jobes et al., 2006; Kertesz, Martinez-Lage, Davidson, & Munoz, 2000).

So, although there is dorsolateral frontal cortical involvement in both PSP and CBD, the frontal dysfunction usually occurs earlier and is more severe in PSP. On the other hand, language is usually more severely affected in CBD.

## Orbitofrontal Circuit

A second area of frontal subcortical circuit involvement, the orbitofrontal circuit, plays an important role in personality and emotional status. It is thought to be significantly, involved in obeying rules of social behavior, the experience of reward and punishment and the interpretation of complex emotions, as determined in functional imaging studies (Brooks & Doder, 2001; Konishi et al., 1999a, 1999b; Rolls, 1996) as well as lesion studies. Lesions within the structures of the orbitofrontal circuit can

**TABLE 27.1. Cognitive Functioning in PSP and CBD**

| | PSP | CBD Corticobasal syndrome | CBD Dementia corticobasal syndrome |
|---|---|---|---|
| Attention/concentration | +++ | ++ | +++ |
| Planning | +++ | + | +++ |
| Problem solving | +++ | + | +++ |
| Concept formation | +++ | + | +++ |
| Concrete thought | +++ | + | +++ |
| Language | + | +/+++ | +/+++ |

*Note.* + mildly impaired; ++ moderately impaired; +++ severely impaired.

result in personality changes, behavioural disinhibition and emotional lability (Chow, 2000; Cummings, 1993).

Patients with PSP frequently exhibit personality changes, often in combination with disinhibition (Table 27.2) characterized by a lack of judgment of consequences of their motor impulsivity (i.e., getting up to pick up something in the floor despite severe postural instability). On the other hand, patients with PSP usually do not talk to or take liberties with strangers as if they know them, or have other inappropriate social behaviors observed in patients with frontal lobe dementias. The orbitofrontal cortex in PSP is only mildly affected; however, the other nuclei of the orbitofrontal circuit are all mildly to moderately involved, likely resulting in the aforementioned personality changes and disinhibitive behavior.

Patients with the corticobasal syndrome, on the other hand, usually exhibit depression (73%) and, less commonly, irritability (20%) and agitation (20%) (Table 27.2) (Litvan et al., 1996; Litvan, Cummings, & Mega, 1998). Neuroimaging and neuropathological studies describe multiple brain regions involved in depression (Baker, Frith, & Dolan, 1997; Frasson et al., 1998; Mayberg et al., 1990; Ring et al., 1994), suggesting a limbic–cortical network (Mayberg, 2003). The orbitofrontal cortex is one of the most important regions linked to depression and is severely affected in these patients (Hattori et al., 2003).

## Medial Frontal Circuit

The medial frontal circuit is associated with initiation and motivation, as determined by neuroimaging (Konishi et al., 1999a, 1999b; Rolls, 1996) and neuropathological studies.

Lesions in one of the structures within this circuit are related with lack of spontaneity, apathy, and paucity of movement.

Neuropsychiatric assessment of PSP patients show a high prevalence of apathy (Table 27.2) not related to disease duration or cognitive impairment. Because apathy shares many behavioral features with depression and is frequently mistaken for a depressive disorder, patients with PSP are often treated, typically unsuccessfully, with antidepressants (Litvan et al., 1996). Neuropathological studies show a mild to moderate involvement of all the structures in the medial frontal circuit of patients with PSP (Hattori et al., 2003). Unilateral or asymmetric involvement of the orbitofrontal circuit is likely prerequisite to manifestation of biological depression, whereas bilateral involvement of the medial frontal circuit is necessary for the presence of apathy (Litvan et al., 1998). This is supported by the fact that asymmetrical cortical involvement is often observed in the corticobasal syndrome but not in PSP.

Only 40% of patients with the corticobasal syndrome exhibit apathy (Litvan et al., 1998), possibly related to anterior cingulate cortex involvement in affected patients. The anterior cingulate cortex shows a highly variable involvement in CBD (Hattori et al., 2003). Neuropsychiatric symptoms are important predictors of future admissions of patients to institutions. Thus, identification and treatment of the associated behavioral abnormalities may be relevant for improving the quality of life of patients and their caregivers.

## Motor Circuit

The basal ganglia motor output nuclei project onto the motor and premotor cortex and exert

### TABLE 27.2. Neuropsychiatric Signs in PSP and CBD

|  | PSP | CBD Corticobasal syndrome | CBD Dementia corticobasal syndrome |
|---|---|---|---|
| Depression (OFC) | 18% | 73% | ? |
| Disinhibition (OFC) | 36% | 20% | ? |
| Anxiety (OFC) | 18% | < 14% | ? |
| Apathy (MFC) | 91% | 40% | +++ |

*Note.* ? unknown; +++ severe; MFC, medial frontal circuit; OFC, orbitofrontal circuit. Data from Litvan, Mega, Cummings, and Fairbanks (1996); Litvan (1994); and Litvan, Cummings, and Mega (1998).

an important influence on our movement activity.

Patients with PSP typically exhibit axial more than limb akinesia, early postural instability, and a lack or transient levodopa (L-dopa) response. These patients usually develop a peculiar wide-based, slow, and unsteady gait that is frequently complicated by early falls or a tendency to fall (Table 27.3) (Josephs & Dickson, 2003; Litvan, 1998). Postmortem studies show severely affected putamen, pallidum, substantia nigra, and premotor and motor cortices, and moderate involvement of the other structures in the motor circuit (Hattori et al., 2003), that together result in akinesia. In addition to the pathological changes described, the involvement of the pedunculopontine nuclei and other brainstem and cerebellar nuclei are likely to account for the severe gait and postural instability. Involvement of the various nigrostriatal frontal subcortical nuclei explain the transient or lack of L-dopa response.

Patients with corticobasal syndrome exhibit an asymmetrical parkinsonism, typically presenting with a slowly progressive, unilaterally jerky, tremulous, akinetic, rigid and apraxic limb, held in a fixed dystonic posture, and eventually display an alien limb syndrome. Neuroimaging (Gerhard et al., 2004; Henkel et al., 2004; Hossain et al., 2003) and neuropathological changes in patients with corticobasal syndrome include severe involvement of premotor and motor cortices, often with asymmetry corresponding to the clinically most affected side. These functional and pathological changes are likely to cause the asymmetrical parkinsonism and contribute to apraxia, dystonia, and alien limb syndrome. Patients may characterize their limb as "having a mind of its own" and may talk about their limb in the third person. Other frequent motor symptoms are mirror movements (involuntary movements of the opposite limb imitating movements in the examined limb), and a postural or action tremor, usually reflecting an underlying myoclonus that increases with action and tactile stimulation (Table 27.3) (Litvan et al., 1997). Several neuroimaging studies have related limb apraxia to the supplementary motor areas and superior parietal regions. Apraxia is thought to be a result of motor, sensorimotor, and cognitive dysfunction (Litvan et al., 1997). The anatomical base for alien limb syndrome is not completely clear given that callosal, medial frontal lobe, and posterior parietal lobe lesions may cause this syndrome and are affected in this disorder. However, in patients with the corticobasal syndrome, neuroimaging studies link motor areas to this symptom (Valls-Sole et al., 2001) and frequently associated mirror movements (Scepkowski & Cronin-Golomb, 2003).

**TABLE 27.3. Motor Signs in PSP and CBD**

| | | CBD | |
| --- | --- | --- | --- |
| | PSP | Corticobasal syndrome | Dementia corticobasal syndrome |
| Parkinsonism | Symmetric | Asymmetric | Symmetric |
| L-Dopa response | Transient/none | Transient/none | ? |
| Axial versus limb involvement | Axial > limb | Limb | ? |
| Tremor | –/+ | Action/postural | – |
| Myoclonus | – | +/+++ | – |
| Balance disturbances | Early | Late (usually) | Late |
| Gait | Wide based, unsteady | Apraxic | Small step |
| Ideomotor apraxia | +/– | +++ | –? |
| Lateralized dystonia | +/– | +++ | –? |
| Axial dystonia | +/+++ | +/– | |
| Mirror movements | +/– | +++ | ? |
| Speech | Spastic, hypokinetic | Apraxic, hypokinetic | |

*Note.* – not present; +/– occasionally present; + mild; +++ severe, ? unknown; –? probably not present.

## Oculomotor Circuit

The different structures involved in the oculomotor circuit are of major importance in eye and eyelid movements.

Supranuclear vertical gaze palsy is a key-feature in diagnosing PSP (Table 27.4); however, it may not be present until 3 to 4 years after symptom onset and can be explained by severe lesions in the superior colliculus and acqueductal gray (Hattori et al., 2003). In addition, blink rate is profoundly diminished in PSP. Not infrequently, eyelid apraxia, lid retraction, and blepharospasm are exhibited as well. This causes a characteristic staring facial expression in PSP (Esteban, Traba, & Prieto, 2004; Rivaud-Pechoux et al., 2000; Vidailhet et al., 1994). Multiple areas are involved with eyelid movements (Esteban et al., 2004), of which the superior colliculus and the red nucleus are severely affected in patients with PSP (Hattori et al., 2003).

In the corticobasal syndrome, oculomotor apraxia typically precedes other oculomotor features (i.e., supranuclear gaze palsy) and impairs initiation of voluntary gaze and saccadic initiation, whereas pursuit and optokinetic nystagmus are preserved. Furthermore, horizontal and vertical gaze abnormalities are usually equally affected in corticobasal syndrome, whereas in PSP, vertical gaze abnormalities precede the horizontal disturbances. In patients with corticobasal syndrome, no lesions were described in either the superior colliculi, acqueductal gray, or the red nucleus in pathological cases (Hattori et al., 2003). Because oculomotor apraxia is one of the most important oculomotor features in corticobasal syndrome, other areas (e.g., superior parietal regions) might contribute to these symptoms.

## PARIETAL CORTICAL INVOLVEMENT

Besides the frontal subcortical circuits, the parietal cortex is also involved in CBD. Symptoms in patients with corticobasal syndrome vary and seem to relate to underlying pathology of cortical more than subcortical structures, which is clearly apparent in parietal involvement. These may be manifested by the severe ideomotor and at times ideatory apraxia, as well as corticosensory disturbances. Involvement of cortical areas in CBD explain the frequently observed motor aphasia in patients with involvement of the dominant hemisphere, and the visuospatial disturbances (neglect) observed when the nondominant hemisphere is more prominently affected (Graham, Bak, & Hodges, 2003). During disease progression, both hemispheres eventually can be affected, with consequent development of a dementia syndrome (Frattali et al., 2000)

## EPILOGUE

Using the frontosubcortical circuits as our guideline, we have discussed commonalities and differences in clinical features of both PSP and CBD, and have related them to findings in neuroimaging and neuropathology. Both disorders show a broad involvement of structures of the different frontal–subcortical pathways, with a diversity of symptoms. Several studies show that the severity of motor and cognitive signs is not related to each other, implicating that the frontosubcortical pathways are not affected in parallel. This explains a diversity of clinical symptoms in the early disease stages, leading to a challenging diagnostic task for clinicians.

## TABLE 27.4. Oculomotor Signs in PSP and CBD

|  | PSP | CBD | |
| --- | --- | --- | --- |
|  |  | Corticobasal syndrome | Dementia corticobasal syndrome |
| Supranuclear gaze palsy | +++ | +/– | ? |
| Saccades | Normal latency, slow | High latency, normal | ? |
| Oculomotor apraxia | – | ++ | –? |

*Note.* + mild; +/– occasionally present; ++ moderate; +++ severe; – not present; ? unknown; –? probably not present.

## REFERENCES

Baker, S. C., Frith, C. D., & Dolan, R. J. (1997). The interaction between mood and cognitive function studied with PET. *Psychological Medicine, 27*(3), 565–578.

Berman, K. F., Ostrem, J. L., Randolph, C., Gold, J., Goldberg, T. E., Coppola, R., et al. (1995). Physiological activation of a cortical network during performance of the Wisconsin Card Sorting Test: a positron emission tomography study. *Neuropsychologia, 33*(8), 1027–1046.

Boeve, B. F., Lang, A. E., & Litvan, I. (2003). Corticobasal degeneration and its relationship to progressive supranuclear palsy and frontotemporal dementia. *Annals of Neurology, 54*(Suppl. 5), S15–S19.

Boeve, B. F., Maraganore, D. M., Parisi, J. E., Ahlskog, J. E., Graff-Radford, N., Caselli, R. J., et al. (1999). Pathologic heterogeneity in clinically diagnosed corticobasal degeneration. *Neurology, 53*(4), 795–800.

Brooks, D. J., & Doder, M. (2001). Depression in Parkinson's disease. *Current Opinion in Neurology, 14*(4), 465–470.

Chow, T. W. (2000). Personality in frontal lobe disorders. *Current Psychiatry Reports, 2*(5), 446–451.

Cummings, J. L. (1993). Frontal–subcortical circuits and human behavior. *Archives of Neurology, 50*(8), 873–880.

Dickson, D. W., Bergeron, C., Chin, S. S., Duyckaerts, C., Horoupian, D., Ikeda, K., et al. (2002). Office of Rare Diseases neuropathologic criteria for corticobasal degeneration. *Journal of Neuropathology and Experimental Neurology, 61*(11), 935–946.

Dubois, B., Slachevsky, A., Pillon, B., Beato, R., Villalponda, J. M., & Litvan, I. (2005). "Applause sign" helps to discriminate PSP from FTD and PD. *Neurology, 64*(12), 2132–2133.

Esteban, A., Traba, A., & Prieto, J. (2004). Eyelid movements in health and disease: The supranuclear impairment of the palpebral motility. *Neurophysiologie Clinique, 34*(1), 3–15.

Frasson, E., Moretto, G., Beltramello, A., Smania, N., Pampanin, M., Stegagno, C., et al. (1998). Neuropsychological and neuroimaging correlates in corticobasal degeneration. *Italian Journal of Neurological Sciences, 19*(5), 321–328.

Frattali, C. M., Grafman, J., Patronas, N., Makhlouf, F., & Litvan, I. (2000). Language disturbances in corticobasal degeneration. *Neurology, 54*(4), 990–992.

Gerhard, A., Watts, J., Trender-Gerhard, I., Turkheimer, F., Banati, R. B., Bhatia, K., et al. (2004). *In vivo* imaging of microglial activation with [$^{11}$C](R)-PK11195 PET in corticobasal degeneration. *Movement Disorders, 19*(10), 1221–1226.

Goedert, M. (2004). Tau protein and neurodegeneration. *Seminars in Cell and Developmental Biology, 15*(1), 45–49.

Grafman, J., & Litvan, I. (1999). Importance of deficits in executive functions. *Lancet, 354,* 1921–1923.

Grafman, J., Litvan, I., Gomez, C., & Chase, T. N. (1990). Frontal lobe function in progressive supranuclear palsy. *Archives of Neurology, 47*(5), 553–558.

Grafman, J., Litvan, I., & Stark, M. (1995). Neuropsychological features of progressive supranuclear palsy. *Brain and Cognition, 28*(3), 311–320.

Graham, N. L., Bak, T. H., & Hodges, J. R. (2003). Corticobasal degeneration as a cognitive disorder. *Movement Disorders, 18*(11), 1224–1232.

Grimes, D. A., Lang, A. E., & Bergeron, C. B. (1999). Dementia as the most common presentation of cortical-basal ganglionic degeneration. *Neurology, 53*(9), 1969–1974.

Hattori, M., Hashizume, Y., Yoshida, M., Iwasaki, Y., Hishikawa, N., Ueda, R., et al. (2003). Distribution of astrocytic plaques in the corticobasal degeneration brain and comparison with tuft-shaped astrocytes in the progressive supranuclear palsy brain. *Acta Neuropathologica (Berlin), 106*(2), 143–149.

Henkel, K., Karitzky, J., Schmid, M., Mader, I., Glatting, G., Unger, J. W., et al. (2004). Imaging of activated microglia with PET and [$^{11}$C]PK 11195 in corticobasal degeneration. *Movement Disorders, 19*(7), 817–821.

Hossain, A. K., Murata, Y., Zhang, L., Taura, S., Saitoh, Y., Mizusawa, H., et al. (2003). Brain perfusion SPECT in patients with corticobasal degeneration: Analysis using statistical parametric mapping. *Movement Disorders, 18*(6), 697–703.

Josephs, K. A., & Dickson, D. W. (2003). Diagnostic accuracy of progressive supranuclear palsy in the Society for Progressive Supranuclear Palsy brain bank. *Movement Disorders, 18*(9), 1018–1026.

Josephs, K. A., Petersen, R. C., Knopman, D. S., Boeve, B. F., Whitwell, J. L., Duffy, J. R., et al. (2006). Clinicopathologic analysis of frontotemporal and corticobasal degenerations and PSP. *Neurology, 66*(1), 41–48.

Kertesz, A., Martinez-Lage, P., Davidson, W., & Munoz, D. G. (2000). The corticobasal degeneration syndrome overlaps progressive aphasia and frontotemporal dementia. *Neurology, 55*(9), 1368–1375.

Konishi, S., Kawazu, M., Uchida, I., Kikyo, H., Asakura, I., & Miyashita, Y. (1999). Contribution of working memory to transient activation in human inferior prefrontal cortex during performance of the Wisconsin Card Sorting Test. *Cerebral Cortex, 9*(7), 745–753.

Konishi, S., Nakajima, K., Uchida, I., Kikyo, H., Kameyama, M., & Miyashita, Y. (1999). Common inhibitory mechanism in human inferior prefrontal cortex revealed by event-related functional MRI. *Brain, 122*(5), 981–991.

Litvan, I. (1994). Cognitive disturbances in progressive supranuclear palsy. *Journal of Neural Transmission: Supplementum, 42,* 69–78.

Litvan, I. (1998). Progressive supranuclear palsy revisited. *Acta Neurologica Scandinavica, 98*(6), 73–84.

Litvan, I. (2004). Update on progressive supranuclear palsy. *Current Neurology and Neuroscience Reports, 4*(4), 296–302.

Litvan, I., Agid, Y., Goetz, C., Jankovic, J., Wenning, G. K., Brandel, J. P., et al. (1997). Accuracy of the clinical diagnosis of corticobasal degeneration: A clinicopathologic study. *Neurology, 48*(1), 119–125.

Litvan, I., Cummings, J. L., & Mega, M. (1998). Neuropsychiatric features of corticobasal degeneration. *Journal of Neurology, Neurosurgery, and Psychiatry, 65*(5), 717–721.

Litvan, I., Grafman, J., Gomez, C., & Chase, T. N. (1989). Memory impairment in patients with progressive supranuclear palsy. *Archives of Neurology, 46*(7), 765–767.

Litvan, I., Mega, M. S., Cummings, J. L., & Fairbanks, L. (1996). Neuropsychiatric aspects of progressive supranuclear palsy. *Neurology, 47*(5), 1184–1189.

Mayberg, H. S. (2003). Modulating dysfunctional limbic–cortical circuits in depression: Towards development of brain-based algorithms for diagnosis and optimised treatment. *British Medical Bulletin, 65*, 193–207.

Mayberg, H. S., Starkstein, S. E., Sadzot, B., Preziosi, T., Andrezejewski, P. L., Dannals, R. F., et al. (1990). Selective hypometabolism in the inferior frontal lobe in depressed patients with Parkinson's disease. *Annals of Neurology, 28*(1), 57–64.

McIntosh, A. R. (2000). Towards a network theory of cognition. *Neural Networks, 13*(8–9), 861–870.

Nagahama, Y., Fukuyama, H., Yamauchi, H., Matsuzaki, S., Konishi, J., Shibasaki, H., et al. (1996). Cerebral activation during performance of a card sorting test. *Brain, 119*(5), 1667–1675.

Pillon, B., Blin, J., Vidailhet, M., Deweer, B., Sirigu, A., Dubois, B., et al. (1995). The neuropsychological pattern of corticobasal degeneration: Comparison with progressive supranuclear palsy and Alzheimer's disease. *Neurology, 45*(8), 1477–1483.

Pillon, B., Deweer, B., Michon, A., Malapani, C., Agid, Y., Dubois, B., et al. (1994). Are explicit memory disorders of progressive supranuclear palsy related to damage to striatofrontal circuits?: Comparison with Alzheimer's, Parkinson's, and Huntington's diseases. *Neurology, 44*(7), 1264–1270.

Pillon, B., & Dubois, B. (2000). Memory and executive processes in corticobasal degeneration. *Advances in Neurology, 82*, 91–101.

Pillon, B., Dubois, B., Lhermitte, F., & Agid, Y. (1986). Heterogeneity of cognitive impairment in progressive supranuclear palsy, Parkinson's disease, and Alzheimer's disease. *Neurology, 36*(9), 1179–1185.

Pillon, B., Dubois, B., Ploska, A., & Agid, Y. (1991). Severity and specificity of cognitive impairment in Alzheimer's, Huntington's, and Parkinson's diseases and progressive supranuclear palsy. *Neurology, 41*(5), 634–643.

Ring, H. A., Bench, C. J., Trimble, M. R., Brooks, D. J., Frackowiak, R. S., & Dolan, R. J. (1994). Depression in Parkinson's disease. A positron emission study. *British Journal of Psychiatry, 165*(3), 333–339.

Rivaud-Pechoux, S., Vidailhet, M., Gallouedec, G., Litvan, I., Gaymard, B., & Pierrot-Deseilligny, C. (2000). Longitudinal ocular motor study in corticobasal degeneration and progressive supranuclear palsy. *Neurology, 54*(5), 1029–1032.

Rolls, E. T. (1996). The orbitofrontal cortex. *Philosophical Transactions of the Royal Society of London: Series B, Biological Sciences, 351*, 1433–1443.

Scepkowski, L. A., & Cronin-Golomb, A. (2003). The alien hand: Cases, categorizations, and anatomical correlates. *Behavioral and Cognitive Neuroscience Reviews, 2*(4), 261–277.

Valls-Sole, J., Tolosa, E., Marti, M. J., Valldeoriola, F., Revilla, M., Pastor, P., et al. (2001). Examination of motor output pathways in patients with corticobasal ganglionic degeneration using transcranial magnetic stimulation. *Brain, 124*(6), 1131–1137.

Vidailhet, M., Rivaud, S., Gouider-Khouja, N., Pillon, B., Bonnet, A. M., Gaymard, B., et al. (1994). Eye movements in parkinsonian syndromes. *Annals of Neurology, 35*(4), 420–426.

Williams, D. R., de Silva, R., Paviour, D. C., Pittman, A., Watt, H. C., Kilford, L., et al. (2005). Characteristics of two distinct clinical phenotypes in pathologically proven progressive supranuclear palsy: Richardson's syndrome and PSP-parkinsonism. *Brain, 128*(6), 1247–1258.

# CHAPTER 28

# Frontal Variant of Alzheimer's Disease

*Julene K. Johnson*
*Arne Brun*
*Elizabeth Head*

Alzheimer's disease (AD) is a progressive neurodegenerative disorder and the most common cause of dementia in older adults. It is accepted that AD typically begins with a progressive memory impairment and later affects language, executive function, visuospatial skills, and daily living functions (Grady et al., 1988; Hodges & Patterson, 1995; Welsh, Butters, Hughes, Mohs, & Heyman, 1991). This clinical progression is believed to reflect the relatively predictable sequence of neurofibrillary neuropathology accumulation beginning in the entorhinal cortex and spreading to the cortical regions (Arnold et al., 1991; Braak & Braak, 1991; Brun & Englund, 1981). The classic AD neuropathology also includes neuron loss, the abnormal accumulation of ß-amyloid in senile plaques with hyperphosphorylated tau proteins, and dystrophic neurites.

Atypical presentations of AD have been also described from clinical, imaging, and neuropathological perspectives. These presentations are considered "atypical" because (1) nonmemory or behavioral changes may be the first symptom, (2) nonmemory or behavioral symptoms may predominate throughout the course of the disease, or (3) the distribution of neuropathology may differ from the typical pattern. Discussion about the heterogeneity of AD began with Alois Alzheimer's first papers (1907, 1907/1987, 1911; Alzheimer, Forstl, & Levy, 1911/1991) and continues to spark debate 100

years later. The prevalence of the atypical presentations of AD is not known, but a few reports suggest that approximately 14–17% of patients with AD may have focal nonmemory presentations (Becker, Huff, Nebes, Holland, & Boller, 1988; Galton, Patterson, Xuereb, & Hodges, 2000).

One could argue that it is important to define both the "typical" and "atypical" presentations of a disease. However, one could also argue that it is not scientifically useful to focus on variations in a clinical or neuropathological presentation that represent one disease, and that these variations do not have an underlying biological basis. Several authors have hypothesized the existence of subgroups in AD (Cummings, 2000; Vogt, Vogt, & Hof, 2001). Because the definitive diagnosis of AD can only be determined at autopsy, an accurate clinical diagnosis of AD remains critical. Until we have a definitive clinical diagnostic test for AD, we are left with improving our clinical tools. As disease-specific therapeutics become available, it will be even more important to diagnose AD accurately.

Our goal in this chapter is to discuss the heterogeneity of AD, with a particular emphasis on the frontal variant of AD. We argue that studying atypical presentations of AD can be useful for understanding brain–behavior relationships and the underlying biological mechanisms of AD.

## EARLY OBSERVATIONS OF HETEROGENEITY IN AD

In the early 1900s, Alois Alzheimer (1906, 1907, 1911) described the clinical and neuropathological findings of two patients who presented with an unusual progressive disorder in later middle life. The first patient, a 51-year-old woman referred to as Auguste D, suddenly developed jealousy toward her husband and shortly thereafter experienced a rapid decline in memory, frequently got lost, and had delusions that people were going to kill her. As described in Perusini (1909, 1909/1987), Alzheimer examined Auguste D and described severe deficits in language, orientation, and memory, as well as delusions and anxiety. He considered the deficits in language to be focal, which contrasted with a relative preservation of motor skills. Alzheimer noted:

> During the course of the disease symptoms appeared which could be considered focal symptoms; sometimes these were prominent and sometimes quite faint. But they were always mild. Mental regression advanced quite steadily. After four and one half years of illness the patient died. (1907/1987, p. 2; original German in Note 1)

He considered the clinical presentation atypical because it did not resemble other, known clinical patterns with an onset in later middle age. At autopsy, Alzheimer found an "evenly affected atrophic brain without macroscopic foci" and the deposition of cored plaques and intracellular fibrils (now known as neurofibrillary tangles). A few years later, Alzheimer (1911) described a second patient, Johann F, a 56-year-old man who first became "quiet and dull," and then 1.5 years later developed symptoms of forgetfulness, getting lost, overeating, poor hygiene, and difficulty performing simple tasks. Alzheimer again considered the presence of focal symptoms (i.e., agnosia, aphasia, apraxia), noting, however, that they were difficult to analyze because of severe language deficits. At autopsy, he discussed the distribution of neuropathology:

> A further peculiarity of the present case was the localization of the alterations. Even if we were dealing with a diffuse disease of the cortex alone, the parietal and temporal lobes bilaterally were unmistakably especially affected and much more so than the frontal brain. In ordinary cases of se-

nile dementia, the frontal brain is the most severely diseased, as has been found only recently by Simchowicz. (1911/1991, p. 92; original German in Note 2)

It is remarkable that Alzheimer noticed a predominance of atrophy in the parietal and temporal lobes, while noting that others, namely Simchowicz (1910), had recently observed prominent atrophy in the frontal cortex. Although he described evenly distributed gross atrophy of Auguste D's brain, Alzheimer observed focal parietal and temporal lobe atrophy in the brain of Johann F. Other early researchers, such as Fischer (1907/1987), Bonfiglio (1908/1987), and Perusini (1909), focused on describing the specific histopathological findings and not the regional distribution of neuropathology. It is clear that Alzheimer thought about both focal symptoms and focal atrophy patterns. His prior interest in dementia in older adults and "general paralysis" (i.e., neurosyphilis) (Alzheimer, 1898, 1899, 1899/1991) provided a good background for differentiating between AD and other mental disorders in elderly individuals.

From these early descriptions through the 1950s, however, AD was known as a global disorder that was secondary to diffuse neuropathological involvement. A disproportionate emphasis was placed on differentiating presenile and senile dementia based on the age of onset (Benson, 1986; Katzman & Bick, 2000). The issue of clinical and pathological heterogeneity was discussed, however, to a lesser degree. A common theme involved differentiating between AD and Pick's disease. For example, Rothschild and Kasanin (1936) described a 49-year-old man who developed changes in behavior (i.e., childish, euphoric, overactive) and cognition that resembled that in Pick's disease. At autopsy, the patient had focal atrophy of the frontal cortex, widespread cell loss and plaques, and tangles characteristic of AD. Delay and Brion (1962) identified three groups with focal atrophy, including one group with focal frontal cortex atrophy. Others also described focal frontal lobe atrophy in patients with AD neuropathology (Abeley, Desclaux, Naudascher, & Suttel, 1945; Divry, Levy, & Titeca, 1935; Kreindler, Hornet, & Appel, 1959; Liebers, 1939; Moyano, 1932; Seitelberger & Jellinger, 1958; Tariska, 1970). Berlin (1949) described a patient who had focal temporal lobe atrophy, a combination of plaques and tangles, but also "inflated cells of Pick." Observations of focal (circumscribed) cerebral atrophy on gross examination of the brain and a combination of both AD and Pick's disease neuropathology in some cases led early clinicians to question whether AD and Pick's disease could be differentiated clinically (Chlopicki & Rzewuska-Szatowska, 1971; Sjogren, Sjogren, & Lindgren, 1952).

In 1957, Lars Gustafson and David Ingvar at the University of Lund (Sweden) began a clinical and metabolic brain imaging study, with the goal of prospectively following the development of symptoms and imaging changes in dementia and ultimately improving diagnostics and therapy (Gustafson, Hagberg, Holley, Risberg, & Ingvar, 1970; Ingvar et al., 1968). This study also allowed for the study of atypical presentations of dementia. The first neuropathological findings from this study were presented at the Seventh International Congress of Neuropathology in Budapest in 1974 (Brun, Gustafson, & Ingvar, 1975), where the authors reported a relationship between neuropathological findings, neuropsychiatric symptoms, and regional cerebral blood flow in presenile dementia. Additional studies addressed the relationship between neuropathology and clinical symptoms. Based on a histological grading of the regional severity of the neuronal degeneration, the team found a predominance of degeneration in the limbic system (i.e., amygdala, hippocampus) and inferior temporal-parietal areas (Gustafson, Brun, & Ingvar, 1977). In addition, a focus on the posterior cingulate cortex was added (Brun & Gustafson, 1976, 1978). This neuropathological pattern was later confirmed by PET imaging (Minoshima, Foster, & Kuhl, 1994; Minoshima et al., 1997), and the regional pattern of pathology was further systematized by Braak and Braak (1991, 1995). In 1970, Lauter discussed the difference between senile and presenile AD, pointing out that senile dementia was more global than presenile dementia, with less pronounced temporoparietal focus and relatively more frontal involvement in the senile form.

Much of the early work on heterogeneity focused on defining the clinical syndromes of AD and Pick's disease. The early researchers also were interested in determining whether AD was a focal or global disorder. These early studies highlight the consideration of both typical and atypical presentations of AD.

## CLINICAL HETEROGENEITY OF AD

After almost 100 years since Alzheimer described his first cases of AD, the issue of clinical heterogeneity still stimulates discussion. In addition to the traditional clinical and neuropathological approaches, new data from neuroimaging and behavioral studies have added to the understanding of AD heterogeneity. A renewed interest in focal presentations of dementia emerged in the 1980s, when several authors hypothesized that AD might underlie a number of focal presentations of dementia (Chui, Teng, Henderson, & Moy, 1985; Kirshner, Webb, Kelly, & Wells, 1984; Mayeux, Stern, & Spanton, 1985). However, only a few were autopsy-confirmed, including patients with AD and pronounced behavioral symptoms (Brun, 1987; Tariska, 1970) or disproportionate impairment on visuospatial (Crystal, Horoupian, Katzman, & Jotkowitz, 1982; Faden & Townsend, 1976; Hof, Bouras, Constantinidis, & Morrison, 1989) or language domains (Pogacar & Williams, 1984). These initial clinicopathological studies also made the point that focal clinical symptoms could be associated with focal and disproportionate neuropathology in corresponding brain regions. For example, patients with pronounced behavioral symptoms were found to have pronounced AD neuropathology in the frontal cortex. Based on the observations of cognitive heterogeneity, several authors proposed the existence of distinct subgroups in AD (Becker et al., 1988; Martin et al., 1986; Mayeux et al., 1985), a concept that has persisted (Black, 1996; Cummings, 2000; Galton et al., 2000; Martin, 1990; Vogt et al., 1999, 2001). In 1987, the National Institutes of Health sponsored a conference that focused on the heterogeneity of AD (Friedland et al., 1988), and an open peer commentary involving several authors was published in 2000 (Cummings, 2000). In a large study of 407 autopsy-confirmed patients with AD, Kanne, Balota, Storandt, McKeel, and Morris (1998) correlated three subgroups with different distributions of neuropathology, including frontal cortex/mental control, temporal cortex/verbal memory, and parietal cortex/visuospatial subgroups.

Clinical heterogeneity of AD has also been studied from a neuroimaging perspective. Metabolic imaging studies suggest a relationship between focal cognitive deficits and metabolic changes in specific brain regions. In one of the first detailed early studies of cognitive and neuroimaging heterogeneity in AD, Foster and colleagues (1983), using positron emission tomography (PET), found that patients with AD who had prominent visuospatial impairment had focal hypometabolism in the right parietal cortex, whereas focal language deficits were associated with marked hypometabolism in the left hemisphere. Martin and colleagues (1986) used factor analysis of cognitive scores and identified patients with probable AD who had prominent language or visuospatial deficits. When correlated with PET, patients with prominent language deficits had greater left temporoparietal hypometabolism, whereas the patients with prominent visuospatial deficits had greater right temporoparietal hypoperfusion. Others confirmed that patients with AD and prominent visuospatial deficits have lower blood flow in the parietal cortex, whereas patients with prominent language deficits have pronounced hypometabolism in the left perisylvian region (Bokde et al., 2001; Celsis, Agniel, Rascol, & Marc-Vergnes, 1987; Chase et al., 1984; Grady et al., 1990; Haxby, Duara, Grady, Cutler, & Rapoport, 1985; Haxby et al., 1988; Mann, Mohr, Gearing, & Chase, 1992; Pietrini et al., 1996). Grady and colleagues (1990) found a subgroup of patients with a combination of temporoparietal and frontal cortex hypometabolism in patients with AD and behavioral disturbances, and Waldemar and colleagues (1994) found frontal hypometabolism in 19 of 25 patients with AD.

Although episodic memory dysfunction is still considered the most prominent cognitive symptom in AD (Lange et al., 2002; Welsh et al., 1991), it is now more widely recognized that AD can present with disproportionate impairment in nonmemory domains, such as executive functioning, visuospatial, and language abilities. However, the National Institute of Neurological and Communicative Disorders and Stroke, and Alzheimer's Disease and Related Disorders Association (NINCDS-ADRDA) criteria (McKhann et al., 1984) require the presence of a memory deficit as one of the affected cognitive domains for a clinical diagnosis of probable or possible AD. The clinical diagnosis of dementia, as outlined in the fourth edition of the *Diagnostic and Statistical Manual of Mental Disorders* (DSM-IV; American Psychiatric Association, 1994), also requires the presence of a memory deficit that is sufficient to produce a functional impairment. These criteria may therefore exclude some atypical presentations of AD (Mayeux et al., 1985) and create a diagnostic challenge for atypical presentations of AD.

## EXECUTIVE FUNCTION IN AD

"Executive function" is cognitive ability that involves the planning and execution of complex, goal-oriented behaviors (Lezak, 1995; Stuss & Knight, 2002). More specifically, executive function includes attentional control, setting of goals, set shifting, abstraction, response monitoring, and flexibility. Executive function can be subdivided into subcomponents based on functional and anatomical bases; however, there is not yet agreement on the best models of executive function. Executive dysfunction is a central feature of several neurodegenerative and psychiatric disorders, such as frontotemporal dementia (FTD), progressive supranuclear palsy, schizophrenia, and major depression. In the early stages of AD, some patients report difficulties with concentration, multitasking, problem solving, and, sometimes, behavior. However, executive dysfunction is traditionally not considered to be a core feature of AD (Nebes & Brady, 1989). Several studies suggest that executive dysfunction occurs later in the course of AD (Nestor, Parasuraman, Haxby, & Grady, 1991; Pillon, Dubois, Lhermitte, & Agid, 1986).

More recent studies suggest that executive dysfunction may be an early feature of AD (Binetti et al., 1996; Collette, Van der Linden, & Salmon, 1999; Cummings & Benson, 1992; Sgaramella et al., 2001). In one of the early longitudinal imaging studies, Grady and colleagues (1988) studied memory, executive function, and language in patients with early AD. The results suggested that executive dysfunction (i.e., Porteus Maze Test, Trail Making Test B, Raven's Progressive Matrices) occurred after memory impairment but before visuospatial and language impairment. Other studies have attempted to identify which subcomponents of executive function are impaired versus preserved in AD (Duke & Kaszniak, 2000; Perry & Hodges, 1999). In another early study, Laflèche and Albert (1995) found that 20 patients with Ad and mild dementia performed significantly worse than controls on measures of executive function that required concurrent manipulation of information (i.e., Trail Making Test B, Self-Ordering Test, verbal fluency [FAS], Hukok Test). Other studies suggest that sustained and divided attention remains intact in early AD, whereas selective attention is impaired (Laflèche & Albert, 1995; Nebes & Brady, 1989; Perry, Watson, & Hodges, 2000). Inhibitory function in early AD is also impaired (Collette, Van der Linden, Delrue, & Salmon, 2002). Perry and colleagues (2000) also argue that selective attention is affected only after an initial amnestic stage in early AD. However, when comparing AD with other frontal lobe dementias, most studies suggest that patients with FTD exhibit greater executive dysfunction than those withAD (Pachana, Boone, Miller, Cummings, & Berman, 1996; Perry & Hodges, 2000; Razani, Boone, Miller, Lee, & Sherman, 2001).

Evidence also suggests that there is a subgroup of AD patients with disproportionate executive impairment and behavioral disturbances. We have discussed early neuropathological studies and further discussion about a frontal variant of AD from a clinical and neuropathological perspective follows. Binetti and colleagues (1996) split patients with mild AD into two groups based on executive function measures: those who scored below one standard deviation of controls on tests of executive function (i.e., Wisconsin Card Sorting Test [WCST], release from proactive interference, verbal fluency, and Stroop) and those who scored within the normal range. The patients with and without executive impairment performed similarly on tests from other cognitive domains (i.e., memory, language, visuospatial), suggesting that a subgroup of patients with disproportionate executive impairment. Others have observed a prominent executive dysfunction with relatively preserved memory in AD (Baddeley, Della Sala, & Spinnler, 1991; Becker, 1988; Becker, Bajulaiye, & Smith, 1992). Below we discuss the clinical and pathological characteristics of a frontal variant of AD.

Thus, executive dysfunction appears to be an important cognitive domain in the understanding of AD. The underlying etiology of executive dysfunction in AD is also not yet known. Cummings (1998) suggests that a disruption in the frontal–subcortical circuits may contribute to executive dysfunction in AD.

## BEHAVIORAL CORRELATES OF EXECUTIVE DYSFUNCTION IN AD

Executive dysfunction in AD has also been linked with behavioral symptoms (e.g., apathy, aggression, depression, and psychosis) and functional impairment. Additional studies using brain imaging have found an association between behavioral disturbances and frontal lobe dysfunction. A few studies have explored the relationship with specific behavioral syndromes, neuropathology, and genetics.

Apathy in AD has been associated with executive dysfunction, functional impairment, and prefrontal hypometabolism. Several studies suggest that patients with AD and apathy perform worse on tests of executive function than patients with AD without apathy (Kuzis, Sabe, Tiberti, Dorrego, & Starkstein, 1999; McPherson, Fairbanks, Tiken, Cummings, & Back-Madruga, 2002). Patients with AD with apathy and prominent executive dysfunction also have more functional impairment on activities of daily living (Boyle et al., 2003; Stout, Wyman, Johnson, Peavy, & Salmon, 2003). A pronounced hypometabolism in prefrontal and anterior temporal cortex in patients with AD and significant apathy (Craig et al., 1996) suggests that frontal lobe dysfunction may be related to the development of apathy.

Executive dysfunction has also been linked with agitation and aggression. For example, Chen, Sultzer, Hinkin, Mahler, and Cummings (1998) found that poor performance on tests of executive function was associated with agitation, disinhibition, and functional impairment. Another study found that patients with AD and poor executive function had more agitation and functional impairment than patients with AD and intact executive function (Back-Madruga et al., 2002; Cummings & Back, 1998). Aggression in AD patients correlates with left frontotemporal hypometabolism (Hirono, Mega, Dinov, Mishkin, & Cummings, 2000; Sultzer et al., 1995) and is associated with an increase in neurofibrillary tangles in the orbitofrontal and anterior cingulate cortex (Tekin et al., 2001). Agitation in AD has been linked to polymorphisms associated with serotonin (Assal et al., 2004; Craig, Hart, Carson, McIlroy, & Passmore, 2004; Sukonick et al., 2001) and the apolipoprotein ε4 allele (Craig, Hart, McCool, McIlroy, & Passmore, 2004).

Finally, psychosis in AD has also been linked with executive dysfunction and frontal hypometabolism. For example, Swanberg, Tractenberg, Mohs, Thal, and Cummings (2004) found a relationship between poor performance on tests of executive function, psychosis, and greater impairment on activities of daily living. Psychosis in AD has also been linked to prefrontal hypometabolism (Mega et al., 2000; Sultzer et al., 1995, 2003). Early studies suggested an increase in frontal cortex neuropathology in patients with AD and psychosis (Zubenko et al., 1991); however, better controlled studies have not found this pattern (Forstl, Burns, Levy, & Cairns, 1994; Sweet et al., 2000). Psychosis in AD is also associated with serotonin polymorphisms (Holmes, Arranz, Powell, Collier, & Lovestone, 1998; Nacmias et al., 2001) and an interleukin promoter polymorphism (Craig, Hart, et al., 2004).

There is clearly an link between executive function, behavior, and functional impairment in AD. The underlying reason for this link is not yet known. However, genetic and neuropathological studies may improve understanding. It appears that patients with AD and prominent executive dysfunction are at risk for poor clinical outcomes.

## FRONTAL VARIANT OF AD

As can be gleaned from a review of the history of AD, there has been a long-standing interest in examining the heterogeneity of AD. Over the years, it became clear that the typical presentation of AD involves an early decline in memory, followed by deficits in other domains and a typical predominance of plaques and tangles in the hippocampal formation and temporoparietal cortex. However, as described earlier, there were early reports of patients with prominent frontal atrophy (on gross examination), AD neuropathology, and sometimes a significant behavioral syndrome.

However, it was not until the work by Brun and Gustafson that the clinicopathological relationship between behavioral dysfunction and a predominance of frontal cortex neuropathology was better linked. Brun (1987) and Gustafson (1987) described the neuropathological findings on 26 patients with a frontal or frontotemporal presentation of dementia. Of these, 16 (62%) had neuropathological evidence of neuron loss, gliosis, and spongiosis in the superficial layers, primarily in the frontal and, to a lesser extent, temporal lobes, currently referred to as dementia lacking distinctive histopathological features (DLDH) or frontotemporal lobar degeneration (FTLD). The insula and cingulate gyrus were also affected. The remaining patients had Pick's disease (*n* = 4), Creutzfeldt–Jakob disease (*n* = 3), AD (*n* = 2), and one patient had thalamic infarctions. Appendix 28.1 includes the clinical summaries for the two patients with AD. Both patients had early and prominent changes in personality, judgment, and memory, and focal frontal hypometabolism on imaging. At autopsy, Brun described a predominance of plaques and tangles, neuronal loss, gliosis, and spongiosis in the frontal cortex when compared with other cortical regions. In these two patients, the topographic pattern for the severity of the AD departed markedly from the predominant temporoparietal pattern, with a far more pronounced degeneration in the prefrontal area than usual. An incomplete white matter infarction could be added, though it was not exclusively frontal. In the second case, there was evidence of a diseased striatum. This may explain the impression of a frontal dysfunction that was possibly reinforced by the frontal blood flow decrement. Thus, these two cases suggest a strong association between the clinical profile, brain imaging, and a predominance of AD neuropathology in the frontal cortex. They also showed that AD can be associated with a FTD-like phenotype.

Later in 1999, Johnson, Head, Kim, Starr, and Cotman were studying an atypical presentation of AD that involved early and prominent impairments on tests of verbal fluency and set shifting. We hypothesized that patients with AD and prominent executive dysfunction in the early stages of dementia would also have a predominance of pathology in the prefrontal cortex. After reviewing pathology-confirmed AD cases with clinical data from the mild stage of AD (i.e., Mini-Mental State Exam [MMSE] ≥ 18), we identified three patients with an impairment on two tests of executive function (i.e., verbal fluency [FAS] and the Trail Making Test). We then compared these patients with three typical patients with AD matched in dementia severity, age, education, and extent of neurofibrillary tangle pathology in the entorhinal cortex (to control for disease severity). The groups did not differ on measures of memory, language, or visuospatial skills. However, the frontal variant AD group had an approximately 10 times greater degree of neurofibrillary tangle pathology in the prefrontal cortex (area 8). We suggested that the correlation between cognitive patterns and neuropathological distribution represented a subgroup of AD with prominent executive dysfunction and greater-than-expected prefrontal cortex neuropathology.

Vogt and colleagues (1999) described an 85-year-old man (FG) who exhibited significant behavioral changes (i.e., paranoia, aggression) and executive dysfunction, and AD neuropathology at autopsy. His first symptom was a severe paranoia related to truck drivers. The plaques and tangles were most prominent in the prefrontal cortex and cingulate. In another study, Johnson, Vogt, Kim, Cotman, and Head (2004) described a nondemented individual with an isolated impairment on a test of executive function and preserved memory, with a predominance of both tangle and plaque neuropathology in the prefrontal cortex when compared to other regions.

There also may exist a relationship with genetics and neurobiology. Several authors have found a presenilin-1 mutation associated with a familial FTD phenotype (Raux et al., 2000; Tang-Wai et al., 2002), including one autopsy-confirmed patient with Pick's disease (Dermaut et al., 2004). Another recent study found a presenilin-1 polymorphism in an autopsy-confirmed patient with AD with an FTD phenotype (Goldman et al., 2005). In terms of underlying biological differences, Talbot and colleagues (2000) found a significant decrease in a marker of membrane function, phospholipase A2, in the frontal cortex when compared with other brain regions and typical patients with AD.

Although there are a number of reports about patients with a frontal or executive presentation of AD, the phenotype is not yet thoroughly described. A combination of cognitive, behavioral, functional, brain imaging, genetic, and neuropathological studies have not yet been done.

## FRONTAL CORTEX NEUROPATHOLOGY IN AGING AND AD

To better understand why the frontal cortex is more affected in some patients with AD, we review the literature about the frontal cortex in healthy aging and AD. The aging brain suffers a general atrophy that is, however, most marked in the white matter and cortex of the frontal lobe, second only to the hippocampus. Frontal white matter may be particularly vulnerable to the aging process as described in studies using *in vivo* imaging procedures, as well as postmortem autopsy experiments (Buckner, 2004). With age, frontal cortical atrophy (Raz, Gunning-Dixon, Head, Dupuis, & Acker, 1998), a loss of white matter integrity (Madden et al., 2004; O'Sullivan et al., 2001), and white matter lesions detected as hyperintensities (de Groot et al., 2000) are all associated with poorer cognition and, specifically, executive function in nondemented older adults. The mechanisms underlying cortical atrophy and white matter loss/dysfunction have not been fully elucidated but may be related to observations in postmortem studies. For example, genes important for maintaining synaptic plasticity, vesicular transport, and mitochondrial function are downregulated in the aged frontal cortex (Lu, 2004). Some studies of protein levels reflecting synapse loss are consistent with gene expression studies and demonstrate synapse protein loss (Liu, Erickson, & Brun, 1996; Masliah, Mallory, Hanson, DeTeresa, & Terry, 1993), but others show no change with age (Haas, Hung, & Selkoe, 1991; Honer, Dickson, Gleeson, & Davies, 1992). A study using unbiased, stereology-based estimates of synapse number in the frontal cortex also suggested that the frontal cortex synapse number appears unaffected with age in nondemented individuals (Scheff, Price, & Sparks, 2001). Variable reports may stem from the cases included in the study, the region of frontal cortex examined, and other possible methodological issues (e.g., types of synapse number and quantification methods). Liu and Brun (1995), on the other hand, found a progressive, age-related loss of frontal cortical synapse density amounting to roughly 40% between ages 20 and 100. Mitochondrial dysfunction observed in the frontal cortex of older adults (Ojaimi, Masters, Opeskin, McKelvie, & Byrne, 1999) and cumulative oxidative damage observed with age (Ames & Shigenaga, 1992) may also be related to neuron dysfunction or losses, and/or cortical atrophy reported in imaging studies, and is consistent with decreased gene expression results. Another sign of frontal pathology is increased astrogliosis (Unger, 1998), and messenger RNA (mRNA) levels for the astrocyte cytoskeletal protein glial fibrillary acidic protein, also increase with age (Nichols, Day, Laping, Johnson, & Finch, 1993). In combination, these results suggest that the frontal cortex is vulnerable to aging, and neurobiological changes may be reflected in impairments in frontal lobe function. Last, from a phylogenetic and ontogenetic point of view, the frontal lobes, with their protracted and late maturation, would be expected to be selectively vulnerable, which is all the more obvious when compared with the adjoining sensorimotor cortex that is old, early, and robust.

In AD, significant frontal cortex pathology is observed, but it is not typically a focus of neuropathology studies. AD is characterized by widespread senile plaque and neurofibrillary tangle (NFT) formation throughout association cortex and within limbic regions, leaving primary sensory or motor cortex relatively intact (Brun & Gustafson, 1976). In 1991, a careful description of a large number of samples in an autopsy study by Braak and Braak led to the description of various stages of either senile plaque or NFT distribution. In this study, cases that had come to autopsy from several hospitals, but not from geriatric psychiatry institutions, were used. Of 83 cases, 29 had a clinical diagnosis of dementia, but 8 subsequently did not have AD pathology, and 4 cases were adults with Down's syndrome; the remaining cases were clinically undescribed. Six stages of NFT formation were observed with the entorhinal cortex and hippocampus affected early in the disease. Although, later in the disease, neocortex accumulates NFT pathology, Braak and Braak staging does not differentiate between frontal cortex and other regions of the brain as being more or less affected. With senile plaque accumulation, only three stages could be consistently categorized due to significant interindividual variability. Stage A was characterized as showing β-amyloid (Aβ) within the basal forebrain (including basal portions of the frontal, temporal and occipital lobes) including weakly stained clouds of Aβ within the presubiculum and entorhinal cortex.

In a more recent study, a series of 51 prospectively followed, clinically characterized patients with autopsies were used to describe four phases of Aβ deposition. In this study, Aβ appears in neocortex (frontal, parietal, temporal, and occipital) early in disease, followed by entorhinal, hippocampus, amygdala, and insular cortex (Thal, Rub, Orantes, & Braak, 2002).

Thus, based on careful descriptions of large autopsy series, the frontal cortex appears to be affected significantly by Aβ, possibly early in AD, but late in disease by NFT accumulation. This contrasts with the hippocampus and underlying cortex, where NFT formation predominates early in disease. Selective memory deficits in mild cognitive impairment (MCI) and more severe memory deficits in AD may be related to early involvement of limbic structures but also possibly to frontal cortex dysfunction. A recent stereology-based study of NFT and neuron counts that included a subregion of the frontal cortex (area 9) demonstrated a significant association between overall dementia severity, measured by MMSE, and frontal cortex pathology, in addition to hippocampal and entorhinal cortex pathology (Sarazin et al., 2003). However, a subset of patients with AD presents with early and predominant executive dysfunction, as described below.

In addition to senile plaques and NFT, white matter pathology also reflects neuronal dysfunction. Frontal cortex infarcts but, in particular, incomplete white matter infarcts (i.e., not associated with complete infarcts) may cause or reinforce a frontal dysfunction. They may be part of more general white matter damage, but the frontal white matter is a common preferential location in AD (Brun & Englund, 1986). Most likely, this preferential frontal white matter damage is caused by repeated episodes of hypoperfusion due to blood pressure drops, in addition to arteriolosclerosis that affects the autoregulatory vascular response. This may develop in discrete steps and may build up in a seemingly progressive course. Incomplete white matter infarcts also surround lacunes in Binswanger's disease when they may engage wide areas, particularly the frontal white substance. The mechanism by which they may cause dysfunction is by partial undermining of the cortex or destroying cholinergic transport routes passing through the white matter on their way from nucleus basalis of Meynert via the extreme capsule to the frontal cortex. This way they may thus add or reinforce a frontal dysfunction in AD and other dementias. In the case of transport blockage, they may explain a beneficiary effect of cholinergic treatment in vascular diseases.

In addition, selective pyramidal neuron loss (Hof, Bouras, Constantinides, & Morrison, 1990), loss of synaptic proteins (Masliah et al., 2001) or reduced expression of genes related to synaptic vesicle trafficking (Yao et al., 2003), loss of synuclein immunoreactivity, and myelin basic protein immunoreactivity (Wang et al., 2004a, 2004b) have all been detected in frontal cortex. Synapse loss in the frontal cortex may be an early event in AD progression, because a 25% loss of synaptophysin has been reported in patients with a Clinical Dementia Rating (CDR) of 0.5 (Masliah et al., 2001). Furthermore, loss of synuclein and myelin basic protein in frontal cortex correlates with deficits in frontal function (Wang et al., 2004a, 2004b). Myelin basic protein loss may be a mechanism underlying reports of significant white matter pathology in AD visualized by *in vivo* imaging.

Establishing the neurobiological mechanisms underlying impaired frontal cortex function in AD is challenging. First, postmortem studies are more heavily weighted toward the examination of end-stage disease cases, which is an unavoidable limitation to studying AD. Less frequent are the number of studies of individuals that came to autopsy earlier in the disease process, when selective cognitive deficits may be apparent. These cases can be invaluable for establishing a link between cognition and neuropathology, but they are infrequent. In a cohort of 210 subjects with possible AD, only nine subjects exhibited atypical signs of prominent frontal dysfunction (Villareal et al., 2003). But these atypical cases can be instructive (Vogt et al., 2001). For example, autopsy studies in nondemented individuals with select and severe impairment in memory (amnestic MCI) provided solid evidence that this is an early form of AD based on significant pathology in the hippocampus and entorhinal cortex (Morris et al., 2001). Focal frontal atrophy was also observed in another case study of a patient with early signs of dysexecutive syndrome and was also linked to diffuse frontal Aß deposition (Vogt et al., 1999). We recently reported a case study of an individual with a selective and severe impairment in executive function that, at autopsy, exhibited significant frontal senile plaque and NFT pathology (Johnson et al., 2004). Second, there may be a bias toward selectively studying

the hippocampus given that AD is commonly associated with memory impairment. Although frontal cortex specimens may be included in these studies, they are less likely to be a focus of the link between cognition and neuropathology in AD. This may, in turn, be due to inherent difficulties with studying the neuropathology of the frontal cortex. The frontal cortex is complex and contains multiple anatomical and functional domains, and selection of key regions of interest is difficult to establish. Based on models of how AD pathology begins and spreads (Braak & Braak, 1991, 1995), it is surprising that executive dysfunction would occur early in AD, because the frontal cortex is affected later in the course.

## CURRENT CONCEPTUALIZATION OF FRONTAL VARIANT OF AD

The key question remains: Does the clinical heterogeneity in AD reflect biologically distinct disorders or variability in the expression of the same disease? It is still not possible to answer this research question definitively. However, 100 years of research about AD has helped to focus the question. There is now more clinical, cognitive, imaging, behavioral, genetic, and neuropathological evidence to suggest that AD is heterogeneous and subgroups are likely. However, the underlying neurobiological basis of the heterogeneity in AD remains a mystery.

Several authors have hypothesized that heterogeneity in AD is highly influenced by the location, degree, and type of neuropathology. Clearly, the pattern of neurodegeneration in AD is not uniform (Brun & Englund, 1981; Vogt et al., 2001), and there is considerable evidence regarding the selective vulnerability of different cortical regions and subregions (Detoledo-Morrell et al., 1997; Morrison & Hof, 2002; Vogt et al., 1999). There is also evidence that cognitive and behavioral deficits vary according to which brain areas are most involved (Kanne et al., 1998). It is not yet known whether there is variability in the location of initial AD neuropathology. The type of AD neuropathology may also affect heterogeneity. Whereas tangles only are increased in some reports of focal presentations of AD, others report an increase in both plaques and tangles. Other neuropathological lesions, such as white matter loss or vascular changes, may also influence the heterogeneity. However, there are not good methods to evaluate the interaction among all these pathological variables. It is also possible that multiple etiologies or comorbid medical conditions could affect the heterogeneous presentation of AD. For example, coexistent Lewy body, cerebrovascular, white matter pathologies can affect the clinical expression of AD (Lopez et al., 2000). It is also plausible that focal deficits are influenced by multiple brain regions. For example, executive dysfunction can arise from both prefrontal cortex or subcortical damage, thus damaging frontal–subcortical circuits or other areas connected with the prefrontal cortex (Collette et al., 2002; Cummings, 1998; Perry & Hodges, 1999).

There are also hints that genetics may influence the heterogeneity in AD. The strongest support for this hypothesis comes from studying in association of genetic polymorphisms and specific behavioral syndromes in AD. Another hypothesis is that developmental or premorbid vulnerabilities may interact with environmental factors to create heterogeneity of disease expression.

It is also important to keep in mind that clinical heterogeneity could reflect diagnostic inaccuracy. In fact, many of the studies we have discussed do not have pathological confirmation of AD. Although diagnostic accuracy at tertiary centers for typical AD is good (> 90% accurate) (Lopez et al., 2000), diagnosis of atypical AD remains difficult. Focal presentations of dementia can be caused by a number of neurodegenerative diseases (Black, 1996; Kramer & Miller, 2000). It is important to study heterogeneity in the preclinical or early stages of dementia.

Thus, the frontal subgroup or variant of AD remains a hypothesis. New clinical, imaging, and genetic approaches to the heterogeneity of AD will improve diagnosis and allow better differentiation from non-AD dementias. Studying the early stages of dementia, such as the frontal presentation of MCI, will also help elucidate the neurobiological basis. The probability of a frontal presentation of AD also expands the need for better differential diagnosis and better comparisons with other neurodegenerative diseases that affect the frontal lobes (e.g., frontotemporal dementia, Huntington's disease, Creutzfeldt–Jakob disease). Future research should combine clinical, cognitive, behavioral, brain imaging, genetics, and neuropathological approaches to studying heterogeneity in AD.

## APPENDIX 28.1. CLINICAL DESCRIPTIONS OF CASES 1 AND 2 OF BRUN (1987)

*Case 1.* An 81-year-old woman (EL) previously in good health started around age 65 to suffer from personality changes with poor judgment, increasing forgetfulness, restlessness, unrest, and general loss of interest. At age 73, she was admitted under the diagnosis of senile dementia. Somatically, her condition was unremarkable. She became increasingly confused and disturbed, aggressive, and talked incoherently. She was disoriented as to time, person, and whereabouts, and could not carry on a conversation. She was unable to manage her daily living activities. She soon became incontinent and bedridden, lying in her bed in a fetal position, now with increased general muscle tone and with a left-sided positive Babinski. She also developed epilepsy, that began with a couple of grand mal seizures and a diffusely coarse, dysrhythmic electroencephalogram (EEG) with a left-sided focus, though later her epilepsy subsided and became less disturbing to the patient and her surroundings. Regional cerebral blood flow recorded 6 years after admission showed bilateral prefrontal hypoperfusion, with a slight left–right asymmetry; 3 years later, it showed marked left-sided frontal and frontotemporal hypoperfusion, yet a year later indicated 20% reduction in left-hemispheric average flow and marked focal decrement frontally and frontotemporally on both sides. The clinical picture was considered somewhat unclear but suggestive of FTD. Her dementia progressed and she died at the age of 81. Autopsy showed pulmonary emboli and bilateral bronchopneumonia as the cause of death. Grossly, the brain weighed 960 grams and showed a general atrophy that was most marked in the frontal lobes. Microscopic examination revealed AD, and in accord with the gross atrophy pattern, the AD changes were most intense in the prefrontal areas. There were no complete infarcts, but there were incomplete infarcts, though more parietally than frontally. The motor cortex was well preserved, as was the calcarine cortex, and the parietal cortex took an intermediate position with regard to severity of microscopic AD changes.

*Case 2.* A woman (BH), age 70 at death, was admitted at age 68 under a suspicion of FTD. Previously healthy, she suffered from memory difficulties from age 65 on. On admission she had urinary incontinence and ate only on command. Her condition rapidly worsened and she became confused and had to be cared for around the clock. Two years after admission, she was completely disoriented but could state her name and answer questions only with a yes. Regional cerebral blood flow studies indicated a frontal dysfunction. She was unconcerned, disoriented, and denied any somatic or psychiatric symptoms. Three years after admission, she was apraxic, with a somewhat staggering, short-paced gait. Computed tomography (CT) showed a general brain atrophy, and a repeat cerebral blood flow study indicated a frontal hypoperfusion; now, in addition, there was a postcentral flow decrement with some side asymmetry. Postmortem, only the brain was available for analysis. It weighed 910 grams, with a general atrophy, though somewhat more pronounced basotemporally. Microscopy revealed AD with an unusually severe involvement of the frontal lobes, including the anterior portion of the cingulate gyrus. Also, somewhat unusually, there was a degeneration of the caudate nucleus with gliosis, though with only scattered plaques. There were also cavitating infarcts underneath the sensorimotor gyri, and a general white matter incomplete infarction that included the frontal lobes.

## NOTES

1. "Im weiteren Verlaufe treten die als Herdsymptome zu deutenden Erscheinungen bald stärker, bald schwächer hervor. Immer sind sie nur leicht. Dagegen macht die allgemeine Verblödung Fortschritte. Nach 4½ jähriger Krankheitsdauer tritt der Tod ein" (Alzheimer, 1907, p. 147).

2. "Eine weitere Besonderheit des vorliegenden Falles lag in der Lokalisation der Veränderungen. Wenn es sich auch um eine diffuse Erkrankung der ganzen Rinde (abgesehen von dem übringen Zentralnervensystem) handelte, so waren doch unverkennbar beiderseits Scheitel- und Schläfenlappen besonders stark und stärker als das Stirnhirn betroffen. Bei den gewöhnlichen Fällen der senilen Demenz ist jedenfalls das Stirnhirn am erheblichsten erkrankt, wie das neuerdings auch wieder Simchowicz gefunden hat" (Alzheimer, 1911, p. 377).

## REFERENCES

Abéley, X., Desclaux, P., Naudascher, J., & Suttel, R. (1945). Maladie d'Alzheimer avec atrophie frontale prédominante [Alzheimer's disease with predominant frontal atrophy]. *Annals Médico-Psychologiques, 1*, 151–157.

Alzheimer, A. (1898). Neuer Arbeiten uber die dementia senilis und die auf atheromatoser Gefasserkrankung basierenden Gehirnkrankheiten [Newer studies on senile dementia and brain diseases caused by atheromatous vascular disease]. *Monatschrift für Psychiatrie und Neurologie, 3*, 101–115.

Alzheimer, A. (1899). Beitrag zur pathologischen Anatomie der Seelenströrungen des Greisenalters [A contribution concerning the pathological anatomy of mental disturbances in old age]. *Allgemeine Zeitschrift für Psychiatrie und psychisch-gerichtliche Medizin, 56*, 272–273.

Alzheimer, A. (1899/1991). A contribution concerning the pathological anatomy of mental disturbances in old age. *Alzheimer Disease and Associated Disorders, 5*, 69–70.

Alzheimer, A. (1906). Uber einen eigenartigen schweren Erkrankungsprozess der Hirnrinde [On an extraordinary, severe disease process of the cerebral cortex]. *Neurologisches Zentralblatt, 25*, 1134.

Alzheimer, A. (1907). Ueber eine eigenartige Erkrankung der Hirnrinde. *Allgemeine Zeitschrift für Psychiatrie und Psychisch-Gerichtliche Medizin, 64*, 146–148.

Alzheimer, A. (1907/1987). A characteristic disease of the cerebral cortex. In K. Bick, L. Amaducci, & G. Pepeu (Eds.), *The early story of Alzheimer's disease.* New York: Raven.

Alzheimer, A. (1911). Ueber eigenartige Krankheitsfalle des spateren Alters. *Zeitschrift für die gesamte Neurologie und Psychiatrie, 4*, 356–385.

Alzheimer, A., Forstl, H., & Levy, R. (1911/1991). On certain peculiar diseases of old age. *History of Psychiatry, 2*, 71–101.

American Psychiatric Association. (1994). *Diagnostic and statistical manual of mental disorders* (4th ed.). Washington, DC: Author.

Ames, B. N., & Shigenaga, M. K. (1992). Oxidants are a major contributor to aging. *Annals of the New York Academy of Sciences, 663*, 85–96.

Arnold, S. E., Hyman, B. T., Flory, J., Damasio, A. R., & Van Hoesen, G. W. (1991). The topographical and neuroanatomical distribution of neurofibrillary tangles and neuritic plaques in the cerebral cortex of patients in Alzheimer's disease. *Cerebral Cortex, 1*, 103–116.

Assal, F., Alarcon, M., Solomon, E. C., Masterman, D., Geschwind, D. H., & Cummings, J. L. (2004). Association of the serotonin transporter and receptor gene polymorphisms in neuropsychiatric symptoms in Alzheimer disease. *Archives of Neurology, 61*, 1249–1253.

Back-Madruga, C., Boone, K. B., Briere, J., Cummings, J., McPherson, S., Fairbanks, L., et al. (2002). Functional ability in executive variant Alzheimer's disease and typical Alzheimer's disease. *Clinical Neuropsychology, 16*, 331–340.

Baddeley, A. D., Della Sala, S., & Spinnler, H. (1991). The two-component hypothesis of memory deficit in Alzheimer's disease. *Journal of Clinical and Experimental Neuropsychology, 13*, 372–380.

Becker, J. T. (1988). Working memory and secondary memory deficits in Alzheimer's disease. *Journal of Clinical and Experimental Neuropsychology, 10*, 739–753.

Becker, J. T., Bajulaiye, O., & Smith, C. (1992). Longitudinal analysis of a two component model of the memory deficit in Alzheimer's disease. *Psychological Medicine, 22,* 437–445.

Becker, J. T., Huff, R. J., Nebes, R. D., Holland, A., & Boller, F. (1988). Neuropsychological function in Alzheimer's disease: Pattern of impairment and rates of progression. *Archives of Neurology, 45,* 263–268.

Benson, D. F. (1986). Alzheimer's disease: The pedigree. In A. B. Scheibel, A. F. Wechsler, & M. A. B. Brazier (Eds.), *The biological substrates of Alzheimer's disease* (pp. 1–7). New York: Academic Press.

Berlin, L. (1949). Presenile sclerosis (Alzheimer's disease) with features resembling Pick's disease. *Archives of Neurology and Psychiatry, 61,* 369–384.

Binetti, G., Magni, E., Padovani, S., Cappa, S. F., Bianchetti, A., & Trabucchi, M. (1996). Executive dysfunction in early Alzheimer's disease. *Journal of Neurology, Neurosurgery, and Psychiatry, 60,* 91–93.

Black, S. E. (1996). Focal cortical atrophy syndromes. *Brain and Cognition, 31,* 188–229.

Bokde, A. L., Pietrini, P., Ibanez, V., Furey, M. L., Alexander, G. E., Graff-Radford, N. R., et al. (2001). The effect of brain atrophy on cerebral hypometabolism in the visual variant of Alzheimer disease. *Archives of Neurology, 58,* 480–486.

Bonfiglio, F. (1908/1987). Concerning special findings in a case of probable cerebral syphilis. In K. Bick, L. Amaducci, & G. Pepeu (Eds.), *The early story of Alzheimer's disease* (pp. 19–31). New York: Raven.

Boyle, P. A., Malloy, P. F., Salloway, S., Cahn-Weiner, D. A., Cohen, R., & Cummings, J. L. (2003). Executive dysfunction and apathy predict functional impairment in Alzheimer disease. *American Journal of Geriatric Psychiatry, 11,* 214–221.

Braak, H., & Braak, E. (1991). Neuropathological stageing of Alzheimer-related changes. *Acta Neuropathologica, 82,* 239–259.

Braak, H., & Braak, E. (1995). Staging of Alzheimer's disease-related neurofibrillary changes. *Neurobiology of Aging, 16,* 271–284.

Brun, A. (1987). Frontal lobe degeneration of non-Alzheimer type: I. Neuropathology. *Archives of Gerontology and Geriatrics, 6,* 193–208.

Brun, A., & Englund, E. (1981). Regional pattern of degeneration in Alzheimer's disease: Neuronal loss and histopathological grading. *Histopathology, 5,* 549–564.

Brun, A., & Englund, E. (1986). A white matter disorder in dementia of the Alzheimer type: A pathoanatomical study. *Annals of Neurology, 19,* 253–262.

Brun, A., & Gustafson, L. (1976). Distribution of cerebral degeneration in Alzheimer's disease: A clinico-pathological study. *Archiv für Psychiatrie und Nervenkrankheiten, 223,* 15–33.

Brun, A., & Gustafson, L. (1978). Limbic lobe involvement in presenile dementia. *Archiv für Psychiatrie und Nervenkrankheiten, 226,* 79–93.

Brun, A., Gustafson, L., & Ingvar, D. H. (1975). Neuropathological findings related to neuropsychiatric symptoms and regional cerebral blood flow in presenile dementia. In *VIIth International Congress of Neuropathology* (pp. 101–105). Amsterdam: Excerpta Medica.

Buckner, R. L. (2004). Memory and executive function in aging and AD: Multiple factors that cause decline and reserve factors that compensate. *Neuron, 44*(1), 195–208.

Celsis, P., Agniel, A., Puel, M., Rascol, A., & Marc-Vergnes, J. P. (1987). Focal cerebral hypoperfusion and selective cognitive deficit in dementia of the Alzheimer type. *Journal of Neurology, Neurosurgery, and Psychiatry, 50,* 1602–1612.

Chase, T. N., Foster, N. L., Fedio, P., Brooks, R., Mansi, L., & Di Chiro, G. (1984). Regional cortical dysfunction in Alzheimer's disease as determined by positron emission tomography. *Annals of Neurology, 15*(Suppl.), S170–S174.

Chen, S. T., Sultzer, D. L., Hinkin, C. H., Mahler, M. E., & Cummings, J. L. (1998). Executive dysfunction in Alzheimer's disease: Association with neuropsychiatric symptoms and functional impairment. *Journal of Neuropsychiatry and Clinical Neurosciences, 10,* 426–432.

Chlopicki, K., & Rzewuska-Szatowska, M. (1971). [Differential diagnosis in Alzheimer–Pick disease]. *Psychiatria Polska, 5,* 363–366.

Chui, H. C., Teng, E. L., Henderson, V. W., & Moy, A. C. (1985). Clinical subtypes of dementia of the Alzheimer type. *Neurology, 35,* 1544–1550.

Collette, F., Van der Linden, M., Delrue, G., & Salmon, E. (2002). Frontal hypometabolism does not explain inhibitory dysfunction in Alzheimer disease. *Alzheimer Disease and Associated Disorders, 16,* 228–238.

Collette, F., Van der Linden, M., & Salmon, E. (1999). Executive dysfunction in Alzheimer's disease. *Cortex, 35,* 57–72.

Craig, A. H., Cummings, J. L., Fairbanks, L., Itti, L., Miller, B. L., Li, J., et al. (1996). Cerebral blood flow correlates of apathy in Alzheimer disease. *Archives of Neurology, 53,* 1116–1120.

Craig, D., Hart, D. J., Carson, R., McIlroy, S. P., & Passmore, A. P. (2004). Allelic variation at the A218C tryptophan hydroxylase polymorphism influences agitation and aggression in Alzheimer's disease. *Neuroscience Letters, 363,* 199–202.

Craig, D., Hart, D. J., McCool, K., McIlroy, S. P., & Passmore, A. P. (2004). Apolipoprotein E ε4 allele influences aggressive behaviour in Alzheimer's disease. *Journal of Neurology, Neurosurgery, and Psychiatry, 75,* 1327–1330.

Crystal, H. A., Horoupian, D. S., Katzman, R., & Jotkowitz, S. (1982). Biopsy-proved Alzheimer disease presenting as a right parietal lobe syndrome. *Annals of Neurology, 12,* 186–188.

Cummings, J. L. (1998). Frontal–subcortical circuits and human behavior. *Journal of Psychosomatic Research, 44,* 627–628.

Cummings, J. L. (2000). Cognitive and behavioral heterogeneity in Alzheimer's disease: Seeking the neurobiological basis. *Neurobiology of Aging, 21*, 845–861.

Cummings, J. L., & Back, C. (1998). The cholinergic hypothesis of neuropsychiatric symptoms in Alzheimer's disease. *American Journal of Geriatric Psychiatry, 6*, S64–S78.

Cummings, J. L., & Benson, D. F. (1992). *Dementia: A clinical approach*. Boston: Butterworth-Heinemann.

de Groot, J. C., de Leeuw, F. E., Oudkerk, M., van Gijn, J., Hofman, A., Jolles, J., et al. (2000). Cerebral white matter lesions and cognitive function: The Rotterdam Scan Study. *Annals of Neurology, 47*(2), 145–151.

Delay, J., & Brion, S. (1962). *Les démences tardives* [Late-onset dementia]. Paris: Masson.

Dermaut, B., Kumar-Singh, S., Engelborghs, S., Theuns, J., Rademakers, R., Saerens, J., et al. (2004). A novel presenilin 1 mutation associated with Pick's disease but not beta-amyloid plaques. *Annals of Neurology, 55*, 617–626.

Detoledo-Morrell, L., Sullivan, M. P., Morrell, F., Wilson, R. S., Bennett, D. A., & Spencer, S. (1997). Alzheimer's disease: *In vivo* detection of differential vulnerability of brain regions. *Neurobiology of Aging, 18*, 463–468.

Divry, P., Ley, J., & Titeca, J. (1935). Maladie d'Alzhiemer avec atrophie frontale predominante [Alzheimer's disease with predominant frontal atrophy]. *Journal Belge de Neurologie et de Psychiatrie, 35*, 495–507.

Duke, L. M., & Kaszniak, A. W. (2000). Executive control functions in degenerative dementias: A comparative review. *Neuropsychology Review, 10*, 75–99.

Faden, A. I., & Townsend, J. J. (1976). Myoclonus in Alzheimer's disease. *Archives of Neurology, 33*, 278–280.

Fischer, O. (1907/1987). Miliary necrosis with nodular proliferation of the neurofibrils, a common change of the cerebral cortex in senile dementia. In K. Bick, L. Amaducci, & G. Pepeu (Eds.), *The early story of Alzheimer's disease* (pp. 5–18). New York: Raven.

Forstl, H., Burns, A., Levy, R., & Cairns, N. (1994). Neuropathological correlates of psychotic phenomena in confirmed Alzheimer's disease. *British Journal of Psychiatry, 165*, 53–59.

Foster, N. L., Chase, T. N., Fedio, P., Patronas, N. J., Brooks, R. A., & Di Chiro, G. (1983). Alzheimer's disease: Focal cortical changes shown by positron emission tomography. *Neurology, 33*, 961–965.

Friedland, R. P., Koss, E., Haxby, J. V., Grady, C. L., Luxenberg, J., Schapiro, M. B., et al. (1988). NIH conference: Alzheimer disease: Clinical and biological heterogeneity. *Annalso of Internal Medicine, 109*, 298–311.

Galton, C. J., Patterson, K., Xuereb, J. H., & Hodges, J. R. (2000). Atypical and typical presentations of Alzheimer's disease: A clinical, neuropsychological, neuroimaging and pathological study of 13 cases. *Brain, 123*(3), 484–498.

Goldman, J. S., Johnson, J. K., McElligott, K.,

Suchowersky, O., Miller, B. L., & Van Deerlin, V. M. (2005). The presenilin 1 Glu318Gly polymorphism: Interpret with caution. *Archives of Neurology, 62*, 1624–1627.

Grady, C. L., Haxby, J. V., Horwitz, B., Sundaram, M., Berg, G., Schapiro, M., et al. (1988). Longitudinal study of the early neuropsychological and cerebral metabolic changes in dementia of the Alzheimer type. *Journal of Clinical and Experimental Neuropsychology, 10*, 576–596.

Grady, C. L., Haxby, J. V., Schapiro, M. B., Gonzalez-Aviles, A., Kumar, A., Ball, M. J., et al. (1990). Subgroups in dementia of the Alzheimer type identified using positron emission tomography. *Journal of Neuropsychiatry and Clinical Neurosciences, 2*, 373–384.

Gustafson, L. (1987). Frontal lobe degeneration of non-Alzheimer type: II. Clinical picture and differential diagnosis. *Archives of Gerontology and Geriatrics, 6*, 209–223.

Gustafson, L., Brun, A., & Ingvar, D. H. (1977). Clinical and neurocirculatory findings in presenile dementia related to neuropathological changes. *Activitas Nervosa Superior, 19*(Suppl. 2), 351–353.

Gustafson, L., Hagberg, B., Holley, J. W., Risberg, J., & Ingvar, D. H. (1970). Regional cerebral blood flow in organic dementia with early onset: Correlations with psychiatric symptoms and psychometric variables. *Acta Neurologica Scandinavica, 46*(Suppl. 43), 74–45.

Haas, C., Hung, A. Y., & Selkoe, D. J. (1991). Processing of beta-amyloid precursor protein in microglia and astrocytes favors an internal localization over constitutive secretion. *Journal of Neuroscience, 11*, 3783–3793.

Haxby, J. V., Duara, R., Grady, C. L., Cutler, N. R., & Rapoport, S. R. (1985). Relations between neuropsychological and cerebral metabolic asymmetries in early Alzheimer's disease. *Journal of Cerebral Blood Flow and Metabolism, 5*, 193–200.

Haxby, J. V., Grady, C. L., Koss, E., Horwitz, B., Schapiro, M., Friedland, M. P. et al. (1988). Heterogeneous anterior–posterior metabolic patterns in dementia of the Alzheimer type. *Neurology, 38*, 1853–1863.

Hirono, N., Mega, M. S., Dinov, I. D., Mishkin, F., & Cummings, J. L. (2000). Left frontotemporal hypoperfusion is associated with aggression in patients with dementia. *Archives of Neurology, 57*, 861–866.

Hodges, J. R., & Patterson, K. (1995). Is semantic memory consistently impaired early in the course of Alzheimer's disease?: Neuroanatomical and diagnostic implications. *Neuropsychologia, 33*, 441–459.

Hof, P. R., Bouras, C., Constantinidis, J., & Morrison, J. H. (1989). Balint's syndrome in Alzheimer's disease: Specific disruption of the occipito-parietal visual pathway. *Brain Research, 493*, 368–375.

Hof, P. R., Bouras, C., Constantinidis, J., & Morrison, J. H. (1990). Selective disconnection of specific visual association pathways in cases of Alzheimer's disease presenting with Balint's syndrome. *Journal of Neuro-pathology and Experimental Neurology, 49*, 168–184.

Holmes, C., Arranz, M. J., Powell, J. F., Collier, D. A., & Lovestone, S. (1998). 5-HT$_{2A}$ and 5-HT$_{2C}$ receptor polymorphisms and psychopathology in late onset Alzheimer's disease. *Human Molecular Genetics, 7*, 1507–1509.

Honer, W. G., Dickson, D. W., Gleeson, J., & Davies, P. (1992). Regional synaptic pathology in Alzheimer's disease. *Neurobiology of Aging, 13*(3), 375–382.

Ingvar, D., Obrist, W., Chivian, E., Cronquist, S., Risberg, J., Gustafson, L., et al. (1968). General and regional abnormalities of cerebral blood flow in senile and "presenile" dementia. *Scandinavian Journal of Clinical and Laboratory Investigation: Supplement, 102*, XII:B.

Johnson, J. K., Head, E., Kim, R., Starr, A., & Cotman, C. W. (1999). Clinical and pathological evidence for a frontal variant of Alzheimer disease. *Archives of Neurology, 56*, 1233–1239.

Johnson, J. K., Vogt, B. A., Kim, R., Cotman, C. W., & Head, E. (2004). Isolated executive impairment and associated frontal neuropathology. *Dementia and Geriatric Cognitive Disorders, 17*, 360–367.

Kanne, S. M., Balota, D. A., Storandt, M., McKeel, D. W., Jr., & Morris, J. C. (1998). Relating anatomy to function in Alzheimer's disease: Neuropsychological profiles predict regional neuropathology 5 years later. *Neurology, 50*, 979–985.

Katzman, R., & Bick, K. (2000). *Alzheimer disease: The changing view.* San Diego, CA: Academic Press.

Kirshner, H. J., Webb, W. G., Kelly, M. P., & Wells, C. E. (1984). Language disturbance: An initial symptom of cortical degenerations and dementia. *Archives of Neurology, 41*, 491–496.

Kramer, J., & Miller, B. (2000). Alzheimer's disease and its focal variants. *Seminars in Neurology, 20*, 447–454.

Kreindler, A., Hornet, T., & Appel E. (1959). Complex forms of cerebral senility. *Rumanian Medical Review, 3*, 43–47.

Kuzis, G., Sabe, L., Tiberti, C., Dorrego, F., & Starkstein, S. E. (1999). Neuropsychological correlates of apathy and depression in patients with dementia. *Neurology, 52*, 1403–1407.

Laflèche, G., & Albert, M. S. (1995). Executive function deficits in mild Alzheimer's disease. *Neuropsychology, 9*, 313–320.

Lange, K. L., Bondi, M. W., Salmon, D. P., Galasko, D., Delis, D. C., Thomas, R. G., et al. (2002). Decline in verbal memory during preclinical Alzheimer's disease: Examination of the effect of APOE genotype. *Journal of the International Neuropsychological Society, 8*, 943–955.

Lauter, H. (1970). Über spätformen der Alzheimerschen Krankheit und ihre Beziehung zur senilen Demenz [Late forms of Alzheimer's disease and their relationship to senile dementia]. *Psychiatria Clinica, 3*, 169–189.

Lezak, M. D. (1995). *Neuropsychological assessment* (3rd ed.). New York: Oxford University Press.

Liebers, M. (1939). Alzheimersche Krankheit mit Pickscher Atrophie der Stirnlappen. *Archiv für Psychiatrie und Nervenkrankheiten, 109*, 363–370.

Liu, X., & Brun, A. (1995). Synaptophysin immunoreactivity is stable 36 h postmortem. *Dementia, 6*, 211–217.

Liu, X., Erikson, C., & Brun, A. (1996). Cortical synaptic changes and gliosis in normal aging, Alzheimer's disease and frontal lobe degeneration. *Dementia, 7*(3), 128–134.

Lopez, O. L., Becker, J. T., Klunk, W., Saxton, J., Hamilton, R. L., Kaufer, D. I., et al. (2000). Research evaluation and diagnosis of possible Alzheimer's disease over the last two decades: II. *Neurology, 55*, 1863–1869.

Lu, T., Pan, Y., Kao, S.-Y., Li, C., Kohane, I., Chan, J., et al. (2004). Gene regulation and DNA damage in the ageing human brain. *Nature, 429*, 883–891.

Madden, D. J., Whiting, W. L., Huettel, S. A., White, L. E., MacFall, J. R., & Provenzale, J. M. (2004). Diffusion tensor imaging of adult age differences in cerebral white matter: Relation to response time. *NeuroImage, 21*(3), 1174–1181.

Mann, U. M., Mohr, E., Gearing, M., & Chase, T. N. (1992). Heterogeneity in Alzheimer's disease: Progression rate segregated by distinct neuropsychological and cerebral metabolic profiles. *Journal of Neurology, Neurosurgery, and Psychiatry, 55*, 956–959.

Martin, A. (1990). Neuropsychology of Alzheimer's disease: The case for subgroups. In M. F. Schwartz (Ed.), *Modular deficits in Alzheimer's type dementia* (pp. 145–175). Cambridge, MA: MIT Press.

Martin, A., Brouwers, P., Lalonde, F., Cox, C., Teleska, P., Fedio, P., et al. (1986). Towards a behavioral typology of Alzheimer's patients. *Journal of Clinical and Experimental Neuropsychology, 8*, 594–610.

Masliah, E., Mallory, M., Hansen, L., DeTeresa, R., & Terry, R. D. (1993). Quantitative synaptic alterations in the human neocortex during normal aging. *Neurology, 43*(1), 192–197.

Masliah, E., Rockenstein, E., Veinbergs, I., Sagara, Y., Mallory, M., Hashimoto, M., et al. (2001). Beta-amyloid peptides enhance alpha-synuclein accumulation and neuronal deficits in a transgenic mouse model linking Alzheimer's disease and Parkinson's disease. *Proceedings of the National Academy of Sciences of the United States of America, 98*, 12245–12250.

Mayeux, R., Stern, Y., & Spanton, S. (1985). Heterogeneity in dementia of the Alzheimer type: Evidence of subgroups. *Neurology, 35*, 453–461.

McKhann, G., Drachman, D., Folstein, M., Katzman, R., Price, D., & Stadlan, E. M. (1984). Clinical diagnosis of Alzheimer's disease: Report of the NINCDS-ADRDA Work Group under the auspices of Department of Health and Human Services Task Force on Alzheimer's Disease. *Neurology, 34*, 939–944.

McPherson, S., Fairbanks, L., Tiken, S., Cummings, J.

L., & Back-Madruga, C. (2002). Apathy and executive function in Alzheimer's disease. *Journal of the International Neuropsychological Society, 8,* 373–381.

Mega, M. S., Lee, L., Dinov, I. D., Mishkin, F., Toga, A. W., & Cummings, J. L. (2000). Cerebral correlates of psychotic symptoms in Alzheimer's disease. *Journal of Neurology, Neurosurgery, and Psychiatry, 69,* 167–171.

Minoshima, S., Foster, N. L., & Kuhl, D. E. (1994). Posterior cingulate cortex in Alzheimer's disease [Letter]. *Lancet, 344,* 895.

Minoshima, S., Giordani, B., Berent, S., Frey, K. A., Foster, N. L., & Kuhl, D. E. (1997). Metabolic reduction in the posterior cingulate cortex in very early Alzheimer's disease. *Annals of Neurology, 42,* 85–94.

Morris, J. C., Storandt, M., Miller, J. P., McKeel, D. W., Price, J. L., Rubin, E. H., et al. (2001). Mild cognitive impairment represents early-stage Alzheimer disease. *Archives of Neurology, 58,* 397–405.

Morrison, J. H., & Hof, P. R. (2002). Selective vulnerability of corticocortical and hippocampal circuits in aging and Alzheimer's disease. *Progress in Brain Research, 136,* 467–486.

Moyano, B. A. (1932). I. Enfermedad de Alzeimer II: Atrofia de Pick [Alzheimer's disease II: Pick atrophy]. *Archivos argentinos de Neurologia, 7,* 231–286.

Nacmias, B., Tedde, A., Forleo, P., Piacentini, S., Guarnieri, B. M., Bartoli, A., et al. (2001). Association between 5-HT(2A) receptor polymorphism and psychotic symptoms in Alzheimer's disease. *Biological Psychiatry, 50,* 472–475.

Nebes, R. D., & Brady, C. B. (1989). Focused and divided attention in Alzheimer's disease. *Cortex, 25,* 305–315.

Nestor, P. G., Parasuraman, R., Haxby, J. V., & Grady, C. L. (1991). Divided attention and metabolic brain dysfunction in mild dementia of the Alzheimer's type. *Neuropsychologia, 29,* 379–387.

Nichols, N. R., Day, J. R., Laping, N. J., Johnson, S. A., & Finch, C. E. (1993). GFAP mRNA increases with age in rat and human brain. *Neurobiology of Aging, 14*(5), 421–429.

Ojaimi, J., Masters, C. L., Opeskin, K., McKelvie, P., & Byrne, E. (1999). Mitochondrial respiratory chain activity in the human brain as a function of age. *Mechisms of Ageing and Development, 111*(1), 39–47.

O'Sullivan, M., Jones, D. K., Summers, P. E., Morris, R. G., Williams, S. C., & Markus, H. S. (2001). Evidence for cortical "disconnection" as a mechanism of age-related cognitive decline. *Neurology, 57*(4), 632–638.

Perry, R. J., & Hodges, J. R. (1999). Attention and executive deficits in Alzheimer's disease: A critical review. *Brain, 122,* 383–404.

Perry, R. J., & Hodges, J. R. (2000). Differentiating frontal and temporal variant frontotemporal dementia from Alzheimer's disease. *Neurology, 54,* 2277–2284.

Perry, R. J., Watson, P., & Hodges, J. R. (2000). The nature and staging of attention dysfunction in early (minimal and mild) Alzheimer's disease: Relationship to episodic and semantic memory impairment. *Neuropsychologia, 38,* 252–271.

Perusini, G. (1909). Uber klinisch und histologisch eigenartige psychische Erkrankungen des spateren Lebensalters. *Histologische und histopathologische Arbeiten uber die Grosshirnrinde, 3,* 297–358.

Perusini, G. (1909/1987). Histology and clinical findings of some psychiatric diseases of older people. In K. Bick, L. Amaducci, & G. Pepeu (Eds.), *The early story of Alzheimer's disease* (pp. 82–128). New York: Raven.

Pietrini, P., Furey, M. L., Graff-Radford, N., Freo, U., Alexander, G. E., Grady, C. L., et al. (1996). Preferential metabolic involvement of visual cortical areas in a subtype of Alzheimer's disease: Clinical implications. *American Journal of Psychiatry, 153,* 1261–1268.

Pillon, B., Dubois, B., Lhermitte, F., & Agid, Y. (1986). Heterogeneity of cognitive impairment in progressive supranuclear palsy, Parkinson's disease, and Alzheimer's disease. *Neurology, 36,* 1179–1185.

Pogacar, S., & Williams, R. S. (1984). Alzheimer's disease presenting as slowly progressive aphasia. *Rhode Island Medical Journal, 67,* 181–185.

Raux, G., Gantier, R., Thomas-Anterion, C., Boulliat, J., Verpillat, P., Hannequin, D., et al. (2000). Dementia with prominent frontotemporal features associated with L113P presenilin 1 mutation. *Neurology, 55,* 1577–1578.

Raz, N., Gunning-Dixon, F. M., Head, D., Dupuis, J. H., & Acker, J. D. (1998). Neuroanatomical correlates of cognitive aging: Evidence from structural magnetic resonance imaging. *Neuropsychology, 12*(1), 95–114.

Razani, J., Boone, K. B., Miller, B. L., Lee, A., & Sherman, D. (2001). Neuropsychological performance of right- and left-frontotemporal dementia compared to Alzheimer's disease. *Journal of the International Neuropsychological Society, 7,* 468–480.

Rothschild, D., & Kasanin, J. (1936). Clinicopathological study of Alzheimer's disease: Relationship to senile conditions. *Archives of Neurology and Psychiatry, 36,* 293–321.

Sarazin, M., Michon, A., Pillon, B., Samson, Y., Canuto, A., Gold, G., et al. (2003). Metabolic correlates of behavioral and affective disturbances in frontal lobe pathologies. *Journal of Neurology, 250,* 827–833.

Seitelberger, F., & Jellinger, K. (1958). Umschriebene Grosshirnatrophie bei Alzheimerscher Krankheit [Circumscribed cerebral atrophy in Alzheimer's disease]. *Deutsche Zeitschrift für Nervenheilkunde, 178,* 365–379.

Sgaramella, T. M., Borgo, F., Mondini, S., Pasini, M., Toso, V., & Semenza, C. (2001). Executive deficits appearing in the initial stage of Alzheimer's disease. *Brain and Cognition, 46,* 264–268.

Simchowicz, T. (1910). Histologische Studien uber die senile Demenz. *Histologische und Histopathologische Arbeiten uber die Grosshirnrinde, 4*, 267–444.

Sjogren, T., Sjogren, H., & Lindgren, A. G. (1952). Morbus Alzheimer and morbus Pick; a genetic, clinical and patho-anatomical study. *Acta Psychiatrica et Neurologica Scandinavica, 82*, 1–152.

Stout, J. C., Wyman, M. F., Johnson, S. A., Peavy, G. M., & Salmon, D. P. (2003). Frontal behavioral syndromes and functional status in probable Alzheimer disease. *American Journal of Geriatric Psychiatry, 11*, 683–686.

Stuss, D. T., & Knight, R. T. (2002). *Principles of frontal lobe function.* Oxford, UK: Oxford University Press.

Sukonick, D. L., Pollock, B. G., Sweet, R. A., Mulsant, B. H., Rosen, J., Klunk, W. E., et al. (2001). The 5-HTTPR*S/*L polymorphism and aggressive behavior in Alzheimer disease. *Archives of Neurology, 58*, 1425–1428.

Sultzer, D. L., Brown, C. V., Mandelkern, M. A., Mahler, M. E., Mendez, M. F., Chen, S. T., et al. (2003). Delusional thoughts and regional frontal/temporal cortex metabolism in Alzheimer's disease. *American Journal of Psychiatry, 160*, 341–349.

Sultzer, D. L., Mahler, M. E., Mandelkern, M. A., Cummings, J. L., Van Gorp, W. G., Hinkin, C. H., et al. (1995). The relationship between psychiatric symptoms and regional cortical metabolism in Alzheimer's disease. *Journal of Neuropsychiatry and Clinical Neurosciences, 7*, 476–484.

Swanberg, M. M., Tractenberg, R. E., Mohs, R., Thal, L. J., & Cummings, J. L. (2004). Executive dysfunction in Alzheimer disease. *Archives of Neurology, 61*, 556–560.

Sweet, R. A., Hamilton, R. L., Lopez, O. L., Klunk, W. E., Wisniewski, S. R., Kaufer, D. I., et al. (2000). Psychotic symptoms in Alzheimer's disease are not associated with more severe neuropathologic features. *International Psychogeriatrics, 12*, 547–558.

Talbot, K., Young, R. A., Jolly-Tornetta, C., Lee, V. M., Trojanowski, J. Q., & Wolf, B. A. (2000). A frontal variant of Alzheimer's disease exhibits decreased calcium-independent phospholipase A2 activity in the prefrontal cortex. *Neurochemistry International, 37*, 17–31.

Tang-Wai, D., Lewis, P., Boeve, B., Hutton, M., Golde, T., Baker, M., et al. (2002). Familial frontotemporal dementia associated with a novel presenilin-1 mutation. *Dementia and Geriatric Cognitive Disorders, 14*, 13–21.

Tariska, I. (1970). Circumscribed cerebral atrophy in Alzheimer's disease: A pathological study. In G. E. W. Wolstenholme & M. O'connor (Eds.), *Alzheimer's disease and related conditions: A CIBA Foundation Symposium* (pp. 51–73). London: Churchill.

Tekin, S., Mega, M. S., Masterman, D. M., Chow, T., Garakian, J., Vinters, H. V., et al. (2001). Orbitofrontal and anterior cingulate cortex neurofibrillary tangle burden is associated with agitation in Alzheimer disease. *Annals of Neurology, 49*, 355–361.

Thal, D. R., Rub, U., Orantes, M., & Braak, H. (2002). Phases of A beta-deposition in the human brain and its relevance for the development of AD. *Neurology, 58*, 1791–1800.

Unger, J. W. (1998). Glial reaction in aging and Alzheimer's disease. *Microscopy Research and Technique, 43*(1), 24–28.

Villareal, D. T., Grant, E., Miller, J. P., Storandt, M., McKeel, D. W., & Morris, J. C. (2003). Clinical outcomes of possible versus probable Alzheimer's disease. *Neurology, 61*(5), 661–667.

Vogt, B. A., Martin, A., Vrana, K. E., Absher, J. R., Vogt, L. J., & Hof, P. R. (1999). Mutifocal cortical neurodegeneration in Alzheimer's disease. *Cerebral Cortex, 14*, 553–601.

Vogt, B. A., Vogt, L. J., & Hof, P. R. (2001). Patterns of cortical neurodegeneration in Alzheimer's disease: Subgroups, subtypes, and implications for staging strategies. In P. R. Hof & C. V. Mobbs (Eds.), *Functional neurobiology of aging* (pp. 111–129). San Diego, CA: Academic Press.

Waldemar, G., Bruhn, P., Kristensen, M., Johnsen, A., Paulson, O. B., & Lassen, N. A. (1994). Heterogeneity of neocortical cerebral blood flow deficits in dementia of the Alzheimer type: A [$^{99m}$Tc]-d,l-HMPAO SPECT study. *Journal of Neurology, Neurosurgery, and Psychiatry, 57*, 285–295.

Wang, D. S., Bennett, D. A., Mufson, E., Cochran, E., & Dickson, D. W. (2004). Decreases in soluble alpha-synuclein in frontal cortex correlate with cognitive decline in the elderly. *Neuroscience Letters, 359*, 104–108.

Wang, D. S., Bennett, D. A., Mufson, E. J., Mattila, P., Cochran, E., & Dickson, D. W. (2004). Contribution of changes in ubiquitin and myelin basic protein to age-related cognitive decline. *Neuroscience Research, 48*, 93–100.

Welsh, K., Butters, N., Hughes, J., Mohs, R., & Heyman, A. (1991). Detection of abnormal memory decline in mild cases of Alzheimer's disease using CERAD neuropsychological measures. *Archives of Neurology, 48*, 278–281.

Yao, P. J., Zhu, M., Pyun, E. I., Brooks, A. I., Therianos, S., Meyers, V. E., et al. (2003). Defects in expression of genes related to synaptic vesicle trafficking in frontal cortex of Alzheimer's disease. *Neurobiology of Disease, 12*, 97–109.

Zubenko, G. S., Moossy, J., Martinez, A. J., Rao, G., Claassen, D., Rosen, J., et al. (1991). Neuropathologic and neurochemical correlates of psychosis in primary dementia. *Archives of Neurology, 48*, 619–624.

# SECTION B

# Other Neurological Disorders

# CHAPTER 29

# Vascular Disease of the Frontal Lobes

*Ae Young Lee*
*Helena Chui*

The frontal cortices are the keystones of numerous distributed networks, including those related to movement, motivation, emotion, and higher intellectual function. The subcortical basal forebrain is an integral component of the medial temporal–diencephalic memory circuit. The anatomical connections underlying frontal-basal ganglia–thalamic networks are outlined in detail in earlier sections of this book. In this chapter, we focus on the vascular systems that supply these frontal–subcortical networks and the clinical disturbances that ensue following circulatory disruption.

For several reasons, it is not possible to make one-to-one correlations between cerebrovascular disease, structural anatomy, and clinical behavior.

1. Anatomically contiguous areas may belong to distinct functional systems. Thus, disruption of blood flow at different points along an arterial tree may be associated with a variety of behavioral disturbances. Various combinations of behavioral, intellectual, motor, or sensory disturbance are seen with lesions of either the anterior cerebral artery (ACA) or middle cerebral artery (MCA), depending upon the site of blood flow disturbance.

2. Integral components of a given functional system are often widely distributed in space. Thus, similar behavioral symptoms may arise when blood supply is disrupted in completely different arterial systems. For example, weakness may result when the ACA or MCA is

blocked, and when a large cortical or deep penetrating branch is affected.

3. Anatomical units, particularly those located in the deeper portions of the brain, may receive their supply from multiple arteries. For example, the head of the caudate is supplied by perforating arteries from both the ACA and MCA; the dorsomedial nucleus of the thalamus is supplied by the tuberothalamic, paramedian thalamic, and posterior medial choroidal arteries. Identification of the vessel involved may be difficult, particularly when the impacted artery is small.

4. Individual variations in the anatomical development of the arterial tree are not uncommon. In some individuals, the right and left ACA, or the right and left paramedian arteries, may arise from a common root. The posterior communicating artery (PCoA) may be congenitally absent or the posterior cerebral artery (PCA) may take its origin from the anterior circulation. Thus, a single arterial lesion may have unexpected consequences, leading to compromise of both cerebral hemispheres or to nontraditional areas.

With these limitations in mind, we review first the vascular supply of frontal–subcortical networks, followed by the behavioral disturbances associated with vascular disease affecting the large and small arteries of the anterior circulation (i.e., ACA and MCA), as well some of the small arteries of the posterior circulation. For larger arteries, we use a vascular approach; for smaller arteries, we switch to an anatomical approach.

## FUNCTIONAL NEUROANATOMY AND CORRESPONDING VASCULAR SUPPLY

To make sense of the signs and symptoms of strokes affecting the frontal lobes and frontal lobe function, it is necessary to understand the vascular supply of the frontal–subcortical networks. The frontal lobes themselves are supplied by the ACA and MCA, whereas the distributed components of frontal lobe networks may be nourished by small branches from the ACA, MCA, and PCA.

- The mesial, superior frontal, and cingulate gyri, and the mesial extension of the precentral gyrus, the paracentral lobule, and orbital sectors are supplied by the anterior branches of the ACA (orbitofrontal, anterior and middle, posterior internal frontal, and paracentral branches) (H. Damasio, 1992; Kumral, Bayulkem, Evyapan, & Yunten, 2002) (Figure 29.1).
- Deep midline structures that are intimately connected with the frontal cortex receive their blood supply from other sources, including penetrating arteries that emanate from the circle of Willis, ACA, MCA, as well as the PCA and basilar arteries.
- The dorsolateral part of the frontal lobe, the inferior and middle frontal gyri, and the lateral sector of the superior frontal gyrus, as well as most of the precentral gyrus, lie in the territory of the anterior branches of the MCA (orbitofrontal, prefrontal, precentral, and central branches) (Figure 29.2).

### Cortical–Basal Ganglia–Thalamocortical Loops

Segregated, but parallel, cortical–basal ganglia––thalamocortical pathways have been tentatively identified in nonhuman primates for each of the major functional divisions (i.e., motor, motivational, emotional, and cognitive) of frontal cortex (Alexander & Crutcher, 1990; Alexander, DeLong, & Strick, 1986). A somatotopic organization is maintained throughout each functional circuit. Each circuit contains multiple, partially overlapping corticostriate inputs to striatum that become progressively integrated as they pass through the pallidum or substantia nigra pars reticulata (SNr) to re-

stricted areas of the thalamus and then back to a single cortical area. The cortical areas that project to striatum within a given functional loop are functionally related and usually interconnected. Thus, the circuits integrate and converge, or "funnel" information, from multiple-related cortical areas back to a single primary cortical area. In this way, the primary cortical area becomes part of a closed feedback loop, whereas the secondary cortical areas contribute to part of an open loop.

The vascular supply for these distributed networks is complex, with tributaries sometimes originating from widely separated arterial trunks and branches. In the discussion that follows, a certain degree of interpolation has been involved in identifying the corresponding vascular supply. Detailed information about anatomical connectivity is derived largely from work in nonhuman primates (Alexander et al., 1986), whereas information about the blood supply comes from studies of humans (Pullicino, 1993; Schlesinger, 1976; Stephens & Stilwell, 1969).

### Motor Circuit

The basal ganglia–thalamocortical circuit is thought to be involved in the control of movement, speed, and amplitude, and possibly in the programming and initiation of internally generated movement. In the motor circuit, corticostriate projections originate from the supplementary motor area (SMA), lateral arcuate premotor area, and primary motor and somatosensory cortices (Brodmann's areas 6, 4 and 3, 1, 2), which are irrigated by branches of the ACA and MCA. Cortical areas located on the mesial side of the cerebral hemisphere are supplied by branches from the ACA (posterior internal frontal branch), whereas those situated on the dorsolateral side are perfused by branches of the MCA (precentral and central branches) (Figures 29.1b and 29.2a).

Axons from these cortical areas terminate primarily in the putamen (which is supplied by the lateral lenticulostriate arteries emanating from the MCA). Neurons in the putamen project to the ventrolateral two-thirds of both the internal and external segments of the globus pallidus (which are fed by medial lenticulostriate arteries) and to the caudolateral portions of the SNr (which are fed by anterolateral branches coming off the basilar artery). Output from the pallidum and SNr projects to the oral part of the ventrolateral nucleus of the thalamus (VL-o) (which is supplied by the tuberothalamic and thalamogeniculate arteries). Finally, VL-o projects back to the SMA. Thus, disturbances of blood flow in the proximal or distal branches of the ACA and MCA, and also branches of the circle of Willis and proximal branches of the PCA, may impact various components of the motor circuit.

### Anterior Cingulate Limbic Circuit

A "limbic" circuit has been identified that is connected in a closed loop with the anterior cingulate gyrus (area 24). The anterior cingulate gyrus plays an important role in attending and responding to the motivational content of internal and external stimuli (Devinsky, Morrell, & Vogt, 1995). Other corticostriate contributions to this circuit originate in the hippocampus, amygdala, and other limbic and paralimbic areas (entorhinal, perirhinal, temporal pole, superior and inferior temporal gyri, and posterior medial orbitofrontal areas [Brodmann's areas 24, 28, 38, 22, 20, 11]).

These iso- and allocortical areas send projections to the ventral striatum (i.e., nucleus accumbens) (supplied anteriorly by the recurrent artery of Heubner and posteriorly by other perforating branches from the ACA). The ventral striatum projects to the rostrolateral internal globus pallidus and the ventral pallidum (also supplied by perforating branches of the ACA), as well as the rostrodorsal SNr. In turn, these nuclei project upon the posterior medial portion of the mediodorsal (MD) nucleus of the thalamus (fed by the posterior medial choroidal artery coming off the proximal PCA). Finally, the MD projects back upon the anterior cingulate area. Thus, the limbic cortical–basal ganglia–thalamocortical loop may be affected by altered blood flow in proximal and distal branches of the ACA, or proximal branches of the PCA. It is notable, that the branches of the MCA do not contribute a significant blood supply to the principal components of the limbic circuit.

### Orbital Limbic Circuit

The lateral orbital limbic circuit is related to emotional and social behavior. Corticostriate projections from the lateral orbitofrontal cortex (Brodmann's area 10) are supplied by the orbitofrontal branches from the ACA and

MCA. Secondary corticostriate projections participating in this circuit originate from auditory and visual association cortices in the temporal lobes (areas 22 and 37).

Axons from the lateral orbitofrontal cortex terminate in the ventromedial sector of the head of the caudate, which is supplied by the recurrent artery of Heubner that arises from the proximal ACA. The ventromedial caudate projects to the medial dorsomedial internal pallidum, which is supplied by the anterior choroidal artery and by perforators from the ACA, as well as rostromedial SNr. Projections continue to the medial portions of the ventral anterior (VA) nucleus of the thalamus, which is fed by the tuberothalamic artery and the magnocellular portion of the medial dorsal (MD-mc) nucleus of the thalamus that is supplied jointly by the tuberothalamic, paramedian thalamic, and posterior medial choroidal arteries. Finally, the thalamic nuclei project back to the lateral orbitofrontal cortex. Thus, the lateral orbital circuit is vulnerable to impaired perfusion in perforating arteries coming from proximal ACA and PCA, as well as the carotid, PCoA, and basilar arteries. In addition, the lateral orbitofrontal cortex itself might be selectively damaged by a strategic occlusion of the orbitofrontal branches of the ACA or MCA.

### Dorsolateral Prefrontal Circuit

The dorsolateral prefrontal circuit is related to higher-order executive function, including supervisory attention, sequencing, planning, decision making, and errors correction. The dorsolateral prefrontal circuit originates from and converges back upon the cortex around the principal sulcus (Brodmann's areas 9, 10), which is supplied by precentral branches of the MCA. Secondary contributions arise from multimodal association areas in the posterior parietal cortex and arcuate premotor areas, which are involved in the analysis of motion and space.

Corticostriate fibers in the dorsolateral prefrontal circuit terminate in the dorsolateral head of the caudate, which is supplied by the lateral lenticulostriate arteries that arise from the proximal MCA. The circuit continues its topographic projection onto the lateral dorsomedial portion of the internal segment of the globus pallidus, which is supplied by the anterior choroidal artery, as well as the rostrolateral SNr, then on to two thalamic nuclei: the ventral anterior pars parvocellularis (VA-pc) and the mediodorsal pars parvocellularis (MD-pc) thalamic nuclei (which are jointly supplied by the tuberothalamic, thalamogeniculate, and paramedian thalamic arteries). To complete the loop, these thalamic nuclei project back upon the dorsolateral prefrontal cortex. Like the motor circuit, the dorsolateral circuit depends for its blood supply upon the MCA, as well as deep penetrating arteries. For the dorsolateral circuit, these include the anterior choroidal artery and arteries near the posterior circle of Willis.

## Medial Temporal–Diencephalic Memory System

The substantia innominata in the basal forebrain represents a relatively small but strategic component of the medial temporal–diencephalic declarative memory system. The substantia innominata includes the septal nuclei, nucleus of the diagonal band (of Broca), and nucleus basalis of Meynert, which are fed by perforating arteries from the ACA and anterior communicating artery (ACoA). The diagonal band of Broca is interconnected with the hippocampus (supplied by the anterior choroidal artery), an area critical for declarative memory and learning. The hippocampus is connected via the fornix to the septal nuclei, mammillary bodies, and the anterior nucleus of the thalamus (supplied by the tuberothalamic artery). The anterior thalamic nucleus projects to the anterior cingulate gyrus (Papez, 1937).

The basolateral amygdala is connected via the ventral amygdalofugal projection to the basal forebrain and then to the lateral preoptic and hypothalamic areas (Carpenter & Sutin, 1983). Other fibers enter the inferior thalamic peduncle and project to the MD-mc nucleus of the thalamus, which is jointly supplied by the tuberothalamic and paramedian thalamic arteries. The dorsomedial thalamic nucleus projects to orbitofrontal cortex. Thus, the hippocampus and amygdala are interlinked with other frontal–subcortical circuits and depend in part upon blood supply from arteries originating from or near the anterior and posterior circle of Willis.

## STROKE AND THE FRONTAL LOBES

Stroke or brain injury due to cerebrovascular disease is the third leading cause of death in most industrialized countries. According to the American Heart Association (1994), there are 3 million survivors of stroke in the United States and nearly 500,000 people have new strokes each year. The incidence of stroke increases exponentially with age. In Rochester, Minnesota, the incidence rate increased 10% per year of age after age 60. Between 1980 and 1984, the age- and sex-adjusted average annual incidence of stroke was 102 per 100,000, and 572 per 100,000 in persons 60–74 years of age (Broderick, Phillips, Whisnant, O'Fallon, & Begstrahl, 1989). In North Manhattan, the incidence rate is significantly higher among Asians and African Americans compared to Caucasians or Hispanics (Sacco, Hauser, & Mohr, 1991).

Cerebrovascular disease causes brain injury by two basic, non-mutually-exclusive, pathophysiological mechanisms, namely, ischemia and hemorrhage. "Ischemia" refers to conditions in which blood flow is insufficient to meet the metabolic needs of the brain tissue. Territorial infarcts result from occlusion of individual arteries. Borderzone infarcts result from hypoperfusion in the terminal zones of two or more arteries. In the frontal lobes, the borderzone between the ACA and MCA can be drawn along the dorsolateral convexity, the frontal centrum semiovale, the head of the caudate, anterior limb of the internal capsule, anterior inferior putamen, and globus pallidus.

"Hemorrhage" refers to the rupture of blood vessel walls and the extravasation of blood into the brain parenchyma (intracerebral hemorrhage, or ICH) or subarachnoid space (subarachnoid hemorrhage, or SAH). Cerebral microbleeds (CMBs), resulting from hemorrhage-prone microangiopathy, can be detected by gradient echo magnetic resonance imaging (MRI) (Fazekas et al., 1999; Greenberg, Finklestein, & Schaefer, 1996; Lee et al., 2004; Tsushima, Tamura, Unno, Kusano, & Endo, 2000). Not including CMBs, in the United States and Europe, approximately 20% of strokes are due to hemorrhage. ICH is twice as common as SAH. In Japan, the percentage of strokes due to hemorrhage is higher because of an increased incidence of ICH.

By virtue of its relative mass and proportionate blood flow from the ACA and superior or upper division of the MCA, the frontal lobe is frequently impacted by stroke. When one considers that (1) occlusion of the ACA virtually affects the frontal lobe, (2) occlusion of the

MCA affects the frontal lobes in the majority of instances, and (3) occlusion of a small penetrating artery usually involves a frontal–subcortical circuit, the frontal lobe or its networks are damaged in over half of all ischemic strokes.

Emboli from the heart tend to lodge in the anterior circulation: about 60% in the MCA and 20% in the ACA versus 20% in the PCA territory (Wijdicks & Jack, 1996). Beyond the stem of the MCA, flow seems equally directed to the two divisions, but the lower division bound for the temporal and temporal–parietal lobes receive the larger share of the emboli (Mohr et al., 2004). Infarcts in the distribution of the ACA or MCA most often result from artery-to-artery emboli from the internal carotid artery rather than from primary stenosis/thrombosis of the ACA and MCA proper. Approximately 20–30% of hemispheric infarcts are small lacunes in the territory of deep-penetrating arteries. Of these, 50–60% fall into the distribution of either the MCA or ACA, and 15–26% fall in the PCA distribution (Hollander et al., 2002; Lindgren, Norrving, Rudling, & Johannson, 1994; Mean, Lewis, Wardlaw, Dennis, & Warlow, 2000).

Spontaneous ICH usually arises in subcortical locations, including the putamen (35–50%), subcortical white matter (30%), and thalamus (10–15%) (Kase, Mohr, & Caplan, 2004). Hemorrhages, however, also occur in more centrifugal lobar locations. Blood collects between the cortex and underlying white matter, separating them and often extending along the white matter pathways. Although the parietal and occipital lobes are the most common sites for lobar hemorrhage overall (Kase, Williams, Wyatt, & Mohr, 1982), 35% of cerebral amyloid angiopathy (CAA)-associated lobar hemorrhages occur in the frontal lobes (Greenberg, 2004; Vinters, 1987).

Finally, SAH from ruptured saccular aneurysms has a predilection for the frontal lobes (Fox, 1983). In an analysis of 5,267 aneurysms, Stehbens (1972) reported that 85 to 95% of aneurysms were located at major branch sites from the anterior circle of Willis, including 38% in internal carotid artery, 31% in ACA, and 20% in MCA. The most common sites were at the bifurcation of the intracranial carotid, the carotid origins of the PCoA or the anterior choroidal artery, the first 3 cm of the MCA, and the region of the ACoA.

The major risk factors for stroke are similar regardless of which lobe of the brain is involved. Age is the strongest risk factor for stroke. There are several genetic forms of cerebrovascular disease. Cerebral autosomal dominant arteriopathy with subcortical infarcts and leukoencephalopathy (CADASIL) is caused by mutations in the *Notch3* gene on chromosome 19q12 (Dichgans, Herzog, & Gasser, 2001; Joutel et al., 1997; Tournier-Lasserve et al., 1993). Autosomal dominant forms of CAA are manifest clinically as recurrent lobar hemorrhage, cognitive deterioration, and ischemic stroke (Vinters, 2001). Deep white matter changes and lacunar infarcts without accompanying hemorrhage are seen on MRI in familial British dementia with amyloid angiopathy (Mead et al., 2000).

Some other risk factors are modifiable, including atrial fibrillation, hypertension, cardiac disease, diabetes mellitus, smoking, alcoholism, and hyperlipidemia (Sacco, 1994; Schonberg & Schulte, 1988; Tell, Crouse, & Fuberg, 1988; Wolf, D'Agostino, Belanger, & Kannel, 1991). Hypertension is the most common risk factor for ICH (found in 72% and 81% of cases, respectively; Broderick, 1994; Kase et al., 2004), followed especially in elderly persons by CAA (Vinters, 1987). Low total cholesterol and high level of high-density lipoprotein, as well as chronic hypertension, are independent risk factors for CMB (Lee et al., 2002). During the past two decades, the death rate due to stroke has declined by 60%, probably in part due to the early detection of risk factors and the institution of appropriate preventive measures (Higgins, 1993).

## ANTERIOR CEREBRAL ARTERY

### Vascular Anatomy

The ACA supplies the anterior four-fifths of the corpus callosum, as well as the anterior and medial portions of the basal forebrain, basal ganglia, and cerebral hemispheres. The proximal A1 segment (average diameter = 2.6 mm, average length = 13 mm) originates from the intracranial carotid artery and gives rise to several small perforating arteries, including the recurrent artery of Heubner (Weir, 1987). These small arteries supply the tuberculum olfactorium, septal nuclei, medial portion of the globus pallidus internus, ventromedial head of the caudate, anterior third of the putamen, and anterior limb of the internal capsule (Critchley, 1930; Pullicino, 1993; see Figure 29.1b and c).

A single, short ACoA joins the right and left ACA in 74% of cases, with variations including rare absence in the remaining cases (Krayenbühl & Yasargil, 1968). The ACA distal to the ACoA arches around the genu and over the body of the corpus callosum. From its concave side, the ACA gives rise to numerous short twigs that supply the genu and body of the corpus callosum, septum pellucidum, medial anterior commissure, and anterior pillars of the fornix. From its convex side, the ACA gives rise to approximately eight major branches (e.g., orbitofrontal, frontopolar, anterior internal frontal, middle internal frontal, posterior inferior frontal, paracentral, superior internal parietal, and inferior internal parietal branches) that supply the medial surface and 2.5 cm deep into the adjacent white matter of the frontal and parietal lobes (Figure 29.1b). Thus, all but the most distal two of the eight centrifugal branches of the ACA supply key structures of the frontal lobe or components of the frontal–subcortical circuit (Table 29.1).

## Vascular Disease

ACA infarction commonly results from vasospasm following rupture of an ACA or ACoA saccular aneurysm. Approximately 25% of saccular aneurysms are found at the ACoA (Weir, 1987). Excluding cases secondary to vasospasm, ACA infarction corresponds to 0.6–3.0% of acute ischemic stroke (Brust & Chamorro, 2004; Kumral et al., 2002). Infarcts involving the ACA are associated with internal carotid artery atherosclerosis (Rodda, 1986), local narrowing or hypoplastic change (Kazui, Sawada, Naritomi, Kuriyama, & Yamaguchi, 1993), and cardiac emboli.

## Symptoms and Signs

Distinct clinical symptoms and signs are noted when the ACA is occluded unilaterally at successive points along its course (Critchley, 1930). Occlusion of the proximal ACA, including Heubner's artery and the ACoA, results in hemiplegia involving both the arm and the leg, sensory loss of the distal leg, ipsilateral deviation of the eyes, ideomotor apraxia of the left

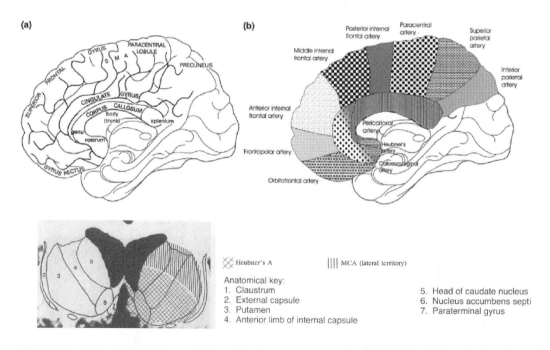

FIGURE 29.1. ACA territory. Schematic representations of anatomy. Superficial (a) and deep (b) branches of ACA, and blood supply of coronal scan through head of caudate (c). (a) and (b) from Pullicino (1993). Copyright 1993 by Lippincott Williams and Wilkins. Adapted by permission. (c) From Kumral, Bayulkam, Evyapan, and Yunten (2002). Copyright 2002 by Lippincott Williams and Wilkins. Adapted by permission.

**TABLE 29.1. Branches of the ACA and Its Territories**

| Branches | Origin | Territories |
|---|---|---|
| HA | A1 | Head of caudate<br>Anterior inferior part of the internal's anterior limb<br>Anterior globus pallidus<br>Putamen |
| OF | A2 | Olfactory bulb<br>Medial part of the orbital surface of the frontal lobe |
| FP | A2 | Medial and lateral surfaces of the frontal lobe |
| AIF | CM | Anterior portion of the superior portion of the superior frontal gyrus |
| MIF | CM or A3 | Middle portions of the medial and lateral surfaces of the superior frontal gyrus |
| PIF | CM or A3 | Posterior third of the superior frontal gyrus<br>Part of the cingulate gyrus |
| PC | A4 | Paracentral lobule |
| SUP | A5, A4 | Superior portion of precuneus |
| IP | A5 | Posterior inferior part of the cuneus and adjacent portions of the cuneus |

*Note.* HA, Heubner's artery; OF, orbitofrontal artery; FP, frontopolar artery; AIF, anterior internal frontal artery; MIF, middle inferior frontal artery; PIF, posteroinferior frontal artery; PC, paracentral artery; SUP, superior parietal artery; IP, inferior parietal artery; CM, callosomarginal artery. From Kumral, Bayulkem, Evyapan, and Yunten (2002). Copyright 2002 by Lippincott Williams & Wilkins. Adapted by permission.

side of the body, some degree of cognitive impairment, and aphasia (if the lesion is in the dominant hemisphere). When occlusion is limited to Heubner's artery, weakness predominantly affects the arm, face, and bulbar musculature (with irritability, forgetfulness, and some emotional incontinence). On the other hand, when occlusion occurs distal to Heubner's artery and the ACoA, weakness and sensory loss predominantly affect the leg. Regardless of the side of the lesion, the left arm is vulnerable to apraxia due to callosal disconnection. The arm contralateral to the lesion, while maintaining good power, may exhibit forced grasping and groping (so-called "alien hand"). Forced grasping is not seen when occlusion of the main trunk occurs distal to the origin of the posterior internal frontal artery. Anosognosia is commonly associated with right-hemispheric ACA lesions and frontal-type emotional incontinence with bilateral frontal involvement (Table 29.2).

### Crural Predominant Weakness

Occlusion of ACA distal to the ACoA leads to greater weakness in the leg compared to the arm (i.e., crural predominant weakness). For several reasons, weakness is greater in the distal compared to proximal lower extremity: (1) The sensorimotor somatotopic representation of the proximal leg is situated either superiorly on the medial hemisphere or on the high convexity, where it may receive collateral blood flow from the MCA, and (2) proximal muscles have substantial representation in the ipsilateral hemisphere (Brust & Chamorro, 2004). In a series of 12 cases, when the lesion involved the medial precentral gyrus, medial premotor cortex, and SMA, the pattern of weakness in the leg was greater distally than proximally, and recovery of function was poor (Schneider & Gautier, 1994). When the precentral gyrus was spared, the leg weakness appeared to be greater proximally than distally, and recovery was better. Hemiparesis with faciobrachiocrural predominance occurred as a result of occlusion of the recurrent artery of Heubner, probably because of the involvement of other A1 segment perforating branches supplying the genu and contiguous limb of the internal capsule (Brust, Sawada, & Kazui, 2001). Crural paresis due to infarction in the ACA may also be associated with homolateral ataxia (Moulin et al., 1995).

### Akinetic Mutism

Bilateral infarction of the medial frontal cortex, particularly the anterior cingulate gyri and the SMA, is associated with akinetic mutism (Freemon, 1971; Kumral et al., 2002;

**TABLE 29.2. Clinical Features Following ACA Infarction**

| Clinical findings | RACA | LACA | BACA |
|---|---|---|---|
| Crural predominant weakness | (+) | (+) | (+) |
| Mutism/akinetic mutism | (+) | (+) | (++) |
| Abulia | (+) | (+) | |
| Motor neglect | (++) | (+) | |
| Decreased verbal fluency | | (+) | |
| Transcortical motor aphasia | (+) | (+) | |
| Affective aprosodia | (+) | | |
| Alien hand | (+) | | |
| Apraxia | (+) | (+) | |
| Amnesia | (+) | (+) | (+) |
| Depression | (+) | (++) | |
| Anosognosia | (+) | | |
| Incontinence | (+) | (+) | (+) |

*Note.* RACA, right anterior cerebral artery; LACA, left anterior cerebral artery; BACA, bilateral cerebral artery.

Nagaratnam, Nagaratnam, Ng, & Diu, 2004). Akinetic mutism is "a state of limited responsiveness to the environment in the absence of gross alteration of sensorimotor mechanisms operating at a more peripheral level" (Segarra, 1970). The SMA is concerned with programming, initiating, and executing movements (Damasio & Vandstensen, 1980) and has strong reciprocal connections with the cingulate gyrus. When both ACAs originate from a common stem, occlusion of the proximal ACA may cause simultaneous infarction of bilateral SMA and cingulate gyri, and a state of akinetic mutism.

Milder forms of diminished emotional motor responsiveness may follow unilateral damage to the anterior cingulate and SMA (Damasio & van Hoesen, 1983) or to components of the "limbic" frontobasal ganglia–thalamic circuit. Abulia or akinetic mutism has been described following ischemic lesions in the right head of caudate (Degos, da Fonseca, Gray, & Cesaro, 1993). Hypokinesia, bradykinesia, and hypometria (reduced range of motion) of the contralateral limbs following right mesial frontal lobe hemorrhage have also been reported (Meador, Watson, Bowers, & Heilman, 1986).

## Aphasia

Several alterations of spoken language may result from interruption of blood supply to mesial hemispheric structures, including the

SMA and proximal regions of cingulate cortex. These structures are supplied by the postero-internal frontal and paracentral arteries—distal branches of the callosal marginal artery. Whereas left-sided medial frontal lesions are associated with transcortical motor aphasia, right medial frontal lesions may induce affective aprosodia (Heilman, Leon, & Rosenbek, 2004).

Transcortical motor aphasia is characterized by limited spontaneous speech, intact repetition, normal articulation, and good auditory comprehension (Freedman, Alexander, & Naeser, 1984; Kumral et al., 2002). Transcortical motor aphasia or "SMA aphasia" is characterized initially by mutism, which often improves except for persistent impairment of speech initiation (Goodglass, 1993). The SMA is considered the most anterior portion of an integrated brain mechanism responsible for the initiation of speech. Destruction of fibers from the SMA to frontal premotor cortex is postulated to disconnect the limbic "starter mechanism" from the cortical regions that control speech (Freedman et al., 1984).

## Callosal Disconnection Signs

Patients with naturally occurring or surgically caused callosal lesions involving the genu and body of the corpus callosum may develop unilateral apraxia of the nondominant limb (Geschwind & Kaplan, 1962; Graff-Radford, Welsh, & Godersky, 1987; Leiguarda, Starkstein, & Berthier, 1989; Liepmann & Maas, 1907; Sweet, 1941; Watson & Heilman, 1983). Liepmann and Maas (1907) proposed that motor centers in the right hemisphere (necessary for controlling movements of the left hand) are disconnected from space–time representations (necessary for skilled movements) located in the left hemisphere. The most enduring callosal-type apraxia is demonstrated for verbal–motor tasks, such as pantomiming to command using the nondominant hand (Graff-Radford et al., 1987; Leiguarda & Marsden, 2000).

"Alien hand" refers to an upper limb that performs autonomous complex movements against the patient's will (Fisher, 2000). Callosal and frontal subtypes have been described. Patients with damage to the anterior corpus callosum may demonstrate intermanual conflict. Coordination between the right and left SMAs during the generation of action plans is disrupted, leaving a "free running" or "alien" nondominant hand (Gasquoine, 1993).

In contrast, the frontal-type "alien hand" affects the dominant hand and results from damage to dominant medial frontal lobe, including premotor, SMA, and the anterior cingulate gyrus. The behaviors of frontal type include grasp reflex, impulsive groping, and compulsive tool manipulation. These are ascribed to frontal release of spontaneous exploratory movements of the dominant hand, coupled with normal inhibition of the nondominant hand (Feinberg, Schindler, Flanagan, & Haber, 1992; Scepkowski & Cronin-Golomb, 2003).

### Amnesia

Neurobehavioral changes observed following rupture of ACoA aneurysms include impaired memory, confabulation, personality change, and impaired executive function. Several stages of behavior typically evolve, beginning with confusion and agitation, followed by confabulation with denial of illness, and evolving to amnesia with personality change. On closer analysis, confabulation can often be related to fragments from the patient's past, strung together in the wrong context and sequence. Over several weeks, confabulation may wane, leaving impaired anterograde memory with other changes in personality (e.g., lack of concern, apathy, irritability, fatuousness, and socially inappropriate behavior). Both the quality of the amnesia and the accompanying personality disturbances are consistent with prefrontal and paralimbic dysfunction.

Damage to the basal forebrain, particularly the medial septum and nucleus of the diagonal band of Broca, is thought to underlie the amnesia observed in a subset of patients with ACoA damage (Böttger, Prosiegel, Steiger, & Yassouridis, 1998; Damasio, Graff-Radford, Eslinger, Damasio, & Kassell, 1985; DeLuca, 1992). The ACoA gives rise to several small, perforating branches that supply the anterior hypothalamus, septal nuclei, lamina terminalis, columns of the fornix, medial ventral corpus callosum, and anterior cingulate (Dunker & Harris, 1976). Several of these structures (i.e., septal nuclei, columns of the fornix, and anterior cingulate) are integral components of the limbic–diencephalic memory system, and injury may contribute to temporary or permanent amnesia. Damage to the basal forebrain, combined with either neostriatal or frontal injury, is deemed necessary for the development of amnesia (Irle, Wowra, Kunert, Hampl, & Kunze, 1992). Generally, for storage processes, long-term memory is more impaired than short-term memory. For retrieval processes, free recall is more affected than cued recall or recognition. In the temporal dimension, anterograde amnesia is more severe than retrograde amnesia, memory spans are preserved, and implicit memory and procedural learning are undisturbed in patients with ACoA rupture (Bötgger et al., 1998).

### Regulation of Mood

Major depression develops in 5–11% of stroke survivors and minor depression in 11–40% (Bodini, Iacoboni, & Lenzi, 2004; Burvill, Johnson, Jamrozik, Anderson, & Stewart-Wynne, 1997; Castillo, Schultz, & Robinson, 1995; Eastwood, Rifat, Nobbs, & Ruderman, 1989; Palomaki et al., 1999). An association between poststroke depression (PSD) and left anterior lesions has frequently been observed (Astrom, Adolfsson, & Asplund, 1993; Morris, Robinson, Raphael, & Hopwood, 1996; Robinson, Starr, & Price, 1984; Vataja et al., 2001). Risk of depression arising during the first 2 months poststroke has been correlated to proximity of the lesion to the left frontal pole (Robinson, 2003).

Branches from the ACA supply a number of cortical and subcortical structures that are implicated in the regulation of mood. Infarcts involving the left head of caudate, supplied by branches of the lenticulostriate artery are associated with secondary depression (Starkstein,

Robinson, Berthier, Parikh, & Price, 1988). Several studies propose the role of frontal–subcortical circuits (Beblo, Wallesch, & Herrmann, 1999), basal ganglia (Steffens, Helms, Krisnan, & Burke, 1999), and limbic lobes, with the mediation of a serotonin hyporegulation (Kim & Choi-Kwon, 2000).

Mania, irritable mood, and disinhibited behaviors have also been reported following stroke to orbitofrontal, basolateral polar temporal areas, as well as head of caudate and thalamus. For mania, a predilection for a right-hemisphere lesion has been noted (Bogousslavsky & Regli, 1990; Cummings & Mendez, 1984; Starkstein, Boston, & Robinson, 1988; Starkstein, Pearlson, Boston, & Robinson, 1987). When anterior cingulate and orbital lesions both exist, the result may be severe social agnosia (Devinsky et al., 1995).

## MIDDLE CEREBRAL ARTERY

### Vascular Anatomy

The MCA is the largest of the major branches of the internal carotid artery. Within the brain, the MCA irrigates not only most of the convex surface of the brain but also almost all of the basal ganglia and capsule, including the extreme capsule, claustrum, putamen, the upper parts of the globus pallidus, the posterior portion of the head and all of the body of the caudate nucleus, and all but the very lowest portions of the anterior and posterior limbs of the internal capsule (Figure 29.2a). The MCA has been divided into four segments: M1, the sphenoidal segment; M2, the insular segment; M3, the opercular segment; and M4, the cortical segment (Figure 29.2b).

The M1 or sphenoidal segment (average diameter = 3 mm, average length = 15 mm) has two components. The first is an undivided MCA stem from which the lenticulostriate branches arise; the second is composed of the short segments from the point of bifurcation of the MCA into its major divisions to their entry into the sylvian fissure (Mohr et al., 2004). The M1 and proximal M2 segments give rise to approximately 10 lenticulostriate arteries (medial and lateral groups) that supply the lateral substantia innominata, lateral anterior commissure, dorsolateral head of the caudate, dorsolateral globus pallidi, and the middle and posterior putmen. These structures are intimately interconnected with frontal cortex.

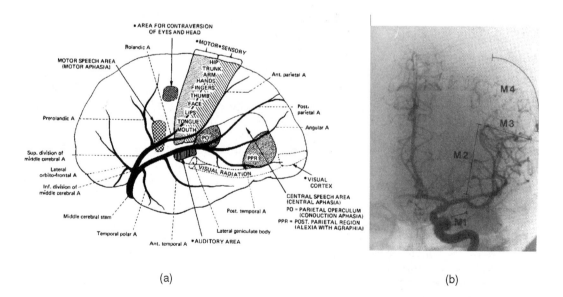

(a)                                        (b)

FIGURE 29.2. MCA circulation. (a) Lateral view of MCA distribution with its corresponding areas of functional localization. (b) Classification of the MCA by segments. (a) From Adams, Hachinski, and Norris (2001). Copyright 2001 by Elsevier. Adapted by permission. (b) From Mohr, Lazar, Marshall, and Hier (2004). Copyright 2004 by Churchill Livingstone. Adapted by permission.

Divided into two or three trunks, the MCA subsequently reaches the insula, where it branches further to supply roughly 12 territories of the lateral frontotemporal lobe: orbitofrontal, prefrontal, precentral, central, anterior parietal, posterior parietal, angular, temporal–occipital, and temporopolar. Altered perfusion in the proximal M1 segment or upper division of the MCA is most likely to affect frontal lobe circuits and functions.

## Vascular Disease

Among the three major cerebral arteries, the MCA is the most common site of symptomatic vascular disease. Embolism is the common cause of occlusion for the major cerebral arteries beyond the circle of Willis. It accounts for between 15 and 30% of strokes, most of which occur in the territory of the MCA (Mohr et al., 2004). Approximately 45% of cardiac emboli find their destination within the MCA territory (Yamaguchi, Minematsu, Choki, & Ikeda, 1984). Approximately 60% of hypertensive hemorrhages originate from weakened lenticulostriate arteries. In a review of 3,110 cases of single saccular aneurysms, Fox (1983) noted that 13% were located at the MCA bi- or trifurcation.

## Symptoms and Signs

Occlusion of the stem of the MCA affects the temporal and parietal, as well as the frontal lobes. When occlusion is limited to the upper division of the MCA, the brunt of injury is borne by the frontal lobes. Ischemia in the territories of the frontal polar, prefrontal, precentral, central, and posterior parietal branch arteries leads to infarction of the lateral prefrontal, lateral premotor, and primary sensorimotor cortices, together with their underlying white matter.

The typical syndrome of an uncollateralized MCA occlusion includes contralateral hemiplegia, deviation of the head and eyes toward the side of the infarct, hemianesthesia, and hemianopsia. The behavioral syndromes associated with MCA strokes are largely determined by the side, as well as the site, of occlusion. Strokes in the dominant hemisphere are associated with greater disturbances in language, whereas strokes in the right hemisphere are associated with greater disturbances in attention.

## Aphasia

In greater than 95% of right-handed and even most left-handed persons, the left hemisphere is dominant for speech and language. Occlusion of the left MCA trunk or upper division produces global disruption of language function. Brust and associates (2001) reported aphasia in 177 (21%) of 850 patients with acute MCA infarction. Fifty-seven (32%) were classified as "fluent" aphasia and 120 (68%) as "nonfluent" aphasia.

The principal cortical area supporting speech output extends posteriorly from Broca's area in the left frontal operculum along the lower frontal lobe to the Rolandic fissure. This area is supplied by the prefrontal and orbitofrontal branches of the upper MCA trunk. Broca's aphasia is characterized by suppression of speech output, agrammatism, limited vocabulary access, and relatively spared comprehension (Benson, 1993; Goodglass, 1993). Although persistent Broca's aphasia has been associated with damage to basal ganglia, it is now believed that complete loss of voluntary speech implies damage to deep white matter pathways supplied by the lenticulostriate branches of the left MCA. These pathways include the subcallosal fasciculus, the middle portion of periventricular white matter adjacent to the lateral ventricle, and the genu of the internal capsule (Goodglass, 1993; Naeser, Palumbo, Helm-Estabrooks, Stiassny-Eden, & Albert, 1989). Lesions in the speech outflow pathway (i.e., the genu of the internal capsule) are characterized by severe dysarthria and dysprosody, but have no linguistic component, and are referred to as "aphemia" or subcortical motor aphasia (Goodglass, 1993).

Transcortical motor aphasia is most often caused by insufficient blood supply to the vascular border zone between left middle and anterior cerebral artery territories, anterior or superior to Broca's area (Goodglass, 1993; Stuss & Benson, 1986). Responsible lesions have been found in the white matter anterolateral to the left frontal horn, caused by infarction or hemorrhage in the upper division of the MCA (Mohr et al., 2004). Transcortical motor aphasia shares features with SMA aphasia, without the accompanying right-sided leg weakness. Freedman and colleagues (1984) proposed that transcortical motor aphasia results from the disconnection of Broca's area from the supplementary motor cortex.

## Inattention or Neglect

Whereas the left hemisphere is specialized for language, the right hemisphere plays a predominant role in directing attention toward extrapersonal space. In concert with the reticular activating system and the inferior parietal lobule, two areas (items 3 and 4 below) of the frontal lobe participate in a distributed cortical network for attention (Mesulam, 1981): (1) the reticular activating system sets the level of arousal and vigilance, (2) the inferior parietal lobe provides an internal sensory map, (3) the cingulate gyrus signals the motivational priority, and (4) the dorsolateral frontal cortex (including the frontal eye field) directs motor exploration.

Although profound unilateral neglect classically follows damage to the right parietal lobule, neglect also emerges subsequent to vascular injury to the medial or dorsolateral frontal lobes (Damasio, Damasio, & Chui, 1980; Heilman & Valenstein, 1972; Mesulam, 1981). Recently, Ringman, Saver, Woolson, Clarke, and Adams (2004) noted that right frontal lesions were associated with neglect as frequently as right parietal lesions, 3 months after stroke.

## Intentional Motor Disorders

Fisher (1956) introduced the term "motor impersistence" to describe the inability to sustain simple acts such as eye closure, breath holding, conjugate gaze deviation, tongue protrusion, and hand gripping. Although Fisher considered motor impersistence to be a nondominant, hemisphere-specific symptom, it can be seen with left- or right-hemispheric infarcts, particularly if the latter are located in the central or frontal regions (Kertesz, Nicholson, Cancelliere, Kassa, & Black, 1985; Levin, 1973). Heilman and Watson (1991) postulated that as part of a cortical–subcortical circuit, the dorsolateral frontal cortices play a key role in intentional motor activity. Sakai, Nakamura, Sakurai, Yamaguchi, and Hirai (2000) proposed that simultanapraxia, a subset of motor impersistence, is associated with the lesions involving the frontal areas 6 and 8 in the right middle cerebral artery territory.

## SMALL ARTERIES AND SUBCORTICAL STROKES

The frontal lobe, together with its intimate connections with the basal ganglia and thalamus, integrates motor, attentional, emotional, and executive responses. The basal ganglia and thalamus are perfused by small penetrating arteries that arise from or near the circle of Willis. In the basal ganglia, the "limbic" and lateral orbital circuits, which subserve attention and emotion, are positioned in the ventromedial caudate and receive their blood supply primarily from perforating branches of the ACA.

The motor and dorsolateral frontal–subcortical circuits, which make major contributions to movement and executive function, are positioned more laterally and are fed predominantly from the lenticulostriate arteries, originating from the M1 segment of the MCA. The vascular supply of these circuits as they pass through the thalamus is overlapping and complex.

Chronic hypertension and diabetes mellitus are the main risk factors for the development of arteriolar sclerosis in these small penetrating arteries. Occlusion leads to small lacunar infarcts (Fisher, 1965, 1979). Rupture leads to deep intracerebral hemorrhages. A wide variety of motor, cognitive, and behavioral deficits manifest, with many having a "frontal lobe" quality.

## Basal Ganglia

### Head of Caudate

The head of the caudate is supplied by penetrating arteries from both the ACA and the MCA (Figure 29.1c). The ACA gives rise to Heubner's arteries, a series of two to four vessels that usually arise from the A2 portion of the ACA. These vessels supply the inferior part of the head of the caudate nucleus, the adjacent anterior limb of the internal capsule, and the subfrontal white matter. Direct penetrating arteries from the ACA (called "medial striate" or "anterior lenticulostriate arteries") supply the anterior portion of the head of the caudate nucleus.

The MCA gives rise to medial lenticulostriate arteries that branch from the proximal M1 portion of that artery and supply a small portion of the lateral border of the caudate head and the adjacent internal capsule. The lateral lenticulostriate arteries branch from the mainstem MCA or its superior division to supply the major portion of the head of the caudate nucleus, as well as the adjacent internal capsule and the anterior half of the putamen (Caplan, 2002). The most commonly involved arterial territories in caudate infarction are the territory of the lateral lenticulostriate arteries from the MCA and the territory of the anterior lenticulostriate arteries from the ACA (Kumral, Evyapan, & Balkir, 1999) (see Figure 29.3).

Infarcts in the territory of the lateral lenticulostriate arteries cause prominent motor and neuropsychological deficits (Kumral et al., 1999). Small infarcts in the caudate or striatum and internal capsule result from small-artery disease, ipsilateral internal carotid or MCA disease, cardiac embolism, and mixed etiologies (Bang, Heo, Kim, Park, & Huh, 2002; Kumral et al., 1999).

Based on anatomical connectivity, three distinct behavioral syndromes are predicted: (1) Lesions in the ventromedial head of the caudate, by virtue of its connections with the orbital frontal cortex, will be associated with irritability and disinhibition; (2) lesions in the dorsolateral head of the caudate, as part of the feedback circuit to the principal sulcus, will be associated with dysexecutive function; and (3) lesions in the nucleus accumbens or ventral striatum, which is closely connected with the anterior cingulate, will be associated with apathy and hypokinesia.

Attempts have also been made to localize the site of a lesion within the head of the caudate. Mendez, Adams, and Lewandowsky (1989) reviewed 12 cases with caudate lesions, 11 unilateral, and 1 bilateral. In seven cases, where neuropsychological testing was available, impairments were noted in planning and sequencing, attention, and recent and remote memory. When the lesions were more extensive and involved most of the head of the caudate, affective disturbances such as anxiety and depression were predominant. When the dorsolateral was more affected than the ventromedial head of the caudate, patients tended to be apathetic and abulic.

In this study, behavioral patterns correlated with the size and location, but not with the side, of the lesions. Clinical brain–behavior correlations correspond in a general way to predictions based on anatomical connectivity in nonhuman primates. Patients with anterior type of striatocapsular hemorrhage, which mainly involves the caudate nucleus, showed similar behavioral features with caudate infarcts, including acute confusion, abulia, and transcortical motor aphasia (Chung et al., 2000).

Side of the lesion correlates with clinical syndrome. Linguistic deficits, including micrographia, verbal memory problems, hypersexuality, decreased attention, and impaired abstract thinking are associated with left-sided lesions, whereas neglect is related to right-sided ones (Bokura & Robinson, 1997; Caplan et al., 1990; Kumral et al., 1999; Mendez et al., 1989; Nagaratnam et al., 2004; Nakamura et al., 2003; Troyer, Black, Armilio, & Moscovitch, 2004). Croisile, Tourniaire, Confavreux, Trillet, and Aimard (1989) reported on a patient who initially presented with apathy, word-finding difficulty, and incoherent writing in association with an infarct in the left head of caudate. These differences correspond with lateralization of these functions following cortical lesions. But the relationship of side of lesion behavioral changes that result is not always consistent because of the involvement of neighboring structures and/or the difference in assessing the behavioral changes.

Behavioral or emotional abnormalities include abulia, restlessness/agitation, depression,

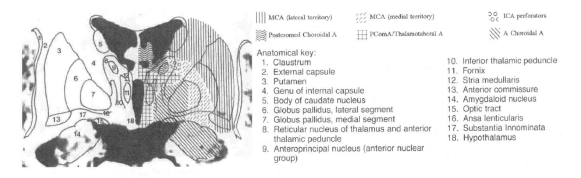

FIGURE 29.3. Blood supply of the basal ganglia; coronal scan through genu of internal capsule. From Pullicino (1993). Copyright 1993 by Lippincott Williams and Wilkins. Adapted by permission.

confusion, and hyperactivity more commonly in case of bilateral damage to the head of the caudate. Richfield, Twyman, and Berent (1987) reported on a woman with bilateral caudate head infarction who showed personality changes, including impulsive behaviors, indifference, hypersexuality, minor criminal acts, low tolerance of frustration, and angry outbursts. Habib and Poncet (1988) described two cases with multiple lacunar lesions in bilateral striatum and caudate. Both showed marked personality changes, including a loss of interest and drive, loss of curiosity, and flattened affect. Thus, the behaviors associated with bilateral infarction of the head of caudate are reminiscent of all three prefrontal syndromes.

### Putamen

The putamen, the major striatal component of the motor system, is largely supplied by the lateral bank of lenticuostriate arteries from the MCA (Figure 29.3). The clinical presentation of pure lenticular infarction includes faciobrachiocrural hemiparesis with ataxia, sensory deficit, and deep pain (Russmann, Vingerhoets, Ghika, Maeder, & Bogousslavsky, 2003). Movement disorders such as chorea and dystonia may be seen (Giroud, Lemesle, Madinier, Billiar, & Dumas, 1997). In the case of striatocapsular hemorrhage, the middle and posterolateral types primarily affect the putamen, and clinical features resemble those of striatocapsular infarcts except for frequent impairment of consciousness (Chung et al., 2000).

Neurocognitive features with infarcts limited to the putamen include transcortical motor or nonfluent aphasia, acute short-term memory deficits, and hemineglect (Damasio et al., 1980; Giroud et al., 1997; Karnath, Ferber, & Himmelbach, 2001; Russmann et al., 2003). Relatively minor degrees of dysexecutive function are reported with lenticular lesions. Godefroy and colleagues (1992) reported on six patients with unilateral subcortical lesions who were impaired in cross-tapping (a motor task) but not in other tasks sensitive to executive dysfunction (e.g., Trail Making Test or Wisconsin Card Sorting Test). Significant executive dysfunctions were only noted in patients who had additional cortical lesions.

Weiller and colleagues (1993) reviewed 57 cases with striatocapsular infarcts and found 12 cases with neglect, all with right-sided lesions predominantly in the putamen. The most severe neglect syndromes were caused by either large caudate–putaminal–capsular infarcts in the distribution of the lateral lenticulostriate branches or smaller infarcts of the capsule and pallidum in the distribution of the anterior choroidal artery. A lesser degree of neglect or extinction was noted with capsular–pallidal lesions in the distribution of the mesial lenticulostriate arteries. Spatial neglect following putaminal lesions may result because of its dense anatomical connectivity with the superior temporal gyrus, which is important for spatial awareness (Karnath et al., 2001; Karnath, Himmelbach, & Rorden, 2002).

In summary, disturbances in movement, language, and spatial attention are commonly reported with striatocapsular lesions. Personality changes and dysexecutive syndrome occur less frequently with lesions in the putamen compared to the head of the caudate. This is in keeping with the pattern of anatomical connectivity: the putamen with the motor system; the head of the caudate with lateral orbital and dorsolateral prefrontal cortices.

### Globus Pallidus

The globus pallidus externus is supplied by the medial lenticulostriate arteries, whereas the globus pallidus internus is fed by the anterior choroidal artery and ACA perforators (Figure 29.3). Behavioral and cognitive disorders are associated with infarction of the globus pallidus (Giroud et al., 1997). Symptoms may include acute abulia and disinhibition, and later, obsessive–compulsive disorders. Akinetic mutism may follow bilateral basal ganglia lesions (LaPlane, Baulac, Widlocher, & Dubois, 1984). Acute verbal short-term memory deficits were observed in patients with globus pallidus infarction with concomitant decreased blood flow in the homolateral temporal area, despite the absence of cortical lesions on MRI (Giroud et al., 1997). Hemorrhage involving the globus pallidus may cause impairment in consciousness and language dysfunction (anomic dysphasia and global aphasia). Personality change has been described following bilateral pallidal hemorrhage (Chung et al., 2000; Strub, 1989).

Experimental evidence indicates that lesions in the external globus pallidus may result in movement or behavioral disorders, depending on the site of focal dysfunction (Grabli et al., 2004). Abnormal movements were observed after microinjections of bicuculine in the posterior sensorimotor territory, whereas behavioral changes followed microinjections into the anterior external globus pallidus. Anatomical studies suggest that neuronal circuits from the globus pallidus are involved in pathologies such as Tourette's syndrome, attention-deficit/hyperactivity disorders, and obsessive–compulsive disorders (François et al., 2004).

## Thalamus

The thalamus represents a key way station in the parallel, but segregated, organization of the frontal–subcortical circuits. The three prefrontal behavioral circuits converge on the anterior thalamic or dorsomedial nucleus. In turn, the anterior thalamic nucleus projects to the anterior cingulate gyrus, whereas the dorsomedial thalamic nucleus projects to dorsolateral and orbitofrontal cortices. The motor circuit projects to the ventral anterior/ventrolateral nucleus of the thalamus, and subsequently back upon the SMA.

The arterial supply to the thalamus can be divided into four territories originating from the circle of Willis and vertebrobasilar system: (1) the tuberothalamic or polar territory; (2) the paramedian territory; (3) the thalamogeniculate or inferolateral territory; and (4) the posterior choroidal territory (Figure 29.4).

### Ventral Anterior and Anterior Thalamus

The ventral anterior thalamic nucleus (VA) participates in two of the three prefrontal circuits (Alexander et al., 1986): (1) The pars parvocellularis projects to the dorsolateral prefrontal cortex, and (2) the pars magnocellularis, to the lateral orbitoprefrontal cortex. The anterior nucleus of the thalamus is an integral component of the limbic–diencephalic memory system. The anterior thalamic nucleus together with portions of the ventrolateral thalamic nucleus (VL) is supplied by the tuberothalamic artery, which arises from the PCoA (Bogousslavsky, Regli, & Uske, 1988). Mild transient hemiparesis or hemisensory deficits (Bogousslavsky & Regli, 1986; Bogousslavsky et al., 1988), facial paresis for emotional movements (Bogousslavsky & Regli, 1986), hemiataxia (Melo, Bogousslavsky, Moulin, Nader, & Regli, 1992), and disappearance of hemiparkinsonian dysfunction (Dubois, Pillon, De Saxcé, Lhermitte, & Agid, 1986) have been reported.

Infarction in the territory of the tuberothalamic artery is characterized by severe neuropsychological dysfunctions, including fluctuating level of consciousness, personality changes, emotional unconcern or disinhibition, executive dysfunction, and impairment of recent memory (Gutierrez, Davalos, Pedraza, Garcia, & Kulisevsky, 2003; Schmahmann,

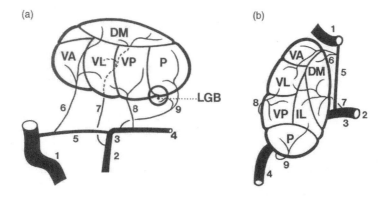

FIGURE 29.4. Thalamic vascular supply. Schematic diagram of lateral (a) and dorsal (b) views of the four major thalamic arteris and the nuclei they irrigate: 1, carotid artery; 2, basilar artery; 3, P1 region of the posterior cerebral artery (mesencephalic artery); 4, posterior cerebral artery; 5, posterior communicating artery; 6, tuberothalamic or polar artery; 7, paramedian artery; 8, thalamogeniculate or inferolateral artery; 9, posterior choroidal artery; DM, dorsomedial nucleus; VA, ventral anterior nucleus; VL, ventral lateral nucleus; VP, ventral posterior nucleus; IL, intralaminar nucleus complex; P, pulvinar; LBG, lateral geniculate body. From de Freitas and Bogousslavsky (2002). Copyright 2002 by Oxford University Press. Adapted by permission.

2003). Impaired planning and motor sequencing, and severe perseverative behaviors were also noted in thinking, spontaneous speech, memory, and executive tasks in the same patients. Daum and Akerman (1994) described frontal-type memory problems, including impaired spatial working memory, increased forgetting rates, poor prospective memory, inadequate elaborative encoding, as well as prefrontal-type personality change (e.g., irritability, liability, disinhibition, inappropriateness, and distractability) following right anterior thalamic infarction.

Memory deficits in tuberothalamic infarcts may represent a disconnection involving two pathways: (1) between anterior thalamic nuclei and hippocampal formation in virtue of the disruption of the mamillothalamic tract, and (2) between amygdala and anterior nuclei by damage to the amygdalothalamic projections passing through the internal medullary lamina (Graff-Radford, Tranel, van Hoesen, & Brandt, 1990; Schott, Crutch, Fox, & Warrington, 2003; von Cramon, Hebel, & Schuri, 1985).

### Dorsomedial Thalamus

The dorsomedial nucleus of the thalamus is interwoven with all three prefrontal–subcortical circuits (Alexander et al., 1986): (1) the pars parvocellularis has reciprocal connections with the dorsolateral prefrontal cortex, (2) the pars magnocellularis has reciprocal connections with orbitofrontal cortex, and (3) the posteromedial dorsomedial nucleus is interconnected with the anterior cingulate (Sandson, Daffner, Carvalho, & Mesulam, 1991). The dorsomedial nucleus is also integrated within the limbic–diencephalic memory system. The principal vascular supplies to the dorsomedial thalamic nuclei are branches of the paramedian artery arising from the basilar artery and, to a lesser degree, branches of the tuberothalamic artery, which arises from the PCoA (de Freitas & Bogousslavksy, 2002).

The behavioral sequelae of dorsomedial thalamic lesions recapitulate all of the principal features of the three prefrontal syndromes (Table 29.3). Lesions including the dorsomedial nucleus, midline nuclei, and/or intralaminar nuclei accompanied executive dysfunction (Ysbrand et al., 2003). Reduced simple processing speed and attention were associated with age, but complex attention deficits followed damage to the intralaminar nucleus.

**TABLE 29.3. Neuropsychological Disturbances of Paramedian Infarcts**

Left-sided
  Dysphasia, aphonia
  Decreased verbal memory
  Amnesia (Korsakoff-like)
Right-sided
  Hemineglect and impaired visuospatial
    processing
  Decreased nonverbal memory
  Apathy, aspontaneity
  Acute confusional state
  Pseudomaniac state
Bilateral
  Amnesia and other disturbances listed above
  Thalamic dementia
  Akinetic mutism
  Loss of psychic self-activation
  Others: palilalia, hallucinosis, utilization
    behavior, bulimia

*Note.* From de Freitas and Bogousslavsky (2002). Copyright 2002 by Oxford University Press. Adapted by permission.

Left-sided lesions are accompanied by deficits in verbal processing and memory, whereas right-sided lesions tend to be associated with hemineglect and visuospatial problems. Behavioral changes include decreased response initiation and inhibition, perseverative behaviors, poor judgment and insight (Baumgartner & Regard, 1993; Sandson et al., 1991), or manic delirium (Bogousslavsky, Ferrazzini, et al., 1988). In a recent study of thalamic structure–function relationships (Ysbrand et al., 2003), deficits of episodic long-term memory with relative sparing of intellectual capacities and short-term memory were associated with the mamillothalamic tract damage.

### Internal Capsule

The blood supply of the fan-shaped internal capsule is highly complex: its anterior limb receives some supply from a large branch of the ACA known as Heubner's artery. Although the MCA supplies the anterior limb in one-third of cases, most of the posterior limb of the internal capsule is fed by the deep, lenticulostriate branches of the MCA, whereas the lowest portion of the posterior limb is supplied by the anterior choroidal artery, which usually arises from the internal carotid artery (Mohr et al., 2004) (see Figure 29.5).

Small deep infarcts, or lacunes, confined to the internal capsule typically cause unilateral

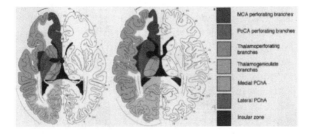

FIGURE 29.5. Arterial territories of internal capsule. From Tatu, Moulin, Bogousslavsky, and Duvernoy (1998). Copyright 1998 by Lippincott Williams & Wilkins. Adapted by permission.

isolated weakness (50%), although other syndromes such as motor–sensory loss (30%) or ataxic hemisparesis (20%) are also seen (Tei, Uchyyama, & Maruyama, 1993). In a series of 72 single capsular infarcts, 71% were in the MCA distribution, 21% were in anterior choroidal, and 8% were in the ACA distribution (Tei et al., 1993).

### Anterior Limb

The anterior limb of the internal capsule conveys axons from the SMA (Fries, Danek, Scheidtmann, & Hamburger, 1993), as well as frontopontine and thalamic peduncles. The anterior limb is usually fed by Heubner's artery, which also supplies the medial head of the caudate. Thus, ischemic lesions usually extend into the medial portion of the head of the caudate, globus pallidus, or putamen ("striatocapsular infarct").

Infarction of the anterior limb is initially associated with hemiparesis, predominantly affecting the arm, face, and bulbar musculature, and causing slow gait, urinary incontinence, or pure dyarthria (Ozaki, Baba, Marita, Matsunaga, & Takebe, 1986). Infarction limited to the anterior limb of the right internal capsule causes motor extinction or motor neglect (de la Sayette et al., 1989; Viader, Cambier, & Pariser, 1982). Bilateral infarction in the anterior limb of the internal capsule produced loss of motivation for speaking (Croisile et al., 1989). Recovery of motor weakness and dysarthria is usually good (Fries et al., 1993; Ozaki et al., 1986).

### Genu

The genu carries fibers that originate from the SMA and course initially through the anterior limb of the internal capsule (Fries et al., 1993).

Infarction of the genu of the internal capsule is associated with contralateral facial or lingual weakness and dysarthria (Bogousslavsky & Regli, 1990). Yamanaka, Fukuyama, and Kimura (1996) reported on two patients with pure abulia, without motor weakness associated with unilateral capsular genu infarction.

The genu and the anterior limb of the internal capsule also contain fibers that originate from the anterior and dorsomedial nuclei of the thalamus through the anterior thalamic peduncle and terminate in the frontal lobe and the cingulate gyrus. Therefore, disconnection of the thalamofrontal fibers due to the infarction of the genu may produce frontal lobe dysfunction such as abulia.

Tatemichi, Desmond, and Mayeux (1992) and Tatemichi, Desmond, and Prohovnik (1995) reviewed six patients who developed confusion, memory loss, or dementia associated with lacunar infarction of the inferior genu of the internal capsule fed by the internal carotid artery or ACA perforators. These authors posited that these lesions strategically disrupted the inferior and medial thalamic peduncles carrying thalamocortical fibers related to cognition and memory.

### Posterior Limb

The superior portion of the posterior limb of the internal capsule is supplied by lenticulostriate arteries, whereas the inferior–posterior portion of the posterior limb is supplied by the anterior choroidal artery. The anterior portion of the posterior limb of the internal capsule contains fibers from dorsolateral premotor cortex, whereas the middle and posterior areas of the posterior limb carry fibers from primary motor cortex (Fries et al., 1993). The pyramidal tract located in the anterior half of the posterior limb intermingles with fibers of the superior thalamic peduncle. Parietal–occipital–pontine fibers are located in the posterior part of the posterior limb (Hubertus & Diedrich, 2000).

Severe motor weakness follows infarction of the middle one-third of posterior limb of the internal capsule. Milder weakness occurs following infarction of the genu, anterior limb, and anterior or posterior one-third of the posterior limb (Misra & Kalita, 1997). Kashihara and Matsumoto (1985) described more favorable recovery of motor function with lesions located more laterally and superiorly compared to those located more posteriorly. Fries and colleagues (1993) noted excellent motor recovery when lesions were confined to the white matter of the posterior limb (e.g., distribution of anterior choroidal artery), but less favorable recovery if the lesion also affected the thalamus. Differences in recovery might reflect the extent of damage to the descending motor pathways, as well as the degree of concomitant sensory loss.

Mild ataxia, with and without hemiparesis or hemisensory loss, has been infrequently reported following small ischemic lesions in the posterior limb of the internal capsule that may extend into the neighboring thalamus (Helgason & Wilbur, 1990; Iragui & McCutchen, 1982; Luijckx, Boiten, Lodder, Heuts-van Raak, & Wilmink, 1994). Hypesthetic ataxic hemiparesis correlated with larger infarcts than those of pure motor and sensory lacunar stroke, and most often were located in the posteromedial superior territory of the anterior choroidal artery (Helgason & Wilbur, 1990). Such lesions are purported to interrupt corticocerebellar pathways, either the ascending dentatorubrothalamocortical or the descending corticopontocerebellar fibers.

Helgason and colleagues (1988) described eight patients with acute pseudobulbar mutism due to bilateral infarction of the posterior limb of the internal capsule. Inability to speak, swallow, or phonate appeared with the onset of a new infarct located in a mirror position, contralateral to an older lesion located in the territory of the anterior choroidal artery.

## SUBCORTICAL ISCHEMIC VASCULAR DEMENTIA (SIVD)

Three dementia syndromes have been described in relation to subcortical ischemic brain injury: (1) strategic-infarct dementia, (2) lacunar state, and (3) Binswanger's syndrome. All of them are characterized by a frontal dysexecutive syndrome.

## Strategic-Infarct Dementia

Strategic-infarct dementia refers to a single stroke that results in a variety of cognitive deficits. These lesions tend to be left-sided or bilateral and located in the caudate and thalamus. Thalamic dementia is characterized by marked apathy, impaired attention and mental control, anterograde and retrograde amnesia, impaired verbal fluency, transcortical aphasia, and disinhibition due to interruption of thalamocortical circuits (Katz, Alexander, & Mandell, 1987; Stuss, Guberman, Nelson, & Larochelle, 1988; Szirmai, Vastagh, Szombathelyi, & Kamondi, 2002). Other strategic locations associated with dementia syndromes include the left angular gyrus, left subcortical frontal lobe, including minor forceps, left basal forebrain, anterior corpus callosum, and medial frontal lobe, together with the anterior corpus callosum (Auchus, Chen, Sodagar, Thong, & Sng, 2002).

## Lacunar State

Lacunar state describes the cases with multiple subcortical infarcts affecting the thalamus, basal ganglia, and deep white matter. Neurological findings include mild pyramidal tract signs, gait disorders (apractic–atactic or small-stepped), urinary incontinence, dysarthria, and extrapyramidal signs. Cognitive and behavioral dysfunction include lack of volition, personality changes, depression, emotional lability, slowing of information processing, and decreased attention (Babikian & Ropper, 1987; Ishii, Nishihara, & Imamura, 1986; Pohjasvaara, Mäntylä, Ylikoski, Kaste, & Erkinjuntti, 2003; Thomas et al., 2002). Psychomotor speed and simple attention are preferentially impaired in subcortical forms of dementia, whereas the higher levels of selective and divided attention are likely more markedly disrupted in AD (Gainotti, Marra, & Villar, 2001). Overall rate of deterioration in subcortical dementia (Aharon-Peretz, Daskovski, Mashiach, & Tomer, 2002), mainly lacunar type (−1.4 ± 2.3 by Mini-Mental State Examination [MMSE] points), is usually less than that of Alzheimer's disease (−3.9 ± 3.7 MMSE points) (Morris et al., 1989).

## Binswanger's Syndrome

Binswanger (1894) described eight patients with slow, progressive mental deterioration and pronounced white matter changes, with secondary dilatation of the ventricles. Alzheimer (1902) described the corresponding microscopic features, including hyalination, intimal fibrosis, and onion skinning of the long medullary arteries, together with severe gliosis of the white matter. Loeb (2000) suggested that the clinicopathological features of Binswanger's syndrome, or "chronic microvascular leukoencephalopathy," may result from various pathogenetic mechanisms. Several non-mutually-exclusive possibilities include (1) chronic ischemia and incomplete infarction (Englund & Person, 1987; Román, 1987), (2) loss of myelinated axons caused by arterial adventitial fibrosis and breakdown of the ventricular lining (Scheltens et al., 1995), (3) combination of myelin loss, axonal loss, scattered microinfarcts, astrogliosis, and dilatation of perivascular spaces (Udaka, Sawada, & Kameyama, 2002), (4) heredity (Carmelli et al., 1998), and (5) apoptosis of oligodendroytes (Brown, Moody, Challa, Thore, & Anstrom, 2002).

The advent of neuroimaging has markedly lowered the threshold for the detection of white matter changes. These are referred to as white matter hyperintensities (WMHs) on T2-weighted MRI or leukoaraiosis (LA, or white matter rarefaction) on computed tomography. WMH is associated with stroke (Inzitari, 2003), multiple lacunes and callosal atrophy (Ferro & Madureira, 2002), and cognitive decline (Breteler et al., 1994; Englund, 2002; Pantoni & Garcia, 1995; Pantoni et al., 1999; Skoog, Berg, Johansson, Palmertz, & Andreasson, 1996).

Anterior WMHs are more relevant for cognitive decline than are posterior WMHs. Frontal WMHs are related to verbal fluency (Fernaeus et al., 2001; Yamauchi, Fukuyama, & Shio, 2000). The Rotterdam Study (de Groot et al., 2000) suggests that periventricular WMHs are more important for cognitive function than are subcortical WMHs, whereas other studies describe a regional difference of WMH that causes cognitive dysfunction (Ferro & Madureira, 2002; Fukui, Sugita, Sato, Takeuchi, & Tsukagoshi, 1994; Garde, Mortensen, Krabbe, Rostrup, & Larsson, 2000). Interestingly, white matter lesions impair frontal lobe function regardless of their location and are associated with frontal glucose metabolism (Tullberg et al., 2004).

## CONCLUSION

Our understanding of the vascular diseases of the frontal lobes reflects a dynamic interplay among clinical observation, experimental studies, and cognitive neuroscience. Early observations in patients with large-vessel strokes outlined the principal features of the major motor, cognitive, and behavioral syndromes. Essentially identical observations are recapitulated in connection with much smaller infarcts located deep in the brain. These similarities make sense once frontal lobe functions are conceptualized as a distributed network—even more so, when segregated but parallel frontal–subcortical circuits are mapped in nonhuman primates. Sensitive and noninvasive neuroimaging tools are now available for brain–behavior correlations. These developments promise a new level of investigation and insight regarding vascular diseases of the frontal lobes.

## REFERENCES

Adams, J. P., Jr., Hachinski, V., & Norris, J. W. (2001). *Ischemic cerebrovascular disease*. New York: Oxford University Press.

Aharon-Peretz, J., Daskovski, E., Mashiach, T., & Tomer, R. (2002). Natural history of dementia associated with lacunar infarction. *Journal of the Neurological Sciences, 203–204,* 53–55.

Alexander, G. E., & Crutcher, M. D. (1990). Functional architecture of basal ganglia circuits: Neural substrates of parallel processing. *Trends in Neurosciences, 13,* 266–271.

Alexander, G. E., DeLong, M. R., & Strick, P. L. (1986). Parallel organization of functionally segregated circuits linking basal ganglia and cortex. *Annual Review of Neuroscience, 9,* 357–381.

Alzheimer, A. (1902). Die Seelenstrorungen auf arteriscleroticcher Grundlage. *Allgemeine Zeitschrift für Psychiatrie und Psychisch-Gerichtlich Medicin, 59,* 695–711.

American Heart Association. (1994). *Heart and stroke facts: Statistical supplement.* Dallas, TX: Author.

Astrom, M., Adolfsson, R., & Asplund, K. (1993). Major depression in stroke patients: A 3-year longitudinal study. *Stroke, 24,* 976–982.

Auchus, A. P., Chen, C., Sodagar, S. N., Thong, M., & Sng, E. (2000). Single stroke dementia: Insights from 12 cases in Singapore. *Journal of the Neurological Sciences, 203–204,* 85–89.

Babikian, V., & Ropper, A. H. (1987). Binswanger's disease: A review. *Stroke, 18,* 2–12.

Bang, O. Y., Heo, J. H., Kim, J. Y., Park, J. H., & Huh, K. (2002). Middle cerebral artery stenosis is a major clinical determinant in striatocapsular small, deep infarction. *Archives of Neurology, 59,* 259–263.

Baumgartner, R. W., & Regard, M. (1993). Bilateral neuropsychological deficits in unilateral paramedian thalamic infarction. *European Neurology, 33,* 195–198.

Beblo, T., Wallesch, C. W., & Herrmann, M. (1999). The crucial role of frontostriatal circuits for depressive disorders in the postacute stage after stroke. *Neuropsychiatry, Neuropsychology, and Behavioral Neurology, 12,* 236–246.

Benson, D. F. (1993). Aphasia. In K. M. Heilman & E. Valenstein (Eds.), *Clinical neuropsychology* (pp. 17–36). New York: Oxford University Press.

Binswanger, O. (1894). Die Abgrenzung der allgemeinen progressiven Paraluse. *Berliner Linnische Wochenschrift, 31,* 1102–1105, 1137–1139.

Bodini, B., Iacoboni, M., & Lenzi, G. L. (2004). Acute stroke effects on emotions: An interpretation through the mirror system. *Current Opinion in Neurology, 17,* 55–60.

Bogousslavsky, J., Ferrazzini, F., Regli, F., Assal, G., Tanabe, H., & Delaloye-Bischof A. (1988). Manic delirium and frontal-like syndrome with paramedian infarction of the right thalamus. *Journal of Neurology, Neurosurgery, and Psychiatry, 51,* 116–119.

Bogousslavsky, J., & Regli, F. (1986). Borderzone infarctions distal to internal carotid artery occlusion: Prognostic implications. *Annals of Neurology, 20,* 346–350.

Bogousslavsky, J., & Regli, F. (1990). Capsular genu syndrome. *Neurology, 40,* 1499–1502.

Bogousslavksy, J., Regli, F., & Uske, A. (1988). Thalamic infarcts: Clinical syndrome, etiology, and prognosis. *Neurology, 38,* 837–848.

Bokura, H., & Robinson, R. (1997). Long-term cognitive impairment associated with caudate stroke. *Stroke, 28,* 970–975.

Böttger, S., Prosiegel, M., Steiger, H. J., & Yassouridis, A. (1998). Neurobehavioral disturbances, rehabilitation outcome, and lesion site in patients after rupture and repair of anterior communicating artery aneurysm. *Journal of Neurology, Neurosurgery, and Psychiatry, 65,* 93–102.

Breteler, M. M. B., van Swieten, J. C., Bots, M. L., Grobbee, D. E., Claus, J. J., van den Hout, J. H., et al. (1994). Cerebral white matter lesions, vascular risk factors, and cognitive function in a population-based study: The Rotterdam study. *Neurology, 44,* 1246–1252.

Broderick, J. P. (1994). Intracerebral hemorrhage. In P. B. Gorelick & M. Alter (Eds.), *Handbook of neuroepidemiology* (pp. 141–164). New York: Marcel Dekker.

Broderick, J. P., Phillips, S. J., Whisnant, J. P., O'Fallon, W. M., & Begstrahl, E. J. (1989). Incidence rates of stroke in the eighties: The end of the decline in stroke? *Stroke, 20,* 577–582.

Brown, W. R., Moody, D. M., Challa, V. R., Thore, C. R., & Anstrom, J. A. (2002). Apoptosis in leuko-araiosis lesions. *Journal of the Neurological Sciences, 203–204,* 169–171.

Brust, J. C., & Chamorro, A. (2004). Anterior cerebral artery disease. In J. P. Mohr, D. W. Choi, J. C. Grotta, B. Weir, & P. A. Wolf (Eds.), *Stroke: Pathophysiology, diagnosis, and management* (4th ed., pp. 101–122). Philadelphia: Churchill Livingstone.

Brust, J. C., Sawada, T., & Kazui, S. (2001). Anterior cerebral artery. In J. Bogousslavsky & L. R. Caplan (Eds.), *Stroke syndromes* (pp. 439–450). Cambridge, UK: Cambridge University Press.

Burvill, P., Johnson, G., Jamrozik, K., Anderson, C., & Stewart-Wynne, E. (1997). Risk factors for post-stroke depression. *International Journal of Geriatric Psychiatry, 12,* 219–226.

Caplan, L. R. (2002). Caudate infarcts. In G. Donnan, B. Norrving, J. Bamford, & J. Bogousslavsky (Eds.), *Subcortical stroke* (2nd. ed., pp. 209–223). New York: Oxford University Press.

Caplan, L. R., Schmahmann, J. D., Kase, C. S., Feldmann, E., Baquis, G., Greenberg, J. P., et al. (1990). Caudate infarcts. *Archives of Neurology, 47,* 133–143.

Carmelli, D., DeCarli, C., Swan, G. E., Jack, L. M., Reed, T., Wolf, P. A., et al. (1998). Evidence for genetic variance in white matter hyperintensity volume in normal elderly male twins. *Stroke, 29,* 1177–1181.

Castillo, C. S., Schultz, S. K., & Robinson, R. G. (1995). Clinical correlates of early-onset and late-onset post-stroke generalized anxiety. *American Journal of Psychiatry, 152,* 1174–1179.

Chung, C. S., Caplan, L. R., Yamamoto, Y., Chang, H. M., Lee, S. J., Song, H. J., et al. (2000). Striato-capsular haemorrhage. *Brain, 123,* 1850–1862.

Critchley, M. (1930). The anterior cerebral artery and its syndromes. *Brain, 53,* 120–165.

Croisile, B., Tourniaire, D., Confavreux, C., Trillet, M., & Aimard, G. (1989). Bilateral damage to the head of the caudate nuclei. *Annals of Neurology, 25,* 313–314.

Cummings, J. L., & Mendez, M. F. (1984). Secondary mania with focal cerebrovascular lesions. *American Journal of Psychiatry, 141,* 1084–1087.

Damasio, A. R., Damasio, H., & Chui, H. (1980). Neglect following damage to frontal lobe or basal ganglia. *Neuropsychologia, 18,* 123–132.

Damasio, A. R., Graff-Radford, N. R., Eslinger, P. J., Damasio, H., & Kassell, N. (1985). Amnesia following basal forebrain lesions. *Archives of Neurology, 42,* 263–271.

Damasio, A. R., & Vandstensen, G. W. (1980). Structure and function of the supplementary motor area. *Neurology, 30,* 300–359.

Damasio, A. R., & van Hoesen, G. W. (1983). Focal lesions of the limbic frontal lobe. In K. M. Heilman & P. Satz (Eds.), *Neuropsychology of human emotion* (pp. 85–110). New York: Guilford Press.

Damasio, H. (1992). Neuroanatomy of frontal lobe in vivo: A comment on methodology. In H. S. Levin, H. M. Eisenberg, & A. L. Benton (Eds.), *Frontal lobe function and dysfunction* (pp. 92–121). New York: Oxford University Press.

Daum, I., & Akerman, H. (1994). Frontal-type memory impairment associated with thalamic damage. *International Journal of Neuroscience, 75,* 153–165.

de Freitas, G. R., & Bogousslavsky, J. (2002). Thalamic infarcts. In G. Donnan, B. Norrving, J. Bamford, & J. Bogousslavsky (Eds.), *Subcortical stroke* (2nd ed., pp. 255–285). New York: Oxford University Press.

Degos, J. D., da Fonseca, N., Gray, F., & Cesaro, P. (1993). Severe frontal syndrome associated with infarcts of the left anterior cingulate gyrus and the head of the right caudate nucleus: A clinico-pathological case. *Brain, 116,* 1541–1548.

de Groot, J. C., De Leeuw, F.-E., Oudkerk, M., van Gijn, J., Hoffman, A., Jolles, J., et al. (2000). Cerebral white matter lesions and cognitive function: The Rotterdam Scan Study. *Annals of Neurology, 47,* 145–151.

de la Sayette, V., Bouvard, G., Eustache, F., Chapon, F., Viader, F., & Lechevalier, B. (1989). Infarct of the anterior limb of the right internal capsule causing left motor neglect: Case report and cerebral blood flow study. *Cortex, 25,* 147–154.

DeLuca, J. (1992). Cognitive dysfunction after aneurysm of the anterior communicating artery. *Journal of Clinical and Experimental Neuropsychology, 14,* 924–934.

Devinsky, O., Morrell, M. J., & Vogt, B. A. (1995). Contributions of the anterior cingulate cortex to behavior. *Brain, 118,* 279–306.

Dichgans, M., Herzog, J., & Gasser, T. (2001). Notch3 mutation involving three cysteine residues in a family with typical CADASIL. *Neurology, 57,* 1714–1717.

Dubois, B., Pillon, B., De Saxcé, H., Lhermitte, F., & Agid, Y. (1986). Disappearance of parkinsonian signs after spontaneous vascular "thalamotomy." *Archives of Neurology, 43,* 815–817.

Dunker, R. O., & Harris, A. B. (1976). Surgical anatomy of the proximal anterior cerebral artery. *Journal of Neurosurgery, 44,* 359–367.

Eastwood, M. R., Rifat, S. L., Nobbs, H., & Ruderman, J. (1989). Mood disorder following cerebrovascular accident. *British Journal of Psychiatry, 154,* 195–200.

Englund, E. (2002). Neuropathology of white matter lesions in vascular cognitive impairment. *Cerebrovascular Disorders, 13*(Suppl. 2), 11–15.

Englund, E., & Person, B. (1987). Correlations between histopathologic white matter changes and proton MR relaxation times in dementia. *Alzheimer Disease and Associated Disorders, 1,* 156–170.

Fazekas, F., Kleinert, R., Roob, G., Kleinert, G., Kapeller, P., Schmidt, R., et al. (1999). Histopathologic analysis of foci of signal loss on gradient-echo T2-weighted MR images in patients with spontaneous intracerebral hemorrhage: Evidence of microangiopathy-related microbleeds. *American Journal of Neuroradiology, 20,* 637–642.

Feinberg, T. E., Schindler, R. J., Flanagan, N. G., & Haber, L. D. (1992). Two alien hand syndromes. *Neurology, 42,* 19–24.

Fernaeus, S. E., Almkvist, O., Bronge, L., Ostberg, P., Hellstrom, A., Winbald, B., et al. (2001). White matter lesions impair initiation of FAS flow. *Dementia and Geriatric Cognitive Disorders, 12,* 52–56.

Ferro, J. M., & Madureira, S. (2002). Age-related white matter changes and cognitive impairment. *Journal of the Neurological Sciences, 203–204,* 221–225.

Fisher, M. (1956). Left hemiplegia and motor impersistence. *Journal of Nervous and Mental Disease, 123,* 201–218.

Fisher, C. M. (1965). Lacunes: Small deep cerebral infarcts. *Neurology, 15,* 774–784.

Fisher, C. M. (1979). Capsular infarcts: The underlying vascular lesions. *Archives of Neurology, 36,* 65–73.

Fisher, C. M. (2000). Alien hand phenomenon: A review with the addition of six personal cases. *Canadian Journal of Neurological Sciences, 27,* 192–203.

Fox, J. L. (1983). *Intracranial aneurysms.* New York: Springer-Verlag.

François, C., Grabli, D., McCairn, K., Jan, C., Karachi, C., Hirsch, E-C., et al. (2004). Behavioral disorders induced by external globus pallidus dysfunction in primates: II. Anatomical study. *Brain, 127,* 2055–2070.

Freedman, R. B., Alexander, M. P., & Naeser, M. A. (1984). The anatomical basis of transcortical motor aphasia. *Neurology, 34,* 409–417.

Freemon, F. R. (1971). Akinetic mutism and bilateral anterior cerebral artery occlusion. *Journal of Neurology, Neurosurgery, and Psychiatry, 34,* 409–417.

Fries, W., Danek, A., Scheidtmann, K., & Hamburger, C. (1993). Motor recovery following capsular stroke. *Brain, 116,* 369–382.

Fukui, T., Sugita, K., Sato, Y., Takeuchi, T., & Tsukagoshi, H. (1994). Cognitive functions in subjects with incidental cerebral hyperintensities. *European Neurology, 4,* 272–276.

Gainotti, G., Marra, C., & Villar, G. (2001). A double dissociation between accuracy and time of execution on attentional tasks in Alzheimer's disease and multi-infarct dementia. *Brain, 124,* 731–738.

Garde, E., Mortensen, E. L., Krabbe, K., Rostrup, E., & Larsson, H. B. W. (2000). Relation between age-related decline in intelligence and cerebral white matter hyperintensities in healthy octogenarians: A longitudinal study. *Lancet, 356,* 628–634.

Gasquoine, P. G. (1993). Alien hand sign. *Journal of Clinical and Experimental Neuropsychology, 15,* 653–667.

Geschwind, N., & Kaplan, E. (1962). A human cerebral disconnection syndrome. *Neurology, 12,* 675–685.

Giroud, M., Lemesle, M., Madinier, G., Billiar, T. H., & Dumas, R. (1997). Unilateral lenticular infarcts: Radiological and clinical syndromes, aetiology, and prognosis. *Journal of Neurology, Neurosurgery, and Psychiatry, 63,* 611–615.

Godefroy, O., Rousseaux, M., Leys, D., Destée, A., Scheltens, P., & Pruvo, J. P. (1992). Frontal lobe dysfunction in unilateral lenticulostriate infarcts: Prominent role of cortical lesions. *Archives of Neurology, 49,* 1285–1289.

Goodglass, H. (1993). *Understanding aphasia.* New York: Academic Press.

Grabli, D., McCairn, K., Hirsch, E. C., Agid, Y., Féger, J., François, C., et al. (2004). Behavioral disorders induced by external globus pallidus dysfunction in primates: I. Behavioral study. *Brain, 127,* 2039–2054.

Graff-Radford, N. R., Tranel, D., van Hoesen, G. W., & Brandt, J. P. (1990). Diencephalic amnesia. *Brain, 113*(1), 1–25.

Graff-Radford, N. R., Welsh, K., & Godersky, J. (1987). Callosal apraxia. *Neurology, 37,* 100–105.

Greenberg, S. M. (2004). Cerebral amyloid angiopathy. In J. P. Mohr, D. W. Choi, J. C. Grotta, B. Weir, & P. A. Wolf (Eds.), *Stroke: Pathophysiology, diagnosis, and management* (4th ed., pp. 693–705). Philadelphia: Churchill Livingstone

Greenberg, S. M., Finklestein, S. P., & Schaefer, P. W. (1996). Petechial hemorrhages accompanying lobar hemorrhages: Detection by gradient-echo MRI. *Neurology, 46,* 1751–1754.

Gutierrez, L., Davalos, A., Pedraza, S., Garcia, S. C., & Kulisevsky, J. (2003). Neuropsychological and behavioral impairments resulting from bilateral thalamic infarct. *Neuropsychologia, 18,* 404–408.

Habib, M., & Poncet, M. (1988). Perte de l'élan vital, de l'intérêt et de l'affectivité (symdrome athymhormique) au cours de lesions lacunaires des corps striés. *Review of Neurology, 144,* 571–577.

Heilman, K. M., Leon, S. A., & Rosenbek, J. C. (2004). Affective aprosodia from a medial frontal stroke. *Brain and Language, 89,* 411–416.

Heilman, K. M., & Valenstein, E. (1972). Frontal neglect in man. *Neurology, 22,* 660–664.

Heilman, K. M., & Watson, R. T. (1991). Intentional motor disorders. In H. S. Levin, H. M. Eisenberg, & A L. Benton (Eds.), *Frontal lobe function and dysfunction* (pp. 200–213). Oxford, UK: Oxford University Press.

Helgason, C. M., & Wilbur, A. C. (1990). Capsular hypesthetic ataxic hemiparesis. *Stroke, 21,* 24–33.

Helgason, C. M., Wilbur, A. C., Weiss, A., Redmond, K. J., & Kingsbury, N. A. (1988). Acute pseudobulbar mutism due to discrete bilateral capsular infarction in the territory of the anterior choroidal artery. *Brain, 111,* 507–524.

Higgins, M. (1993). Proceedings of the National Heart, Lung and Blood Institute Conference on the decline in stroke mortality. *Annals of Epidemiology, 3,* 453–575.

Hollander, M., Bots, M. L., Del Sol, A. I., Koudstaal, P. J., Witteman, J. C. M., Grobbee, D. E., et al. (2002). Carotid plaques increase the risk of stroke and subtypes of cerebral infarction in asymptomatic elderly: The Rotterdam study. *Circulation, 105,* 2872–2877.

Hubertus, A., & Diedrich, G. K. (2000). Mapping of fiber orientation in human internal capsule by means of polarized light and confocal scanning laser microscopy. *Journal of Neuroscience Methods, 94,* 165–175.

Inzitari, D. (2003). Leukoaraiosis: An independent risk factor for stroke? *Stroke, 34,* 2067–2071.

Iragui, V. J., & McCutchen, C. B. (1982). Capsular ataxic hemiparesis. *Archives of Neurology, 39,* 528–529.

Irle, E., Wowra, B., Kunert, H. J., Hampl, J., & Kunze, S. (1992). Memory disturbances following anterior communicating artery rupture. *Annals of Neurology, 31,* 473–480.

Ishii, N., Nishihara, Y., & Imamura, T. (1986). Why do frontal lobe symptoms predominate in vascular dementia with lacunes? *Neurology, 36,* 340–345.

Joutel, A., Vahedi, K., Corpechot, C., Troesch, A., Chabriat, H., Vayssiere, C., et al. (1997). Strong clustering and stereotyped nature of mutations in CADASIL patients. *Lancet, 350,* 1511–1515.

Karnath, H.-O., Ferber, S., & Himmelbach, M. (2001). Spatial awareness is a function of the temporal not the posterior parietal lobe. *Nature, 411,* 950–953.

Karnath, H.-O., Himmelbach, M., & Rorden, C. (2002). The subcortical anatomy of human spatial neglect: Putamen, caudate nucleus and pulvinar. *Brain, 125,* 350–360.

Kase, C. S., Mohr, J. P., & Caplan, L. R. (2004). Intracerebral hemorrhage. In J. P. Mohr, D. W. Choi, J. C. Grotta, & B. Weir (Eds.), *Stroke: Pathophysiology, diagnosis, and management* (4th ed., pp. 327–376). Philadelphia: Churchill Livingstone

Kase, C. S., Williams, J. P., Wyatt, D. A., & Mohr, J. P. (1982). Lobar intracerebral hematomas: Clinical and CT analysis of 22 cases. *Neurology, 32,* 1146–1150.

Kashihara, M., & Matsumoto, K. (1985). Acute capsular infarction, location of lesions and the clinical features. *Neuroradiology, 27,* 248–253.

Katz, D. I., Alexander, M. P., & Mandell, A. M. (1987). Dementia following strokes in the mesencephalon and diencephalons. *Archives of Neurology, 44,* 1127–1133.

Kazui, S., Sawada, T., Naritomi, H., Kuriyama, Y., & Yamaguchi, T. (1993). Angiographic evaluation of brain infarction limited to the cerebral artery territory. *Stroke, 24,* 549–553.

Kertesz, A., Nicholson, I., Cancelliere, A., Kassa, K., & Black, S. E. (1985). Motor impersistence: A right-hemisphere syndrome. *Neurology, 35,* 662–666.

Kim, J. S., & Choi-Kwon, S. (2000). Poststroke depression and emotional incontinence: Correlation with lesion location. *Neurology, 54,* 1805–1810.

Kumral, E., Bayulkem, G., Evyapan, D., & Yunten, N. (2002). Spectrum of anterior cerebral artery territory infarction: Clinical and MRI findings. *European Journal of Neurology, 9,* 615–624.

Kumral, E., Evyapan, D., & Balkir, K. (1999). Acute caudate vascular lesions. *Stroke, 30,* 100–108.

LaPlane, D., Baulac, M., Widlocher, D., & Dubois, B.

(1984). Pure psychic akinesia with bilateral lesions of basal ganglia. *Journal of Neurology, Neurosurgery, and Psychiatry, 47*, 377–385.

Lee, S. H., Bae, H. J., Kwon, S. J., Kim, H., Kim, Y. H., Yoon, B. W., et al. (2004). Cerebral microbleeds are regionally associated with intracerebral hemorrhage. *Neurology, 62*, 72–76.

Lee, S. H., Bae, H. J., Yoon, B. W., Kim, H., Kim, D. E., & Roh, J. K. (2002). Low concentration of serum total cholesterol is associated with multifocal signal loss lesions on gradient-echo magnetic resonance imaging: Analysis of risk factors for multifocal signal loss lesions. *Stroke, 33*, 2845–2849.

Leiguarda, R. C., & Marsden, C. D. (2000). Limb apraxias: Higher-order disorders of sensorimotor integration. *Brain, 123*, 860–879.

Leiguarda, R. C., Starkstein, S., & Berthier, M. (1989). Anteiror callosal haemorrhage: A partial interhemispheric disconnection syndrome. *Brain, 112*, 1019–1037.

Levin, H. S. (1973). Motor impersistence and proprioceptive feedback in patients with unilateral cerebral disease. *Neurology, 23*, 833–841.

Liepmann, H., & Maas, O. (1907). Fall von linksseiteger Agraphie und Apraxie bei rechtseitiger Lähmung. *Zeitung für Psychologie und Neurologie, 10*, 214–227.

Lindgren, A., Norrving, B., Rudling, O., & Johannson, B. B. (1994). Comparison of clinical and neuroradiological findings in first-ever stroke. *Stroke, 25*, 1371–1377.

Loeb, C. (2000). Binswanger's disease is not a single entity. *Neurological Sciences, 21*, 343–348.

Luijckx, G. J., Boiten, J., Lodder, J., Heuts-van Raak, L., & Wilmink, J. (1994). Isolated hemiataxia after supratentorial brain infarction. *Journal of Neurology, Neurosurgery, and Psychiatry, 57*, 742–744.

Mead, S., James-Galton, M., Revesz, T., Doshi, R. B., Harwood, G., Pan, E. L., et al. (2000). Familial British dementia with amyloid angiopathy: Early clinical, neuropsychological, and imaging findings. *Brain, 123*, 975–991.

Meador, K. L., Watson, R. T., Bowers, D., & Heilman, K. M. (1986). Hypometria with hemispatial and limb motor neglect. *Brain, 109*, 293–305.

Mean, G. E., Lewis, S. C., Wardlaw, J. M., Dennis, M. S., & Warlow, C. P. (2000). How well does the Oxfordshire Community Stroke Project classification predict the site and size of the infarct on brain imaging? *Journal of Neurology, Neurosurgery, and Psychiatry, 68*, 558–562.

Melo, T. P., Bogousslavksy, J., Moulin, T., Nader, J., & Regli, F. (1992). Thalamic ataxia. *Journal of Neurology, 239*, 331–337.

Mendez, M. F., Adams, N. L., & Lewandowsky, K. (1989). Neurobehavioral changes associated with caudate lesions. *Neurology, 39*, 349–354.

Mesulam, M. M. (1981). A cortical network for directed attention and unilateral neglect. *Annals of Neurology, 10*, 309–325.

Misra, U. K., & Kalita, J. (1997). Central motor conduction studies in internal capsule and corona radiate infarction. *Journal of Neurology, 244*, 579–585.

Mohr, J. P., Lazar, R. M., Marshall, R. S., & Hier, D. (2004). Middle cerebral artery disease. In J. P. Mohr, D. W. Choi, J. C. Grotta, B. Weir, & P. A. Wolf (Eds.), *Stroke: Pathophysiology, diagnosis, and management* (4th ed., pp. 123–166). Philadelphia: Churchill Livingstone.

Morris, J. C., Heyman, A., Mohs, R. C., Hughes, J. P., van Belle, G., Fillenbaum, G., et al. (1989). The Consortium to Establish a Registry for Alzheimer's Disease (CERAD): Part I. Clinical and neuropsychological assessment of Alzheimer's disease. *Neurology, 39*, 1159–1165.

Morris, P. L. P., Robinson, R. G., Raphael, B., & Hopwood, M. J. (1996). Lesion location and poststroke depression. *Journal of Neuropsychiatry and Clinical Neuroscience, 8*, 399–403.

Moulin, T., Bogousslavsky, J., Chopard, J. L., Ghika, J., Crepin-Leblond, T., Martin, V., et al. (1995). Vascular ataxic hemiparesis: A re-evaluation. *Journal of Neurology, Neurosurgery, and Psychiatry, 58*, 422–427.

Naeser, M. A., Palumbo, C. L., Helm-Estabrooks, N., Stiassny-Eden, D., & Albert, M. L. (1989). Severe nonfluency in aphasia: Role of the medial subcallosal fasciculus and other white matter pathways in recovery of spontaneous speech. *Brain, 112*, 1–38.

Nagaratnam, N., Nagaratnam, K., Ng, K., & Diu, P. (2004). Akinetic mutism following stroke. *Journal of Clinical Neuroscience, 11*, 25–30.

Nakamura, M., Hamamoto, M., Uchida, S., Nagayama, H., Amemiya, S., Okubo, S., et al. (2003). A case of micrographia after subcortical infarction: Possible involvement of frontal lobe function. *European Journal of Neurology, 10*, 593–596.

Ozaki, I., Baba, M., Marita, S., Matsunaga, M., & Takebe, K. (1986). Pure dysarthria due to anterior internal capsule and corona radiate infarction: A report of five cases. *Journal of Neurology, Neurosurgery, and Psychiatry, 49*, 1435–1437.

Palomaki, H., Kaste, M., Berg, A., Lonnqvist, R., Lonnqvist, J., Lehtihalmes, M., et al. (1999). Prevention of poststroke depression: 1 year randomized placebo controlled double blind trial of mianserin with 6 month follow up after therapy. *Journal of Neurology, Neurosurgery, and Psychiatry, 66*, 490–494.

Pantoni, L., & Garcia, J. (1995). The significance of cerebral white matter abnormalities 100 years after Binswanger's report: A review. *Stroke, 26*, 1293–1301.

Pantoni, L., Leys, D., Fazekas, F., Longstreth, W. T., Jr., Inzitari, D., Wallin, A., et al. (1999). Role of white matter lesions in cognitive impairment of vascular origin. *Alzheimer Disease and Associated Disorders, 13*(Suppl. 3), S49–S54.

Papez, J. W. (1937). A proposed mechanism of emotion. *Archives of Neurology and Psychiatry, 38*, 725–743.

Pohjasvaara, T., Mäntylä, R., Ylikoski, R., Kaste, M., &

Erkinjuntti, T. (2003). Clinical features of MRI-defined subcortical vascular disease. *Alzheimer Disease and Associated Disorders, 17,* 236–242.

Pullicino, P. M. (1993). Diagrams of perforating artery territories in axial, coronal, and sagittal planes. In P. M. Pullicino, L. R. Caplan, & M. Hommel (Eds.), *Advances in neurology* (Vol. 62, pp. 41–72). New York: Raven.

Richfield, E. K., Twyman, R., & Berent, S. (1987). Neurological syndrome following bilateral damage to the head of the caudate. *Annals of Neurology, 22,* 768–771.

Ringman, J. M., Saver, J. L., Woolson, R. F., Clarke, W. R., & Adams, H. P. (2004). Frequency, risk factors, anatomy, and course of unilateral neglect in an acute stroke cohort. *Neurology, 63,* 468–474.

Robinson, R. G. (2003). Poststroke depression: Prevalence, diagnosis, treatment, and disease progression. *Biological Psychiatry, 54,* 376–387.

Robinson, R. G., Starr, L. B., & Price, T. R. (1984). A two-year longitudinal study of post-stroke mood disorders: Dynamic changes in associated variables over the first six months of follow-up. *Stroke, 15,* 510–517.

Rodda, R. A. (1986). The arterial patterns associated with internal carotid disease and cerebral infarcts. *Stroke, 17,* 69–75.

Román, G. C. (1987). Senile dementia of the Binswanger type: A vascular form of dementia in the elderly. *Journal of the American Medical Association, 258,* 1782–1788.

Russmann, H., Vingerhoets, F., Ghika, J., Maeder, P., & Bogousslavsky, J. (2003). Acute infarction limited to the lenticular nucleus: Clinical, etiologic, and topographic features. *Archives of Neurology, 60,* 351–355.

Sacco, R. (1994). Ischemic stroke. In P. B. Gorelick & M. Alter (Eds.), *Handbook of neuroepidemiology* (pp. 77–119). New York: Marcel Dekker.

Sacco, R. L., Hauser, W. A., & Mohr, J. P. (1991). Hospitalized stroke incidence in blacks and Hispanics in northern Manhattan. *Stroke, 22,* 1491–1496.

Sakai, Y., Nakamura, T., Sakurai, A., Yamaguchi, H., & Hirai, S. (2000). Right frontal areas 6 and 8 are associated with simultanapraxia, a subset of motor impersistence. *Neurology, 54,* 522–524.

Sandson, T. A., Daffner, K. R., Carvalho, P. A., & Mesulam, M.-M. (1991). Frontal lobe dysfunction following infarction of the left-sided and medial thalamus. *Archives of Neurology, 48,* 1300–1302.

Scepkowski, L. A., & Cronin-Golomb, A. (2003). The alien hand: Cases, categorizations, and anatomical correlates. *Behavioral and Cognitive Neuroscience Reviews, 2,* 261–277.

Scheltens, P., Barkhof, F., Leys, D., Wolters, E., Ravid, R., & Kamphorst, W. (1995). Histopathologic correlates of white matter changes on MRI in Alzheimer's disease and normal aging. *Neurology, 45,* 883–888.

Schlesinger, B. (1976). *The upper brainstem in the human.* Berlin: Springer-Verlag.

Schmahmann, J. D. (2003). Vascular syndromes of the thalamus. *Stroke, 34,* 2264–2278.

Schneider, R., & Gautier, J. C. (1994). Leg weakness due to stroke: Site of lesions, weakness patterns, and causes. *Brain, 117,* 347–354.

Schoenberg, B. S., & Schulte, B. P. M. (1988). Cerebrovascular disease: Epidemiology and geopathology. In P. J. Vinken, G. W. Bruyn, & H. L. Klawans (Eds.), *Handbook of clinical neurology, vascular disease, Part I* (Vol. 53, pp. 1–26). Amsterdam: Elsevier.

Schott, J. M., Crutch, S. J., Fox, N. C., & Warrington, E. K. (2003). Development of selective verbal memory impairment secondary to a left thalamic infarct: A longitudinal case study. *Journal of Neurology, Neurosurgery, and Psychiatry, 74,* 255–257.

Segarra, J. M. (1970). Cerebral vascular disease and behavior: I. The syndrome of the mesencephalic artery (basilar artery bifurcation). *Archives of Neurology, 22,* 408–418.

Skoog, I., Berg, S., Johansson, B., Palmertz, B., & Andreasson, L. A. (1996). The influence of white matter lesions on neuropsychological functioning in demented and non-demented 85-year-olds. *Acta Neurologica Scandinavica, 93,* 142–148.

Starkstein, S. E., Boston, J. D., & Robinson, R. G. (1988). Mechanisms of mania after brain injury: 12 case report and review of the literature. *Journal of Nervous Mental Disease, 176,* 87–100.

Starkstein, S. E., Pearlson, G. D., Boston, J., & Robinson, R. G. (1987). Mania after brain injury: A controlled study of causative factors. *Archives of Neurology, 44,* 1069–1073.

Starkstein, S. E., Robinson, R. G., Berthier, M. L., Parikh, R. M., & Price, T. R. (1988). Differential mood changes following basal ganglia vs. thalamic lesions. *Archives of Neurology, 45,* 725–730.

Stehbens, W. E. (1972). Intracranial arterial aneurysms. In W. E. Stehbens (Eds.), *Pathology of the cerebral blood vessels* (pp. 351–470). St. Louis, MO: Mosby.

Steffens, D. C., Helms, M. J., Krishnan, K. R., & Burke, G. L. (1999). Cerebrovascular disease and depression symptoms in the Cardiovascular Health Study. *Stroke, 30,* 2159–2166.

Stephens, R. B., & Stilwell, D. L. (1969). *Arteries and veins of the human brain.* Springfield, IL: Thomas.

Strub, R. L. (1989). Frontal lobe syndrome in patient with bilateral globus pallidus lesions. *Archives of Neurology, 46,* 1024–1027.

Stuss, D. T., & Benson, D. F. (1986). *The frontal lobes.* New York: Raven.

Stuss, D. T., Guberman, A., Nelson R., & Larochelle, S. (1988). The neuropsychology of paramedian thalamic infarction. *Brain and Cognition, 8,* 348–378.

Szirmai, I., Vastagh, I., Szombathelyi, É., & Kamondi, A. (2002). Strategic infarcts of the thalamus in vascular dementia. *Journal of the Neurological Sciences, 203–204,* 91–97.

Tatemichi, T. K., Desmond, D. W., & Mayeux, R. (1992). Dementia after stroke: Baseline frequency, risks, clinical features in a hospitalized cohort. *Neurology*, 42, 1185–1193.

Tatemichi, T. K., Desmond, D. W., & Prohovnik, I. (1995). Strategic infarcts in vascular dementia: A clinical and brain imaging experience. *Drug Research*, 45, 371–385.

Tatu, L., Moulin, T., Bogousslavsky, J., & Duvernoy, H. (1998). Arterial territories of the human brain: Cerebral hemispheres. *Neurology*, 50, 1699–1708.

Tei, H., Uchiyama, D., & Maruyama, S. (1993). Capsular infarcts: Location, size, and etiology of pure motor hemiparesis, sensorimotor stroke, and ataxic hemiparesis. *Acta Neurologica Scandinavica*, 88, 264–268.

Tell, G., Crouse, J., & Furberg, C. (1988). Relation between blood lipids, lipoproteins, and cerebrovascular atherosclerosis: A review. *Stroke*, 19, 423–430.

Thomas, A. J., O'Brien, J. T., Davis, S., Ballard, C., Barber, R., Kalaria, R. N., et al. (2002). Ischemic basis for deep white matter hyperintensities in major depression. *Archives of General Psychiatry*, 59, 785–792.

Tournier-Lasserve, E., Joutel, A., Melki, J., Weissenbach, J., Lathrop, M., Chabriat, H., et al. (1993). Cerebral autosomal dominant arteriopathy with infarcts and leukoencephalopathy maps to chromosome 19q12. *Nature Genetics*, 3, 256–259.

Troyer, A. K., Black, S. E., Armilio, M. L., & Moscovitch, M. (2004). Cognitive and motor functioning in a patient with selective infarction of the left basal ganglia: Evidence for decreased non-routine response selection and performance. *Neuropsychologia*, 42, 902–911.

Tsushima, Y., Tamura, T., Unno, Y., Kusano, S., & Endo, K. (2000). Multifocal low signal brain lesions on T2-weighted gradient-echo imaging. *Neuroradiology*, 42, 499–504.

Tullberg, M., Fletcher, E., DeCarli, C., Mungas, D., Reed, B. R., Harvey, D. J., et al. (2004). White matter lesions impair frontal lobe function regardless of their location. *Neurology*, 63, 246–253.

Udaka, F., Sawada, H., & Kameyama, M. (2002). White matter lesions and dementia: MRI–pathological correlation. *Annals of the New York Academy of Sciences*, 977, 411–415.

Vataja, R., Pohjasvaara, T., Leppavuori, A., Mantyla, R., Aronen, H. J., Salonen, O., et al. (2001). Magnetic resonance imaging correlates of depression after ischemic stroke. *Archives of General Psychiatry*, 58, 925–931.

Viader, F., Cambier, J., & Pariser, P. (1982). Left motor extinction due to an ischemic lesion on the anterior limb of the internal capsule. *Revue Neurologique (Paris)*, 138, 213–217.

Vinters, H. V. (1987). Cerebral amyloid angiopathy: A critical review. *Stroke*, 18, 311–324.

Vinters, H. V. (2001). Cerebral amyloid angiopathy: A microvascular link between parenchymal and vascular dementia? *Annals of Neurology*, 49, 691–693.

von Cramon, D. Y., Hebel, N., & Schuri, U. (1985). A contribution to the anatomical basis of thalamic amnesia. *Brain*, 108(4), 993–1008.

Weiller, C., Willnes, K., Reiche, W., Thron, C. I., Buell, U., & Rigelstein, E. B. (1993). The case of aphasia or neglect after striatocapsular infarction. *Brain*, 16, 1509–1525.

Weir, B. (1987). *Aneurysms affecting the nervous system*. Baltimore: Williams & Wilkins.

Wijdicks, E. F., & Jack, C. R. (1996). Coronary artery bypass grafting-associated ischemic stroke: A clinical and neuroradiological study. *Journal of Neuroimaging*, 6, 20–22.

Wolf, P. A., D'Agostino, R. B., Belanger, A. J., & Kannel, W. B. (1991). Probability of stroke: A risk profile from the Framingham Study. *Stroke*, 22, 312–318.

Yamaguchi, H., Fukuyama, H., & Shio, H. (2000). Corpus callosum atrophy in patients with leukoaraiosis may indicate global cognitive impairment. *Stroke*, 31, 1515–1520.

Yamaguchi, T., Minematsu, K., Choki, J., & Ikeda, M. (1984). Clinical and neurradiological analysis of thrombotic and embolic cerebral infarction. *Japan Circulation Journal*, 48, 50–58.

Yamanaka, K., Fukuyama, H., & Kimura, J. (1996). Abulia from unilateral capsular genu infarction: Report of two cases. *Journal of Neurological Sciences*, 143, 181–184.

Ysbrand, D., Van der Werf, Y. D., Scheltens, P., Lindeboom, J., Witter, M. P., Uylings, H. B. M., et al. (2003). Deficits of memory, executive functioning and attention following infarction in the thalamus: A study of 22 cases with localized lesions. *Neuropsychologia*, 41, 1330–1344.

# CHAPTER 30

# Parkinson's Disease with and without Dementia and Lewy Body Dementia

*Bruno Dubois*
*Bernard Pillon*
*Ian G. McKeith*

This chapter reviews the clinical and pathological aspects of Parkinson's disease (PD) with and without dementia and of dementia with Lewy bodies (DLB), with particular reference to frontal lobe involvement.

## PD WITHOUT DEMENTIA

Several cognitive changes have been regularly reported in nondemented patients with PD. They are usually referred as "specific cognitive changes," although the term "specific" is not semantically correct, because most of these changes are not exclusively found in PD. Another difficulty is that impaired performance on a given test cannot be readily associated with a single cognitive function or to a given neural structure. For example, the Wisconsin Card Sorting Test is usually considered a test of impaired concept abstraction following lesions of the frontal lobes, although several cognitive processes and several brain areas are in fact involved in execution of the test. In a similar way, poor performance on visuospatial tests is generally considered to result from impaired visuospatial perception secondary to lesions of the right parietal lobe, whereas planning disorders, more related to frontal lobe function, may also make a significant contribution. Finally, whenever the "specificity" of cognitive deficits in PD is discussed, it must also be kept in mind that any disease of the central nervous system (CNS) that limits attention resources may also impair performance in cognitive tasks when compared to controls.

With these caveats in mind, in this section we review the literature concerning impairment of executive functions, memory, visuospatial perception, and speech, and demonstrate that most of these changes result from a frontal lobe dysfunction that characterizes PD.

### The Dysexecutive Syndrome

The term "executive functions" refers to the mental processes involved in the realization of goal-directed behavior, whether expressed through a mental or a motor act. They are generally thought to control formulation, planning, carrying out, and effective performance of goal-oriented actions (Lezak, 1995). Executive functions are often disturbed following frontal lobe damage (Tranel, Anderson, & Benton, 1994). Studies show that executive functions can also be disturbed after damage to other, related parts of the brain, particularly the basal ganglia (Laplane et al., 1989). This underscores the close relationship between the prefrontal cortex and some subcortical structures that belong to the "striatofrontal system." Table 30.1 lists the tests most frequently used to evaluate executive functions in patients with PD.

## Wisconsin Card Sorting Test

Among tests, the Wisconsin Card Sorting Test (WCST) is the most widely used, probably because it requires the participation of all the cognitive processes needed for executive functions: set elaboration, maintaining, and shifting. It is therefore possible to determine several indices of performance: the number of categories achieved (a measure of the subject's concept or set formation ability); the number of perseverative errors (a measure of the patient's ability to "get out" of the previous category and to shift from one sorting principle to another); and the number of nonperseverative errors (a measure of attention deficits). Thus, the WCST allows one to evaluate conceptual ability and behavioral regulation, but to a different extent, according to the administration procedure. In Milner's (1963) original report, the subject has to discover the categories in a predetermined order. This procedure highlights "concept formation" ability. In the Nelson (1976) procedure, the order of selection of categories is freely determined by the subject. For that

reason, the Nelson procedure mainly evaluates the ability to shift from one category to another and to maintain a category.

Bowen, Kamieny, Burns, and Yahr (1975) were the first to study the WCST in patients with PD and to demonstrate a decreased number of categories and an increased number of total and nonperseverative errors. Her results were confirmed by subsequent studies that mainly showed a significant decrease of the number of categories achieved. These findings suggest a deficit either in conceptual ability or in behavioral regulation in PD. The deficit was found from the earliest stages of the disease, even in untreated patients and in subjects with preserved intellectual functions (Lees & Smith, 1983; Taylor, Saint-Cyr, & Lang, 1986). Thus, the difficulty encountered by patients with PD seems to be a specific phenomenon related to the pathology of the disease. Indeed, the specificity of these patients' cognitive difficulty in elaborating new concepts in response to environmental demands, evidenced on the WCST, was confirmed in a large study investigating the cognitive patterns seen in various CNS degenerative diseases, including Alzheimer's disease (AD), Huntington's disease (HD), progressive supranuclear palsy (PSP), and PD, with subjects matched for level of intellectual deterioration (Pillon, Dubois, Ploska, & Agid, 1991). When the level of global intellectual efficiency was normal, a deficit on the WCST was the only cognitive alteration in the PD group. In other studies, only a significant increase in errors was reported, either perseverative (Cooper, Sagar, Jordan, Harvey, & Sullivan, 1991), as in patients with selective focal lesions of the frontal lobes or with frontal lobectomies, or nonperseverative, suggesting that maintaining set may be more difficult than shifting set in PD (Partiot et al., 1996). Indeed, errors of maintenance are rarely observed in de novo patients (Cooper et al., 1991), but their number may increase with the progression of the disease (Taylor et al., 1986). This emphasizes the importance of the analysis of error patterns to better understand the difficulties of patients with PD.

Several arguments favor a frontal dysfunction as an explanation of the poor performance of patients with PD in the WCST: (1) the number of trials required for them to complete the first category is increased; (2) they often verbalize but do not execute the correct response; and (3) they are also impaired on other tests known to assess frontal lobe function.

**TABLE 30.1. The Dysexecutive Syndrome of PD: Main Standard Tests and References**

1. Wisconsin Card Sorting Test (Taylor et al., 1986; Cooper et al., 1991)
2. Other conceptual tasks and set regulation
   - California Card Sorting Test (Dimitrov et al., 1999)
   - Odd Man Out Test (Richards et al., 1993)
   - Intra- and extradimensional set shifting (Gauntlett-Gilbert et al., 1999)
   - Verbal fluency (Lees & Smith, 1983)
   - Trail Making Test (Hietanen & Teräväinen, 1986)
   - Stroop test (Dujardin et al., 1999)
   - Delayed response tasks (Partiot et al., 1996)
3. Planning and execution of action
   - Tower tasks (Owen et al., 1995)
   - Maze task (Wallesch et al., 1990)
   - Script ordering (Zalla et al., 1998)
   - Concurrent motor tasks (Malapani et al., 1994)
4. Frontal behaviors (Pillon et al., 1991)
5. Temporal structuring (Vriezen & Moscovitch, 1990)

*Other Conceptual Tasks and Set Regulation*

Patients with PD tend to test fewer hypotheses, to achieve fewer correct solutions, to have difficulty suppressing prepotent responses, to use less appropriate lose–shift strategies following negative feedback, and to share longer response times in other conceptual or sorting tasks. Verbal fluency, reported to be sensitive to frontal lobe damage (Lezak, 1995), is reduced in patients with PD (Bondi, Kaszniak, Bayles, & Vance, 1993), even in the early stages of the disease (Lees & Smith, 1983). Here again the difficulties of patients with PD can be analyzed in terms of impaired ability to maintain a mental set. Gotham, Brown, and Marsden (1988), using an alternative fluency task in which subjects are asked to name examples alternatively from two different categories (e.g., boys' names and fruits), showed that patients with PD were more severely impaired in the alternating condition, suggesting that self-generated strategies are less required in fluency tasks that are based upon access to stored information than in sorting tasks in which the instructions do not indicate how to solve the problem (Van Spaendonck, Berger, Horstink, Buytenhuijs, & Cools, 1996).

The difficulty that patients with PD show in alternating between conceptual categories raises the question of a set-shifting deficit. Aptitude for shifting was studied by Cools, Van Der Bercken, Horstink, Van Spaendonck, and Berger (1984) using motor and nonmotor tasks divided into two successive phases. The first phase tested patients' concept formation ability. The second phase evaluated the capacity to shift to new categories. Patients with PD performed worse in the shifting phase, and their decreased shifting aptitude occurred at different levels of behavioral organization, including motor aspects, as indicated by the reduced capacity for shifting set from one sequence of movements to another. This impairment of cognitive shifting in PD was postulated to be associated with the severity of motor symptoms, particularly with rigidity (Van Spaendonck et al., 1996).

Shifting abilities have been further studied of patients with PD with the Trail Making and Stroop Tests. Several studies have found that patients with PD are impaired on the Trail Making Test part B (Hietanen & Teräväinen, 1986; Pirozzolo, Hansch, Mortimer, Webster, & Kuskowski, 1982), even in patients with early and untreated PD. This finding is consistent with the set-shifting deficit reported by Cools and colleagues (1984). Results of the Stroop test (1935) in patients with PD can also be interpreted in terms of decreased cognitive flexibility, especially in the third condition (interference), where the subject must inhibit the strong tendency to read the word. It has been known for some years that patients with PD are significantly impaired on this test (Brown & Marsden, 1988; Dujardin, Degreef, Rogelet, Defebvre, & Destée, 1999), indicating a deficit in shifting aptitude.

This deficit may also explain the difficulties encountered by patients in executing concurrent activities, such as simultaneous and competing motor or cognitive tasks (Malapani, Pillon, Dubois, & Agid, 1994; Schwab, Chafetz, & Walker, 1954), and in a test of attentional set-shifting designed by Robbins and his group. This test was aimed at investigating various aspects of shifting: set-shifting formation, reversal shifting, intradimensional shifting (IDS, in which shifts are made to different exemplars of the same rule or perceptual dimension), and extradimensional shifting (EDS, in which shifts are made to different perceptual dimensions). Patients with PD revealed not only a specific EDS deficit (Downes et al., 1989) but also set-elaboration (Owen et al., 1992) and "learned irrelevance" difficulties (Owen & Robbins, 1993). "Learned irrelevance" was defined as an inability to shift to a dimension that was previously irrelevant. A new study led to the conclusion that learned irrelevance was not sufficient to explain the shifting deficit of patients with PD (Gauntlett-Gilbert, Roberts, & Brown, 1999). To better distinguish switching from set-elaboration deficits, an "alternating-runs" task was devised. Subjects were required to switch between letter- and digit-naming tasks on every second trial. Switch costs were calculated by subtracting performance (reaction times and errors) on nonswitch trials from performance on switch trials. In this complex paradigm, patients with PD did not show increased switch costs, but did show progressively increasing error costs as the task proceeded (Rogers et al., 1998), suggesting a deficit in the maintaining of attention for patients with PD.

Failure to shift attention between competing dimensions may therefore reflect a deficit in cognitive mechanisms not directly related to perseverations of an attention set. It may well be conceived within the larger framework of overall behavioral control. Patients with PD are able to form workable hypothesis but tend to abandon them prematurely when they have to choose between a range of equally possible options. They have difficulty not only changing sets but also maintaining mental sets. The Odd Man Out Test (Flowers & Robertson, 1985; Richards, Cote, & Stern, 1993) is a sorting task with two rules of classification that should be alternated on successive trials. Patients with PD tend, after the first shift, to return to the incorrect category, indicating difficulty in maintaining attention to the relevant attribute. The instability of cognitive set revealed by the Odd Man Out Test brings to mind the performance of patients with PD on the Necker cube (Talland, 1962), which is characterized by a high rate of spontaneous reversal of perspective. It is also reminiscent of the performance of patients with PD on motor tasks with a new manual skill (Frith, Bloxham, & Carpenter, 1986), which is thought to result from a disturbance in the acquisition and maintenance of motor sets. In summary, patients with PD have reduced control over reversals on cognitive (Odd Man Out Test), perceptual (Necker test), and motor tasks, suggesting a general difficulty with set regulation.

The acquisition of a set refers to the capacity to ameliorate the processing of information through the repetition of an event. Difficulty in acquisition or generation of sets can be demonstrated in mental, motor (planning), or even perceptual (attention) functions. Indeed, impaired performance of patients with PD on some tests believed to assess visuospatial functions can be interpreted as a failure of elaboration of mental set (Stern, 1987). For example, the errors made by patients with PD in the Aubert paradigm (Danta & Hilton, 1975) were attributed to subjects' failure to preset their sensory systems to account for body tilt.

### Planning and Execution of Action

"Planning" may be defined as the ability to organize behavior in relation to time and space. This ability is required when a goal must be achieved through a series of intermediate steps, particularly in novel situations. The Tower of London task, with its specific constraints, is considered very sensitive for investigating planning capacities (Shallice, 1988). On a computerized version of the Tower of London, patients with PD solved the problem as well as controls in terms of number of moves (Morris et al., 1988), but their planning time was longer, even after researchers controlled for the actual movement time. This indicates that patients with PD were accurate but not as efficient as the control group. The increased response time rather results from a specific planning disorder rather than a nonspecific slowing of processing. In a more complex version of the task, nonmedicated patients with PD with mild clinical symptoms were significantly impaired in terms of both accuracy and latency of performance (Owen et al., 1995). Saint-Cyr, Taylor, and Lang (1988) showed that patients with PD used significantly more moves than the normal control subjects in a variant task, the Tower of Toronto. This result was interpreted by the authors as a procedural learning deficit, as discussed later, although an increased number of moves during the first block of trials favors the hypothesis of an associated problem-solving deficit in this group. A computerized version allowed only partial vision of a maze requiring plan generation. Patients with PD showed a response bias that favored repetition of the previous action and slowed planning (Wallesch et al., 1990). Planning was also investigated by measuring patients' capacity to organize script that requires the ability to order predetermined sequences of familiar events when sequence, boundary, and means–end constraints have to be taken into account. In this situation, patients with PD committed errors of sequence and inserted actions not related to the script goal (Zalla et al., 1998). These errors disappeared when similar scripts had to be generated spontaneously (Zalla et al., 2000), suggesting that the difficulties of patients with PD were due to an impairment of behavioral control rather than a deficit of script "syntax" knowledge.

Planning deficits of patients with PD were also reported in the execution of sequential motor tasks, resulting in the inability to elaborate or maintain a global motor plan of action and to control its execution (Gentilucci & Negrotti, 1999; Marsden, 1982). These deficits are more evident when the sequential movements are driven by internal rather than external cues (Richards et al., 1993). Ability to generate random movement sequences was impaired in patients with PD by the intrusion of unwanted systematic strategies (Ebersbach, Hattig, Schlelosky, Wissel, & Poewe, 1994).

This is in agreement with Flowers's work (1978) on behavioral anticipation ability of subjects with PD. In tracking a moving target, patients do not show the normal tendency to predict the immediate future movement of the target they are tracking. They do not spontaneously use prediction as readily as normal subjects in controlling their actions, but tend to be related more directly to current sensory information, responding to events rather than anticipating them. Patients' dependency on the environment and on environmental stimulation may represent an attempt to compensate for their deficit in self-generated programming (Stern, 1987).

This dependency on the environment may be responsible for the presence of pathological behaviors such as prehension, utilization, and imitation (Pillon, Dubois, Lhermitte, & Agid, 1986). These behaviors express a spontaneous tendency to prehend the objects presented in front of them, to use them, or to imitate the examiner's gestures, in the absence of a verbal order to do so. They result from the lack of inhibition, normally exerted by the frontal lobes, on the automatic activation of patterns of prehension or imitation induced by sensory stimuli. This syndrome of environmental dependency is characteristic of frontal lesions or dysfunction (Lhermitte, Pillon, & Serdaru, 1986) and is never observed in normal controls.

### Temporal Structuring

The critical role of the prefrontal cortex in temporal organization of behavior has been demonstrated (Fuster, 1989). Like patients with frontal lobe lesions, patients with PD have trouble in temporal–structural formation. Their performance is impaired in delayed response tasks (Freedman & Oscar-Berman, 1986; Partiot et al., 1996; Taylor et al., 1986). A temporal ordering deficit in PD has also been demonstrated by Sagar, Sullivan, Gabrieli, Corkin, and Growdon (1988) and Vriezen and Moscovitch (1990). Moreover, patients with PD are impaired in their capacity to date past public events despite preserved ability to recognize these events (Sagar, Cohen, Sullivan, Corkin, & Growdon, 1988).

Overall, these studies show a reliable deficit of executive functions in PD that is not the mirror image of that associated with a direct frontal lesion (Partiot et al., 1996). Executive func-

tions of patients with PD are impaired only when an internal set of rules or cues govern the selection of the response and the patient has to switch between alternatives. As we discuss later, the dysexecutive syndrome of PD, which is expressed in a great number of apparently different processes or tests, might result from the perturbation of some fundamental mechanisms intervening in the allocation of attention resources in the absence of an external, explicit cue (Brown & Marsden, 1988; Taylor et al., 1986). Such fundamental mechanisms might also intervene in other cognitive domains such as learning, retrieval, syntactic comprehension, and visuospatial organization. Although some authors consider that PD results in a constellation of cognitive symptoms (Beatty, Dennis-Staton, Weir, Monzon, & Whitaker, 1989), we favor the hypothesis of underlying unifying mechanisms, at least in patients without dementia. The expression of these mechanisms in different cognitive domains is responsible for the apparent heterogeneity of cognitive symptoms.

### Frontal-Related Memory Disorders

Memory is not unitary, but must be parceled according both to the temporal organization of information storage (i.e., short- and long-term memory; Squire, 1989), and to underlying mechanisms, with four essential components: (1) a frontal lobe component "working with memory" on strategic explicit tests; (2) a medial temporal–hippocampal component that mediates encoding, storage, and retrieval on associative cue-dependent explicit memory tests; (3) a basal ganglia component intervening in tests of sensorimotor procedural memory; and (4) a nonfrontal neocortical component involving various perceptual and semantic modules and mediating performance on item-specific implicit memory tests (Moscovitch, 1994). Given the underlying neuropathological features of PD, a relative specificity of memory disorders may be expected. Table 30.2 summarizes the specific pattern of memory disorders of patients with PD.

### Short-Term Memory Deficits

According to Squire (1989), "primary memory" refers to the information to be remembered that is the focus of current attention. Compared to "short-term memory," it places

**TABLE 30.2. PD and Memory Processes**

| Preserved memory components | | Impaired memory components | |
|---|---|---|---|
| Medial temporal | Retro-Rolandic neocortical | Frontal related | Basal ganglia related |
| 1. Learning curves<br>2. Verbal and spatial recognition<br>3. Cued recall<br>4. Delayed information<br>5. Remote memory | 1. Verbal and spatial short-term reproduction<br>2. Semantic memory<br>3. Priming | 1. Verbal and spatial working memory<br>2. Random generation<br>3. Word-list acquisition and recall<br>4. Visuospatial acquisition and recall<br>5. Trial-and-error learning<br>6. Recency discrimination and temporal ordering | 1. Procedural learning |

*Note.* For references, see text.

more emphasis on the role of attention, conscious processing, and memory capacity. "Working memory" describes a workspace that maintains information while it is being processed: It consists of a number of interrelated systems, the three principal components of which are the central executive system (CES), the articulatory loop system (ALS), and the visuospatial scratchpad (VSSP) (Baddeley, 1996). The ALS permits recycling of verbal information while it is being processed. The VSSP permits temporary storage and manipulation of visuospatial informations. Finally, the CES, assumed to function like a "limited-capacity attentional system," controls and coordinates the other subsystems by selecting strategies and integrating information.

Attention deficits of patients with PD are a function of the tests used. They are not observed at a basic level. For instance, the passive and immediate repetition of a digit series (Hietanen & Teravainen, 1988) and the immediate tapping of a block array (Morris et al., 1988) are usually preserved even in patients with late onset of the disease (Dubois, Pillon, Sternic, Lhermitte, & Agid, 1990), with poor response to L-dihydroxyphenylalanine (L-dopa) treatment (Taylor, Saint-Cyr, & Lang, 1987), or with dementia (Huber, Shuttleworth, & Freidenberg, 1989). Difficulties may appear with the use of interfering stimuli, intended to prevent rehearsal of the to-be-remembered items, as in the Peterson and Peterson (1959) procedure (Cooper, Sagar, & Sullivan, 1993; Marié et al., 1995). In the Digit Ordering Test,

in which subjects are required to reorder in ascending fashion a random selection of seven digits maintained in working memory, de novo patients with PD were significantly impaired, whereas they had a normal forward digit span (Cooper et al., 1991; Stebbins, Gabrieli, Masciari, Monti, & Goetz, 1999). This impairment was sensitive to L-dopa therapy (Cooper et al., 1992), suggesting that working memory could be one of the few cognitive processes supported by dopaminergic transmission. In the Sternberg (1975) paradigm, the subject must decide whether or not probe digits belong to a set of a variable number of digits held in a short-term memory. Wilson, Kaszniak, Klawans, and Garron (1980) found that scanning speed was lower for the older patients. This phenomenon of cognitive slowing could explain why patients with PD are impaired at the shortest but not at the longest intervals in recognition (Sagar, Sullivan, et al., 1988) and matching to sample (Sahakian et al., 1988) tasks.

Spatial working memory has also been found to be impaired (Owen, Beksinska, et al., 1993; Pillon et al., 1998; Postle, Jonides, Smith, Corkin, & Growdon, 1997), even when the response was performed by eye movements (Vermersch et al., 1994). A specific impairment of visuospatial working memory was postulated by Bradley, Welch, and Dick (1989). In the visuospatial task, patients were shown a videotape of a road and were asked to imagine that road and report the direction of all turns, starting mentally from one extremity of the road. They were also administered a verbal memory task that involved memorizing a short sentence, then making decisions about initial letters of the words in the phrases. The reaction times of patients with PD were much slower on the visuospatial task than on the verbal task, even though a level of difficulty cannot be excluded as a contributory factor.

The visuospatial working memory deficit of patients with PD may be either modality-specific, in relation to a disturbance of the visuospatial sketchpad (Bradley et al., 1989), or dependent on the required level of attentional resources, in relation to a disturbance of the central executive (Pillon et al., 1998). The similar effect of visuospatial versus verbal interference in a spatial working memory task in patients with PD suggests that the visuospatial sketchpad was not specifically impaired (Le Bras, Pillon, Damier, & Dubois, 1999). In contrast, significant correlation between the visuospatial span and performance on tests of executive functions suggests a deficiency of the central executive. Therefore, reduced working memory resources at the level of the central executive may account for impaired performance in different working memory tasks in relation to difficulties in initiating or sustaining appropriate strategies. In agreement with this hypothesis is the impaired performance of patients with PD in the Pattern Span Test (Fournet, Moreaud, Roulin, Naegele, & Pellat, 1996; Pillon et al., 1998), in which subjects must elaborate their own visuospatial organization of the stimulus to be able to reproduce it after the delay, but not in the Corsi Block Span Test (Levin, Labre, & Weiner, 1989), in which the organization of the material to be memorized is set up by the examiner. It should be noted, however, that dissociation was also reported as a function of the modality. According to some authors, spatial but not visual or verbal working memory tasks were impaired in the early stages of PD (Owen, Iddon, Hodges, Summers, & Robbins, 1997; Postle, Jonides, et al., 1997), although others reported impaired verbal working memory (Cooper et al., 1991) and preserved spatial working memory (Owen, Beksinska, et al., 1993) in de novo patients with PD. Whatever the interpretation, the spatial working memory deficit of these patients affects not only the maintenance of the representation in short-term memory but also its monitoring at the encoding and response pro-

gramming steps (Le Bras et al., 1999), suggesting that striatofrontal circuits intervene at all steps of working memory processing in human, as in nonhuman primates. In conclusion, most if not all these deficits would be independent of the modality of the stimulus (verbal vs. nonverbal) insofar as the tests require equal working memory demands (Gabrieli, Singh, Stebbins, & Goetz, 1996; Pillon et al., 1998).

## Episodic Memory Retrieval Deficits

Early clinical studies fostered the general impression that impaired memory is one of the cognitive consequences of PD (El-Awar, Becker, Hammond, & Boller, 1987; Pirozzolo et al., 1982). The recall deficit was present in early-onset PD (Levin et al., 1989) and was not significantly worse in the late-onset form of the disease (Dubois, Pillon, Sternic, et al., 1990). Thus, it could not be interpreted as a nonspecific effect of aging. Because the recall deficit was also observed in untreated patients with PD (Cooper et al., 1991), neither could it be due to a nonspecific effect of treatment. El-Awar and colleagues (1987) suggested that several patterns of memory impairment can be discerned among patients with PD. In fact, despite this apparent diversity, there is a relative specificity of memory disorders in these patients, as we see now.

First, the medial temporal–hippocampal component that mediates the more automatic aspects of encoding, storage, and retrieval tends to be preserved in PD:

1. Recognition, the more "passive" paradigm of declarative memory was found to be normal in PD for verbal and visuospatial material (El-Awar et al., 1987; Gabrieli et al., 1996; Vriezen & Moscovitch, 1990).
2. The slope of the learning curves was also found to be normal in patients with PD without loss of information after delay (Massman, Delis, Butters, Levin, & Salmon, 1990; Pillon et al., 1998; Taylor, Saint-Cyr, & Lang, 1990).
3. Explicit guidelines can abolish performance deficits in patients with PD (Pillon, Deweer, Agid, & Dubois, 1993).
4. Finally, a dissociation may be observed between impaired incidental learning and preserved intentional learning, suggesting the influence of attention resources in the memory deficits of patients with PD (Cooper &

Sagar, 1993; Ivory, Knight, Longmore, & Caradoc-Davies, 1999).

By contrast, the frontal lobe component that mediates the more strategic aspects of explicit tests tends to be impaired in PD. Recognition may be impaired when tasks require patients to scan mentally, manipulate the material, or organize actively a response (Stebbins et al., 1999; Taylor et al., 1990). Recall requires a greater demand upon strategic operations than recognition because the participant must develop an internally generated strategy to guide memory search. In PD, story recall and paired-associate learning are impaired (El-Awar et al., 1987; Pirozzolo et al., 1982). The impairment is even more severe when the material to be learned is not semantically organized, as in word-list acquisition (Weingartner, Burns, Diebel, & Lewitt, 1984), in the Rey Auditory Verbal Learning Test (Taylor et al., 1986), or in the Buschke Selective Reminding Test (Helkala, Laulumaa, Soininen, & Riekkinen, 1989). Furthermore, when the task contains an implicit semantic organization, patients with PD do not use it spontaneously, as in the California Verbal Learning Test (Delis, Kramer, Kaplan, & Ober, 1987). Explicit cues enhance the performance of these patients by replacing defective internally generated cues. This is the case with the procedure of Grober and Buschke (1987): By allowing control of both encoding and retrieval by the same semantic cues, it normalizes not only cued recall but also free recall in patients with PD (Pillon, Ertle, et al., 1996). The weakness of internal processing in PD also explains that patients' performance was normal on paired-associate learning but impaired when trial-and-error learning was required (Vriezen & Moscovitch, 1990).

Visuospatial explicit memory has been less studied than verbal explicit memory. Visual recognition of patients with PD may be impaired (Stebbins et al., 1999; Taylor et al., 1990), as well as visual recall (Boller et al., 1984), and spatial recall and recognition (Pillon, Ertle, et al., 1996). Is the visuospatial memory impairment of patients with PD specific to this domain of information or dependent on "strategic" processes? This issue is still a matter of debate. When compared on spatial and object variants of conditional associative learning, the performance of patients was found to be selectively impaired in the spatial condition (Postle, Locascio, Corkin, & Growdon, 1997). By contrast, even newly presenting, untreated patients with PD were as severely impaired in verbal as in spatial conditional associative learning, suggesting that the required strategic processes were likely more important than the nature of the information to be treated (Pillon et al., 1998). If this last hypothesis is true, the visuospatial learning deficit may disappear once attention resources are taken into account, since storage is preserved in PD, as mentioned previously. In agreement with this interpretation, the pattern span, evaluating attention resources, was found to be impaired in PD, but not visuospatial supraspan learning, which is adapted to the individual pattern span (Pillon et al., 1998).

In conclusion, all memory tasks thought to be sensitive to frontal lobe dysfunction have been found to be impaired in PD. Although the magnitude of memory deficits depends on the severity of the disease, they are less marked than those in frontal lobe lesions. They include recency discrimination (Taylor et al., 1986), temporal ordering (Vriezen & Moscovitch, 1990), dating capacity (Sagar, Cohen, et al., 1988), source memory (Taylor et al., 1990), subject-ordered pointing (Gabrieli et al., 1996), conditional associative learning (Pillon et al., 1998), and the shifting phase of an associative learning task (Goldenberg, Podreka, Muller, & Deecke, 1989). All these tasks require the ability to generate spontaneously efficient strategies and to use internally guided behavior. A correlation between the severity of memory disorders and that of the dysexecutive syndrome has been observed (Pillon et al., 1993), and the memory performance of nondemented patients with PD no longer differed from that of elderly controls once the score on a series of frontal tests was covaried (Bondi et al., 1993). These results suggest that the impaired explicit memory of patients with PD, like their dysexecutive syndrome, results from the perturbation of some fundamental mechanisms intervening in the allocation of attention resources in the absence of an external explicit cue. Although agreeing with the hypothesis of a specific impairment of the "frontal" memory component at the early stages of PD, some authors suggest the additional participation of the "temporal" component at more advanced stages (Owen, Beksinska, et al., 1993). We discuss this later in relation to dementia in PD.

## Frontal-Related Procedural Memory Deficits

Neuropsychological evidence for multiple implicit memory systems has been provided by Heindel, Salmon, Shults, Wallcke, and Butters (1989). Procedural learning is the ability to acquire a perceptual or motor skill, or a cognitive routine, through repeated exposures to a specific activity constrained by invariant rules (Cohen & Squire, 1980). Although the anatomical substrate of procedural learning is not established, the neostriatum, especially the caudate nucleus, is thought to play a key role. Conflicting results have been reported in patients with PD as a function of the nature of the task and the severity of the dysexecutive or motor syndrome. These results may be considered as a critique of the habit-learning hypothesis, which states that only the basal ganglia subserve procedural learning and nondeclarative memory (Wise, Murray, & Gerfen, 1996). Several interpretations may explain these conflicting results:

1. There is no unique procedural system: Several subcortical–frontal circuits have been described (Alexander, De Long, & Strick, 1986) and each of these circuits may support specific procedural memory processes. For instance, the caudate nucleus and connected structures may be more involved in cognitive procedural learning and the putamen, in motor procedural learning (Dubois, Défontaines, Deweer, Malapani, & Pillon, 1995). Alternatively, the circuits involved may vary with the level of automatization of the task (Seitz, Roland, Bohm, Gretiz, & Stone-Elander, 1990).

2. Procedural learning can be considered as multiple steps and consequently may involve different processes: more strategic processes in the first stages when the subject is confronted with a new challenging situation, and more automatic processes later, with the repetition of the situation (Sarazin, Deweer, Pillon, Merkl, & Dubois, 2001). The fact that serial reaction time learning was found to be impaired in patients with a "frontal lobe" or dysexecutive syndrome (Jackson, Jackson, Harrison, Henderson, & Kennard, 1995) and that only patients with executive difficulties were impaired in mirror reading (Sarazin et al., 2002) support this interpretation. Indeed, strategic and attentional resource factors of the "frontal" component intervene in the earlier stages of many tasks considered as investigating procedural memory.

## Frontal-Related Impairment of Instrumental Functions

Visuospatial function may be impaired in PD, even when intellectual efficiency is preserved and tests require few motor components (Boller et al., 1984; Hovestadt, De Jong, & Meerwaldt, 1987). Although some authors believe that there is a genuine visuospatial deficit in PD, most of them attribute impaired performance to the high cognitive demand usually required by these tasks. Indeed, except for difficulties in discriminating line orientation, the deficits are mainly observed in paradigms requiring set shifting (Brown & Marsden, 1986; Raskin, Borod, & Tweedy, 1992), self-elaboration of the response (Ransmayr et al., 1987), or forward planning capacity (Ogden, Growdon, & Corkin, 1990). In a study that used both visuospatial and frontal-related tasks, visuospatial deficits disappeared once performance on the frontal-related tasks was statistically covaried (Bondi et al., 1993). It can be concluded that visuospatial disorders in PD result from a decrease in central processing resources rather than a specific alteration of visuospatial function.

Among the various speech and language difficulties encountered in patients with PD, frontal-related changes mainly involve word-finding difficulties (Beatty & Monzon, 1989). Patients with PD were also impaired in sentence completion and grammatical comprehension (Grossman et al., 1993), but only in a subgroup of patients, and for complex constructions, for instance, final relative clauses or multiclausal constructions. This would suggest that the sentence comprehension impairment in PD results from a disturbance of the central executive component of working memory. Patients' decreased verbal fluency, which we discussed, is in agreement with this hypothesis.

## Are the Cognitive Changes of PD Really Specific?

May the cognitive deficits of nondemented patients with PD be considered to be specific? On the one hand, deficits are observed in all cognitive domains: executive functions, memory, visuospatial perception, and speech. On the other hand, they are mainly observed when an internal set of rules or cues govern the selection of the response, requiring the intervention of the central executive component of working memory and attentional resources. This pattern is reminiscent of that observed in frontal lobe lesions but is less severe than that observed in PD with dementia, HD, PSP, or diffuse Lewy body disease (Pillon, Dubois, & Agid, 1996). It differs from corticobasal degeneration by the absence of aphasia or apraxia. It is close to—and difficult to distinguish from— the pattern of multiple system atrophy, although some subtle differences are observed in the Tower of London test, the spatial working memory task, and the attentional set-shifting paradigm of the Cambridge Neuropsychological Test Automated Battery (CANTAB; Owen & Robbins, 1993). Taken together, it can be concluded that PD provokes rather specific cognitive deficits, in keeping with the specific neuronal lesions of the disease.

In conclusion, several cognitive changes are frequently observed in PD, even at the earliest stages of the disease. They may appear in all cognitive domains but result from dysfunction of processes that are commonly considered to be controlled by the prefrontal cortex. This frontal dysfunction is considered to result from lesion of the basal ganglia via the striatofrontal circuits, the mesocorticolimbic dopaminergic, and other ascending neuromodulator systems that arise from subcortical structures and project to cortical, mainly frontal areas.

## PD WITH DEMENTIA

The development of dementia in a patient with PD is a very significant event. The most frequently cited reasons for patients' transfer to institutional care are the triple aggregate of dementia, incontinence, and sleep disorders. Determining precisely when the cognitive deficits of PD, as described earlier, become sufficient to qualify as a dementia can be difficult. Conventional definitions of the dementia syndrome include the need for cognitive dysfunction to impair significantly personal, social, or occupational function, but this criterion cannot easily be applied to patients with PD who may already have severe functional disabilities caused by motor dysfunction. Fully operationalized diagnostic criteria for PD dementia are still lacking, and the term, as it is currently used, probably includes variable groups of patients.

## Prevalence and Risk Factors

Most contemporary authors agree that in an unselected population of patients with PD, the prevalence of dementia is greater than in age-matched control subjects. Cummings (1988) has shown that estimates of the prevalence of dementia vary widely among different sources. A longitudinal study of newly diagnosed patients separated late- (> 70 years) from early-onset (< 70 years) PD and concluded that, in untreated patients, dementia was found in 8% of patients with early onset and 32% in those with late onset (Reid et al., 1990). At the 3-year follow-up, 18% of the early-onset group and 83% of the late-onset group were classified as demented, on the basis of formal neuropsychological tests. In contrast, other studies estimate a lower percentage (10–15%) of dementia in PD (Brown & Marsden, 1984; Mayeux et al., 1988), but generally the percentage remains greater than that in control subjects.

The risk factors for dementia in PD are far from clearly known. Aging seems to play a major role, as suggested by the positive correlation between cognitive impairment and age of disease onset (Lieberman et al., 1979). Early-onset patients do not acquire severe cognitive impairment even with disease duration of over 20 years (Schrag, Ben-Schlomo, Brown, Marsden, & Quinn, 1998). The influence of age of disease onset on cognitive status has been confirmed by studies comparing intellectual performance of early- and late-onset forms of the disease (Dubois, Pillon, Sternic, et al., 1990; Reid et al., 1990). Severity and duration of motor symptoms may also be considered as risk factors: Prospective data for 191 patients showed that no patient with PD in Stage 1 of Hoehn and Yahr's scale (unilateral symptoms only) had dementia, whereas 35% of those in Stage 4 and 57% of those in Stage 5 had dementia (Growdon, Corkin, & Rosen, 1990). Among the motor symptoms, rigidity and akinesia have been proposed as the best predictors (Mortimer, Pirozzolo, Hansch, & Webster, 1982), although other studies have emphasized the frequency of gait disorders in patients with PD and dementia (Pillon, Dubois, Cusimano, et al., 1989). In a hypothesis based on this last finding, dementia in PD is associated with symptoms that respond poorly to L-dopa and are therefore related to nondopaminergic lesions of the brain. Additionally, in a longitudinal, community-based, epidemiological study, poor performance on verbal fluency was associated with incident dementia and may be considered a characteristic of the preclinical phase of dementia in PD (Jacobs et al., 1995). In contrast, duration of illness and of L-dopa treatment were not predictors of dementia; nor was apolipoprotein ε4, which suggests that the biological bases of dementia in PD and AD may differ.

## Neuropsychological Profile

Dementia may be difficult to recognize or assess in PD. When "off" L-dopa treatment, patients can be severely akinetic, with slowing, hypophonic, and slurred speech that may affect their performance in tests with motor or verbal output. When "on" L-dopa, patients may be inattentive and hampered by uncontrolled dyskinesias. Depression, observed in about 40% of patients with PD, may induce attention and memory disorders, and impair cognitive functions, especially those of the executive system. Another confounding factor is the presence of anticholinergic medications that may specifically impair the cognitive performance of patients with PD because of (1) neuronal loss in the nucleus basalis of Meynert of patients with dementia almost as severe as that in patients with AD; and (2) 50% reduction in choline acetyltransferase activity in the nucleus basalis of Meynert, and in all its target cortical areas.

The neuropsychological profile of demented patients with PD is less clearly established than one would expect, in part because, in many published studies, the diagnosis of dementia relied simply on clinical judgment or on simple, informal tests. Other authors used the Wechsler Adult Intelligence Scale (WAIS) or other standard tests and found, in addition to a decreased IQ, a tendency for the Performance Scale to be significantly lower than the Verbal Scale, an exaggeration of the effect usually found in normal aging. Unfortunately, these earlier studies did not include the assessment of executive functions such as concept formation, problem solving, shifting aptitude, maintenance of mental sets, or elaboration of strategies. The criteria of the fourth edition of the *Diagnostic and Statistical Manual of Mental Disorders* (DSM-IV) more appropriately detect dementia in PD than the previous editions, because they include the presence of a dysexecutive syndrome. Dementia in PD can be recognized in the case of a severe dysexecutive syndrome, with memory deficits in the absence of aphasia, apraxia or agnosia.

In recent papers, cognitive status in patients with PD has been more critically examined. Loss of intellectual ability is well evaluated by global scales such as the Mattis (1988) Dementia Rating Scale. This scale is more appropriate than Folstein's Mini-Mental State Exam (MMSE) for subcortical disorders, because it includes tests assessing attention and executive functions. Such tools provide cutoff scores that allow a psychometric approach to dementia. A deficit in learning new information, the hallmark for the diagnosis of dementia, is regularly reported in demented patients with PD, although it is less severe than in AD (Helkala et al., 1989; Pillon et al., 1991). The nature of the memory deficit was specified with the Grober and Buschke procedure (1987), designed to control for the effective encoding of verbal items. Despite a marked deficit in free recall, the performance of demented patients with PD was dramatically improved by semantic cueing, which triggered efficient retrieval processes (Pillon et al., 1993). This result suggests that the recall deficit is primarily due to a memory disruption, because the ability to register, store, and consolidate information is preserved, rather than to difficulties in activating the neuronal processes involved in the functional use of memory stores. Correlation analysis showed that the memory scores in this task were strongly related to performance in tests of executive functions, favoring the role of frontal lobe dysfunction in the defective activation of memory processes. The existence of a dysexecutive syndrome in patients with PD with dementia, although less severe than in PSP (Pillon et al., 1991), is in agreement with this interpretation. Beside this severe dysexecutive syndrome, which is the main characteristic of dementia in PD, instrumental activities are on the whole preserved. Linguistic difficulties, however, have been described. They include word-finding difficulties, decreased information content of spontaneous speech, diminished word-list generation, and impaired strategies in sentence comprehension (Cummings, Darkins, Mendez, Hill, & Benson, 1988). Moreover, poor performance on tests of verbal fluency is thought to be predictive of dementia in PD (Jacobs et al., 1995). Praxis disorders may also be observed, although their nature is still a matter of debate. As a rule, these instrumental deficits are less severe than those in AD and may be related to frontal lobe dysfunction. As underlined by Girotti and colleagues (1988), cognitive deficits are more severe and widespread in demented than in nondemented patients with PD, but affect particularly those tests that already distinguished nondemented patients from controls. Is this pattern of dementia specific to PD?

## Is the Dementia of PD Specific?

The cognitive deficits of PD dementia differ from those of AD: (1) Instrumental activities, such as language, praxis and gnosis, are never defective, as in AD; (2) executive dysfunction is significantly greater; and (3) explicit memory is affected differently: AD amnesia is characterized by rapid forgetting and a severe recall deficit slightly improved by cueing, whereas recall in demented patients with PD can be normalized by the same semantic cues that were given to control encoding. In PD dementia, the ability to register and store information is preserved: Only functional use of memory stores is defective. Thus, memory functions dependent upon the integrity of the temporal lobe function may be relatively well preserved in patients with PD, unlike those with AD. The severe executive dysfunction and the profile of memory deficits in demented patients with PD evoke a subcorticofrontal type of dementia. More dramatic planning, monitoring, and recall deficits are, however, observed in PSP and HD, associated with a severe environmental dependency syndrome (prehension, utilization, and imitation behaviors) in PSP, and more severe attention disorders in HD. Signs of cortical involvement are observed early in corticobasal degeneration (CBD) and diffuse Lewy body disease (DLBD), with asymmetric instrumental disorders in CBD (praxic and linguistic or visuospatial deficits) and more severe dementia and visuospatial disorders in DLBD.

## DEMENTIA WITH LEWY BODIES

DLB is probably the second most prevalent cause of degenerative dementia in older people; only AD is more common. It has carried a variety of diagnostic labels during the last two decades, including diffuse Lewy body disease (DLBD) (Kosaka, Yoshimura, Ikeda, & Budka, 1984), Lewy body dementia (LBD) (Gibb, Luthert, Janota, & Lantos, 1989), the Lewy body variant of Alzheimer's disease (LBVAD) (Hansen et al., 1990), senile dementia of Lewy body type (SDLT) (Perry, Irving, Blessed, Perry, & Fairbairn, 1989), and dementia associated with cortical Lewy bodies (DCLB) (Byrne et al., 1991).

## Clinical Picture

The core clinical features by which DLB is recognized are summarized in Table 30.3 (McKeith et al., 1996).

## Neuropsychological Profile

The profile of neuropsychological impairments in patients with DLB differs from that of AD and other dementia syndromes, reflecting the combined involvement of cortical and subcortical pathways and relative sparing of the

---

**TABLE 30.3. Core Clinical Features of DLB**

1. Central feature
   - Progressive cognitive decline of sufficient magnitude to interfere with normal social and occupational function. Prominent or persistent memory impairment may not necessarily occur in the early stages but is usually evident with progression. Deficits on tests of attention and of frontal–subcortical skills and visuospatial ability may be especially prominent.

2. Core features (two core features essential for a diagnosis of *probable*, one for *possible* DLB)
   - Fluctuating cognition, with pronounced variations in attention and alertness
   - Recurrent visual hallucinations that are typically well formed and detailed
   - Spontaneous features of parkinsonism

3. Supportive features
   - Repeated falls
   - Syncope
   - Transient loss of consciousness
   - Neuroleptic sensitivity
   - Systematized delusions
   - Hallucinations in other modalities
   - Rapid eye movement (REM) sleep behavior disorder
   - Depression

4. Features less likely to be present
   - History of stroke
     Any other physical illness or brain disorder sufficient enough to interfere with cognitive performance

*Note.* Data from McKeith et al. (1996).

hippocampus. Patients with DLB perform better than those with AD on tests of verbal memory (McKeith, Perry, Fairbairn, Jabeen, & Perry, 1992) but worse on tests of visual perception (Calderon et al., 2001; Lambon et al., 2001; Mori et al., 2000), tests that require drawing and copying (Aarsland, Andersen, Larsen, Lolk, & Kragh-Sorensen, 2003; Gnanalingham, Byrne, Thornton, Sambrook, & Bannister, 1997; Salmon & Galasko, 1996) and tests of attention and executive functions. Fifty patients with autopsy-verified DLB performed significantly worse than 95 patients with autopsy-verified AD on tests of visuospatial ability, verbal fluency, psychomotor speed, and abstract reasoning (Salmon & Hamilton, 2005). The groups did not differ, however, on tests of global cognitive functioning (i.e., the MMSE) or on specific tests of confrontation naming, general semantic knowledge, attention, or episodic memory. A logistical regression model designed to distinguish between patients with DLB and AD on the basis of scores achieved on tests of verbal fluency (i.e., the Phonemic Fluency Test), visuospatial ability (i.e., the Wechsler Intelligence Scale for Children—Revised [WISC-R] Block Design Test, the Clock Drawing Test), psychomotor speed (i.e., Part A of the Trail Making Test), and general semantic knowledge (the Number Information Test) was highly significant and correctly classified approximately 60% of patients with DLB and 88% of patients with AD.

Sahgal and colleagues carried out a series of investigations using CANTAB, which includes tests of recognition memory, sensitive to temporal lobe (cortical, hippocampal) damage. Other tests require intact frontal or frontostriatal structures and circuitry necessary to execute efficiently attentional, strategic planning, and certain memory functions. Patient with DLB and AD matched for age, estimated premorbid Verbal IQ, and global severity of dementia were compared with each other and with elderly normal subjects. Nondemented patients with PD and age-matched controls were also tested (Sahgal, Galloway, McKeith, Edwardson, & Lloyd, 1992; Sahgal, Galloway, McKeith, Lloyd, et al., 1992; Sahgal, Lloyd, et al., 1992). The demented groups were similarly impaired on a simple test of recognition memory, but patients with DLB required more trials in a conditional pattern-location–paired-associate learning task in which they were required to identify the location of a target stimulus that had previously been presented in one of six possible locations in a spatial array. This test is sensitive to right-sided hippocampal damage, and the conditional element also has potential to detect evidence of frontal lobe dysfunction. Both demented groups performed worse than controls under conditions of simultaneous matching to sample (no delay) and did not differ from one another. Patients with DLB performed significantly worse than patients with AD in a delayed matching to sample task, and did so at all delay intervals. The investigators speculated that the exceptionally marked impairment demonstrated by patients with DLB, who were unable to tolerate even very short delays, reflects relatively severe posterior temporal cortical degeneration at an early stage of the disease. Patients with DLB were also significantly impaired on a visual search task testing focal attentional ability and requiring intact frontostriatal circuits for efficient performance, whereas patients with AD performed at or about control levels. Interestingly, patients with PD were not impaired on this task compared to their controls. On a more complex visual–attentional discrimination (set shifting) problem, indirectly related to the WCST, and designed to be sensitive to frontal lobe damage, both DLB and AD groups performed much worse than controls. None of the patients with DLB solved an intradimensional shift stage within the test, and at this level their performance was significantly worse than that of the AD group. This is the level of the task at which efficient attentional capacity, mediated by frontal lobe structures, is particularly necessary. Finally, patients with DLB made more errors than patients with AD on a spatial working memory task that assessed both spatial working memory and the ability to use an efficient search strategy. Patients with PD also performed poorly on this test, which represents a development of the radial maze techniques used to assess memory in rodents and is known to be affected by temporal and especially frontal lobe damage. In an extension to these studies, the Cognitive Drug Research Computerized Assessment System (COGDRAS) has been used not only to record attentional performance (speed and accuracy) (Wesnes et al., 2002) but also to measure cognitive fluctuation, which is the core feature of DLB that has until very recently proved difficult to quantify by other means (Bradshaw, Saling, Hopwood,

Anderson, & Brodtmann, 2004; Ferman et al., 2004; Walker et al., 2000a, 2000b). Patients with DLB and PD with dementia show similar attentional slowing on the COGRAS choice reaction time test compared with patients with AD and PD without dementia, and also show greater between-test variability (a measure of fluctuation) when the choice reaction time paradigm is repeatedly presented at 3-second intervals.

## PROPOSED MODELS FOR THE COGNITIVE CHANGES ASSOCIATED WITH PD

### Cognitive Mechanisms

#### Slowing of Cognitive Processes

Slowing of cognitive processes has been proposed to explain cognitive changes in patients with PD without dementia, and indeed, bradyphrenia is often considered one of the cognitive symptoms of PD (Rogers, Lees, Smith, Trimble, & Stern, 1987). Yet the very existence of bradyphrenia in PD is controversial and not formally established, and the exact meaning of the concept is still far from precise. The slowing of thoughts has been interpreted in two ways. According to some authors, it is a purely clinical entity that includes a series of symptoms typically present in PD: apathy, intellectual inertia, slow use of previously acquired notions, and even disorders of attention. In that sense, bradyphrenia is reminiscent of the concept of "subcortical dementia" (Albert, Feldman, & Willis, 1974). In contrast, other authors look at bradyphrenia in a semantically narrower sense, viewing it as a symptom defined as a measurable lengthening of normal information-processing time. It is then considered a physiological parameter that can be quantified experimentally.

One problem often encountered in the clinical evaluation of cognitive slowing concerns its differentiation from the depressive and motor slowing so frequently present in PD. Patients with bradyphrenia are often the most akinetic, the most depressed, or both. Rogers and colleagues (1987) found that the cognitive slowing observed in a group of 30 newly diagnosed patients with PD was correlated with affective disturbance assessed by the Hamilton Depression Scale. Cognitive slowing was also observed in a group of 30 patients with primary depressive illness, and in both cases was improved after treatment with dopaminergic agonists, in relation to improvement in the affective symptoms. For these authors, this finding indicates a close relation between cognitive slowing and affective disturbances, which may be based on a common dopaminergic mechanism. Similarly, motor slowing may influence the clinical evaluation of intellectual slowing. Most mental operations require a motor output. It may therefore be difficult to evaluate clinically the cognitive component of response-time slowing. The frequent association of these two elements justifies the clinical concept of psychomotor slowing.

REACTION TIME

Reaction time (RT) procedures allow one to compare the performance of patients with PD with that of matched normal control subjects in tasks with different levels of complexity but with the same motor response. For instance, the difference between choice RT and simple RT performance gives information on central processing time needed for decision making. In most of the studies, the increase of central processing time in patients with PD was either the same (Jahanshahi, Brown, & Marsden, 1992) or even shorter (Pullman, Watts, Juncos, Chase, & Sanes, 1988) relative to control subjects. This unexpected finding suggests that additional processing needed for the selection and formulation of central programs is normal in PD, at least for processing involved in motor programming. Two possible explanations can be offered for the normal performance of patients with PD: The central component of the response in perceptuomotor choice–RT can be given out between the initiation time and the increased movement time phases of the response (Brown & Marsden, 1986); alternatively, perceptuomotor choice–RT may be too simple to reveal a specific impairment in PD.

For that reason, slowing of thought processing can be better investigated with the use of more complex tasks with higher cognitive demands. Even under those conditions, cognitive slowing has not always been clearly demonstrated, even on tests that require a high level of processing. For instance, Dubois, Pillon, Legault, Agid, and Lhermitte (1988) found no difference in their multiple-square experiment, an RT procedure with a cognitive component that varies in two different tasks. Indeed, the performance of patients with PD depends on the complexity of the task (Cooper, Sagar, Tidswell, & Jordan, 1994): A significant increase in response time was reported on a computerized version of the Tower of London task (Owen et al., 1992, 1995), on the Stroop test (Brown & Marsden, 1988), and on the 15-Objects Test, a visual discrimination task of 15 superimposed images of objects (Pillon, Dubois, Bonnet, et al., 1989). In these more complex tasks, the greater time required by patients may indicate a disturbance in cognitive strategy rather than a true slowing of central processing. For instance, the performance slowing on the 15-Objects Test increased from the first to the 12th object identified, as the task became more difficult. The slowest patients identified objects randomly, extracted details without reference to the global shape, and repeated previous identifications, indicating inappropriate maintenance of a category of activity. Thus, the slowing of cognitive processing demonstrated in this study seems to be partly a by-product of defective strategy, suggesting frontal lobe dysfunction.

An increase in thinking time was also observed on the Trail Making Test, even when the influence of motor speed was eliminated (difference in time B–A), but only for a subgroup of patients with PD who had a poor response to L-dopa therapy (Taylor et al., 1987). The fact that cognitive slowing was observed in the poor responders suggests that cognitive slowing is not supported by dopaminergic lesions, contrary to the observations of Rogers and colleagues (1987). This hypothesis is in agreement with the lack of effect of L-dopa treatment on the 15-Objects Test score (Pillon, Dubois, Bonnet, et al., 1989) and on planning time in the Tower of London task (Owen et al., 1995). Taken together, the results may indicate that cognitive slowing is rather related to abnormalities of nondopaminergic neuronal systems in the brain.

In conclusion, bradyphrenia in PD is a valid and useful concept from a clinical standpoint. There are also enough data to suggest that there is a lengthening of response time in some cognitive tasks, even after controlling for the motor component. However, cognitive slowing, the most genuine expression of bradyphrenia, is only found on complex tasks that have in common the participation of executive functions supposed to be under the control of the frontal system. This explanation applies in particular to the Trail Making Test (shifting aptitude), the Tower of London (planning ability), and the 15-Objects Test (self-elaboration and maintenance of strategy). The more complex a task from the point of view of requiring the elaboration of a strategy and specific behavioral regulation, the greater the cognitive slowing.

### Behavioral Regulation and Planning Deficits

Patients with PD have difficulty maintaining or shifting sets in response to environmental cues. This fundamental deficit may account for cognitive disorders (altered performance on the WCST) and more generally for behavioral disorders encountered in these patients. Resolution of complex neuropsychological tasks requires mental flexibility as a function of environmental cues. This theory has been criticized by Brown and Marsden (1988) because a shifting deficit is not generalizable to all tasks. This does not imply that patients with PD do not have a behavioral regulation deficit; rather, their performance is often related to the complexity of the task.

#### PLANNING DEFICITS

The performance of patients with PD on the Tower of London task (Morris et al., 1988; Owen et al., 1995), and to a lesser extent on the Tower of Toronto task (Saint-Cyr et al., 1988), points to a deficit in planning and programming. These deficits are often mild. A planning deficit has also been suggested by Flowers and Robertson (1985) to explain the difficulties these patients have on the Odd Man Out Test: Subjects can apply the rules once they are made, and it must be in their initial formulation that the parkinsonian impairment lies. Difficulty in self-elaboration of programmed plans may explain the strategy deficit observed in many studies. Patients with PD appear to be unable to elaborate an appropriate adaptive behavior because of a difficulty in integrating the pertinent information. This impairment, in turn, may be explained in terms of the attentional model of Shallice (1988). The supervisory attentional system (SAS) represents a general programming device that controls planning and decision making in nonroutine tasks or novel situations. Disorders of patients with PD may therefore result from either a deficit in the SAS itself or a limited internal storage capacity for information needed to elaborate a response. The vulnerability of these patients' performance to task characteristics favors the hypothesis of a limited capacity for processing resources.

### Task Demands and Resource Capacities

Whether or not performance is impaired in the PD group seems to hinge on the degree to which internally organized guidelines are required to succeed. This point was made by Taylor and colleagues (1986), who found that the neuropsychological tests that distinguished between patients with PD and normal control subjects shared the common feature of requiring spontaneous generation of task-specific strategies. The influence of external cues in PD performance was confirmed by Brown and Marsden (1988), who showed that patients were unimpaired in a cued version of the Stroop test but were impaired on a parallel task, in which they had to rely on their own, internal cues to perform the test. The distinction between external and internal cues may be crucial for understanding the deficits of patients with PD in executive tasks. Patients are impaired in tasks that require the use of internal cues for the control of attention. This hypothesis explains WCST performance, because subjects must focus their attention and define a strategy relying only on self-generated internal control. This hypothesis may also explain the inability of patients to use an internal model in a tracking procedure (Flowers, 1978).

The second, pertinent task-related factor is the complexity of the task. Patients with PD performed normally on the three-bead phase of the Tower of Toronto task (Saint-Cyr et al., 1988), indicating preserved problem-solving ability. They were impaired in the same task at a higher level of complexity (four beads). In both cases (i.e., noncued and complex tasks), performance was impaired because the demands of the task were too great, and exceeded the attentional resources of the patient. For that reason, patients with PD can succeed or fail in tasks according to whether they are more or less resource demanding. This interpretation is in line with the Shiffrin and Schneider (1977) model of attention, which distinguishes between effort demanding and automatic tasks, and which explains some cognitive deficits observed in PD, especially in learning and memory.

Besides the voluntary control of attention, based on internal explicit cues, some more fundamental mechanism, such as the automatic allocation of attention in response to external cues, may also intervene in the cognitive deficits of PD. In the Posner paradigm, subjects must engage their attention to an explicit cue indicating the direction in which an impending stimulus will appear. If the directional cue is valid, the attention may be engaged automatically. If the directional cue is invalid (the impending stimulus appearing in the direction opposite to that indicated by the cue), attention must be disengaged and rerouted to the alternate location. In patients with PD, valid cueing significantly improved reaction times, as in normal controls, but the cost of invalid cueing was low, suggesting instability in the process of attentional maintenance (Wright, Burns, Geffen, & Geffen, 1990). Other studies confirm an abnormally rapid disengagement of attention in PD or a rapid decay of inhibition that usually serves to bias subjects from shifting attention to an uncued stimulus or location (Filoteo et al., 1997; Sharpe, 1990). This impairment might intervene in cognitive deficits in PD, such as visuoperceptual or learning deficits. An automatic maintaining of attention is also likely required by the automatization of procedures and is probably a marker of basal ganglia function.

### A Functional Model for the Frontal-Related Cognitive Changes in PD

When a new task is proposed, executive functions and the conscious allocation of attentional resources required to build up a new strategy need the intervention of the prefrontal cortex (Shallice, 1988). With repetition of the task, the executive and conscious processes may be progressively relayed by more automatic and implicit processes. The automatic engagement and maintenance of attention and proceduralization of response schemas might be controlled by the basal ganglia (Doyon et al., 1998; Graybiel, 1998; Partiot et al., 1996). Therefore, PD might intervene in two different components of cognitive and behavioral control: an implicit and automatic "basal ganglia" component, and an explicit and voluntary "frontal" component. The dopaminergic system would contribute to both components. The intervention of the basal ganglia component is indispensable to free the attentional resources of the SAS (Shallice, 1988). In case of basal ganglia dysfunction, the lack of automatic engagement and maintenance of attention and acquisition of procedures impose the constant maintenance of the voluntary control of attention and thus limit the attentional resources of the SAS. Such a model might explain the differences observed between the effects of frontal lesions that would intervene only on the voluntary control of attention and those of the subcortical–frontal dysfunction of PD that would intervene both on the automatic (basal ganglia) and voluntary (frontal cortex) allocation of attentional resources. This intervention at both levels may be explained by the neuronal correlates of cognitive changes in PD.

## Neuronal Mechanisms

During the past three decades, our knowledge concerning the frequency and nature of cognitive changes associated with PD, on the one hand, and the type and extent of neuronal loss in the brains of patients on the other, has progressed significantly. PD thus represents a good model for studying the relationships between specific cognitive disorders and defined lesions of the CNS. However, it should be remembered that cognitive changes in PD do not comprise a monolithic picture that is identical in all patients. As previously reviewed, a spectrum of intellectual disorders can be observed, ranging from a few limited frontal signs to dementia. Moreover, the identification of biochemical changes in PD is far from complete, and new data may well render present theories obsolete. Neuronal interactions underlying brain functions are far too complex for such an approach to provide all the answers. They are, however, a place to start.

### Subcortical Lesions

From the pathologist's point of view, PD is mainly characterized by degeneration of subcortical neuronal systems. In typical cases, cortical abnormalities are limited and tend to occur late in the course of the disease. For this reason, histological changes in cortical neurons are not considered to play a significant role in the onset of cognitive disorders. Whether the same can be said of DLB is unclear, because cortical pathology may occur earlier and may predominate. Among the subcortical neuronal systems, nigrostriatal dopaminergic neurons are known to be the most affected by the disease, justifying the definition of PD as a "striatal dopamine deficiency" syndrome (Hornykiewicz, 1975). The dopaminergic avenue, therefore, is explored first and in greatest detail.

### DOPAMINERGIC SYSTEMS

Most dopaminergic systems are affected in PD (Javoy-Agid & Agid, 1980) and have been considered to account for most of the motor symptoms. We next review the main attempts that have been made to implicate dopaminergic lesions in the occurrence of cognitive symptoms.

*The Primate Model.* If one acknowledges a contribution of dopaminergic striatal depletion to cognitive disabilities, one must ask by which means the loss of dopaminergic input to the striatum leads to the particular cognitive profile of PD. At least a part of the cognitive syndrome seen in parkinsonian patients may result from a functional alteration of the corticostriatal loops. Indeed, the loss of nigral dopaminergic input to the striatum may lead to a cascade of dysfunctions throughout the basal ganglia system and to a functional alteration of specific cerebral regions (mainly the prefrontal cortex) to which it is connected. Frontostriatal connections are organized in relatively segregated circuits (Alexander et al., 1986; Strick, Dum, & Picard,1995). For instance, projections from the dorsolateral prefrontal cortex in the monkey (DLPFC, Walker's areas 9 and 46) target the dorsomedial parts of the head of the caudate nucleus, with a caudal extension shaping a rostrocaudal longitudinal strip (Selemon & Goldman-Rakic, 1985). The caudate subregion, which receives from the DLPFC, is also the recipient of the frontal eye field (FEF; area 8) and subregions from the posterior parietal cortex (Cavada & Goldman-Rakic, 1991), suggesting some role in spatial cognition. This suggested role of the dorsal part of the head of the caudate nucleus in spatial cognition raised by anatomical findings is partly confirmed by lesions and metabolic studies using the 2-deoxyglucose technique in the monkeys performing various spatial working memory tasks, such as the delayed spatial alternation tasks (Levy, Friedman, Davachi, & Goldman-Rakic, 1997). The orbitoventral parts of the prefrontal cortex are connected to more ventral regions of striatum, mostly the so-called "limbic" striatum or ventral striatum, which also receive connections from the amygdala (Haber, Kunishio, Mizobuchi, & Lynd-Balta, 1995). Recent electrophysiological works in the monkeys suggest a particular role of this structure in motivational aspects of behavior such as adaptation throughout the reinforcement system (Schultz et al., 1995). Finally, findings from anatomical and functional studies reveal that the posterior part of the caudate nucleus (mainly the tail) and the posterior putamen are likely involved in cognitive processes based on visual discrimination (Levy et al., 1997). Taken as a whole, these data could lead to the conclusion that there is a relative anatomical and functional dissociation of cognitive functions within the caudate nucleus. Indeed, recent studies suggest that parkinsonian patients at early stages of the disease have particular difficulties in tasks (mainly working memory tasks) in which the visuospatial domain is triggered (Owen et al., 1997; Postle, Jonides, et al., 1997). However, there are as yet only few data indicating that the dopaminergic denervation is more severe in the head than in the body or tail of the caudate nucleus. The relative segregation of the corticobasal ganglia loops is maintained throughout the basal ganglia system. Thus, Strick and colleagues have demonstrated in a series of experiments in the monkey, using neurotropic viruses as retrograde trans-synaptic tracers, targeted by different portions of the globus pallidus interna/substantia nigra recticularis (GPi/SNr) complex, via the GPi/SNpr–thalamic and then the thalamocortical pathways, different subregions of the prefrontal cortex (for review, see Middleton & Strick, 2000).

In summary, the particular functional and anatomical organization of the basal ganglia system suggests that specific circuits within the basal ganglia (including the input and output structures) are closely related to associative cortices and contribute to cognitive processes in close relationship with the prefrontal cortex, to which they are more densely connected. Consequently, it is easily conceivable that functional dysfunction of these circuits may lead to cognitive disorders similar to those observed after direct prefrontal lesions. And indeed, such a dysfunction is likely to occur after the progressive loss of dopaminergic neurons, such as that seen in PD.

The use of the neurotoxin MPTP (N-methyl-4-phenyl-1,2,3,6-tetrahydropyridine) in monkeys has given new impetus to the study of cognitive deficits after lesion of the nigrostriatal dopaminergic neurons. MPTP is known to selectively destroy these neurons. Taylor, Elsworth, Roth, Sladek, and Redmond (1990) have shown that MPTP-exposed monkeys exhibit cognitive deficits in an object retrieval task that tests planning ability. The treated animals made an increased number of perseverative errors that might be likened to a frontal-type deficit similar to that observed in patients with PD. Schneider, Sun, and Roeltgen (1994) have also demonstrated in motor asymptomatic monkeys intoxicated with chronic and low doses of MPTP, a decrease of performance in several tasks such as delayed response, discrimination, reversal and object retrieval tasks. The influence of reduced dopaminergic transmission on cognition also might be mediated by the mesocorticolimbic dopaminergic pathway. Specific lesions of this system in experimental animals produced marked behavioral disturbances (Simon & Le Moal, 1984): hypoexploration, disruption of behavioral inhibition, and delayed alternation, indicative of frontal dysfunction. This is not surprising given the target areas of these neurons that project to cortex (mainly prefrontal) and to limbic structures, such as the amygdala, hippocampus, and septal nuclei, known to be implicated in mental processes and behavioral regulation.

In conclusion, the review of experimental studies in animals supports the hypothesis that lesions of dopaminergic neuronal pathways may be responsible for cognitive changes by affecting the function of the deafferented structures.

*Correlations between Cognitive Impairment and Motor Symptoms.* Correlation between the degree of motor disability, thought to reflect damage to the nigrostriatal dopaminergic system, and intellectual impairment supports a relationship between dopamine depletion and cognitive disorders in PD. Among the classic triad of motor symptoms, intellectual impairment usually correlates best with akinesia, a symptom considered to be a marker of dopaminergic lesions (Martilla & Rinne, 1976), even in untimed tests (Mortimer et al., 1982). It must be stressed, however, that correlations indicate nothing about causality. In early-onset PD, characterized by severe akinesia and marked response to L-dopa and considered to reflect pure degeneration of dopaminergic neurons, no significant cognitive impairment is observed even after many years of the disease. A new approach to analysis by correlation was devised, in which the motor symptoms were distinguished according to their response to L-dopa (Pillon, Dubois, Cusimano, et al., 1989). Cognitive dysfunction correlated strongly with motor symptoms that respond little, if at all, to L-dopa, such as gait disorders or dysarthria, and weakly with motor symptoms that respond well, suggesting that cognitive disorders may be related to the dysfunction of nondopaminergic neuronal systems, in accordance with other studies (Taylor et al., 1987).

*Studies of Patients with Hemiparkinsonism.* PD motor symptoms usually start on one side of the body and often remain lateralized during the early and middle stages of the disease. This asymmetry, considered to reflect an asymmetrical striatal dopamine deficiency, has been partially confirmed by position emission tomography (PET) (Garnett, Nahmias, & Firnau, 1984). If the striatal dopamine deficiency plays a role in cognitive disorders, specialized hemispheric functions contralateral to the motor symptoms should be altered selectively in patients with hemiparkinsonism, providing a unique opportunity to study the effect of asymmetrical subcortical degeneration on cognitive function. The results of such studies have, however, been controversial. Some authors have found specific differences (Starkstein, Leiguarda, Gershanik, & Berthier, 1987), whereas others have not (St. Clair, Borod, Slivinski, Cote, & Stern, 1998). Methodological biases may account for some of these discrepancies, and adjustment for symptom severity resulted in the disappearance of differences between groups (Riklan, Stellar, & Reynolds, 1990). When methodological pitfalls are avoided, patterns of cognitive changes do not differ with respect to the lateralization of motor symptoms. Correlational analyses with motor symptoms do not provide unequivocal evidence of a primary, isolated, dopaminergic mechanism underlying cognitive changes in PD.

*In Vivo Metabolic Studies in Patients with PD. In vivo* studies, focused on the intensity of nigrostriatal denervation, may help to determine whether the striatal dopaminergic depletion contributes to cognitive dysfunction in PD. In this approach, the relationship is not straightforward, because it is based on an indirect marker of striatal dopaminergic deficiency, the level of fluorodopa ($^{18}$[F]dopa) uptake. Results of these studies remain a matter of debate. Brousolle, Dentresangle, and Landais (1999) concluded that cognitive disabilities in patients with PD were not associated with changes in striatal $^{18}$[F]dopa uptake, suggesting that cognitive dysfunction may not be related to striatal dopaminergic depletion. By contrast, Rinne and colleagues (2000) found that low performances in working memory, verbal fluency, and attention tasks were correlated to reduced $^{18}$[F]dopa uptake in the caudate nucleus. Future approaches in the field may benefit from modern imaging techniques such as functional magnetic resonance imaging (fMRI) coupled with cognitive paradigms in patients with PD at different stages of the disease.

*Correlations between Cognitive Changes and Postmortem Markers of Dopaminergic Neurons.* Such correlations are difficult to establish, because (1) degeneration of the nigrostriatal dopaminergic system is massive in all patients, reaching 90% by the time the patient dies, and (2) studies are generally performed on hospitalized patients with severe cognitive impairment that largely exceeds the subtle cognitive changes considered to be specific to the disease and related to loss of well-defined neuronal systems. Indeed, the late-onset cognitive deterioration observed in these patients can result from additional lesions of other neuronal systems or histological changes in the cortex, which would obscure putative correlations between specific cognitive deficits and dopaminergic lesions. The principal correlations observed in postmortem studies are, indeed, with nondopaminergic lesions, since PD dementia has been attributed variously to (1) coexisting AD (Boller, Mizutani, Roessmann, & Gambetti, 1980); (2) the presence of AD-type pathology, primarily in the hippocampus (Dubois et al., 1985); (3) neuronal loss in the nucleus basalis of Meynert (Whitehouse, Hedreen, White, & Price, 1983); and (4) decreased choline acetyltransferase (CAT) activity (Dubois, Ruberg, Javoy-Agid, Ploska, & Agid, 1983) or somatostatin-like immunoreactivity in the cerebral cortex (Epelbaum et al., 1983).

Striatal dopamine concentrations were shown to decrease severely and to the same extent in demented and nondemented patients with PD (Ruberg & Agid, 1988). Furthermore, a comparison of the neuronal loss in the substantia nigra of 18 demented and 14 nondemented patients with PD showed no correlation with dementia (Gaspar & Gray, 1984). However, in a study of 12 patients with PD, Rinne, Rummukainen, Paljärui, and Rinne (1989) found a significant correlation between the degree of dementia and neuronal loss in the medial part of the substantia nigra, that is, the part that projects more specifically to the caudate nucleus, suggesting that degeneration of nigral projections may in itself contribute to dementia in PD via deafferentation of the caudate nucleus. This observation needs to be confirmed in a larger series of patients, because it contradicts previous studies. Degeneration of the mesocortical dopaminergic system may also be implicated in the cognitive changes, because the decrease in dopamine levels in neocortical areas is greater in demented than in nondemented patients with PD (Agid et al., 1989).

*MPTP in Humans.* MPTP intoxication produces a parkinsonian syndrome in humans, provoked by specific damage to the nigrostriatal dopaminergic pathway. Patients with MPTP-induced parkinsonism were compared to drug-addicted controls (Stern, Tetrud, Martin, Kutner, & Langston, 1990). The patients performed worse in some memory tasks, drawing, category naming, and the Stroop Word–Color Test. Although the battery used in this study was not extensive, the deficits observed in the patients resembled those of patients with idiopathic PD, characterized by memory deficits and frontal lobe-like symptoms, supporting the idea that the dopaminergic system mediates a specific set of cognitive functions.

*Effects of Levodopa on Cognition.* If the cognitive functions that deteriorate in PD are mediated by a dopaminergic mechanism, improvement with L-dopa analogous to the response of dopamine-dependent motor signs might be expected. The main conclusion of the review of the literature on this topic is that in general the effects of L-dopa therapy on cognition are much more limited and specific than previously thought, even in the early stages. By contrast with motor or mood disorders, there is no evidence that cognitive performance fluctuates in response to L-dopa in patients with on–off phenomena. This may be interpreted in two ways: (1) cognitive changes are mediated by a dopaminergic mechanism but are unresponsive to L-dopa for pharmacodynamic reasons that are not yet understood, or (2) cognitive changes are mediated, at least in part, by lesions of nondopaminergic neuronal systems, in which case L-dopa would not be expected to be effective.

OTHER NEUROTRANSMITTER SYSTEMS

In addition to dopaminergic systems, other neuronal lesions have been described in PD, mainly confined to subcortical nuclei in the mesencephalic and diencephalic region: nucleus basalis of Meynert, locus coeruleus, and raphe nuclei. The neurons in these nuclei (cholinergic, noradrenergic, and serotoninergic, respectively) project to the cerebral cortex. Each of these neuronal systems has been implicated in cognitive processing by experimental and pharmacological studies.

*Lesions of Cholinergic Neurons and Cognitive Changes.* Decreases in the activity of CAT—an index of cholinergic innervation—in the cerebral cortex and in the substantia innominata support the contention that the innominatocortical cholinergic system is lesioned in patients with PD (Perry et al., 1985). This assumption is confirmed by evidence of neuronal loss in the nucleus basalis of Meynert (Gaspar & Gray, 1984; Whitehouse et al., 1983). Neuronal loss was found to be greater in demented (60–77%) than in nondemented (34–49%) patients with PD (Jellinger, 1987), in accordance with biochemical measures in the cortical projection areas. Even in patients with PD without dementia, CAT activity was reduced in the frontal, parietal, and occipital cortex, and in the hippocampus, although to a lesser extent than in patients with intellectual impairment (Dubois et al., 1985; Perry et al., 1985).

Blockade of cholinergic transmission with drugs consistently results in learning and memory deficits in different species. Atropine and scopolamine, muscarinic receptor antagonists, have been shown to impair memory acquisition, storage, retrieval, and free recall in humans (Sunderland, Tariot, & Newhouse, 1988). In rodents ibotenic acid injections in the nucleus basalis, which resulted in a cortical cholinergic deficiency, induced a severe behavioral syndrome consisting of impaired spatial learning (in T maze, radial maze, and Morris water maze) and avoidance learning (Dubois, Mayo, Agid, Le Moal, & Simon, 1985). In addition, nicotinic agonists have been considered to improve performance in working memory tasks in rodents and primates (for review, see Levin & Simon, 1998).

Studies of patients with PD confirm that loss of these cholinergic neurons might play a role in their cognitive disorders. First, there is a tendency for the severity of intellectual decline to correlate with the magnitude of the cortical cholinergic deficiency (Dubois et al., 1985). Second, cholinergic receptor antagonists regularly induce cognitive deficits in patients with PD, particularly when they are old or already show intellectual impairment (De Smet et al., 1982). In the same vein, it is noteworthy that patients with PD without any sign of intellectual or memory impairment shared a selective vulnerability to low doses of scopolamine in a double-blind, crossover study with matched controls (Dubois et al., 1987). To further investigate the contribution of cholinergic denervation to cognitive disorders in PD, the neuropsychological performance of patients treated with anticholinergics was compared to that of a group of patients matched for all the variables of parkinsonism, but who received no anticholinergic drugs (Dubois, Pillon, Lhermitte, & Agid, 1990). At the dose used, the performance of the two groups differed only on the frontal lobe tests, suggesting that the central cholinergic deficit demonstrated postmortem in PD may be implicated in the subcortical–frontal behavioral impairment characteristic of the disease. Rivastigmine, an acetylcholinesterase inhibitor, significantly improved cognitive performance of subjects with PD and dementia in a large, double-blind, placebo-controlled study (Emre et al., 2004), confirming the influence of the cholinergic deficiency in the occurrence of dementia in PD.

*Lesion of Noradrenergic and Serotoninergic Systems and Cognitive Changes in PD.* The noradrenergic and serotoninergic systems are of particular importance to cognition. In PD, the dorsal noradrenergic bundle that originates in the locus coeruleus is severely damaged. Both neuronal loss and noradrenaline depletion in the locus coeruleus were significantly more severe in patients with dementia (Cash et al., 1987). Noradrenaline concentrations also were reduced in the neocortex and in limbic structures, such as the nucleus accumbens,

amygdala, and hippocampus (Scatton, Javoy-Agid, Rouquier, Dubois, & Agid, 1983), although no difference between demented and nondemented patients with PD could be detected. Levels of 3-methoxy-d-hydroxyphenylglycol (MHPG) in the cerebrospinal fluid (CSF) of patients with PD were correlated with a measure of general intellectual ability and with performance on RT and attentional tasks (Stern, Mayeux, & Cote, 1984). Degeneration of noradrenergic coeruleocortical neurons may contribute to cognitive changes in PD. Pharmacological studies that used noradrenergic agonists improved significantly the cognitive performance of patients with PD (Bédard et al., 1998). A role in the depression observed in patients with PD is also substantiated. In accordance with the noradrenergic hypothesis of depression, tricyclic antidepressants that are potent noradrenaline uptake blockers have been shown to be efficacious in treatment of depressed patients with PD (Strang, 1976).

The same analysis can be made for the ascending serotoninergic neurons. These neurons are partially destroyed in PD, judging from neuronal loss in the raphe nuclei and decreased serotonin concentrations in the striatopallidal complex and in certain cortical areas (Scatton et al., 1983). The decrease was greater in the hippocampus and frontal cortex. No difference between patients with and without dementia was observed. The central serotoninergic deficiency may be implicated in cognitive processes. It seems, however, that, like the noradrenergic deficiency, the serotoninergic deficit is more likely to be implicated in depressive states in patients with PD: 5-HIAA (5-hydroxyindoleacetic acid) concentrations in the CSF are lower in depressed patients with PD than in the others (Mayeux, Stern, Cote, & Williams, 1984), and imipramine-like drugs, which are inhibitors of serotonin uptake, have significant antidepressant activity in patients with PD.

In addition to massive involvement of the nigrostriatal dopaminergic pathway and partial degeneration of the long ascending subcorticocortical systems, dysfunction of other neuronal circuitry also may be implicated directly or indirectly in the genesis of cognitive symptomatology in PD. Examples include loss of neurons both in the basal ganglia, as suggested by the dysfunction of various peptidergic and amino acid–containing neurons and in the brainstem, where cell loss in the pedunculopontine tegmental nucleus has been found in some patients (review in Agid et al., 1989).

## Cortical Lesions

Alterations of neurons in the cerebral cortex (i.e., diffuse Lewy body inclusions and AD-like histological changes) probably occur in most PD dementia cases, suggesting that intrinsic cortical pathology may account for some of the cognitive deficits and behavioral features. The extent to which these various cortical lesions contribute to the clinical picture remains controversial.

### Alzheimer Pathology

Are the dementia-related symptoms in patients with PD the expression of superimposed AD? At first glance, several arguments in the literature might favor this hypothesis (see Braak et al., 1997). It seems unlikely that these observations result from concomitant AD, however, because, as previously discussed, the cognitive deficits differ in the two diseases: The severe executive dysfunction and the profile of memory deficits observed in demented patients with PD evoke a subcortical–frontal type of dementia. Moreover, instrumental functions, such as language, praxis, or gnosis, are never as severely impaired as in patients with AD.

A large number of senile plaques (SPs) and/or neurofibrillary tangles (NFTs) are found postmortem in the hippocampus and neocortex of patients with PD (Boller et al., 1980), but they are not correlated with dementia. A high level of abnormal tau proteins is detected in temporal and prefrontal cortices of patients with PD and dementia (Vermersch, Delacourte, Javoy-Agid, Haw, & Agid, 1993), although the pattern and intensity of immunostaining is different from that in AD. Marked posterior hypoperfusion is reported in single-photon emission computed tomography (SPECT) studies of PD with dementia, although less than in AD (Spampinato et al., 1991). Taken together these findings have led some researchers to suggest that dementia in PD might result from a coexisting superimposed AD. However, other authors disagree. To some extent, this is a matter of definition. Out of a subgroup of 38 autopsied patients with PD, only two fulfilled the "criteria for coexistence" of PD and AD (Xuereb et al., 1989). This figure is based on reports from the same group showing that "a large number of neuritic plaques" could be found in subjects who seemed to have been intellectually normal. For that reason, they consider that only the combined presence of SPs and neurofibrillary tangles NFTs warrant the firm diagnosis of AD. This criterion differs from the guidelines recommended by the National Institutes of Health (NIH) panel (Khachaturian, 1985), according to which the diagnosis relies mainly on the number of SPs, particularly in elderly subjects. Xuereb and colleagues (1989) point out that, by following the NIH guidelines, the figure for patients with PD demonstrating AD-like neuropathological lesions would rise to 20%. The most recent (National Institute on Aging–Reagan Institute) guidelines for the pathological diagnosis of AD require suprathreshold plaque and tangle counts in neocortical areas (Hyman & Trojanowski, 1997). Thus, by modern standards, only a minority (< 10%) of patients with PD and dementia have coexistent AD at autopsy (Apaydin, Ahlskog, Parisi, Boeve, & Dickson, 2002).

Although the frequency and significance of the cortical changes are still controversial, there is a definite overlap between PD, PD with dementia, and AD. Patients with PD without dementia sometimes show cortical, AD-like changes in the cerebral cortex. As in AD, a significant decrease in ChAT activity has been found in the cortex and in the nucleus basalis of Meynert, associated with reduced levels of somatostatin concentration in the cortex of demented patients with PD. By contrast, Lewy bodies are found in the substantia nigra of a significant number of patients with AD (Ditter & Mirra, 1987). This overlap has been confirmed by De la Monte, Wells, Hedley-White, and Growdon (1989), who compared the histological features of demented patients with PD and those showing PD and AD.

### The Neural Basis of DLB and the Role of Cortical Lewy Bodies

Most DLB cases coming to autopsy show the coexistence of a-synuclein–positive Lewy bodies (LBs) and Lewy neurites (LNs), together with abundant AD-type pathology, predominantly in the form of amyloid plaques. Tau-positive inclusions and neocortical NFTs sufficient to meet NIA-Reagan criteria or Braak Stages V or VI occur in only a minority of cases. AD pathology is not a prerequisite for the existence of dementia, however, because patients with "pure" LB disease may present clinically with cognitive impairment and other neuropsychiatric features. Nor is the number of cortical LB robustly correlated with either the severity or duration of dementia (Gómez-Tortosa et al., 1999; Harding & Halliday, 2001) although associations have been reported with LB and plaque density in midfrontal cortex (Samuel, Galasko, Masliah, & Hansen, 1996). LNs and neurotransmitter deficits are suggested as more likely correlates of clinical symptom symptoms (Gómez-Tortosa et al., 1999; Perry et al., 2003).

In DLB, frontal lobe function may be compromised in at least two ways. First, there is diffuse cortical LB and LN pathology that includes frontal cortex, although the burden is less than in temporal regions (Harding & Halliday, 2001). Second, and probably more importantly, there is disruption of frontostriatal, frontothalamic, and other circuits linking the frontal cortex with subcortical structures. Only a limited amount is known about the precise neuroanatomical and neurochemical pathology impacting on these systems, but there are certainly major reductions in striatal dopamine and cortical acetylcholine (Perry et al., 1993). Although reductions in cortical ChAT in DLB correlate with severity of cognitive impairment (Samuel et al., 1996), this is unlikely to be the sole explanation for the neuropsychiatric features. Attentional dysfunction and/or disturbances in consciousness may, for example (McKeith et al., 2003), be related to loss in cholinergic activity in the reticular formation of thalamus, reflecting loss of pedunculopontine neurones. Cortical ChAT reductions also relate to visual hallucinations (Perry et al., 2003). The $\alpha$-7 nicotinic receptor is reported to be lower in hallucinating compared with non-hallucinating patients with DLB (Court et al., 1999), and visual hallucinations, which are experienced by up to 80% of patients with DLB, may therefore arise as a result of disruptions in the integration of visual perception and memory, related to defective cholinergic transmission. Although the substantia nigra neuronal loss is less than that in PD, dopamine concentration in DLB is reduced in the striatum by almost as much as in PD (Piggott et al., 1999); this reduction is sufficient to account for the extrapyramidal features. Frontocortical dopaminergic systems are implicated in working memory performance, and dopamine receptors

are also expressed in temporal cortex. Limited investigations in PD have shown no change in cortical dopamine ($D_1$) receptors in early disease or in experimental parkinsonism, but in advanced PD, PET imaging has shown $D_2$ receptors to be reduced by 40% in frontal cortex. The mesocortical dopamine system is also affected in DLB, with reduced $D_2$ receptors in temporal cortex and slightly raised $D_1$ receptors in orbitofrontal cortex, but with no change in cortical dopamine transporter.

In summary, there are at least two separate pathological mechanisms with the potential to compromise frontal lobe function in DLB: One is cortical and the other, subcortical, in origin. Diffuse cortical LB formation and neuronal loss involves frontocortical regions, reflected by reductions in measures of cortical cholinergic activity. The extent to which these local pathological changes are manifest as frontal signs or symptoms is not yet known. Patients with DLB do not present with the behavioral changes typically seen in the primary frontal lobe atrophies. The major functional correlate of cortical pathology in DLB appears to be the genesis of persistent visual hallucinations, with temporal and occipital association cortex being the regions most strongly implicated. The second element contributing to frontal dysfunction is a consequence of nigrostriatal degeneration that in DLB is similar to, but not so severe as, that seen in PD. Experimental evidence has demonstrated attentional and executive impairment in DLB that is indicative of frontostriatal dysfunction. Similar deficits are seen in patients with PD, but not in those with AD. By contrast, patients with DLB show less impairment on tests of recognition memory than patients with AD, reflecting the relative sparing of the hippocampus and related structures in DLB.

### How Are DLB and PD Dementia Related to One Another?

The relationships between DLB and PD with dementia are controversial and may be regarded as either simple or complex. The simple explanation is that the two disorders are different clinical manifestations of a common disease process (LB disease) and differ only in the temporal sequence in which symptoms appear, and in the relative severity of motor and cognitive symptoms (McKeith et al., 1996). In this model, an arbitrary "1-year rule" proposes that onset of dementia within 12 months of parkinsonism qualifies as DLB, and parkinsonism for more than 12 months before dementia qualifies as PD with dementia. Certainly there is a growing literature to support the view that DLB and PD with dementia may have similar endpoints on a common disease spectrum (Aarsland et al., 2003; Emre, 2003), particularly with respect to fluctuating neuropsychological function (Ballard et al., 2002), neuropsychiatric features (Aarsland, Ballard, Larsen, & McKeith, 2001), and extrapyramidal motor features (Aarsland, Ballard, McKeith, Perry, & Larsen, 2001). An alternative interpretation is that DLB results from a different anatomical and temporal distribution of pathological lesions (LB- and AD-related) than does PD with dementia. Indeed, the pattern of cognitive changes may be different in typical cases (more severe dysexecutive syndrome in PD with dementia; more severe visuospatial deficits in DLB).

Issues related to the clinical and pathological diagnosis and classification of DLB and its clinical management have recently been systematically reviewed and are not repeated exhaustively here (McKeith et al., 2004). The International Consortium on DLB will shortly be recommending updates and revisions to their previous guidance (McKeith et al., 2005).

## A Proposed Neuroanatomical Model for the Cognitive Changes of PD

It is hazardous to attempt a theory of the neuronal basis of cognitive disorders in the absence of prospective anatomical–clinical studies. The dopamine hypothesis is certainly attractive, because it takes into account the most severe lesions reported in the disease. Indeed, dopamine depletion, which is the first biochemical deficiency to appear, probably plays a primary role in the genesis of the basal ganglia and frontal lobe dysfunction observed in the early stages of the disease. Impaired performance on the WCST, Stroop test, and Trail Making Test has been reported in the beginning of the disease, even in untreated de novo patients, that is, in patients with isolated lesions of the nigrostriatal dopaminergic pathway. This assumption is consistent with the presence of frontal lobe–like cognitive disorders in MPTP-induced parkinsonism.

What is the anatomical substrate for the dopamine theory? Recent data provide a coherent description of the interaction between the dopaminergic innervation of the striatum and frontal lobe. The striatum, particularly the caudate nucleus, and various associative areas of the frontal cortex are linked by parallel and more or less independent neuronal circuits (Alexander et al., 1986). These circuits are dependent on a dopaminergic mechanism via the nigrostriatal or the mesocorticolimbic dopaminergic neurons. Disruption of caudate outflow (resulting from involvement of the nigrostriatal dopaminergic system) would be expected to alter the functioning of these circuits, as would depletion of dopamine within the frontal cortex or limbic structures (resulting from involvement of the mesocorticolimbic dopaminergic system). In conclusion, it may be postulated that striatal dopaminergic depletion plays a role in the frontal lobe–like syndrome observed in early stages of the disease. The lack of a reliable correlation with motor symptoms may result from the fact that the dopamine depletion in the caudate is not as great as in the putamen, as shown *in vivo* by PET (Nahmias, Garnett, Firnau, & Lang, 1985).

However, the explanation for the absence of improvement of cognitive changes under L-dopa treatment has long been a challenge. Recent data may be helpful in suggesting that the dopaminergic nigrostriatal lesions may not be as precocious as initially thought. Indeed, neuropathological data suggest that lesions of the nucleus basalis of Meynert might be present in the early stages of the disease and may be responsible for the cognitive changes as well. During the course of the disease, patients become increasingly handicapped as motor symptoms become unresponsive to L-dopa (e.g., gait disorders, or dysarthria, appear and cognitive disorders worsen). All these symptoms may correspond to the aggravation of nondopaminergic lesions, notably of the cholinergic, noradrenergic, and serotoninergic ascending systems. The respective roles of each of these additional pathological alterations remain, however, difficult to establish. These systems are thought to modulate cell activity in regions of projection involved in specific functions rather than transmitting specific information themselves. Furthermore, they do not act separately, but contribute in parallel or by mutual interaction to the expression of integrated behaviors. Despite these caveats, one is tempted to propose that cholinergic lesions, which denervate the hippocampus and cerebral cortex, affect memory function, attention, and frontal lobe activity, and that the noradrenergic lesion of the locus coeruleus may contribute to attentional disorders and, with serotoninergic dysfunction, to depressive mood.

If, as the evidence suggests, cognitive disorders in PD result mainly from lesions of subcortical origin, cognitive programs intrinsic to the cortex are not necessarily damaged but rather are deactivated. Deactivation may occur beyond a certain threshold of denervation when a single neuronal system is involved or when more than one system is damaged. For example, it has been shown that degeneration of cholinergic neurons, which is severe in patients with mental impairment, is present in all patients with PD even in the absence of intellectual and memory disorders. This suggests that there are two phases in the degeneration of cholinergic input to the cerebral cortex: a moderate and asymptomatic phase, and a second phase in which neuronal loss becomes sufficient for memory deficits to appear. Intellectual impairment occurs when synaptic adjustments (hyperactivity of the remaining neurons or supersensitivity of muscarinic receptors) are no longer sufficient to compensate for neuronal loss.

Alternatively, deactivation may occur only when destruction of several ascending neuronal pathways reaches the necessary threshold. This has been demonstrated in experimental studies (Nilsson, Strecker, Daszuta, & Bjorklund, 1988). If these results can be transposed to humans, they suggest that disorders of cognition mediated by ascending subcorticocortical systems may be observed in PD, either when there is sufficient partial destruction of several ascending neuronal pathways, or when there is a severe and selective lesion of one of them.

Age of onset of the disease may influence the threshold at which neuronal lesions become symptomatic. The compounding effect of aging on cognitive disturbances has been demonstrated by comparing the neuropsychological performance of early-onset and late-onset patients with PD to age-matched controls, suggesting that additional, age-related brain lesions may adversely affect compensatory mechanisms (Dubois, Pillon, Sternic, et al., 1990). This could explain the high frequency of dementia in older patients with PD. In a small number of patients, dementia defined according to DSM-IV criteria is observed. In these cases, neuronal loss or AD-like histological changes and/or LB inclusion in cortical neurons

may play a crucial role in the intellectual deterioration, in addition to subcortical lesions. The role of cortical lesions in PD is not, however, clearly established. Some cases of this type of dementia have been reported in the absence of apparent cortical lesions (Perry et al., 1985), suggesting that subcortical lesions may be sufficiently severe to cause overt dementia, at least in some patients. Conversely, AD-like changes or LB inclusions have been observed in the cortex of patients with PD without evidence of dementia.

The foregoing hypotheses based on clinical, pathological, and experimental observations are certainly oversimplifications. Nevertheless, they may have the merit of stimulating further experiments, particularly longitudinal studies aimed at establishing objective correlates of the clinical observations.

## REFERENCES

Aarsland, D., Andersen, K., Larsen, J. P., Lolk, A., & Kragh-Sorensen, P. (2003). Prevalence and characteristics of dementia in Parkinson disease: An 8-year prospective study. *Archives of Neurology, 60,* 387–392.

Aarsland, D., Ballard, C., Larsen, J. P., & McKeith, I. (2001). A comparative study of psychiatric symptoms in dementia with Lewy bodies and Parkinson's disease with and without dementia. *International Journal of Geriatric Psychiatry, 16,* 528–536.

Aarsland, D., Ballard, C., McKeith, I., Perry, R. H., & Larsen, J. P. (2001). Comparison of extrapyramidal signs in dementia with Lewy bodies and Parkinson's disease. *Journal of Neuropsychiatry and Clinical Neurosciences, 13,* 374–379.

Agid, Y., Cervera, P., Hirsch, E. C., Javoy-Agid, F., Lehericy, S., Raisman, R., et al. (1989). Biochemistry of Parkinson's disease 28 years later: A critical review. *Movement Disorders, 4*(Suppl. 1), 126–144.

Alexander, G. E., De Long, M. R., & Strick, P. L. (1986). Parallel organization of functionally segragated circuits linking basal ganglia and cortex. *Annual Review of Neuroscience, 9,* 357–381.

Albert, M. L., Feldman, R. G., & Willis, A. L. (1974). The subcortical dementia of progressive supranuclear palsy. *Journal of Neurology, Neurosurgery, and Psychiatry, 37,* 121–130.

Apaydin, H., Ahlskog, J. E., Parisi, J. E., Boeve, B. F., & Dickson, D. W. (2002). Parkinson's disease neuropathplogy: Later-developing dementia and loss of the levodopa response. *Archives of Neurology, 59,* 102–112.

Baddeley, A. D. (1996). The fractionation of working memory. *Proceedings of the National Academy of Sciences of the United States of America, 93,* 13468–13472.

Ballard, C. G., Aarsland, D., McKeith, I. G., O'Brien, J., Gray, A., Cormack, F., et al. (2002). Fluctuations in attention: PD dementia vs. DLB with parkinsonism. *Neurology*, 59, 1714–1720.

Beatty, W. W., Dennis-Staton, R., Weir, W. S., Monzon, N., & Whitaker, H. A. (1989). Cognitive disturbances in Parkinson's disease. *Journal of Geriatric Psychiatry and Neurology*, 2, 22–33.

Beatty, W. W., & Monzon, N. (1989). Lexical processing in Parkinson's disease and multiple sclerosis. *Journal of Geriatric Psychiatry and Neurology*, 2, 145–152.

Bédard, M. A., El Massioui, F., Malapani, C., Dubois, B., Pillon, B., Renault, B., et al. (1998). Attentional deficits in Parkinson's disease: Partial reversibility with naphtoxazine (SD NVI-085), a selective noradrenergic a1 agonist. *Clinical Neuropharmacology*, 21, 108–117.

Boller, F., Mizutani, T., Roessmann, U., & Gambetti, P. (1980). Parkinson's disease, dementia and Alzheimer's disease: Clinicopathological correlations. *Annals of Neurology*, 7, 329–335.

Boller, F., Passafiume, D., Keefe, N. C., Rogers, K., Morrow, L., & Kim, Y. (1984). Visuospatial impairment in Parkinson disease: Role of perceptual and motor factors. *Archives of Neurology*, 41, 485–490.

Bondi, M. W., Kaszniak, A. W., Bayles, K. A., & Vance, K. T. (1993). Contribution of frontal system dysfunction to memory and perceptual abilities in Parkinson's disease. *Neuropsychology*, 7, 89–102.

Bowen, F. P., Kamieny, R. S., Burns, M. M., & Yahr, M. D. (1975). Parkinsonism: Effects of levodopa on concept formation. *Neurology*, 25, 701–704.

Braak, H., Braak, F., Ylmazer, D., de Vos, R. A., Jansen, E. N., & Bohl, J. (1997). Neurofibrillary tangles and neuropil threads as a cause of dementia in Parkinson's disease. *Journal of Neural Transmission: Supplementum*, 51, 49–55.

Bradley, V. A., Welch, J. L., & Dick, D. J. (1989). Visuospatial working memory in Parkinson's disease. *Journal of Neurology, Neurosurgery, and Psychiatry*, 52, 1228–1235.

Bradshaw, J., Saling, M., Hopwood, M., Anderson, V., & Brodtmann, A. (2004). Fluctuating cognition in dementia with Lewy bodies and Alzheimer's disease is qualitatively distinct. *Journal of Neurology, Neurosurgery, and Psychiatry*, 75, 382–387.

Brousolle, E., Dentresangle, C., & Landais, P. (1999). The relation of putamen and caudate nucleus 18F-Dopa uptake to motor and cognitive performances in Parkinson's disease. *Journal of Neurological Sciences*, 166, 141–145.

Brown, R. G., & Marsden, C. D. (1984). How common is dementia in Parkinson's disease? *Lancet*, 2, 1262–1265.

Brown, R. G., & Marsden, C. D. (1986). Visuospatial function in Parkinson's disease. *Brain*, 109, 987–1002.

Brown, R. G., & Marsden, C. D. (1988). Internal versus external cues and the control of attention in Parkinson's disease. *Brain*, 111, 323–345.

Byrne, E. J., Lennox, G., Godwin-Austen, R. B., Jefferson, D., Lowe, J., Mayer, R. J., et al. (1991). Dementia associated with cortical Lewy bodies: Proposed diagnostic criteria. *Dementia*, 2, 283–284.

Calderon, J., Perry, R. J., Erzinclioglu, S. W., Berrios, G. E., Dening, T. R., & Hodges, J. R. (2001). Perception, attention, and working memory are disproportionately impaired in dementia with Lewy bodies compared with Alzheimer's disease. *Journal of Neurology, Neurosurgery, and Psychiatry*, 70, 157–164.

Cash, R., Dennis, T., L'Heureux, R., Raisman, R., Javoy-Agid, F., & Scatton, B. (1987). Parkinson's disease and dementia: Norepinephrine and dopamine in locus ceruleus. *Neurology*, 37, 42–46.

Cavada, C., & Goldman-Rakic, P. S. (1991). Topographic segregation of corticostriatal projections from parietal subdivisions in the macaque rhesus. *Neuroscience*, 42, 683–696.

Cohen, J., & Squire, L. R. (1980). Preserved learning and retention of pattern analysing skill in amnesia: Dissociation in knowing how and knowing that. *Science*, 210, 207–209.

Cools, A. R., Van Der Bercken, J. H., Horstink, M. W., Van Spaendonck, K. P., & Berger, H. J. (1984). Cognitive and motor shifting aptitude disorder in Parkinson's disease. *Journal of Neurology, Neurosurgery, and Psychiatry*, 47, 443–453.

Cooper, J. A., & Sagar, H. J. (1993). Incidental and intentional recall in Parkinson's disease: An account based on diminished attentional resources. *Journal of Clinical and Experimental Neuropsychology*, 15, 713–731.

Cooper, J. A., Sagar, H. J., Doherty, S. M., Jordan, N., Tidswell, P., & Sullivan, E. V. (1992). Different effects of dopaminergic and anticholinergic therapies on cognitive and motor function in Parkinson's disease: A follow-up study of untreated patients. *Brain*, 115, 1701–1725.

Cooper, J. A., Sagar, H. J., Jordan, N., Harvey, N. S., & Sullivan, E. V. (1991). Cognitive impairment in early, untreated Parkinson's disease and its relationship to motor disability. *Brain*, 114, 2095–2122.

Cooper, J. A., Sagar, H. J., & Sullivan, E. V. (1993). Short-term memory and temporal ordering in early Parkinson's disease: Effects of disease chronicity and medication. *Neuropsychologia*, 31, 933–949.

Cooper, J. A., Sagar, H. J., Tidswell, P., & Jordan, N. (1994). Slowed central processing in simple and go/no-go reaction time tasks in Parkinson's disease. *Brain*, 117, 517–529.

Court, J., Spurden, D., Lloyd, S., McKeith, I., Ballard, C., Cairns, N., et al. (1999). Neuronal nicotinic receptors in dementia with Lewy bodies and schizophrenia: ?-bungarotoxin and nicotine binding in the thalamus. *Journal of Neurochemistry*, 73, 1590–1597.

Cummings, J. L. (1988). Intellectual impairment in Parkinson's disease: Clinical, pathological and biochemical correlates. *Journal of Geriatric Psychiatry and Neurology, 1,* 24–36.

Cummings, J. L., Darkins, A., Mendez, M., Hill, M. A., & Benson, D. F. (1988). Alzheimer's disease and Parkinson's disease: Comparison of speech and language alterations. *Neurology, 38,* 680–684.

Danta, G., & Hilton, R. C. (1975). Judgement of the visual vertical and horizontal in patients with parkinsonism. *Neurology, 25,* 43–47.

De la Monte, S. M., Wells, S. E., Hedley-White, T., & Growdon, J. H. (1989). Neuropathological distinction between Parkinson's dementia and Parkinson's plus Alzheimer's disease. *Annals of Neurology, 26,* 309–320.

Delis, D. C., Kramer, J. H., Kaplan, E., & Ober, B. A. (1987). *California Verbal Learning Test: Research edition.* New York: Psychological Corporation.

De Smet, Y., Ruberg, M., Serdaru, M., Dubois, B., Lhermitte, F., & Agid, Y. (1982). Confusion, dementia and anticholinergics in Parkinson's disease. *Journal of Neurology, Neurosurgery, and Psychiatry, 45,* 1161–1164.

Dimitrov, M., Grafman, J., Soares, A. H., & Clark, K. (1999). Concept formation and concept shifting in frontal lesions and Parkinson's disease patients assessed with the California Card Sorting Test. *Neuropsychology, 13,* 135–143.

Ditter, S. M., & Mirra, S. S. (1987). Neuropathologic and clinical features of Parkinson's disease in Alzheimer's disease patients. *Neurology, 37,* 754–760.

Downes, J. J., Roberts, A. C., Sahakian, B. J., Evenden, J. L., Morris, R. G., & Robbins, T. W. (1989). Impaired extra-dimensional shift performance in medicated and unmedicated Parkinson's disease: Evidence for a specific attentional dysfunction. *Neuropsychologia, 27,* 1329–1343.

Doyon, J., Laforce, R., Bouchard, G., Gaudreau, D., Roy, J., Poirie, M., et al. (1998). Role of the striatum, cerebellum and frontal lobes in the automatization of a repeated visuomotor sequence of movements. *Neuropsychologia, 36,* 625–641.

Dubois, B., Danze, F., Pillon, B., Cusimano, G., Agid, Y., & Lhermitte, F. (1987). Cholinergic-dependent cognitive deficits in Parkinson's disease. *Annals of Neurology, 22,* 26–30.

Dubois, B., Défontaines, B., Deweer, B., Malapani, C., & Pillon, B. (1995). Cognitive and behavioral changes in patients with focal lesions of the basal ganglia. In W. J. Weiner & A. E. Lang (Eds.), *Behavioral neurology of movement disorders* (Vol. 65, pp. 29–41). New York: Raven Press.

Dubois, B., Hauw, J. J., Ruberg, M., Serdaru, M., Javoy-Agid, F., & Agid, Y. (1985). Démence et maladie de Parkinson: Corrélations biochimiques et anatomocliniques. *Revue Neurologique, 141,* 184–193.

Dubois, B., Mayo, W., Agid, Y., Le Moal, M., & Simon, H. (1985). Profound disturbances of spontaneous and learned behaviors following lesions of the nucleus basalis magnocellularis in the rat. *Brain Research, 338,* 249–258.

Dubois, B., Pillon, B., Legault, F., Agid, Y., & Lhermitte, F. (1988). Slowing on cognitive processing in progressive supranuclear palsy. *Annals of Neurology, 45,* 1194–1199.

Dubois, B., Pillon, B., Lhermitte, F., & Agid, Y. (1990). Cholinergic deficiency and frontal dysfunction in Parkinson's disease. *Annals of Neurology, 28,* 117–121.

Dubois, B., Pillon, B., Sternic, N., Lhermitte, F., & Agid, Y. (1990). Age-induced cognitive disturbances in Parkinson's disease. *Neurology, 40,* 38–41.

Dubois, B., Ruberg, M., Javoy-Agid, F., Ploska, A., & Agid, Y. (1983). A subcortico-cortical cholinergic system is affected in Parkinson's disease. *Brain Research, 288,* 213–218.

Dujardin, K., Degreef, J. F., Rogelet, P., Defebvre, L., & Destée, A. (1999). Impairment of the supervisory attentional system in early untreated patients with Parkinson's disease. *Journal of Neurology, 246,* 783–788.

Ebersbach, G., Hattig, H., Schlelosky, L., Wissel, J., & Poewe, P. (1994). Perseverative motor behaviour in Parkinson's disease. *Neuropsychologia, 32,* 799–804.

El-Awar, M., Becker, J. T., Hammond, K. M., & Boller, F. (1987). Learning deficits in Parkinson's disease: Comparison with Alzheimer's disease and normal aging. *Archives of Neurology, 44,* 180–184.

Emre, M. (2003). Dementia associated with Parkinson's disease. *Lancet: Neurology, 2*(4), 229–237.

Emre, M., Arsland, D., Albanese, A., Byrne, E. J., Deuschl, G., De Deyn, P. P., et al. (2004). Rivastigmine for dementia associated with Parkinson's disease. *New England Journal of Medicine, 351,* 2509–2518.

Epelbaum, J., Ruberg, M., Moyse, E., Javoy-Agid, F., Dubois, B., & Agid, Y. (1983). Somatostain and dementia in Parkinson's disease. *Brain Research, 278,* 376–379.

Ferman, T. J., Smith, G. E., Boeve, B. F., Ivnik, R. J., Petersen, R. C., Knopman, D., et al. (2004). DLB fluctuations: Specific features that reliably differentiate from AD and normal aging. *Neurology, 62,* 181–187.

Filoteo, J. V., Delis, D. C., Demadura, T. L., Salmon, D. P., Roman, M. J., & Shults, C. W. (1997). An examination of the nature of attentional deficits in patients with Parkinson's disease: Evidence from a spatial orienting task. *Journal of the International Neuropsychological Society, 3,* 337–347.

Flowers, K. A. (1978). Lack of prediction in the motor behavior of parkinsonism. *Brain, 101,* 35–52.

Flowers, K. A., & Robertson, C. (1985). The effects of Parkinson's disease on the ability to maintain a mental set. *Journal of Neurology, Neurosurgery, and Psychiatry, 48,* 517–529.

Fournet, N., Moreaud, O., Roulin, J. L., Naegele, B., & Pellat, J. (1996). Working memory in medicated patients with Parkinson's disease: The central executive seems to work. *Journal of Neurology, Neurosurgery, and Psychiatry, 60,* 313–317.

Freedman, M., & Oscar-Berman, M. (1986). Selective delayed response deficits in Parkinson's and Alzheimer's disease. *Archives of Neurology, 43,* 886–890.

Frith, C. D., Bloxham, C. A., & Carpenter, K. M. (1986). Impairments in the learning and performance of a new manual skill in patients with Parkinson's disease. *Journal of Neurology, Neurosurgery, and Psychiatry, 49,* 661–668.

Fuster, J. M. (1989). *The prefrontal cortex: Anatomy, physiology and neuropsychology of the frontal lobe.* New York: Raven.

Gabrieli, J. D., Singh, J., Stebbins, G. T., & Goetz, C. G. (1996). Reduced working memory span in Parkinson's disease: Evidence for the role of a frontostriatal system in working and strategic memory. *Neuropsychology, 10,* 322–332.

Garnett, E. S., Nahmias, C., & Firnau, G. (1984). Central dopaminergic pathways in hemiparkinsonism examined by positron emission tomography. *Canadian Journal of Neurological Sciences, 11,* 174–179.

Gaspar, P., & Gray, F. (1984). Dementia in idiopathic Parkinson's disease. *Acta Neuropathologica, 64,* 43–52.

Gauntlett-Gilbert, J., Roberts, R. C., & Brown, V. J. (1999). Mechanisms underlying attentional set-shifting in Parkinson's disease. *Neuropsychologia, 37,* 605–616.

Gentilucci, M., & Negrotti, A. (1999). Planning and executing an action in Parkinson's disease. *Movement Disorders, 14,* 69–79.

Gibb, W. R. G., Luthert, P. J., Janota, I., & Lantos, P. L. (1989). Cortical Lewy body dementia: Clinical features and classification. *Journal of Neurology, Neurosurgery, and Psychiatry, 52,* 185–192.

Girotti, F., Soliveri, P., Carella, F., Piccolo, I., Caffarra, P., Musicco, M., et al. (1988). Dementia and cognitive impairment in Parkinson's disease. *Journal of Neurology, Neurosurgery, and Psychiatry, 51,* 1498–1502.

Gnanalingham, K. K., Byrne, E. J., Thornton, A., Sambrook, M. A., & Bannister, P. (1997). Motor and cognitive function in Lewy body dementia: Comparison with Alzheimer's and Parkinson's diseases. *Journal of Neurology, Neurosurgery, and Psychiatry, 62,* 243–252.

Goldenberg, G., Podreka, I., Muller, C., & Deecke, L. (1989).The relationship between cognitive deficits and frontal lobe function in patients with Parkinson's disease: An emission computerized tomography study. *Behavioral Neurology, 2,* 79–87.

Gómez-Tortosa, E., Newell, K., Irizarry, M. C., Albert, M., Growdon, J. H., & Hyman, B. T. (1999). Clinical and quantitative pathological correlates of dementia with Lewy bodies. *Neurology, 53,* 1284–1291.

Gotham, A. M., Brown, R. G., & Marsden, C. D. (1988). "Frontal" cognitive function in patients with Parkinson's disease "on" and "off" levodopa. *Brain, 111,* 299–321.

Graybiel, A. M. (1998). The basal ganglia and chunking of action repertoires. *Neurobiology of Learning and Memory, 70,* 119–136.

Grober, E., & Buschke, H. (1987). Genuine memory deficits in dementia. *Developmental Neuropsychology, 3,* 13–36.

Grossman, M., Carvell, S., Gollomp, S., Stern, M. B., Reivitch, M., Morrison, D., et al. (1993). Cognitive and physiological substrates of impaired sentence processing in Parkinson's disease. *Journal of Cognitive Neuroscience, 5,* 480–498.

Growdon, J. H., Corkin, S., & Rosen, J. T. (1990). Distinctive aspects of cognitive dysfunction in Parkinson's disease. In M. Streifler (Ed.), *Parkinson's disease* (Vol. 53, pp. 365–376). New York: Raven.

Haber, S. N., Kunishio, K., Mizobuchi, M., & Lynd-Balta, E. (1995). The orbital and medial prefrontal circuit through the primate basal ganglia. *Journal of Neuroscience, 15,* 4851–4867.

Hansen, L., Salmon, D., Galasko, D., Masliah, E., Katzman, R., DeTeresa, R., et al. (1990). The Lewy body variant of Alzheimer's disease: A clinical and pathologic entity. *Neurology, 40,* 1–8.

Harding, A. J., & Halliday, G. M. (2001). Cortical Lewy body pathology in the diagnosis of dementia. *Acta Neuropathologica, 102,* 355–363.

Heindel, W. C., Salmon, D. P., Shults, C. W., Wallcke, P. A., & Butters, N. (1989). Neuropsychological evidence for multiple implicit memory systems: A comparison of Alzheimer's and Parkinson's disease patients. *Journal of Neuroscience, 9,* 582–587.

Helkala, E. L., Laulumaa, U., Soininen, H., & Riekkinen, P. J. (1989). Different error pattern of episodic and semantic memory in Alzheimer's disease and Parkinson's disease with dementia. *Neuropsychologia, 27,* 1241–1248.

Hietanen, M., & Teräväinen, H. (1986). Cognitive performance in early Parkinson's disease. *Acta Neurologica Scandinavica, 73,* 151–159.

Hietanen, M., & Teräväinen, H. (1988). The effect of age of disease onset on neuropsychological performance in Parkinson's disease. *Journal of Neurology, Neurosurgery, and Psychiatry, 51,* 244–249.

Hornykiewicz, O. (1975). Parkinson's disease and its chemotherapy. *Biochemical Pharmacology, 24,* 1061–1065.

Hovestadt, A., De Jong, J. G., & Meerwaldt, J. D. (1987). Spatial disorientation as an early symptom of Parkinson's disease. *Neurology, 37,* 485–487.

Huber, S. J., Shuttleworth, E. C., & Freidenberg, D. O. (1989). Neuropsychological differences between dementia of Alzheimer's and Parkinson's disease. *Archives of Neurology, 46,* 1287–1291.

Hyman, B. T., & Trojanowski, J. Q. (1997). Consensus recommendations for the postmortem diagnosis of Alzheimer disease from the National Institute on Aging and the Reagan Institute Working Group on diagnostic criteria for the neuropathological assessment of Alzheimer disease. *Journal of Neuropathology and Experimental Neurology, 56,* 1095–1097.

Ivory, S. J., Knight, R. G., Longmore, B. E., & Caradoc-Davies, T. (1999). Verbal memory in non-demented patients with idiopathic Parkinson's disease. *Neuropsychologia, 37,* 817–828.

Jackson, G. M., Jackson, S. R., Harrison, J., Henderson, L., & Kennard, K. (1995). Serial reaction time learning and Parkinson's disease: Evidence for a procedural learning deficit. *Neuropsychologia, 33,* 577–593.

Jacobs, D., Marder, K., Cote, L., Sano, M., Stern, Y., & Mayeux, R. (1995). Neuropsychological characteristics of preclinical dementia in Parkinson's disease. *Neurology, 45,* 1691–1696.

Jahanshahi, M., Brown, R. G., & Marsden, C. D. (1992). Simple and choice reaction time and the use of advance information for motor preparation in Parkinson's disease. *Brain, 115,* 539–564.

Javoy-Agid, F., & Agid, Y. (1980). Is the mesocortical dopaminergic system involved in Parkinson's disease? *Neurology, 30,* 1326–1330.

Jellinger, K. (1987). The pathology of parkinsonism. In C. D. Marsden & S. Fahn (Eds.), *Movement disorders: Vol. 2. Neurology* (pp. 124–165). London: Butterworth.

Khachaturian, Z. (1985). Diagnosis of Alzheimer's disease. *Archives of Neurology, 42,* 1097–1105.

Kosaka, K., Yoshimura, M., Ikeda, K., & Budka, H. (1984). Diffuse type of Lewy body disease: Progressive dementia with abundant cortical Lewy bodies and senile changes of varying degree—A new disease? *Clinical Neuropathology, 3,* 185–192.

Lambon, R. M. A., Powell, J., Howard, D., Whitworth, A. B., Garrard, P., & Hodges, J. R. (2001). Semantic memory is impaired in both dementia with Lewy bodies and dementia of Alzheimer's type: A comparative neuropsychological study and literature review. *Journal of Neurology, Neurosurgery, and Psychiatry, 70,* 149–156.

Laplane, D., Levasseur, M., Pillon, B. Dubois, B., Baulac, M., Mazoyer, B., et al. (1989). Obsessive–compulsive and other behavioral changes with bilateral basal ganglia lesions: A neuropsychological, magnetic resonance imaging and positron tomography study. *Brain, 112,* 699–725.

Le Bras, C., Pillon, B., Damier, P., & Dubois, B. (1999). At which steps of spatial working memory processing do striatofrontal circuits intervene in humans? *Neuropsychologia, 37,* 83–90.

Lees, A. J., & Smith, E. (1983). Cognitive deficits in the early stages of Parkinson's disease. *Brain, 106,* 257–270.

Levin, B. E., Labre, M. M., & Weiner, W. J. (1989). Cognitive impairments associated with early Parkinson's disease. *Neurology, 39,* 557–561.

Levin, E. D., & Simon, B. B. (1998). Nicotinic acetylcholine involvement in cognitive function in animals. *Psychopharmacology, 138,* 217–230.

Levy, R., Friedman, H. R., Davachi, L., & Goldman-Rakic, P. S. (1997). Differential activation of the caudate nucleus in primates performing spatial and nonspatial working memory tasks. *Journal of Neuroscience, 17,* 3870–3882.

Lezak, M. D. (1995). *Executive functions: Neuropsychological assessment.* Oxford, UK: Oxford University Press.

Lhermitte, F., Pillon, B., & Serdaru, M. (1986). Human autonomy and the frontal lobes: I. Imitation and utilization behaviors: A neuropsychological study of 75 patients. *Annals of Neurology, 19,* 326–334.

Lieberman, A., Dziatolowski, M., Kupersmith, M., Serby, M., Goodgold, A., Korein, J., et al.(1979). Dementia in Parkinson disease. *Annals of Neurology, 6,* 355–359.

Malapani, C., Pillon, B., Dubois, B., & Agid, Y. (1994). Impaired simultaneous cognitive task performance in Parkinson's disease: A dopamine-related dysfunction. *Neurology, 44,* 319–326.

Marié, R. M., Rioux, P., Eustache, F., Travère, J. M., Lechevalier, B., & Baron, J. C. (1995). Clues about the functional anatomy of verbal working memory: A study of resting brain glucose metabolism in Parkinson's disease. *European Journal of Neurology, 2,* 83–94.

Martilla, R. J., & Rinne, U. K. (1976). Dementia in Parkinson's disease. *Acta Neurologica Scandinavica, 54,* 431–441.

Marsden, C. D. (1982). The mysterious motor function of the basal ganglia: The Robert Wartenberg Lecture. *Neurology, 32,* 514–539.

Massman, P. J., Delis, D. C., Butters, N., Levin, D. E., & Salmon, D. P. (1990). Are all subcortical dementias alike?: Verbal learning and memory in Parkinson's and Huntington's disease patients. *Journal of Clinical and Experimental Neuropsychology, 12,* 729–744.

Mattis, S. (1988). *Dementia Rating Scale.* Odessa, FL: Psychological Assessment Resources.

Mayeux, R., Stern, Y., Cote, L., & Williams, J. B. (1984). Altered serotonin metabolism in depressed patients with Parkinson's disease. *Neurology, 34,* 642–646.

Mayeux, R., Stern, Y., Rosenstein, I., Marder, K., Hauser, A., Cote, L., et al. (1988). An estimate of the prevalence of dementia in idiopathic Parkinson's disease. *Archives of Neurology, 45,* 260–262.

McKeith, I., Dickson, D., Lowe, M., Emre, M., Feldman, H., Cummings, J. L., et al. (2005). Dementia with Lewy bodies: Diagnosis and management: Third Report of the DLB Consortium. *Neurology, 65,* 1863–1872.

McKeith, I., Mintzer, J., Aarsland, D., Burn, D., Chiu, H., Cohen-Mansfield, J., et al. (2004). Dementia with Lewy bodies. *Lancet: Neurology, 3,* 19–28.

McKeith, I. G., Burn, D. J., Ballard, C. G., Collerton, D., Jaros, E., Morris, C. M., et al. (2003). Dementia with Lewy bodies. *Seminars in Clinical Neuropsychiatry, 8,* 46–57.

McKeith, I. G., Galasko, D., Kosaka, K., Perry, E. K., Dickson, D. W., Hansen, L. A., et al. (1996). Consensus guidelines for the clinical and pathologic diagnosis of dementia with Lewy bodies (DLB): Report of the consortium on DLB international workshop. *Neurology*, 47, 1113–1124.

McKeith, I. G., Perry, R. H., Fairbairn, A. F., Jabeen, S., & Perry, E. K. (1992). Operational criteria for senile dementia of Lewy body type (SDLT). *Psychological Medicine*, 22, 911–922.

Milner, B. (1963). Effects of different brain lesions on card sorting: The role of the frontal lobes. *Archives of Neurology*, 9, 90–100.

Mori, E., Shimomura, T., Fujimori, M., Hirono, N., Imamura, T., Hashimoto, M., et al. (2000). Visuoperceptual impairment in dementia with Lewy bodies. *Archives of Neurology*, 57, 489–493.

Morris, R., Downes, J. J., Sahakian, B. J., Evenden, J. L., Heald, A., & Robbins, T. W. (1988). Planning and spatial working memory in Parkinson's disease. *Journal of Neurology, Neurosurgery, and Psychiatry*, 51, 757–766.

Mortimer, J. A., Pirozzolo, F. J., Hansch, E. C., & Webster, D. D. (1982). Relationship of motor symptoms to intellectual deficits in Parkinson disease. *Neurology*, 32, 133–137.

Moscovitch, M. (1994). Memory and working with memory: Evaluation of a component process model and comparisons with other models. In D. L. Schacter & E. Tulving (Eds.), *Memory systems* (pp. 269–310). Cambridge, MA: MIT Press.

Nahmias, C., Garnett, E. S., Firnau, G., & Lang, A. (1985). Striatal dopamine distribution in Parkinsonian patients during life. *Journal of Neurological Science*, 69, 223–230.

Nelson, H. E. (1976). Modified card sorting test sensitive to frontal lobe defects. *Cortex*, 12, 313–324.

Nilsson, O. E., Strecker, R. E., Daszuta, A., & Bjorklund, A. (1988). Combined cholinergic and serotonergic denervation of the forebrain produces severe deficits in a special learning task in the rat. *Brain Research*, 453, 235–246.

Ogden, J. A., Growdon, J. H., & Corkin, S. (1990). Deficits on visuospatial tests involving forward planning in high-functioning parkinsonians. *Neuropsychiatry, Neuropsychology and Behavioral Neurology*, 3, 125–139.

Owen, A. M., Beksinska, M., James, M., Leigh, P. N., Summers, B. A., Marsden, C. D., et al. (1993). Visuospatial memory deficits at different stages of Parkinson's disease. *Neuropsychologia*, 31, 627–644.

Owen, A. M., Iddon, J. L., Hodges, J. R., Summers, B. A., & Robbins, T. W. (1997). Spatial and non-spatial working memory at different stages of Parkinson's disease. *Neuropsychologia*, 35, 519–532.

Owen, A. M., James, M., Leigh, P. N., Summers, B. A., Marsden, C. D., Quinn, N. P., et al. (1992). Frontostriatal cognitive deficits at different stages of Parkinson's disease. *Brain*, 115, 1727–1751.

Owen, A. M., & Robbins, T. W. (1993). Comparative neuropsychology of parkinsonian syndromes. In E.

C. Wolters & P. Scheltens (Eds.), *Mental dysfunction in Parkinson's disease* (pp. 221–241). Amsterdam: Vrije Universiteit.

Owen, A. M., Roberts, A. C., Hodges, J. R., Summers, B. A., Polkey, C. H., & Robbins, T. W. (1993). Contrasting mechanisms of impaired attentional set-shifting in patients with frontal lobe damage or Parkinson's disease. *Brain*, 116, 1159–1175.

Owen, A. M., Sahakian, B. J., Summers, B. A., Hodges, J. R., Polkey, C. E., & Robbins, T. W. (1995). Dopamine-dependent frontostriatal planning deficits in early Parkinson's disease. *Neuropsychology*, 9, 126–140.

Partiot, A., Vérin, M., Pillon, B., Teixeira-Ferreira, C., Agid, Y., & Dubois, B. (1996). Delayed response task in basal ganglia lesions in man: Further evidence for a striato-frontal cooperation in behavioral adaptation. *Neuropsychologia*, 34, 709–721.

Perry, E. K., Curtis, M., Dick, D. J., Candy, J. M., Atack, J. R., Bloxham, C. A., et al. (1985). Cholinergic correlates of cognitive impairment in Parkinson's disease: Comparisons with Alzheimer's disease. *Journal of Neurology, Neurosurgery, and Psychiatry*, 48, 413–421.

Perry, E. K., Marshall, E., Thompson, P., McKeith, I. G., Collerton, D., Fairbairn, A. F., et al. (1990). Monoaminergic activities in Lewy body dementia: Relation to hallucinosis and extrapyramidal features. *Journal of Neural Transmission*, 6, 167–177.

Perry, E. K., Piggott, M. A., Johnson, M., Ballard, C. G., McKeith, I. G., Perry, R., et al. (2003). Neurotransmitter correlates of neuropsychiatric symptoms in dementia with Lewy bodies. In M. A. Bedard, Y. Agid, S. Chouinard, S. Fahn, A. D. Korczyn, & P. Lesperance (Eds.), *Mental and behavioral dysfunction in movement disorders* (pp. 285–294). Totowa, NJ: Humana Press.

Perry, R. H., Irving, D., Blessed, G., Perry, E. K., & Fairbairn, A. F. (1989). Senile dementia of Lewy body type and spectrum of Lewy body disease. *Lancet*, 13, 1088.

Piggott, M. A., Marshall, E. F., Thomas, N., Lloyd, S., Court, J. A., Jaros, E., et al. (1999). Striatal dopaminergic markers in dementia with Lewy bodies, Alzheimer's and Parkinson's diseases: Rostrocaudal distribution. *Brain*, 122, 1449–1468.

Pillon, B., Deweer, B., Agid, Y., & Dubois, B. (1993). Explicit memory in Alzheimer's, Huntington's and Parkinson's diseases. *Archives of Neurology*, 50, 374–379.

Pillon, B., Deweer, B., Vidailhet, M., Bonnet, A. M., Hahn-Barma, V., & Dubois, B. (1998). Is impaired memory for spatial location in Parkinson's disease domain specific or dependent on "strategic" processes? *Neuropsychologia*, 36, 1–9.

Pillon, B., Dubois, B., & Agid, Y. (1996). Testing cognition may contribute to the diagnosis of movement disorders. *Neurology*, 46, 329–333.

Pillon, B., Dubois, B., Bonnet, A. M., Esteguy, M., Guimaraes, J., Vigouret, J. M., et al. (1989). Cognitive "slowing" in Parkinson's disease fails to respond to levodopa treatment; "The 15 objects test." *Neurology, 39,* 762–768.

Pillon, B., Dubois, B., Cusimano, G., Bonnet, A. M., Lhermitte, F., & Agid, Y. (1989b). Does cognitive impairment in Parkinson's disease result from nondopaminergic lesions? *Journal of Neurology, Neurosurgery, and Psychiatry, 52,* 201–206.

Pillon, B., Dubois, B., Lhermitte, F., & Agid, Y. (1986). Heterogeneity of cognitive impairment in progressive supranuclear palsy, Parkinson's disease and Alzheimer's disease. *Neurology, 36,* 1179–1185.

Pillon, B., Dubois, B., Ploska, A., & Agid, Y. (1991). Neuropsychological specificity of dementia in Alzheimer's, Huntington's, Parkinson's diseases and progressive supranuclear palsy. *Neurology, 41,* 634–643.

Pillon, B., Ertle, S., Deweer, B., Sarazin, M., Agid, Y., & Dubois, B. (1996). Memory for spatial location is affected in Parkinson's disease. *Neuropsychologia, 34,* 77–85.

Pirozzolo, F. J., Hansch, E. C., Mortimer, J. A., Webster, D. D., & Kuskowski, M. A. (1982). Dementia in Parkinson disease: A neuropsychological analysis. *Brain and Cognition, 1,* 71–83.

Postle, B. R., Jonides, J., Smith, E., Corkin, S., & Growdon, J. H. (1997). Spatial, but not object, delayed response is impaired in early Parkinson's disease. *Neuropsychology, 11,* 171–179.

Postle, B. R., Locascio, J. J., Corkin, S., & Growdon, J. H. (1997). The time course of spatial and object learning in Parkinson's disease. *Neuropsychologia, 35,* 1413–1422.

Pullman, S. L., Watts, R. L., Juncos, J. L., Chase, T. N., & Sanes, J. N. (1988). Dopaminergic effects on simple and choice reaction time performance in Parkinson's disease. *Neurology, 38,* 249–254.

Ransmayr, G., Schmidhuber-Eiler, B., Karamat, E., Engler-Plörer, S., Poewe, W., & Leidlmair, K. (1987). Visuoperception and visuospatial and visuorotational performance in Parkinson's disease. *Journal of Neurology, 235,* 99–101.

Raskin, S. A., Borod, J. C., & Tweedy, J. R. (1992). Set-shifting and spatial orientation in Parkinson's disease. *Journal of Clinical and Experimental Neuropsychology, 14,* 801–821.

Reid, W. G., Broe, G. A., Hely, M. A., Morris, J. G., Genge, S. A., Moss, N. G., et al. (1990). *The evolution of dementia in idiopathic Parkinson's disease: Neuropsychological and clinical evidence in support of subtypes.* Paper presented at the First International Congress of Movement Disorders, Washington, DC.

Richards, M., Cote, L. J., & Stern Y. (1993). Executive functions in Parkinson's disease: Set-shifting or set-maintenance? *Journal of Clinical and Experimental Neuropsychology, 15,* 266–279.

Riklan, M., Stellar, S., & Reynolds, C. (1990). The relationship of memory and cognition in Parkinson's disease to lateralisation of motor symptoms. *Journal of*

*Neurology, Neurosurgery, and Psychiatry, 53,* 359–360.

Rinne, J. O., Portin, R., Ruottinen, H., Nurmi, E., Bergman, J., Haaparanta, M., et al. (2000). Cognitive impairment and the brain dopaminergic system in Parkinson disease: [$^{18}$F]fluorodopa positron emission tomographic study. *Archives of Neurology, 57,* 470–475.

Rinne, J. O., Rummukainen, J., Paljärui, L., & Rinne U. K. (1989). Dementia in Parkinson's disease is related to neuronal loss in the medial substantia nigra. *Annals of Neurology, 26,* 47–50.

Rogers, D., Lees, A. J., Smith, E., Trimble, M., & Stern, G. M. (1987). Bradyphrenia in Parkinson's disease and psychomotor retardation in depressive illness: An experimental study. *Brain, 110,* 761–776.

Rogers, R. D., Sahakian, B. J., Hodges, J. R., Polkey, C. E., Kennard, C., & Robbins, T. W. (1998). Dissociating executive mechanisms of tasks control following frontal lobe damage and Parkinson's disease. *Brain, 121,* 815–842.

Ruberg, M., & Agid, Y. (1988). Dementia in Parkinson's disease. In L. Iversen, S. D. Iversen, & S. H. Snyder (Eds.), *Handbook of psychopharmacology: Vol. 20. Psychopharmacology of the aging nervous system* (pp. 157–206). New York: Plenum Press.

Sagar, H. J., Cohen, N. J., Sullivan, E. V., Corkin, S., & Growdon, J. H. (1988). Remote memory function in Alzheimer's disease and Parkinson's disease. *Brain, 111,* 185–206.

Sagar, H. J., Sullivan, E. V., Gabrieli, J. D., Corkin, S., & Growdon, J. H. (1988). Temporal ordering and short-term memory deficits in Parkinson's disease. *Brain, 111,* 525–535.

Sahgal, A., Galloway, P. H., McKeith, I. G., Edwardson, J. A., & Lloyd, S. (1992). A comparative study of attentional deficits in senile dementias of Alzheimer and Lewy body types. *Dementia, 3,* 350–354.

Sahgal, A., Galloway, P. H., McKeith, I. G., Lloyd, S., Coo, J. H., Ferrier, I. N., et al. (1992). Matching-to-sample deficits in senile dementias of Alzheimer and Lewy body types. *Archives of Neurology, 49,* 1043–1046.

Sahgal, A., Lloyd, S., Wray, C. J., Galloway, P. H., Robbins, T. W., Sahakian, B. J., et al. (1992). Does visuospatial memory in senile dementia of the Alzheimer type depend upon the severity of the disorder? *International Journal of Geriatric Psychiatry, 7,* 427–436.

Sahakian, B. J., Morris, R. G., Evenden, J. L., Heald, A., Levy, R., Philpot, M., et al. (1988). A comparative study of visuospatial memory and learning in Alzheimer's-type dementia and Parkinson's disease. *Brain, 111,* 695–718.

Saint-Cyr, J. A., Taylor, A, E., & Lang, A. E. (1988). Procedural learning and neostriatal dysfunction in man. *Brain, 111,* 941–959.

Salmon, D., & Galasko, D. (1996). Neuropsychological aspects of Lewy body dementia. In R. Perry, I.

McKeith, & E. Perry (Eds.), *Dementia with Lewy bodies* (pp. 99–113). New York: Cambridge University Press.

Salmon, D., & Hamilton, J. M. (2005). Neuropsychological features of dementia with Lewy bodies. In J. T. O'Brien, D. Ames, I. McKeith, & E. Chiu (Eds.), *Dementia with Lewy bodies*. London: Martin Dunitz.

Samuel, W., Galasko, D., Masliah, E., & Hansen, L. A. (1996). Neocortical Lewy body counts correlate with dementia in the Lewy body variant of Alzheimer's disease. *Journal of Neuropathology and Experimental Neurology, 55,* 44–52.

Sarazin, M., Deweer, B., Merkl, A., Von Pose, N., Pillon, B., & Dubois B. (2002). Procedural learning and striatofrontal dysfunction in Parkinson's disease. *Movement Disorders, 17,* 265–273.

Sarazin, M., Deweer, B., Pillon, B., Merkl, A., & Dubois, B. (2001). Procedural learning and Parkinson's disease: Implication of striato-frontal loops. *Revue Neurologique, 157,* 1513–1518.

Scatton, B., Javoy-Agid, F., Rouquier, L., Dubois, B., & Agid, Y. (1983). Reduction of cortical dopamine, noradrenaline, serotonin and their metabolites in Parkinson's disease. *Brain Research, 275,* 321–328.

Schneider, J. S., Sun, Z. Q., & Roeltgen, D. P. (1994). Effect of dopamine agonists on delayed response performance in chronic low-dose MPTP-treated monkeys. *Pharmacology, Biochemistry, and Behavior, 48,* 235–240.

Schrag, A., Ben-Schlomo, Y., Brown, R., Marsden, C. D., & Quinn, N. (1998). Young-onset Parkinson's disease revisited—clinical features, natural history, and mortality. *Movement Disorders, 13,* 885–894.

Schultz, W., Romo, R., Ljungberg, J., Mirenowicz, J., Hollerman, J., & Dickinson, A. (1995). Reward-related signals carried by dopamine neurons. In J. C. Houk, J. L. Davis, & D. G. Beiser (Eds.), *Models of information processing in the basal ganglia* (pp. 233–248). Cambridge, MA: MIT Press.

Schwab, R. S., Chafetz, M. E., & Walker, S. (1954). Control of two simultaneous voluntary motor acts in normal and in parkinsonism. *Archives of Neurology and Psychiatry, 75,* 591–598.

Seitz, R. J., Roland, P. E., Bohm, C., Gretiz, T., & Stone-Elander, S. (1990). Motor learning in man: Positron emission tomography study. *NeuroReport, 1,* 17–20.

Selemon, L. D., & Goldman-Rakic, P. S. (1985). Longitudinal topography and interdigitation of corticostriatal projections in the rhesus monkeys. *Journal of Neuroscience, 5,* 776–794.

Shallice, T. (1988). The allocation of processing resources: Higher-level control. In T. Shallice, *From neuropsychology to mental structure* (pp. 328–352). Cambridge, UK: Cambridge University Press.

Sharpe, M. H. (1990). Distractibility in early Parkinson's disease. *Cortex, 26,* 239–246.

Shiffrin, R. M., & Schneider, W. (1977). Controlled and automatic human information processing: II. Perceptual learning, automatic attending, and a general theory. *Psychological Review, 84,* 127–192.

Simon, H., & Le Moal, M. (1984). Mesencephalic dopaminergic neurons: Functional role. In E. Usdin, A. Carlsson, A. Liahlstrom, & J. Engel (Eds.), *Catecholamines: Neuropharmacology and central nervous system–theoretical aspects* (pp. 293–308). New York: Liss.

Spampinato, U., Habert, M. O., Mas, J. L., Bourdel, M. C., Ziegler, M., De Recondot, J., et al. (1991). HMPAO SPECT and cognitive impairment in Parkinson's disease: A comparison with dementia of the Alzheimer type. *Journal of Neurology, Neurosurgery, and Psychiatry, 54,* 787–792.

Squire, L. R. (1989). Memory and its disorders. In F. Boller & J. Grafman (Eds.), *Handbook of neuropsychology* (Vol. 3). Amsterdam: Elsevier.

St. Clair, J., Borod, J. C., Slivinski, M., Cote, L. J., & Stern, Y. (1998). Cognitive and affective functioning in Parkinson's disease patients with lateralized motor signs. *Journal of Clinical and Experimental Neuropsychology, 20,* 320–327.

Starkstein, S., Leiguarda, R., Gershanik, O., & Berthier, M. (1987). Neuropsychological disturbances in hemiparkinson's disease. *Neurology, 37,* 1762–1764.

Stebbins, G. T., Gabrieli, J. D., Masciari, F., Monti, L., & Goetz, C. G. (1999). Delayed recognition memory in Parkinson's disease: A role for working memory? *Neuropsychologia, 37,* 503–510.

Stern, Y. (1987). The basal ganglia and intellectual function. In J. Schneider & T. Lidsky (Eds.), *Basal ganglia and behavior: Sensory aspects of motor functioning* (pp. 169–174). Amsterdam: Hans Huber.

Stern, Y., Mayeux, R., & Cote, L. (1984). Reaction time and vigilance in Parkinson's disease: Possible role of norepinephrine metabolism. *Archives of Neurology, 41,* 1086–1089.

Stern, Y., Tetrud, J. W., Martin, W. R., Kutner, S. J., & Langston, J. W. (1990). Cognitive changes following MPTP exposure. *Neurology, 40,* 261–264.

Sternberg, S. (1975). Memory scanning: New finding and current controversies. *Quarterly Journal of Experimental Psychology, 27,* 1–32.

Strang, R. R. (1976). Imipramine in treatment of parkinsonism: A double blind placebo study. *British Medical Journal, 2,* 33–34.

Strick, P. L., Dum, R. P., & Picard, N. (1995). Macroorganization of the circuits connecting the basal ganglia and the cortical motor areas. In J. C. Houk, J. L. Davis, & D. G. Beiser (Eds.), *Models of information processing in the basal ganglia* (pp. 117–130). Cambridge, MA: MIT Press.

Stroop, J. R. (1935). Studies of interferences in serial verbal reactions. *Journal of Experimental Neurology, 18,* 643–662.

Sunderland, R., Tariot, P., & Newhouse, P. (1988). Differential responsivity of mood, behavior, and cognition to cholinergic agents in elderly neuropsychiatric population. *British Research Review, 13,* 371–389.

Talland, G. A. (1962). Cognitive function in Parkinson's disease. *Journal of Nervous and Mental Disease, 135,* 196–205.

Taylor, A. E., Saint-Cyr, J. A., & Lang, A. E. (1986). Frontal lobe dysfunction in Parkinson's disease. *Brain, 109,* 845–883.

Taylor, A. E., Saint-Cyr, J. A., & Lang, A. E. (1987). Parkinson's disease: Cognitive changes in relation to treatment response. *Brain, 110,* 35–51.

Taylor, A. E., Saint-Cyr, J. A., & Lang, A. E. (1990). Memory and learning in early Parkinson's disease: Evidence for a "frontal lobe syndrome." *Brain and Cognition, 13,* 211–232.

Taylor, J. R., Elsworth, J. D., Roth, R. H., Sladek, J. R., & Redmond, D. E. (1990). Cognitive and motor deficits in the acquisition of an object retrieval/detour task in MPTP-treated monkeys. *Brain, 113,* 617–637.

Tranel, D., Anderson, S. W., & Benton, A. (1994). Development of the concept of "executive function" and its relationship to the frontal lobes. In F. Boller & J. Grafman (Eds.), *Handbook of neuropsychology* (Vol. 9, pp. 125–148). Amsterdam: Elsevier Science.

Van Spaendonck, K. P., Berger, H. J., Horstink, M. W., Buytenhuijs, E. L., & Cools, A. R. (1996). Executive functions and disease characteristics in Parkinson's disease. *Neuropsychologia, 34,* 617–626.

Vermersch, A., Rivaud, S., Vidailhet, M., Bonnet, A. M., Gaymard, B., Agid, Y., et al. (1994). Sequences of memory guided saccades in Parkinson's disease. *Annals of Neurology, 35,* 487–490.

Vermersch, P., Delacourte, A., Javoy-Agid, F., Haw, J. J., & Agid, Y. (1993). Dementia in Parkinson's disease: Biochemical evidence for cortical involvement using the immunodetection of abnormal tau protein. *Annals of Neurology, 33,* 445–450.

Vriezen, E. R., & Moscovitch, M. (1990). Memory for temporal order and conditional associative learning in patients with Parkinson's disease. *Neuropsychologia, 28,* 1283–1293.

Walker, M. P., Ayre, G. A., Cummings, J. L., Wesnes, K., McKeith, I. G., O'Brien, J. T., et al. (2000a). The clinician assessment of fluctuation and the One Day Fluctuation Assessment Scale: Two methods to assess fluctuating confusion in dementia. *British Journal of Psychiatry, 177,* 252–256.

Walker, M. P., Ayre, G. A., Cummings, J. L., Wesnes, K., McKeith, I. G., O'Brien, J. T., et al. (2000b). Quantifying fluctuation in dementia with Lewy bodies, Alzheimer's disease and vascular dementia. *Neurology, 54,* 1616–1624.

Wallesch, C. W., Karnath, H. O., Papagno, C., Zimmerman, P., Deuschl, G., & Lucking, C. H. (1990). Parkinson's disease patients behaviour in a covered maze learning task. *Neuropsychologia, 28,* 839–849.

Weingartner, H., Burns, S., Diebel, R., & Lewitt, P. A. (1984). Cognitive impairment in Parkinson's disease: Distinguishing between effort-demanding and autonomic cognitive processes. *Psychiatry Research, 11,* 223–235.

Wesnes, K. A., McKeith, I. G., Ferrara, R., Emre, M., del Ser, T., Spano, P. F., et al. (2002). Effects of rivastigmine on cognitive function in dementia with Lewy bodies: A randomised placebo-controlled international study using the Cognitive Drug Research computerised assessment system. *Dementia and Geriatric Cognitive Disorders, 13,* 183–192.

Whitehouse, P. J., Hedreen, J. C., White, C. L., & Price, D. L. (1983). Basal forebrain neurons in the dementia of Parkinson disease. *Annals of Neurology, 13,* 243–248.

Wilson, R. S., Kaszniak, A. W., Klawans, H. L., & Garron, D. C. (1980). High speed memory scanning in parkinsonism. *Cortex, 16,* 67–72.

Wise, S. P., Murray, E. A., & Gerfen, G. R. (1996). The frontal cortex–basal ganglia system in primates. *Critical Review of Neurobiology, 10,* 317–356.

Wright, M. J., Burns, G. M., Geffen, G. M., & Geffen, L. B. (1990). Covert orientation of visual attention in Parkinson's disease. *Neuropsychologia, 28,* 151–159.

Xuereb, J., Perry, E. K., Irving, D., Blessed, G., Tomlinson, B. E., & Perry, R. H. (1989). Cortical and subcortical pathology in Parkinson's disease: Relationship to parkinsonian dementia. In F. Boller & L. A. Amaducci (Eds.), *Clinico-pathological correlations of dementia in Parkinson's disease.* Report of the Symposium Farmitalia Carlo Erba, Milano, Italy.

Zalla, T., Sirigu, A., Pillon, B., Dubois, B., Agid, Y., & Grafman, J. (2000). How do patients with Parkinson's disease retrieve and manage cognitive event knowledge? *Cortex, 36,* 163–179.

Zalla, T., Sirigu, A., Pillon, B., Dubois, B., Grafman, J., & Agid, Y. (1998). Deficit in evaluating predetermined sequences of script events in patients with Parkinson's disease. *Cortex, 34,* 621–628.

# CHAPTER 31

# Neurosurgical Intervention for Psychiatric Illness

## PAST, PRESENT, AND FUTURE

*Anthony P. Weiss*
*Scott L. Rauch*
*Bruce H. Price*

Neurosurgical intervention to relieve mental distress is the oldest known form of psychiatric therapy, dating back to the documented use of trephining in the Late Paleolithic Period, 10,000 years ago (Gross, 1999). The modern rebirth of the neurosurgical approach to psychiatric illness, in the form of prefrontal leucotomy, was widely hailed as a safe and effective form of treatment for mental disorders and led to the 1949 Nobel Prize for its developer, Dr. Egas Moniz. Despite this august beginning, the use of neurosurgery for psychiatric illness (aka "psychosurgery") dropped precipitously, and for the past 50 years these techniques have been performed in only a handful of clinics worldwide. Even the term "psychosurgery," given its association with long-abandoned blind, freehand, neurosurgical techniques, has fallen out of favor, replaced by the terms "psychiatric neurosurgery" or "limbic system surgery." Indeed, the rise and fall of psychosurgery is one of the most interesting chapters in modern medicine.

Whereas most discussions of this topic have been written in retrospective fashion, often in the tone of a cautionary tale, we aim to provide in this chapter a forward-looking approach. While not neglecting the past, and the important scientific and ethical lessons it provides, we also discuss the present and future use of this therapeutic modality. There is a renewed interest in psychiatric neurosurgery, inspired by the use of focally ablative magnetic resonance imaging (MRI)-guided techniques and the recent application of deep brain stimulation (DBS) for psychiatric indications (Cosgrove, 2004; Greenberg et al., 2003; Husted & Shapira, 2004; Kopell, Greenberg, & Rezai, 2004; Rauch, Greenberg, & Cosgrove, 2005). We hope to encourage others to consider how the thoughtful application of these surgical approaches could be used to improve the lives of those suffering from the mental anguish of psychiatric illness.

## HISTORICAL OVERVIEW

The history of the modern era of psychiatric neurosurgery has been well documented, serving as the basis of two large monographs (Pressman, 1998; Valenstein, 1986) and several reviews (Braslow, 1999; Fins, 2003; Kopell & Rezai, 2003). We highlight aspects of this story that we find most relevant in considering the current and future use of this practice.

To understand the enthusiasm generated by the early uses of neurosurgery for psychiatric indications in the 1930s, one must consider the historical context of that era. Prior to the 20th century, the role of the psychiatrist was largely curatorial, because there were no effective treatments for patients plagued by depression or insanity. Arguably the most important developments during this premodern era revolved around the encouragement of humane treatment of the mentally ill, including the work of Pinel (1801) in France and Connolly (1830) in England, both of whom recommended the abolishment of mechanical restraints and chains. Scientific reports of the day were largely observational, and as a result, most of the writing was taxonomic or nosological in nature.

The development of the "malaria cure" for general paresis of the insane (tertiary neurosyphilis) by Julius Wagner-Jauregg first demonstrated the ability to actually treat, and even cure, chronically ill patients within the asylum. Conceived in 1887, first attempted in 1917, and described formally in 1920, Wagner-Jauregg's malaria treatment led to remission of syphilitic infection and its mental concomitant, through the induction of spirochete-killing fevers in the afflicted patients. Although eventually phased out due to the development of penicillin in the 1940s, the malaria cure was widely used and highly effective, and for his efforts, Wagner-Jauregg was awarded the 1927 Nobel Prize in Medicine.

Although this procedure benefited a great number of patients, many more remained untreatable in the asylums, including those with primary affective or psychotic illnesses. A number of therapies were attempted over the next couple of decades, including hydrotherapy (baths and wet blankets) and Sakel's insulin shock treatment, but none led to the safe and effective cure needed to empty the overflowing psychiatric wards.

It was in this context that the use of neurosurgery to treat patients with severe mental illness took root. The inspiration for this development is typically dated to August 1935, at the Second International Neurological Congress in London. As part of a full-day symposium on the frontal lobes, Yale physiologists Carlyle Jacobsen and John F. Fulton presented their findings on bilateral frontal lobe ablation in two chimpanzees, "Becky" and "Lucy" (Fulton & Jacobsen, 1935; Jacobsen, 1936). Using a delayed matching to sample memory task, Jacobsen and Fulton demonstrated substantial impairment on task performance, approximately at chance levels, following frontal

lesioning. Perhaps more interestingly, the behavioral pattern in response to these errors was markedly altered: Presurgically, one of the chimps (Becky) would become agitated after an incorrect choice; this behavior acquiesced after the frontal lobe surgery. Curiously, however, the other chimp (Lucy) demonstrated an opposite response, changing from docile to violent.

The esteemed professor and Chair of Neurology at Lisbon, Egas Moniz, in attendance at this lecture, was intrigued by these behavioral findings—at least those demonstrated by the chimp Becky. Within 4 months of the conference, Moniz (with the aid of neurosurgeon Almeida Lima) began testing the use of prefrontal leucotomy on patients with "certain psychoses." Initially performed by injecting alcohol into the subcortical white matter, Moniz and Lima then modified the procedure by using a steel leucotome to sever the white matter pathways within the prefrontal cortex (Moniz, 1937).

Walter Freeman, Professor of Neurology at George Washington University, was also in attendance at the 1935 International Neurological Congress. Once he became aware of Moniz's initial report, he quickly pursued the use of this procedure in the United States. He and a collaborator, neurosurgeon James Watts, performed their first procedure (now dubbed "frontal lobotomy") in mid-1936 (Freeman & Watts, 1937). By 1942, they had used this technique to treat 200 patients and had published their results in a large monograph (Freeman & Watts, 1942). Their results suggested that this procedure proved helpful in a large percentage of their surgical patients, though they did note the presence of adverse events in a significant number of cases, including seizures and apathy.

The use of neurosurgery for psychiatric indications escalated, in large part due to the enthusiasm of Freeman, who became increasingly vocal in touting the benefits of this procedure (Kopell & Rezai, 2003). In seeking a way to perform the procedure more efficiently, he came across the work of Amarro Fiamberti (1937), who had been performing transorbital lobotomies by injecting alcohol or formalin into the prefrontal white matter paths. Freeman modified Fiamberti's procedure by using an ordinary ice pick (and later a specially crafted surgical leucotome) to break through the orbital bone and sever the prefrontal cortex immediately above it. After practicing on cadavers, Freeman then began performing his "ice pick lobotomy" on patients in his private office, using electroconvulsive therapy as the only form of anesthesia. When Watts became aware of this, he was aghast, and broke off relations with his colleague. Indeed, although the second edition of their monograph was published jointly in 1950, Watts included the following disclaimer after the description of the transorbital approach:

> It is Walter Freeman's opinion that transorbital lobotomy is a minor operation. . . . It is my opinion that any procedure involving cutting of the brain tissue is a major surgical operation, no matter how quickly or atraumatically one enters the intracranial cavity. Therefore, it follows, logically, that only those who have been schooled in neurosurgical technics [*sic*] and can handle complications which may arise, should perform the operation. (Freeman & Watts, 1950, pp. 58–61)

The dissonance with Watts over this new approach did little to dissuade Freeman from the potential benefit of the procedure. He began touring the country to perform this transorbital procedure, often with media fanfare.

Enthusiasm regarding neurosurgery as a psychiatric treatment soon reached its peak, however, and in the early 1950s, began a steep decline in popularity (Figure 31.1). Although there are several likely explanations for this rapid descent, two are perhaps most important: (1) the development of chlorpromazine and other medications for the treatment of severe psychiatric illness, and (2) increasing concern over the cognitive and conative effects of frontal lobe ablation.

The 1953 discovery of chlorpromazine and its quieting effect on the patient with acute psychosis represented the beginning of the end for the widespread use of psychosurgery. For the first time, one could selectively treat the agitation and tension associated with schizophrenia and affective psychoses. Because surgery was thought to act primarily on these symptoms, providing little benefit for the other aspects of the schizophrenic syndrome, the *raison d'etre*

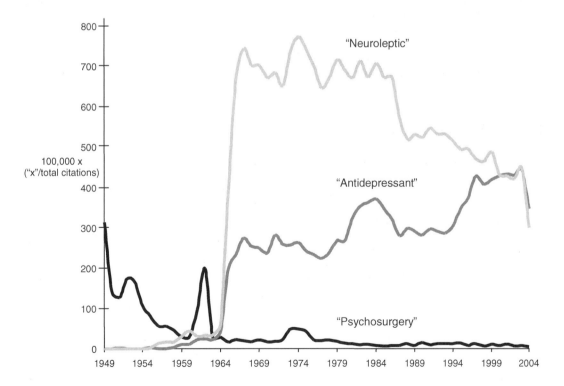

FIGURE 31.1. The decline in psychosurgery as depicted by citation rate. Total number of Medline citations for "psychosurgery" per year (1949–2004), corrected for the total number of MEDLINE citations in a given year. Results are displayed over time, with data on "antidepressant" and "neuroleptic" included for comparison.

of psychosurgery was now in question. Chlorpromazine was followed by the development of similar psychopharmacological breakthroughs for other illnesses, including anxiety and affective disorders. Armed with these new treatments, psychosurgery was pushed to the background and used only in patients deemed treatment refractory.

Even prior to the development of chlorpromazine, the unabashed enthusiasm for the frontal lobotomy within the psychiatric community at large began to wane, as reports of its effects on cognitive processing and emotional drive (among other adverse events) became more well known. Although hindsight affords us the opportunity to note evidence for cognitive effects in even the earliest papers describing the use of psychosurgery, this realization was delayed across the field as a whole. With the benefit of better longitudinal follow-up, and with greater understanding of the precise functions of the frontal lobes in mediating cognitive processes and emotional drive, the damage caused by full-scale frontal lobotomy became more readily apparent. In addition, these cognitive deficits were unmasked as many surgically treated patients left the "dull and sheltered atmosphere of the chronic hospital ward" (Strom-Olsen & Tow, 1949; Tow, 1955) and had to face the complexities of the outside world.

## THE DEVELOPMENT OF CURRENT TREATMENTS

As these limitations became apparent, physicians began to examine whether smaller, focal lesions could replicate the benefits of the prefrontal leucotomy without concomitant adverse sequelae. This work focused on patients with severe (treatment refractory) obsessive–compulsive disorder (OCD) and major depressive disorder (MDD). Although many cerebral regions have been considered as appropriate targets for neurosurgical intervention, three have received the most study: the anterior cingulate gyrus (with its associated white matter tract, the cingulum bundle), the basal forebrain, and the anterior limb of the internal capsule. In this section, we briefly review the literature that led to the development of these specific procedures, summarize the data concerning the efficacy and adverse sequelae of lesions in these areas, and discuss any known literature concerning the use of DBS at these sites.

A number of caveats need to be mentioned when considering the efficacy data for all of the procedures described in this chapter. As noted by Greenberg and colleagues (2003) in a recent review, the efficacy of psychosurgical procedures is difficult to assess for several reasons:

1. The criteria for psychiatric diagnoses have changed over time, becoming more rigidly codified only after the release of the third edition of the *Diagnostic and Statistical Manual of Mental Disorders* (DSM-III) in 1980.
2. The use of standardized disease-severity scales is a relatively new phenomenon, with the vast majority of the literature defining outcome on nominal scales (e.g., *improved, moderately improved, markedly improved*).
3. With the development of an extensive array of pharmaceutical therapies for these illnesses, the concept of "treatment-refractory illness" has changed over time, with the current patients undergoing surgery likely to be more ill than those in the past.
4. The procedures are performed on a limited basis at only a few specialized centers around the world, leading to efficacy reports with notoriously small sample sizes.
5. There are few prospective reports, and given concerns about the ethical nature of "sham" psychosurgery, no known studies using adequate control groups.

### Anterior Cingulate

*Development of the Cingulotomy*

The function of the anterior cingulate gyrus remained relatively unclear until the middle of the 20th century. It had long been considered to be a component of the rhinencephalon, with a role in olfaction, despite evidence of a fully developed cingulate gyrus in some anosmic mammals (e.g., dolphin and porpoise) (Smith, 1945). Papez (1937), closely following Broca's (1878) model of *le grand lobe limbique*, considered the cingulate to be an important component of the neural circuitry producing emotion. Experimental evidence for this proposed role came within the next decade, when both Smith (1945) and Ward (1948) demonstrated the impact of anterior cingulate ablation on autonomic function, the physiological correlate of emotional excitation, in the monkey. Both authors also noted that anterior cingulectomy led to significant relaxation of muscle tension, prompting Ward to wonder whether the severing of cingulofrontal efferents during standard lobotomy might account for the beneficial effect of this procedure.

In 1948, at least four separate groups began to translate these experimental primate findings into therapeutic neurosurgical procedures for severe psychiatric illness. Bockoven and Greenblatt, as part of the Second Lobotomy Project of Boston Psychopathic Hospital (Greenblatt & Solomon, 1953), modified the bilateral prefrontal lobotomy of Poppen (1948) into a bimedial lobotomy, with the expressed interest in specifically interrupting those efferent fibers situated near the cingulate. In a randomized outcome study of 116 consecutive patients with psychoses, this bimedial approach was demonstrated to be more effective (60% showed *marked* or *moderate* improvement) than either the standard bilateral lobotomy (46%) or a unilateral frontal lobotomy (28%) (Greenblatt & Solomon, 1953). They concluded that "since bimedial operation was followed by clinical changes more favorable than standard bilateral operation, it may be assumed that the destruction in bilateral [frontal lobes] is excessive and unnecessary" (p. 390).

William Scoville (1949), also citing the work of Ward (1948), attempted a new approach with a less destructive form of lobotomy through "cortical undercutting," a method that separated gray matter from white at the gray–white junction. In addition to orbital surface undercutting (which ultimately led to subcaudate tractotomy, see below), Scoville also performed cingulate gyrus undercutting for "mental disease," again hoping to specifically interrupt the efferents extending from this region. Though his initial report is largely a methodological description, he did note that results were favorable enough to continue to explore this form of limited frontal ablation.

LeBeau and Pecker (1949), followed closely thereafter by Whitty, Duffield, Tow, and Cairns (1952), performed the first limited resection of the anterior cingulate gyrus itself, a cingulectomy. LeBeau (1954) accurately noted that "the operation is much more precise anatomically than any other psychosurgical technique" (p. 269). Both groups reported positive outcomes in samples of 50 and 24 patients, respectively. Importantly, Whitty and colleagues (1952) concluded that "the operation has little place in the treatment of advanced psychotics,

but where anxiety and obsessions in a basically well-preserved personality are so intransigent and disabling as to require consideration of psychosurgery, cingulectomy clearly calls for further trial" (p. 475).

The modern stereotactic cingulotomy was developed by Foltz and White (1961) for treatment of the emotional component of chronic pain. Their approach used pneumoencephalography for localization of the lateral ventricles, a technique also used by Ballantine, Cassidy, Flanagan, and Marino (1967), who widened the application to patients suffering from depression and OCD. In current practice, cingulotomy is performed with use of a stereotactic frame, with the target in the anterior cingulate (20–25 mm posterior to the tip of the frontal horn, 7 mm from the midline, and 1 mm above the roof of the lateral ventricle) guided by MRI. It is important to note that this current procedure is as much a "cingu*lum*otomy" as a cingulotomy; in creating the surgical lesion, the thermocoagulative electrode passes through the cingulate cortex to ablate the underlying white matter fasciculus (the cingulum bundle), resulting in a lesion approximately 2 cm in height and 8–10 mm in diameter (Cosgrove, 2000; Rauch et al., 2000) (Figure 31.2). It is at this point unknown whether it is the gray and/or white matter component of this procedure that results in its efficacy.

### Efficacy of Cingulotomy

Jenike and colleagues (1991) published the largest retrospective assessment of the efficacy of cingulotomy for OCD using modern diagnostic criteria and outcomes measures (33 patients). Using conservative criteria, they estimated that 25–30% of patients received substantial benefit from the procedure. The largest prospective study in OCD was reported by Dougherty and colleagues (2002) in a cohort of 44 patients with well-characterized, treatment-refractory illness. With a mean follow-up assessment at 32 months postoperatively, 14 of the 44 patients (32%) were determined to be treatment responders (i.e., 35% decrease in Yale–Brown Obsessive Compulsive Scale (Y-BOCS) score and a Clinical Global Improvement (CGI) rating ≤ 2. The overall mean reduction in Y-BOCS score for the entire cohort was 28.7%.

Ballantine and colleagues periodically published large retrospective reports of the efficacy

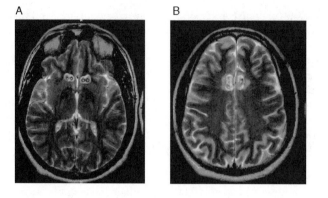

FIGURE 31.2. Limbic leukotomy lesion location. T2-weighted axial MRIs demonstrating bilateral surgical lesions within the subcaudate territory (A) and the cingulum bundle (B).

of cingulotomy, including its effect on patients with affective illness (Ballantine, Bouckoms, Thomas, & Giriunas, 1987; Ballantine, Levy, Dagi, & Giriunas, 1977). In a 1977 chapter describing the results in 154 patients, they indicated that 97% of this cohort reported symptoms of depression preoperatively, whereas only 40% reported depressive symptoms after cingulotomy, making depression one of the symptoms most responsive to this procedure (Ballantine et al., 1977). Spangler and colleagues (1996) indicated that 53% of their patients with major affective illness (both unipolar and bipolar depression) reported to be *very much improved* or *much improved* following cingulotomy. The largest prospective study on the effects of cingulotomy on MDD (13 patients), reported by Dougherty and colleagues (2003), demonstrated a mean decrease in the total Beck Depression Inventory score of 33%.

### Adverse Effects of Cingulotomy

Since Ballantine's first use of the procedure in 1962, over 1,000 stereotactic anterior cingulotomies have been performed at Massachusetts General Hospital (MGH) in Boston. Overall, the procedure has never been directly implicated in a patient's death, and of the 156 MRI-guided procedures performed since 1991, only two patients have experienced severe adverse events: one with hemorrhagic stroke and cerebral abscess, the other with cerebral abscess and hydrocephalus. Three broad categories of adverse events appear to be most common: seizures, urinary difficulties, and mild cognitive impairment (Cosgrove, 2000;

Cosgrove & Rauch, 1995; Greenberg et al., 2003; Marino & Cosgrove, 1997; Rauch et al., 2005). Postoperative seizures occur in approximately 1–5% of patients and are almost always a transient phenomenon; in Ballantine's series of 238 patients, only two required long-term antiseizure therapy postcingulotomy. Urinary incontinence or retention appears to a bit more common but is, again, almost always transient. With regard to cognitive impairment, three large reports that used thorough neuropsychological batteries similarly concluded that the adverse effects of cingulotomy across a cohort are negligible (Corkin, 1980; Corkin, Twitchell, & Sullivan, 1979; Long, Pueschel, & Hunter, 1978). Indeed, 68% of the patients reported by Long and colleagues (1978) demonstrated improvements in cognitive function postoperatively. There are, however, some reports of deficits in high-level visual processing and attention (Cohen, Kaplan, Moser, Jenkins, & Wilkinson, 1999; Cohen, Kaplan, Zuffante, et al., 1999; Ochsner et al., 2001), and a recent report describing deficits on a reward-based task (Williams, Bush, Rauch, Cosgrove, & Eskandar, 2004) following cingulotomy, but the extent to which these effects endure beyond the intraoperative period or impair daily functioning are as yet unclear.

### Cingulate Deep Brain Stimulation

To our knowledge, no published reports document the use of DBS within the anterior cingulate gyrus. As indicated by early reports (Smith, 1945; Ward, 1948) stimulation of the anterior cingulate leads to autonomic effects in both monkeys and humans, including respiratory slowing and bradycardia. Foltz and White (1961) also reported that cingulate stimulation immediately prior to coagulation in two patients led to "a striking increase in agitation, and evidences of fear and apprehension, but neither patient could describe the sensation" (p. 91). Without further detail regarding the exact stimulus location and the nature of the electrical stimulation, it is difficult to know how these findings would extrapolate to the modern DBS procedure. It is also difficult to know whether cingulate DBS would be able to replicate the success of cingulate ablation, because the size of the cingulotomy lesions far exceeds the volume of affected tissue in the conventional uses of DBS for movement disorders such as Parkinson's disease. Perhaps this is why initial attempts at DBS for psychiatric indications have targeted smaller gray matter territories or the internal capsule.

## Basal Forebrain

### Development of the Subcaudate Tractotomy

Unlike the development of surgical procedures within the cingulate, which were based on theory and experimental findings in primates, the development of the basal forebrain as a surgical target for psychiatric indications was empirically derived, and actually preceded our understanding of the role of this region in emotional processing. This work was an extension, literally and figuratively, of the limited surgical ablation of the orbitofrontal cortex, first performed by Scoville (1949), using a cortical undercutting approach. At a 1960 meeting of the Royal Society of Medicine in London, Knight first described a modified version of Scoville's procedure, one that confined the incision to the medial aspect of the orbital gyrus, and extended the incision an additional centimeter posteriorly. He reported, "There is a specific area which when cut produces maximum benefit. In 10 cases a first operation with a 5-cm cut failed, but a second operation extending the cut posteriorly for a further centimetre [sic] produced success in 6" (p. 31).

Knight (1964, 1969) went on to refine the procedure further, ultimately confining it to this posteriormost territory (the substantia innominata) felt to be so critical to the operation's success. This "subcaudate tractotomy" was then performed stereotactically, at first via the implantation of yttrium seeds, and later through electrical thermocoagulation. Through the work of Nauta (1982), Heimer (2003), and others, we have now come to understand the important role of this region, often referred to as "the extended amygdala," in emotional processing.

### Efficacy of Subcaudate Tractotomy

Based on the collective experience of Knight's London group, subcaudate tractotomy appears to be more effective in patients with MDD than in those with OCD, a pattern similar to the effects of cingulotomy. Goktepe, Young, and Bridges (1975), for example, reported response rates of 68% in depressed patients compared to 50% response rates in those with obsessional neurosis. A more recent review examining the response in all 249 tractotomies done from 1979–1995 at that center indicated that 34% were well 1-year postoperatively (Hodgkiss, Malizia, Bartlett, & Bridges, 1995).

We recently reported our experience at MGH with limbic leucotomy, a procedure that includes bilateral lesions in both the anterior cingulate and the basal forebrain (Montoya et al., 2002). In a retrospective assessment of 21 patients (15 with OCD and 6 with MDD), depending on the criteria used to define response, approximately 36–50% of these patients would be considered to have had a positive outcome. Interestingly, whereas 62% of patients with OCD rated themselves as *very much improved* or *much improved*, only 17% of patients with a primary diagnosis of MDD noted this level of response.

### Adverse Effects of Subcaudate Tractotomy

Reported adverse sequelae from subcaudate tractotomy include transient headache, confusion/disinhibition, and/or somnolence. Personality changes were present in 6.7% of surgical patients, and seizures were noted in 2.2% (Greenberg et al., 2003). In terms of cognitive effects, a 1991 prospective study using a thorough neuropsychological battery indicated that although there were decrements in recognition memory and performance on tasks sensitive to frontal lobe functioning during the early postoperative period, there was no evidence for significant, long-term cognitive deficits associated with this procedure (Kartsounis, Poynton, Bridges, & Bartlett, 1991).

## Basal Forebrain Deep Brain Stimulation

To our knowledge, there are two published reports of the use of DBS within the basal forebrain for the treatment of psychiatric illness (Aouizerate et al., 2004; Sturm et al., 2003). The first describes the implantation of electrodes within the right nucleus accumbens in four patients with severe OCD and anxiety disorders (Sturm et al., 2003). Significant symptom reduction was reported in three of the four patients. The second report involves a 56-year-old man with chronic and severe OCD (Aouizerate et al., 2004). In this patient, the deepest contacts were located within the nucleus accumbens, whereas the two superficial contacts were located within the ventromedial aspect of the head of the caudate. The addition of these latter contacts seemed to provide the greatest therapeutic benefit. Interestingly, the patient showed a rapid improvement in depressive and anxiety symptoms, as measured by the Hamilton depression and anxiety scales, respectively. Only after the 9-month postoperative period did the obsessive symptoms begin to abate. The patient noted no adverse events, and a thorough cognitive battery conducted pre- and postoperatively did not evince any adverse effects due to the procedure.

## Anterior Limb of the Internal Capsule

### Development of the Anterior Capsulotomy

Freeman had long posited that the beneficial aspect of lobotomy came from the severing of thalamocortical connections, particularly those emanating from the medial thalamic nuclei. Indeed, there was some postmortem anatomical evidence describing downstream degeneration of the medial thalamic nuclei following frontal leucotomy (Meyer, Beck, & McLardy, 1947). Based on Freeman's theory, and on the thalamic theory of emotions as described by Walter Cannon (1931), Spiegel and Wycis attempted to interrupt these connections in psychiatric patients by directly lesioning the dorsomedial nuclei bilaterally (Spiegel, Wycis, Freed, & Orchinik, 1951, 1956). These thalamotomies were performed using a self-built stereotactic frame, based on the 1908 description of the frame used by Horsley and Clarke for their work in animals. These psychosurgical procedures therefore represented the first use of stereotactic surgery in humans, as described in their widely cited 1947 paper in *Science* (Spiegel, Wycis, Marks, & Lee, 1947). Although their results were disappointing in patients with schizophrenia, they did indicate some positive benefit for patients with anxiety and depression.

The Swedish neurosurgeon, Lars Leksell, using his own version of the stereotactic frame, attempted to replicate these findings but found the bilateral dorsomedial thalamotomy to be ineffective (Herner, 1961). There were other potential ways to interrupt this thalamocortical pathway, and following a 1949 report by Talairach, Hecaen, and David, Leksell decided to shift to a target site in the anterior aspect of the internal capsule. Originally performed using thermocoagulation, and later with gamma irradiation (Gamma Knife), this anterior capsulotomy continues to be used (Greenberg et al., 2003; Mindus, 1993).

### Efficacy of Anterior Capsulotomy

Early data from Leksell's group indicated good efficacy in both OCD and MDD, with reported response rates of 50% and 48%, respectively (Herner, 1961). More recently, however, this procedure has been used primarily for patients with intractable OCD. Mindus and Jenike (1992), in a large retrospective review, reported a response rate of 64% (137/213). The largest prospective study of anterior capsulotomy indicated a response rate of 70% (Mindus, Rasmussen, & Lindquist, 1994). A more recent prospective report also indicated good efficacy for OCD, with 53% of these 15 severely and chronically ill patients showing evidence of response (as defined by a 33% drop in Y-BOCS score) (Oliver et al., 2003).

### Adverse Effects of Anterior Capsulotomy

As with the other procedures described in this chapter, capsulotomy can cause transient postoperative side effects, including headache, incontinence, and/or confusion. Postoperative weight gain, with an average increase of 10%, has been reported (Mindus, 1991). Persisting seizures requiring treatment are uncommon, occurring in 1/24 and 1/15 patients in two prospective reports (Mindus, 1991; Oliver et al., 2003). There is no evidence for a consistent pattern of cognitive impairment or alteration in personality, though rare reports of behavioral dyscontrol (Oliver et al., 2003), diminution in self-care (Mindus, 1991), and amotivational states (Greenberg et al., 2003; Ruck et al., 2003) have been described.

*Anterior Capsular Deep Brain Stimulation*

In 1999, Nuttin, Cosyns, Demeulemeester, Gybels, and Meyerson from Leuven, Belgium, collaborated with Bjorn Meyerson, from the Karolinska Institute in Stockholm to describe the first use of DBS for a psychiatric indication: implanting electrodes in the anterior limb of the interior capsule in four patients with severe OCD. In this original report, they describe beneficial effects occurring in three of the four patients. Positive results in an additional six patients have now also been reported by this group (Gabriels, Cosyns, Nuttin, Demeulemeester, & Gybels, 2003; Nuttin, Gabriels, Cosyns, et al., 2003; Nuttin, Gabriels, van Kuyck, & Cosyns, 2003). Overall there have been no notable side effects, though the high current amplitude required for optimal therapeutic benefit seems to necessitate frequent (e.g., up to yearly) stimulator replacement. Anderson and Ahmed (2003) at Loyola University in Illinois recently reported significant benefit from anterior capsular DBS in a 35-year-old woman with chronic, treatment-refractory OCD. Importantly, they obtained these results using a current amplitude less than half of that required by the group in Belgium, though at this point, only 10-month outcome data on this patient are available. DBS in the anterior internal capsule is now under way in tandem multicenter trials in patients with OCD or MDD, respectively. Early reports of the outcome in patients with OCD look promising, with four of 10 patients meeting strict criteria for response (Greenberg, 2004).

## WHAT LIES AHEAD?

What is old is new again. With the recently developed use of DBS for OCD and MDD, interest in and optimism about psychiatric neurosurgery is running high. There is good reason to be hopeful: The development of a truly reversible, effective, and safe therapy for patients with otherwise refractory and debilitating mental illness would be a tremendous accomplishment. The history of psychosurgery was built

on the work of some of the greatest surgeons and scientists of the 20th century: Fulton, Moniz, Papez, Cannon, Talairach, Spiegel, Wycis, Scoville, and Leksell, to name just a few. The backlash against the excessive and inappropriate use of surgery in the late 1940s and 1950s had a chilling effect on scientific progress in this area. It is our hope that this current interest in DBS will encourage a new generation of physician-scientists to become involved in the development of biologically based psychiatric therapies.

Clearly, however, a number of outstanding scientific questions need to be addressed regarding the use of neurosurgical approaches that entail either ablation of tissue or reversible stimulation in treating psychiatric illness:

1. *Who* is the optimal patient for this psychiatric neurosurgery? At least at present, these procedures are reserved for patients with the severest illness, who have been refractory to most (if not all) available therapies. Some of these patients with "malignant" mental illness (Mindus & Jenike, 1992) will likely be better candidates than others based on symptom profile alone. In addition, one could conceivably augment this phenomenological profile with the use of specific psychophysiological or neuroimaging biomarkers that portend good surgical outcomes (Rauch, 2003). As an example, using positron emission tomography (PET), our group has demonstrated specific patterns of presurgical cerebral activity that were highly correlated with outcome in patients with OCD (Rauch et al., 2001) and MDD (Dougherty et al., 2003; Rauch et al., 2001). Similar projects assessing the cerebral patterns associated with DBS outcomes in these populations are currently under way. These types of prognostic aids would be extremely useful, so that large numbers of patients do not unnecessarily undergo procedures that are unlikely to be of benefit to them.

2. *What* is the optimal frequency and amplitude of DBS stimulation? As noted by McIntyre, Savasta, Walter, and Vitek (2004) in a recent discussion of the mechanism of DBS action, the therapeutic stimulation parameters for the use of DBS in movement disorders are found largely by trial and error, and can vary substantially from patient to patient. In the movement disorders domain, this trial-and-error approach is feasible given the instanta-

neous and readily observable changes induced by stimulation adjustment. This is unlikely to be the case for DBS in OCD or MDD. Better understanding of the "usually effective" stimulation frequency, pulse width, and amplitude will be critical to avoid months of ineffective stimulation.

3. *Where* is the optimal target location for these procedures, and *why* are they effective in treating psychiatric illness? These questions, so critical to our ability to improve upon current techniques, are unfortunately the most elusive to answer given our current state of knowledge. Although it is believed that both ablative surgery and DBS act by perturbing in some way the aberrant limbic pathways involved in psychopathology, the specific details by which this occurs, and the differences between ablation and stimulation, are only cursorily understood. The typical 3- to 12-month delay between ablation and maximal benefit suggests that neuronal reorganization plays an important role in efficacy. As described earlier, the targets chosen for the standard ablative procedures were based on well-supported theories regarding the neurological basis of emotion. In fact, there is historically a wonderful synergy between this area of clinical neuroscience and experimental neuroscience, with findings from each supporting the other. The study of these patients, both intraoperatively and postsurgically, continues to provide an exciting and unique perspective into the workings of the human brain, advancing our understanding of neuroanatomy (Rauch et al., 2000), neurophysiology (Rauch, 2003), and neuropsychology (Williams et al., 2004). As in the past, it is important for us once again to apply reciprocally the remarkable insights gained in the many areas of modern experimental neuroscience to advance the quality of our clinical practice.

As a first pass, the field has decided to place DBS electrodes in the same locations where historically useful ablative lesions were made, including the basal forebrain and the anterior limb of the internal capsule. Certainly this makes sense at present given the historic experience in operating at these sites, the data indicating the benefit of these ablative procedures, and the underlying theories implicating these areas in the development of affective and behavioral disorders. Yet it is unclear whether these truly are the optimal locations for best

therapeutic effect. Indeed, at first blush, it is somewhat counterintuitive to think that stimulation would be done at the same site as ablation, though the underlying mechanisms of DBS may tell us why this approach is effective.

4. *When* can the stimulator be turned off? As with the stimulation frequency, it is unclear whether there is an optimal pattern of stimulation that lends the most benefit; that is, perhaps continuous stimulation is unwise (or unnecessary) and a pulsed daily or weekly approach (à la electroconvulsive therapy or repetitive transcranial magnetic stimulation) makes more sense. It is also unclear whether DBS responders need to continue stimulation ad infinitum. Perhaps the stimulation resets the neural networks, making long-term stimulation unnecessary in those who show good response over the first year.

5. *How* can the psychiatric patient with DBS implants be managed best in the clinic? A new breed of biologically sophisticated neuropsychiatrists will be required to help in the preoperative assessment and long-term management of the patient with implanted DBS. As nicely described by Poppen (1948) over 50 years ago, a collaborative approach to care of these patients is required:

> I feel strongly that it is the neurosurgeon's duty to perform the operation as safely and accurately as possible, but that the burden of deciding whether a mental patient should be subjected to the procedure falls on the shoulders of competent neuropsychiatrists who have had an opportunity to study many patients before and after operation. No neurosurgeon wishes to be a technician only. In many instances, however, the neurosurgeon has not had the proper training nor has he the time to devote the many weeks and perhaps months of intimate contact with the patient and his relatives. (pp. 519–520)

Experience tells us that early optimism does not always correlate with ultimate success. Indeed, excessive enthusiasm can impair our collective scientific vision, and lead us down paths that are damaging both to individual patients and to the field as a whole. As recently described by Kopell and Rezai (2003), psychiatric neurosurgery will continue to be the battleground of two guiding medical principles: *primum non nocere* (first do no harm) and *melius anceps remdium quam nullum* (better an unknown cure than nothing at all).

## REFERENCES

Anderson, D., & Ahmed, A. (2003). Treatment of patients with intractable obsessive–compulsive disorder with anterior capsular stimulation. *Journal of Neurosurgery*, 98, 1104–1108.

Aouizerate, B., Cuny, E., Martin-Guehl, C., Guehl, D., Amieva, H., Benazzouz, A., et al. (2004). Deep brain stimulation of the ventral caudate nucleus in the treatment of obsessive–compulsive disorder and major depression: Case report. *Journal of Neurosurgery*, 101(4), 682–686.

Ballantine, H. T., Bouckoms, A. J., Thomas, E. K., & Giriunas, I. E. (1987). Treatment of psychiatric illness by stereotactic cingulotomy. *Biological Psychiatry*, 22, 807–819.

Ballantine, H. T., Cassidy, W. C., Flanagan, N. B., & Marino, R. (1967). Stereotaxic anterior cingulotomy for neuropsychiatric illness and intractable pain. *Journal of Neurosurgery*, 26, 488–495.

Ballantine, H. T., Levy, B. S., Dagi, T. F., & Giriunas, I. B. (1977). Cingulotomy for psychiatric illness: Report of 13 years' experience. In W. H. Sweet, S. Obrader, & J. G. Martín-Rodríguez (Eds.), *Neurosurgical treatment in psychiatry, pain, and epilepsy* (pp. 333–353). Baltimore: University Park Press.

Braslow, J. T. (1999). History and evidence-based medicine: Lessons from the history of somatic treatments from the 1900s to the 1950s. *Mental Health Services Research*, 1, 231–240.

Broca, P. (1878). Anatomie comparée des circonvolutions cérébrales. Le grand lobe limbique et la scissure limbique dans le série des mammifères. *Revue Anthropologie*, 7, 385–498.

Cannon, W. B. (1931). The James–Lange and the thalamic theories of emotions. *Psychological Review*, 38, 281.

Cohen, R. A., Kaplan, R. F., Moser, D. J., Jenkins, M. A., & Wilkinson, H. (1999). Impairments of attention after cingulotomy. *Neurology*, 53(4), 819–824.

Cohen, R. A., Kaplan, R. F., Zuffante, P., Moser, D. J., Jenkins, M. A., Salloway, S., et al. (1999). Alteration of intention and self-initiated action associated with bilateral anterior cingulotomy. *Journal of Neuropsychiatry and Clinical Neurosciences*, 11(4), 444–453.

Connolly, J. (1830). *An inquiry concerning the indications of insanity, with suggestions for the better protection and care of the insane*. London: J. Taylor.

Corkin, S. (1980). A prospective study of cingulotomy. In E. S. Valenstein (Ed.), *The psychosurgery debate* (pp. 164–204). San Francisco: Freeman.

Corkin, S., Twitchell, T., & Sullivan, E. (1979). Safety and efficacy of cingulotomy for pain and psychiatric disorders. In E. Hitchcock & H. Ballantine (Eds.), *Modern concepts in psychiatric neurosurgery* (pp. 253–272). New York: Elsevier/North-Holland Biomedical Press.

Cosgrove, G. R. (2004). Deep brain stimulation and psychosurgery. *Journal of Neurosurgery*, 101(4), 574–575; discussion, 575–576.

Cosgrove, G. R., & Rauch, S. L. (1995). Psychosurgery. *Neurosurgery Clinics of North America*, 6(1), 167–176.

Cosgrove, G. S. (2000). Surgery for psychiatric disorders. *CNS Spectrums*, 5(10), 43–53.

Dougherty, D. D., Baer, L., Cosgrove, G. R., Cassem, E. H., Price, B. H., Nierenberg, A., et al. (2002). Prospective long-term follow-up of 44 patients who received cingulotomy for treatment-refractory obsessive–compulsive disorder. *American Journal of Psychiatry*, 159, 269–275.

Dougherty, D. D., Weiss, A. P., Cosgrove, G. R., Alpert, N. M., Cassem, E. H., Nierenberg, A. A., et al. (2003). Cerebral metabolic correlates as potential predictors of response to anterior cingulotomy for treatment of major depression. *Journal of Neurosurgery*, 99(6), 1010–1017.

Fiamberti, A. M. (1937). Proposta di una tecnica operatoria modificata e semplificata per gli interventi alla Moniz sui lobi prefrontali in malati di mente. *Rassegna di studi psichiatrici*, 26, 797.

Fins, J. J. (2003). From psychosurgery to neuromodulation and palliation: History's lessons for the ethical conduct and regulation of neuropsychiatric research. *Neurosurgery Clinics of North America*, 14, 303–319.

Foltz, E. L., & White, L. E. (1961). Pain "relief" by frontal cingulumotomy. *Journal of Neurosurgery*, 19, 89–100.

Freeman, W., & Watts, J. W. (1937). Prefrontal lobotomy in the treatment of mental disorders. *Southern Medical Journal*, 30, 23–31.

Freeman, W., & Watts, J. W. (1942). *Psychosurgery: Intelligence, emotion and social behavior following prefrontal lobotomy for mental disorders*. Springfield, IL: Charles C. Thomas.

Freeman, W., & Watts, J. W. (1950). *Psychosurgery: In the treatment of mental disorders and intractable pain* (2nd ed.). Springfield, IL: Charles C. Thomas.

Fulton, J. F., & Jacobsen, C. F. (1935). *Fonctions des lobes frontaux: Etude comparee chez l'homme et les singes chimpanzes*. Paper presented at the International Neurological Congress, London.

Gabriels, L., Cosyns, P., Nuttin, B., Demeulemeester, H., & Gybels, J. (2003). Deep brain stimulation for treatment-refractory obsessive–compulsive disorder: Psychopathological and neuropsychological outcome in three cases. *Acta Psychiatrica Scandinavica*, 107(4), 275–282.

Goktepe, E. O., Young, L. B., & Bridges, P. K. (1975). A further review of the results of stereotactic subcaudate tractotomy. *British Journal of Psychiatry*, 126, 270–280.

Greenberg, B. D. (2004, June). *Deep brain stimulation in intractable OCD, and preliminary results in intractable depression*. Paper presented at the New

Clinical Drug Evaluation Unit Meeting, Phoenix, AZ.

Greenberg, B. D., Price, L. H., Rauch, S. L., Friehs, G., Noren, G., Malone, D., et al. (2003). Neurosurgery for intractable obsessive–compulsive disorder and depression: Critical issues. *Neurosurgery Clinics of North America, 14,* 199–212.

Greenblatt, M., & Solomon, H. C. (Eds.). (1953). *Frontal lobes and schizophrenia.* New York: Springer.

Gross, C. G. (1999). "Psychosurgery" in Renaissance art. *Trends in Neurosciences, 22,* 429–431.

Heimer, L. (2003). A new anatomical framework for neuropsychiatric disorders and drug abuse. *American Journal of Psychiatry, 160*(10), 1726–1739.

Herner, T. (1961). Treatment of mental disorders with frontal stereotaxic thermo-lesions. *Acta Psychiatrica Scandinavica, 36*(Suppl. 158), 7–140.

Hodgkiss, A. D., Malizia, A. L., Bartlett, J. R., & Bridges, P. K. (1995). Outcome after the psycho-surgical operation of stereotactic subcaudate tractotomy, 1979–1991. *Journal of Neuropsychiatry and Clinical Neurosciences, 7,* 230–234.

Husted, D. S., & Shapira, N. A. (2004). A review of the treatment for refractory obsessive–compulsive disorder: From medicine to deep brain stimulation. *CNS Spectrums, 9,* 833–847.

Jacobsen, C. F. (1936). Studies of cerebral function in primates: I. The functions of the frontal association areas in monkeys. *Comparative Psychology Monographs, 13,* 3–60.

Jenike, M. A., Baer, L., Ballentine, H. T., Martuza, R. L., Tynes, S., Giriunas, I., et al. (1991). Cingulotomy for refractory obsessive–compulsive disorder: A long-term follow-up of 33 patients. *Archives of General Psychiatry, 48,* 548–555.

Kartsounis, L. D., Poynton, A., Bridges, P. K., & Bartlett, J. R. (1991). Neuropsychological correlates of stereotactic subcaudate tractotomy: A prospective study. *Brain, 114,* 2657–2673.

Knight, G. (1960). Cases of restricted orbital cortex undercutting. *Proceedings of the Royal Academy of Medicine, 53,* 728–732.

Knight, G. (1964). The orbital cortex as an objective in the surgical treatment of mental illness. *British Journal of Surgery, 51,* 114–124.

Knight, G. C. (1969). Bi-frontal stereotactic tractotomy: an atraumatic operation of value in the treatment of intractable psychoneurosis. *British Journal of Psychiatry, 115,* 257–266.

Kopell, B. H., Greenberg, B., & Rezai, A. R. (2004). Deep brain stimulation for psychiatric disorders. *Journal of Clinical Neurophysiology, 21*(1), 51–67.

Kopell, B. H., & Rezai, A. R. (2003). Psychiatric neurosurgery: A historical perspective. *Neurosurgery Clinics of North America, 14,* 181–197.

LeBeau, J. (1954). Anterior cingulectomy in man. *Journal of Neurosurgery, 11,* 268–276.

LeBeau, J., & Pecker, J. (1949). La topectomie pericalleuse anterieure dans certaines formes d'agitation psychomotrice au cours de l'epilepsie et de l'arrieration mentale. *Revue Neurologie, 81,* 1039–1041.

Long, C. J., Pueschel, K., & Hunter, S. E. (1978). Assessment of the effects of cingulate gyrus lesions by neuropsychological techniques. *Journal of Neurosurgery, 49,* 264–271.

Marino, R., & Cosgrove, G. R. (1997). Neurosurgical treatment of neuropsychiatric illness. *Psychiatric Clinics of North America, 20*(4), 933–943.

McIntyre, C. C., Savasta, M., Walter, B. L., & Vitek, J. L. (2004). How does deep brain stimulation work?: Present understanding and future questions. *Journal of Clinical Neurophysiology, 21*(1), 40–50.

Meyer, A., Beck, E., & McLardy, T. (1947). Prefrontal leucotomy: A neuro-anatomical report. *Brain, 70,* 18–49.

Mindus, P. (1991). *Capsulotomy in anxiety disorders: A multidisciplinary study.* Stockholm: Caslon Press.

Mindus, P. (1993). Present-day indications for capsulotomy. *Acta Neurochirurgica: Supplementum, 58,* 29–33.

Mindus, P., & Jenike, M. A. (1992). Neurosurgical treatment of malignant obsessive compulsive disorder. *Psychiatric Clinics of North America, 15,* 921–938.

Mindus, P., Rasmussen, S. A., & Lindquist, C. (1994). Neurosurgical treatment for refractory obsessive–compulsive disorder: Implications for understanding frontal lobe function. *Journal of Neuropsychiatry and Clinical Neurosciences, 6*(4), 467–477.

Moniz, E. (1937). Prefrontal leucotomy in the treatment of mental disorders. *American Journal of Psychiatry, 93,* 1379–1385.

Montoya, A., Weiss, A. P., Price, B. H., Cassem, E. H., Dougherty, D. D., Nierenberg, A. A., et al. (2002). Magnetic resonance imaging-guided stereotactic limbic leukotomy for treatment of intractable psychiatric disease. *Neurosurgery, 50*(5), 1043–1049.

Nauta, W. J. (1982). Limbic innervation of the striatum. *Advances in Neurology, 35,* 41–47.

Nuttin, B., Cosyns, P., Demeulemeester, H., Gybels, J., & Meyerson, B. (1999). Electrical stimulation in anterior limbs of internal capsules in patients with obsessive–compulsive disorder. *Lancet, 354,* 1526.

Nuttin, B. J., Gabriels, L. A., Cosyns, P. R., Meyerson, B. A., Andreewitch, S., Sunaert, S. G., et al. (2003b). Long-term electrical capsular stimulation in patients with obsessive–compulsive disorder. *Neurosurgery, 52*(6), 1263–1272; discussion, 1272–1264.

Nuttin, B. J., Gabriels, L., van Kuyck, K., & Cosyns, P. (2003a). Electrical stimulation of the anterior limbs of the internal capsules in patients with severe obsessive–compulsive disorder: Anecdotal reports. *Neurosurgery Clinics of North America, 14*(2), 267–274.

Ochsner, K. N., Kosslyn, S. M., Cosgrove, G. R., Cassem, E. H., Price, B. H., Nierenberg, A. A., et al. (2001). Deficits in visual cognition and attention following bilateral anterior cingulotomy. *Neuropsychologia, 39*(3), 219–230.

Oliver, B., Gascon, J., Aparicio, A., Ayats, E., Rodriguez, R., Maestro De Leon, J. L., et al. (2003). Bilateral anterior capsulotomy for refractory obsessive–compulsive disorders. *Stereotactic and Functional Neurosurgery, 81*(1–4), 90–95.

Papez, J. W. (1937). A proposed mechanism of emotion. *Archives of Neurology and Psychiatry, Chicago, 38,* 725–743.

Pinel, P. (1801). *Traité médico-philosophique sur l'aléniation mentale ou la manie.* Paris: Richard, Caille, & Ravier.

Poppen, J. L. (1948). Technic of prefrontal lobotomy. *Journal of Neurosurgery, 5,* 514–520.

Pressman, J. D. (1998). *Last resort: Psychosurgery and the limits of medicine.* New York: Cambridge University Press.

Rauch, S. L. (2003). Neuroimaging and neurocircuitry models pertaining to the neurosurgical treatment of psychiatric disorders. *Neurosurgical Clinics of North America, 14,* 213–224.

Rauch, S. L., Dougherty, D. D., Cosgrove, G. R., Cassem, E. H., Alpert, N. M., Price, B. H., et al. (2001). Cerebral metabolic correlates as potential predictors of response to anterior cingulotomy for obsessive compulsive disorder. *Biological Psychiatry, 50*(9), 659–667.

Rauch, S. L., Greenberg, B. D., & Cosgrove, G. R. (2005). Neurosurgical treatments and deep brain stimulation. In B. J. Sadock & V. Sadock (Eds.), *Comprehensive textbook of psychiatry* (8th ed., pp. 2983–2990). Philadelphia: Lippincott, Williams & Wilkins.

Rauch, S. L., Kim, H., Makris, N., Cosgrove, G. R., Cassem, E. H., Savage, C. R., et al. (2000). Volume reduction in the caudate nucleus following stereotactic placement of lesions in the anterior cingulate cortex in humans: A morphometric magnetic resonance imaging study. *Journal of Neurosurgery, 93*(6), 1019–1025.

Ruck, C., Andreewitch, S., Flyckt, K., Edman, G., Nyman, H., Meyerson, B. A., et al. (2003). Capsulotomy for refractory anxiety disorders: Long-term follow-up of 26 patients. *American Journal of Psychiatry, 160*(3), 513–521.

Scoville, W. B. (1949). Selective cortical undercutting as a means of modifying and studying frontal lobe function in man. *Journal of Neurosurgery, 6,* 65–73.

Smith, W. K. (1945). The functional significance of the rostral cingular cortex as revealed by its responses to electrical excitation. *Journal of Neurophysiology, 8,* 241–255.

Spangler, W. J., Cosgrove, G. R., Ballantine, H. T., Cassem, E. H., Rauch, S. L., Nierenberg, A., et al. (1996). Magnetic resonance image-guided stereotactic cingulotomy for intractable psychiatric disease. *Neurosurgery, 38,* 1071–1078.

Spiegel, E. A., Wycis, H. T., Freed, H., & Orchinik, C. (1951). The central mechanism of the emotions (experiences with circumscribed thalamic lesions). *American Journal of Psychiatry, 108,* 426–432.

Spiegel, E. A., Wycis, H. T., Freed, H., & Orchinik, C. W. (1956). A follow-up study of patients treated by thalamotomy and by combined frontal and thalamic lesions. *Journal of Nervous and Mental Disease, 124,* 399–404.

Spiegel, E. A., Wycis, H. T., Marks, M., & Lee, A. J. (1947). Stereotaxic apparatus for operations on the human brain. *Science, 106,* 349–350.

Strom-Olsen, R., & Tow, P. M. (1949). Late social results of prefrontal leucotomy. *Lancet, 1,* 87–90.

Sturm, V., Lenartz, D., Koulousakis, A., Treuer, H., Herholz, K., Klein, J. C., et al. (2003). The nucleus accumbens: A target for deep brain stimulation in obsessive–compulsive and anxiety disorders. *Journal of Chemical Neuroanatomy, 26*(4), 293–299.

Talairach, J., Hecaen, H., & David, M. (1949). *Lobotomie prefrontale limitee par electrocoagulation des fibres thalamo-frontales a leur emergence du bras anterieur de la capsule interne.* Paper presented at the 4th Congress of Neurology International, Paris.

Tow, P. M. (1955). Personality changes following frontal leucotomy. In *Oxford medical publications* (pp. 41–61). London: Oxford University Press.

Valenstein, E. S. (1986). *Great and desperate cures: The rise and decline of psychosurgery and other radical treatments for mental illness.* New York: Basic Books.

Ward, A. A. (1948). The cingular gyrus: Area 24. *Journal of Neurophysiology, 11,* 13–23.

Whitty, C. W. M., Duffield, J. E., Tow, P. M., & Cairns, H. (1952). Anterior cingulectomy in the treatment of mental disease. *Lancet, 1,* 475–481.

Williams, Z. M., Bush, G., Rauch, S. L., Cosgrove, G. R., & Eskandar, E. N. (2004). Human anterior cingulate neurons and the integration of monetary reward with motor responses. *Nature Neuroscience, 7,* 1370–1375.

# CHAPTER 32

# Infectious, Inflammatory, and Demyelinating Disorders

*Douglas W. Scharre*

Infectious, inflammatory, and demyelinating disorders often affect widespread brain regions. Whereas certain conditions appear to have a predilection for involving the frontal lobes, such as brain abscesses, almost all of these afflictions produce pathology in the frontal lobes. Symptoms and signs differ depending on the frontal region(s) involved: orbital, dorsolateral, posterior, or mesial. Involvement of the frontal white matter tracts may cause disconnection syndromes disrupting frontal neural circuits to the temporal, parietal, occipital, or limbic lobes. In fact, many destructive conditions can affect "frontal lobe" functioning at a distance by undermining frontal neural networks and resulting in symptoms displaying "frontal" features. The great variety of neuropsychiatric manifestations due to frontal lobe dysfunction caused by these disorders is not only immensely fascinating but also very characteristic and directs the clinician to suspect frontal lobe impairment. In this chapter, I discuss some of the more common or interesting infectious, inflammatory, and demyelinating disorders of the brain, and describe the features that are applicable to frontal lobe involvement.

## INFECTIOUS DISORDERS

Certain central nervous system (CNS) infections occur more commonly in the young, whereas others occur more often in the aged. These infections can affect focal brain regions or be widespread. Table 32.1 lists the main types of infections affecting the brain. The frontal lobes are a favorite site of involvement for many of these disorders. In this section, I further discuss some of these infections and their impact on the frontal lobes.

## Prion Infections

Prions are made of protein and have no functional nucleic acid. They can cause transmissible diseases, can be inherited in 10–15% of individuals on chromosome 20, or may occur sporadically (DeArmond & Prusiner, 2003). The normal prion protein is converted post-translationally from an $\alpha$-helix to an abnormal $\beta$-sheet conformation that is insoluble to detergents and tends to aggregate. The abnormal configuration can induce normal prion proteins to change their conformation to the abnormal form, causing accumulation of prions to sufficient levels to cause a progressive neurodegenerative disease state (Prusiner & Hsiao, 1994).

### Creutzfeldt–Jakob Disease

Creutzfeldt–Jakob disease (CJD) has a worldwide incidence of approximately one per million individuals (Masters et al., 1979). About 90% of the cases arise sporadically; 5–15% are

**TABLE 32.1. Types of CNS Infections Affecting the Frontal Lobes**

| | |
|---|---|
| **Prions** | **Bacteria** |
| Creutzfeldt–Jakob disease (CJD) | Acute bacterial meningitis |
| Variant Creutzfeldt–Jacob disease (vCJD) | Tuberculosis meningitis |
| Gerstmann–Sträussler–Scheinker syndrome (GSS) | Brain abscess |
| Fatal familial insomnia (familial thalamic dementia) | Subdural empyema |
| Kuru | Whipple's disease |
| | |
| **Virus** | **Fungus** |
| Acute | Chronic meningitis |
|   Herpes simplex encephalitis | |
|   West Nile encephalitis | **Spirochetes** |
|   Other meningoencephalitides | Neurosyphilis |
| Chronic | Lyme disease |
|   Human immunodeficiency virus—type 1 (HIV-1) | |
|   Progressive multifocal leukoencephalopathy (PML) | **Parasites** |
| | Toxoplasma |
| | Cysticercosis |
| | Amoeba |

familial, with an autosomal dominant inheritance, and only rarely have cases been transmitted (Lang, Schuler, Engelhardt, Spring, & Brown, 1995; Rappaport, 1987; Will et al., 1996). The clinical course is typically very rapid, with death occurring usually within several months to 1 year. Occasionally, individuals have survived for several years.

Initially, the patient has complaints of generalized fatigue, neurovegetative symptoms, and forgetfulness. After a few weeks, a progressive dementia ensues, with aphasia, amnesia, apraxia, and agnosia. Myoclonus, chorea, tremor, ataxia, cerebellar signs, pyramidal signs, spasticity, rigidity, and seizures typically occur after the dementia has started (Brown, Cathala, Castaigne, & Gajdusek, 1986; Cummings & Benson, 1992). The frontal lobes are involved as part of the widespread cortical and subcortical multifocal process and contribute to the cognitive deficits, aphasia, and motor abnormalities. Akinetic mutism, a frequent clinical feature in the end stage, is suggestive of mesial frontal lobe involvement.

Pathology shows a spongiform state in the cortical and subcortical gray matter, with loss of neurons and gliosis. Frontal, temporal, and occipital lobes may be more affected than parietal lobes. Magnetic resonance imaging (MRI) diffusion-weighted imaging (DWI) shows multifocal cortical and subcortical hyperintensities in the gray matter (Mendez, Shang, Jungreis, & Kaufer, 2003). Positron emission tomography (PET) and single-photon emission computed tomography (SPECT) show multiple diffuse areas of hypometabolism or hypoperfusion in both cortical and subcortical regions (Goldman et al., 1993; Watanabe et al., 1996). Cerebrospinal fluid (CSF) showing a positive immunoassay for the 14-3-3 brain protein is supportive of CJD, but neuronal injury from other conditions may cause spurious results, and many patients with autopsy-proven CJD are negative for this protein (Hsich, Kenney, Gibbs, Lee, & Harrington, 1996; Geschwind et al., 2003) (Table 32.2). The electroencephalogram (EEG) shows background slowing and a very characteristic periodic polyspike discharge (Chiofalo, Fuentes, & Galvez, 1980). Diagnosis can be made by the clinical features, neuroimaging, EEG, and CSF, and is confirmed by brain biopsy if the features are atypical. Treatment is not available except for supportive care.

### Variant Creutzfeldt–Jakob Disease

First presenting in the United Kingdom in 1994, this still rare condition is caused by dietary exposure to meat that contain brain or spinal cord tissue infected with the prion responsible for bovine spongiform encephalopathy (Croes & van Duijn, 2003). In contrast to CJD, behavioral symptoms including dysphoria, insomnia, apathy, and withdrawal start first and suggest early frontal lobe involve-

**TABLE 32.2. CSF Profiles of Various Conditions**

| Infection | White cells (cells/mm$^3$) | Protein (mg/dl) | Glucose (mg/dl) | Miscellaneous |
|---|---|---|---|---|
| Creutzfeldt–Jakob disease | 0–15 lymphocytosis | NL, 50–120 | NL | Occ IgG Inc, 14-3-3 brain protein |
| Herpes simplex encephalitis | 50–1,000 lymphocytosis | 50–400 | NL | Culture, PCR |
| West Nile encephalitis | 0–1,800 lymphocytosis | 45–80 | NL | IgM ELISA for West Nile |
| Aseptic meningoencephalitis | 5–1,000 lymphocytosis | 45–80 | 20–40, NL | Culture |
| HIV-1 dementia complex | 0–8 lymphocytosis | < 80 | Occ dec | IgG inc, culture |
| PML | 0–8 lymphocytosis | < 80 | NL | PCR for *JC* virus DNA |
| Acute bacterial meningitis | 100–60,000 PMN | 100–1,000 | 5–40 | Culture, antigen detection |
| Brain abscess | 0–500 PMN, lymphocytes | 40–100 | Occ dec | |
| Fungal meningitis | 5–800 lymphocytosis | 45–500 | 10–40, NL | Culture, crypto ag, crypto PCR |
| Neurosyphilis | 5–1,000 lymphocytosis | 50–100 | < 40, NL | VDRL, IgG inc |
| Neuroborreliosis (Lyme) | 0–150 lymphocytosis | 40–100 | NL | IgG inc, PCR, intrathecal antibodies |
| Isolated angiitis of the CNS | 0–800 lymphocytosis | 40–600 | Occ dec | Occ IgG inc |
| Lymphomatoid granulomatosis | 0–225 atypical lymphocytes | 40–780 | NL | Occ OGB |
| Behcet's syndrome | 0–500 lymphocytosis | NL–160 | NL | Occ IgG inc, BBB |
| SLE | 0–50 lymphocytosis | NL–100 | NL | OCB, IgG inc, BBB, antineuronal antibodies |
| Sjogren's syndrome | Mild lymphocytosis | NL–100 | NL | OCB, IgG inc |
| MS | 0–20 lymphocytosis | NL–100 | NL | OCB, IgG inc |
| Acute disseminated encephalomyelitis | 10–4,000 PMN, lymphocytes | NL–344 | NL | Inc pressure, Occ OCB |

*Note.* BBB, blood–brain barrier breakdown; crypto ag, cryptococcal antigen; dec, decrease; ELISA, enzyme-linked immunoabsorbent assay; IgG, immunoglobulin G; inc, increased; NL, normal; Occ, occasional; OGB, oligoclonal bands; PCR, polymerase chain reaction; PMN, polymorphonuclear cells. Data compiled from multiple sources: Alexander (1993); Ashwal (1995); Bale (1991); Brink and Miller (1996); Bushunow et al. (1996); Fishman (1992); Geerts et al. (1991); Halperin et al. (1991); Hsich et al. (1996); Kirschbaum (1968); Kleinschmidt-DeMasters et al. (1992); Levy, Bredesen, and Rosenblum (1985); Marshall et al. (1988); McLean et al. (1995); Navia, Jordan, and Price (1986); Pachner (1995); Paschoal et al. (2004); Sampathkumar (2003); Schmidt (1989); West et al. (1995); Whitley and Lakeman (1995); Younger et al. (1988).

ment. A few months later, dementia, gait imbalance, dysarthria, and sensory symptoms occur (Spencer, Knight, & Will, 2002). Bilateral hyperintensities on MRI in the pulvinar regions of the thalami are characteristic (Collie et al., 2001). Neuropathology shows florid plaques with vacuoles (Ironside, 2000). The key is prevention of transmission by contaminated meat products or blood transfusions from infected persons (Llewelyn et al., 2004).

### Gerstmann–Sträussler–Scheinker Disease

Gerstmann–Sträussler–Scheinker disease (GSS) is a rare autosomal dominant disorder with onset between 40 and 60 years of age. There are eight known point mutations in the prion protein gene that can result in the GSS syndrome (Panegyres et al., 2001; Prusiner, 1996). GSS is characterized by a mild dementia with pyramidal, extrapyramidal, and cerebellar signs

(Farlow et al., 1989). Marked frontal atrophy on MRI and neuronal loss with severe gliosis in the frontal lobes have been described in the codon 105 mutation form (Kitamoto et al., 1993; Kubo, Nishimura, Shikata, Kokubun, & Takasu, 1995).

### Fatal Familial Insomnia

Fatal familial insomnia (FFI), sometimes referred to as familial thalamic dementia, is inherited and does not appear to be transmissible (Medori et al., 1992; Petersen et al., 1992). There is a *D178N* mutation of the prion protein gene. FFI has a course and presentation similar to CJD, with the addition of progressive insomnia and dysautonomia. Although the neuropathology in FFI seems mostly restricted to the anterior and dorsomedial thalamic nuclei (gliosis), these nuclei have tremendous connections with specific frontal lobe regions, and neuropsychological evaluation of these patients reveals "frontal" dysfunction, with difficulties in working memory, sequencing, and planning abilities (Gallassi, Morreale, Montagna, Gambetti, & Lugaresi, 1992). PET imaging shows prominent reduced glucose metabolism in bilateral thalami (Bar et al., 2002; Harder et al., 2004).

## Viral Infections

Viral infections can be classified as either acute, with a rapid onset of symptoms, or chronic, with a slower course over months to years (Table 32.1). The clinical features of an infection relate to the selective vulnerability of certain cell types to the particular virus (Johnson, 1982). Some infections have a predilection for the frontal lobes.

### Herpes Simplex Encephalitis

Temporal and frontal lobes are often attacked with this acute infection and although treatable, mortality is high (Kapur et al., 1994; Schmutzhard, 2001).

Initial clinical features include headache, fever, stiff neck, and photophobia. This progresses over a few days to produce lethargy, mental status changes, personality changes, memory impairment, aphasia, focal neurological deficits, seizures, and eventually coma (Whitley, 1991). Recovery may be complete or partial. Frontal lobe injury may cause grasp re-

flexes, frontal release signs, motor impersistence, disinhibition, impulsivity, confabulation, psychomotor hyperactivity, hyperoral behavior, apathy, echolalia, mutism, anomia, inattention, and utilization behaviors (Brazzelli, Colombo, Della Sala, & Spinnler, 1994). Temporal lobe damage often results in amnesia, and if bilateral, the Klüver–Bucy syndrome. Aphasia or dementia may also be permanent (Cummings & Benson, 1992).

Hemorrhagic necrosis and petechial hemorrhages are seen in the brain at autopsy. In the frontal lobes, the mesial, prefrontal, and basal forebrain regions are more affected than dorsolateral regions (Kapur et al., 1994). Periodic lateralized epileptiform discharges (PLEDs), the usual focal EEG abnormality, are seen in 80% of patients (Bale, 1991). MRI scan often shows focal areas of increased T2 signal in the temporal/insular or frontal regions. Lumbar puncture usually suggests a viral infection, and application of polymerase chain reaction (PCR) has allowed for a specific diagnosis of herpes simplex virus infection in the brain (Whitley & Lakeman, 1995) (Table 32.2). Brain biopsy has been replaced by PCR due to the 3% risk of serious morbidity. Therapy with acyclovir (10–15 mg/kg every 6–8 hours for 10–14 days) is started empirically and immediately, because the toxic effects are minimal and mortality is reduced from 70% to 19% (Whitley, 1991).

### West Nile Encephalitis

West Nile virus is caused by a flavivirus; humans are typically infected by a mosquito bite. West Nile virus causes a meningoencephalitis in one out of every 150 cases. Adults over age 50 are most susceptible. Typical clinical features include encephalopathy, acute flaccid paralysis, myelitis involving the anterior gray matter, optic neuritis, tremors, myoclonus, ataxia, postural instability, and seizures (Guharoy, Gilroy, Noviasky, & Ference, 2004). Thalami and basal ganglia are most frequently involved, but frontal lobe impairment is also seen, with personality changes and agitation. CSF shows lymphocytic predominant pleocytosis, mild to moderately elevated protein, and normal glucose. CSF West Nile virus immunoglobulin M is diagnostic (Sampathkumar, 2003) (Table 32.2). Treatment with intravenous immunoglobulin (IVIG) has been suggested (Roos, 2004) but primary prevention can be achieved with DEET-containing insect repellants.

## Human Immunodeficiency Virus—Type 1

Human immunodeficiency virus—type 1 (HIV-1) is a retrovirus that preferentially infects T-helper cells (Pantaleo, Graziosi, & Fauci, 1993). As the number of T-helper cells decline, acquired immunodeficiency syndrome (AIDS) occurs, making the individual susceptible to numerous opportunistic infections (Centers for Disease Control and Prevention, 1992). The most common signs and symptoms of HIV-1 infection include lymphadenopathy, diarrhea, fever, night sweats, weight loss, and lethargy (Bale, 1991). Neurological symptoms occur early, and opportunistic infections account for many additional clinical syndromes.

Direct HIV-1 infection can cause aseptic meningitis, minor cognitive/motor disorder, dementia, myelopathy, a variety of peripheral neuropathies, and myopathy. Opportunistic infections, CNS lymphoma, metastatic neoplasms, cerebrovascular events, metabolic disturbances, and medication effects can also affect the brain. Frontal lobe involvement is common and can occur in any of the conditions affecting the brain.

At the time of seroconversion, some individuals develop a primary HIV-1 meningitis, consisting of fever, headache, meningismus, and CSF pleocytosis (Cooper et al., 1985). Once systemic findings appear (lymphadenopathy syndrome or AIDS-related complex), 50% of patients have neurological signs or symptoms and 50% have abnormalities on neuropsychological testing (Janssen et al., 1988). Mental and motor slowness (Kieburtz & Schiffer, 1989) suggesting disruption of frontal–subcortical circuits is referred to as the HIV-1–associated minor cognitive/motor disorder and is the most common abnormality (American Academy of Neurology AIDS Task Force, 1991).

HIV-1–associated dementia (HIVD) has been described by many names, including subacute encephalopathy, HIV encephalopathy, or AIDS dementia complex. HIVD affects 15–20% of patients with AIDS (Power & Johnson, 1995). It is characterized by progression over weeks to months of a subcortical dementia syndrome with mental slowness, impaired concentration, forgetfulness, cognitive abnormalities, apathy, social withdrawal, slowed motor skills, ataxia, and weakness, potentially resulting in severe global cognitive dysfunction, paraplegia, mutism, and incontinence (American Academy of Neurology AIDS Task Force, 1991; Price,

Sidtis, Navia, Pumarola-Sune, & Ornitz, 1988). Neuropsychological testing reveals deficits particularly in nonverbal tasks and frontal lobe tasks, including Trail Making Test B and verbal fluency (Hestad et al., 1993; Power & Johnson, 1995), which suggest frequent frontal lobe involvement. Computed tomography (CT) and MRI show generalized cerebral atrophy and periventricular white matter abnormalities (Ekholm & Simon, 1988; Navia, Jordan, & Price, 1986). CSF is abnormal but nonspecific (Marshall et al., 1988; Navia, Jordan, & Price, 1986) (Table 32.2). The pathology of the HIVD complex consists of reactive gliosis and microglial nodules especially in the subcortical white and gray matter (Masliah et al., 1992; Navia, Cho, Petito, & Price, 1986). Loss of cortical neurons occur in the orbitofrontal, temporal, and parietal cortical regions but do not correlate well with the severity of dementia (Ketzler, Weis, Huag, & Budka, 1990; Masliah, Ge, Achim, Hansen, & Wiley, 1992). Since the advent of zidovudine and subsequent treatments, it appears that HIVD occurs less frequently, and its progression is slowed (Atkinson & Grant, 1994; Chang & Tyring, 2004; Schmitt et al., 1988). Using combinations of newer antiviral agents, including nucleoside, nucleotide, and non-nucleoside reverse transcriptase inhibitors, as well as protease and fusion inhibitors, the treatment of the neurological complications of AIDS has dramatically improved (Chang & Tyring, 2004; Henry, 1995).

The common opportunistic diseases that frequently involve the frontal lobes include cryptococcal meningitis, CMV encephalitis, cerebral toxoplasmosis, primary CNS lymphoma, and progressive multifocal leukoencephalopathy (PML) (Price, 1996). Cryptococcal meningitis and PML are discussed below. CMV encephalitis in its severe forms cause diffuse, bilateral cerebral dysfunction with impaired alertness. Neuroimaging can occasionally show subependymal enhancement (Price, 1996). Cerebral toxoplasmosis and primary CNS lymphoma can be diagnosed by clinical presentation, neuroimaging, and a treatment trial, or occasionally a brain biopsy (Bale, 1991). Cerebral toxoplasmosis evolves in only a few days, with focal neurological findings and ring-enhancing lesions with mass effect and edema on MRI. Primary CNS lymphoma also causes focal neurological deficits but progresses more slowly, and MRI lesions are more diffuse in the deep white matter. Treatment with zidovudine lowers the frequency and mortality of opportunistic infections (Schmitt et al., 1988). Specific treatments are also available for many of the opportunistic infections and neoplasms (Bale, 1991).

### Progressive Multifocal Leukoencephalopathy

Progressive multifocal leukoencephalopathy (PML), caused by the papovavirus, JC virus, typically occurs in patients with deficits in cell-mediated immunity (Berger & Major, 1999). Onset is usually between ages 30 and 70, and typically progresses over several weeks or months to death in less than 1 year.

The frontal lobes are commonly affected as part of the multifocal brain involvement. Typical neurological manifestations include deficits in attention, visuospatial skills, memory, language, calculation, motor speed, strength, sensation, vision, and coordination (Berger, Kaszovitz, Post, & Dickinson, 1987; Cummings & Benson, 1992). Fever or other systemic signs are not present.

Pathologically multifocal demyelination is found in the subcortical white matter particularly in the frontal or parietal–occipital regions (Whiteman et al., 1993). MRI shows areas of demyelination without mass effect or contrast enhancement (Berger et al., 1987; Brink & Miller, 1996). CSF may confirm PML by detection of the CSF JC virus DNA (Brink & Miller, 1996) (Table 32.2). Diagnosis is also made by brain biopsy, and treatment is supportive.

## Bacterial Infections

### Acute Bacterial Meningitis

The incidence of bacterial meningitis is five per 100,000 individuals per year. Frontal lobe involvement is fairly common and most often occurs from direct intracranial extension of paranasal sinusitis, orbital cellulitis, otitis media, dental abscesses, facial and skull fractures, head trauma, endonasal sinus surgery, and neurosurgical procedures (Dolan & Chowdhury, 1995; Weber et al., 1996). Typical organisms causing acute bacterial meningitis in the newborn are gram-negative bacilli, Group B streptococci, and *Listeria monocytogenes*; in children are *Haemophilus influenzae* type B, *Neisseria meningitidis*, *Streptococcus pneumoniae*; and in adults are *S. pneumoniae*, *N. meningitidis*, and *H. influenzae* type B (Ashwal, 1995; Durand et al., 1993).

Fever, headache, stiff neck, photophobia, nausea, and occasionally vomiting are the initial symptoms of bacterial meningitis. Agitation, lethargy, and acute confusional states follow. Focal neurological deficits and seizures are usually due to cerebrovascular complications or acute obstructive hydrocephalus (Durand et al., 1993). When the frontal lobes are involved, long-term sequelae include dementia, aphasia, hemiparesis, anger control problems, disinhibition, and other personality changes.

CT or MRI may show evidence of hydrocephalus, edema, or infarct (Figure 32.1). CSF is diagnostic, revealing increased intracranial pressure, polymorphonuclear pleocytosis, elevated protein, hypoglycorrhachia, positive cultures, and bacterial antigen detection (Ashwal, 1995) (Table 32.2). Early antibiotic use improves outcomes. Routine adjunctive steroid use with the first dose of antibiotics reduces both mortality and neurological deficits in bacterial meningitis (van de Beek, de Gans, McIntyre, & Prasad, 2004). Vaccination for *N. meningitidis* and *H. influenzae* type B are available and potentially cost-effective (Getsios, Caro, El-Hadi, & Caro, 2004; Hanna, 2004). Flu shots for those at highest risks for exposure to influenza (elderly persons, children, health care workers, and day care workers) may protect against disease (Handa, Teo, & Booy, 2004).

### Brain Abscess

The incidence of brain abscess is four individuals per million per year. Abscesses commonly occur in the frontal lobes because of direct intracranial extension of paranasal sinusitis, orbital cellulitis, otitis media, dental abscesses, neoplasms eroding through facial bones, chronic intranasal abuse of cocaine, facial and skull fractures, cranial trauma from penetrating wounds, and neurosurgical procedures (Dolan & Chowdhury, 1995; Richter, 1993; Wispelwey & Scheld, 1992). *Staphylococcus aureus*, anaerobic bacteria, and gram-negative organism infections are frequent causes of brain abscesses due to extension from a frontal sinusitis or middle ear infection (Luby, 1992). Less commonly seen are *Streptococcus*, *Bacteroides*, *Fusobacterium*, and *Clostridium* species. In immunocompromised individuals, various fungal species, cysticercosis, and toxo-

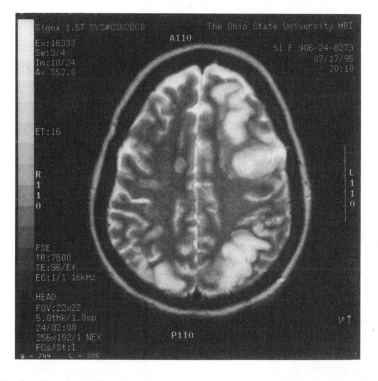

FIGURE 32.1. MRI of a 51-year-old woman with *Streptococcus pneumoniae* meningitis, showing multiple areas of cortical edema and underlying white matter changes. The frontal lobes are prominently involved. CSF revealed 10,000 cells/mm³ (99% polymorphonuclear cells), protein 1000 mg/dl, low glucose, and detection of pneumococcal antigen.

plasmosis are prevalent (Wispelwey & Scheld, 1992).

Headache, fever, mental status changes, and focal neurological signs are common initial symptoms (Wispelwey & Scheld, 1992). Seizures, papilledema, focal neurological deficits, and neuropsychiatric manifestations may suggest frontal lobe involvement. Enhanced MRI is very helpful in diagnosing brain abscesses (Sze & Zimmerman, 1988), and EEG usually shows focal δ activity. Lumbar puncture may precipitate a herniation syndrome and is contraindicated in brain abscesses (Table 32.2). Treatments for brain abscesses include broad-coverage antibiotics and occasionally surgical drainage (Wispelwey & Scheld, 1992).

## Fungal Infections

Individuals with depressed immune systems or chronic debilitation account for half of all chronic fungal meningitis (Cummings & Benson, 1992). Cryptococcal meningitis is the most frequently seen (Jones & Nathwani,

1995). Other causative organisms include *Coccidioides*, *Histoplasma*, *Candida* species, *Blastomyces*, and *Aspergillus*.

Fungal meningitis often begins insidiously and progresses slowly over weeks to months. Although headache, fever, and stiff neck are common, they may not always be present. Mental status changes occur frequently, and executive impairments suggest frontal lobe dysfunction. Many fungal infections involve the basal meninges, often resulting in focal neurological deficits, cranial nerve dysfunction, gait imbalance, or hydrocephalus (Cummings & Benson, 1992). Cryptococcal antigen and PCR for cryptococcosis in the CSF is specific for cryptococcal meningitis (Fishman, 1992; Paschoal et al., 2004) (Table 32.2). Cultures or titers are necessary for diagnosis of other infections. Fluconazole or combination of antifungal agents is safe and effective as first-line therapies without the severe toxicity seen with amphotericin B (Lewis & Kontoyiannis, 2001; Slavoski & Tunkel, 1995).

## Spirochete Infections

### Neurosyphilis

Syphilis, caused by the spirochete *Treponema pallidum*, is spread by intimate contact, and although CNS invasion may occur, most patients are asymptomatic (Scheck & Hook, 1994). Increasingly, HIV-1 patients are getting syphilis (Fox, Hawkins, & Dawson, 2000). The three forms of tertiary neurosyphilis are meningovascular, paretic, and tabetic, and they present anywhere from 1 to 50 years after the primary infection. The tabetic form does not involve the brain, and the meningovascular form manifests by causing strokes.

General paresis results from syphilitic invasion into the brain parenchyma. Prior to penicillin treatment, general paresis accounted for up to 20% of all admissions to mental hospitals (Hook & Marra, 1992) but now it is extremely uncommon. Many of the clinical features of general paresis suggest frontal lobe involvement and include inattention, dementia, tremulous speech, impaired judgment, irritability, pseudobulbar palsy, paralysis, tremor, ataxia, incontinence, optic atrophy, and Argyll Robertson pupils. Mania is seen in 20–40% of patients, and psychosis with grandiose delusions, paranoia, and hallucinations in 3% to 6% (Cummings & Benson, 1992). MRI shows bilateral frontal and/or temporal lobe atrophy and subcortical abnormalities (Zifko et al., 1996). *T. pallidum* organisms are found most abundantly in the frontal lobes. Neuronal loss, gliosis, inflammatory infiltrates, and, rarely, gumma formations are also seen (Cummings & Benson, 1992).

Screening for neurosyphilis should be done with the Florescent Treponemal Antibody Absorption (FTA-ABS) test, because other screening tests may become nonreactive in tertiary syphilis (Simon, 1985). If the FTA-ABS is positive, a lumbar puncture is indicated. CSF in neurosyphilis shows lymphocytic pleocytosis, elevated protein, and positive Venereal Disease Research Laboratory (VDRL) test (Table 32.2). Penicillin is the treatment of choice for all forms of syphilis, with the intravenous route and longer duration of treatments required for patients with neurosyphilis and syphilis associated with HIV-1 (Hook & Marra, 1992).

### Lyme Disease

Lyme disease is caused by the tick-borne spirochete *Borrelia burgdorferi*. After the tick bite, an acute localized erythema chronicum migrans (ECM) rash and a viral-like syndrome occur. Dissemination occurs within a few weeks to months, with symptoms including a multifocal ECM rash, acute arthritis, cardiac conduction block, myocarditis, myositis, hepatitis, meningitis, or radiculoneuritis. Some individuals develop a chronic course leading to chronic arthritis, radiculoneuritis, seventh cranial nerve palsies, encephalomyelitis, or encephalopathy.

The encephalopathy typically results in mild dementia, depression, sleep disturbances, fatigue, and irritability. Deficits in executive function, attention, working memory, organization, initiation, abstract concept formation, and verbal fluency are typical and suggest frontal lobe dysfunction (Fallon & Nields, 1994; Waniek, Prohovnik, Kaufman, & Dwork, 1995). Neuropathological findings include vasculitis, focal demyelination, and, in the late stages, neuronal loss, gliosis, and signs of brain parenchyma infection. MRI may reveal multifocal regions of increased signal in the white matter consistent with demyelination (Halperin, Volkman, & Wu, 1991). Diagnosis is made with a positive serology in the setting of appropriate clinical findings. Demonstration of intrathecal antibody production and CSF PCR for the spirochete may help with diagnosis (Pachner, 1995) (Table 32.2). Intravenous antibiotics, usually with ceftriaxone or cefotaxime, can prevent or halt the neurological complications and may lead to significant improvement (Hengge et al., 2003). Long-term antibiotic treatment is sometimes necessary but needs more study.

## INFLAMMATORY DISORDERS

Inflammatory disorders affecting the brain include the vasculitides, the collagen vascular diseases, and paraneoplastic conditions. Most have systemic manifestations and they directly impact the frontal lobes as part of a more widespread process of brain dysfunction. In some cases, the frontal lobes are the primary site of involvement. Table 32.3 lists the main causes of inflammatory disorders involving the brain. Of the collagen vascular diseases, scleroderma, rheumatoid arthritis, and Cogan's syndrome only rarely affect the CNS. Neoplastic-related disorders are discussed elsewhere in this book.

**TABLE 32.3. Causes of Inflammatory Disorders Involving the Frontal Lobes of the Brain**

Vasculitides

Isolated angiitis of the central nervous system
Polyarteritis nodosa
Churg–Strauss angiitis
Wegener's granulomatosis
Lymphomatoid granulomatosis
Giant cell (temporal) arteritis
Takayasu's arteritis
Behcet's syndrome

Collagen vascular diseases

Systemic lupus erythematosus (SLE)
Antiphospholipid antibody syndrome
Sneddon's syndrome
Sjogren's syndrome
Scleroderma
Rheumatoid arthritis
Cogan's syndrome
Mixed connective tissue disease

Other

Acute disseminated encephalomyelitis
Neoplastic-related disorders
Infectious-related disorders
Drug/toxin-induced
Sarcoid

## Vasculitides

### Isolated Angiitis of the CNS

This rare vasculitis of unknown etiology is confined to the CNS and routinely involves the frontal lobes. Lymphoma, sarcoidosis, and herpes zoster conditions have occasionally been associated with this vasculitis. Constitutional symptoms of fever and weight loss are observed in 25% of patients. In most cases, there is an initial subacute presentation with severe headache and encephalopathy, gradually followed by focal deficits caused by strokes, and progressing to a vascular dementia syndrome affecting medium and small vessels (Vollmer, Guarnaccia, Harrington, Pacia, & Petroff, 1993). Both cortical and subcortical frontal regions may be involved, leading to headache, seizures, aphasia, hemiparesis, psychosis, and behavioral changes (Block & Reith, 2000). Supranuclear cranial nerve palsies, cerebellar signs, and myelopathy have also been reported. Increased intracranial pressure may occur, leading to papilledema and coma.

A segmental vasculitis with necrosis and giant cells is typically found. The sedimentation rate is increased in 60% of the patients but only to a mean of about 35 mm/hour. CT or MRI may be normal or reveal focal, occasionally enhancing lesions, hemorrhage, or edema, which are found most commonly in the temporal and frontal cortical regions. SPECT tends to show patchy frontal hypoperfusion (Vollmer et al., 1993). Angiography may show vasculopathy, but usually does not. CSF findings are nonspecific (Table 32.2). Diagnosis is made clinically and should be confirmed as early as possible by brain biopsy. Treatment with prednisone and cyclophosphamide is often ineffective, and there is an 87% mortality rate, with death occurring a mean of 6 months after onset of symptoms (Alreshaid & Powers, 2003; Younger, Hays, Brust, & Rowland, 1988).

### Polyarteritis Nodosa

Polyarteritis nodosa (PAN) characterizes a group of acute, systemic, necrotizing vasculitides that includes Churg–Strauss angiitis. Immune complex deposition in PAN causes a relapsing and remitting vasculitis that eventually leads to infarction or hemorrhage in multiple organs. Common systemic findings include fever, weight loss, headache, anorexia, asthma, dyspnea, proteinuria, hypertension, arthralgias, skin rash, congestive heart failure, and gastrointestinal pain.

Neurological manifestations occur in up to 80% of cases, mostly resulting from peripheral nervous system involvement giving rise to mononeuritis multiplex, polyneuropathy, cranial neuropathy, or myopathy. CNS involvement, including frontal lobe dysfunction, is seen in about 40% of cases and typically occurs later in the course, causing dementia, encephalopathy, attentional deficits, hypoarousal, psychosis, seizures, or strokes (Moore & Calabrese, 1994).

Pathology shows a necrotizing vasculitis of the small and medium muscular arteries. Diagnosis is made clinically and confirmed by tissue biopsy (muscle, skin, nerve, or kidney) and angiography. Corticosteroids and immunosuppressive agents are the treatments of choice and often lead to remissions or recovery (Bonsib, 2001).

### Wegener's Granulomatosis

Wegener's granulomatosis is a systemic necrotizing granulomatosis vasculitis that always affects the respiratory tract and often the kidneys. Typical systemic clinical manifestations include fever, weight loss, sinusitis, otitis media, saddlenose deformity, cough, hemoptysis, pleuritis, glomerulonephritis, visual symptoms, ulcerative or papular skin lesions, arthralgias, myalgias, and pericarditis, (Duna, Galperin, & Hoffman, 1995).

Neurological involvement consists mostly of cranial and peripheral neuropathies, including mononeuritis multiplex. The frontal lobes can be affected by ischemic or hemorrhagic stroke, diffuse periventricular white matter lesions, meningeal inflammation, or granulomatous mass lesions. Seizures, focal deficits, and encephalopathy often result (Duna et al., 1995). Contiguous extension of granulomatous inflammation from the paranasal sinuses to the frontal lobes is also seen (Geiger, Garrison, & Losh, 1992).

Vasculitis, necrosis, and granulomas are seen pathologically on biopsy. Diagnosis is made by cytoplasmic antineutrophil cytoplasmic antibodies (c-ANCA), with a sensitivity and specificity of about 90% (Duna et al., 1995). Angiography is not very helpful, neuroimaging is useful but nonspecific, and CSF can rule out infection. Corticosteroids and cytotoxic agents are needed for successful treatment.

### Lymphomatoid Granulomatosis

This rare condition typically affects the lungs, skin, and nervous system. It is a B-cell lymphoproliferative disorder related to Epstein–Barr virus infection (Mizuno et al., 2003). In 60% of cases, a malignant large B-cell lymphoma does develop (Bushunow, Casas, & Duggan, 1996). Common manifestations include fever, weight loss, cough, chest pain, skin ulcers and papules, and peripheral neuropathies.

CNS dysfunction occurs in 20% to 40% of cases and includes a broad spectrum of deficits, including monocular blindness, internuclear ophthalmoplegia, dysphagia, dysarthria, spasticity, paraparesis, hemiparesis, seizures, ataxia, aphasia, encephalopathy, and dementia. Common behavioral symptoms, including personality change, irritability, disinhibition, impulsivity, distractibility, mood disturbance, and memory loss, suggest frontal lobe involvement (Bushunow et al., 1996; Kleinschmidt-DeMasters, Filley, & Bitter, 1992).

CSF shows pleocytosis with atypical cells (Bushunow et al., 1996) (Table 32.2). Angi-

ography may show a vasculitic pattern, and neuroimaging may show mass lesions, enhancement, or white matter changes. Treatment with prednisone and cyclophosphamide is usually necessary to maintain prolonged remissions. Adjunctive radiotherapy or chemotherapy can also be effective.

### Giant Cell (Temporal) Arteritis

This systemic vasculitis nearly always occurs in patients over age 50 and affects women twice as often as men (Calvo-Romero, 2003). Constitutional symptoms are prominent and include fever, weight loss, anorexia, and malaise. Headache, jaw claudication, scalp tenderness, and tenderness and nodularity of the superior temporal artery are common. Fifty percent of patients also get pain and stiffness in the neck, shoulders, and pelvic regions.

Except for visual disturbances, CNS involvement is infrequent. Blurred vision, amaurosis fugax, and diplopia are reported, with blindness occurring, usually without warning, in 8–23% of patients (Caselli & Hunder, 1993). Multiple infarcts, more common in the posterior circulation territories, have been reported, but dementia syndromes involving frontal lobe function that is unexplained by strokes are also seen (Caselli, 1990).

Pathology frequently involves the branches of the external carotid, ophthalmic, and vertebral arteries. Anemia is common and an elevated Westergren sedimentation rate (over 50 and often over 100 mm/hour), is almost always found. A superior temporal artery biopsy is positive in about 70% of cases (Nadeau & Watson, 1990). Prednisone, typically in doses of 40–60 mg per day, is an effective treatment.

### Behcet's Syndrome

Behcet's syndrome, an inflammatory disorder of uncertain etiology, is characterized by recurrent oral and genital ulcers, uveitis, thrombophlebitis, and arthritis (Kurokawa & Suzuki, 2003). Fever and gastrointestinal complaints are also common.

The nervous system is affected in approximately 40% of cases, most often in the form of a relapsing focal meningoencephalitis affecting the brainstem, with headache, cranial neuropathies, dysarthria, long-tract signs, and bulbar and pseudobulbar palsies (Siva, Altintas, & Saip, 2004). Increased intracranial pressure and even seizures can develop. Symptoms of frontal lobe dysfunction are frequently reported and may include dementia, personality change, disinhibition, apathy, emotional disturbance, and akinetic mutism (Yamamori et al., 1994).

A chronic, small-vessel vasculitis is seen pathologically, often involving the frontal white matter (Totsuka, Hattori, Yazaki, Nago, & Mizoshima, 1985; Yamamori et al., 1994). MRI sometimes reveals venous thrombosis and frequently shows subcortical abnormalities (Al Kawi, Bohlega, & Banna, 1991). SPECT may show cortical hypoperfusion, including frontal lobe involvement (Arai et al., 1994; Watanabe et al., 1995). Angiography is usually normal, whereas CSF is abnormal but nonspecific (McLean, Miller, & Thompson, 1995) (Table 32.2). Diagnosis is based on clinical features. Treatment for CNS disease includes high-dose steroids, immunosuppressive agents, and possibly interferon α (Kotter, Gunaydin, Zierhut, & Stubiger, 2004).

## Collagen Vascular Diseases

### Systemic Lupus Erythematosus

Systemic lupus erythematosus (SLE) is an inflammatory disorder of uncertain cause. Systemic manifestations may include fever, anorexia, rash, lymphadenopathy, arthralgias, pericarditis, valvular disease, pleuritis, Raynaud's phenomenon, alopecia, renal insufficiency, nephrotic syndrome, and hypertension (Nadeau & Watson, 1990).

Neuropsychiatric and focal neurological manifestations, often occurring early in the disease course, are seen in 40% to 75% of SLE cases and represent the highest incidence for any of the collagen vascular disorders. CNS dysfunction may occur from primary involvement of the brain or secondarily from complications of the disease, including infection, embolism from endocarditis, steroid treatment toxicity, and severe hypertension. Disturbances of frontal and frontal–subcortical circuits are common in SLE and result in acute confusional states/delirium, dementia, psychosis, depression, mania, phobias, and anxiousness (West, 1994). Executive impairment on neuropsychological tests reveals deficits in information processing, cognitive flexibility, working memory, attention, and verbal fluency (Denburg, Denburg, Carbotte, Fisk, & Hanly, 1993). Seizures, strokes, supranuclear cranial nerve deficits, chorea, ataxia, parkinsonism, transverse myelitis, and focal paresis are present in 10–35% of cases (West, 1994).

The antiphospholipid antibody syndrome, occasionally associated with SLE, consists of the presence of antiphospholipid (APL) antibodies (particularly the lupus anticoagulant and anticardiolipin antibodies), venous or arterial thrombotic strokes or ischemia, recurrent abortions, and thrombocytopenia (Brey, Gharavi, & Lockshin, 1993). APL antibodies are present in up to 50% of patients with SLE. Sneddon's syndrome, recurrent strokes often causing dementia in patients with livedo reticularis, is also associated with APL antibodies.

Diagnosis of SLE is based on clinical features, a positive antinuclear antibody (ANA) test, and other specific antibody tests (Tan et al., 1982). The main pathological feature of SLE is a small-vessel vasculopathy that angiography usually is unable to identify. An autoimmune process with antineuronal antibodies may be an important cause of neuropsychiatric CNS involvement, and serum antiribosomal-P antibodies are often seen in patients with cerebral disease and neuropsychiatric symptoms of psychosis and depression (Reichlin, 2003). Routine MRI is useful in localizing strokes, but its sensitivity is low for detecting pathology in neuropsychiatric lupus unless there is an acute flare up of symptoms. However, magnetization transfer imaging appears to show correlation with cognitive dysfunction and diffusion-weighted MRI may be able to differentiate ischemic changes from inflammatory lesions (Peterson, Howe, Clark, & Axford, 2003). SPECT scanning is very sensitive, with focal cortical hypoperfusion found most often in the frontal regions, followed by the parietal and temporal regions (Colamussi et al., 1995). Nearly all individuals with neuropsychiatric CNS involvement have an abnormal CSF immunoglobulin G (IgG) index, oligoclonal bands, CSF antineuronal antibodies, and/or serum antiribosomal-P antibodies, which may improve with response to therapy (West, Emlen, Wener, & Kotzin, 1995) (Table 32.2). Treatments include nonsteroidal anti-inflammatory agents, steroids, and immunosuppressive agents. Plasmapheresis is used in refractory cases and intrathecal methotrexate with dexamethasone have been successful in patients with severe CNS disease (Sanna, Bertolaccini,

& Mathieu, 2003). Oral anticoagulants are advisable to prevent the recurrent thrombotic events seen with APL antibodies and may be more successful than immunotherapies for focal thrombotic disease (Sanna et al., 2003). Aspirin is given in those that are asymptomatic and have the APL antibodies. Neuroleptics are used for psychosis, antidepressants for mood symptoms, and anticonvulsants for seizures.

### Sjogren's Syndrome

Sjogren's syndrome, a systemic autoimmune disorder seen mostly in women, is characterized by symptoms of dry eyes and dry mouth, and may involve the lung, liver, kidney, heart, blood vessels, skin, muscles, joints, peripheral nerves, spinal cord, and the brain. CNS manifestations, reported in up to 25% of patients in some centers (Alexander, 1993) and rarely observed in others (Moutsopoulos, Sarmas, & Talal, 1993), include migraine, focal neurological deficits, intracerebral hemorrhage, subarachnoid hemorrhage, seizures, myelitis, aseptic meningitis, dementia, and psychiatric symptoms (Alexander, 1993).

The frontal lobes are commonly affected, mostly by subcortical pathology. A subcortical dementia syndrome occurs, with deficits in attention, concentration, memory, executive abilities, and mood disturbances, depression, and obsessive–compulsive traits (Alexander, 1993; Belin et al., 1999; Moutsopoulos et al., 1993). In a SPECT study of 32 subjects with Sjogren's syndrome, 28% had frontal hypoperfusion (Chang, Shiau, Wang, Ho, & Kao, 2002).

The dry eyes and mouth are due to a lymphocytic infiltration of the exocrine glands. Sjogren's syndrome causes a vasculopathy involving mostly the smaller caliber cerebral vessels, so only in 20% of patients does angiography reveal evidence of vasculitis (Alexander, 1993). Laboratory evaluations are frequently positive for ANAs and occasionally for anti-SS-A (Ro; Sjogren syndrome antibodies seen with more serious CNS disease) and anti-SS-B (La) antibodies. Autoantibodies to cerebral muscarinic acetylcholine receptors may play a role in cognitive impairment (Reina, Sterin-Borda, Orman, & Borda, 2004). Biopsy of a minor salivary gland is diagnostic. MRI shows nonspecific subcortical and periventricular white matter lesions in 80% of cases. SPECT is a more sensitive tool, and shows cortical hypoperfusion in regions where

MRI is normal in those patients with neuropsychiatric dysfunction (Chang et al., 2002). Corticosteroids and, rarely, other immunosuppressive agents are used for treatment.

## DEMYELINATING DISORDERS

A comprehensive list of white matter disorders involving the frontal lobes is presented in Table 32.4. Primary demyelination involves the loss of the myelin sheath, leaving the axon intact but denuded. Dysmyelination, mostly seen in hereditary–metabolic disturbances, is due to impairment in the formation or development of the myelin sheath. Although I will not specifically discuss dysmyelinating disorders, they share many clinical features with the demyelinating conditions. Vascular and neoplastic causes of demyelinating disorders are discussed in other chapters in this volume and many of the autoimmune and infectious causes were discussed earlier in this chapter.

### Autoimmune Disorders

#### Multiple Sclerosis

Multiple sclerosis (MS) is the most common demyelinating disorder of the CNS. It is rare in the tropics, but its frequency increases in more northern latitudes, and women are affected more than men are by a 2:1 ratio. The clinical course has several forms, all of which show lesion dissemination in time and space: relapsing–remitting, secondary progressive, and primary progressive, and benign.

Brainstem and spinal cord regions are frequently affected and may cause internuclear ophthalmoplegia, trigeminal neuralgia, myelopathy, acute transverse myelitis, bladder dysfunction, sensory disturbances, gait imbalance, and pain syndromes. Brain demyelination often results in weakness, sensory dysfunction, visual impairment, gait disturbance, ataxia, movement disorders, and neuropsychiatric syndromes. Treatment with steroids or other medications can complicate and contribute to the cognitive and psychiatric disturbances.

Frontal lobe involvement typically causes cognitive dysfunction, neuropsychiatric symptoms, and impaired motor control. About 30–50% of patients with MS develop cognitive dysfunction (Fennell & Smith, 1990; Rao, Leo,

**TABLE 32.4. Causes of Demyelinating Disorders Involving the Frontal Lobes of the Brain**

| Autoimmune | Hereditary–metabolic |
|---|---|
| Multiple sclerosis (MS) | Metachromatic leukodystrophy (MLD) |
| Behcet's syndrome | Adrenoleukodystrophy (ALD) |
| Systemic lupus erythematosus (SLE) | Cerebrotendinous xanthomatosis |
| Sjogren's syndrome | Membranous lipodystrophy |
| Acute disseminated encephalomyelitis | Hereditary adult-onset leukodystrophy |
| | Globoid cell leukodystrophy, late onset |
| **Vascular** | |
| Binswanger's disease | **Infectious** |
| | HIV-1 associated cognitive/motor complex |
| **Toxic–metabolic** | Progressive multifocal leukoencephalopathy (PML) |
| Marchiafava–Bignami disease | Lyme disease |
| Vitamin $B_{12}$ deficiency | |
| Folate deficiency | **Neoplastic** |
| Thiamine deficiency (vitamin $B_1$) | Lymphoma of the central nervous system |
| Vitamin $B_6$ deficiency | Paraneoplastic syndromes |
| Vitamin E deficiency | |
| Anoxic–hypoxic leukoencephalopathy | |
| Radiation leukoencephalopathy | |
| Chemotherapy-related leukoencephalopathy | |

Bernardin, & Unverzagt, 1991) typical of a subcortical dementia syndrome, manifested by slowed information-processing speed, retrieval memory deficits, visuospatial difficulties, and frontal–executive dysfunction (Rao, 1986). Neuropsychological testing shows specific frontal lobe dysfunctioning in 33% of patients with MS (McIntosh-Michaelis et al., 1991; Mendozzi, Pugnetti, Saccani, & Motta, 1993), including deficits in verbal fluency, conceptual reasoning, the Wisconsin Card Sorting Test, planning abilities, organizational skills, sustained attention, and set shifting (Fennell & Smith, 1990; Mendozzi et al., 1993). Corpus callosal atrophy on MRI and increased plaque volume correlate with the severity of cognitive impairment (Huber et al., 1992b; Swirsky-Sacchetti et al., 1992). Individuals with demyelination of frontal–subcortical circuits in MS on MRI performed worse on tasks of conceptual reasoning abilities (Wisconsin Card Sorting Test) and had more perseverative errors than others without significant frontal involvement but with similar overall white matter burden (Arnett et al., 1994). Frontal white matter lesions are also correlated with apathy, diminished spontaneity of speech, executive dysfunction, and slowed information-processing speed (Comi et al., 1995; Huber et al., 1992a).

Behavioral and psychiatric symptoms in MS are common and include emotional lability, depression, euphoria, mania, psychosis, personal-

ity changes, fatigue, and sexual dysfunction. Frontal cognitive impairment has been shown to be significantly related to depression symptoms, suggesting involvement of shared anatomical circuits (Filippi et al., 1994). Euphoria, seen in about 25% of patients with MS, is a cheerful affect inappropriate to the situation (Rabins, 1990). Euphoria has been associated with bilateral subfrontal demyelination (Minden & Schiffer, 1990) and with a higher rate of neurological and cognitive deficits (Rabins, 1990). Patients with symptoms of pathological laughter and crying do worse on frontal lobe measures, including the Stroop test, verbal fluency, and the Wisconsin Card Sorting Test (Feinstein, O'Connor, Gray, & Feinstein, 1999). Apathy, lack of concern over their disabilities, lack of initiation, impaired insight, irritability, and poor judgment are personality changes observed in as many as 40% of patients with MS (Mahler, 1992) and may be related to frontal lobe dysfunction (Mendez, 1995).

Impaired motor function caused by frontal lobe dysfunction in MS has also been described and includes weakness, loss of motor control, frontal gait apraxia, and frontal release signs (Franklin, Nelson, Filley, & Heaton, 1989; Mendez, 1995).

MS is believed to be caused by an immune-mediated response triggered by exposure to an unknown environmental agent in the genetically predisposed individual. This results in multifocal, discrete demyelinated areas scattered throughout the white matter, which can often be seen as plaques on MRI (Figure 32.2). The plaques are typically seen in the periventricular white matter, corpus callosum, near the gray–white junction, and spinal cord (Bakshi, Hutton, Miller, & Radue, 2004). Gadolinium contrast can distinguish active from inactive plaques (Bastianello et al., 1990). Cortical brain atrophy, most often seen in the frontal lobes on MRI, occurs in 33% of patients (Bekiesinska-Figatowska, Walecki, & Stelmasiak, 1996). In fact, normalized measures of frontal lobe atrophy in subjects with MS show very strong correlations with neuropsychological impairment and disability (Locatelli, Zivadinov, Grop, & Zorzon, 2004). Cortical hypoperfusion in the frontal lobes on SPECT (Pozzilli et al., 1991), especially in the chronic progressive form (Lycke, Wikkelso, Bergh, Jacobsson, & Andersen, 1993), may represent frontal disconnection from other subcortical and cortical regions. Diagnosis is aided by finding increased immunoglobulin production and oligoclonal bands in the CSF (Table 32.2), and

by evoked potentials reflecting a delay between a stimulus and resulting brain activity.

Prednisone, methylprednisolone, and adrenocorticotropic hormone (ACTH) appear to speed the recovery of an acute exacerbation. Reduction of the frequency of clinical relapses in patients with relapsing–remitting MS have been shown with immunotherapies including intravenous immune globulin (Achiron et al., 1996), glatiramer acetate (Johnson et al., 1995), and interferon β-1b (IFNB Multiple Sclerosis Study Group & University of British Columbia MS/MRI Analysis Group, 1995; Lublin et al., 1996). Interferon β-1a agents have also been shown to delay the accumulation of physical disability in those patients (Clanet, Kappos, Hartung, & Hohlfeld, 2004; Jacobs et al., 1996; Panitch et al., 2002). Mitoxantrone has demonstrated reduction of neurological disability and/or the frequency of clinical relapses in patients with secondary progressive, progressive relapsing, or worsening relapsing–remitting MS (Millefiorini et al., 1997). The first selective adhesion molecule inhibitor for MS, natalizumab (Miller et al., 2003; O'Connor et al., 2004), a monoclonal

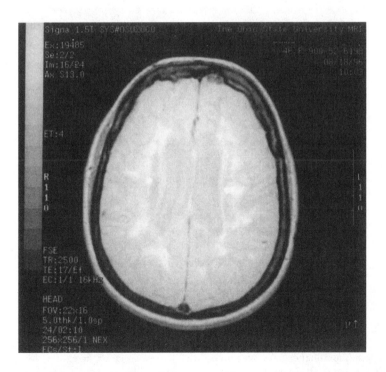

FIGURE 32.2. Proton density–weighted MRI of a 46-year-old woman with chronic progressive multiple sclerosis affecting the frontal lobes, showing bilateral, multiple regions of increased signal in the periventricular and deep white matter of the corona radiata.

antibody designed to prevent immune cells from escaping into the tissue of the brain, was recently pulled due to development of cases of PML.

Treatments for the neuropsychiatric manifestations are also available. Cognitive impairment may be helped with cholinesterase inhibitors (Krupp et al., 2004; Leo & Rao, 1988; Parry, Scott, Palace, Smith, & Matthews, 2003) or the use of memory aids, lists, routinization of daily activities, and other cognitive retraining strategies (LaRocca, 1990). Depression and mood disturbances are treated with antidepressants, antimanic agents, support groups, and psychotherapy.

### Acute Disseminated Encephalomyelitis

Disseminated encephalomyelitis and its many variations, including acute necrotizing hemorrhagic, postinfectious, postvaccinal, multiphasic, and recurrent, represent an immune-mediated condition resulting in CNS demyelination. It is typically, but not exclusively, a monophasic, acute illness presenting with fever,

headache, and altered consciousness, and typically preceded days or weeks earlier by either a viral syndrome, or other illness or vaccination (Geerts, Dehaene, & Lammens, 1991). Hemiparesis, sensory deficits, seizures, dysarthria, or dysphasia may be present initially (Geerts et al., 1991). Frontal lobe dysfunction contributes to a subcortical dementia syndrome, similar to that seen in MS. Inflammation, demyelination, and variable hemorrhage occur in the white matter. Neuroimaging studies show multifocal abnormalities, occasionally including large lesions that often involve the cortex, with very little periventricular or callosal involvement (Kesselring et al., 1990) (Figure 32.3). CSF cultures are negative (Table 32.2). A brain biopsy may be required to rule out infection or tumor. Treatment is supportive and may require reduction of increased intracranial pressure. Immunosuppression has been used with some success (Seales & Greer, 1991) and, in those not responding, combinations with IVIG (Straussberg, Schonfield, Weitz, Karmazyn & Harel, 2001) or plasmapheresis may help (Lin, Jeng, & Yip, 2004).

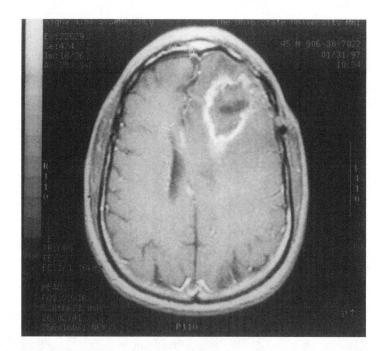

FIGURE 32.3. Gadolinium-enhanced T1-weighted MRI shows a large, irregular, heterogeneous, ring-enhancing lesion in the left frontal lobe causing some midline shift. This 45-year-old man with postinfectious, acute, disseminated encephalomyelitis had three other foci of abnormal signal in the white matter, negative CSF cultures, and two brain biopsies that did not reveal tumor or infection.

## Toxic–Metabolic Disorders

### Marchiafava–Bignami Disease

Marchiafava–Bignami disease is characterized by demyelination of the corpus callosum and adjacent white matter. It is rare and occurs mostly in male, chronic alcoholics, in middle to late adult life. Many individuals exhibit a chronic dementia syndrome that progresses over months to years. Remissions are possible. Severe cases present in stupor or coma and die rapidly.

CNS manifestations include frontal lobe dysfunction, dementia, dysarthria, incontinence, aphasia, hemiparesis, seizures, and signs of corpus callosum interhemispheric disconnection, including left-sided limb apraxia, left-hand anomia, and agraphia (Lechevalier, Andersson, & Morin, 1977; Victor, 1993). The frontal lobe involvement frequently precipitates apathy, slow information processing, frontal release signs (grasp and suck), paratonia, and frontal-related apraxic gait with incontinence (Victor, 1993). Personality changes, violence, and sexual deviations have also been reported.

Demyelination of the anterior commissure and corpus callosum, with relative sparing of the splenium and absence of inflammatory changes, is the characteristic pathology. Interruption of callosal fibers is thought to cause occurrences of frontal cortical (layer 3) neuronal loss and gliosis (Lechevalier et al., 1977; Victor, 1993). Frontal lobe dysfunction may therefore be the result of direct frontal pathology or a frontal disconnection syndrome. PET studies have shown hypometabolism in frontal and posterior association cortices (Pappata, Chabriat, Levasseur, Legault-Demare, & Baron, 1994), perhaps reflecting this cortical gliosis. However, MRI scans show demyelination essentially limited to the callosum, with severity of involvement correlating to severity of the clinical course (Heinrich, Runge, & Khaw, 2004). Alcohol abstinence and proper nutrition are recommended. In a few cases, acute steroid treatment showed initial clinical improvement (Gerlach et al., 2003).

### Vitamin B$_{12}$ Deficiency

Vitamin B$_{12}$ deficiency may be secondary to pernicious anemia, malabsorption syndromes, acquired immunodeficiency, stomach or small bowel resections, stomach acid–reducing agents, or, rarely, from a dietary B$_{12}$ deficiency (Swain, 1995). Both folate and vitamin B$_{12}$ deficiency can produce a megaloblastic anemia and demyelination in the spinal cord and brain, causing peripheral neuropathy, myelopathy, gait disturbance, incontinence, visual impairment, and neuropsychiatric syndromes.

Symptoms suggestive of frontal lobe involvement include slow reaction time, dementia, apathy, confusion, perseveration, aggressiveness, depression, psychosis, and personality changes (Clementz & Schade, 1990; Cummings & Benson, 1992; Lindenbaum et al., 1988).

The dorsal and lateral columns of the spinal cord and the white matter in the brain show areas of spongiform degenerative demyelination. A low serum B$_{12}$ level is usually diagnostic. Serum methylmalonic acid and homocysteine are good confirmatory tests, and malabsorption is demonstrated by performing a Schilling test. Administration of vitamin B$_{12}$ may reverse or stop the progression of the neurological symptoms and dementia.

## REFERENCES

Achiron, A., Barak, Y., Goren, M., Gabbay, U., Miron, S., Rotstein, Z., et al. (1996). Intravenous immune globulin in multiple sclerosis: Clinical and neuro-radiological results and implications for possible mechanisms of action. *Clinical and Experimental Immunology, 104*(Suppl. 1), 67–70.

Alexander, E. L. (1993). Neurologic disease in Sjogren's syndrome: Mononuclear inflammatory vasculopathy affecting central/peripheral nervous system and muscles, a clinical review and update of immunopathogenesis. *Rheumatic Disease Clinics of North America, 19*, 869–908.

Al Kawi, M. Z., Bohlega, S., & Banna, M. (1991). MRI findings in neuro-Behcet's disease. *Neurology, 41*, 405–408.

Alreshaid, A. A., & Powers, W. J. (2003). Prognosis of patients with suspected primary CNS angiitis and negative brain biopsy. *Neurology, 61*, 831–833.

American Academy of Neurology AIDS Task Force. (1991). Nomenclature and research case definitions for neurologic manifestations of human immunodeficiency virus–type 1 (HIV-1) infection. *Neurology, 41*, 778–785.

Arai, T., Mizukami, K., Sasaki, M., Tanaka, Y., Shiraishi, H., Horiguchi, H., et al. (1994). Clinico-pathological study on a case of neuro-Behcet's disease: In special reference to MRI, SPECT and neuropathological findings. *Japanese Journal of Psychiatry and Neurology, 48*, 77–84.

Arnett, P. A., Rao, S. M., Bernardin, L, Grafman, J.,

Yetkin, F. Z., & Lobeck, L. (1994). Relationship between frontal lobe lesions and Wisconsin Card Sorting Test performance in patients with multiple sclerosis. *Neurology, 44*(3, Pt. 1), 420–425.

Ashwal, S. (1995). Neurologic evaluation of the patient with acute bacterial meningitis. *Neurologic Clinics, 13*(3), 549–577.

Atkinson, J. H., & Grant, I. (1994). Natural history of neuropsychiatric manifestations of HIV disease. *Psychiatric Clinics of North America, 17*(1), 17–33.

Bakshi, R., Hutton, G. J., Miller, J. R., & Radue, E.-W. (2004). The use of magnetic resonance imaging in the diagnosis and long-term management of multiple sclerosis. *Neurology, 63*(Suppl. 5), S3–S11.

Bale, J. F., Jr. (1991). Encephalitis and other virus-induced neurologic disorders. In A. B. Baker & R. J. Joynt (Eds.), *Clinical neurology* (pp. 1–56). New York: Harper & Row.

Bar, K.-J., Hager, F., Nenadic, I., Opfernabb, T., Brodhun, M., Tauber R. F., et al. (2002). Serial positron emission tomographic findings in an atypical presentation of fatal familial insomnia. *Archives of Neurology, 59*, 1815–1818.

Bastianello, S., Pozzilli, C., Bernardi, S., Bozzao, L., Fantozzi, L. M., Buttinelli, C., et al. (1990). Serial study of gadolinium-DPTA MRI enhancement in multiple sclerosis. *Neurology, 40*, 591–595.

Bekiesinska-Figatowska, M., Walecki, J., & Stelmasiak, K. (1996). The value of magnetic resonance imaging in diagnosis and monitoring of treatment in multiple sclerosis. *Acta Neurobiologiae Experimentalis, 56*, 171–176.

Belin, C., Moroni, C., Caillat-Vigneron, N., Debray, M., Baudin, M., Dumas, J. L., et al. (1999). Central nervous system involvement in Sjogren's syndrome: Evidence from neuropsychological testing and HMPAO-SPECT. *Annales de Médecine Interne, 50*, 598–604.

Berger, J. R., Kaszovitz, B., Post, J. D., & Dickinson, G. (1987). Progressive multifocal leukoencephalopathy associated with human immunodeficiency virus infection. *Annals of Internal Medicine, 107*, 78–87.

Berger, J. R., & Major, E. O. (1999). Progressive multifocal leukoencephalopathy. *Seminars in Neurology, 19*, 193–200.

Block, F., & Reith, W. (2003). Isolated vasculitis of the central nervous system. *Der Radiologe, 40*, 1090–1097.

Bonsib, S. M. (2001). Polyarteritis nodosa. *Seminars in Diagnostic Pathology, 18*, 14–23.

Brazzelli, M., Colombo, N., Della Sala, S., & Spinnler, H. (1994). Spared and impaired cognitive abilities after bilateral frontal damage. *Cortex, 30*, 27–51.

Brey, R. L., Gharavi, A. E., & Lockshin, M. D. (1993). Neurologic complications of antiphospholipid antibodies. *Rheumatic Disease Clinics of North America, 19*(4), 833–850.

Brink, N. S., & Miller, R. F. (1996). Clinical presentation, diagnosis and therapy or progressive multifocal leukoencephalopathy. *Journal of Infection, 32*, 97–102.

Brown, P., Cathala, F., Castaigne, P., & Gajdusek, D. C. (1986). Creutzfeldt–Jakob disease: Clinical analysis of a consecutive series of 230 neuropathologically verified cases. *Annals of Neurology, 20*, 597–602.

Bushunow, P. W., Casas, V., & Duggan, D. B. (1996). Lymphomatoid granulomatosis causing central diabetes insipidus: Case report and review of the literature. *Cancer Investigation, 14*, 112–119.

Calvo-Romero, J. M. (2003). Giant cell arteritis. *Postgraduate Medical Journal, 79*, 511–515.

Caselli, R. J. (1990). Giant cell (temporal) arteritis: A treatable cause of multi-infarct dementia. *Neurology, 40*, 753–755.

Caselli, R. J., & Hunder, G. G. (1993). Neurologic aspects of giant cell (temporal) arteritis. *Rheumatic Disease Clinics of North America, 19*(4), 941–953.

Centers for Disease Control and Prevention. (1992). 1993 revised classification system for HIV infection and expanded surveillance case definition for AIDS among adolescents and adults. *Morbidity and Mortality Weekly Report, 41*(RR-17), 1–19.

Chang, C. P., Shiau, Y. C., Wang, J. J., Ho, S. T., & Kao, A. (2002). Abnormal regional cerebral blood flow on 99mTc ECD brain SPECT in patients with primary Sjogren's syndrome and normal findings on brain magnetic resonance imaging. *Annals of the Rheumatic Disease, 61*, 774–778.

Chang, Y. C., & Tyring, S. K. (2004). Therapy of HIV infection. *Dermatologic Therapy, 17*, 449–464.

Chiofalo, N., Fuentes, A., & Galvez, S. (1980). Serial EEG findings in 27 cases of Creutzfeldt–Jakob disease. *Archives of Neurology, 37*, 143–145.

Clanet, M., Kappos, L., Hartung, H. P., & Hohlfeld, R. (2004). Interferon beta-1a in relapsing remitting multiple sclerosis: Four-year extension of the European IFNbeta-1a Dose Comparison Study. *Multiple Sclerosis, 10*, 139–144.

Clementz, G. L., & Schade, S. G. (1990). The spectrum of vitamin $B_{12}$ deficiency. *American Family Physician, 41*, 150–162.

Colamussi, P., Giganti, M., Cittanti, C., Dovigo, L., Trotta, F., Tola, M. R., et al. (1995). Brain single-photon emission tomography with 99mTc-HMPAO in neuropsychiatric systemic lupus erythematosus: Relations with EEG and MRI findings and clinical manifestations. *European Journal of Nuclear Medicine, 22*, 17–24.

Collie, D. A., Sellar, R. J., Zeidler, M., Colchester, A. C., Knight, R., & Will, R. G. (2001). MRI of Creutzfeldt-Jakob disease: Imaging features and recommended MRI protocol. *Clinical Radiology, 56*, 726–739.

Comi, G., Filippi, M., Martinelli, V., Campi, A., Rodegher, M., Alberoni, M., et al. (1995). Brain MRI correlates of cognitive impairment in primary and secondary progressive multiple sclerosis. *Journal of the Neurological Sciences, 132*, 222–227.

Cooper, D. A., Gold, J., MacLean, P., Donovan, B., Finlayson, R., Barnes, T. G., et al. (1985). Acute AIDS retrovirus infection. *Lancet, 1*, 537–540.

Croes, E. A., & van Duijn, C. M. (2003). Variant Creutzfeldt–Jakob disease. *European Journal of Epidemiology, 18*, 473–477.

Cummings, J. L., & Benson, D. F. (1992). *Dementia: A clinical approach* (2nd ed.). Stoneham, MA: Butterworth.

DeArmond, S. J., & Prusiner, S. B. (2003). Perspectives on prion biology, prion disease pathogenesis, and pharmacologic approaches to treatment. *Clinics in Laboratory Medicine, 23*(1), 1–41.

Denburg, S. D., Denburg, J. A., Carbotte, R. M., Fisk, J. D., & Hanly, J. G. (1993). Cognitive deficits in systemic lupus erythematosus. *Rheumatic Disease Clinics of North America, 19*(4), 815–831.

Dolan, R. W., & Chowdhury, K. (1995). Diagnosis and treatment of intracranial complications of paranasal sinus infections. *Journal of Oral and Maxillofacial Surgery, 53*, 1080–1087.

Duna, G. F., Galperin, C., & Hoffman, G. S. (1995). Wegener's granulomatosis. *Rheumatic Disease Clinics of North America, 21*(4), 949–986.

Durand, M. L., Calderwood, S. B., Weber, D. J., Miller, S. I., Southwick, F. S., Caviness, V. S., Jr., et al. (1993). Acute bacterial meningitis in adults: A review of 493 episodes. *New England Journal of Medicine, 328*, 21–28.

Ekholm, S., & Simon, J. H. (1988). Magnetic resonance imaging and the acquired immunodeficiency syndrome dementia complex. *Acta Radiologica, 29*, 227–230.

Fallon, B. A., & Nields, J. A. (1994). Lyme disease: A neuropsychiatric illness. *American Journal of Psychiatry, 151*, 1571–1583.

Farlow, M. R., Yee, R. D., Dlouhy, S. R., Conneally, P. M., Azzarelli, B., & Ghetti, B. (1989). Gerstmann–Straussler–Scheinker disease: I. Extending the clinical spectrum. *Neurology, 39*, 1446–1452.

Feinstein, A., O'Connor, P., Gray, T., & Feinstein, K. (1999). Pathological laughing and crying in multiple sclerosis: A preliminary report suggesting a role for the prefrontal cortex. *Multiple Sclerosis, 5*, 69–73.

Fennell, E. B., & Smith, M. C. (1990). Neuropsychological assessment. In S. M. Rao (Ed.), *Neurobehavioral aspects of multiple sclerosis* (pp. 63–81). New York: Oxford University Press.

Filippi, M., Alberoni, M., Martinelli, V., Sirabian, G., Bressi, S., Canal, N., et al. (1994). Influence of clinical variables on neuropsychological performance in multiple sclerosis. *European Neurology, 34*, 324–328.

Fishman, R. A. (1992). *Cerebrospinal fluid in diseases of the nervous system* (2nd ed.). Philadelphia: Saunders.

Fox, P. A., Hawkins, D. A., & Dawson, S. (2000). Dementia following an acute presentation of meningovascular neurosyphilis in an HIV-1 positive patient. *AIDS, 14*, 2062–2063.

Franklin, G. M., Nelson, L. M., Filley, C. M., & Heaton, R. K. (1989). Cognitive loss in multiple scle-rosis: Case reports and review of the literature. *Archives of Neurology, 46*, 162–167.

Gallassi, R., Morreale, A., Montagna, P., Gambetti, P., & Lugaresi, E. (1992). "Fatal familial insomnia": Neuropsychological study of a disease with thalamic degeneration. *Cortex, 28*, 175–187.

Geiger, W. J., Garrison, K. L., & Losh, D. P. (1992). Wegener's granulomatosis. *American Family Physician, 45*, 191–196.

Geerts, Y., Dehaene, I., & Lammens, M. (1991). Acute hemorrhagic leucoencephalitis. *Acta Neurologica Belgica, 91*, 201–211.

Gerlach, A., Oehm, E., Wattchow, J., Ziyeh, S., Glocker, F.-X., & Els, T. (2003). Use of high-dose cortisone in a patient with Marchiafava–Bignami disease. *Journal of Neurology, 250*, 758–760.

Geschwind, M. D., Martindale, J., Miller, D., DeArmond, S. J., Uyehara-Lock, J., Gaskin, D., et al. (2003). Challenging the clinical utility of the 14-3-3 protein for the diagnosis of sporadic Creutzfeldt–Jakob disease. *Archives of Neurology, 60*, 813–816.

Getsios, D., Caro, I., El-Hadi, W., & Caro, J. J. (2004). Assessing the economics of vaccination for *Neisseria meningitidis* in industrialized nations: A review and recommendations for further research. *International Journal of Technology Assessment in Health Care, 20*, 280–288.

Goldman, S., Liard, A., Flament-Durand, J., Luxen, A., Bidaut, L. M., Stanus, E., et al. (1993). Positron emission tomography and histopathology in Creutzfeldt–Jakob disease. *Neurology, 43*, 1828–1830.

Guharoy, R., Gilroy, S. A., Noviasky, J. A., & Ference, J. (2004). West Nile virus infection. *American Journal of Health-System Pharmacy, 61*, 1235–1241.

Halperin, J. J., Volkman, D. J., & Wu, P. (1991). Central nervous system abnormalities in Lyme neuroborreliosis. *Neurology, 41*, 1571–1582.

Handa, R., Teo, S., & Booy, R. (2004). Influenza: Current evidence and informed predictions. *Expert Review of Vaccines, 3*, 443–451.

Hanna, J. N. (2004). Impact of *Haemophilus influenzae* type b (Hib) vaccination on Hib meningitis in children in Far North Queensland, 1989 to 2003. *Communicable Diseases Intelligence, 28*, 255–257.

Harder, A., Gregor, A., Wirth, T., Kreuz, F., Schulz-Schaeffer, W. J., Windle, O., et al. (2004). Early age of onset in fatal familial insomnia: Two novel cases and review of the literature. *Journal of Neurology, 251*, 715–724.

Heinrich, A., Runge, U., & Khaw, A. V. (2004). Clinicoradiolgic subtypes of Marchiafava–Bignami disease. *Journal of Neurology, 251*, 1050–1059.

Hengge, U. R., Tannapfel, A., Tyring, S. K., Erbel, R., Arendt, G., & Ruzicka, T. (2003). Lyme borreliosis. *Lancet Infectious Diseases, 3*, 489–500.

Henry, K. (1995). Management of HIV infection: A 1995–96 overview for the clinician. *Minnesota Medicine, 78*, 17–24.

Hestad, K., McArthur, J. H., Dal Pan, G. J., Selnes, O. A., Nance-Sproson, T. E., Aylward, E., et al. (1993).

Regional brain atrophy in HIV-1 infection: Association with specific neuropsychological test performance. *Acta Neurologica Scandinavica, 88,* 112–118.

Hook, E. W., III., & Marra, C. M. (1992). Acquired syphilis in adults. *New England Journal of Medicine, 326,* 1060–1069.

Hsich, G., Kenney, K., Gibbs, C. J., Lee, K. H., & Harrington, M. G. (1996). The 14-3-3 brain protein in cerebrospinal fluid as a marker for transmissible spongiform encephalopathies. *New England Journal of Medicine, 335,* 924–930.

Huber, S. J., Bornstein, R. A., Rammohan, K. W., Christy, J. A., Chakeres, D. W., & McGhee, R. B., Jr. (1992a). Magnetic resonance imaging correlates of executive function impairments in multiple sclerosis. *Neuropsychiatry, Neuropsychology, and Behavioral Neurology, 5,* 33–36.

Huber, S. J., Bornstein, R. A., Rammohan, K. W., Christy, J. A., Chakeres, D. W., & McGhee, R. B. (1992b). Magnetic resonance imaging correlates of neuropsychological impairment in multiple sclerosis. *Journal of Neuropsychiatry and Clinical Neurosciences, 4,* 152–158.

IFNB Multiple Sclerosis Study Group and the University of British Columbia MS/MRI Analysis Group. (1995). Interferon beta-1b in the treatment of multiple sclerosis: Final outcome of the randomized controlled trial. *Neurology, 45,* 1277–1285.

Ironside, J. W. (2000). Pathology of variant Creutzfeldt–Jakob disease. *Arch Virol: Supplementum, 16,* 143–151.

Jacobs, L. D., Cookfair, D. L., Rudick, R. A., Herndon, R. M., Richert, J. R., Salazar, A. M., et al. (1996). Intramuscular interferon beta-1a for disease progression in relapsing multiple sclerosis. *Annals of Neurology, 39,* 285–294.

Janssen, R. S., Saykin, A. J., Kaplan, J. E., Spira, T. J., Pinsky, P. F., Sprehn, G. C., et al. (1988). Neurological complication of human immunodeficiency virus infection in patients with lymphadenopathy syndrome. *Annals of Neurology, 23,* 49–55.

Johnson, K. P., Brooks, B. R., Cohen, J. A., Ford, C. C., Goldstein, J., Lisak, R. P., et al. (1995). Copolymer 1 reduces relapse rate and improves disability in relapsing–remitting multiple sclerosis: Results of a phase III multicenter, double-blind, placebo-controlled trial. *Neurology, 45,* 1268–1276.

Johnson, R. T. (1982). Viruses and chronic neurologic diseases. *Johns Hopkins Medical Journal, 150,* 132–140.

Jones, G. A., & Nathwani, D. (1995). Cryptococcal meningitis. *British Journal of Hospital Medicine, 54,* 439–445.

Kapur, N., Barker S., Burrows, E. H., Ellison, D., Brice, J., Illis, L. S., et al. (1994). Herpes simplex encephalitis: Long term magnetic resonance imaging and neuropsychological profile. *Journal of Neurology, Neurosurgery, and Psychiatry, 57,* 1334–1342.

Kesselring, J., Miller, D. H., Robb, S. A., Kendall, B. E.,

Moseley, I. F., Kingsley, D., et al. (1990). Acute disseminated encephalomyelitis: MRI findings and the distinction from multiple sclerosis. *Brain, 113,* 291–302.

Ketzler, S., Weis, S., Huag, H., & Budka, H. (1990). Loss of neurons in the frontal cortex in AIDS brains. *Acta Neuropathology, 80,* 92–94.

Kieburtz, K., & Schiffer, R. B. (1989). Neurologic manifestations of human immunodeficiency virus infections. *Neurologic Clinics, 7,* 447–468.

Kirschbaum, W. R. (1968). *Jakob–Creutzfeldt disease.* New York: Elsevier.

Kitamoto, T., Amano, N., Terao, Y., Nakazato, Y., Isshiki, T., Mizutani, T., et al. (1993). A new inherited prion disease (PrP-P105L mutation) showing spastic paraparesis. *Annals of Neurology, 34,* 808–813.

Kleinschmidt-DeMasters, B. K., Filley, C. M., & Bitter, M. A. (1992). Central nervous system angiocentric, angiodestructive T-cell lymphoma (lymphomatoid granulomatosis). *Surgical Neurology, 37,* 130–137.

Kotter, I., Gunaydin, I., Zierhut, M., & Stubiger, N. (2004). The use of interferon alpha in Behcet's disease: Review of the literature. *Seminars in Arthritis and Rheumatism, 33,* 320–325.

Krupp, L. B., Christodoulou, C., Melville, R. N., Scherl, W. F., McAllister, W. S., & Elkin, L. E. (2004). Donepezil improved memory in multiple sclerosis in a randomized clinical trial. *Neurology, 63,* 1579–1585.

Kubo, M., Nishimura, T., Shikata, E., Kokubun, Y., & Takasu, T. (1995). [A case of variant Gerstmann–Straussler–Scheinker disease with the mutation of codon P105L]. *Rinsho Shinkeigaku: Clinical Neurology, 35,* 873–877.

Kurokawa, M. S., & Suzuki, N. (2003). Behcet's disease. *Clinical and Experimental Medicine, 3,* 10–20.

Lang, C. J., Schuler, P., Engelhardt, A., Spring, A., & Brown, P. (1995). Probable Creutzfeldt–Jakob disease after a cadaveric dural graft. *European Journal of Epidemiology, 11,* 79–81.

LaRocca, N. G. (1990). A rehabilitation perspective. In S. M. Rao (Ed.), *Neurobehavioral aspects of multiple sclerosis* (pp. 215–229). New York: Oxford University Press.

Lechevalier, B., Andersson, J. C., & Morin, P. (1977). Hemispheric disconnection syndrome with a "crossed avoiding" reaction in a case of Marchiafava-Bignami disease. *Journal of Neurology, Neurosurgery, and Psychiatry, 40,* 483–497.

Leo, G. J., & Rao, S. M. (1988). Effects of intravenous physostigmine and lecithin on memory loss in multiple sclerosis: Report of a pilot study. *Journal of Neurological Rehabilitation, 2,* 123–129.

Levy, R. M., Bredesen, D. E., & Rosenblum, M. L. (1985). Neurological manifestations of the acquired immunodeficiency syndrome (AIDS): Experience at UCSF and review of the literature. *Journal of Neurosurgery, 62,* 475–495.

Lewis, R. E., & Kontoyiannis, D. P. (2001). Rationale

for combination antifungal therapy. *Pharmacotherapy, 21*, 149S–164S.

Lin, C.-H., Jeng, J.-S., & Yip, P.-K. (2004). Plasmapheresis in acute disseminated encephalomyelitis. *Journal of Clinical Apheresis, 19*, 154–159.

Lindenbaum, J., Healton, E. B., Savage, D. G., Brust, J. C. M., Garrett, T. J., Podell, E. R., et al. (1988). Neuropsychiatric disorders caused by cobalamin deficiency in the absence of anemia or macrocytosis. *New England Journal of Medicine, 318*, 1720–1728.

Llewelyn, C. A., Hewitt, P. E., Knight, R. S. G., Amar, K., Cousens, S., Mackenzie, J., et al. (2004). Possible transmission of variant Creutzfeldt–Jakob disease by blood transfusion. *Lancet, 363*, 417–421.

Locatelli, L., Zivadinov, R., Grop, A., & Zorzon, M. (2004). Frontal parenchymal atrophy measures in multiple sclerosis. *Multiple Sclerosis, 10*, 562–568.

Lublin, F. D., Whitaker, J. N., Eidelman, B. H., Miller, A. E., Arnason, B. G. W., & Burks, J. S. (1996). Management of patients receiving interferon beta-1b for multiple sclerosis: Report of a consensus conference. *Neurology, 46*, 12–18.

Luby, J. P. (1992). Southwestern Internal Medicine Conference: Infections of the central nervous system. *American Journal of the Medical Sciences, 304*, 379–391.

Lycke, J., Wikkelso, C., Bergh, A. C., Jacobsson, L., & Andersen, O. (1993). Regional cerebral blood flow in multiple sclerosis measured by single photon emission tomography with technetium-99m hexamethylpropyleneamine oxime. *European Neurology, 33*, 163–167.

Mahler, M. E. (1992). Behavioral manifestations associated with multiple sclerosis. *Psychiatric Clinics of North America, 15*, 427–438.

Marshall, D. W., Brey, R. L., Cahill, W. T., Houk, R. W., Zajac, R. A., & Boswell, R. N. (1988). Spectrum of cerebrospinal fluid findings in various stages of human immunodeficiency virus infection. *Archives of Neurology, 45*, 954–958.

Masliah, E., Achim, C. L., Ge, N., DeTeresa, R., Terry, R. D., & Wiley, C. A. (1992). Spectrum of human immunodeficiency virus-associated neocortical damage. *Annals of Neurology, 32*, 321–329.

Masliah, E., Ge, N., Achim, C. L., Hansen, L. A., & Wiley, C. A. (1992). Selective neuronal vulnerability in HIV encephalitis. *Journal of Neuropathology and Experimental Neurology, 51*, 585–593.

Masters, C. L., Harris, J. O., Gajdusek, D. C., Gibbs, C. J., Jr., Bernoulli, C., & Asher, D. M. (1979). Creutzfeldt–Jakob disease: Patterns of worldwide occurrence and the significance of familial and sporadic clustering. *Annals of Neurology, 5*, 177–188.

McIntosh-Michaelis, S. A., Roberts, M. H., Wilkinson, S. M., Diamond, I. D., McLellan, D. L., Martin, J. P., et al. (1991). The prevalence of cognitive impairment in a community survey of multiple sclerosis. *British Journal of Clinical Psychology, 30*(4), 333–348.

McLean, B. N., Miller, D., & Thompson, E. J. (1995). Oligoclonal banding of IgG in CSF, blood–brain barrier function, and MRI findings in patients with sarcoidosis, systemic lupus erythematosus, and Behcet's disease involving the nervous system. *Journal of Neurology, Neurosurgery, and Psychiatry, 58*, 548–554.

Medori, R., Tritschler, H.-J., LeBlanc, A., Villare, F., Manetto, V., Chen, H. Y., et al. (1992). Fatal familial insomnia, a prion disease with a mutation at codon 178 of the prion protein gene. *New England Journal of Medicine, 326*, 444–449.

Mendez, M. F. (1995). The neuropsychiatry of multiple sclerosis. *International Journal of Psychiatry in Medicine, 25*, 123–130.

Mendez, O. E., Shang, J., Jungreis, C. A., & Kaufer, D. I. (2003). Diffusion-weighted MRI in Creutzfeldt–Jakob disease: A better diagnostic marker than CSF protein 14-3-3? *Journal of Neuroimaging, 13*, 147–151.

Mendozzi, L., Pugnetti, L., Saccani, M., & Motta, A. (1993). Frontal lobe dysfunction in multiple sclerosis as assessed by means of Lurian tasks: Effect of age at onset. *Journal of the Neurological Sciences, 115*(Suppl.), S42–S50.

Millefiorini, E., Gasperini, C., Pozzilli, C., D'Andrea, F., Bastianello, S., Trojano, M., et al. (1997). Randomized placebo-controlled trial of mitoxantrone in relapsing–remitting multiple sclerosis: 24-month clinical and MRI outcome. *Journal of Neurology, 244*, 153–159.

Miller, D. H., Khan, O. A., Sheremata, W. A., Blumhardt, L. D., Rice, G. P. A., Libonati, M. A., et al. (2003). A controlled trial of natalizumab for relapsing multiple sclerosis. *New England Journal of Medicine, 348*, 15–23.

Minden, S. L., & Schiffer, R. B. (1990). Affective disorders in multiple sclerosis: Review and recommendations for clinical research. *Archives of Neurology, 47*, 98–104.

Mizuno, T., Takanashi, Y., Onodera, H., Shigeta, M., Tanaka, N., Yuya, H., et al. (2003). A case of lymphomatoid granulomatosis/angiocentric immunoproliferative lesion with a long clinical course and diffuse brain involvement. *Journal of the Neurological Sciences, 213*, 67–76.

Moore, P. M., & Calabrese, L. H. (1994). Neurologic manifestations of systemic vasculitides. *Seminars in Neurology, 14*, 300–306.

Moutsopoulos, H. M., Sarmas, J. H., & Talal, N. (1993). Is central nervous system involvement a systemic manifestation of primary Sjogren's syndrome? *Rheumatic Disease Clinics of North America, 19*(4), 909–912.

Nadeau, S. E., & Watson, R. T. (1990). Neurologic manifestations of vasculitis and collagen vascular syndromes. In A. B. Baker & R. J. Joynt (Eds.), *Clinical neurology.* New York: Harper & Row.

Navia, B. A., Cho, E.-S., Petito, C. K., & Price, R. W. (1986). The AIDS dementia complex: II. Neuropathology. *Annals of Neurology, 19*, 525–535.

Navia, B. A., Jordan, B. D., & Price, R. W. (1986). The AIDS dementia complex: I. Clinical features. *Annals of Neurology, 19,* 517–524.

O'Conner, P. W., Goodman, A., Willmer-Hulme, A. J., Libonati, M. A., Metz, L., Murray, R. S., et al. (2004). Randomized multicenter trial of natalizumab in acute MS relapses: Clinical and MRI effects. *Neurology, 62,* 2038–2043.

Pachner, A. R. (1995). Early disseminated Lyme disease: Lyme meningitis. *American Journal of Medicine, 98*(Suppl. 4A), 30S–37S.

Panegyres, P. K., Toufexis, K., Kakulas, B. A., Cerbevakova, L., Brown, P., Ghetti, B., et al. (2001). A new PRNP mutation (G131V) associated with Gerstmann–Straussler–Scheinker disease. *Archives of Neurology, 58,* 1899–1902.

Panitch, H., Goodin, D. S., Francis, G., Chang, P., Coyle, P. K., O'Connor, P., et al. (2002). Randomized, comparative study of interferon beta-1a treatment regimens in MS: The EVIDENCE Trial. *Neurology, 59,* 1496–1506.

Pantaleo, G., Graziosi, C., & Fauci, A. S. (1993). The immunopathogenesis of human immunodeficiency virus infection. *New England Journal of Medicine, 328,* 327–335.

Pappata, S., Chabriat, H., Levasseur, M., Legault-Demare, F., & Baron, J. C. (1994). Marchiafava–Bignami disease with dementia: Severe cerebral metabolic depression revealed by PET. *Journal of Neural Transmission: Parkinsons and Dementia Section, 8,* 131–137.

Parry, A. M., Scott, R. B., Palace, J., Smith, S., & Matthews, P. M. (2003). Potentially adaptive functional changes in cognitive processing for patients with multiple sclerosis and their acute modulation by rivastigmine. *Brain, 126,* 2750–2760.

Paschoal, R. C., Hirata, M. H., Hirata, R. C., Melhem, M. S., Dias, A. L., & Paula, C. R. (2004). Neurocryptococcosis: Diagnosis by PCR method. *Revista do Instituto de Medicina Tropical de Sao Paulo, 46,* 203–207.

Petersen, R. B., Tabaton, M., Berg, L., Schrank, B., Torack, R. M., Leal, S., et al. (1992). Analysis of the prion protein gene in thalamic dementia. *Neurology, 42,* 1859–1863.

Peterson, P. L., Howe, F. A., Clark, C. A., & Axford, J. S. (2003). Quantitative magnetic resonance imaging in neuropsychiatric systemic lupus erythematosus. *Lupus, 12,* 897–902.

Power, C., & Johnson, R. T. (1995). HIV-1 associated dementia: Clinical features and pathogenesis. *Canadian Journal of Neurological Sciences, 22,* 92–100.

Pozzilli, C., Passafiume, D., Bernardi, S., Pantano, P., Incoccia, C., Bastianello, S., et al. (1991). SPECT, MRI and cognitive functions in multiple sclerosis. *Journal of Neurology, Neurosurgery, and Psychiatry, 54,* 110–115.

Price, R. W. (1996). Neurological complications of HIV infection. *Lancet, 348,* 445–452.

Price, R. W., Sidtis, J. J., Navia, B. A., Pumarola-Sune, T., & Ornitz, D. B. (1988). The AIDS dementia complex. In M. L. Rosenblum, R. M. Levy, & D. E. Bredesen (Eds.), *AIDS and the nervous system* (pp. 203–219). New York: Raven.

Prusiner, S. B. (1996). Human prion diseases and neurodegeneration. *Current Topics in Microbiology and Immunology, 207,* 1–17.

Prusiner, S. B., & Hsiao, K. K. (1994). Human prion diseases. *Annals of Neurology, 35,* 385–395.

Rabins, P. V. (1990). Euphoria in multiple sclerosis. In S. M. Rao (Ed.), *Neurobehavioral aspects of multiple sclerosis* (pp. 180–185). New York: Oxford University Press.

Rappaport, E. B. (1987). Iatrogenic Creutzfeldt–Jakob disease. *Neurology, 37,* 1520–1522.

Rao, S. M. (1986). Neuropsychology of multiple sclerosis: A critical review. *Journal of Clinical and Experimental Neuropsychology, 8,* 503–542.

Rao, S. M., Leo, G. J., Bernardin, L., & Unverzagt, F. (1991). Cognitive dysfunction in multiple sclerosis: I. Frequency, patterns, and prediction. *Neurology, 41,* 685–691.

Reichlin, M. (2003). Ribosomal P antibodies and CNS lupus. *Lupus, 12,* 916–918.

Reina, S., Sterin-Borda, L., Orman, B., & Borda, E. (2004). Autoantibodies against cerebral muscarinic cholinoceptors in Sjogren syndrome: Functional and pathological implications. *Journal of Neuroimmunology, 150,* 107–115.

Richter, R. W. (1993). Infections other than AIDS. *Neurologic Clinics, 11*(3), 591–603.

Roos, K. L. (2004). West Nile encephalitis and myelitis. *Current Opinion in Neurology, 17,* 343–346.

Sampathkumar, P. (2003). West Nile virus: Epidemiology, clinical presentation, diagnosis, and prevention. *Mayo Clinic Proceedings, 78,* 1137–1144.

Sanna, G., Bertolaccini, M. L., & Mathieu, A. (2003). Central nervous system lupus: A clinical approach to therapy. *Lupus, 12,* 935–942.

Scheck, D. N., & Hook, E. W., III. (1994). Neurosyphilis. *Infectious Disease Clinics of North America, 8*(4), 769–795.

Schmidt, R. P. (1989). Neurosyphilis. In A. B. Baker & R. J. Joynt (Eds.), *Clinical neurology.* New York: Harper & Row.

Schmitt, F. A., Bigley, J. W., McKinnis, R., Logue, P. E., Evans, R. W., Drucker, J. L., et al. (1988). Neuropsychological outcome of zidovudine (AZT) treatment of patients with AIDS and AIDS-related complex. *New England Journal of Medicine, 319,* 1573–1578.

Schmutzhard, E. (2001). Viral infections of the CNS with special emphasis on *Herpes simplex* infections. *Journal of Neurology, 248,* 469–477.

Seales, D., & Greer, M. (1991). Acute hemorrhagic leukoencephalitis: A successful recovery. *Archives of Neurology, 48,* 1086–1088.

Simon, R. P. (1985). Neurosyphilis. *Archives of Neurology, 42,* 606–613.

Siva, A., Altintas, A., & Saip, S. (2004). Behcet's syndrome and the nervous system. *Current Opinion in Neurology, 17,* 347–357.

Slavoski, L. A., & Tunkel, A. R. (1995). Therapy of fungal meningitis. *Clinical Neuropharmacology, 18,* 95–112.

Spencer, M. D., Knight, R. S. G., & Will, R. G. (2002). First hundred cases of variant Creutzfeldt–Jakob disease retrospective case note review of early psychiatric and neurological features. *British Journal of Medicine, 324,* 1479–1482.

Straussberg, R., Schonfeld, T., Weitz, R., Karmazyn, B., & Harel, L. (2001). Atypical acute disseminated encephalomyelitis and intravenous immunoglobuin. *Pediatric Neurology, 24,* 139–143.

Swain, R. (1995). An update of vitamin $B_{12}$ metabolism and deficiency states. *Journal of Family Practice, 41,* 595–600.

Swirsky-Sacchetti, T., Mitchell, D. R., Seward, J., Gonzales, C., Lublin, F., Knobler, R., et al. (1992). Neuropsychological and structural brain lesions in multiple sclerosis: A regional analysis. *Neurology, 42,* 1291–1295.

Sze, G., & Zimmerman, R. D. (1988). The magnetic resonance imaging of infections and inflammatory diseases. *Radiology Clinics of North America, 26,* 839–859.

Tan, E. M., Cohen, A. S., Fries, J. F., Masi, A. T., McShane, D. J., Rothfield, N. F., et al. (1982). The 1982 revised criteria for the classification of systemic lupus erythematosus. *Arthritis and Rheumatism, 25,* 1271–1277.

Totsuka, S., Hattori, T., Yazaki, M., Nago, K., & Mizushima, S. (1985). Clinicopathologic studies on neuro-Behcet's disease. *Folia Psychiatrica et Neurologica Japonica, 39,* 155–166.

van de Beek, D., de Gans, J., McIntyre, P., & Prasad, K. (2004). Steroids in adults with acute bacterial meningitis: A systematic review. *Lancet Infectious Diseases, 4,* 139–143.

Victor, M. (1993). Persistent altered mentation due to ethanol. *Neurologic Clinics, 11,* 639–661.

Vollmer, T. L., Guarnaccia, J., Harrington, W., Pacia, S. V., & Petroff, O. A. C. (1993). Idiopathic granulomatous angiitis of the central nervous system. *Archives of Neurology, 50,* 925–930.

Waniek, C., Prohovnik, I., Kaufman, M. A., & Dwork, A. J. (1995). Rapidly progressive frontal-type dementia associated with Lyme disease. *Journal of Neuropsychiatry and Clinical Neurosciences, 7,* 345–347.

Watanabe, N., Seto, H., Sato, S., Simizu, M., Wu, Y. W., Kageyama, M., et al. (1995). Brain SPECT with neuro-Behcet disease. *Clinical Nuclear Medicine, 20,* 61–64.

Watanabe, N., Seto, H., Shimizu, M., Tanii, Y., Kim, Y.-D., Shibata, R., et al. (1996). Brain SPECT of Creutzfeldt–Jakob disease. *Clinical Nuclear Medicine, 21*(3), 236–241.

Weber, R., Keerl, R., Draf, W., Schick, B., Mosler, P., & Saha, A. (1996). Management of dural lesions occurring during endonasal sinus surgery. *Archives of Otolaryngology, 122,* 732–736.

West, S. G. (1994). Neuropsychiatric lupus. *Rheumatic Disease Clinics of North America, 20*(1), 129–158.

West, S. G., Emlen, W., Wener, M. H., & Kotzin, B. L. (1995). Neuropsychiatric lupus erythematosus: A 10-year prospective study on the value of diagnostic tests. *American Journal of Medicine, 99,* 153–163.

Whiteman, M. L., Post, M. J., Berger, J. R., Tate, L. G., Bell, M. D., & Limonte, L. P. (1993). Progressive multifocal leukoencephalopathy in 47 HIV-seropositive patients: Neuroimaging with clinical and pathologic correlation. *Radiology, 187,* 233–240.

Whitley, R. J. (1991). Herpes simplex virus infections of the central nervous system: Encephalitis and neonatal herpes. *Drugs, 42,* 406–427.

Whitley, R. J., & Lakeman, F. (1995). *Herpes simplex* virus infections of the central nervous system: Therapeutic and diagnostic considerations. *Clinical Infectious Diseases, 20,* 414–420.

Will, R. G., Ironside, J. W., Zeidler, M., Cousens, S. N., Estibeiro, K., Alperovitch, A., et al. (1996). A new variant of Creutzfeldt–Jakob disease in the UK. *Lancet, 347,* 921–925.

Wispelwey, B., & Scheld, W. M. (1992). Brain abscess. *Seminars in Neurology, 12,* 273–278.

Yamamori, C., Ishino, H., Inagaki, T., Seno, H., Iijima, M., Torii, I., et al. (1994). Neuro-Behcet disease with demyelination and gliosis of the frontal white matter. *Clinical Neuropathology, 13,* 208–215.

Younger, D. S., Hays, A. P., Brust, J. C., & Rowland, L. P. (1988). Granulomatous angiitis of the brain: An inflammatory reaction of diverse etiology. *Archives of Neurology, 45,* 514–518.

Zifko, U., Wimberger, D., Lindner, K., Zier, G., Grisold, W., & Schindler, E. (1996). MRI in patients with general paresis. *Neuroradiology, 38,* 120–123.

# CHAPTER 33

# Traumatic Brain Injury

*Judith Aharon-Peretz*
*Rachel Tomer*

The frontal cortex constitutes nearly half of the cerebral mantle. It is reciprocally connected to virtually all cortical and subcortical structures. Due to its relative mass and extensive connectivity, traumatic brain injury (TBI) is a major cause of frontal networks damage. In this chapter we describe the consequences of traumatic frontal damage as they relate to cognition and personality in the chronic stages.

TBI denotes a clinical syndrome ranging from purely focal to diffuse brain damage resulting from a combination of neural and vascular events brought about by the mechanical distortion of the head (Gennarelli & Graham, 1998). TBI can result from closed-head injury, penetrating-head injury, or a combination of both. Penetrating-head injury may involve any part of the brain. Damage following closed-head injury is always diffuse. Diffuse brain injury occurs via rapid cranial acceleration–deceleration, with or without impact (Adams, Graham, Murray, & Scott, 1982). The main form of diffuse injury is diffuse axonal injury, which affects white matter tracts and may be the cause of widespread axonal disruption (Holbourn, 1943; Singleton & Povlishock, 2004; Strich, 1956). Diffuse injury may trigger transport failure in axons, dysfunction of neuronal cell bodies, diffuse vascular injury, ischemic–hypoxic injury, and brain swelling (Adams et al., 1982). Consequently, surrounding tissue deafferentation may occur. Damage is usually most evident at the surface of the brain. When impact is severe enough to produce loss of consciousness, both cortical and subcortical systems are already involved (Ommaya & Gennarelli, 1974). Mild injuries typically result in diffuse axonal damage, showing no additional signs of neuronal or vascular changes (Povlishock, 1993). Moderate to severe injuries, on the other hand, frequently result in added neuronal and vasculature damage (Gaetz, 2004). Diffuse axonal injury most commonly involves the white matter of the frontal lobes, the corpus callosum, and the corona radiata (Gentry, Godersky, & Thompson, 1988). Accordingly, frontal dysfunction is the most common acquired manifestation following diffuse axonal injury, especially during later phases of recovery (Levine, Katz, Dade, & Blach, 2002). In young children, in addition to the acquired damage, diffuse axonal injury may also disrupt development of connectivity and constrain the development of networks that mediate prefrontal cognitive and behavioral skills (Anderson, Damasio, Tranel, & Damasio, 2000; Eslinger, Grattan, Damasio, & Damasio, 1992). Focal brain injuries occur in the form of contusions (disruption of brain tissue) and bleedings. Hemorrhages and hematomas occur in the extradural, subarachnoid, and intracerebral areas (Gennarelli, 1993). Contusions typically occur at the apex of the gyri and appear as multiple punctuate hemorrhages or streaks with eventual progression of bleeding to the adjacent white matter (Gennarelli & Graham, 1998). The common sites of cerebral contusions are the ventral and polar frontal and temporal regions (Courville, 1937; Gennarelli & Graham, 1998) because of excessive strain in these areas against the ridges of the anterior and middle fossa. Contusions occur beneath fractures, under the site of impact (coup), or at a distance from the impact (contrecoup) and may also be associated with herniation.

Delayed or secondary complication following traumatic brain injury may also disrupt the frontal cortex. Secondary damage to the frontal systems may result from delayed neuronal injury, herniation syndromes, such as frontal trans-falcine herniation which may impair anterior cerebral artery perfusion and compromise medial frontal lobes (Bullock, Maxwell, Graham, Teasdale, & Adams, 1991; Gennarelli & Graham, 1998), hydrocephalus which typically compromises white matter tracts adjacent to the lateral and third ventricles, and chronic subdural hematomas.

The relationship between the trauma and the ensuing cognitive and behavioral manifestations is not always clear. The functional defects usually exceed the structural damage. The clinical appearance in the individual survivor of TBI is determined by trauma-associated parameters (impact severity; focal or diffuse damage; size, depth, and laterality of the lesion; associated complication, such as shock; or respiratory problems), and host-related parameters such as age and preinjury personality.

Civilian head injuries are commonly associated with closed-head injury. At least a temporary loss of consciousness (concussion) frequently occurs, and even though the skull is not penetrated, the brain may suffer gross damage.

## POSTTRAUMATIC COGNITIVE AND BEHAVIORAL SYNDROMES

Many individuals who survive a TBI continue to experience debilitating cognitive and emotional problems long after their injury. The typical posttraumatic brain injury syndrome comprises slower information processing; deficits in attention (Ponsford & Kinsella, 1992; Spikman, van Zomeren, & Deelman, 1996; Stuss et al., 1989; van Zomeren & Brouwer, 1994), memory (Crosson, Novack, Trenerry, & Craig, 1988; Levin & Goldstein, 1986), and executive functions (Bohnen, Jolles, & Twijnstra, 1992; Chen et al., 2004; Hinton-Bayre, Geffen, & McFarland, 1997; Newcombe, Rabbitt, & Briggs, 1994); and problems in controlling behavior (Rappaport,

Herrero-Backe, Rappaport, & Winterfield, 1989). These problems, together with headaches, sleep disturbances, dizziness, irritability, and heightened sensitivity to noise, are referred to as "postconcussion syndrome."

In the normal human individual, the cortical surface of the frontal lobe evolves prenatally throughout the fourth decade of life (Grattan & Eslinger, 1991). This growth is associated with evolving cognitive and behavioral stages through the first 16 years of life (Grattan & Eslinger, 1991). As a result, the consequence of TBI in children may not only cause impairment of function but also prevent development of abilities, such as personality, planning, executive functions, and social skills that come into play later in development.

Following TBI, the effect of damage to the frontal lobes on cognitive performance often depends on the demands of the task (Stuss, 1996). Cognitive tasks that require working memory, maintaining attentional set or shifting attention between response sets, inhibiting inappropriate responses, planning and selecting the appropriate responses (all of which have been termed "executive functions") may be impaired and cause difficulties not only in performing a given cognitive task but also in daily living.

## Attention

Attentional and concentration impairments are common residual deficits following TBI in adults and in children (Fenwick & Anderson, 1999; Lezak, 1978). Attention comprises an important component of the executive functions. It can be described as a limited process that allows the preferential processing of certain sensory or imagined information at the expense of other stimuli (Andrewes, 2001).

Attention is mediated by a neural network involving the ascending reticular activating system exerting bottom-up regulation and the heteromodal prefrontal, parietal, and limbic cortices regulating top-down influences (Mesulam, 2000). The ascending reticular activating system influences attention globally, without displaying selectivity for sensory modality or cognitive domain. The prefrontal cortex, together with the parietal and limbic cortices, on the other hand, mediates the attentional responses in ways that are sensitive to context, motivation, acquired significance, and conscious volition (Mesulam, 2000). Following

TBI, patients often report difficulties in paying attention to more than one thing at a time, make mistakes because of not paying attention properly, miss important details, and have difficulties in concentrating (Gronwall, 1987; Lezak, 1978; Ponsford & Kinsella, 1992). In cognitive terms, these complaints represent deficits in several aspects of attention, which are discussed in detail below.

### Sustained Attention (Vigilance)

The ascending reticular activating system is a critical structure for sustained attention (Mesulam, 1985; Posner & Petersen, 1990; Stuss & Benson, 1986). Dysfunction of the brainstem ascending reticular activating system may cause coma following severe insult or drifting of alertness and attention when the damage is less severe. Recent functional imaging studies imply that sustained attention (as measured by continuous performance tasks) is mediated by a distributed network in which midfrontal regions, predominantly of the right hemisphere, play a major role (Cohen, Nordahl, Semple, Andreason, & Pickar, 1998; Lewin et al., 1996; Pardo, Fox, & Raichle, 1991; Rueckert & Grafman, 1996; Strakowski, Adler, Holland, Mills, & DelBello, 2004). Sustained attention has two aspects: time over which a certain performance can be maintained (time-on-task) and the consistency of performance over that period (intraindividual variability). Compared to healthy individuals, patients with frontal lesions tend to show longer reaction times, miss more targets on continuous performance tests, and demonstrate a tendency toward slips into inconsistent, unintended actions (Chan, 2001; Robertson, Manly, Andrade, Baddeley, & Yiend, 1997; Stuss et al., 1989).

### Selective Attention

The phenomenon of "selective attention" is the ability to focus only on the object or scene of interest, while disregarding irrelevant stimuli and suppressing interference by automatic responses (Kandel, 2000; Schneider & Shiffrin, 1977). Although a few studies report that selective attention is unaffected (Anderson, Fenwick, Manly, & Robertson, 1998; Rieger & Gauggel, 2002, other studies document that interference tasks are particularly sensitive to the effects of TBI. Bate, Mathias, and Craw-

ford (2001) studied patients following severe head injury and reported that the modified color–word subtest of the Stroop test was one of only two tasks that were best able to discriminate between the patients and control groups. Similar deficits have been also reported in patients with milder TBI, where the presence of diffuse axonal injury was correlated with behavioral and cognitive symptoms of frontal lobe dysfunction, especially in interference tasks such as go/no-go and Stroop (Wallesch, Curio, Galazky, Jost, & Synowitz, 2001).

### Divided Attention

The ability to perform effectively on more than one task simultaneously is determined by the speed and efficiency of information processing (the amount of information being processed in a given time) and the ability to shift the focus of attention between subtasks that cannot be executed simultaneously (van Zomeren & Brouwers, 1994). Neuroimaging studies reveal that divided attention is associated with activation of the dorsolateral prefrontal, cingulate, and superior parietal cortices (Kondo et al., 2004; Loose, Kaufmann, Auer, & Lange, 2003; Szameitat, Schubert, Muller, & Von Cramon, 2002). Divided attention is commonly impaired following TBI (Stuss et al., 1989). Neuropsychological studies have depicted significant slowing in processing speed while performing dual tasks procedures (Cicerone, 1996; Leclercq et al., 2000; McDowell, Whyte, & D'Esposito, 1997) and deficits in task shifting, response inhibition, error detection, and conflict monitoring—all necessary ingredients for effective divided attention (Cicerone, 1996; Leclercq et al., 2000; McDowell, Whyte, & D'Esposito, 1997).

## Memory

Memory impairment, a common complaint following TBI, is frequently associated with medial temporal or diencephalic pathology. In this chapter, we review only those syndromes associated with TBI that manifest frontal networks–related impairment of memory. Damage to the medial temporal lobes or diencephalic structures usually results in anterograde amnesia, characterized by impaired recall and recognition. In contrast, frontal lobe damage does not typically produce general memory loss. Following frontal lobe damage, patients are impaired when recall depends on self-initiated cues, organization, search selection, and verification of the stored information (Moscovitch & Winocur, 1995). These patients usually perform within normal limits on tests of cued recall and recognition.

Closed-head injuries are usually followed by a transient state of confusion and disorientation, during which patients fail to learn and recall information from memory, and occasionally confabulate (van Zomeren & Saan, 1990). This initial interval between injury and regaining continuous day-to-day memory with intact orientation is referred to as "posttraumatic amnesia" (Brooks, 1972; Levin, 1992). Patients who recover from posttraumatic amnesia either do not recall the period or perceive details from it as if it were a dream. The duration of posttraumatic amnesia correlates with the severity and outcome of TBI (Ellenberg, Levin, & Saydjari, 1996; Katz & Alexander, 1994; Levin, Benton, & Grossman, 1982; Russel, 1971). Posttraumatic amnesia may subside despite persistence of memory impairment (Levin, 1992). The mechanism of posttraumatic amnesia has not been elucidated yet. Similar manifestations may occur following rupture of an anterior communicating artery aneurism (Damasio, Graff-Radford, Eslinger, Damasio, & Kassell, 1985), in the acute stages of the Wernicke–Korsakoff syndrome (Victor, Adams, & Collins, 1989) and following bilateral thalamic (Guberman & Stuss, 1983) or thalamic–frontal infarctions (Schnider, Gutbrod, Hess, & Schroth, 1996).

Temporal context confusion, and the occurrence of spontaneous confabulation in the posttraumatic period, has been shown to correlate with lesions in the medial orbitofrontal cortex or its connection (Schnider, von Daniken, & Gutbrod, 1996), whereas damage in nonconfabulating amnestics involved the posterior medial temporal lobe (Schnider, Ptak, von Daniken, & Remonda, 2000). The observation that temporal orientation is the most prominent and prolonged deficit in posttraumatic amnesia and the occurrence of spontaneous confabulation suggest that the core features of posttraumatic amnesia emanate from damage or disconnection to the orbitofrontal cortex, at least in patients who confabulate. Following the resolution of posttraumatic amnesia, patients may experience deficits in working memory, acquisition and retention of new information (anterograde amnesia), and impaired recall of information acquired prior to the onset of injury (retrograde amnesia).

## Working Memory

Working memory (Baddeley, 1992), the ability to maintain and manipulate information temporarily over a period of seconds, is particularly vulnerable to disruption following TBI. Working memory is an attention supported, age-dependent ability related to frontal lobe maturation. It is important in the development and function of a wide variety of cognitive skills, such as planning, problem solving, reading, auditory language comprehension, and arithmetic, and is essential to memory acquisition and adaptive behavior (Levin et al., 2002). Working memory normally relies on processing in brain regions that are often selectively damaged by TBI. Working memory is divided into two processes: the attentional online maintenance of information (the phonological loop and the visuospatial sketchpad) and its volitional manipulation, the "central executive" (D'Esposito et al., 1995). Functional imaging provides evidence that the neuroanatomical substrate of the "online maintenance" involves both the prefrontal and posterior parietal cortices, whereas that of the "central executive" involves principally the dorsolateral prefrontal cortex (D'Esposito et al., 1995; D'Esposito, Postle, Ballard, & Lease, 1999; Postle & D'Esposito, 1999). Tasks that emphasize maintaining goals and products of one task while performing another (executive functions) activate principally the anterior prefrontal cortices (Burgess, Veitch, de Lacy Costello, & Shallice, 2000; Postle & D'Esposito, 1999). Functional neuroimaging illustrates that relative to healthy controls, patients with posttraumatic brain injury exhibit altered patterns of activation in working memory–related brain regions characterized by increased dispersion, and increased activation in the right prefrontal and right parietal cortices (Christodoulou et al., 2001). Examination of the pattern of behavioral responding and the temporal course of activation suggests that working memory deficits following moderate-to-severe TBI are usually due to associative or strategic aspects of working memory, and not impairments in active maintenance of the stimulus (Perlstein et al., 2004; Scheibel et al., 2003), suggesting that the "central executive" component is affected in these cases.

## Long-Term Memory

Long-term memory, the ability to retain information for long periods, is assessed by tasks that require retrieval of remote information. In a study that assessed retrieval in patients with posttraumatic brain injury (Levine, 2002), the functional anatomy of retrieval was similar in healthy individuals and patients with posttraumatic brain injury and involved the right frontal, temporal, occipital, subcortical, and cerebellar regions. Yet patients showed higher activation of frontal polar and anterior cingulate regions, including recruitment of left frontal regions, which suggests that TBI causes reorganization of the memory systems.

Long-term memory is classified into semantic memory, the factual knowledge about the world or oneself, and episodic (autobiographical) memory, which comprises subjective memories of past episodes from a specific place and time (Tulving, 1972; Wheeler, Stuss, & Tulving, 1997). Selective episodic memory impairment has been described in patients with right anterior temporal and ventral frontal lobe damage. Affected patients consistently report an inability to reexperience events as part of their own subjective past, although their ability to acquire new memories and recall factual knowledge may be intact. These patients experience the feeling that the events might just as well have happened to someone else (De Renzi & Lucchelli, 1993; Goldberg et al., 1981; Hunkin et al., 1995; Mattioli et al., 1996). Functional imaging has demonstrated the preferential involvement of the right prefrontal cortex in episodic memory retrieval (Fletcher, Frith, & Rugg, 1997; Nyberg et al., 1996). Additional memory impairment in patients with frontal damage includes their tendency to forget how information was acquired, a deficit called "source amnesia." Because the ability to associate a piece of information with the time and place where it was acquired is at the core of how accurately we remember the individual episodes of our lives, a deficit in source information interferes dramatically with the recall of episodic knowledge (Kandel, Kupfermann, & Iversen, 2000).

## Procedural Memory

Procedural memory may also be affected following frontal trauma. "Procedural memory" refers to the learning of perceptual motor skills (tested by tasks such as mirror reading or rotor-pursuit tracking), and acquisition of rules and sequences (tested by serial reaction time tests). Procedural memory is usually implicit (independent of conscious recollection). It is processed within a network that includes the cerebellum (Molinari et al., 1997), the basal ganglia (Soliveri, Brown, Jahanshahi, Caraceni, & Marsden, 1997), and the dorsolateral prefrontal cortex (Gomez-Beldarrain, Grafman, Pascual-Leone, & Garcia-Monco, 1999). Impairment in the performance of procedural learning tasks may occur following prefrontal cortical injury or damage to the fiber pathways connecting the dorsolateral prefrontal cortex to the basal ganglia.

## Personality and Emotional/Behavioral Changes

In this chapter, "emotion" is defined as a feeling state with psychic, somatic, and behavioral components that is related to mood and affect; "affect" denotes the observed expression of emotion (prosody and facial expression); and "mood" designates the subjective experience (Benson, 1984; Kaplan, Sadock, & Grebb, 1991).

"Personality" is defined as the totality of emotional and behavioral traits that characterize the person in day-to-day living under ordinary conditions, and it is influenced by learned and inherent qualities against which mental alteration reacts (Kaplan et al., 1991).

Following TBI, feeling and expression of emotion may be affected, and posttraumatic emotional and personality changes are usually associated with frontal lobe injury. Fifty to 76% of patients show persistent changes of personality and emotion up to 15 years after injury (Brooks & McKinlay, 1983; Thomsen, 1984). Emotional and personality changes are usually associated with poor social and vocational outcome (Brooks, Campsie, Symington, Beattie, & McKinlay, 1986; Thomsen, 1984), and present a heavier burden for the caregivers than do patients' physical disabilities and residual cognitive deficits.

The etiology of the emotional and behavioral disturbances occurring after brain injury has not been elucidated as yet, but it can be conceptualized as the product of a person's preinjury personality, the sequelae of the injury itself, the individual's response to the trauma and its consequences, and the social environment within which the person is located after injury.

Following frontal damage, patients may have poor emotional control and dysfunctional social behavior. They may alternate between being disinterested and apathetic to being outspoken, bombastic, and tactless—behavioral styles referred to by Blumer and Benson (1975) as pseudodepressed and pseudopsychopathic personalities, respectively. However, the pseudodepressed patient need not necessarily suffer from depressed mood; rather, he or she may occasionally appear to be depressed because of lack of spontaneity and apathy. The pseudopsychopaths are usually not psychopathic or sociopathic by intention; rather, these patients lack awareness and sensitivity to the feeling of others (Andrewes, 2001) and fail to use their past experience to register in advance the consequences of their doings.

The spectrum of the behavioral changes associated with frontal lobe trauma was concisely summarized in the case of Phineas Gage, probably the first published, carefully analyzed patient with frontal lobe injury (Harlow, 1868). Gage, a reliable and upright man, became profane, hot-tempered, and irresponsible following an accident in which an iron rod penetrated his frontal lobe. Consequent to the injury, his personality changed profoundly, and he experienced alterations in strategic thinking, emotional integration, and behavior, whereas his language, memory, and motor–sensory functions remained relatively intact.

## The Spectrum of Posttraumatic Emotional and Behavioral Changes

### Anxiety

Emergence of disorders of anxiety (the feeling of apprehension caused by anticipation of danger; Kaplan et al., 1991), including generalized anxiety, panic, phobias, and stress disorders, is frequently reported after TBI (Bryant & Harvey, 1998). Patients' anxiety symptoms were found to correlate with preinjury anxiety attitudes and damage to the medial prefrontal cortex (Blumer & Benson, 1975; Vasa et al., 2002). Although both exaggerated (Astrom, 1996; Castillo, Starkstein, Fedoroff, Price, & Robinson, 1993; Grafman, Vance, Weingartner, Salazar, & Amin, 1986) and decreased anxiety have been reported, most recent lesion-based imaging studies suggest that patients with damage to the orbitofrontal cortex

are less likely to develop anxiety (Bechara, Damasio, & Damasio, 2000; Vasa et al., 2004).

Posttraumatic stress disorder, a condition associated with intrusive recollections of a traumatic event, hyperarousal, avoidance of clues associated with the trauma, and psychological numbing, has also been associated with a neural circuitry involving frontal, especially medial and inferior frontal, regions (Nutt & Malizia, 2004; Tanev, 2003; Williams, Evans, Wilson, & Needham, 2002). It has been repeatedly documented, however, that victims of accidents are less likely to develop the posttraumatic stress syndrome if the impact to the head resulted in an extended period of unconsciousness (Glaesser, Neuner, Lutgehetmann, Schmidt, & Ebert, 2004; Klein, Caspi, & Gil, 2003).

### Apathy

"Apathy" is defined as the lack of goal-directed behavior due to reduced motivation that is not caused by cognitive deterioration, emotional distress, or reduced consciousness (Marin, 1991). It has been described in 23–43% of patients following TBI (Andersson & Bergedalen, 2002; Oddy, Coughlan, Tyerman, & Jenkins, 1985; van Zomeren & van den Burg, 1985). Apathy is commonly associated with damage to dorsolateral and medial frontal regions, and frontal–subcortical dopaminergic pathways. The dorsolateral damage is the most likely cause of the "pseudodepressive" syndrome described by Blumer and Benson (1975), and is characterized by passivity, flattened affect, reduced verbal output, and slowness to initiate a response. Patients with apathy are impaired when facing novel situations (Godefroy & Rousseaux, 1997). Apathy is associated with poor recovery and rehabilitation.

### Obsessive–Compulsive Disorder

Obsessive–compulsive disorder is a rare complication of TBI (Berthier, Kulisevsky, Gironell, & Lopez, 2001). It is usually associated with dysfunction of the frontostriatal–pallidofrontal circuit (Graybiel & Rauch, 2000; Lacerda et al., 2003; Stein, 2000). The clinical and neuropsychological phenomenology of posttraumatic obsessive–compulsive disorder is similar to that of the idiopathic condition (Berthier et al., 2001) and is often associated with non-obsessive–compulsive anxiety and heightened emotional arousal such as stress reactions and posttraumatic stress (Berthier et al., 2001).

## Major Depression

Major depression, a frequent complication among patients who have TBI (Jorge et al., 2004; Kreutzer, Seel, & Gourley, 2001), is associated with executive dysfunction, negative affect, and anxiety, and frequently also with aggressive behavior (Jorge et al., 2004). The cognitive abnormalities observed in patients with TBI and major depression are consistent with left lateral prefrontal dysfunctions. Neuroimaging reveals a similar pattern of reduced left ventrolateral and dorsolateral prefrontal gray matter volumes (Jorge et al., 2004; Stuss, Gow, & Hetherington, 1992). Patients with major depression are more likely to have a history of mood and anxiety disorder that antedates injury.

## Social Behavior

Impairment in interpersonal relationships is a common and devastating consequence of frontal trauma. Patients with lesions in the ventromedial prefrontal cortex are particularly impaired and tend to exercise poor judgment in decision making, which is especially manifested in the disadvantageous choices they make in their personal lives and in the ways they relate to others (Blair & Cipolotti, 2000; Damasio, 1994; Dias, Robbins, & Roberts, 1996; Eslinger & Damasio, 1985; Stuss & Benson, 1986). Although neither the neural networks nor the cognitive and emotional mechanisms underlying social behavior are fully understood, constructs such as empathy, the ability to make inferences regarding the mental state of others (theory of mind), "perspective-taking ability" (Price, Daffner, Stowe, & Mesulam, 1990), and the ability to register in advance the consequences of one's actions all seem to contribute to inappropriate interpersonal behavior, and all have been described as impaired following frontal trauma.

## Empathy

"Empathy" refers to the reaction of one individual to the observed experience of another (Davis, 1980) and reflects cognitive processes such as the ability to make inference regarding the mental state of others (Baron-Cohen, 1995;

Premack & Woodruff, 1978), "perspective taking" (Price et al., 1990), and the ability to recognize, experience, share, and express emotions (Mehrabian & Epstein, 1972). The ability to experience an appropriate empathic response depends on cognitive flexibility (Cicerone, Lazar, & Shapiro, 1983) and working memory (Eslinger, 1998), faculties commonly associated with dorsolateral prefrontal cortex. It also depends on emotional processing and episodic memory, which are associated with the intact functioning of the orbitofrontal cortex. Indeed, prefrontal damage often results in impaired empathic abilities, especially when the damage involves the ventromedial regions of the prefrontal cortex and affects the right hemisphere (Shamay-Tsoory, Tomer, Berger, & Aharon-Peretz, 2003).

In addition, patients with ventromedial damage often fail to identify vocal and facial emotional expressions (Blonder, Bowers, & Heilman, 1991; DeKosky, Heilman, Bowers, & Valenstein, 1980) and are impaired on face memory and recognition (Rapcsak et al., 2001), which may further enhance their difficulty in recognizing another's affect and perspective. Aberrant behavior following damage to the right ventromedial prefrontal cortex may also occur secondary to impairment in retrieval of episodic memories, resulting in inability to reactivate past memories and relate them to the other person's experience.

Damasio, Tranel, and Damasio (1991) put forward the "somatic marker hypothesis" to account for changes in social conduct, planning, and decision making that characterize patients with ventromedial prefrontal damage. This hypothesis suggests that by integrating information regarding body states (including emotional states) evoked by positive and negative experiences, together with the outcomes of these experiences, the ventromedial prefrontal region acquires the capacity to use emotion and feelings to guide behavior. According to the "somatic marker" theory, when a person is confronted with situations that call for decision making, the emotional memory of previous, similar situations is reactivated, and a decision regarding the most appropriate behavior is then undertaken. Efficient decision making requires simultaneously holding, comparing, and manipulating the various alternatives for option outcomes, to allow effective ability to register the consequences of behaviors in advance. Without somatic markers, response options and outcomes become more or less equalized. The process of decision making and response selection would then depend on logical operations over many potential alternatives, without taking into account previous experiences, and might become random or impulsive. The somatic marker hypothesis also helps explain why too little emotion may be as bad for decision making as too much emotion (Bechara, Damasio, Tranel, & Anderson, 1998). This theory may account for the inexplicable violent and aggressive behaviors occasionally seen in patients with ventromedial frontal lobe damage and also for the developmental sociopathy following early life injury to these areas (Grafman et al., 1986). Most patients with frontal lobe injury, however, do not develop violent and aggressive behaviors.

## SUMMARY

The natural history following frontal trauma is characterized by cognitive, behavioral, and emotional changes. Personal and social recovery depends on the amount of damage to the frontal lobes and their subcortical connections. Patients may alternate between apathy and inappropriate bouts of aggression and irritability, between distractibility and stimulus boundness. Their memory may be impaired, affecting their ability to use previous personal knowledge for recent problem solving. These patients may be impaired when facing novel situation and especially when the context necessitates perspective taking and decision making while facing parallel processing of multiple considerations, or while interacting with other individuals. Being cognitively affected and emotionally impaired, patients usually lose their premorbid occupational and social status. In patients with early-acquired frontal lobe damage, appropriate emotional and social faculties may not develop at all, and socially deviant behaviors such as sociopathy may develop instead.

## REFERENCES

Adams, J. H., Graham, D. I., Murray, L. S., & Scott, G. (1982). Diffuse axonal injury due to nonmissile head injury in humans: An analysis of 45 cases. *Annals of Neurology, 12,* 557–563.

Anderson, S. W., Damasio, H., Tranel, D., & Damasio, A. R. (2000). Long-term sequelae of prefrontal cortex damage acquired in early childhood. *Developmental Neuropsychology, 18,* 281–296.

Anderson, V., Fenwick, T., Manly, T., & Robertson, I. (1998). Attentional skills following traumatic brain injury in childhood: A componential analysis. *Brain Injury, 12,* 937–949.

Andersson, S., & Bergedalen, A. M. (2002). Cognitive correlates of apathy in traumatic brain injury. *Neuropsychiatry, Neuropsychology, and Behavioral Neurology, 15,* 184–191.

Andrewes, D. G. (2001). Disorders of attention. In *Neuropsychology: From theory to practice* (pp. 139–206). Philadelphia: Psychology Press.

Astrom, M. (1996). Generalized anxiety disorder in stroke patients. A 3-year longitudinal study. *Stroke, 27,* 270–275.

Baddeley, A. (1992). Working memory. *Science, 255,* 556–559.

Baron-Cohen, S. (1995). *Mindblindness: An essay on autism and theory of mind.* Cambridge, MA: MIT Press.

Bate, A. J., Mathias, J. L., & Crawford, J. R. (2001). Performance on the Test of Everyday Attention and standard tests of attention following severe traumatic brain injury. *Clinical Neuropsychology, 3,* 405–422.

Bechara, A., Damasio, H., & Damasio, A. R. (2000). Emotion, decision making and the orbitofrontal cortex. *Cerebral Cortex, 10,* 295–307.

Bechara, A., Damasio, H., Tranel, D., & Anderson, S. W. (1998). Dissociation of working memory from decision making within the human prefrontal cortex. *Journal of Neurosciences, 18,* 428–437.

Benson, D. F. (1984). The neurology of human emotion. *Bulletin of Clinical Neurosciences, 49,* 23–42.

Berthier, M. L., Kulisevsky, J. J., Gironell, A., & Lopez, O. L. (2001). Obsessive compulsive disorder and traumatic brain injury: Behavioral, cognitive, and neuroimaging findings. *Neuropsychiatry, Neuropsychology, and Behavioral Neurology, 14,* 23–31.

Blair, R. J., & Cipolotti, L. (2000). Impaired social response reversal: A case of "acquired sociopathy." *Brain, 123,* 1122–1141.

Blonder, L. X., Bowers, D., & Heilman, K. M. (1991). The role of the right hemisphere in emotional communication. *Brain, 114,* 1115–1127.

Blumer, D., & Benson, D. F. (1975). Personality changes with frontal and temporal lobe lesions. In *Psychiatric aspects of neurologic disease* (pp. 151–170). New York: Grune & Stratton.

Bohnen, N., Jolles, J., & Twijnstra, A. (1992). Neuropsychological deficits in patients with persistent symptoms six months after mild head injury. *Neurosurgery, 30,* 692–695.

Brooks, D. N. (1972). Memory and head injury. *Journal of Nervous and Mental Disease, 155,* 350–355.

Brooks, D. N., & McKinlay, W. (1983). Personality and behavioural change after severe blunt head injury—a relative's view. *Journal of Neurology, Neurosurgery, and Psychiatry, 46,* 336–344.

Brooks, N., Campsie, L., Symington, C., Beattie, A., & McKinlay, W. (1986). The five year outcome of severe blunt head injury: A relative's view. *Journal of Neurology, Neurosurgery, and Psychiatry, 49,* 764–770.

Bryant, R. A., & Harvey, A. G. (1998). Relationship between acute stress disorder and posttraumatic stress disorder following mild traumatic brain injury. *American Journal of Psychiatry, 155,* 625–629.

Bullock, R., Maxwell, W. L., Graham, D. I., Teasdale, G. M., & Adams, J. H. (1991). Glial swelling following human cerebral contusion: An ultrastructural study. *Journal of Neurology, Neurosurgery, and Psychiatry, 54,* 427–434.

Burgess, P. W., Veitch, E., de Lacy Costello, A., & Shallice, T. (2000). The cognitive and neuroanatomical correlates of multitasking. *Neuropsychologia, 38,* 848–863.

Castillo, C. S., Starkstein, S. E., Fedoroff, J. P., Price, T. R., & Robinson, R. G. (1993). Generalized anxiety disorder after stroke. *Journal of Nervous and Mental Disease, 181,* 100–106.

Chan, R. C. (2001). Attentional deficits in patients with post-concussion symptoms: A componential perspective. *Brain Injury, 15,* 71–94.

Chen, J. K., Johnston, K. M., Frey, S., Petrides, M., Worsley, K., & Ptito, A. (2004). Functional abnormalities in symptomatic concussed athletes: An f-MRI study. *NeuroImage, 22,* 68–82.

Christodoulou, C., DeLuca, J., Ricker, J. H., Madigan, N. K., Bly, B. M., Lange, G., et al. (2001). Functional magnetic resonance imaging of working memory impairment after traumatic brain injury. *Journal of Neurology, Neurosurgery, and Psychiatry, 71,* 161–168.

Cicerone, K. D. (1996). Attention deficits and dual task demands after mild traumatic brain injury. *Brain Injury, 10,* 79–89.

Cicerone, K. D., Lazar, R. M., & Shapiro, W. R. (1983). Effects of frontal lobe lesions on hypothesis sampling during concept formation. *Neuropsychologia, 21,* 513–524.

Cohen, R. M., Nordahl, T. E., Semple, W. E., Andreason, P., & Pickar, D. (1998 ). Abnormalities in the distributed network of sustained attention predict neuroleptic treatment response in schizophrenia. *Neuropsychopharmacology, 19,* 36–47.

Courville, C. B. (1937). *Pathology of the central nervous system* (Part 4). Mountain View, CA: Pacific Press.

Crosson, B., Novack, T. A., Trenerry, M. R., & Craig, P. L. (1988). California Verbal Learning Test (CVLT) performance in severely head-injured and neurologically normal adult males. *Journal of Clinical and Experimental Neuropsychology, 10,* 754–768.

Cummings, J. L. (1993). Frontal–subcortical circuits and human behavior. *Archives of Neurology, 50,* 873–880.

Damasio, A. R. (1994). *Descartes' error: Emotion, reason and the human brain.* New York: Avon Books.

Damasio, A. R., Graff-Radford, N. R., Eslinger, P. J., Damasio, H., & Kassell, N. (1985). Amnesia following basal forebrain lesions. *Archives of Neurology, 42,* 263–271.

Damasio, A. R., Tranel, D., & Damasio, H. C. (1991). Somatic markers and guidance of behavior: Theory and preliminary testing. In H. S. Levin, H. M. Eisenberg, & A. L. Benton (Eds.), *Frontal lobe function and dysfunction* (pp. 217–229). New York: Oxford University Press.

De Renzi, E., & Lucchelli, F. (1993). Dense retrograde amnesia, intact learning capability and abnormal forgetting rate: A consolidation deficit? *Cortex, 29,* 449–466.

DeKosky, S. T., Heilman, K. M., Bowers, D., & Valenstein, E. (1980). Recognition and discrimination of emotional faces and pictures. *Brain and Language, 9,* 206–214.

D'Esposito, M., Detre, J. A., Alsop, D. C., Shin, R. K., Atlas, S., & Grossman, M. (1995). The neural basis of the central executive system of working memory. *Nature, 378,* 279–281.

D'Esposito, M., Postle, B. R., Ballard, D., & Lease, J. (1999). Maintenance versus manipulation of information held in working memory: An event-related f-MRI study. *Brain and Cognition, 41,* 66–86.

Dias, R., Robbins, T. W., & Roberts, A. C. (1996). Dissociation in prefrontal cortex of affective and attentional shifts. *Nature, 380,* 69–72.

Ellenberg, J. H., Levin, H. S., & Saydjari, C. (1996). Posttraumatic amnesia as a predictor of outcome after severe closed head injury: Prospective assessment. *Archives of Neurology, 53,* 782–791.

Eslinger, P. J. (1998). Neurological and neuropsychological bases of empathy. *European Journal of Neurology, 39,* 193–199.

Eslinger, P. J., & Damasio, A. R. (1985). Severe disturbance of higher cognition after bilateral frontal lobe ablation: Patient EVR. *Neurology, 35,* 1731–1741.

Eslinger, P. J., Grattan, L. M., Damasio, H., & Damasio, A. R. (1992). Developmental consequences of childhood frontal lobe damage. *Archives of Neurology, 49,* 764–769.

Fenwick, T., & Anderson, V. (1999). Impairments of attention following childhood traumatic brain injury. *Neuropsychology, Development and Cognition: Section C, Child Neuropsychology, 5,* 213–223.

Fletcher, P. C., Frith, C. D., & Rugg, M. D. (1997). The functional neuroanatomy of episodic memory. *Trends in Neurosciences, 20,* 213–218.

Gaetz, M. (2004). The neurophysiology of brain injury. *Clinical Neurophysiology, 115,* 4–18.

Gennarelli, T. A. (1993). Mechanisms of brain injury. *Journal of Emergency Medicine, 11*(Suppl. 1), 5–11.

Gennarelli, T. A., & Graham, D. I. (1998). Neuropathology of the head injuries. *Seminars in Clinical Neuropsychiatry, 3,* 160–175.

Gentry, L. R., Godersky, J. C., & Thompson, B. (1988). MR imaging of head trauma: Review of the distribution and radiopathologic features of traumatic lesions. *American Journal of Roentgenology, 150,* 663–672.

Glaesser, J., Neuner, F., Lutgehetmann, R., Schmidt, R., & Elbert, T. (2004). Posttraumatic stress disorder in patients with traumatic brain injury. *BMC Psychiatry, 4, 5.*

Godefroy, O., & Rousseaux, M. (1997). Novel decision making in patients with prefrontal or posterior brain damage. *Neurology, 49,* 695–701.

Goldberg, E., Antin, S. P., Bilder, R. M., Jr., Gerstman, L. J., Hughes, J. E., & Mattis, S. (1981). Retrograde amnesia: Possible role of mesencephalic reticular activation in long-term memory. *Science, 213,* 1392–1394.

Gomez-Beldarrain, M., Grafman, J., Pascual-Leone, A., & Garcia-Monco, J. C. (1999). Procedural learning is impaired in patients with prefrontal lesions. *Neurology, 52,* 1853–1860.

Grafman, J., Vance, S. C., Weingartner, H., Salazar, A. M., & Amin, D. (1986). The effects of lateralized frontal lesions on mood regulation. *Brain, 109,* 1127–1148.

Grattan, L. M., & Eslinger, P. J. (1991). Frontal lobe damage in children and adults: A comparative review. *Developmental Neuropsychology, 7,* 283–326.

Graybiel, A. M., & Rauch, S. L. (2000). Toward a neurobiology of obsessive–compulsive disorder. *Neuron, 28,* 343–347.

Gronwall, D. (1987). Advances in the assessment of attention and information processing after head injury. In H. S. Levin, J. Grafman, & H. M. Eisenberg (Eds.), *Neurobehavioral recovery from head injury* (pp. 355–371). New York: Oxford University Press.

Guberman, A., & Stuss, D. (1983). The syndrome of bilateral paramedian thalamic infarction. *Neurology, 33,* 540–546.

Harlow, J. M. (1868). Recovery from the passage of an iron bar through the head. *Publication of the Massachusetts Medical Society, 2,* 327–346.

Hinton-Bayre, A. D., Geffen, G., & McFarland, K. (1997). Mild head injury and speed of information processing: A prospective study of professional rugby league players. *Journal of Clinical and Experimental Neuropsychology, 19,* 275–289.

Holbourn, A. H. S. (1943). Mechanism of head injury. *Lancet, 2,* 438.

Hunkin, N. M., Parkin, A. J., Bradley, V. A., Burrows, E. H., Aldrich, F. K., Jansari, A., et al. (1995). Focal retrograde amnesia following closed head injury: A case study and theoretical account. *Neuropsychologia, 33,* 509–523.

Jorge, R. E., Robinson, R. G., Moser, D., Tateno, A., Crespo-Facorro, B., & Arndt, S. (2004). Major depression following traumatic brain injury. *Archives of General Psychiatry, 61,* 42–50.

Kandel, E. R. (2000). From nerve cells to cognition: The internal cellular representation required for perception and action. In E. R. Kandel, J. H. Schwartz, & T. M. Jessell (Eds.), *Principles of neural sciences* (4th ed., pp. 381–403). New York: McGraw-Hill.

Kandel, E. R., Kupfermann, I., & Iversen, S. (2000). Learning and memory. In E. R. Kandel, J. H. Schwartz, & T. M. Jessell (Eds.), *Principles of neural sciences* (4th ed., pp. 1227–1246). New York: McGraw-Hill.

Kaplan, H. I., Sadock, B. J., & Grebb, J. A. (1991). *Synopsis of psychiatry.* Baltimore: Williams & Wilkins.

Katz, D. I., & Alexander, M. P. (1994). Traumatic brain injury: Predicting course of recovery and outcome for patients admitted to rehabilitation. *Archives of Neurology, 51,* 661–670.

Klein, E., Caspi, Y., & Gil, S. (2003). The relation between memory of the traumatic event and PTSD: Evidence from studies of traumatic brain injury. *Canadian Journal of Psychiatry, 48,* 28–33.

Kondo, H., Morishita, M., Osaka, N., Osaka, M., Fukuyama, H., & Shibasaki, H. (2004). Functional roles of the cingulo-frontal network in performance on working memory. *NeuroImage, 21,* 2–14.

Kreutzer, J. S., Seel, R. T., & Gourley, E. (2001). The prevalence and symptom rates of depression after traumatic brain injury: A comprehensive examination. *Brain Injury, 15,* 563–576.

Lacerda, A. L., Dalgalarrondo, P., Caetano, D., Haas, G. L., Camargo, E. E., & Keshavan, M. S. (2003). Neuropsychological performance and regional cerebral blood flow in obsessive–compulsive disorder. *Progress in Neuropsychopharmacology and Biological Psychiatry, 27,* 657–665.

Leclercq, M., Couillet, J., Azouvi, P., Marlier, N., Martin, Y., Strypstein, E., et al. (2000). Dual task performance after severe diffuse traumatic brain injury or vascular prefrontal damage. *Journal of Clinical and Experimental Neuropsychology, 22,* 339–350.

Levin, H. S. (1992). Head injury and its rehabilitation. *Current Opinion in Neurology and Neurosurgery, 5,* 673–676.

Levin, H. S., Benton, A. L., & Grossman, R. G. (1982). *Neurobehavioral consequences of closed head injury.* New York: Oxford University Press.

Levin, H. S., & Goldstein, F. C. (1986). Organization of verbal memory after severe closed-head injury. *Journal of Clinical and Experimental Neuropsychology, 8,* 643–656.

Levin, H. S., Hanten, G., Chang, C. C., Zhang, L., Schachar, R., Ewing-Cobbs, L., et al. (2002). Working memory after traumatic brain injury in children. *Annals of Neurology, 52,* 82–88.

Levine, B., Katz, D. I., Dade, L., & Black, S. E. (2002). Novel approaches to the assessment of frontal damage and executive deficits in traumatic brain injury. In D. T. Stuss & R. T. Knight (Eds.), *Principles of frontal lobe function* (pp. 448–450). New York: Oxford University Press.

Lewin, J. S., Friedman, L., Wu, D., Miller, D. A., Thompson, L. A., Klein, S. K., et al. (1996). Cortical localization of human sustained attention: Detection with functional MR using a visual vigilance paradigm. *Journal of Computer Assisted Tomography, 20,* 695–701.

Lezak, M. D. (1978). Subtle sequelae of brain damage: Perplexity, distractibility, and fatigue. *American Journal of Physical Medicine and Rehabilitation, 57,* 9–15.

Loose, R., Kaufmann, C., Auer, D. P., & Lange, K.W. (2003). Human prefrontal and sensory cortical activity during divided attention tasks. Human *Brain Mapping, 18,* 249–259.

Marin, R. S. (1991). Apathy: A neuropsychiatric syndrome. *Journal of Neuropsychiatry and Clinical Neuroscience, 3,* 243–254.

Mattioli, F., Grassi, F., Perani, D., Cappa, S. F., Miozzo, A., & Fazio, F. (1996). Persistent post-traumatic retrograde amnesia: A neuropsychological and ($^{18}$F)FDG PET study. *Cortex, 32,* 121–129.

McDowell, S., Whyte, J., & D'Esposito, M. (1997). Working memory impairments in traumatic brain injury: Evidence from a dual-task paradigm. *Neuropsychologia, 35,* 1341–1353.

Mehrabian, A., & Epstein, N. (1972). A measure of emotional empathy. *Journal of Personality, 40,* 523–543.

Mesulam, M. M. (1985). Attention, confusional states and neglect. In M. M. Mesulam (Ed.), *Principles of behavioral neurology* (pp. 125–168). Philadelphia: Davis.

Mesulam, M. M. (2000). Attentional networks, confusional states and neglect syndromes. In *Principles of behavioral neurology* (2nd ed., pp. 187–192). New York: Oxford University Press.

Molinari, M., Leggio, M. G., Solida, A., Ciorra, R., Misciagna, S., Silveri, M. C., et al. (1997). Cerebellum and procedural learning: Evidence from focal cerebellar lesions. *Brain, 120,* 1753–1762.

Moscovitch, M., & Winocur, G. (1995). Frontal lobes, memory, and aging. *Annals of the New York Academy of Sciences, 15,* 119–150.

Newcombe, F., Rabbitt, P., & Briggs, M. (1994). Minor head injury: Pathophysiological or iatrogenic sequelae? *Journal of Neurology, Neurosurgery, and Psychiatry, 57,* 709–716.

Nutt, D. J., & Malizia, A .L. (2004). Structural and functional brain changes in posttraumatic stress disorder. *Journal of Clinical Psychiatry, 65*(Suppl. 1), 111–117.

Nyberg, L., McIntosh, A. R., Cabeza, R., Habib, R., Houle, S., & Tulving, E. (1996). General and specific brain regions involved in encoding and retrieval of events: What, where, and when. *Proceedings of the National Academy of Sciences of the United States of America, 93,* 11280–11285.

Oddy, M., Coughlan, T., Tyerman, A., & Jenkins, D. (1985). Social adjustment after closed head injury: A further follow-up seven years after injury. *Journal of Neurology, Neurosurgery, and Psychiatry, 48,* 564–568.

Ommaya, A. K., & Gennarelli, T. A. (1974). Cerebral concussion and traumatic unconsciousness: Correlation of experimental and clinical observations of blunt head injuries. *Brain, 97,* 633–654.

Pardo, J. V., Fox, P. T., & Raichle, M. E. (1991). Localization of a human system for sustained attention by positron emission tomography. *Nature, 349,* 61–64.

Perlstein, W. M., Cole, M. A., Demery, J. A., Seignourel, P. J., Dixit, N. K., Larson, M. J., et al. (2004). Parametric manipulation of working memory load in traumatic brain injury: Behavioral and neural correlates. *Journal of the International Neuropsychological Society, 10,* 724–741.

Plum, F., & Posner, J. B. (1980). *The diagnosis of stupor and coma.* Philadelphia: Davis.

Ponsford, J., & Kinsella, G. (1992). Attentional deficits following closed head injury. *Journal of Experimental and Clinical Neuropsychology, 14,* 822–838.

Posner, M. I., & Petersen, S. E. (1990). The attention system of the human brain. *Annual Review of Neuroscience, 13,* 25–42.

Postle, B. R., & D'Esposito, M. (1999). "What"-then-"where" in visual working memory: An event-related fMRI study. *Journal of Cognitive Neuroscience, 11,* 585–597.

Povlishock, J. T. (1993). Pathobiology of traumatically induced axonal injury in animals and man. *Annals of Emergency Medicine, 22,* 980–986.

Premack, D., & Woodruff, G. (1978). Chimpanzee problem-solving: A test for comprehension. *Science, 202,* 532–535.

Price, B. H., Daffner, K. R., Stowe, R. M., & Mesulam, M. M. (1990). The comportmental learning disabilities of early frontal lobe damage. *Brain, 113,* 1383–1393.

Rapcsak, S. Z., Nielsen, L., Littrell, L. D., Glisky, E. L., Kaszniak, A. W., & Laguna, J. F. (2001). Face memory impairments in patients with frontal lobe damage. *Neurology, 57,* 1168–1175.

Rappaport, M., Herrero-Backe, C., Rappaport, M. L., & Winterfield, K. M. (1989). Head injury outcome up to ten years later. *Archives of Physical Medicine and Rehabilitation, 70,* 885–892.

Rieger, M., & Gauggel, S. (2002). Inhibition of ongoing responses in patients with traumatic brain injury. *Neuropsychologia, 40,* 76–85.

Robertson, I. H., Manly, T., Andrade, J., Baddeley, B. T., & Yiend, J. (1997). "Oops!": Performance correlates of everyday attentional failures in traumatic brain injured and normal subjects. *Neuropsychologia, 35,* 747–758.

Rueckert, L., & Grafman, J. (1996). Sustained attention deficits in patients with right frontal lesions. *Neuropsychologia, 34,* 953–963.

Russel, W. R. (1971). *The traumatic amnesias.* New York: Oxford University Press.

Scheibel, R. S., Pearson, D. A., Faria, L. P., Kotrla, K. J., Aylward, E., Bachevalier, J., et al. (2003). An f-MRI study of executive functioning after severe diffuse TBI. *Brain Injury, 17,* 919–930.

Schneider, W., & Shiffrin, R. M. (1977). Controlled and automatic human information processing: I. Detection, search and attention. *Psychological Review, 84,* 1–66.

Schnider, A., Gutbrod, K., Hess, C. W., & Schroth, G. (1996). Memory without context: Amnesia with confabulations after infarction of the right capsular genu. *Journal of Neurology, Neurosurgery, and Psychiatry, 61*, 186–193.

Schnider, A., Ptak, R., von Daniken, C., & Remonda, L. (2000). Recovery from spontaneous confabulations parallels recovery of temporal confusion in memory. *Neurology, 55*, 74–83.

Schnider, A., von Daniken, C., & Gutbrod, K. (1996). The mechanisms of spontaneous and provoked confabulations. *Brain, 119*, 1365–1375.

Shamay-Tsoory, S. G., Tomer, R., Berger, B. D., & Aharon-Peretz, J. (2003). Characterization of empathy deficits following prefrontal brain damage: The role of the right ventromedial prefrontal cortex. *Journal of Cognitive Neuroscience, 15*, 324–337.

Singleton, R. H., & Povlishock, J. T. (2004). Identification and characterization of heterogeneous neuronal injury and death in regions of diffuse brain injury: Evidence for multiple independent injury phenotypes. *Journal of Neuroscience, 24*, 3543–3553.

Soliveri, P., Brown, R. G., Jahanshahi, M., Caraceni, T., & Marsden, C. D. (1997). Learning manual pursuit tracking skills in patients with Parkinson's disease. *Brain, 120*, 1325–1337.

Spikman, J. M., van Zomeren, A. H., & Deelman, B. G. (1996). Deficits of attention after closed-head injury: Slowness only? *Journal of Clinical and Experimental Neuropsychology, 18*, 755–767.

Stein, D. J. (2000). Neurobiology of the obsessive–compulsive spectrum disorders. *Biological Psychiatry, 47*, 296–304.

Strakowski, S. M., Adler, C. M., Holland, S. K., Mills, N., & DelBello, M. P. (2004). A preliminary f-MRI study of sustained attention in euthymic, unmedicated bipolar disorder. *Neuropsychopharmacology, 29*, 1734–1740.

Strich, S. J. (1956). Diffuse degeneration of the cerebral white matter in severe dementia following head injury. *Journal of Neurochemistry, 19*, 163–185.

Stuss, D. T. (1996). Frontal lobes. In J. G. Beaumont, P. M. Kenealy, & M. J. C. Rogers (Eds.), *The Blackwell dictionary of neuropsychology* (pp. 3346–3530). Oxford, UK: Blackwell.

Stuss, D. T., & Benson, D. F. (1986). *The frontal lobes*. New York: Raven Press.

Stuss, D. T., Gow, C. A., & Hetherington, C. R. (1992). "No longer Gage": Frontal lobe dysfunction and emotional changes. *Journal of Consulting and Clinical Psychology, 60*, 349–359.

Stuss, D. T., Stethem, L. L., Hugenholtz, H., Picton, T., Pivik, J., & Richard, M. T. (1989). Reaction time after head injury: Fatigue, divided and focused attention, and consistency of performance. *Journal of Neurology, Neurosurgery, and Psychiatry, 52*, 742–748.

Szameitat, A. J., Schubert, T., Muller, K., & Von Cramon, D. Y. (2002). Localization of executive functions in dual-task performance with f-MRI. *Journal of Cognitive Neuroscience, 14*, 1184–1199.

Tanev, K. (2003). Neuroimaging and neurocircuitry in post-traumatic stress disorder: What is currently known? *Current Psychiatry Reports, 5*, 369–383.

Thomsen, I. V. (1984). Late outcome of very severe blunt head trauma: A 10–15 year second follow-up. *Journal of Neurology, Neurosurgery, and Psychiatry, 47*, 260–268.

Tulving, E. (1972). Episodic and semantic memory. In E. Tulving & W. Donaldson (Eds.), *Organization of memory* (pp. 382–403). New York: Academic Press.

van Zomeren, A. H., & Brouwer, W. H. (1994). *Clinical neuropsychology of attention*. New York: Oxford University Press.

Van Zomeren, A. H., & Saan, R. J. (1990). Psychological and social sequelae of severe head injury. In R. Braakman (Ed.), *Handbook of clinical neurology: Head injury* (Vol. 57, pp. 397–420). Amsterdam: Elsevier Science.

van Zomeren, A. H., & van den Burg, W. (1985). Residual complaints of patients two years after severe head injury. *Journal of Neurology, Neurosurgery, and Psychiatry, 48*, 21–28.

Vasa, R. A., Gerring, J. P., Grados, M., Slomine, B., Christensen, J. R., Rising, W., et al. (2002). Anxiety after severe pediatric closed head injury. *Journal of the American Academy of Child and Adolescent Psychiatry, 41*, 148–156.

Vasa, R. A., Grados, M., Slomine, B., Herskovits, E. H., Thompson, R. E., Salorio, C., et al. (2004). Neuroimaging correlates of anxiety after pediatric traumatic brain injury. *Biological Psychiatry, 55*, 208–216.

Victor, M., Adams, R. D., & Collins, G. H. (1989). *The Wernicke–Korsakoff syndrome* (2nd ed.). Philadelphia: Davis.

Wallesch, C. W., Curio, N., Galazky, I., Jost, S., & Synowitz, H. J. (2001). The neuropsychology of blunt head injury in the early postacute stage: Effects of focal lesions and diffuse axonal injury. *Neurotrauma, 18*, 11–20.

Wheeler, M. A., Stuss, D. T., & Tulving, E. (1997). Toward a theory of episodic memory: The frontal lobes and autonoetic consciousness. *Psychological Bulletin, 121*, 331–354.

Williams, W. H., Evans, J. J., Wilson, B. A., & Needham, P. (2002). Brief report: Prevalence of post-traumatic stress disorder symptoms after severe traumatic brain injury in a representative community sample. *Brain Injury, 16*, 673–679.

# CHAPTER 34

# Adult-Onset Genetic Disorders
# Involving the Frontal Lobes

*Michael D. Geschwind*
*Grace Yoon*
*Jill Goldman*

We discuss adult-onset genetic disorders of the frontal lobes in this chapter. Most of the diseases covered here affect many cortical areas, but all result in frontal dysfunction either through direct involvement of, or connections to, the frontal lobes (see Chow & Cummings, Chapter 3, this volume).

The diseases in this chapter are separated into three areas based on regions of most prominent involvement on magnetic resonance imaging (MRI): gray matter, white matter, and mixed (gray and white matter involvement). Gray matter conditions are divided into neurodegenerative, triplet repeats, and metabolic diseases. Mixed disorders are separated into mitochondrial and metabolic subtypes. Although this division is somewhat arbitrary, the purpose is to facilitate clinical evaluation and assessment of patients with frontal lobe disorders of potential genetic etiology. Table 34.1 summarizes the conditions discussed in this chapter and their division by MRI findings.

Importantly, it is not possible in this chapter to cover in a comprehensive manner every genetic condition that involves the frontal lobe in adulthood. Rather, this chapter is meant as a guide to the recognition of common disorders of the frontal lobes; therefore, rarer disorders receive less attention. Also, some conditions here are also discussed by Scharre (Chapter 32, this volume) and may only be briefly mentioned here for consideration in the differential.

## GRAY MATTER DISEASES

### Neurodegenerative Conditions

#### Alzheimer's Disease

Although Alzheimer's disease (AD) is classically a condition that affects the hippocampus and parietal lobes, frontal lobes can also be involved, and frontal variants or presentations of AD occur and are sometimes mistaken clinically for frontotemporal dementia (FTD). The etiology and risk of AD is multifactorial. As with many other neurodegenerative diseases, the vast majority of late-onset AD (LOAD) is sporadic. Although genetic factors contribute to the overall risk of LOAD (see discussion below), early-onset AD (EOAD) is much more likely to have a genetic etiology. Four genes have been associated with AD. Three of these, presenilin 1 (PSEN1) (Schellenberg et al., 1992; Sherrington et al., 1995) and presenilin 2 (PSEN2) (Levy-Lahad, Wasco, et al., 1995; Levy-Lahad, Wijsman, et al., 1995; Rogaev et al., 1995), and the amyloid precursor protein gene (APP) (Goate et al., 1991) are autosomal

## TABLE 34.1. Adult-Onset Genetic Disorders of the Frontal Lobes

| Disease | Predominant MRI findings |
| --- | --- |
| **Gray matter** | |
| Alzheimer's disease | Predominantly parietal and hippocampal atrophy |
| Frontotemporal dementia | Frontal and temporal atrophy |
| Creutzfeldt–Jakob disease | DWI and FLAIR cortical, basal ganglia, and/or thalamus hyperintensity |
| McLeod neuoracanthocytosis syndrome | BG (few cases have white matter) |
| Autosomal recessive choreoacanthocytosis | BG and SN atrophy |
| Wilson's disease | Cortical and brainstem atrophy; T1 BG hypodensity (white matter tracts may be T2 hyperintense); DWI hyperintense in BG |
| Dentatorubropallidoluysian atrophy | Cerebellar atrophy (rarely white matter involvement) |
| Huntington's disease | Caudate atrophy |
| PANK2 (Hallervorden–Spatz disease) | Eye of the tiger sign in BG |
| Gaucher's disease—type 3 | Mild cerebral atrophy |
| Spinocerebellar ataxias | Cerebellar, olivocerebellar, or global atrophy |
| Kufs' disease (adult neuronal ceroid lipofuscinosis) | Cerebral or cerebellar atrophy |
| Neimann–Pick disease—type C | Late cerebral atrophy (rare white matter abnormalities) |
| Adult Tay–Sachs disease (adult hexosaminodase A deficiency) | Cerebellar atrophy |
| **White matter** | |
| Adrenal leukodystrophy | Early, predominantly posterior white matter |
| Adult polyglucosan body disease | Patchy white matter hyperintensity often with lesions |
| Krabbe's disease (globoid cell leukodystrophy) | Posterior predominant leukoencephalopathy |
| Adult orthochromatic leukodystrophy | Varied; typically diffuse white matter changes sparing U-fibers |
| Pelizaeus—Merzbacher disease/spastic paraplegia 2 | Diffuse leukoencephalopathy |
| Metachromatic leukodystrophy | White matter leukoencephalopathy, moving anterior to posterior, initially sparing U-fibers |
| Vanishing white matter disease | Diffuse leukoencephalopathy involving U-fibers and vermian atrophy |
| X-linked adrenoleukodystrophy/ adrenomyelopathy | Parietal–occipital predominant leukoencephaloloapthy with enhancing margins and U-fiber involvement |
| Fabry's disease | Symmetric white matter involvement of frontal and parietal lobes; vascular dementia |
| **Mixed** | |
| Cerebral autosomal dominant arteriopathy with subcortical infarcts and leukoencephalopathy | Predominantly white matter disease, initially involving anterior temporal lobes; subcortical infarcts involve white and gray matter |
| Cerebrotendinous xanthomatosis | T2 hyperintensity in dentate nuclei, cerebral, and cerebellar white matter |
| Mitochondrial diseases | T2 white matter hyperintensities, diffuse atrophy |
| Nasu–Hakola disease | Frontal atrophy and white matter abnormalities; BG calcifications |
| Alexander's disease | Extensive, frontal predominant, white matter disease; periventricular rim of decreased signal on T2-weighted MRI and increased signal on T1-weighted MRI; BG and brainstem abnormalities; contrast enhancement |

*Note.* BG, basal ganglia; SN, substantia nigra; DWI, diffusion-weighted imaging; FLAIR, fluid-attenuated inversion recovery.

dominant, causative genes, whereas the apolipoprotein E gene (APOE) is strongly associated with the risk for AD and is thus only a susceptibility gene. Whereas less than 5% of all AD is due to autosomal dominant inheritance, a significant amount of the risk of AD and the early age of onset may be due to APOE genotype. Many other linkage sites are being investigated as possible additional susceptibility loci (Bertram & Tanzi, 2004b).

Most cases of LOAD are not genetic and are due to the accumulation of β-amyloid protein, especially Aβ42, which is derived from cleavage of its larger parent protein, APP. APP has three cleavage sites: α, β, and γ. Depending on which sites are cleaved, three different protein products of APP are produced. If the β/γ secretase pathway predominates, a greater amount of Aβ42 is produced, leading eventually to the development of AD.

## AUTOSOMAL DOMINANT AD

Autosomal dominant AD is caused by mutations involving genes that metabolize the APP protein. These mutations result in the misprocessing of APP and the accumulation of β-amyloid. The presenilin proteins appear to be a part of the γ secretase complex involved in the cleavage of APP.

Up to 50% of autosomal dominant AD is due to mutations in *PSEN1*, a gene located on chromosome 14. More than 130 mutations have been found in *PSEN1*. The gene is thought to be strongly penetrant, but phenotypic expression can be variable, even within families. Onset ranges from ages 24 to 60, with a mean age of 44 years (Bertram & Tanzi, 2004b). The majority of AD cases caused by *PSEN1* cannot be distinguished from sporadic AD. However, certain mutations can lead to unusual features, including FTD, myoclonus, parkinsonism, spastic paraparesis, and epilepsy (Brooks et al., 2003; Furuya et al., 2003; Queralt et al., 2002; Raux et al. 2000; Rippon et al., 2003).

Mutations in *PSEN2* (on chromosome 1) are much rarer than those in *PSEN1*, accounting for less than 1% of hereditary AD. Only nine mutations in this gene have been reported from 15 kindreds. The majority of cases can be traced to a founder mutation in a Volga German family. Unlike *PSEN1* and *APP*, *PSEN2* appears to be less than 100% penetrant. A few individuals carrying mutations in the gene have

lived to as old as 85 without becoming symptomatic. The onset of disease is also quite variable, ranging from ages 46 to 71, with a mean age of 57 years (Bertram & Tanzi, 2004a, 2004b).

*APP* mutations are extremely rare. Approximately 15 mutations have been reported from 40 families. Age of onset ranges from 35 to 60 years, with a mean age of 52. Most mutations in this gene result in a phenotype similar to sporadic AD. However, certain *APP* mutations result in hereditary cerebral hemorrhage with amyloidosis. Of note, the triple dose of APP located on chromosome 21 is thought to be the reason for AD in persons with Down's syndrome.

Currently, clinical genetic testing is available for *PSEN1* and *PSEN2*. APP testing is available on a research basis only. Genetic testing can provide definitive diagnosis and provide families with an understanding of disease etiology and the opportunity for presymptomatic genetic testing of other family members. (See final section, "Genetic Testing and Counseling.")

## SUSCEPTIBILITY GENES

The *APOE4* gene is thought to be responsible for as much as 20% of AD (Cruts & Van Broeckhoven, 1998; Slooter et al., 1998). The mechanism for the increased risk is still unknown, although APOE4 has been implicated in impaired cholesterol transport. Three different APOE alleles (2, 3, and 4) code for three isoforms of this protein. Of these, APOE4 has been strongly associated with the risk for AD, particularly before age 70 (Corder et al., 1993; Duara et al., 1996). The APOE2 allele may be protective against AD. The APOE-related risk of AD is dose dependent. A single APOE4 allele increases risk by two to three times that of the general population, whereas APOE4 homozygosity increases risk by 8- to 15-fold. The APOE effect differs by gender (Farrer et al., 1995; Soragna et al., 2003). Heterozygous women seem to develop AD at an earlier age than heterozygous men (Farrer et al., 1995). Most, but not all, data suggest that the risk of the APOE4 allele differs by ethnic group (Green et al., 2002; Harwood, Barker, Ownby, Mullan, & Duara, 2004).

Unlike the autosomal dominant genes, genetic testing for susceptibility genes such as APOE is the subject of much debate. Because approximately 15% of the general population carries the APOE4 gene without developing AD, an APOE test cannot be definitive for diagnosis of AD. Currently, because of its predictive uncertainty, presymptomatic APOE testing is not recommended (Greely, 1999). The multicenter Risk Evaluation and Education for Alzheimer's disease study (REVEAL) is using APOE genotyping and family history to derive reliable lifetime risk estimates (Cupples et al., 2004). Additionally, it is studying the impact of offering information about personal risk of AD (LaRusse et al., 2005; Zick et al., 2005).

Research studies have implicated many other chromosomal linkages, including chromosomes 10, 12, and 19, as containing possible AD autosomal genes and susceptibility factors (for review, see Bertram & Tanzi, 2004b; Wijsman et al., 2004). Further studies are needed to confirm and clarify their contribution to AD.

### Frontotemporal Lobar Degeneration

Studies on the heritability of frontotemporal lobar degeneration (FTLD) have found that between 30 and 50% of cases have a positive family history of dementia (Binetti et al., 2003) and 10–40% are autosomal dominant. The *tau* gene on chromosome 17 accounts for up to 18% of the autosomal dominant cases (Binetti et al., 2003; Bird et al., 2003; Poorkaj et al., 1998; Stanford et al., 2004). Collectively these cases are known as FTD-17 or frontotemporal dementia and parkinsonism (FTDP-17) because of the frequent presence of parkinsonian symptoms. At least five other gene regions have been linked to FTLD.

### FTD-17

More than 25 mutations have been found in *tau* (van Swieten et al., 2004). These mutations cause destabilization of neuronal microtubules because of tau dysfunction or altered tau splicing, leading to abnormal distribution of tau isoforms. Whereas normally 3R and 4R tau proteins are equally present, certain *tau* mutations cause too much 3R tau (Pick's disease) or too much 4R tau (progressive supranuclear palsy [PSP] and corticobasal degeneration [CBD]; Arai et al., 2001; Spillantini et al., 2000). Inter- and intrafamilial phenotypic variation is considerable (Stanford et al., 2004; van Swieten et al., 2004). Age of onset ranges from ages 29 to 75 (Alzheimer's Research Forum, www.alzforum.org), with a mean age of 56 (Chow et al., 1999). Some members of FTD-17 families have symptoms of FTD, whereas others present with CBD or PSP (Bird et al., 1999; Bugiani et al., 1999; Soliveri et al., 2003). As with autosomal dominant AD, cognitive and behavioral changes may begin early in life, well before the development of the full-blown disease (Geschwind et al., 2001). Limited clinical genetic testing is available for *tau* mutations, but several labs are conducting research testing. Finding a *tau* mutation is highly unlikely in persons without an autosomal dominant family history of dementia.

### OTHER GENES

The combination of FTD and amyotrophic lateral sclerosis (ALS) is frequently found in families with autosomal dominant inheritance patterns without *tau* mutations. Autopsy diagnoses of motor neuron disease are not uncommon in such families, even when symptoms of motor neuron disease are not apparent. Linkages to chromosomes 3, 9, and a non*tau* region of chromosome 17 have been discovered for some kindreds (Brown et al., 2004; Gydesen et al., 2002; Hosler et al., 2000; Wilhelmsen et al., 2004).

Still other families with autopsy-confirmed FTD have been found to have *PSEN1* mutations (Dermaut et al., 2004; Halliday et al., 2005; Tang-Wai et al. 2002). Last, two syndromes have been described that include FTD and bone abnormalities. The valosin-containing protein gene on chromosome 9p has been found to cause inclusion body myopathy associated with Paget's disease of the bone and frontotemporal dementia (Kovach et al., 2001; Watts et al., 2004). This autosomal dominant disorder has a highly variable phenotype. Of individuals with mutations, 82% will have myopathy and 49% will have Paget disease of the bone, whereas only 30% present with FTD. The second syndrome, Nasu–Hakola disease, is an autosomal recessive disease with bone cysts and sclerosing leukoencephalopathic presenile dementia. It is due to mutations in two genes, *TYROBP* and *TREM2* (Soragna et al., 2003). Finally, a new gene on chromosome 3, involved with endosomal processing, has been reported in an autosomal dominant form of FTD (Skibinski et al., 2005).

## SUSCEPTIBILITY FACTORS

Currently no definitive gene has been associated with increased susceptibility to sporadic FTLD. Studies of APOE have had mixed results. Most reports have found little to no association between FTLD and the APOE4 allele, whereas others have found a weak association with the APOE2 allele (Geschwind, Karrim, Nelson, & Miller, 1998; Gustafson, Abrahamson, Grubb, Nilsson, & Fex, 1997; Ingelson et al., 2001; Nielsen, Ravid, Kamphorst, & Jorgensen, 2003; Verpillat et al., 2002).

The strongest association between FTLD spectrum diseases and a chromosomal region is found with the H1 haplotype of the *tau* gene. *Tau* has two different haplotypes formed by linkage disequilibrium, H1 and H2 (Baker et al., 1999). The 3R tauopathies, CBD and PSP, are strongly associated with homozygosity of the H1 *tau* haplotype (Houlden et al., 2001; Pittman et al., 2005). Research is being conducted to discover other susceptibility loci.

### Prion Diseases

About 10–15% of prion diseases are familial, or genetic, in origin. More than 50 mutations have been identified in the prion gene, *Prnp*, on chromosome 20. Genetic prion diseases are all autosomal dominant and have been divided into three forms based on their clinical–pathological phenotype: familial Creutzfeldt–Jakob disease (fCJD), Gerstmann–Sträussler–Scheinker syndrome (GSS), and fatal familial insomnia (FFI). Genetic forms of prion disease differ from sporadic CJD (sCJD) in that they tend to have much longer duration. Median survival in sCJD is approximately 7–8 months, with 90% of patients living less than 1 year, whereas disease duration can be years in genetic prion diseases. In genetic prion diseases, the mutation causes the nascent prion protein to become more susceptible to changing conformation to an abnormal shaped (disease-causing) protein. It is not clear when during life this transformation of protein shape occurs, but presumably it is in adulthood, shortly before symptom onset.

All forms of familial prion diseases can have varied presentations, sometimes even within a family. fCJD can present identically to sCJD, with rapid onset and progression of cognitive, motor, and behavioral symptoms, and death occurring after just a few months. fCJD can also present more slowly, lasting years with dementia, parkinsonism, and/or ataxia. Patients with GSS typically have onset in their 40s or 50s, with either parkinsonism or ataxia; even within the same family, one family member may have a parkinsonian disorder, while another an ataxic disorder with minimal parkinsonism. GSS can also rarely present as a spastic paraparetic disorder. FFI, an exceedingly rare prion disorder, is characterized by insomnia and dysautonomia, leading to dementia. Psychiatric symptoms are also common (Kong et al., 2004).

Cognitive features of prion diseases are incredibly varied, depending upon where the prions are accumulating in the brain. Cognitive dysfunction in genetic prion diseases often seems to be due to disruption of frontal–subcortical circuits—particularly connections of the basal ganglia with the frontal lobes. Patients often have frontal–executive deficits. Psychiatric and behavioral problems are common and often the first symptoms. In fact, some recently identified genetic prion diseases were initially mistaken for Huntington's disease, due to onset of an adult psychiatric or behavioral disturbance, followed by neurological problems and dementia (Laplanche et al., 1999; Moore et al., 2001). Unless aphasia is an early or presenting symptom, language function may be spared in many cases until later stages of the disease (M. Geschwind, unpublished data).

In animal models of prion disease, the prions appear to spread from the thalamus to the cortex along thalamic–cortical fibers. However, in these animal models, prions are inoculated into the peritoneum or the thalamus, thus making it likely that prions would affect the subcortical structures first as they spread to the cortex. In human forms, it is difficult to know whether prions first accumulate in the cortex and then spread to subcortical structures. On diffusion-weighted imaging (DWI), it is more common initially to see the cortex involved than the basal ganglia and/or thalamus. If solely the cortex is involved initially on MRI, when patients are followed serially, eventually the basal ganglia and/or thalamus become involved (M. Geschwind, 2006; Shiga et al., 2004; Young et al., 2005). These data suggest that prions often accumulate first in the cortex, followed later by involvement of subcortical structures such as the basal ganglia and thalamus.

## Triplet-Repeat Neurodegenerative Diseases

### Huntington's Disease

Huntington's disease (HD) is an autosomal dominant, genetic neurodegenerative condition typically characterized by a hyperkinetic, ataxic movement disorder with prominent psychiatric and cognitive features. Frontal lobe dysfunction is a key feature of HD. Prominent motor symptoms include chorea, ataxia, and dystonia. Onset of motor symptoms typically occurs from ages 30–50. Psychiatric and subtle cognitive symptoms often occur before obvious motor dysfunction (Paulsen, Ready, Hamilton, Mega, & Cummings, 2001). In rare, juvenile-onset cases, patients often present with a parkinsonian rather than a choreoform disorder. Many patients have a known family history of HD; however, sometimes patients are not aware of their family history (Gusella & MacDonald, 1995).

There is a great deal of literature regarding frontal lobe involvement, both clinically and pathologically, in HD. One theory as to why there is so much frontal cortical dysfunction in HD is that caudate degeneration leads to loss of activity and eventually degeneration of cortical–thalamic–striatal connections, ultimately leading to atrophy of the frontal cortex (Selemon, Rajkowska, & Goldman-Rakic, 2004). Significantly increased numbers of mitochondrial DNA deletions have been found in the frontal and temporal lobes of patients with HD (Horton et al., 1995).

The gene for HD on chromosome 4, coding for the protein huntingtin, was identified in 1993, and genetic testing is now widely available (Huntington's Disease Collaborative Research Group, 1993). HD is part of a family of neurological diseases called triplet repeat diseases, caused by an increased number of repeats of three nucleotides, or a codon, in a gene. In HD, mutations are due to an excessive number of repeats of a CAG codon, which codes for glutamine. Hence, HD is often referred to as a "polyglutamine" disease. The *huntingtin* gene normally has a polyglutamine region with typically about 15 CAG repeats; a normal variation of this repeat number is typically between 9 and 36. Repeats of 37 or greater CAGs result in HD, although rarely patients with a CAG repeat of 37 may not develop symptoms. Another interesting phenomenon of triple repeat diseases is "anticipation":

expansion to a longer repeat length, causing earlier onset of the disease. For example, juvenile-onset cases may have repeats approaching 100 or greater. For reasons that are not entirely known, anticipation occurs more commonly in paternal than in maternal transmission (Gusella & MacDonald, 1995; Zuhlke, Riess, Bockel, Lange, & Thies, 1993).

Clinical diagnosis of HD is based on a constellation of symptoms, including clumsiness, chorea, ataxia, and psychiatric or behavioral disturbance. MRI typically reveals atrophy of the caudate, resulting in a "boxcar" appearance of the frontal horns of the lateral ventricles. Genetic testing confirms the diagnosis. Some other conditions to consider in the differential include Huntington disease–like 2 (Holmes et al., 2001), neuroacanthocytosis (Danek, Tison, et al., 2001), McLeod's chorea acanthocytosis (Danek, Rubio, et al., 2001; Walker et al., 2003), spinocerebellar ataxias (SCAs), Wilson's disease, prion disease (Moore et al., 2001), and other causes of ataxia. Because HD is an autosomal dominant disorder, identification of a mutation has profound repercussions for the patient and biologically related relatives. (See the section "Genetic Testing and Counseling.")

### HD-Like 2

HD-Like 2 is an adult-onset autosomal dominant, neurodegenerative disorder characterized by a progressive hyperkinetic movement disorder, dementia, and psychiatric features. The disease is very similar to HD but is caused by a *CTG/CAG* mutation expansion in chromosome 16q24.3 in the gene coding for junctophilin-3. The range of normal and abnormal repeats is similar to those for HD. Pathology is similar to HD, with striatal and cortical atrophy with intranuclear inclusions. This disease has been found almost exclusively in African Americans (Bauer et al., 2002; Margolis, Rudnicki, & Holmes, 2005).

### Spinocerebellar Ataxias

SCAs are a heterogeneous group of neurological disorders with varied clinical presentation and genetic etiology. Approximately 25 SCAs have been described as of 2005. Genes have been identified for the majority and are generally due to increased number of triplet repeats.

The clinical presentations of SCAs are varied but often include motor, psychiatric, and cognitive impairment (Manto, 2005). Patients typically present with a gradual-onset cerebellar disorder. Psychiatric and cognitive features are quite common, and patients often exhibit frontal executive dysfunction. It is suspected that frontal deficits are due to disruption of connections between the cerebellum and frontal lobes (Manto, 2005). SCAs with prominent frontal executive cognitive impairment include SCA 1, 2, 3 (Burk et al., 2003), 6 (Globas et al., 2003), 17 (Manto, 2005), and 19 (Schelhaas et al., 2003). Additional symptoms can include extrapyramidal disorders, peripheral neuropathy, and seizures (Manto, 2005). Most SCAs have adult onset, although some, such as SCA 13, have childhood onset (Manto, 2005; Stevanin, Durr, Benammar, & Brice, 2005).

Currently, there are no cures for SCAs. Treatment remains symptomatic. The list of conditions with similar presentations to the SCAs is large. Autosomal dominant disorders may include HD, dentatorubropallidoluysian atrophy (DRPLA), episodic ataxias (EAs), hereditary spastic paraplegias (HSPs), and prion diseases, to name a few. Some other conditions to consider in the differential include fragile X syndrome, fragile X–associated tremor–ataxia syndrome (FXTAS), leukodystrophies, mitochondrial diseases, Friedreich's ataxia (Manto, 2005) and multiple-system atrophy (MSA). MRI shows three distinct patterns: pure cerebellar atrophy, olivopontocerebellar atrophy, or global brain atrophy (Manto, 2005).

### Dentatorubropallidoluysian Atrophy

DRPLA is a rare, autosomal recessive disorder characterized in adults by chorea, ataxia, behavioral changes, and dementia. Onset of DRPLA is typically in the 20s or 30s but can occur in infancy through late adulthood. With onset before age 20, presenting symptoms typically differ from those of adults and include progressive seizures, myoclonus, and progressive cognitive decline. Cognitive and behavioral dysfunction is quite common in DRPLA, possibly due to disturbance of white matter tracks involving frontal–subcortical circuits. Behavioral or psychiatric disturbance, including psychosis, may be the presenting symptoms (Naito & Oyanagi, 1982).

Like HD, DPRLA is a polyglutamine triplet repeat disease. The gene involved in DRPLA on chromosome 12 is called *ATN-1*, coding for the protein atrophin-1, and typically has 6–25 CAG repeats; in DRPLA, CAG repeat lengths of 48–93 cause disease. Significant anticipation is common. The disease is mostly commonly found in Japan, where "mutable normal alleles" (CAG repeat lengths of 20–35) are common. Although mutable normal alleles are not disease causing, this repeat number can through anticipation expand in the next generation to ≥ 48 repeats, thereby causing disease (Ikeuchi et al., 1995; Nagafuchi, Yanagisawa, Ohsaki, et al., 1994; Nagafuchi, Yanagisawa, Sato, et al., 1994; Naito & Oyanagi, 1982; Neumann, 1959; Smith, Gonda, & Malamud, 1958).

Clinical diagnosis is suspected with onset of an ataxic, choreiform, and cognitive and/or behavioral disorder after age 20 or so. Diagnosis can be difficult due to varied clinical presentation, even within genetic subtypes. Additionally, there is considerable phenotypic overlap with the SCAs. Several years after onset of clinical symptoms, MRI may show significant white matter T2 hyperintensities and cerebellar atrophy (Koide et al., 1997).

## Metabolic Diseases

### McLeod Neuroacanthocytosis Syndrome

Neuroacanthocytosis is an X-linked disorder involving the hematological, neuromuscular, and central nervous systems. Men often have a progressive neurological disorder with features overlapping HD with chorea, psychiatric symptoms (psychosis), and cognitive decline. Women carriers rarely manifest symptoms. Neuropathy and myopathy may be very mild or subclinical. Seizures can occur. Cognitive testing often reveal deficits in working memory and frontal lobe dysfunction (Danek, Tierney, Sheesley, & Grafman, 2001). Blood analysis reveals McLeod phenotype, red blood cell acanthocytes (erythrocytes with multiple protrusions) and compensated hemolysis (hemolysis without anemia). Appropriate testing must be done to identify acanthocytes properly (Jung, Danek, & Dobson-Stone, 2004). Cardiomyopathy is common. Age of onset range is 25–57 years, with chorea occurring in the fifth or sixth decade (Danek, Rubio, et al., 2001).

Clinical diagnosis can be made based on the constellation of symptoms in conjunction with various laboratory testing. Creatine kinase (CK) may be slightly elevated. Electromyographic nerve conduction studies (EMG/NCS) may reveal a mild sensorimotor axonal neuropathy. MRI often shows caudate and putaminal atrophy (Danek, Rubio, et al., 2001). In a few cases, mild T2-weighted and fluid-attenuated inversion recovery (FLAIR) white matter hyperintensities have also been reported (Danek, Rubio, et al., 2001; Nicholl et al., 2004). FDG-PET ([$^{18}$F]b-fluoro-2-deoxy-glucose) imaging may reveal caudate or frontal hypometabolism, even before a clinically evident movement disorder (Danek, Tison, et al., 2001).

The disease is caused by a mutation in the *XK* gene encoding for the protein KX found in erythrocytes. KX normally forms a complex with the endothelin-3–processing Kell protein in erythrocytes and brain cells (Danek, Rubio, et al., 2001).

Other neurological diseases that may also show acanthocytes include abetalipoproteinemia (Bassen–Kornszweig syndrome), autosomal recessive neuroacanthocytoses, and partothenate kinase-associated neurodegeneration (PKAN) (Danek, Rubio, et al., 2001).

## Autosomal Recessive Choreoacanthocytosis

Choreoacanthocytosis, an autosomal recessive disorder, is genetically distinct from but has significant clinical overlap with McLeod neuroacanthocytosis. Choreoacanthocytosis is due to a mutation in the *CHAC* gene on chromosome 9q21, encoding the chorein protein, which is involved in intracellular protein sorting. Symptoms include chorea often involving the face/buccal area and parkinsonism. Both forms of acanthocytosis may show neuromuscular involvement with abnormal EMG/NCS and elevated CKs. Oculomotor abnormalities, such as progressive supranuclear palsy and eyelid opening apraxia, have been found. Seizures are more common than for McLeod neuroacanthocytosis, and cardiomyopathy does not generally occur. MRI shows caudate, putaminal, as well as substantia nigra atrophy (Danek, Tison, et al., 2001). Cognitive testing may reveal deficits in memory, visuoconstruction, and verbal

fluency, whereas some patients have problems in tasks of frontal–executive function (Danek, Tierney, et al., 2001).

## Wilson's Disease (Hepatolenticular Degeneration)

Wilson's disease is an autosomal recessive disorder of copper (Cu) metabolism due to a mutation on chromosome 13, causing increased absorption of Cu in ceruloplasmin and decreased biliary Cu excretion. Onset is usually in infancy, with peak onset in the late teens, but several patients with onset as late as their 50s have been reported (Danks, Metz, Sewell, & Prewett, 1990; Gow et al., 2000; Ross, Jacobson, Dienstag, & Martin, 1985). Most common symptoms are liver and central nervous system (CNS) dysfunction (Kinnear Wilson, 1912). Psychiatric features, including intellectual deterioration, behavioral disturbances, and psychoses, are common. The most frequent presenting neurological motor symptoms include dysarthria and loss of coordination. Cognitive function is reportedly normal in asymptomatic patients, whereas patients with neurological involvement have problems with frontal–executive ability, memory, and visuospatial processing (Seniow, Bak, Gajda, Poniatowska, & Czlonkowska, 2002). Oculomotor problems occur frequently. Involuntary movements, such as dystonia, tremor, and titubation, can occur. Deposition of Cu within Descemet's membrane at the limbus of the cornea causes Kayser–Fleischer (KF) rings, which are rarely visible with the naked eye but can be seen with the ophthalmoscope, and always by slit lamp. KF rings are present in virtually all patients with neurological disease. Lab findings include greatly reduced serum ceruloplasmin, low serum Cu (this reflects total Cu; because ceruloplasmin is not carrying it, the amount is decreased), increased free Cu, increased urine Cu (100–1,000 mcg/24 hours, whereas normal adults excrete less than 40 mcg/24 hours). Occasionally, these lab studies may be normal, and if the diagnosis is strongly suspected, the gold standard is liver biopsy.

T1-weighted MRI reveals cortical and brainstem atrophy (which, remarkably, may be reversible with treatment) and hypodensity in the lenticular, thalamic, and caudate nuclei. T2-weighted MRI may show hyperintensity of white matter tracks and basal ganglia (rarely hyperintense in basal ganglia) (Alanen, Komu,

Penttinen, & Leino, 1999; van Wassenaer-van Hall, van den Heuvel, Jansen, Hoogenraad, & Mali, 1995). DWI MRI often shows abnormality in the basal ganglia consistent with either vasogenic or cytotoxic edema (Sener, 2003). Treatment is highly effective and includes a low-copper diet (avoids liver, nuts, chocolate, coffee, and shellfish [especially lobster]), copper chelators (trientine, D-penicillamine, and others), zinc, and albumin infusions for acute treatment. D-Penicillamine should be avoided in patients presenting with neurological symptoms due to risk of worsening symptoms (Brewer, 2005; Brewer & Askari, 2005).

### Pantothenate Kinase–Associated Neurodegeneration (Hallervorden–Spatz Disease)

This condition, formerly eponymously referred to as Hallervorden–Spatz disease, was recently found, in most cases, to be due to mutations in the pantothenate kinase gene (PANK2). This enzyme catalyzes the first step in coenzyme A synthesis. The PANK2 gene is found in brain mitochondria. Mutations lead to abnormal neuronal mitochondrial lipid metabolism. PANK2 has been divided into two phenotypes—an early-onset, rapidly progressive (classic) form and a later-onset, slowly progressive (atypical) form. The atypical form has onset in the second to third decade, with speech problems, neuropsychiatric issues, corticospinal tract involvement, and an extrapyramidal disorder characterized by dystonia, dysarthria, and rigidity. Due to deposition of iron in the basal ganglia, T2-weighted MRI often reveals the classic "eye of the tiger" sign (Hayflick et al., 2003).

### Gaucher's Disease—Type 3

Gaucher's disease is a relatively common lipid storage disease. It may present at any age, and clinical severity ranges from a lethal perinatal form to an asymptomatic form. It has been subdivided into at least three major clinical subtypes: types 1, 2, and 3. Type 1 affects bone and other organ systems, but spares the CNS. Types 2 and 3 are predominantly neurological disorders that likely represent a spectrum of a single disorder. Type 2, generally referred to as the acute and fatal or infantile form beginning before age 2, often lacks bone involvement. Type 3, the subacute or juvenile form, typically occurs after age 2 and is more slowly progres-

sive, with patients often living into their third or fourth decade. Types 2 and 3 primarily affect the nervous system but often have hepatosplenomegaly, anemia, thrombocytopenia, and/or skeletal involvement. The main neurological findings are bulbar signs, pyramidal signs, oculomotor apraxia, ataxia, seizures, and dementia later in the disease course. All forms are due to autosomal recessive mutations in the gene for beta-glucocerebrosidase and subsequent decreased activity in this enzyme, resulting in the accumulation of the glycolipid glucocerebroside in the lysosomes of macrophages. These lipid-laden macrophages are also called "Gaucher's cells" (Altarescu et al., 2001; Pastores, 2000). Gaucher's disease may be mistaken for PSP due to limitation of gaze (Patterson et al., 1993). Mutations in glucocerebrosidase, even in heterozygotes, have been linked to increased risk of developing parkinsonism (Aharon-Peretz, Rosenbaum, & Gershoni-Baruch, 2004; Sidransky, 2005). MRI may only show mild cerebral atrophy (Pastores, 2000). Clinical findings alone are not diagnostic. Diagnosis is made by showing Gaucher's cells on bone biopsy and decreased β-glucocerebrosidase activity in white cells; clinical genetic testing for the more common mutations in the glucocerebrosidase gene on chromosome 1q21 is available (Altarescu et al., 2001; Pastores, 2000). Type 1 is especially common among the Ashkenazi Jewish population.

### Adult Neuronal Ceroid Lipofuscinosis (Kufs' Disease)

Neuronal ceroid lipofuscinoses (NCLs) are a group of lysosomal storage diseases with varying ages of onset. There are three forms: I (infantile), II (juvenile or Batten's disease), and III (adult or Kufs' disease). Here we only discuss the adult-onset form, adult neuronal ceroid lipofuscinosis (ANCL), which comprises 10% of all NCLs. Most cases are due to autosomal recessive inheritance, although rare cases of autosomal dominant inheritance have been reported. Age of onset varies from the third decade to the seventh, but typically begins in the fourth decade and lasts for about 10 years (Nardocci et al., 1995). Presentation is variable in Kufs' disease, although initial clinical symptoms are often behavioral or psychiatric. Some researchers have classified ANCL into two predominant clinical presentations: Type A, with progressive myoclonic epilepsy, dementia, and ataxia, followed later by pyramidal and extrapyramidal (parkinsonism) symptoms (and sometimes photosensitivity), and Type B, with prominent behavioral problems and dementia, which may be associated with motor decline, ataxia, and extrapyramidal and bulbar problems (Constantinidis, Wisniewski, & Wisniewski, 1992; Wisniewski, 2001). All patients with ANCL eventually develop dementia, ataxia, and motor signs. The dementia often involves subcortical–frontal circuits (Hinkebein & Callahan, 1997). Many patients develop seizures, often myoclonic in type. Movement disorders may include chorea, dystonia, ataxia, and spasticity (Hinkebein & Callahan, 1997). MRI findings are generally nonspecific but often reveal cerebral and cerebellar atrophy within a few years of onset (Nardocci et al., 1995; Wisniewski, 2001). White matter lesions and basal ganglia iron deposition, although uncommon, have also been reported (Hammersen, Brock, & Cervos-Navarro, 1998; Schreiner, Becker, & Wiegand, 2000; Tomiyasu et al., 2000).

The diagnosis of ANCL is based on clinical and pathological findings, whereas some of the other forms can also be diagnosed by enzymatic assay and molecular genetic testing. Ultrastructural (electron microscopic) studies must be performed to confirm the presence and nature of lysosomal storage material (fingerprint or curvilinear profiles, or granular osmiophilic deposits) in blood or punch biopsies (e.g., skin, rectal, eccrine sweat glands, or conjunctiva); if positive, then enzyme and genetic testing can be pursued (Nardocci et al., 1995; Schreiner et al., 2000). The genes for ANCL have not yet been identified (Wisniewski, 2001). Some other diseases to consider in the differential would include MLD, HD, Wilson's disease, progressive myoclonic epilepsy, and early-onset dementia with Lewy bodies (Nardocci et al., 1995).

### Niemann–Pick Disease—Type C

Niemann–Pick disease—type C is an autosomal recessive disorder of cholesterol metabolism (lipid storage disease) that presents in infants, children, and adults. Niemann–Pick type C is caused by a mutation to either of the *NPC1* or *NPC2* genes involved in intracellular cycling of sterols, leading to an accumulation of cholesterol in neurons, and resulting in axonal and neuronal loss in the corpus callo-

sum, cerebellum, and hippocampus. The classic presentation in childhood often involves insidious onset of cognitive decline, ataxia, and vertical supranuclear ophthalmoplegia (Patterson et al., 1993). Psychiatric features, including a schizophrenia-like illness, can begin several years before the onset of other symptoms. Adults typically have slower progression and begin with psychiatric symptoms or dementia, often followed by ataxia and splenomegally. Other common neurological features include dysarthria and dystonia. Vertical supranuclear ophthalmoplegia is often absent in adults (Shulman, David, & Weiner, 1995). MRI is often normal until late stages, when there is general cerebral atrophy. A few cases have revealed frontal lobe atrophy (Klunemann et al., 2002). An adult case with white matter changes mimicking multiple sclerosis has been reported (Grau et al., 1997). Magnetic resonance spectroscopy (MRS) shows abnormalities primarily in the frontal lobes and centrum semiovale, but also in the parietal cortex and caudate (Tedeschi et al., 1998). Frontal lobe hypoperfusion can be seen on single-photon emission computed tomography (SPECT).

Definitive diagnosis can be made by identifying abnormal intracellular cholesterol metabolism (decreased cholesterol esterification and filipin staining) in cultured fibroblasts. Bone marrow aspirate may show so-called "sea blue" histiocytes (Klunemann et al., 2002; Shulman et al., 1995).

### Adult GM2 Gangliosidoses: Hexosaminidase A Deficiency

Hexosaminidase A deficiency, also called Tay–Sachs disease, causes a group of neurodegenerative disorders due to intralysosomal storage of glycosphingolipid GM2 ganglioside. Hexosaminidase A deficiencies are autosomal recessive and are classified into infantile, juvenile, chronic, and adult-onset forms. The infantile form is a relentlessly progressive neurodegenerative disease with onset between 3 and 6 months of age, and death typically by age 4. Late-onset hexosaminidase A deficiencies have slower progression and more variable presentation than earlier-onset forms. Patients with adult-onset disease may have progressive dystonia, spinocerebellar degeneration, motor neuron disease, which may mimic amyotrophic lateral sclerosis (ALS), and/or psychosis. At least 30% of patients develop psychiatric disturbance (bipolar disorder, psychosis, agitation, disorganized thought, delusions, hallucinations, paranoia) without dementia (Kaback, 1999; Navon, Argov, & Frisch, 1986). In the adult form, MRI reveals only severe cerebellar atrophy (Grosso et al., 2003; Neudorfer et al., 2005). Pathology shows accumulation of glycolipid in neurons of the hippocampus, brainstem, and spinal cord. The cortex is remarkably spared, in contrast with the infantile and juvenile forms (Grosso et al., 2003).

Laboratory diagnosis is made by showing decreased activity of hexosaminidase A levels in white cells. The disease is caused by a mutation in the *HEXA* gene that encodes the α-chain of the heterodimeric protein, β-hexosaminidase A (HEX A); HEX A is also called GM2 gangliosidase. Younger onset, more severe forms are due to mutations that cause absence of *HEXA*, whereas older forms are due to mutations that result in a severe deficiency. A high proportion of patients are of Ashkenazi Jewish or French Canadian heritage. Adult patients often have muscle wasting, weakness, and fasciculations (Kaback, 1999). This disorder should be considered in adults with late-onset psychoses, particularly those with a family history of neuromuscular symptoms or late-onset psychiatric disease (Kaback, 1999; Navon et al., 1986). Other disorders, particularly with neuromuscular involvement, in the differential might include ALS, Friedreich ataxia, spinal muscular atrophy, and Kufs' disease (Kaback, 1999; Navon et al., 1986).

## WHITE MATTER DISEASES

### Adult Polyglucosan Body Disease

Adult polyglucosan body disease (APBD) is a rare, adult-onset, glycogen storage disease of the central and peripheral nervous systems typically characterized by a quadrad of urinary incontinence, gait disorder, length-dependent peripheral neuropathy, and eventually dementia. Other symptoms may include upper motor neuron signs, cardiomyopathy, cerebellar ataxia, and extrapyramidal symptoms. Although the etiology of APBD is likely heterogeneous, most cases of APBD are probably due to a deficiency of glycogen-branching enzyme (GBE), which is critical in the branching of glycogen (Bruno et al., 1993). In the majority of cases, autosomal recessive mutations have been iden-

tified in the gene encoding for GBE (Klein et al., 2004). The most common mutation, a tyrosine to serine substitution at codon 329, is more common among Ashkenazi Jews (Lossos et al., 1991, 1998). Patients often start with urinary incontinence, followed by a gait disorder, then neuropathy, and eventually cognitive impairment. The disease typically progresses slowly over many years (Okamoto, Llena, & Hirano, 1982; Peress, DiMauro, & Roxburgh, 1979; Robitaille, Carpenter, Karpati, & DiMauro, 1980; Suzuki, David, & Kutschman, 1971).

Although cognitive deficits are common in APBD, unfortunately, they have generally not been well-documented or reported. When cognitive impairment occurs, memory is almost always affected (Boulan-Predseil et al., 1995; Peress et al., 1979; Rifai et al., 1994; Stam, Wigboldus, & Bots, 1980; Suzuki et al., 1971). The dementia is often due a combination of cortical and subcortical features (Rifai et al., 1994). Some patients have amnestic disorders with relative sparing of other cognitive domains. Others may present with more isolated frontal executive dysfunction (Boulan-Predseil et al., 1995).

Clinical diagnosis of APBD can be difficult, because it can be mistaken for many other conditions. The constellation of clinical findings, including a combination of urinary incontinence, neuropathy, gait disorder, and/or cognitive impairment, should make physicians consider APBD in their differential. Brain MRI often shows a leukoencephalopathy and cortical atrophy (Berkhoff, Weis, Schroth, & Sturzenegger, 2001; Boulan-Predseil et al., 1995). Basal ganglia T2 hyperintensities have also been reported (Rifai et al., 1994). Spinal cord atrophy is commonly seen on MRI (Berkhoff et al., 2001). Nerve conduction studies may show evidence of a neuropathy, often length dependent, with greater motor than sensory involvement. Levels of GBE, typically measured in cultured skin fibroblasts, are reduced. Premortem pathological diagnosis is made by identifying polyglucosan bodies on biopsy of sural nerve, axilla skin (Milde, Guccion, Kelly, Locatelli, & Jones, 2001), or rarely, the brain (Boulan-Predseil et al., 1995). Genetic diagnosis can be made by identifying mutations in the gene for GBE in blood leukocytes (Lossos et al., 1998). At postmortem, autopsy will identify extensive polyglucosan bodies in the brain and peripheral nerves.

It is not known why the nervous system is preferentially affected in APBD, whereas in other, related disorders of GBE, other organs such as liver and heart may be more affected. For example, glycogen storage disease (GSD)—type IV (Andersen's disease), an autosomal recessive disease involving deficiency of the same GBE enzyme, manifests in infancy with various systemic manifestations. It is not known why the same enzyme deficiency and, in some cases, even the same *GBE* gene mutation, presents so differently in APBD (Ziemssen et al., 2000). This may possibly be due to other, unidentified modifier genes. In more severely affected, younger patients the disease may be due to a complete absence of GBE (Schroder, May, Shin, Sigmund, & Nase-Huppmeier, 1993). Unfortunately, at present no treatments are available for APBD. A potential mouse model has been developed and could be an important step toward potential cures (Raben et al., 2001).

### Krabbe's Disease (Globoid Cell Leukodystrophy)

Krabbe's disease is an autosomal recessive genetic disorder caused by a mutation in the *GALC* gene encoding for galactocerebrosidase. About 85–90% of cases occur in infants, with about 10–15% of cases occurring in older children and, rarely, adults up to their 40s. Later-onset forms tend to be more slowly progressive, with weakness, vision loss due to optic atrophy, painful neuropathy, and, in many but not all cases, cognitive decline (Kolodny, Raghavan, & Krivit, 1991; Wenger & Coppola, 2000). Late-onset and adult forms of Krabbe's disease are generally due to mutations at the 5' end of the gene, versus early-onset, more severe forms being associated with mutations at the 3' end (Jardim et al., 1999).

Brain MRI often reveals evidence of a demyelinating disease, predominantly a posterior leukoencephalopathy, although more diffuse involvement, including the frontal white matter, can sometimes occur. There is often involvement of brainstem, cerebellum, and even subcortical white matter. Over time there is global cerebral atrophy (Jardim et al., 1999; Wenger & Coppola, 2000). One family with adult-onset Krabbe's disease presenting as a spastic paraplegia had apparently normal MRIs (Bajaj, Waldman, Orrell, Wood, & Bhatia, 2002). Definitive diagnosis is made by finding 0–5% of normal activity of galacto-cerebrosidase in blood leukocytes or cultured skin fibroblasts (Jardim et al., 1999; Kolodny et al., 1991).

### Pelizaeus–Merzbacher Disease/ Spastic Paraplegia 2

Pelizaeus–Merzbacher disease (PMD) and spastic paraplegia 2 (SPG2) are X-linked recessive allelic disorders due to mutations in the gene for proteolipid protein 1 (*PLP1*), which is involved in myelin formation. Depending on the mutation, the illness can present along a spectrum between PMD and SPG2 (Warshawsky, Rudick, Staugaitis, & Natowicz, 2005). PMD usually presents in infancy or childhood, with nystagmus, hypotonia, and severe developmental delay. SPG2 is typically a less severe form of the disorder, with spastic paraparesis, ataxia, demyelinating peripheral neuropathy, and cognitive deficits, including dementia, as the major features. Autonomic dysfunction and ataxia also occur. Extrapyramidal signs are a rare feature (Garbern, Krajewski, & Hobson, 1999). As in most X-linked recessive disorders, women are typically unaffected; however, possibly due to X-inactivation, carriers from families with severely affected males are generally not affected, whereas carriers from families with mildly affected males are usually affected. A reported case described an adult carrier around 40 years old, with a 10-year illness consistent with primary progressive multiple sclerosis, with a progressive spastic gait disorder, dysarthria, and nocturia, who was found to have a novel *PLP1* mutation. Unfortunately, the patient's cognitive status was not discussed (Warshawsky et al., 2005).

Most cases of PMD reveal a diffuse leukoencephalopathy on T2-weighted MRI, involving white matter of the cerebral hemispheres, cerebellum, and brainstem. SPG2 may have milder MRI findings or show diffuse leukoencephalopathy. Molecular diagnostic testing is available (Garbern et al., 1999).

### Vanishing White Matter Disease/Childhood Ataxia with Central Nervous System Hypomyelination

Vanishing white matter disease (VWMD) is an illness characterized by ataxia, spasticity, and variable optic atrophy that occurs in several forms, including a rare adult form. Early-onset forms tend to be very rapid, leading to death. Adult-onset forms tend to be milder, with behavioral problems in adolescence and slow cognitive decline; initial motor and cognitive development may be normal or delayed. Eventually there is the gradual onset of ataxia, spasticity, and pyramidal signs. In all phenotypes, progression can be accelerated by trauma or other illness. Regardless of severity, brain MRI reveals a diffuse leukoencephalopathy involving U-fibers and cerebellar vermian atrophy. Definitive genetic diagnosis can be made by identification of a mutation in one of the five causative genes encoding the five subunits of the eukaryotic translation initiation factor, eIF2B (Schiffmann, Fogli, Van der Knaap, & Boespflug-Tanguy, 2003).

## X-Linked Adrenoleukodystrophy/ Adrenomyeloneuropathy

Classical X-linked adrenoleukodystrophy (X-ALD) is a perixosomal disease largely affecting the white matter and adrenal glands. It comes in three phenotypes: childhood, adrenomyeloneuropathy, and "Addison's disease only." The childhood form usually presents in boys with symptoms that include behavioral difficulties, progressive decline in vision, hearing, and motor function, and complete disability within 2 years of disease onset. The adult-onset form of X-ALD, called adrenomyeloneuropathy (AMN), has a typical age of onset in the second or third decade. Typical symptoms of AMN include progressive spastic paraparesis, difficulties with sphincter control, and sexual dysfunction. The disorder affects primarily males; however, approximately 20% of carrier females are affected, typically with spastic paraparesis, albeit of later onset (after age 35) and a milder course. Approximately 70% of patients with AMN have involvement of the adrenal gland, requiring replacement therapy. Between 10 and 20% of patients develop progressive behavioral disturbance and dementia. MRI of the brain typically shows symmetric T2 and FLAIR signal hyperintensity in the parietal–occipital regions, often with enhancement at the margins, and involvement of cortical U-fibers. Clinical diagnosis is made by identifying elevated plasma very long-chain fatty acid (VLCFA) levels in men. In women, VLCFAs can be measured in serum or skin fibroblasts. The clinical phenotype of X-ALD can vary greatly regardless of VLCFA levels, and even within a family. Adult men with X-ALD can present less commonly with other symptoms, such as headache, focal neurological deficits (hemiparesis, visual field deficits), behavioral problems, dementia, ataxia, and neurogenic bowel and bladder. Patients may not become symptomatic until middle age or later. Testing for mutations in the *ABCD1* gene can confirm the diagnosis in men and identify female carriers. Bone marrow transplant may be a treatment option for young patients with mild neurological disease. Lorenzo's oil, a mixture of various oils, can lower plasma levels of VLFCAs but does not stop or slow neurological decline. One large noncontrolled, prospective, observational study suggests that Lorenzo's oil in combination with dietary fat restriction can prevent the onset of neurological disease (Moser, Moser, Steinberg, & Raymond, 1999; Moser et al., 2005).

## Metachromatic Leukodystrophy

Metachromatic Leukodystrophy (MLD), an autosomal recessive lipid storage disease caused by a deficiency of the lysosomal enzyme arylsulfatase A (cerebroside sulfatase A), was first described in 1925. This deficiency leads to certain sulfatides not being cleaved and therefore accumulating in Schwann cells and oligodendrocytes. MLD occurs in two main forms, juvenile and adult, although there is also a less common, but more severe, infantile form. The term "metachromatic" is used because the lipid material accumulating in neurons and glia stains brown or gold with toluidine blue. MLD is a systemic disease involving multiple organs and the nervous system (von Figura, Gieselmann, & Jaeken, 2001). In the adult form, dementia develops between the third and fourth decade, although onset as late as age 63 has been reported (Bosch & Hart, 1978). Typical symptoms include progressive cognitive decline and neuropathy, as well as cortibobulbar, corticospinal, and cerebellar abnormalities. Behavioral symptoms often suggest frontal lobe involvement, with apathy, poor judgment, and disinhibition (Shapiro, Lockman, Knopman, & Krivit, 1994). Patients may present with psychiatric disease, including depression psychosis and other schizophrenic-like symptoms (Hyde, Ziegler, & Weinberger, 1992). Because MLD is a demyelinating disease, visual and somatosensory evoked potentials are delayed, and nerve conduction velocities are often markedly slowed.

Brain MRI usually reveals diffuse T2 hyperintensity in the white matter, particularly periventricular, and generalized atrophy. The white matter typically moves from anterior to posterior, initially sparing the connecting subcortical U-fibers. Life expectancy after onset is typically 10–20 years, although survival varies widely, from 1 to 44 years; survival has been reported into the seventh decade (Bosch & Hart, 1978; von Figura et al., 2001).

Diagnosis can be made by identifying decreased arylsulfatase A activity in tissues (skin fibroblasts and leukocytes) and elevated sulfatides in the urine (Marcao et al., 2005). Adult-onset cases of MLD may often be mistaken for multiple sclerosis, isolated neuropathy, or psychiatric disease.

### Adult-Onset Orthochromatic Leukodystrophy

Nonmetachromatic (orthochromatic) leukodystrophies (OLDs) are a heterogeneous group of disorders with no identified enzyme deficiency. Sudan red staining usually reveals lipid accumulation in macrophages (sudanophilic). They are often sporadic, but some families have been reported. They can be a pigmentary type of OLD associated with cerebellar ataxia and dementia or a form mimicking chronic multiple sclerosis (cerebellar ataxia, pyramidal dysfunction, disturbance of autonomic nervous system) and related to chromosome 5q31.7. A recent description of a new OLD, apparently dominantly inherited, included two family members (ages 57 and 38 at presentation) who developed dementia progressing to death over 2–3 years. One patient had severe frontal dysfunction on neuropsychological testing, with frontal and corpus callosal atrophy with minimal subcortical white matter changes on MRI; the other had a more diffuse cognitive pattern, with extensive white matter hypodensity on head computed tomography (CT). The histopathology revealed bilateral, symmetrical, demyelinating lesions with macrophages containing sudanophilic lipids. In both patients, cortical U–fibers were spared, and one patient had an unusual posterior predominance of the pathology (Letournel, Etcharry-Bouyx, Verny, Barthelaix, & Dubas, 2003).

### Fabry's Disease (Anderson–Fabry Disease)

Anderson–Fabry disease is an X-linked, recessive, lysosomal storage disease caused by a deficiency of the enzyme $\alpha$-galactosidase A, resulting in widespread accumulation of globo-triaosylceramide in various cells. The classical form of Fabry's disease typically presents in adolescent (or younger) males with acroparesthesias (crises of severe extremity pain), angiokeratomas, hypohidrosis, and corneal/lenticular opacities. Renal failure, cardiac (cardiomyopathy) and cerebrovascular disease occur during the third to fifth decades. Patients may develop vascular dementia as a consequence of cerebrovascular disease, and in rare cases this may be the presenting symptom. Manifestations of CNS dysfunction are due in most part to multifocal small vessel involvement, and include thrombosis, transient ischemic attacks (TIAs), basilar artery ischemia, seizures, hemiplegia, aphasia, and cerebral hemorrhage. Involvement of the gastrointestinal and pulmonary systems is also common.

Brain MRI may reveal asymmetric, widespread, deep white matter T2-weighted hyperintensities predominantly in frontal and parietal lobes. When neurological involvement is present, MRI findings may suggest multiple sclerosis or vascular dementia. Diagnosis is made by assaying for levels of the enzyme in plasma, white cells, or fibroblasts. The disease should be considered in men under the age of 65 with vascular dementia (Mendez, Stanley, Medel, Li, & Tedesco, 1997). Enzyme replacement therapy is now available in Europe and is being tested in the United States through the National Institutes of Health (Mehta, 2002).

## MIXED GRAY AND WHITE MATTER DISEASES

### Cerebral Autosomal Dominant Arteriopathy with Subcortical Infarcts and Leukoencephalopathy

Cerebral autosomal dominant arteriopathy with subcortical infarcts and leukoencephalopathy (CADASIL) is an autosomal dominant disease causing problems with the small arteries in the brain, resulting in subcortical strokes. Patients with CADASIL typically develop symptoms between their 30s to 50s and then progress over several years. About 30–40% of patients have migraine headaches (often with auras), which are often an early feature of the disease. Migraines may be complicated with focal neurological signs. As the name implies, patients with CADASIL eventually develop leukoencephalopathy due to recurrent ischemia. Most patients will have TIAs, and all patients eventually have strokes, often in midadulthood, leading to dementia and pseudobulbar palsy, and eventually significant neurological debilitation. Other neurological features include gait disturbance and pyramidal signs (Dichgans et al., 1998).

White matter abnormalities can be seen on MRI often before a patient with CADASIL becomes clinically symptomatic, and almost always by the age of 35 (Chabriat et al., 1998). MRI findings typically include symmetric, T2-weighted white matter hyperintensities, particularly in the frontal and temporal lobes (preferentially affecting periventricular areas), subinsular white matter, internal and external capsules, as well as the basal ganglia. Approximately 45% of patients have brainstem involvement. Lacunar infarcts are found in the white matter (particularly periventricular) and basal ganglia (Chabriat et al., 1998). Early on, MRI white matter lesions in CADASIL may be mistaken for multiple sclerosis.

CADASIL is caused by a mutation in the Notch3 gene on chromosome 19. Notch3, a transmembrane protein involved in developmental cell fate, has an intraceullar and an extracellular domain. Many disease-causing mutations have been identified in various regions of the gene; thus far, most involve cysteine residues in the epidermal-like growth factor 2 (EGF2) domains. It is not yet known precisely how mutations affect Notch3 function. Disease results from abnormalities in the wall of small vessels, although the precise mechanism is not fully elucidated. One key pathological hallmark of the disease is granular osmiophilic material (GOM) in the small-vessel walls in the skin and brain, as well as in other areas (Peters, Opherk, Bergmann, et al., 2005).

The white matter arteriopathy and resulting leukoencephalopathy and subcortical infarcts in CADASIL lead to mild cognitive impairment characterized by significant frontal–executive dysfunction, likely due to involvement of frontal–subcortical pathways eventually resulting over time in a vascular dementia syndrome. Patients' initial cognitive symptoms involve executive function, problems with attention, processing speed and verbal fluency, and other frontal lobe tasks (Dichgans et al., 2002; Peters, Opherk, Danek, et al., 2005). Even patients without dementia have subtle frontal lobe cognitive deficits that do not necessarily correlate with the amount of lesions on brain MRI (Taillia et al., 1998). There is evidence from one postmortem case that there may be a cholinergic deficit in CADASIL (Mesulam, Siddique, & Cohen, 2003).

Probable diagnosis of CADASIL is based on clinical history, symptoms, and MRI findings. Definitive diagnosis can be made by detection of a gene mutation or by skin biopsy that shows intimal loss, degeneration of vascular smooth muscle cells, and fibrosis. Misdiagnosis of CADASIL is common. Other common misdiagnoses include multiple sclerosis and Binswanger's syndrome. Due to often prominent psychiatric symptoms, particularly early in the disease, patients with CADASIL can present with depression and/or bipolar disease (Chabriat et al., 1998; Peters, Opherk, Danek, et al., 2005).

Curiously, the Notch3 gene in CADASIL is very close to another gene locus, 19p13, where mutations cause an overlapping neurological disorder, familial hemiplegic migraine (FHM). Like CADASIL, FHM is an autosomal dominant disorder characterized by migraines with hemiparesis; unlike patients with CADASIL, however, patients with FHM do not develop additional symptoms.

There is currently no cure for CADASIL; treatment is symptom-specific, with some preventive care, such as antiplatelet agents (e.g., aspirin). Research studies are under way to improve treatment and find a cure. Management of CADASIL involves and treatment of symptoms such as migraines.

## Alexander's Disease

Alexander's disease is an autosomal dominant disease due to mutation in the gene for glial fibrillary acid protein (GFAP), which is found in astrocytes. It typically presents in infancy or childhood with hydrocephalus, seizures, spastic quadraparesis, developmental delay, and death within 10 years of disease onset. Adult-onset forms of the disease with GFAP mutations have been identified. Neurological symptoms are highly variable, even within families, but are typically characterized by a combination of bulbar and pseudobulbar signs (palatal myoclonus, dysphagia, dysphonia, dysarthria), progressive spastic paraparesis, mild to moderate ataxia and other cerebellar signs, autonomic dysfunction (bladder dysfunction, constipation, orthostasis), sleep problems, and seizures (Namekawa et al., 2002; Stumpf et al., 2003). Most adult-onset patients with GFAP mutations have been reportedly cognitively normal, although it does not appear that cognitive function has been well studied (Okamoto et al., 2002).

Although MRI criteria have been established for the childhood form, the adult form may be more variable and less specific. The MRI in the childhood form of Alexander's disease reveals extensive white matter abnormalities with frontal lobe predominance, as well as involvement of gray matter structures, such as basal ganglia and thalami, and atrophy of the brainstem, optic tract, and fornix (van der Knaap et al., 2001). Adult-onset forms generally show significant medulla oblongata and spinal cord atrophy due to GFAP mutations, with sparing of the pons and some cerebellar atrophy. Some cases have diffuse white matter hyperintensities on T2-weighted MRI (Okamoto et al., 2002), but many do not have white matter involvement (Namekawa et al., 2002; Stumpf et al., 2003). Cerebrospinal fluid (CSF) may show mildly elevated protein. Diagnosis can be made by identification of mutations in the GFAP gene.

### Nasu–Hakola Disease (Polycystic Lipomembranous Osteodysplasia with Sclerosing Leukoencephalopathy)

The autosomal recessive Nasu–Hakola disease, or polycystic lipomembranous osteodysplasia with sclerosing leukoencephalopathy (PLOSL), usually presents by age 30 with fractures due to bone cysts, followed by a frontal dementia with upper motor neuron symptoms and seizures. Choreoathetosis or myoclonus may occur. Subtle memory deficits, often due to executive dysfunction, accompany personality changes; however, this remains mild until the last stage of the disease. Patients eventually progress to frank dementia (motor apraxia, aphasia, agraphia, acalculia), with immobility and death in their 40s. The disease is worldwide, but many cases have been reported in Japan and Finland (Montalbetti et al., 2004). Brain imaging shows progressive cerebral atrophy (mostly frontal), basal ganglia calcifications, and T2-hyperintensities, predominantly in the frontal white matter, sparing the arcuate fasciculis. Two different genes have been linked to this disease, *DAP12* on chromosome 19, and *TREM2* (Kondo et al., 2002; Paloneva et al., 2001; Soragna et al., 2003). Although an autosomal recessive disorder, heterozygotes for a *TREM2* mutation showed deficits in visuo-spatial memory and hypoperfusion of the basal ganglia on SPECT study (Montalbetti et al., 2005). This condition should be suspected in any patient with bone cysts and dementia or neuropsychiatric disease.

### Cerebrotendinous Xanthomatosis

Cerebrotendinous xanthomatosis (CTX) is an autosomal recessive, gradually progressive disorder with characteristic findings at various ages. Diarrhea occurs in infancy, cataracts in childhood, tendon xanthomas usually in adolescence or late teens, and neurological dysfunction in the 20s. The main neurological features include dementia; psychiatric disturbance; pyramidal, extrapyramidal, and cerebellar signs; and seizures. Dementia with slow deterioration tends to start in the second or third decades and affects over half of patients. The psychiatric disturbance is characterized by personality change, hallucinations, agitation, aggressive behavior, and depression. Pyramidal and/or cerebellar signs present in patients between 20 and 30 years of age. Peripheral neuropathy may rarely occur. MRI shows bilateral T2-wieghted hyperintensity of the dentate nuclei and focal cerebral and cerebellar white matter lesions. Diffuse cerebral and cerebellar atrophy appear later in the disease course. MRS often shows decreased *N*-acetylaspartate (NAA) and increased lactate signal in abnormal areas on MRI. Laboratory testing, such as elevated plasma cholesterol, elevated levels of urine and plasma bile alcohols, and related glycoconjugates, can help to differentiate between CTX and other disorders with xanthomas. Nerve biopsy reveals primary axonal degeneration and demyelination (Federico & Dotti, 2003).

### Mitochondrial Disorders

Mitochondrial disorders may present at any age and often have a prominent neurological, especially myopathic, component. The main neurological findings include ptosis, external ophthalmoplegia, sensorineural deafness, proximal myopathy, encephalopathy, seizures, dementia, migraine, stroke-like episodes, ataxia, and spasticity. Multiple organ systems are often involved, and the clinical presentation is markedly variable. Common nonneurological features of mitochondrial disease include cardiomyopathy, optic atrophy, pigmentary retinopathy, and diabetes. Despite the degree of clinical heterogeneity, many patients have symptoms that can be recognized as discrete syndromes. Entities that specifically involve the frontal lobes include the following:

- Kearns–Sayre syndrome (KSS)—progressive external ophthalmoplegia, pigmentary retinopathy, deafness, myopathy, diabetes, hypoparathyroidism, and dementia.
- Mitochondrial encephalomyopathy with lactic acidosis and stroke-like episodes (MELAS)—stroke-like episodes, seizures, dementia, cardiomyopathy, deafness, cerebellar ataxia, and pigmentary retinopathy.
- Myoclonic epilepsy with ragged-red fibers (MERRF)—myoclonus, seizures, myopathy, cerebellar ataxia, dementia, optic atrophy, deafness, spasticity, peripheral neuropathy, cardiomyopathy, and lipomas.

MRI typically reveals T2 hyperintensities, usually in the occipital cortex, but may be generalized. There is often cortical and cerebellar atrophy. MRS reveals abnormalities as well. Laboratory investigations can show elevated lactate (> 3 mmol/liter), elevated CSF lactate (1.5 mmol/liter), elevated lactate:pyruvate ratio (> 20), as well as abnormal plasma amino acids (elevated alanine and threonine), acylcarnitine profile, increased urine organic acids, and ketones. Electromyography and nerve conduction velocities (EMG/NCV) and electrocardiogram (EKG) may also reveal abnormalities. Muscle biopsy can reveal ragged-red fibers, deficiencies in the mitochondrial respiratory chain. Mutations of nuclear or mitochondrial DNA can sometimes be identified. Only certain mutations can be tested for clinically. Inheritance is often maternal, with point mutations and duplications in mitochondrial DNA. However, inheritance may be autosomal, either dominant or recessive (nuclear DNA mutations). *De novo* mutations, often due to large deletions in mitochondrial DNA, can also occur (Chinnery, 2000; Sartor, Loose, Tucha, Klein, & Lange, 2002).

## GENETIC TESTING AND COUNSELING

Genetic testing can often provide a definitive diagnosis and provide families with an understanding of disease etiology and the opportunity for presymptomatic genetic testing of other family members. However, genetic testing should never be undertaken without education and informed consent of the patient (if possible) and other family members. Some families might prefer to live without a diagnosis of a hereditary condition. Because of the emotional impact and potentially life-altering outcome, predictive testing should be performed only after extensive genetic counseling, preferably within a protocol similar to that used with Huntington's disease predictive testing. Current guidelines recommend against testing children or adolescents (International Huntington Association and the World Federation of Neurology Research Group on Huntington's Chorea, 1994). It should be noted that studies have found early cognitive changes in family members of mutation carriers in some conditions such as familial FTD (Geschwind et al., 2001).

## REFERENCES

Aharon-Peretz, J., Rosenbaum, H., & Gershoni-Baruch, R. (2004). Mutations in the glucocerebrosidase gene and Parkinson's disease in Ashkenazi Jews. *New England Journal of Medicine, 351*(19), 1972–1977.

Alanen, A., Komu, M., Penttinen, M., & Leino, R. (1999). Magnetic resonance imaging and proton MR spectroscopy in Wilson's disease. *British Journal of Radiology, 72*(860), 749–756.

Altarescu, G., Hill, S., Wiggs, E., Jeffries, N., Kreps, C., Parker, C. C., et al. (2001). The efficacy of enzyme replacement therapy in patients with chronic neuronopathic Gaucher's disease. *Journal of Pediatrics, 138*(4), 539–547.

Arai, T., Ikeda, K., Akiyama, H., Shikamoto, Y., Tsuchiya, K., Yagishita, S., et al. (2001). Distinct isoforms of tau aggregated in neurons and glial cells in brains of patients with Pick's disease, corticobasal degeneration and progressive supranuclear palsy. *Acta Neuropathologica (Berlin), 101*(2), 167–173.

Bajaj, N. P., Waldman, A., Orrell, R., Wood, N. W., & Bhatia, K. P. (2002). Familial adult onset of Krabbe's disease resembling hereditary spastic paraplegia with normal neuroimaging. *Journal of Neurology, Neurosurgery, and Psychiatry, 72*(5), 635–638.

Baker, M., Litvan, I., Houlden, H., Abramson, J., Dickson, D., Perez-Tur, J., et al. (1999). Association of an extended haplotype in the tau gene with progressive supranuclear palsy. *Human Molecular Genetics, 8*(4), 711–715.

Bauer, I., Gencik, M., Laccone, F., Peters, H., Weber, B. H., Feder, E. H., et al. (2002). Trinucleotide repeat expansions in the junctophilin-3 gene are not found in Caucasian patients with a Huntington's disease-like phenotype. *Annals of Neurology, 51*(5), 662.

Berkhoff, M., Weis, J., Schroth, G., & Sturzenegger, M. (2001). Extensive white-matter changes in case of adult polyglucosan body disease. *Neuroradiology*, *43*(3), 234–236.

Bertram, L., & Tanzi, R. E. (2004a). Alzheimer's disease: One disorder, too many genes? *Human Molecular Genetics*, *13*, R135–R41.

Bertram, L., & Tanzi, R. E. (2004b). The current status of Alzheimer's disease genetics: What do we tell the patients? *Pharmacological Research*, *50*(4), 385–396.

Binetti, G., Nicosia, F., Benussi, L., Ghidoni, R., Feudatari, E., Barbiero, L., et al. (2003). Prevalence of TAU mutations in an Italian clinical series of familial frontotemporal patients. *Neuroscience Letters*, *338*(1), 85–87.

Bird, T., Knopman, D., VanSwieten, J., Rosso, S., Feldman, H., Tanabe, H., et al. (2003). Epidemiology and genetics of frontotemporal dementia/Pick's disease. *Annals of Neurology*, *54*(Suppl. 5), S29–S31.

Bird, T., Nochlin, D., Poorkaj, P., Cherrier, M., Kaye, J., Payami, H., et al. (1999). A clinical pathological comparison of three families with frontotemporal dementia and identical mutations in the tau gene (P301L). *Brain*, *122*(4), 741–756.

Bosch, E. P., & Hart, M. N. (1978). Late adult-onset metachromatic leukodystrophy: Dementia and polyneuropathy in a 63-year-old man. *Archives of Neurology*, *35*(7), 475–477.

Boulan-Predseil, P., Vital, A., Brochet, B., Darriet, D., Henry, P., & Vital, C. (1995). Dementia of frontal lobe type due to adult polyglucosan body disease. *Journal of Neurology*, *242*(8), 512–516.

Brewer, G. J. (2005). Neurologically presenting Wilson's disease: Epidemiology, pathophysiology and treatment. *CNS Drugs*, *19*(3), 185–192.

Brewer, G. J., & Askari, F. K. (2005). Wilson's disease: Clinical management and therapy. *Journal of Hepatology*, *42*(Suppl. 1), S13–S21.

Brooks, W. S., Kwok, J. B., Kril, J. J., Broe, G. A., Blumbergs, P. C., Tannenberg, A. E., et al. (20030. Alzheimer's disease with spastic paraparesis and "cotton wool" plaques: Two pedigrees with PS-1 exon 9 deletions. *Brain*, *126*(Pt. 40, 783–791.

Brown, J., Gydesen, S., Johannsen, P., Gade, A., Skibinski, G., Chakrabarti, L., et al. (2004). Frontotemporal dementia linked to chromosome 3. *Dementia and Geriatric Cognitive Disorders*, *17*(4), 274–276.

Bruno, C., Servidei, S., Shanske, S., Karpati, G., Carpenter, S., McKee, D., et al. (1993). Glycogen branching enzyme deficiency in adult polyglucosan body disease. *Annals of Neurology*, *33*(1), 88–93.

Bugiani, O., Murrell, J. R., Giaccone, G., Hasegawa, M., Ghigo, G., Tabaton, M., et al. (1999). Frontotemporal dementia and corticobasal degeneration in a family with a P301S mutation in tau. *Journal of Neuropathology and Experimental Neurology*, *58*(6), 667–677.

Burk, K., Globas, C., Bosch, S., Klockgether, T., Zuhlke, C., Daum, I., et al. (2003). Cognitive deficits in spinocerebellar ataxia type 1, 2, and 3. *Journal of Neurology*, *250*(2), 207–211.

Chabriat, H., Levy, C., Taillia, H., Iba-Zizen, M. T., Vahedi, K., Joutel, A., et al. (1998). Patterns of MRI lesions in CADASIL. *Neurology*, *51*(2), 452–457.

Chinnery, P. F. (2000). Mitochondrial disorders overview. In *GeneReviews: GeneTests: Medical Genetics Information Resource* (online database). University of Washington, Seattle, 1997–2005.

Chow, T. W., Miller, B. L., Hayashi, V. N., & Geschwind, D. H. (1999). Inheritance of frontotemporal dementia. *Archives of Neurology*, *56*(7), 817–822.

Constantinidis, J., Wisniewski, K. E., & Wisniewski, T. M. (1992). The adult and a new late adult forms of neuronal ceroid lipofuscinosis. *Acta Neuropathologia (Berlin)*, *83*(5), 461–468.

Corder, E. H., Saunders, A. M., Strittmatter, W. J., Schmechel, D. E., Gaskell, P. C., Small, G. W., et al. (1993). Gene dose of apolipoprotein E type 4 allele and the risk of Alzheimer's disease in late onset families. *Science*, *261*, 921–923.

Cruts, M., & Van Broeckhoven, C. (1998). Molecular genetics of Alzheimer's disease. *Annals of Medicine*, *30*(6), 560–565.

Cupples, L. A., Farrer, L. A., Sadovnick, A. D., Relkin, N., Whitehouse, P., & Green, R. C. (2004). Estimating risk curves for first-degree relatives of patients with Alzheimer's disease: The REVEAL study. *Genetics in Medicine*, *6*(4), 192–196.

Danek, A., Rubio, J. P., Rampoldi, L., Ho, M., Dobson-Stone, C., Tison, F., et al. (2001). McLeod neuroacanthocytosis: Genotype and phenotype. *Annals of Neurology*, *50*(6), 755–764.

Danek, A., Tierney, M., Sheesley, L., & Grafman, J. (2001). Cognitive function in patients with chorea-acanthocytosis. Abstract at 1st International Symposium on mental and behavioral dysfunction in movement disorders, Montreal, Canada. *Movement Disorders*, *16*(Suppl. 1), S30–S31.

Danek, A., Tison, F., Rubio, J., Dechsner, M., Kalckreuth, W., & Monaco, A. P. (2001). The chorea of McLeod syndrome. *Movement Disorders*, *16*(5), 882–889.

Danks, D. M., Metz, G., Sewell, R., & Prewett, E. J. (1990). Wilson's disease in adults with cirrhosis but no neurological abnormalities. *British Medical Journal*, *301*, 331–332.

Dermaut, B., Kumar-Singh, S., Engelborghs, S., Theuns, J., Rademakers, R., Saerens, J., et al. (2004). A novel presenilin 1 mutation associated with Pick's disease but not beta-amyloid plaques. *Annals of Neurology*, *55*(5), 617–626.

Dichgans, M., Holtmannspotter, M., Herzog, J., Peters, N., Bergmann, M., & Yousry, T. A. (2002). Cerebral microbleeds in CADASIL: A gradient-echo magnetic resonance imaging and autopsy study. *Stroke*, *33*(1), 67–71.

Dichgans, M., Mayer, M., Uttner, I., Bruning, R.,

Muller-Hocker, J., Rungger, G., et al. (1998). The phenotypic spectrum of CADASIL: Clinical findings in 102 cases. *Annals of Neurology, 44*(5), 731–739.

Duara, R., Barker, W. W., Lopez-Alberola, R., Loewenstein, D. A., Grau, L. B., Gilchrist, D., et al. (1996). Alzheimer's disease: Interaction of apolipoprotein E genotype, family history of dementia, gender, education, ethnicity, and age of onset. *Neurology, 46*(6), 1575–1579.

Farrer, L. A., Cupples, L. A., van Duijn, C. M., Kurz, A., Zimmer, R., Muller, U., et al. (1995). Apolipoprotein E genotype in patients with Alzheimer's disease: Implications for the risk of dementia among relatives. *Annals of Neurology, 38*(5), 797–808.

Federico, A., & Dotti, M. T. (2003). Cerebrotendinous Xanthomatosis In *GeneReviews: GeneTests: Medical Genetics Information Resource* (online database). University of Washington, Seattle, 1997–2005.

Furuya, H., Yasuda, M., Terasawa, K. J., Tanaka, K., Murai, H., Kira, J., et al., (2003). A novel mutation (L250V) in the presenilin 1 gene in a Japanese familial Alzheimer's disease with myoclonus and generalized convulsion. *Journal of Neurological Sciences, 209*(1–2), 75–77.

Garbern, J. Y., Krajewski, K., & Hobson, G. (1999). PLP1-related disorders. In *GeneReviews: GeneTests: Medical Genetics Information Resource* (online database). University of Washington, Seattle, 1997–2005.

Geschwind, D., Karrim, J., Nelson, S. F., & Miller, B. (1998). The apolipoprotein E epsilon4 allele is not a significant risk factor for frontotemporal dementia. *Annals of Neurology, 44*(1), 134–138.

Geschwind, D. H., Robidoux, J., Alarcon, M., Miller, B. L., Wilhelmsen, K. C., Cummings, J. L., et al. (2001). Dementia and neurodevelopmental predisposition: Cognitive dysfunction in presymptomatic subjects precedes dementia by decades in frontotemporal dementia. *Annals of Neurology, 50*(6), 741–746.

Globas, C., Bosch, S., Zuhlke, C., Daum, I., Dichgans, J., & Burk, K. (2003). The cerebellum and cognition: Intellectual function in spinocerebellar ataxia type 6 (SCA6). *Journal of Neurology, 250*(12), 1482–1487.

Goate, A., Chartier-Harlin, M., Mullan, M., Brown, J., Crawford, F., Fidani, L., et al. (1991). Segregation of a missense mutation in the amyloid precursor protein gene with familial Alzheimer's disease. *Nature, 349*, 704–706.

Gow, P. J., Smallwood, R. A., Angus, P. W., Smith, A. L., Wall, A. J., & Sewell, R. B. (2000). Diagnosis of Wilson's disease: An experience over three decades. *Gut, 46*(3), 415–419.

Grau, A. J., Brandt, T., Weisbrod, M., Niethammer, R., Forsting, M., Cantz, M., et al. (1997). Adult Niemann–Pick disease type C mimicking features of multiple sclerosis. *Journal of Neurology, Neurosurgery, and Psychiatry, 63*(4), 552.

Greely, H. T. (1999). Special issues in genetic testing for Alzheimer disease. *Genetic Testing, 3*(1), 115–119.

Green, R. C., Cupples, L. A., Go, R., Benke, K. S., Edeki, T., Griffith, P. A., et al. (2002). Risk of dementia among white and African American relatives of patients with Alzheimer disease. *Journal of the American Medical Association, 287*(3), 329–336.

Grosso, S., Farnetani, M. A., Berardi, R., Margollicci, M., Galluzzi, P., Vivarelli, R., et al. (2003). GM2 gangliosidosis variant B1 neuroradiological findings. *Journal of Neurology, 250*(1), 17–21.

Gusella, J. F., & MacDonald, M. E. (1995). Huntington's disease: CAG genetics expands neurobiology. *Current Opinion in Neurobiology, 5*(5), 656–662.

Gustafson, L., Abrahamson, M., Grubb, A., Nilsson, K., & Fex, G. (1997). Apolipoprotein-E genotyping in Alzheimer's disease and frontotemporal dementia. *Dementia and Geriatric Cognitive Disorders, 8*(4), 240–243.

Gydesen, S., Brown, J. M., Brun, A., Chakrabarti, L., Gade, A., Johannsen, P., et al. (2002). Chromosome 3 linked frontotemporal dementia (FTD-3). *Neurology, 59*(10), 1585–1594.

Halliday, G. M., Song, Y. J., Lepar, G., Brooks, W. S., Kwok, J. B., Kersaitis, C., et al. (2005). Pick bodies in a family with presenilin-1 Alzheimer's disease. *Annals of Neurology, 57*(1), 139–143.

Hammersen, S., Brock, M., & Cervos-Navarro, J. (1998). Adult neuronal ceroid lipofuscinosis with clinical findings consistent with a butterfly glioma: Case report. *Journal of Neurosurgery, 88*(2), 314–318.

Harwood, D. G., Barker, W. W., Ownby, R. L., Mullan, M., & Duara, R. (2004). No association between subjective memory complaints and apolipoprotein E genotype in cognitively intact elderly. *International Journal of Geriatric Psychiatry, 19*(12), 1131–1139.

Hayflick, S. J., Westaway, S. K., Levinson, B., Zhou, B., Johnson, M. A., Ching, K. H., et al. (2003). Genetic, clinical, and radiographic delineation of Hallervorden–Spatz syndrome. *New England Journal of Medicine, 348*(1), 33–40.

Hinkebein, J. H., & Callahan, C. D. (1997). The neuropsychology of Kuf's disease: A case of atypical early onset dementia. *Archives of Clinical Neuropsychology, 12*(1), 81–89.

Holmes, S. E., O'Hearn, E., Rosenblatt, A., Callahan, C., Hwang, H. S., Ingersoll-Ashworth, R. G., et al. (2001). A repeat expansion in the gene encoding junctophilin-3 is associated with Huntington disease-like 2. *Nature Genetics, 29*(4), 377–378.

Horton, T. M., Graham, B. H., Corral-Debrinski, M., Shoffner, J. M., Kaufman, A. E., Beal, M. F., et al. (1995). Marked increase in mitochondrial DNA deletion levels in the cerebral cortex of Huntington's disease patients. *Neurology, 45*(10), 1879–1883.

Hosler, B. A., Siddique, T., Sapp, P. C., Sailor, W., Huang, M. C., Hossain, A., et al. (2000). Linkage of familial amyotrophic lateral sclerosis with frontotemporal dementia to chromosome 9q21-q22. *Jour-*

*nal of the American Medical Association, 284*(13), 1664–1669.

Houlden, H., Baker, M., Morris, H. R., MacDonald, N., Pickering-Brown, S., Adamson, J., et al. (2001). Corticobasal degeneration and progressive supranuclear palsy share a common tau haplotype. *Neurology, 56*(12), 1702–1706.

Huntington's Disease Collaborative Research Group. (1993). A novel gene containing a trinucleotide repeat that is expanded and unstable on Huntington's disease chromosomes. *Cell, 72*(6), 971–983.

Hyde, T. M., Ziegler, J. C., & Weinberger, D. R. (1992). Psychiatric disturbances in metachromatic leukodystrophy: Insights into the neurobiology of psychosis. *Archives of Neurology, 49*(4), 401–406.

Ikeuchi, T., Onodera, O., Oyake, M., Koide, R., Tanaka, H., & Tsuji, S. (1995). Dentatorubralpallidoluysian atrophy (DRPLA): Close correlation of CAG repeat expansions with the wide spectrum of clinical presentations and prominent anticipation. *Seminars in Cell Biology, 6*(1), 37–44.

Ingelson, M., Fabre, S. F., Lilius, L., Andersen, C., Viitanen, M., Almkvist, O., et al. (2001). Increased risk for frontotemporal dementia through interaction between tau polymorphisms and apolipoprotein E epsilon4. *NeuroReport, 12*(5), 905–909.

International Huntington Association and the World Federation of Neurology Research Group on Huntington's Chorea. (1994). Guidelines for the molecular genetics predictive test in Huntington's disease. *Journal of Medical Genetics, 31*(7), 555–559.

Jardim, L. B., Giugliani, R., Pires, R. F., Haussen, S., Burin, M. G., Rafi, M. A., et al. (1999). Protracted course of Krabbe disease in an adult patient bearing a novel mutation. *Archives of Neurology, 56*(8), 1014–1017.

Jung, H. H., Danek, A., & Dobson-Stone, C. (2004). McLeod neuroacanthocytosis syndrome. In *GeneReviews: GeneTests: Medical Genetics Information Resource* (online database). University of Washington, Seattle, 1997–2005.

Kaback, M. M. (1999). Hexosaminidase A deficiency. In *GeneReviews: GeneTests: Medical Genetics Information Resource* (online database). University of Washington, Seattle, 1997–2005.

Kinnear Wilson, S. (1912). Progressive lenticular degeneration: A familial nervous disease associated with cirrhosis of the liver. *Brain, 34*, 295–509.

Klein, C. J., Boes, C. J., Chapin, J. E., Lynch, C. D., Campeau, N. G., Dyck, P. J., et al. (2004). Adult polyglucosan body disease: Case description of an expanding genetic and clinical syndrome. *Muscle and Nerve, 29*(2), 323–328.

Klunemann, H. H., Elleder, M., Kaminski, W. E., Snow, K., Peyser, J. M., O'Brien, J. F., et al. (2002). Frontal lobe atrophy due to a mutation in the cholesterol binding protein HE1/NPC2. *Annals of Neurology, 52*(6), 743–749.

Koide, R., Onodera, O., Ikeuchi, T., Kondo, R., Tanaka,

H., Tokiguchi, S., et al. (1997). Atrophy of the cerebellum and brainstem in dentatorubral pallidoluysian atrophy: Influence of CAG repeat size on MRI findings. *Neurology, 49*(6), 1605–1612.

Kolodny, E. H., Raghavan, S., & Krivit, W. (1991). Late-onset Krabbe disease (globoid cell leukodystrophy): Clinical and biochemical features of 15 cases. *Developmental Neuroscience, 13*(4–5), 232–239.

Kondo, T., Takahashi, K., Kohara, N., Takahashi, Y., Hayashi, S., Takahashi, H., et al. (2002). Heterogeneity of presenile dementia with bone cysts (Nasu–Hakola disease): Three genetic forms. *Neurology, 59*(7), 1105–1107.

Kong, Q. K., Surewicz, W. K., Petersen, R. B., Zou, W., Chen, S. G., Gambetti, P., et al., (2004). Inherited prion diseases. In S. B. Pruisner (Ed.), *Prion biology and disease* (pp. 673–776). Cold Spring Harbor, NY: Cold Spring Harbor Laboratory Press.

Kovach, M. J., Waggoner, B., Leal, S. M., Gelber, D., Khardoni, R., Levenstein, M. A., et al. (2001). Clinical delineation and localization to chromosome 9p13.3-p12 of a unique dominant disorder in four families: Hereditary inclusion body myopathy, Paget disease of bone, and frontotemporal dementia. *Molecular Genetics and Metabolism, 74*(4), 458–475.

Laplanche, J. L., Hachimi, K. H., Durieux, I., Thuillet, P., Defebvre, L., Delasnerie-Laupretre, N., et al. (1999). Prominent psychiatric features and early onset in an inherited prion disease with a new insertional mutation in the prion protein gene. *Brain, 122*(12), 2375–2386.

LaRusse, S., Roberts, J. S., Marteau, T. M., Katzen, H., Linnenbringer, E. L., Barber, M., et al. (2005). Genetic susceptibility testing versus family history-based risk assessment: Impact on perceived risk of Alzheimer disease. *Genetics in Medicine, 7*(1), 48–53.

Letournel, F., Etcharry-Bouyx, F., Verny, C., Barthelaix, A., & Dubas, F. (2003). Two clinicopathological cases of a dominantly inherited, adult onset orthochromatic leucodystrophy. *Journal of Neurology, Neurosurgery, and Psychiatry, 74*(5), 671–673.

Levy-Lahad, E., Wasco, W., Poorkaj, P., Romano, D. M., Oshima, J., Pettingell, W. H., et al. (1995). Candidate gene for the chromosome 1 familial Alzheimer's disease locus. *Science, 269*, 973–977.

Levy-Lahad, E., Wijsman, E. M., Nemens, E., Anderson, L., Goddard, K. A., Weber, J. L., et al. (1995). A familial Alzheimer's disease locus on chromosome 1. *Science, 269*, 970–973.

Lossos, A., Barash, V., Soffer, D., Argov, Z., Gomori, M., Ben-Nariah, Z., et al. (1991). Hereditary branching enzyme dysfunction in adult polyglucosan body disease: A possible metabolic cause in two patients. *Annals of Neurology, 30*(5), 655–662.

Lossos, A., Meiner, Z., Barash, V., Soffer, D., Schlesinger, I., Abramsky, O., et al. (1998). Adult polyglucosan body disease in Ashkenazi Jewish patients carrying the Tyr329Ser mutation in the glycogen-branching enzyme gene. *Annals of Neurology*, *44*(6), 867–872.

Manto, M. U. (2005). The wide spectrum of spinocerebellar ataxias (SCAs). *Cerebellum*, *4*(1), 2–6.

Marcao, A. M., Wiest, R., Schindler, K., Wiesman, U., Weis, J., Schroth, G., et al. (2005). Adult onset metachromatic leukodystrophy without electroclinical peripheral nervous system involvement: A new mutation in the ARSA gene. *Archives of Neurology*, *62*(2), 309–313.

Margolis, R. L., Rudnicki, D. D., & Holmes, S. E. (2005). Huntington's disease like-2: Review and update. *Acta Neurologica (Taiwan)*, *14*(1), 1–8.

Mehta, A. (2002). New developments in the management of Anderson–Fabry disease. *Quarterly Journal of Medicine*, *95*(10), 647–653.

Mendez, M. F., Stanley, T. M., Medel, N. M., Li, Z., & Tedesco, D. T. (1997). The vascular dementia of Fabry's disease. *Dementia and Geriatric Cognitive Disorders*, *8*(4), 252–257.

Mesulam, M., Siddique, T., & Cohen, B. (2003). Cholinergic denervation in a pure multi-infarct state: Observations on CADASIL. *Neurology*, *60*(7), 1183–1185.

Milde, P., Guccion, J. G., Kelly, J., Locatelli, E., & Jones, R. V. (2001). Adult polyglucosan body disease. *Archives of Pathology and Laboratory Medicine*, *125*(4), 519–522.

Montalbetti, L., Ratti, M. T., Greco, B., Aprile, C., Moglia, A., & Soragna, D. (2005). Neuropsychological tests and functional nuclear neuroimaging provide evidence of subclinical impairment in Nasu–Hakola disease heterozygotes. *Functional Neurology*, *20*(2), 71–75.

Montalbetti, L., Soragna, D., Ratti, M. T., Bini, P., Buscone, S., & Moglia, A. (2004). Nasu–Hakola disease: A rare entity in Italy. Critical review of the literature. *Functional Neurology*, *19*(3), 171–179.

Moore, R. C., Xiang, F., Monaghan, J., Han, D., Zhang, Z., Edstrom, L., et al. (2001). Huntington disease phenocopy is a familial prion disease. *American Journal of Human Genetics*, *69*(6), 1385–1388.

Moser, H. W., Moser, A. B., Steinberg, S. J., & Raymond, G. V. (1999). X-linked adrenal leukodystrophy. In *GeneReviews: GeneTests: Medical Genetics Information Resource* (online database). University of Washington, Seattle, 1997–2005.

Moser, H. W., Raymond, G. V., Lu, S. E., Muenz, L. R., Moser, A. B., Xu, J., et al. (2005). Follow-up of 89 asymptomatic patients with adrenoleukodystrophy treated with Lorenzo's oil. *Archives of Neurology*, *62*(7), 1073–1080.

Nagafuchi, S., Yanagisawa, H., Ohsaki, E., Shirayama, T., Tadokoro, K., Inoue, T., et al. (1994). Structure and expression of the gene responsible for the triplet repeat disorder, dentatorubral and pallidoluysian atrophy (DRPLA). *Nature Genetics*, *8*(2), 177–182.

Nagafuchi, S., Yanagisawa, H., Sato, K., Shirayama, T., Ohsaki, S., Bundo, M., et al. (1994). Dentatorubral and pallidoluysian atrophy expansion of an unstable CAG trinucleotide on chromosome 12p. *Nature Genetics*, *6*(1), 14–18.

Naito, H., & Oyanagi, S. (1982). Familial myoclonus epilepsy and choreoathetosis: Hereditary dentatorubral--pallidoluysian atrophy. *Neurology*, *32*(8), 798–807.

Namekawa, M., Takiyama, Y., Aoki, Y., Takayashiki, N., Sakoe, K., Shimazaki, H., et al. (2002). Identification of GFAP gene mutation in hereditary adult-onset Alexander's disease. *Annals of Neurology*, *52*(6), 779–785.

Nardocci, N., Verga, M. L., Binelli, S., Zorzi, G., Angelini, L., & Bugiani, O. (1995). Neuronal ceroid-lipofuscinosis: A clinical and morphological study of 19 patients. *American Journal of Medical Genetics*, *57*(2), 137–141.

Navon, R., Argov, Z., & Frisch, A. (1986). Hexosaminidase A deficiency in adults. *American Journal of Medical Genetics*, *24*(1), 179–196.

Neudorfer, O., Pastores, G. M., Zeng, B. J., Gianutsos, J., Zaroff, C. M., & Kolodny, E. H. (2005). Late-onset Tay–Sachs disease: Phenotypic characterization and genotypic correlations in 21 affected patients. *Genetics in Medicine*, *7*(2), 119–123.

Neumann, M. A. (1959). Combined degeneration of globus pallidus and dentate nucleus and their projections. *Neurology*, *9*(6), 430–438.

Nicholl, D. J., Sutton, I., Dotti, M. T., Supple, S. G., Danek, A., & Lawden, M. (2004). White matter abnormalities on MRI in neuroacanthocytosis. *Journal of Neurology, Neurosurgery, and Psychiatry*, *75*(8), 1200–1201.

Nielsen, A. S., Ravid, R., Kamphorst, W., & Jorgensen, O. S. (2003). Apolipoprotein E epsilon 4 in an autopsy series of various dementing disorders. *Journal of Alzheimer's Disease*, *5*(2), 119–125.

Okamoto, K., Llena, J. F., & Hirano, A. (1982). A type of adult polyglucosan body disease. *Acta Neuropathologica*, *58*(1), 73–77.

Okamoto, Y., Mitsuyama, H., Jonosono, M., Hirata, K., Arimura, K., Osame, M., et al. (2002). Autosomal dominant palatal myoclonus and spinal cord atrophy. *Journal of Neurological Sciences*, *195*(1), 71–76.

Paloneva, J., Autti, T., Raininko, R., Partanen, J., Salonen, O., Puranen, M., et al. (2001). CNS manifestations of Nasu–Hakola disease: A frontal dementia with bone cysts. *Neurology*, *56*(11), 1552–1558.

Pastores, G. M. (2000). Gaucher disease. In *GeneReviews: GeneTests: Medical Genetics Information Resource* (online database). University of Washington, Seattle, 1997–2005.

Patterson, M. C., Horowitz, M., Abel, R. R., Currie, J. N., Yu, K. T., Kaneski, C., et al. (1993). Isolated horizontal supranuclear gaze palsy as a marker of severe systemic involvement in Gaucher's disease. *Neurology*, *43*(10), 1993–1997.

Paulsen, J. S., Ready, R. E., Hamilton, J. M., Mega, M. S., & Cummings, J. L. (2001). Neuropsychiatric aspects of Huntington's disease. *Journal of Neurology, Neurosurgery, and Psychiatry, 71*(3), 310–314.

Peress, N. S., DiMauro, S., & Roxburgh, V. A. (1979). Adult polysaccharidosis: Clinicopathological, ultrastructural, and biochemical features. *Archives of Neurology, 36*(13), 840–845.

Peters, N., Opherk, C., Bergmann, T., Castro, M., Herzog, J., & Dichgans, M. (2005). Spectrum of mutations in biopsy-proven CADASIL: Implications for diagnostic strategies. *Archives of Neurology, 62*(7), 1091–1094.

Peters, N., Opherk, C., Danek, A., Ballard, C., Herzog, J., & Dichgans, M. (2005). The pattern of cognitive performance in CADASIL: A monogenic condition leading to subcortical ischemic vascular dementia. *American Journal of Psychiatry, 162*(11), 2078–2085.

Pittman, A. M., Myers, A. J., Abou-Sleiman, P., Fung, H. C., Kaleem, M., Marlowe, L., et al. (2005). Linkage disequilibrium fine-mapping and haplotype association analysis of the tau gene in progressive supranuclear palsy and corticobasal degeneration. *Journal of Medical Genetics, 42*(11), 837–846.

Poorkaj, P., Bird, T. D., Wijsman, E., Nemens, E., Garroto, R. M., Anderson, L., et al. (1998). Tau is a candidate gene for chromosome 17 frontotemporal dementia. *Annals of Neurology, 43*(6), 815–825.

Queralt, R., Ezquerra, M., Lleo, A., Castellvi, M., Gelpi, J., Ferrer, I., et al. (2002). A novel mutation (V89L) in the presenilin 1 gene in a family with early onset Alzheimer's disease and marked behavioural disturbances. *Journal of Neurology, Neurosurgery, and Psychiatry, 72*(2), 266–269.

Raben, N., Danon, M., Lu, N., Lee, E., Shliselfeld, L., Skurat, A. V., et al. (2001). Surprises of genetic engineering: A possible model of polyglucosan body disease. *Neurology, 56*(12), 1739–1745.

Raux, G., Gantier, R., Thomas-Anterion, C., Boulliat, J., Verpillat, P., Hannequin, D., et al. (2000). Dementia with prominent frontotemporal features associated with L113P presenilin 1 mutation. *Neurology, 55*(10), 1577–1578.

Rifai, Z., Klitzke, M., Tawil, R., Kazee, A. M., Shanske, S., DiMauro, S., et al. (1994). Dementia of adult polyglucosan body disease: Evidence of cortical and subcortical dysfunction. *Archives of Neurology, 51*(1), 90–94.

Rippon, G. A., Crook, R., Baker, M., Halvorsen, E., Chin, S., Hutton, M., et al. (2003). Presenilin 1 mutation in an African American family presenting with atypical Alzheimer dementia. *Archives of Neurology, 60*(6), 884–888.

Robitaille, Y., Carpenter, S., Karpati, G., & DiMauro, S. D. (1980). A distinct form of adult polyglucosan body disease with massive involvement of central and peripheral neuronal processes and astrocytes: A report of four cases and a review of the occurrence of polyglucosan bodies in other conditions such as Lafora's disease and normal ageing. *Brain, 103*(2), 315–336.

Rogaev, E. I., Sherrington, R., Rogaeva, E. A., Levesque, G., Ikeda, M., Liang, Y., et al. (1995). Familial Alzheimer's disease in kindreds with missense mutations in a gene on chromosome 1 related to the Alzheimer's disease type 3 gene. *Nature, 376*, 775–778.

Ross, M. E., Jacobson, I. M., Dienstag, J. L., & Martin, J. B. (1985). Late-onset Wilson's disease with neurological involvement in the absence of Kayser–Fleischer rings. *Annals of Neurology, 17*(4), 411–413.

Sartor, H., Loose, R., Tucha, O., Klein, H. E., & Lange, K. W. (2002). MELAS: A neuropsychological and radiological follow-up study: Mitochondrial encephalomyopathy, lactic acidosis and stroke. *Acta Neurologica Scandinavica, 106*(5), 309–313.

Schelhaas, H. J., van de Warrenburg, B. P., Hageman, G., Ippel, E. E., van Hout, M., & Kremer, B. (2003). Cognitive impairment in SCA-19. *Acta Neurologica Belgique, 103*(4), 199–205.

Schellenberg, G. D., Bird, T. D., Wijsman, E. M., Orr, H. T., Anderson, L., Nemens, E., et al. (1992). Genetic linkage evidence for a familial Alzheimer's disease locus on chromosome 14. *Science, 258*, 668–671.

Schiffmann, R., Fogli, A., Van der Knaap, M. S., & Boesplfug-Tanguy, O. (2003). Childhood ataxia with central nervous system hypomyelination/vanishing white matter. In *GeneReviews: GeneTests: Medical Genetics Information Resource* (online database). University of Washington, Seattle, 1997–2005.

Schreiner, R., Becker, I., & Wiegand, M. H. (2000). [Kufs disease: A rare cause of early-onset dementia]. *Nervenarzt, 71*(5), 411–415.

Schroder, J. M., May, R., Shin, Y. S., Sigmund, M., & Nase-Huppmeier, S. (1993). Juvenile hereditary polyglucosan body disease with complete branching enzyme deficiency (type IV glycogenosis). *Acta Neuropathologica (Berlin), 85*(4), 419–430.

Selemon, L. D., Rajkowska, G., & Goldman-Rakic, P. S. (2004). Evidence for progression in frontal cortical pathology in late-stage Huntington's disease. *Journal of Comparative Neurology, 468*(2), 190–204.

Sener, R. N. (2003). Diffusion MRI findings in Wilson's disease. *Computerized Medical Imaging and Graphics, 27*(1), 17–21.

Seniow, J., Bak, T., Gajda, J., Poniatowska, R., & Czlonkowska, A. (2002). Cognitive functioning in neurologically symptomatic and asymptomatic forms of Wilson's disease. *Movement Disorders, 17*(5), 1077–1083.

Shapiro, E. G., Lockman, L. A., Knopman, D., & Krivit, W. (1994). Characteristics of the dementia in late-onset metachromatic leukodystrophy. *Neurology, 44*(4), 662–665.

Sherrington, R., Rogaev, E. I., Liang, Y., Rogaeva, E. A.,

Levesque, G., Ikeda, M., et al. (1995). Cloning of a gene bearing missense mutations in early-onset familial Alzheimer's disease. *Nature, 375*, 754–760.

Shiga, Y., Miyazawa, K., Sato, S., Fukushima, R., Shibuya, S., Sato, Y., et al. (2004). Diffusion-weighted MRI abnormalities as an early diagnostic marker for Creutzfeldt–Jakob disease. *Neurology, 63*, 443–449.

Shulman, L. M., David, N. J., & Weiner, W. J. (1995). Psychosis as the initial manifestation of adult-onset Niemann–Pick disease type C. *Neurology, 45*(9), 1739–1743.

Sidransky, E. (2005). Gaucher disease and parkinsonism. *Molecular Genetics and Metabolism, 84*(4), 302–304.

Skibinski, G., Parkinson, N. J., Brown, J. M., Chakrabarti, L., Lloyd, S. L., Hummerich, H., et al. (2005). Mutations in the endosomal ESCRTIII-complex subunit CHMP2B in frontotemporal dementia. *Nature Genetics, 37*(8), 806–808.

Slooter, A. J., Cruts, M., Kalmijn, S., Hofman, A., Breteler, M. M., Van Broeckhoven, C., et al. (1998). of dementia by apolipoprotein E genotypes from a population-based incidence study: The Rotterdam Study. *Archives of Neurology, 55*(7), 964–968.

Smith, J. K., Gonda, V. E., & Malamud, N. (1958). Unusual form of cerebellar ataxia: Combined dentato-rubral and pallido-Luysian degeneration. *Neurology, 8*(3), 205–209.

Soliveri, P., Rossi, G., Monza, D., Tagliavini, F., Piacentini, S., Albanese, A., et al. (2003). A case of dementia parkinsonism resembling progressive supranuclear palsy due to mutation in the tau protein gene. *Archives of Neurology, 60*(10), 1454–1456.

Soragna, D., Papi, L., Ratti, M. T., Sestini, R., Tupler, R., & Montalbetti, L. (2003). An Italian family affected by Nasu–Hakola disease with a novel genetic mutation in the TREM2 gene. *Journal of Neurology, Neurosurgery, and Psychiatry, 74*(6), 825–826.

Spillantini, M. G., Van Swieten, J. C., & Goedert, M. (2000). Tau gene mutations in frontotemporal dementia and parkinsonism linked to chromosome 17 (FTDP-17)." *Neurogenetics, 2*(4), 193–205.

Stam, F. C., Wigboldus, J. M., & Bots, G. T. (1980). Presenile dementia—a form of Lafora disease. *Journal of American Geriatric Society, 28*(5), 237–240.

Stanford, P. M., Brooks, W. S., Teber, E. T., Hallupp, M., McLean, C., Halliday, G. M., et al. (2004). Frequency of tau mutations in familial and sporadic frontotemporal dementia and other tauopathies. *Journal of Neurology, 251*(9), 1098–1104.

Stevanin, G., Durr, A., Benammar, N., & Brice, A. (2005). Spinocerebellar ataxia with mental retardation (SCA13). *Cerebellum, 4*(1), 43–46.

Stumpf, E., Masson, H., Duquette, A., Berthelet, F., McNabb, J., Lortie, A., et al. (2003). Adult Alexander disease with autosomal dominant transmission: A distinct entity caused by mutation in the glial fibrillary acid protein gene. *Archives of Neurology, 60*(9), 1307–1312.

Suzuki, K., David, E., & Kutschman, B. (1971). Presenile dementia with "Lafora-like" intraneuronal inclusions. *Archives of Neurology, 25*(1), 69–80.

Taillia, H., Chabriat, H., Kurtz, A., Verin, M., Levy, C., Vahedi, K., et al. (1998). Cognitive alterations in non-demented CADASIL patients. *Cerebrovascular Diseases, 8*(2), 97–101.

Tang-Wai, D., Lewis, P., Boeve, B., Hutton, M., Golde, T., Baker, M., et al. (2002). Familial frontotemporal dementia associated with a novel presenilin-1 mutation. *Dementia and Geriatric Cognitive Disorders, 14*(1), 13–21.

Tedeschi, G., Bonavita, S., Barton, N. W., Betolino, A., Frank, J. A., Patronas, N. J., et al. (1998). Proton magnetic resonance spectroscopic imaging in the clinical evaluation of patients with Niemann–Pick type C disease. *Journal of Neurology, Neurosurgery, and Psychiatry, 65*(1), 72–79.

Tomiyasu, H., Takahashi, W., Ohta, T., Yoshii, F., Shibuya, M., & Shinohura, Y. (2000). [An autopsy case of juvenile neuronal ceroid-lipofuscinosis with dilated cardiomyopathy]. *Rinsho Shinkeigaku, 40*(4), 350–357.

van der Knaap, M. S., Naidu, S., Breiter, S. N., Blaser, S., Stroink, H., et al. (2001). Alexander disease: Diagnosis with MR imaging. *American Journal of Neuroradiology, 22*(3), 541–552.

van Swieten, J. C., Rosso, S. M., Van Herpen, E., Kamphorst, W., Ravid, R., & Heutink, P. (2004). Phenotypic variation in frontotemporal dementia and parkinsonism linked to chromosome 17. *Dementia and Geriatric Cognitive Disorders, 17*(4), 261–264.

van Wassenaer-van Hall, H. N., van den Heuvel, A. G., Jansen, G. H., Hoogenraad, T. U., & Mali, W. P. (1995). Cranial MR in Wilson disease: Abnormal white matter in extrapyramidal and pyramidal tracts. *American Journal of Neuroradiology, 16*(10), 2021–2027.

Verpillat, P., Camuzat, A., Hannequin, D., Thomas-Anterion, C., Puel, M., Belliard, S., et al. (2002). Apolipoprotein E gene in frontotemporal dementia: An association study and meta-analysis. *European Journal of Human Genetics, 10*(7), 399–405.

von Figura, K., Gieselmann, V., & Jaeken, J. (2001). Metachromatic leukodystrophy. In C. Scriver, A. Beaudet, W. Sly, & D. Valle (Eds.), *The metabolic and molecular basis of inherited disease* (8th ed., pp. 3695–3724). New York: McGraw-Hill.

Walker, R. H., Rasmussen, A., Rudnicki, D., Holmes, S. E., Alonso, E., Matsuura, T., et al. (2003). Huntington's disease-like 2 can present as chorea-acanthocytosis. *Neurology, 61*(7), 1002–1004.

Warshawsky, I., Rudick, R. A., Staugaitis, S. M., & Natowicz, M. R. (2005). Primary progressive multiple sclerosis as a phenotype of a PLP1 gene mutation. *Annals of Neurology, 58*(3), 470–473.

Watts, G. D., Wymer, J., Kovach, M. J., Mehta, S. G., Mumm, S., Darvish, D., et al. (2004). Inclusion body myopathy associated with Paget disease of bone and frontotemporal dementia is caused by mutant valosin-containing protein. *Nature Genetics, 36*(4), 377–381.

Wenger, D. A., & Coppola, S. (2000). Krabbe disease. In *GeneReviews: GeneTests: Medical Genetics Information Resource* (online database). University of Washington, Seattle, 1997–2005.

Wijsman, E. M., Daw, E. W., Yu, C. E., Payami, H., Steinbart, E. J., Nochlin, D., et al. (2004). Evidence for a novel late-onset Alzheimer disease locus on chromosome 19p13.2. *American Journal of Human Genetics, 75*(3), 398–409.

Wilhelmsen, K. C., Forman, M. S., Rosen, H. J., Alving, L. I., Goldman, J., Feiger, J., et al. (2004). 17q-linked frontotemporal dementia-amyotrophic lateral sclerosis without tau mutations with tau and alpha-synuclein inclusions. *Archives of Neurology, 61*(3), 398–406.

Wisniewski, K. E. (2001). Neuronal ceroid-lipofuscinoses. In *GeneReviews: GeneTests: Medical Genetics Information Resource* (online database). University of Washington, Seattle, 1997–2005.

Young, G. S., Geschwind, M. D., Fischbein, N. J., Martindale, J. L., Henry, R. G., Liu, S., et al. (2005). Diffusion-weighted and fluid-attenuated inversion recovery imaging in Creutzfeldt–Jakob disease: High sensitivity and specificity for diagnosis. *American Journal of Neuroradiology, 26*(6), 1551–1562.

Zick, C. D., Mathews, C. J., Roberts, J. S., Cook-Deegan, R., Pokorski, R. J., & Green, R. C. (2005). Genetic testing for Alzheimer's disease and its impact on insurance purchasing behavior. *Health Affairs (Project Hope), 24*(2), 483–490.

Ziemssen, F., Sindern, E., Schroder, J. M., Shin, Y. S., Zange, J., Kilimann, M. W., et al. (2000). Novel missense mutations in the glycogen-branching enzyme gene in adult polyglucosan body disease. *Annals of Neurology, 47*(4), 536–540.

Zuhlke, C., Riess, O., Bockel, B., Lange, H., & Thies, U. (1993). Mitotic stability and meiotic variability of the (CAG)n repeat in the Huntington disease gene. *Human Molecular Genetics, 2*(12), 2063–2067.

# CHAPTER 35

# Frontal Lobe Development in Childhood

*Carol Samango-Sprouse*

Enormous strides have been made in our understanding of brain and behavior relationships, and the function of the frontal lobes through the use of advanced technology such as magnetic resonance imaging (MRI), functional magnetic resonance imaging (fMRI), and magnetic resonance spectroscopy (MRS) (Giedd, Bluementhal, Molloy, & Castellanos, 2001; Reiss, Eliez, Schmitt, Patwardhan, & Haberecht, 2000). Within the last 5 years, the evolution of brain development throughout childhood, as well as gender and age differences in brain architecture, has now been well described (Rose et al., 2004). As the relationship between brain–behavior and intellectual capabilities is further elucidated, our ability to discern the genotypic–phenotypic relationships in specific neurogenetic disorders has improved immensely and affords the opportunity to see the linkage from gene to behavior to learning style and performance (Greicius, 2003; Reiss & Denckla, 1996; Reiss et al., 2000).

In this chapter, the relationship between frontal lobe functions, selected neurogenetic disorders, and learning is discussed. Neuroimaging techniques combined with our knowledge of the neurocognitive profile of neurogenetic disorders have increased our understanding the nature versus nurture issues of disorders and, equally important, fostered the development of targeted treatment for childhood disorders (Durston et al., 2001). Targeted treatments result in improved rehabil-

itation and, in selected cases, recovery for some children.

Our understanding of frontal lobe function has blossomed significantly as knowledge of the role of specific brain functions has improved and the influence of these variations on phenotypic characteristics has become available to both scientists and clinicians. As we understand the global function of the brain (white matter vs. gray matter) and the regional variations in brain function, the neuropsychological underpinnings of the specific disorder and also the generalities of these functions to children become more apparent (Giedd, 2003, 2004; Herbert et al., 2002, 2004). Brain maturation and regional differences within normal childhood have allowed for correlations between neurocognitive and neuroimaging to be elucidated. These studies have permitted us to observe without surgery the evolution of learning and brain maturation throughout childhood.

## DEVELOPMENT OF THE FRONTAL LOBE

Brain development is an exquisite process that is orchestrated from conception through adulthood in a very harmonious manner to facilitate learning, the growth of intelligence, and the unfolding of an organism from a dependent and diffuse infant to an independent and complex young adult (Hoon & Melhem, 2000). The development of the brain is both temporally and spatially directed from 1 month of gestation onward. White matter of the brain progresses in a linear fashion, with growth equally distributed between the four major lobes: frontal, temporal, parietal, and occipital (Castellanos et al., 2003; Giedd, 2004). The brain is adult size by 6 years of age, with the male brain approximately 12% larger than the female brain. Although a 6-year-old child has the brain size of an adult, the head circumference is markedly smaller, because there is significant increase in skull thickness over the next 20 years rather than actual brain growth (Giedd, 2004; Giedd et al., 1996).

Cortical gray matter of the frontal lobe has a different growth pattern than white matter. Gray matter grows in an inverted U-pattern rather than linearly (Giedd et al., 1996, 1999). The frontal lobe reaches maximum thickness by adulthood but varies based on gender. Females reach peak frontal lobe thickness by 11 years of age, whereas males reach peak thickness at 12.1 years (Gogtay, Giedd, & Rapoport, 2002). In contrast, the temporal lobe cortical gray matter reaches maturity in females at 17.7 years and in males at 16 years. Motor and sensory areas of the brain mature in the first 2 years of life (Gogtay et al., 2002), and the frontal poles mature early. The dorsal prefrontal cortex (DPFC) is the last area of the frontal lobe to mature and is not fully developed until 10 years after puberty, or 25 years of age (Gogtay et al., 2004). The DPFC is responsible for inhibiting impulses, weighing consequences of decisions, and most importantly, prioritizing and strategizing to obtain a solution to the presenting problem (Fuster, 2002). This blossoming of the DPFC in the mid-20s may explain the clinical presentation classically described as "the late bloomer syndrome."

## EXECUTIVE FUNCTION IN CHILDREN

Executive function is the ability to organize, plan, and execute a complex and discrete action (Espy, 2004; Fuster, 2002; Powell & Voeller, 2004; Sapolsky, 2004). It is intimately connected to the maturation of frontal lobe and has primary connections with other cortical regions of the brain. Executive function is the behavioral response that reflects frontal lobe integrity or dysfunction. Historically, executive function was believed to come "online"

developmentally at 6 or 7 years of age (Casey, Giedd, & Thomas, 2000; Wolfe & Bell, 2004). However, recent neurodevelopmental studies have revealed that in selected cases, executive function can be observed in toddlers as young as 2 years of age (Scerif, Cornish, Wilding, Driver, & Karmiloff-Smith, 2004). The importance of executive function cannot be overstated, because it relates to neurodevelopmental competency and success in the educational, interpersonal, and employment areas. Just as the frontal lobes serve as the governor of the brain and organize input from every other region of the brain, executive function enables an individual to synthesize information, organize, and plan an appropriate strategy, then complete the action (Samango-Sprouse, 1999). The frontal lobes are massive in both size and structure, and communicate through complex pathways with the other regions of the brain (Samango-Sprouse, 1999). It is this synthesis and integration that defines executive function and allows an individual to develop higher associative learning patterns (Casey et al., 2000; Fuster, 2002). Intellectual ability is the basis for learning; however, executive function is the basis for the organization that enables success in life.

Executive function has three primary components: attention, working memory, and inhibition (Casey et al., 2000; Fuster, 2002). Working memory is the ability to retain the memory of an event, an action, or a word for the short term, then to use that memory for the development of a goal. It is distinct and different from short-term memory, which is the recall of a past event or occurrence. Attention is another facet of executive function. The attention is selective and well sustained when functioning appropriately. Attention is discriminating and in some ways biased toward achieving an end or desired goal (Samango-Sprouse, 1999). Inhibition is also mediated by the prefrontal cortex (PFC), as are working memory and attention (Powell & Voeller, 2004). PFC serves as a form of superego, so to speak, in Freudian terms, because it suppresses impulsive behavior in both the form of thoughts and actions (Sapolsky, 2004). In summary, executive function comprise four targets, which are typically assessed by more than 60 measures (Samango-Sprouse, 1999). The four behaviors include planning, decision making, goal selection in a self-directed manner, and supervision and adaptation of that ongoing behavior. Working memory, inhibition, and attention all subserve these behaviors (Casey et al., 2000; Fuster, 2002).

## NEUROGENETIC DISORDERS

Maudsley eloquently described behavioral neurogenetics before DNA, brain imaging, or chromosomal disorders were even a consideration (Harris, 1998). Now, more than 100 years later, behavioral neurogenetics is emerging as an effective and appropriate method to investigate the relationship between human behavior and brain function. Behavioral neurogenetics is predicated on the underlying assumption that neurodevelopmental dysfunction is the result of a complex pathway, including differences in brain, behavioral, and neurocognitive function (Reiss et al., 2000). Behavioral neurogenetics is the investigation of homogeneous populations of children or adults with unique neurogenetic entities from both neuroimaging and neurodevelopmental perspectives. It provides scientists the opportunity to draw conclusions regarding the specific disorder, brain function, and the neuropsychological profile because of the homogeneity of the disorder. Proceeding "from gene to brain to cognitive architecture to manifest learning disabilities" is reliable and more effective with homogeneous populations than with etiologically diverse groups of children, in which confounding variables can cloud the findings (Denckla, 1994).

In this chapter, the frontal lobe function of the various disorders is explored, each with its characteristic signature of brain, neurobehavioral, and neurodevelopmental differences. Frontal lobe dysfunction is common to the majority of neurogenetic disorders, yet each disorder has a unique presentation with behavioral and neurocognitive characteristics. These differences demonstrate the influence and the variability of genetic dosage that makes the field of behavioral neurogenetics simultaneously challenging, rewarding, and frustrating for neuroscientists.

## XXY (Klinefelter Syndrome)

Dr. Harry S. Klinefelter described Klinefelter syndrome in 1942 as an endocrine disorder with features including tall stature, a feminized body with rounded hips, pendulous breasts, and adipose fat in the abdomen (Klinefelter, Reifenstein, & Albright, 1942). Chromosomal configuration of a supernumerary X was identified in 1956 with the development of karyotyping (Bradbury, Bunge, & Boccabella, 1956). Size of the Phallus is reduced in 50% of cases of XXY, although it is not a classic micropenis (Simpson et al., 2003; Simpson, Graham, Samango-Sprouse, & Swerdloff, 2004). Later, it was discovered that boys with XXY were deficient in testosterone, and this deficiency caused the onset of feminized appearance and the disruption in the pubertal development (Laron & Hochman, 1971; Simpson et al., 2004). XXY is the most common cause of male hypogonadism, and it occurs in 8% of the men referred for male infertility (Simpson et al., 2004; Winter, 1990).

### Neurobehavioral Phenotype

XXY occurs in one out of every 600 live births and is one of the most common causes for learning disabilities, dyslexia, and behavioral disturbances in children (Bender, Harmon, Linden, & Robinson, 1995; Linden, Binder, & Robinson, 1996; Neilsen & Wohlert, 1991; Samango-Sprouse, 2001; Simpson et al., 2003; Visootsak, Alystock, & Graham, 2001). XXY is the most frequently occurring of the sex chromosome disorders (SCDs), which also include XXX (triple X), XYY, and XO (Turner's syndrome). XXY occurs more commonly than Down's syndrome or cystic fibrosis, but 66% of boys with XXY are never identified in their lifetime, despite developmental disturbances as early as 12 months of age (Ross et al., 2005; Samango-Sprouse & Rogol, 2002; Samango-Sprouse, Jsang, & Huddleston, 2002).

The diagnosis for these boys is elusive for several reasons. First, there is diminished awareness of the disorder at every stage of life. Boys' parents are often dismissed with "Boys develop slower" or "It is just a developmental delay. Don't you worry." Because of the lack of awareness, XXY is rarely considered in the diagnostic workup for learning or language disabilities, even if there are multiple and complex delays such as dyslexia, attention-deficit/hyperactivity disorder (ADHD), or inappropriate school behaviors. Because chromosomal disorders are usually associated with mental retardation and atypical appearance, boys with XXY are not dysmorphic and often are quite attractive, so medical professionals do not think of this disorder or chromosomal analysis when doing a medical workup (Simpson et al., 2004).

XXY occurs with other neurogenetic disorders and has been reported in association with Prader–Willi syndrome (Butler et al., 1997). Fragile X and XXY have a high comorbidity (Fryns & Van den Berghe, 1988). XXY and trisomy 21 have been described with the characteristics of mental retardation and delayed development typical of trisomy 21 but of few symptoms of XXY (Samango-Sprouse, 1998, unpublished data). There are some common of symptoms between autism spectrum disorder (ASD) and XXY both behaviorally and in brain architecture, and several anecdotal reports suggest an increased association between these two disorders. My associates and I, using the Gilliam Autism Rating Scale, screened for ASD in 65 boys with XXY diagnosed prenatally, and no association was found (Samango-Sprouse, 2005, unpublished data).

Early studies in the 1970s documented an increased incidence of criminal behavior in patients with XXY but these studies were clouded by small sample size and ascertainment bias (Casey, Segall, Street, & Blank, 1966). Recent research studies on XXY have demonstrated language based learning disabilities with executive dysfunction, graphomotor deficits and decreased processing speed (Simpson et al., 2003, 2004). Spatial cognition is enhanced particularly in visual perceptual and visual closure skills (Linden et al., 1996; Neilsen & Wohlert, 1991; Samango-Sprouse, 2001; Simpson et al., 2003; Visootsak et al., 2001). Developmental disturbances have been identified in speech, language, auditory processing, written composition and sensory dysfunction (Robinson, Bender, & Linden, 1991; Salbenblatt, Meyers, Bender, Linden, & Robinson, 1987; Samango-Sprouse & Rogol, 2002).

Infants with XXY have an atypical profile that may present as early as the first 6 months of life (Samango-Sprouse & Rogol, 2002; Visootsak et al., 2001). Infantile presentation of developmental dyspraxia (IDD) occurs in 80% of children with XXY and may be an early indicator of frontal lobe dysfunction and executive function differences (Samango-Sprouse & Rogol, 2002). This neurodevelop-

mental profile consists of discrepancies from typically developing peers in motor, speech, and attention, originating from sensory-based motor deficits in planning and execution as early as 12 months of age (Samango-Sprouse et al., 2002). They have truncal hypotonia with gross motor delay and joint laxity. Balance difficulties with sensory integration dysfunction are evident by the third year of life (Salbenblatt, Meyers, Bender, Linden, & Robinson, 1987; Samango-Sprouse, 2002). There is decreased phonemic repertoire and delayed expressive language skills in comparison to receptive language skills. There are deficits in imitation of nonverbal movements and speech sounds, and in planning novel motor schemes. The young child with XXY usually presents with decreased muscle tonus in upper extremities and trunk, and less frequently in lower extremities (Samango-Sprouse, 2005, unpublished data). In the early childhood years, the neurodevelopmental profile includes dyspraxia or motor planning deficits. This planning dysfunction causes delays in gross and fine motor skills, with postural instability. The deficits observed in the young child may be early indicators of later frontal lobe differences with executive dysfunction, because there is increased incidence of executive dysfunction in older children and adults with XXY (Boone-Brauer et al., 2001; Temple & Sanfilippo, 2003). Speech is delayed secondary to planning deficits and dyspraxia, but skills in receptive vocabulary and auditory comprehension are age appropriate. Children identified through prenatal diagnosis have milder presentations, but still require 80% early intervention services to reduce developmental deficits and to optimize their neurodevelopmental outcome (Samango-Sprouse & Rogol, 2002; Simpson et al., 2004). Children diagnosed postnatally may be more delayed because of the more complex presentation, delayed identification or lack of appropriate and timely early intervention services (Simpson et al., 2004).

As preschoolers, these boys have language formulation issues with word retrieval deficits, and auditory short-term memory problems with residual difficulties imitating novel motor schemes and oral motor movements (Samango-Sprouse, 2001; Samango-Sprouse & Law, 2001; Simpson et al., 2003). As they grow older, there is increased incidence of attentional difficulties and distractibility for verbally mediated tasks (Boone-Brauer et al., 2001; Simpson et al., 2004). Conversely, there are enhanced visual–perceptual and spatial–cognition skills, with excellent attention for these types of tasks.

At school age, the child with XXY has a constellation of differences in auditory attention, reading comprehension with balance differences. Language formulation and written composition are problematic in boys with XXY, and MRI findings support differences in temporal lobe and auditory cortex (Giedd, 2004; Patwardhan, Eliez, Bender, Linden, & Reiss, 2000). Executive dysfunction has been identified in two small studies in boys and men with XXY (Boone-Brauer et al., 2001; Geschwind, Boone, Miller, & Swerdloff, 2000). I have extensively studied the neuro-developmental profile of school-age boys with XXY and have found three cognitive profiles that mirror the Boone-Brauer and associates (2001) results in men with XXY (Samango-Sprouse, 2005, unpublished data). The preponderance of these boys have enhanced spatial cognition, with Performance IQ significantly increased. However, there is a small group in which Verbal IQ and Performance IQ are reversed, with verbal capabilities increased. A very small group of boys have similar Performance and Verbal IQs. This variability in neurocognitive function in boys with XXY suggests that there is more heterogeneity of neurocognitive function in this chromosomal disorder than previously described. The relationship between brain development and neurocognitive variation in this disorder is not well understood, but it is important to discern these underpinnings if we are to target medical and developmental treatment programs for these boys.

### Neuroimaging Findings

Imaging studies of boys with XXY have revealed an evolving, characteristic signature that is consistent with their phenotypic presentation and neurocognitive profile. Findings by Giedd and others revealed diminished frontal lobe capacity, with enhanced parietal lobe volume (Giedd, 2004; Patwardhan et al., 2002). The temporal lobe is diminished, with overall decreased brain volume noted in both studies. The latest quantitative volumetric study conducted by Giedd (2004) revealed caudate abnormalities consistent with the MRI abnormal-

ities observed in children with (ADHD). These caudate abnormalities may explain the presentation in boys with XXY, of auditory inattention and impulsivity with distractibility that resembles but does not meet complete criteria for attention deficit disorder.

Previously, prepubertal boys with XXY were believed to have normal production of testosterone (Ferguson-Smith, 1959; Salbenblatt et al., 1987). Recent studies have indicated that infants with XXY have decreased testosterone levels as early as the newborn period (Lahlou, Fennoy, Carel, & Roger, 2004; Ross et al., 2005). Brain maturation and learning maybe affected by this hormonal insufficiency. Padwardhan and associates (2002), in a small study of adult men, revealed that those treated with hormone replacement had improved neuropsychological function compared to untreated men. There was significant increase in the volumes of the temporal and frontal lobes in treated men. This small study supports the concept that brain maturation and neuropsychological performance may be more normalized with hormone replacement. Samango-Sprouse and Wilson (2005, unpublished data) described a 5-year-old child diagnosed with ASD and XXY who had a very positive response to administration of six shots of testosterone. The patient had dramatic improvement in speech, gaining 3½ years' progress in 12 months' time after the administration of the testosterone. There was improvement in social interactions, organization, and overall well-being. These preliminary results, coupled with results by Padwardhan and colleagues (2002), Lahlou and colleagues (2004), and Ross and colleagues (2005), suggest that hormone replacement may influence brain evolution, as well as neurocognitive function; however, further investigation is essential.

The variance in time of diagnosis in XXY provides an excellent opportunity to compare phenotypic presentation, neuroimaging findings, and neurodevelopmental performance. This could be helpful in understanding the neuroplasticity of children with XXY, as well as the development of frontal lobe function and the effect of early intervention services. Boys with XXY provide an excellent opportunity to study the evolution of executive dysfunction from preschool through adolescence, because 10% of children with this disorder are identified prior to birth (Abramsky & Chappel,

1997; Simpson et al., 2004). Correlation between the natural progression of frontal lobe function and hormonal development could be quite helpful in further understanding gender differences. The relationship between hormone insufficiency, learning dysfunction, and brain variation could enlighten our understanding of why there is a preponderance of males with learning differences.

## Summary

XXY occurs in one in 500 boys, with more than 65% of the children unidentified (Abramsky & Chapple, 1997). More than 90% of children identified through prenatal diagnosis have some type of developmental delay and require special services for several years. Neuroimaging findings reveal regional differences in brain development that correlate with neurodevelopmental findings. These brain variations are highly intriguing, and their relationship to hormone insufficiency and learning warrants further investigation.

## Autism Spectrum Disorder

ASD is a neurobiological disorder that affects more than 1 million children presently (Filipek et al., 1999). ASD is evenly distributed among all racial, ethnic, and socioeconomic groups, and the male predominance is four to one (Ozonoff, 2004). A genetic mechanism for this neurodevelopmental disorder has yet to be identified. Twin studies reveal that it is highly inheritable, with 60% concordance of ASD in monozygotic twins (Folstein & Rosen-Sheidley, 2001). Autism is commonly associated with many neurogenetic disorders, such as Down's syndrome, tuberous sclerosis, neurofibromatosis, and fragile X syndrome, among others (Filipek et al., 1999). The core features of ASD are deficits of social and emotional interactions, repetitive and stereotypical body movements, and severe expressive and receptive language disorder (American Psychiatric Association, 1994). Associated symptoms include gross and fine motor dyspraxia, sensory disturbances, attentional deficits, and executive dysfunction (Filipek et al., 1999). Because of the complexity of the disorder and the wide variability in presentation, identification of subtypes, as well as distinct phenotypic presentations, ASD continues to be perplexing.

## Executive Dysfunction

Executive dysfunction has been studied for more than 20 years in children with ASD (Hill, 2004). Numerous studies demonstrate deficiencies in planning, flexibility, and inhibition in children with ASD (Hill, 2004; Ozonoff & Jensen, 1999; Pennington & Ozonoff, 1996). Planning is one of the more complicated operations for humans, because it is an intricate process and requires the development of a specific, planned action, surveillance of the identified action, the alteration of the existing plan, if necessary, then the execution of the action (Hill, 2004). The Tower of London task is a well-recognized neuropsychological assessment of executive function. In children, adolescents, and adults with ASD, the test reveals impaired function that is consistent with planning deficits and decreased frontal lobe function (Hill, 2004; Ozonoff & Jensen, 1999; Pennington & Ozonoff, 1996). Planning deficits remain constant with time in ASD, although the behavioral manifestations may appear quite different with age (Hill, 2004).

Mental flexibility, a form of executive function, is extremely challenging for children with ASD. Their lack of flexibility is demonstrated by their perservation and stereotypical behaviors, and adherence to very rigid routines (Hill, 2004). This lack of mental flexibility compromises both learning and the acquisition of most aspects of adaptive functioning. Mental inflexibility is evident in the difficulty with transitions and perservation of thoughts, actions, and words. These behaviors have constancy over time, as well as across cultures (Hill, 2004).

Assessment of inhibition processes in children with ASD reveals a task-specific pattern, with some areas within limits normal for their peers, and unimpaired in comparison to other neurodevelopmental disorders such as ADHD (Hill, 2003). The children with ASD perform within normal limits on negative priming and go/no-go tasks. In contrast, their skills were deficient in those tasks demanding cognitive flexibility and "rules to be determined" (Hill, 2004). The complexity of the executive dysfunction in ASD has become clearer in the last decade. Children with ASD have an uneven profile, with select intact components of executive function. There are also several facets of executive dysfunction associated with ASD (Hill & Frith, 2003). This variability in executive function and its correlation to the overgrowth of the brain regions in children with ASD warrants further investigation, so that our understanding of both clinical presentation and the neuropsychological capabilities of children with ASD is improved. It is equally important to discern the underpinnings to the areas of strength versus weaknesses in executive function and the relationship to regional differences in brain development.

## Neuroanatomical Abnormalities

Historically, our understanding of brain abnormalities in ASD has been evolving slowly since the 1980s. Early studies were diffuse in their investigation of brain differences in children with ASD because of limited neuroimaging technology and decreased recognition of the importance of behavioral phenotypes. Damasio and Maurer (1978) revealed damage in the frontal cortex in boys with ASD. Several studies revealed depressed blood flow to right frontal cortex, as well as atypical metabolism in frontal lobe (Gillberg & Rasmussen, 1994; Sherman, Nass, & Shapiro, 1984). Abnormalities have been noted in most cortical structures within the brain architecture of children with ASD, including temporal lobes, cerebellum, basal ganglia, parietal and frontal lobes, hippocampus, and amygdala (Bailey et al., 1998; Belmonte et al., 2004; Carper & Courchesne, 2000; Courchesne, Townsend, & Saitoh, 1994; Herbert et al., 2003).

Neuroimaging studies within the last 5 years have identified several salient features of brain architecture and their relevance to neurocognitive and neurobehavioral aspects of ASD. Regional variations in brain growth in children with ASD have been identified, and these findings are promising for both diagnosis and treatment. Children with ASD begin life with head circumference within the normal range (Courchesne, Redcay, & Kennedy, 2004; Dementieva et al., 2005; Torrey, Dhavale, Lawlor, & Yolken, 2004). The acceleration of head growth begins between ages 6 and 12 months by anthropomorphic measurements and is associated with increased brain volumes. Carper, Moses, Tigue, and Corchesne (2002) detected differences in both gray and white matter in children with ASD with significant enlargement in the prefrontal cerebral cortex volume. This abnormal overgrowth in frontal cortical areas may explain the neurodevelopmental disturbances of executive functioning, planning, integration, and synthesizing. In a landmark study by Herbert and colleagues (2004), using a unique parcellation technique on MRIs of children with developmental language disorder (DLD) and ASD, there was overgrowth in both white and gray matter in the brains of children with ASD and DLD when compared to typically developing peers. This study confirmed previous findings on cerebellum completed by Carper and Courchesne (2000) and Carper and colleagues (2002). The brain differences in children with ASD were more severe in comparison to those with DLD and controls in every parameter. Children with ASD had greater overgrowth in the frontal and temporal lobe white matter than children with DLD. Clinical correlation in ASD populations is evident, because the severe disruption in their speech and language development is well correlated to temporal lobe dysfunction. There was frontal lobe overgrowth in children with DLD and ASD; however, the overgrowth was significantly larger in children with ASD. Executive dysfunction and language disturbances have been identified in ASD, and these skills are subserved by the frontal lobes. These findings suggest that brain function in ASD and DLD are highly related, and the anatomical differences are related to the severity of overgrowth in specific regions of the brain, but not the location of the overgrowth. These findings further suggest that DLD and ASD may have significant overlap in both brain architecture and phenotypic presentation. More investigation is needed into neurocognitive variations in children with DLD and ASD in comparison to their parents and siblings to understand the underlying mechanism of the phenotypic differences and regional brain differences.

Another intriguing MRI finding is the markedly abnormal brain asymmetry in boys with ASD (Herbert et al., 2005). The right frontal region was increased by 27% in boys with ASD, in sharp contrast to typically developing males who had greater volume in the left frontal region. This brain asymmetry is not well understood, but it is interesting to postulate that the lack of integration in higher associative functions and in language formulation is secondary to these cortical differences and asymmetry. The frontal asymmetry may be helpful in augmenting our understanding of the origin of language differences in ASD and DLD, and in developing more syndrome-specific treatment for children with DLD and ASD.

It is also interesting to hypothesize about the influence of gender on the evolution of these brain structures, because in most studies, few females were represented because of the low incidence of ASD in females (Filipek et al., 1999). Studies in ADHD did not find architectural differences based on gender, and more males than females have this disorder as well (Gogtay et al., 2002). However, girls with ASD are usually more severely impaired than their male counterparts, so the study of regional brain variations and the pattern of growth of both white and gray matter could be very helpful in understanding the pathogenesis of this disorder.

The concept of reduced connectivity in regions of the brain as the cause of the developmental differences in ASD has been entertained for a variety of reasons. The atypical connectivity in ASD intuitively makes sense because of the variability of children's performances, the breadth of the phenotypic presentation, and the inconsistencies of the neuropsychological findings. Several recent studies in motor dysfunction have shed some light on the neural circuitry in ASD. Generalized motoric abnormalities in children with ASD have been described in the literature for more than two decades, including gross and fine motor clumsiness and delays, dyspraxia, and hypotonia of trunk and lower extremities (Damasio & Mauer, 1978; Minshew, Sung, Jones, & Furman, 2005). However, the significance of these pervasive motor differences and their relationship to brain dysfunction has not been well appreciated until recently. In one prospective study by Minshew and associates (2005), postural stability responses in children with ASD were abnormal and related more to generalized central nervous system (CNS) dysfunction than abnormal muscle tonus. These findings suggest a more sweeping effect on neural circuitry and brain than simply the core symptoms of atypical social interaction, complex speech and language dysfunction, and repetitive movements would indicate. Postural stability demands a more formalized, complex integration of several systems, because motoric skills range from praxis to sequencing to executive function of a skilled motor sequence. This study suggests an interconnection between postural stability, neural circuitry, and ASD.

Further supporting the pervasiveness of motor dysfunction in ASD are several studies completed by Teitelbaum and colleagues (2004) with infants who have ASD or Asperger's syndrome (AS). Abnormal postural responses in infants in both groups were identified in a retrospective review demonstrating the early onset of motoric dysfunction and persistence of primitive reflexes. These motor deficiencies were distinct and different in presentation in infants depending on whether the diagnosis was AS or ASD. These findings are tantalizing, because these disturbances are associated with postural instability and support the concept of a more global effect on the evolving CNS than the core symptoms indicate. Additionally, these articles suggest that abnormalities associated with ASD are evident as early as 4 months of age; therefore, the motor system may provide a window of opportunity to diagnose children early, as well as to foster insights of the brain and behavior issues associated with ASD.

With the identification of postural stability abnormalities, atypical motor movements in infancy, and the realization that brain overgrowth occurs as early as 6–12 months of age, early identification of infants with ASD without a biological marker becomes feasible. Additionally, the concept of connectivity abnormalities within the brain as a causative factor to explain the differences in ASD seems quite applicable. A basic neural system dysfunction with brain overgrowth goes awry early in brain development, and the timing and degree of this brain overgrowth may explain the variance within the children. Hypothetically, children with ASD are more impaired, because these brain abnormalities occur earlier and have a more pervasive effect on neural systems that are less mature and underdeveloped. This results in a more deleterious effect on the neurodevelopmental performance of the child, because the infant's repertoire of skills is quite primitive. In contrast, when brain overgrowth occurs later in development, the neurodevelopmental profile is affected, but its presentation is milder, because some skills sets are established. These latest findings are tantalizing from the perspectives of both neuroscience and clinical research.

## Summary

ASD is a neurobiological disorder in which motor dysfunction is evident as early as the first year of life and continues throughout the child's life. The core symptoms include receptive and expressive language deficits, atypical social interactions, and repetitive behaviors (Filipek et al., 1999). There are associated deficits of sensory, attentional, and executive dysfunction as well. Recent MRI findings indicate an overgrowth of both gray and white matter, with regional variations in brain architecture that correlate with neuropsychological function (Herbert et al., 2004). The genetic etiology of ASD is not well understood; however, twin studies demonstrate that this is highly inheritable disorder. Although the research studies have reported varying degrees of mental retardation, from 25 to 75%, the intellectual capabilities of the child with ASD are difficult to discern, because the complexity of the disorder both behaviorally and communicatively decreases the effectiveness and validity of standardized assessments for this population.

## Williams' Syndrome

Williams' syndrome (WS) occurs one in 20,000 births and was originally described in 1961 by Williams, Barratt-Boyes, and Lowe. The chromosomal variation was identified in 1995, and is characterized by a contiguous gene deletion of 7q11.23, which includes an elastin gene defect within this large region (Lowery et al., 1995; Osborne et al., 1996). Children with WS have a distinctive facial appearance, previously described as "elfin-like" (Hovis & Butler, 1997). Features include cardiac anomalies, including supravalvular aortic stenosis and pulmonary stenosis; hypocalcemia; and growth retardation with an uneven neurocognitive profile (Hagerman, 1999). The majority of the children function with mild to moderate retardation, but there are reports of normal intellectual abilities. In spite of the retardation, there are areas of acceleration and enhancement in several domains.

In infancy, the neurodevelopmental profile of a child with WS includes hypotonia in the oral facial musculature, trunk, and extremities. As the child becomes older, this hypotonia progresses to increasing stiffness in joints, with decreased range of motion (Mervis et al., 1999). Typically, fingers, knees, and ankles are most affected. The elastin gene defect is believed to be the causative factor in the tonal change over time (Hagerman, 1999). Motor planning defi-

cits are highly associated with this disorder, and more than 70% of the children have praxis deficits (Chapman, du Plessis, & Pober, 1995). Sensory integration dysfunction is evident within the newborn period. The marked hyperacusis throughout patients' lives is now believed to be associated with hyperexcitability in the primary auditory cortex (Holinger et al., 2005).

The neurocognitive profile is quite variable in children with WS (Bellugi, Lichtenberger, Jones, Lai, & St. George, 2000; Osborne & Pober, 2001). Typically, it includes severe visuospatial deficits, and enhanced facial processing and emotionality (Atkinson et al., 2003; Mobbs et al., 2004; Reiss et al., 2004). Some aspects of language processing are enhanced in spite of the neurocognitive deficits. A recent study of 31 individuals with WS demonstrated greater cognitive heterogeneity than has been previously described. Phonological processing in tests of nonverbal reasoning was within normal limits and revealed the possibility of subgroups within WS (Porter & Colthart, 2005). The variability of the phenotype with correlation to brain differences could increase our understanding of genotypic influence and the effect of elastin on motor function, as well as the variability in the neurocognitive function.

### Toddlers with WS and Executive Function

Executive function and visual search in toddlers with WS, fragile X syndrome (FRAX) and typically developing toddlers was studied (Scerif et al., 2004). Although executive dysfunction has been described as a distinct phenotypic presentation consistent in older children and adolescents with WS and FRAX, it has not been investigated in toddlers. Toddlers with WS and FRAX had significantly more executive dysfunction than the control groups. This is one of the first studies to capture executive function in toddlers, as well as to discern differences between two neurogenetic disorders that both feature frontal lobe dysfunction. Toddlers with WS had more errors related to visual distraction than children with either FRAX or the control group. These findings that suggest deficits in visual attention rather than inhibition are present in WS in spite of enhanced visuospatial skills. Visuoperceptual skills in WS may not be intact in early years as believed, or perhaps there is an evolution to accelerated visual skills at school age in WS. Equally intriguing is the possibility that children with WS may be proficient through the auditory channel for some selected tasks that have not been appreciated. This study also reveals that executive dysfunction and frontal lobe integrity can be evaluated in young children with WS (Scerif et al., 2004). This data further applies to regions of brain dysfunction within different neurogenetic disorders but phenotypic variability with some overlap. This is exciting, because it affords the possibility for natural history studies in the evolution of frontal lobe function in the early years of development. Attentional characteristics of infants with WS have shown intriguing results. In a recent study of triadic interactions, infants with WS showed unique attentional capacities with strangers that may predict later personality and temperament traits (Mervis et al., 1999). This study also reveals the variance in arousal in young children with WS, which is related to later frontal lobe function and executive skills.

In summary, WS is a neurogenetic disorder characterized by a homozygous chromosomal deletion of 7q11.23 that has an evolving, characteristic phenotypic presentation that includes mild to moderate mental retardation, with enhanced function in facial processing and emotionality. Frontal lobe dysfunction is evident, with atypical skills in the auditory cortex, resulting in uneven sensitivity to sounds and tone. The frontal–executive function differences have been shown in young children, but further comprehensive studies are necessary to understand the subtleties of the complex gene–behavior interaction.

### Neuroimaging Findings

A common neuroanatomical finding in adults with WS is a large cerebellum in comparison to a small cerebrum (Jones et al., 2002). In a small study of nine children (mean age 21 months) with WS, results revealed enlarged cerebellums, similar in size to those of children with ASD. WS and ASD can co-occur, further suggesting that there is some phenotypic commonality in the two disorders. Now neuroanatomical abnormalities have been identified in the enlarged cerebellum; however, a large cerebellum is not exclusive to either of these disorders. Other studies also suggest that the cerebellum plays a more intricate role in cognition than was previ-

ously appreciated (Lincoln, Lai, & Jones, 2002). Frontal lobe dysfunction in children with WS has been suspected because of attention deficits, planning weaknesses, and executive dysfunction. Several studies have substantiated frontal lobe dysfunction, particularly when associated with facial interactive responses. Atkinson and colleagues (2003) demonstrated that the specific aspects of processing are deficient, which suggests that deficits in frontal parietal circuitry may be deficient, as well as altered. Facial processing findings in children with WS suggest atypical brain activation compared to that of typically developing peers. Children with WS have increased activation in the right fusiform gyrus in selective frontal and temporal regions. Activation was more extensive than in control groups in the right inferior, superior, and medial frontal gyri, as well as the caudate and thalamus. This may account for the atypical clinical presentation of gaze aversion and withdrawal in children with WS in selective circumstances. It is tantalizing to hypothesize that children avoid direct gaze as a self-protective mechanism because of their overarousal. This type of gaze aversion behavior when over aroused has been well described by Als, Butler, Kosta, and McAnulty (2005) for more than 15 years in premature infants. Reiss and colleagues (2004) recently completed a study of individuals with WS. They evaluated the neuroanatomical differences in both volume and density in brain regions related to areas of acceleration in WS. Finding of neuroanatomical differences were highly correlated with neurodevelopmental performances. Patients with WS had reduced volumes in both thalamic and occipital gray matter when compared to controls. Thalamic and occipital areas are highly correlated with the human visuospatial shell development. There was an increase in both density and volume in cortical regions associated with areas of enhancement in WS, especially emotion and face processing. Several regions of the brain, including amygdala, anterior cingulate, and medial prefrontal cortices, had increased volumes, and these correlate to the behavioral and phenotypic presentation of WS.

### Summary

WS is an intriguing disorder because of the variability of the phenotypic presentation, the unevenness of the profile, and the personality differences, which correlate with neuroanatomical variation. Because of the chromosomal deletion associated with the elastic gene deficit, investigation into the disorder may not only enhance our understanding of the genotypic–phenotypic interaction but also increase our comprehension of the elastic gene deficit and its effect on the condition. WS has an evolving neurocognitive profile that is unique and variable at the same time.

## Attention-Deficit/Hyperactivity Disorder

### Neurobehavioral Phenotype

ADHD is a neurobiological disorder that affects developmental processes, school performance, job employment, and family function. It affects about 4.4 million children, according to the latest reports from the Centers for Disease Control and Prevention (2005). Four features of this disorder are atypical and decreased attention span, and impulsivity with distractibility and inappropriate overactivity, usually in the motor domain (American Psychiatric Association, 1994). One of the defining features of ADHD is the predictability of symptoms across diverse situations, including home and school. Prevalence is estimated at 3–5% of children, with a male predominance of seven to one. It occurs in all races, ethnic, and socioeconomic groups (Cantwell, 1996; Swanson et al., 1998). Although studies are not conclusive on the prevalence of ADHD in adults, recent studies indicate that symptoms persist into adulthood in about 30–70% of cases (Karatekin, 2001).

Executive dysfunction with associated frontal lobe abnormalities is one of the hallmarks of the neuropsychological presentation (Carte, Nigg, & Hinshaw, 1996; Karatekin & Asarnow, 1999; Pennington & Ozonoff, 1996; Shallice et al., 2002; Wiers, Gunning, & Sergeant, 1998). The core dysfunction is in inhibition and attention capacities (Munoz, Broughton, Goldring, & Armstrong, 1998; Nigg, 1999; Oosterlaan, Logan, & Sargeant, 1998; Pennington & Ozonoff, 1996). Studies have shown atypical function in various measures of executive processes; however, inconsistencies persist across studies and within the population. The possibility of distinct subtypes

of ADHD has been entertained (Andreasen, 1999). Conversely, because ADHD is highly inheritable, it is possible that parental learning disabilities and learning styles also affect the child with ADHD (Biederman & Faraone, 2002; Johnson et al., 2001).

With increased awareness and identification of children with ADHD, the time of diagnosis is earlier. Typically, symptoms of ADHD present in preschool years; diagnosis has been made consistently between ages 6 and 8 until recently. Within the last 5 years, diagnosis and treatment of preschoolers with ADHD has increased dramatically (Connor, 2002). Executive function in typically developing preschoolers is not well understood. Equally challenging for the research community is discerning the dysfunction of the ADHD versus normal preschool behavior that is characteristically impulsive and distractible (Fraser, 2002). The phenotypic presentation of ADHD in preschoolers is not well established, and efficacy of treatment has been problematic (Connor, 2002).

The neurodevelopmental profile of the child with ADHD evolves with age and can look quite different from preschool to high school (Cantwell, 1996; Karatekin, 2001). Prefrontal cortex abnormalities, as well as several subcortical systems, are associated with ADHD and affect learning styles, educational success, and interpersonal skills (Ernst, Zametkin, Matochik, Jons, & Cohen, 1998; Faraone & Biederman, 1998; Tannock, 1998). Ernst and associates (1998) have postulated evolving neuroimaging findings in ADHD, dependent on the age of the child and maturation. In young children, the primary deficit of the brain is evident in the basal ganglia, whereas the adult with ADHD shows the deficits in the prefrontal cortex (Ernst et al., 1998; Kaplan & Stevens, 2002). It seems highly plausible that there would be different areas of brain activation with maturity, because developmental maturation demands diverse skills sets as the individual matures from infancy to young adulthood (Kaplan & Stevens, 2002).

### Neurobiology

It is now recognized that millions of children and adults have ADHD and some with associated learning differences and executive dysfunction; however, the neurobiology of ADHD remains unclear (Kaplan & Stevens, 2002; Spencer, Beiderman, Wilens, & Faraone, 2002). Candidate genes, inheritance patterns, and risk factors in the prenatal and perinatal periods have been identified in the last 5 years (Spencer et al., 2002). Increased inheritability rates have been demonstrated in family, adoption, and twin studies (Faraone & Beiderman, 1998; Hechtman, 1994; Tannock, 1998). The inheritability rates in monozygotic twin studies indicate that approximately 60–95% of ADHD presentation is related to the genetics of this neurodevelopmental disorder. In recent years, specific candidate genes have been studied as an etiological link to ADHD. Dopamine, a neurotransmitter, has been associated with ADHD because of both structural abnormalities in the brain and pharmacological responses of children with ADHD. Polymorphisms in both the *DAT I* and *DRD 4* candidate genes reveal high linkage to ADHD, further confirming the role of neurotransmission and its interaction with ADHD. Although no neurobiological markers confirm the presence of ADHD, the inheritability of ADHD has been substantiated, and identification of specific candidate genes provides encouragement that the genetics of this disorder will be revealed (Castellanos et al., 2003).

ADHD is a heterogeneous condition with neuroimaging abnormalities of frontal lobe and related subcortical systems. Comorbidity with ASD, FRAX, SCD, and other developmental disorders has been identified. The homogeneity of the neurogenetic disorders and the increased association with ADHD provides an opportunity to study the pathophysiology of ADHD in very select populations. From these studies, some generalities may be applied to the more heterogeneous population of people with ADHD. Conversely, reducing the variance in studies on children with ADHD would be helpful in the effort to tease out the phenotypic features of the disorder.

### Neuroimaging Findings

Neuroimaging studies of people with ADHD have revealed differences in brain structures, metabolism, cerebral blood flow, and volumes within specific brain regions (Kaplan & Stevens, 2002; Trip, Ryan, & Peace, 2002). Some of the early studies by Hynd and colleagues (1990) reveal asymmetry in the frontal lobe, with decreased interior cortexes. Later studies reveal caudate nucleus reduction and calossal abnormalities (Hynd et al., 1993). Recent studies focus on volumetric measures across brain regions and the relationships to clinical presentation ADHD, as well as altered structure in selected regions. Frontal and striatal regions have been identified as atypical in children with ADHD, and their anatomical findings correlate well the neuropsychological findings (Lou, Henriksen, & Bruhn, 1984; Zametkin et al., 1990). Quantitative analysis reveals that boys and girls with ADHD have significantly altered structures in frontal lobes, caudate nucleus, and corpus callosum, specifically, the rostrum (Castellanos et al., 1996, 2001; Giedd et al., 1994). Brain volume is reduced in both girls and boys with ADHD when compared to typically developing peers (Castellanos et al., 2001, 2002). Although there is a predominance in boys, neuropsychological aspects and neuroimaging manifestations of ADHD are consistent across gender (Giedd, Blumenthal, Molloy, & Castellanos, 2001). Consistency in findings across neuroimaging studies reveal involvement in frontal lobes, basal ganglia, corpus callosum, and cerebellum (Giedd et al., 2001). Clinical correlations between brain architecture and behavioral symptoms have been more elusive because of the heterogeneity of the disorder, as well as the breadth of the spectrum, from mild to severe. Recent studies, both in singleton and twin studies, have supported prefrontal striatal circuitry dysfunction (Castellanos et al., 2003). Further neuroimaging investigations are needed to discern the variability of presentation and the etiological link between specific inheritance patterns and ADHD.

Family studies may be helpful in further understanding the genetics of ADHD and the link between brain architecture and behavioral manifestations. A primary caregiver with ADHD affects an at-risk child's learning and development performance because of the chaotic environment and decreased parenting ability. The synergistic effect between the genetics of this disorder and the environment is complex, but it warrants comprehensive investigation to formulate more syndrome-specific treatment protocols, both pharmacologically and behaviorally.

## Summary

ADHD, a common neurobiological developmental disorder, occurs in 3–5% of the population across racial and ethnic groups. The core symptoms of inattention, impulsivity, and motor activity are highly correlated with neuroanatomical differences. The symptoms are associated with executive dysfunction and frontal lobe abnormalities. Neuroimaging findings have correlated brain and behavior manifestations. Further investigation of the subtypes of ADHD and anatomical differences is warranted.

## ACKNOWLEDGMENTS

Funding for this chapter was partially supported from the JV Foundation (2005). Teresa Sadeghin, Shannon Bailey, and Samantha Rosenson were instrumental in assisting with the typing and editing of the manuscript. Finally, my patients continue to enlighten me with their dedication and devotion to their children in spite of the challenges and frustrations of their life.

## REFERENCES

Abramsky, L., & Chapple, J. (1997). 47, XXY (Klinefelter syndrome) and 47, XYY: Estimated rates of and indication for postnatal diagnosis with implications for prenatal counseling. *Prenatal Diagnosis, 17*(4), 363–368.

Als, H., Butler, S., Kosta, S., & McAnulty, G. (2005). The Assessment of Preterm Infants' Behavior (APIB): Furthering the understanding and measurement of neurodevelopmental competence in preterm and full-term infants. *Mental Retardation and Developmental Disabilities Research Reviews, 11*(1), 94–102.

American Psychiatric Association. (1994). *Diagnostic and statistical manual of mental disorders* (4th ed.). Washington, DC: Author.

Andreasen, N. C. (1999). A unitary model of schizophrenia: Bleuler's "fragmented phrene" as schizencephaly. *Archives of General Psychiatry, 56*, 781–787.

Atkinson, J., Braddick, O., Anker, S., Curran, W., Andrew, R., Wattam-Bell, J., et al. (2003). Neurobiological models of viuospatial cognition in children with Williams syndrome: Measure of dorsal-stream and frontal function. *Developmental Neuropsychology, 23*(1–2), 139–172.

Bailey, D. B., Jr., Mesibov, G. B., Hatton, D. D., Clark, R. D., Roberts, J. E., & Mayhew, L. (1998). Autistic behavior in young boys with fragile X syndrome. *Journal Autism and Developmental Disorders, 28*, 499–508.

Bellugi, U., Lichtenberger, L., Jones, W., Lai, Z., & St. George, M. (2000). The neurocognitive profile of Williams syndrome: A complex pattern of strengths and weaknesses. *Journal of Cognitive Neuroscience, 12*(Suppl. 1), 7–29.

Belmonte, M. K. Allen, G., Beckel-Mitchener, A., Boulanger, L. M., Carper, R. A., & Webb, S. J. (2004). Autism and abnormal development of brain connectivity. *Journal of Neuroscience, 24*, 9228–9231.

Belmonte, M. K., Cook, E. H., Jr., Anderson, G. M., Rubenstein, J. L., Greenough, W. T., Beckel-Mitchener, A., et al. (2004). Autism as a disorder of neural information processing: Directions for research and targets of therapy. *Molecular Psychiatry, 9* 646–663.

Bender, B. G., Harmon, R. J., Linden, M. G., & Robinson, A. (1995). Psychosocial adaptation of 39 adolescents with sex chromosome abnormalities. *Pediatrics, 96*, 302–308.

Biederman, J., & Faraone, S. V. (2002). Current concepts on the neurobiology on attention-deficit/hyperactivity disorder. *Journal of Attention Disorders, 6*(Suppl. 1), S7–S16.

Boone-Brauer, K., Swerdloff, R. S. Miller, R. S., Geschwind, D. H., Razani, J., Lee, A., et al. (2001). Neuropsychological profiles of adults with Klinefelter syndrome. *Journal of the International Neuropsychological Society, 7*, 446–456.

Bradbury, J. T., Bunge, R. G., & Boccabella, R. A. (1956). Chromatin test in Klinefelter's syndrome. *Journal of Clinical Endocrine Metabolism, 16*, 689.

Butler, M. G., Hedges, L. K., Rogan, P. K., Seip, J. R., Cassidy, S. B., & Moeschler, J. B. (1997). Klinefelter and trisomy X syndromes in patients with Prader–Willi syndrome and uniparental maternal disomy of chromosome 15—a coincidence? [Letter to the editor]. *American Journal of Medical Genetics, 72*(1), 111–114.

Cantwell, D. P. (1996). Classification of child and adolescent psychopathology. *Journal of Child Psychology and Psychiatry, 37*, 3–12.

Carper, R. A., & Courchesne, E. (2000). Inverse correlation between frontal lobe and cerebellum sizes in children with autism. *Brain, 123*(4), 836–844.

Carper, R. A., & Courchesne, E. (2005). Localized enlargement of the frontal cortex in early autism. *Biological Psychiatry, 57*(2), 126–133.

Carper, R. A., Moses, P., Tigue, Z. D., & Courchesne, E. (2002). Cerebral lobes in autism: Early hyperplasia and abnormal age effects. *NeuroImage, 16*(4), 1038–1051.

Carte, E. T., Nigg, J. T., & Hinshaw, S. P. (1996). Neuropsychological functioning, motor speed, and language processing in boys with and without ADHD. *Journal of Abnormal Child Psychology, 24*, 481–498.

Casey, B. J., Giedd, J. N., & Thomas, K. M. (2000). Structural and functional brain development and its relation to cognitive development. *Biological Psychology, 54*, 241–257.

Casey, M. D., Segall, L. J., Street, D. R., & Blank, C. E. (1966). Sex chromosome abnormalities in two state hospitals for patients requiring special security. *Nature, 209*, 641–642.

Castellanos, F. X., Giedd, J. N., Berquin, P. C., Walter, J. M., Sharp, W., Tran, T., et al. (2001). Quantitative brain magnetic resonance imaging in girls with attention-deficit/hyperactivity disorder. *Archives of General Psychiatry, 58*(3), 289–295.

Castellanos, F. X., Giedd, J. N., Marsh, W. L., Hamburger, S. D., Vaituzis, A. C., Dickstein, D. P., et al. (1996). Quantitative brain magnetic resonance imaging in attention-deficit hyperactivity disorder. *Archives of General Psychiatry, 53*(7), 607–616.

Castellanos, F. X., Lee, P. P., Sharp, W., Jeffries, N. O., Greenstein, D. K., Clasen, L. S., et al. (2002). Developmental trajectories of brain volume abnormalities in children and adolescents with attention-deficit/hyperactivity disorder. *Journal of the American Medical Association, 288*(14), 1740–1748.

Castellanos, F. X., Sharp, W. S., Gottesman, R. F., Greenstein, D. K., Giedd, J. N., & Rapoport, J. L. (2003). Anatomic brain abnormalities in monozygotic twins discordant attention deficit hyperactivity disorder. *American Journal of Psychiatry, 160*(9), 1693–1696.

Centers for Disease Control and Prevention. (2005, September 20). *Attention-deficit/hyperactivity disorder (ADHD)*. Atlanta, GA: Author. Retrieved from www.cdc.gov/ncbddd/adhd

Chapman, C. A., du Plessis, A., & Pober, B. (1995). Neurologic findings in children and adults with Williams syndrome. *Journal of Child Neurology, 10*, 63–65.

Connor, D. F. (2002). Preschool attention deficit hyperactivity disorder: A review of prevalence, diagnosis, neurobiology, and stimulant treatment. *Journal of Developmental and Behavioral Pediatrics, 23*(Suppl. 1), S1–S9.

Courchesne, E., Redcay, E., & Kennedy, D. P. (2004). The autistic brain: Birth through adulthood. *Current Opinion in Neurology, 17*(4), 489–496.

Courchesne, E., Townsend, J., & Saitoh, O. (1994). The brain in infantile autism: Posterior fossa structures are abnormal. *Neurology, 44*(2), 214–223.

Damasio, A. R., & Maurer, R. G. (1978). A neurological model for childhood autism. *Archives of Neurology, 35*, 777–786.

Dementieva, Y. A., Vance, D. D., Donnelly, S. L., Elston, L. A., Wolpert, C. M., Ravan, S. A., et al. (2005). "Accelerated head growth in early development of individuals with autism. *Pediatric Neurology, 32*(2), 102–108.

Denckla, M. B. (1994). Measurement of executive functioning." In G. R. Lyon (Ed.), *Frames of reference for the assessment of learning disabilities: New views on measurement issues* (pp. 117–142). Baltimore: Brooks.

Durston, S., Hulshoff Pol, H. E., Casey, B. J., Giedd, J. N., Buitelaar, J. K., & van Engeland, H. (2001). Anatomical MRI of the developing human brain: What have we learned? *Journal of the American Academy of Child and Adolescent Psychiatry, 40*(9), 1012–1020.

Ernst, M., Zametkin, A. J., Matochik, J. A., Jons, P. H., & Cohen, R. M. (1998). DOPA decarboxylase activity in attention deficit hyperactivity disorder adults: A [18F] fluorodopa positron emission tomographic study. *Journal of Neuroscience, 18*, 5901–5907.

Espy, K. A. (2004). Using developmental, cognitive, and neuroscience approaches to understand executive control in young children. *Developmental Neuropsychology, 26*(1), 379–384.

Faraone, S. V., & Biederman, J. (1998). Neurobiology of attention-deficit hyperactivity disorder. *Biological Psychiatry, 44*, 951–958.

Ferguson-Smith, M. A. (1959). The prepubertal testicular lesion in chromatin-positive Klinefelter's syndrome (primary micro-orchidism) as seen in mentally handicapped children. *Lancet, 1*, 219–222.

Filipek, P. A., Accardo, P. J., Baranek, G. T., Cook, E. H., Jr., Dawson, G., Gordon, B., et al. (1999). The screening and diagnosis of autistic spectrum disorders. *Journal of Autism and Developmental Disorders, 29*(6), 439–484.

Folstein, S. E., & Rosen-Sheidley, B. (2001). Genetics of autism: Complex aetiology for a heterogeneous disorder. *Nature Reviews Genetics, 2*, 943–955.

Fraser, K. M. (2002). Too young for attention deficit disorder?: Views from preschool. *Journal of Development and Behavior in Pediatrics, 23*(1, Suppl.), 46–50.

Fryns, J. P., & Van den Berghe, H. (1988). The concurrence of Klinefelter syndrome and fragile X syndrome. *American Journal of Medical Genetics, 30*, 109–113.

Fuster, J. (2002). Frontal lobe and cognitive development. *Journal of Neuropsychology, 31*, 373–385.

Geschwind, D. H., Boone, K. B., Miller, B. L., & Swerdloff, R. S. (2000). Neurobehavioral phenotype of Klinefelter syndrome. *Mental Retardation and Developmental Disabilities Research Reviews, 6*, 107–116.

Giedd, J. N. (2003). The anatomy of mentalization: A view from developmental neuroimaging. *Bulletin of the Menninger Clinic, 67*(2), 132–142.

Giedd, J. N. (2004). Structural magnetic resonance imaging of the adolescent brain. *Annals of the New York Academy of Sciences, 1021*, 77–85.

Giedd, J. N., Blumenthal, J., Jeffries, N. O., Castellanos, F. X., Liu, H., Zijdenbos, A., et al. (1999). Brain development during childhood and adolescence: A longitudinal MRI study. *Nature Neuroscience, 2,* 861–863.

Giedd, J. N., Blumenthal, J., Molloy, E., & Castellanos, F. X. (2001). Brain imaging of attention deficit/hyperactivity disorder. *Annals of the New York Academy of Sciences, 931,* 33–49.

Giedd, J. N., Castellanos, F. X., Casey, B. J., Kozuch, P., King, A. C., Hamburger, S. D., et al. (1994). Quantitative morphology of the corpus callosum in attention deficit hyperactivity disorder. *American Journal of Psychiatry, 151*(5), 665–669.

Giedd, J. N., Snell, J. W., Lange, N., Rajapakse, J. C., Casey, B. J., Kozuch, P. L., et al. (1996). Quantitative magnetic resonance imaging of human brain development: Ages 4–18. *Cerebral Cortex, 6*(4), 551–560.

Gillberg, L., & Rasmussen, P. (1994). Four case histories and a literature review of Williams syndrome and autistic behavior. *Journal of Autism and Developmental Disorder, 24,* 381–393.

Gogtay, N., Giedd, J. N., Lusk, L., Hayashi, K. M., Greenstein, D., & Vaituzis, A. C. (2004). Dynamic mapping of human cortical development during childhood through early adulthood. *Proceedings of the National Academy of Sciences of the United States of America, 101*(21), 8174–8179.

Gogtay, N., Giedd, J., & Rapoport, J. L. (2002). Brain development in healthy, hyperactive, and psychotic children. *Archives of Neurology, 59*(8), 1244–1248.

Greicius, M. D. (2003). Neuroimaging in developmental disorders. *Current Opinion in Neurology, 16*(2), 143–146.

Hagerman, R. J. (1999). *Neurodevelopmental disorders: Diagnosis and treatment.* New York: Oxford University Press.

Harris, J. C. (1998). *Developmental neuropsychiatry: Fundamentals* (Vol. 1). New York: Oxford University Press.

Hechtman, L. (1994). Genetic and neurobiological aspects of attention deficit hyperactive disorder: A review. *Journal of Psychiatry and Neuroscience, 19*(3), 193–201.

Herbert, M. R., Harris, G. J., Adrien, K. T., Ziegler, D. A., Makris, N., Kennedy, D. N., et al. (2002). Abnormal asymmetry in language association cortex in autism. *Annals of Neurology, 52*(5), 588–596.

Herbert, M. R., Ziegler, D. A., Deutsch, C. K., O'Brien, L. M., Kennedy, D. N., & Filipek, P. A. (2005). Brain asymmetries in autism and developmental language disorder: A nested whole-brain analysis. *Brain, 128*(Pt. 1), 213–226.

Herbert, M. R., Ziegler, D. A., Deutsch, C. K., O'Brien, L. M., Lange, N., & Bakardjiev, A. (2003). Dissociations of cerebral cortex, subcortical and cerebral white matter volumes in boys. *Brain, 126*(Pt. 5), 1182–1192.

Herbert, M. R., Ziegler, D. A., Makris, N., Filipek, P. A., Kemper, T. L., Normandin, J. J., et al. (2004). Localization of white matter volume increase in autism and developmental language disorder. *Annals of Neurology, 55,* 530–540.

Hill, E. L. (2003). Understanding autism: Insights from mind and brain. *Philosophical Transactions of the Royal Society of London, Series B, Biological Sciences, 28,* 281–289.

Hill, E. L. (2004). Executive dysfunction in autism. *Trends in Cognitive Sciences, 8*(1), 26–32.

Hill, E. L., & Frith, U. (2003). Understanding autism: Insights from mind and brain. *Philosophical Transactions of the Royal Society of London, B, Biological Sciences, 358,* 281–289.

Holinger, D. P., Bellugi, U., Mills, D. L., Korenberg, J. R., Reiss, A. L., Sherman, G. F., et al. (2004). Relative sparing of primary auditory cortex in Williams syndrome. *Brain Research, 1037,* 35–42.

Hoon, A. H., & Melhem, E. R. (2000). "Neuroimaging: Applications in disorders of early brain development. *Developmental and Behavioral Pediatrics, 21*(4), 291–302.

Hovis, C. L., & Butler, M. G. (1997). "Photoanthropometric study of craniofacial traits in individuals with Williams syndrome. *Clinical Genetics, 51*(6), 379–387.

Hynd, G. W., Hern, K. L., Novey, E. S., Eliopulos, D., Marshall, R., Gonzalez, J. J., et al. (1993). Attention deficit-hyperactivity disorder and asymmetry of the caudate nucleus. *Journal of Child Neurology, 8*(4), 339–447.

Hynd, G. W., Semrud-Clikeman, M., Lorys, A. R., Novey, E. S., Eliopulos, D. (1990). Brain morphology in developmental dyslexia and attention deficit disorder/hyperactivity. *Archives of Neurology, 47,* 919–925.

Johnson, D. E., Epstein, J. N., Waid, L. R., Latham, P. K., Voronin, K. E., & Anton, R. F. (2001). Neuropsychological performance deficits in adults with attention deficit/hyperactivity disorder. *Archives of Clinical Neuropsychology, 16*(6), 587–604.

Jones, W., Hesselink, J., Courchesne, C., Duncan, T., Matsuda, K., & Bellugi, U. (2002). Cerebellar abnormalities in infants and toddlers with Williams syndrome. *Developmental Medicine and Child Neurology, 44*(10), 688–694.

Kaplan, R. F., & Stevens, M. (2002). A review of adult ADHD: A neuropsychological and neuroimaging perspective. *CNS Spectrums, 7*(5), 355–362.

Karatekin, C. (2001). Developmental disorders of attention." In C. A. Nelson & M. Luciana (Eds.), *Handbook of developmental cognitive neuroscience* (pp. 561–576). London: MIT Press.

Karatekin, C., & Asarnow, R. F. (1999). "Exploratory eye movements to pictures in childhood-onset schizophrenia and attention deficit/hyperactivity disorder

(ADHD). *Journal of Abnormal Child Psychology, 27,* 35–49.

Klinefelter, H. F., Reifenstein, E. C., & Albright, F. (1942). Syndrome characterized by gynecomasia, aspermatogenesis without aleydigism and increased excretion of follicle-stimulating hormone. *Journal of Clinical Endocrinology and Metabolism, 2,* 615–627.

Lahlou, N., Fennoy, I., Carel, J.-C., & Roger, M. (2004). Inhibin B and anti-Müllerian hormone, but not testosterone levels, are normal in infants with nonmosaic Klinefelter syndrome. *Journal of Clinical Endocrinology and Metabolism, 89*(4), 1864–1868.

Laron, Z., & Hochman, I. H. (1971). Small testes in prepubetal boys with Klinefelter's syndrome. *Journal of Clinical Endorcrinology and Metabolism, 32,* 671–672.

Lincoln, A., Lai, Z., & Jones, W. (2002). Shifting attention and joint attention dissociation in Williams syndrome: Implications for the cerebellum and social deficits in autism. *Neurocase, 8*(3), 226–232.

Linden, M. G., Bender, B. G., & Robinson, A. (1996). Intrauterine diagnosis of dex chromosome aneuploidy. *Obstetrics and Gynecology, 87*(3), 468–475.

Lou, H. C., Henriksen, L., & Bruhn, P. (1984). Focal cerebral hypoperfusion in children with dysphasia and/or attention deficit disorder. *Archives of Neurology, 41*(8), 825–829.

Lowery, M. C., Morris, C. A., Ewart, A., Brothman, L. J., Zhu, X. L., Leonard, C. O., et al. (1995). Strong correlation of elastin deletions, detected by FISH, with Williams syndrome: Evaluation of 235 patients. *American Journal of Human Genetics, 57*(1), 49–53.

Mervis, C. B., Morris, C. A., Klein-Tasman, B. P., Bertrand, J., Kwitney, S., & Appelbaum, L. G. (1999). Attentional characteristics of infants and toddlers with Williams syndrome during triadic interactions. *Developmental Neuropsychology, 23*(1), 243–268.

Minshew, N. J., Sung, K., Jones, B. L., & Furman, J. M. (2005). Underdevelopment of the postural control system in autism. *Neurology, 63,* 2056–2061.

Mobbs, D., Garrett, A. S., Menon, V., Rose, F. E., Bellugi, U., & Reiss, A. L. (2004). Anomalous brain activation during face and gaze processing in Williams syndrome. *Neurology, 62*(11), 2070–2076.

Munoz, D. P., Broughton, J. R., Goldring, J. E., & Armstrong, I. T. (1998). Age-related performance of human subjects on saccadic eye movement tasks. *Experimental Brain Research, 121,* 391–400.

Neilsen, J., & Wohlert, M. (1991). Sex chromosome abnormalities found among 34,910 newborn children: Results from a 13-year study in Århus, Denmark." *Birth Defects: Original Article Series, 26*(4), 209–223.

Oosterlaan, J., Logan, G. D., & Sergeant, J. A. (1998). Response inhibition in AD/HD, CD, comorbid AD/HD + CD, anxious, and control children: A meta-analysis of studies with the Stop task. *Journal of Child Psychology and Psychiatry, 39,* 411–425.

Osborne, L. R., Martindale, D., Scherer, S. W., Shi, X. M., Huizenga, J., & Heng, H. H. (1996). Identification of genes from a 500-kb region at 7 q11.23 that is commonly deleted in Williams syndrome patients. *Genomics, 36*(2), 328–336.

Osborne, L., & Pober, B. (2001). Genetics of childhood disorders: XXVII. Genes and cognition in Williams syndrome. *Journal of the American Academy of Child and Adolescent Psychiatry, 40*(6), 732–735.

Ozonoff, S. (2004). Advances in the cognitive neuroscience of autism. In C. A. Nelson & M. Luciana (Eds.), *Handbook of developmental cognitive neuroscience* (pp. 537–548). London: MIT Press.

Ozonoff, S., & Jensen, J. (1999). Brief report: Specific executive function profiles in three neurodevelopmental disorders. *Journal of Autism and Developmental Disorders, 29*(2), 171–177.

Patwardhan, A. J., Brown, W. E., Bender, B. G., Linden, M. G., Eliez, S., & Reiss, A. L. (2002). Reduced size of the amygdala in individuals with 47, XXY and 47, XXX karyotypes. *American Journal of Medical Genetics, 114,* 93–98.

Patwardhan, A. J., Eliez, S., Bender, B., Linden, M. G., & Reiss, A. L. (2000). Brain morphology in Klinefelter syndrome: Extra X chromosomes and testosterone supplementation. *Neurology, 54*(12), 2218–2222.

Pennington, B. F., & Ozonoff, S. (1996). Executive functions in developmental psychopathology. *Journal of Child Psychology and Psychiatry, 37,* 51–87.

Porter, M. A., & Coltheart, M. (2005). Cognitive heterogeneity in Williams syndrome. *Developmental Neuropsychology, 27*(2), 275–306.

Powell, K. B., & Voeller, K. K. (2004). Prefrontal executive function syndromes in children. *Journal of Child Neurology, 19*(10), 785–797.

Reiss, A. L., & Denckla, M. B. (1996). The contribution of neuroimaging: Fragile X syndrome, Turner syndrome, and neurofibromosis-1. In G. R. Lyon & J. M. Rumsey (Eds.), *Neuroimaging* (pp. 147–168). Baltimore: Brookes.

Reiss, A. L., Eckert, M. A., Rose, F. E., Karchemskiy, A., Kesler, S., Chang, M., et al. (2004). An experiment of nature: Brain anatomy parallels cognition and behavior in Williams syndrome. *Journal of Neuroscience, 24*(21), 5009–5015.

Reiss, A. L., Eliez, S., Schmitt, J. E., Patwardhan, A., &

Haberecht, M. (2000). Brain imaging in neurogenetic conditions: Realizing the potential of behavioral neurogenetics research. *Mental Retardation and Developmental Disabilities Research Reviews, 6*(3), 186–197.

Robinson, A., Bender, B., & Linden, M. G. (1991). Summary of clinical findings in children and young adults with sex chromosome abnormalities. In J. A. Evans, J. L. Hamerton, & A. Robinson (Eds.), *Children and young adults with sex chromosome aneuploidy: Follow-up, clinical, and molecular studies* (pp. 225–228). New York: Wiley-Liss.

Rose, A. B., Merke, D. P., Clasen, L. S., Rosenthal, M. A., Wallace, G. L., Vaituzis, A. C., et al. (2004). Effects of hormones and sex chromosomes on stress-influenced regions of the developing pediatric brain. *Annals of the New York Academy of Sciences, 1032,* 231–241.

Ross, J. L., Samango-Sprouse, C., Lahlou, N., Kowal, K., Elder, F. F., & Zinn, A. (2005). Early androgen deficiency in infants and young boys with 47,XXY Klinefelter syndrome. *Hormone Research, 64*(1), 39–45.

Salbenblatt, J. A., Meyers, D. C., Bender, B. G., Linden, M. G., & Robinson, A. (1987). Gross and fine motor development in 47, XXY and 47, XYY males. *Pediatrics, 80*(2), 240–244.

Samango-Sprouse, C. (1999). Frontal lobe development in childhood. In B. L. Miller & J. L. Cummings (Eds.), *The human frontal lobes: Functions and disorders* (pp. 584–604). New York: Guilford Press.

Samango-Sprouse, C. A. (2001). The mental development in polysomy X Klinefelter syndrome (47 XXY; 48 XXXY): Effects of incomplete X-activation. *Seminars in Reproductive Medicine, 9*(2), 93–202.

Samango-Sprouse, C. A., Jsang, T., & Huddleston, J. (2002). Further characterization and expansion of the neurobehavioral phenotype of the child with sex chromosome variations (SCV). *American Journal of Human Genetics, 71*(4), 197.

Samango-Sprouse, C., & Law, P. (2001). The neurocognitive profile of the young child with XXY. *European Journal of Human Genetics, 9*(Suppl. 1), 193.

Samango-Sprouse, C., & Rogol, A. (2002). The hidden disability and prototype for an infantile presentation of developmental dyspraxia (IDD). *Infants and Young Children, 15,* 11–18.

Sapolsky, R. M. (2004). The frontal cortex and the criminal justice system. *Philosophical Transactions of the Royal Society of London, Series B, Biological Sciences, 359,* 1787–1796.

Scerif, G., Cornish, K., Wilding, J., Driver, J., & Karmiloff-Smith, A. (2004). Visual search in typically developing toddlers and toddlers with fragile X or Williams syndrome. *Developmental Science, 7*(1), 116–130.

Shallice, T., Marzocchi, G. M., Coser, S., DelSavio, M., Meuter, R. F., & Rumiati, R. I. (2002). Executive function profile of children with attention deficit hyperactivity disorder. *Developmental Neuropsychology, 21*(1), 43–71.

Sherman, M., Nass, R., & Shapiro, T. (1984). Brief report: Regional cerebral blood flow in autism. *Journal of Autism and Developmental Disorders, 14*(4), 439–446.

Simpson, J. L., de la Cruz, F., Swerdloff, R. S., Samango-Sprouse, C., Skakkebaek, N. E., Graham, J. M., Jr., et al. (2003). Klinefelter syndrome: Expanding the phenotype and identifying new research directions. *Genetics in Medicine, 5*(6), 1–39.

Simpson, J. L., Graham, J. M., Jr., Samango-Sprouse, C., & Swerdloff, R. (2004). Klinefelter syndrome. In S. S. Cassidy & J. Allanson (Eds.), *Management of genetic syndromes* (pp. 323–333). New York: Wiley.

Spencer, T. J., Biederman, J., Wilens, T. E., & Faraone, S. V. (2002). Overview and neurobiology of attention-deficit/hyperactivity disorder. *Journal of Clinical Psychiatry, 63*(Suppl. 12), 3–9.

Swanson, J. M., Sergeant, J. A., Taylor, E., Sonuga-Barke, E. J., Jensen, P. S., & Cantwell, D. P. (1998). Attention deficit hyperactivity disorder and hyperkinetic disorder. *Lancet, 351,* 429–433.

Tannock, R. (1998). Attention deficit hyperactivity disorder: Advances in cognitive, neurobiological, and genetic research. *Journal of Child Psychology and Psychiatry, 39,* 65–99.

Teitelbaum, O., Benton, T., Shah, P., Prince, A., Kelly, J. L., & Teitelbaum, P. (2004). Eshkol–Wachman movement notation in diagnosis. *Proceedings of the National Academy of Sciences of the United States of America, 101*(32), 11909–11914.

Temple, C. M., & Sanfilippo, P. M. (2003). Executive skills in Klinefelter's syndrome. *Neuropsychologia, 41,* 1547–1559.

Torrey, E. F., Dhavale, D., Lawlor, J. P., & Yolken, R. H. (2004). Autism and head circumference in the first year of life. *Biological Psychiatry, 56*(11), 892–894.

Trip, G., Ryan, J., & Peace, K. (2002). Neuropsychological functioning in children with DSM-IV combined type attention deficit hyperactivity disorder. *Australian and New Zealand Journal of Psychiatry, 36*(6), 771.

Visootsak, J., Alystock, M., & Graham, J. M., Jr. (2001). Klinefelter syndrome and its variants: An update and review for the primary pediatrician. *Clinical Pediatrics, 40,* 639–691.

Wiers, R. W., Gunning, W. B., & Sergeant, J. A. (1998). Is a mild deficit in executive functions in boys related to childhood ADHD or to parental mulitgenerational alcoholism? *Journal of Abnormal Child Psychology, 26,* 415–430.

Williams, J. C. P., Barratt-Boyes, B. G., & Lowe, J. B.

(1961). Supravalvular aortic stenosis. *Circulation*, 24, 1311–1318.

Winter, J. S. D. (1990). Androgen therapy in Klinefelter syndrome during adolescence. In J. A. Evans, J. L. Hamerton, & A. Robinson (Eds.), *Children and young adults with sex chromosome aneuploidy* (pp. 235–245). New York: Wiley.

Wolfe, C. D., & Bell, M. A. (2004). Working memory and inhibitory control in early childhood: Contributions from physiology, temperament, and language. *Developmental Psychobiology*, 44(1), 68–83.

Zametkin, A. J., Nordahl, T. E., Cross, M., King, A. C., Semple, W. E., Rumsey, J., et al. (1990). Cerebral glucose metabolism in adults with hyperactivity of childhood onset. *New England Journal of Medicine, 323*, 1361–1366.

# PART VII

## PSYCHIATRIC DISEASES

# CHAPTER 36

# Frontal Lobe Functioning in Schizophrenia

## EVIDENCE FROM NEUROPSYCHOLOGY, COGNITIVE NEUROSCIENCE, AND PSYCHOPHYSIOLOGY

*Susan A. Legendre Ropacki*
*William Perry*

Since Kraepelin's first clinical account of schizophrenia in 1896, a vast body of scientific inquiry has attempted to understand the diverse pathophysiological processes that underlie this complex brain disorder. The past several decades have brought significant advances in our understanding of possible structural and functional central nervous system abnormalities in patients with schizophrenia. For example, early morphological studies led to the suggestion that many individuals with schizophrenia have enlarged ventricles (Johnstone, Crow, Frith, Husband, & Kreel, 1976; Suddath et al., 1989). More recent work has found evidence of diffuse neocortical atrophy (Lawrie et al., 1997) and structural abnormalities of mesial temporal and subcortical nuclei in the brains of patients with schizophrenia (Andreasen et al., 1994; Bogerts, Mertz, Schonfeldt, & Bausch, 1985; Jernigan et al., 1991; Suddath, Christison, Torrey, Casanova, & Weinberger, 1990). Although the evidence for an underlying neuropathology in schizophrenia is compelling, neuroanatomical abnormalities have not been observed in all patients with schizophrenia, undermining the argument that a single, common neuropathophysiology exists. The emphasis in schizophrenia research, as is true of other heterogeneous disorders, is thus placed on under-

standing dysfunctions within particular brain circuits rather than focal brain regions. Study of brain circuitry has, in turn, provided a rich appreciation for the putative biological mechanisms that regulate the signs and symptoms of schizophrenia. An extensive body of research has demonstrated that the diverse pathophysiological processes that characterize schizophrenia produce a "common final pathway" of typical clinical manifestations subserved by the frontal lobes. The emphasis in schizophrenia research, as is true of other heterogeneous disorders, is thus placed on understanding dysfunctions within particular brain circuits that produce a "common final pathway" of typical clinical manifestations subserved by the frontal lobes. Indeed, from times dating back to Kraepelin (1919) in the early 20th century, the frontal lobes have been the area of primary focus in schizophrenia research. Kraepelin's emphasis on the role of the frontal lobes in schizophrenia was based on the observation that there is considerable accord between negative symptoms (e.g., avolition, emotional flattening) and planning difficulties in schizophrenia, and the behavioral disturbances observed after frontal lobe damage (see Fuster, 1989). This chapter reviews some of the most critical and compelling data from neuropsychology, cognitive neuroscience, and psychophysiology that support the role of frontal lobe abnormalities underlying schizophrenia. This chapter is not intended to be an exhaustive account of the immense body of work that has been conducted in the area of frontal lobes and schizophrenia, nor do we imply that only the frontal lobes are involved in the pathophysiology of schizophrenia. Rather, we provide representative works from a variety of areas that collectively speak to the prominence of frontal lobe deficits in schizophrenia research.

## NEUROPSYCHOLOGY

Neuropsychology has proven to be a valuable tool for studying the nature and severity of frontal lobe dysfunction in schizophrenia. With neuropsychological tests, the higher cognitive processes thought to reflect the integrity of the frontal lobes may be assessed. Several higher cognitive processes are thought to be mediated by the frontal lobes (Lezak, 1995), including executive functions (e.g., planning, problem solving, alternating between two or more tasks), working memory, attention, perseveration, inhibition, and verbal fluency. These processes are by no means orthogonal; rather, they overlap and are heuristically useful in the assessment of the frontal lobes.

### Executive Functions

The term "executive functions" was developed in an attempt to describe the "higher" functions of the frontal cortex (Luria, 1966; Milner, 1964). Executive functions are commonly considered to include skills such as conceptual flexibility, planning, abstract reasoning, maintenance and shifting of cognitive sets, hypothesis testing, problem solving, and self-monitoring of goal-directed behavior (Green, 1998; Palmer & Heaton, 2000). Executive functions have gained considerable attention in the schizophrenia literature over the past decade given that they are considered a core neurocognitive abnormality of the disorder (Chen, Chen, Chan, Lam, & Lieh-Mak, 2000; Chen, Lam, Chen, Nguyen, & Chan, 1996; Elliott, McKenna, Robbins, & Sahakian, 1995; Evans, Chua, McKenna, & Wilson, 1997; Green & Braff, 2001; Weinberger, Aloia, Goldberg, & Berman, 1994). Reed, Harrow, Herbener, and Martin (2002) examined performance on measures of executive function in 42 people with schizophrenia, with and without psychosis, 42 people with other psychotic disorders (e.g., bipolar disorder, depression with psychosis), and 73 inpatients with nonpsychotic psychiatric disorders. Those with schizophrenia demonstrated significantly more deficits on executive functioning tests than the other groups. Patients with schizophrenia also had more executive functioning impairment regardless of whether they were psychotic at the time of assessment, supporting the position that executive function deficits are a core component of schizophrenia rather than a direct consequence of symptoms or treatment effects, such as those resulting from the use of antipsychotic medications.

Deficits in executive functioning have most often been associated with the negative symptom/deficit syndrome subtype of schizophrenia (Addington, Addington, & Maticka-Tyndale, 1991; Basso, Nasrallah, Olson, & Bornstein, 1998; Buchanan et al., 1994; Collins, Remington, Coulter, & Birkett, 1997; Nieuwenstein, Aleman, & de Haan, 2001). The relationship between executive dysfunction and negative symptoms is important, because negative symptoms (e.g., inattention, poverty of speech) are clinically observed among a family of frontally impaired patients. Mahurin, Velligan, and Miller (1998) studied the relationship between executive abilities and symptom subtypes of schizophrenia. They administered a battery of executive function tests to patients with schizophrenia and assessed patients' symptoms using the expanded version of the Brief Psychiatric Rating Scale (BPRS). Scores from nine items on the BPRS were factor-analyzed to determine underlying dimensions of symptom expression. The factor analysis resulted in three symptom dimensions: withdrawal–retardation, conceptual disorganization, and reality distortion. Patients were then assigned to one of these groups based on their BPRS ratings. Results showed that the patients with schizophrenia had significant impairment across all executive–frontal tests. Those in the withdrawal–retardation subgroup, however, showed dysfunction across the greatest number of tests. Similarly, Heydebrand and colleagues (2004) tested 307 people with either schizophrenia, schizophreniform disorder, or schizoaffective disorder. They found a strong relationship between negative (but not positive) symptomatology as measured by the Positive and Negative Syndromes Scale

(PANSS) and executive function measures, as well as verbal fluency, psychomotor speed, and memory. Donohoe and Robertson (2003) reviewed the relationship between clinical symptoms and neurocognitive impairment in schizophrenia. These authors reported that 10 of the 11 studies reviewed found negative and disorganized symptoms most strongly associated with executive functioning impairment, whereas no study reported a correlation with positive symptoms.

Among the most widely utilized neuropsychological tests of executive functioning is the Wisconsin Card Sorting Test (WCST; Berg, 1948; Heaton, Chelune, Talley, Kay, & Curtiss, 1993). The WCST requires abstract reasoning and problem-solving skills, as well as an ability to shift strategies according to feedback, all of which are considered to be cornerstone executive functions (Lezak, 1995). In addition, the WCST is one of the few tests that has shown specific sensitivity to frontal lobe lesions (Heaton, 1981), making it an ideal test of potential underlying frontal lobe pathology in schizophrenia. In a seminal series of studies, Weinberger and colleagues (Berman, Zec, & Weinberger, 1986; Weinberger, Berman, & Zec, 1986) demonstrated the role of the frontal lobes in schizophrenia by comparing WCST performances of a group of patients with chronic schizophrenia, who, because of the chronicity of their illnesses, were expected to perform poorly on the task compared to a group of normal, healthy subjects (Goldberg, Weinberger, Berman, Pliskin, & Podd, 1987). Regional cerebral blood flow (rCBF) of patients with schizophrenia and the healthy comparison subjects was measured while each performed an automated, computerized version of the WCST. Patients with schizophrenia exhibited reduced rCBF in the dorsolateral prefrontal cortex (DLPFC) during the task, whereas the healthy comparison subjects showed activation in the same region. Using similar methodology, Liu, Tam, Xie, and Zhao (2002) compared rCBF in 21 inpatients and outpatients with schizophrenia with negative symptoms to 12 healthy, normal comparison subjects while each performed the WCST. Results revealed no differences between the groups at rest. However, during task activation, the patients with schizophrenia showed significantly less increase in rCBF in the left prefrontal region compared to the healthy comparison group.

The nature of cognitive deficits associated with schizophrenia and the particular role of the frontal lobes has also been illustrated by comparing the WCST performance of patients with schizophrenia to that of patients with brain injuries (Pantelis & Nelson, 1994). Haut and colleagues (1996) compared the WCST performance of 12 individuals with schizophrenia to patients with right or left low-grade frontal lobe tumors, patients with nonfrontal high-grade tumors, and healthy normal subjects. On the WCST, those with schizophrenia and patients with right frontal low-grade tumors performed similarly. Each had poorer conceptualization of the task compared to the other groups, as well as a greater number of perseverations and longer strings of perseverations. Thus, the role of frontal lobe dysfunction in schizophrenia was supported.

Subsequent research on WCST performance in schizophrenia considered whether poor WCST performance among patients with schizophrenia was due not to frontal lobe dysfunction but rather to behavioral factors inherent to the disease, such as inattention, poor cooperation, or lack of motivation. To test this possibility, Goldberg and colleagues (1987) examined whether patients with schizophrenia could learn the task and thus improve their performance. These patients were administered the WCST under two conditions: In one condition, patients were told of the sorting rules (e.g., to sort based on matching color, form, or number); in the other condition, patients were provided with instruction after each card placement they made. Although those in the first condition were told of the sorting rules, they failed to improve their performance on the task and continued to commit a high number of perseverative errors. Those who were provided instruction after each card placement, in contrast, did show improved performance. When asked to complete the task again without instruction, however, the same individuals returned to their baseline level of (poor) functioning. In conjunction with findings that patients *were* able to learn to perform other tasks *not* dependent on the frontal lobes, Goldberg and colleagues concluded that patients with schizophrenia were unable to learn the WCST; thus, deficits on this test were due to dysfunction of the DLPFC and not simply a reflection of behavioral factors.

Goldberg and colleagues' (1987) conclusion was challenged on the basis that the study paradigm did not provide adequate behavioral contingencies to promote active participation or motivation. For two decades since that study was published, there has been an effort to assess whether WCST performance may be remediable among patients with schizophrenia. Several investigators have demonstrated that these patients' typically poor WCST performance is indeed remediable with training, suggesting that the deficit may not be fixed (Bellack, Mueser, Morrison, Tierney, & Podell, 1990; Everett, Lavoie, Gagnon, & Gosselin, 2001; Goldman, Axelrod, & Tompkins, 1992; Green, Ganzell, Satz, & Vaclav, 1990; Green, Satz, Ganzell, & Vaclav, 1992; Metz, Johnson, Pliskin, & Luchins, 1994; Nisbet, Siegert, Hunt, & Fairley, 1996; Summerfelt et al., 1991; Vollema, Geurtsen, & van Voorst, 1995). One methodological approach included monetary feedback to determine whether reinforcement could reduce the number of perseverative errors made by patients with schizophrenia (Summerfelt et al., 1991). Although monetary feedback was often successful, several researchers found that additional incentives did not effectively improve performance beyond that of detailed instruction (Bellack et al., 1990; Green et al., 1992; Nisbet et al., 1996).

In a study examining several different types of reinforcement contingencies and their stability over time, Vollema and colleagues (1995) repeatedly tested 34 inpatients with schizophrenia who were selected based on their poor performance (as in the original study by Weinberger et al., 1986). Subjects were randomly assigned to receive standard instructions, to receive instructions on the sorting rules and on the occurrence of shifting sets, or to receive instructions on the sorting rules and on the occurrence of shifting sets plus 25 cents for each correct response. Subjects were administered the WCST at baseline and then 2 weeks later. At the 2-week time point, the task was administered once in standard fashion and once immediately after with the intervention. Additional administrations then took place 10 minutes later, 1 day later, and 2 weeks later. Those patients with marked deficits on the WCST benefited from training; some, in fact, achieved normal performance. Furthermore, the improvements were still evident upon retesting 2 weeks later. The addition of monetary reinforcement to the instructions resulted in an increase in the number of categories completed,

but the gain was less than that observed after instructions without the monetary reinforcement. The authors speculated that the addition of a monetary incentive distracted the patients or resulted in too much information for the patients to process at one time.

Using similar methodology, Everett and colleagues (2001) assessed the extent to which patients with schizophrenia could improve their performance with card-by-card instructions and continuous verbal reinforcement. Subjects included 30 individuals with schizophrenia and 30 healthy controls. Each subject was administered the WCST with standard procedures. After a break of up to 10 minutes, those willing to be tested again were readministered the test. During the retest, card-by-card instructions (such as questioning errors or reminding the patient that the sorting principle changes) and continuous reinforcement (e.g., encouragement after a mistake or congratulatory comments after a correct sort) were given. As expected, before being given instruction and reinforcement, patients with schizophrenia achieved few categories and made a high number of perseverative errors. When provided with verbal explanation and feedback, however, these patients committed significantly fewer perseverative errors. As suggested by Goldman (1994), if an impairment is modifiable and providing cues or other performance strategies helps to improve performance, that improvement may indicate residual neurobehavioral plasticity and provide insight into the nature or "density" of the executive functioning deficit of the patient with schizophrenia. Goldberg and Weinberger (1994), however, also pointed out that although patients in many of these studies improved their performance with advanced instruction and/or verbal reinforcement, they often did not achieve normal perseveration scores. Moreover, they argued that provision of instructions changed the integrity of the test, such that it was no longer assessing planning, hypothesis testing, sequencing, and other executive functions.

In response to the work of Goldman (1994) and Goldberg and Weinberger (1994), Perry, Potterat, and Braff (2001) employed a methodology that actively required subjects to employ executive functions while performing the WCST without significantly altering the integrity of the WCST. These authors tested two groups of patients with schizophrenia using an executive function aid. Half of these patients were administered the first 64 cards of the WCST with the standard instructions, whereas the other half of the patients were simply asked, "Why did you put that card there?" following their sort, without any other instructions or reinforcement to aid in their sorting. The conditions were then switched for the remaining 64 cards. Those subjects who were originally asked to verbalize their strategies following their sort performed similarly to age- and education-matched normal subjects. In the group that was provided the aid for the first 64 cards, the effect continued to the second deck, even though they were no longer asked to verbalize their strategy. The group that was not given the aid for the first 64 cards but was asked about card placement for the second 64 cards also improved during the second deck. These patients did not, however, demonstrate as dramatic a result as did the patients exposed to the aid from the outset. The authors suggested that, consistent with Goldman's work, once the patient with schizophrenia learned a strategy, that strategy was more resistant to new input, whether or not it increased positive results. The authors concluded that patients with schizophrenia have a deficit in initiating and maintaining executive functions, and forcing them to verbalize their responses activated the otherwise fractured executive functions, such as attention, working memory, and planning, that were necessary to complete the task.

## Working Memory

A growing body of evidence suggests that some of the symptoms of schizophrenia reflect dysfunction of the frontal lobes and related medial temporal and diencephalic regions, which are viewed as the neuroanatomical basis of working memory functions (Frith & Dolan, 1996; Goldman-Rakic, 1994). Support for the role of the frontal lobes in working memory comes from a variety of clinical and experimental domains, including lesion and physiological studies in nonhuman primates (e.g., Funuhashi, Bruce, & Goldman-Rakic, 1989, 1993; Goldman-Rakic, 1987, 1991; Wilson, Scalaidhe, & Goldman-Rakic, 1993), human neuropsychological and cognitive psychological studies (e.g., Gold, Carpenter, Randolph, Goldberg, & Weinberger, 1997; Keefe et al., 1995; Pantelis et al., 2004), and brain lesion and functional brain imaging studies (e.g., D'Esposito et al., 1998; Owen, 1997, 2000; Perlstein, Carter,

Noll, & Cohen, 2001). One of the most recognized models of working memory was described by Baddeley (1992) as a process of maintaining a cognitive representation when an interference or noise attempts to disrupt it. Baddeley and Hitch (1974) divided working memory into a "central executive" and two subordinate "slave systems." Together, the central executive and slave systems store information transiently, conduct active rehearsal, transfer it to permanent storage, allocate attentional resources, and manipulate cognitive representations to guide behavior (Baddeley, 1986, 1992; Frith & Dolan, 1996; Goldman-Rakic, 1994).

Both verbal and visuospatial working memory deficits have been found in patients with schizophrenia and their first-degree relatives (Bressi, Miele, Bressi, & Astori, 1996; Delahunty & Morice, 1996; Gold et al., 1997; Huguelet, Zanello, & Nicastro, 2000; Pantelis et al., 1999; Perry, Heaton, et al., 2001), which supports the notion that the prefrontal cortex is involved in the neuropathology of schizophrenia spectrum disorders (Park & Holtzman, 1992; Park, Holzman, & Goldman-Rakic, 1995). Goldberg and colleagues (1993), for example, compared patients with schizophrenia to their unaffected twin on digit span forward and backward tests. The patients and their twins performed similarly on the digit span forward task, but the patients demonstrated significantly poorer performance on the digits backward task. The authors posited that the latter differences reflected impaired working memory in schizophrenia, because the digits backward task required that numbers be held in working memory, manipulated, and recalled in reverse order as opposed to the forward task, which was a simpler "hold and repeat" task. Conklin, Clayton, Katsanis, and Iacono (2000) also used the digit span task to examine verbal working memory in patients with schizophrenia. They compared 52 patients with schizophrenia to 56 of their first-degree relatives and 73 nonpsychiatric comparison subjects. Relatives showed no impairment on the forward digit span task, purported to be a measure of general attention, but did show impairment on the backward digit span task. In contrast to previous findings, however, patients with schizophrenia showed impairment on both the forward and backward digit span tasks, indicative of both simple attentional deficits and working memory impairment.

Conflicting results on working memory tasks prompted subsequent research examining whether working memory impairments were impacted by general attentional deficits or other factors, such as intellectual level. One objective of a study conducted by Pukrop and colleagues (2003), for example, was to examine whether working memory performance of patients with schizophrenia was poorer than that of nonpatients due to a generally lower IQ in patients with schizophrenia. They studied working memory performance in 66 patients with schizophrenia using eight working memory tests, and found that patients indeed scored lower on the Verbal IQ measure (a multiple-choice vocabulary test) and showed significantly greater impairments across the working memory tests than nonpatients. Performance was not systematically influenced by symptoms or general psychopathology. When differences in intelligence scores were controlled, patients with schizophrenia continued to demonstrate deficits on all working memory tests, with the exception of the WCST. Thus, the data revealed that although patients with schizophrenia may generally score lower on Verbal IQ tests, their working memory deficits were not a result of a lower intellectual level.

In addition to the potentially confounding roles of attention and intellectual level on working memory performance, another fundamental problem in assessing working memory arises from differences in how the term "working memory" is used and defined. Perry, Heaton, and colleagues (2001) proposed a basic distinction between a concept of "transient online storage working memory" and a concept of "executive-functioning memory." Transient online storage occurs when short-term information storage is the primary requirement of the task and there is little manipulation of the stored material. Executive-functioning working memory applies when information is stored in short-term memory and subsequently manipulated via the central executive component. Perry, Heaton, and colleagues examined their proposed distinction between transient online storage and executive-functioning memory, as well as the role of factors such as attention and intellectual level on working memory, by comparing the performance of patients with schizophrenia and nonpsychiatric comparison subjects on a battery of both proposed types of working memory tests (Digit Span subtest, Spa-

tial Span subtest, Letter–Number Sequencing subtest, WCST, Auditory Consonant Trigrams, Category Test, Tower of Hanoi), an attention task, and a verbal intelligence measure. In a series of four studies, they found that patients with schizophrenia demonstrated equally impaired performance on tests of both transient online storage tasks and more complex executive-functioning working memory tasks. Results also suggested that patients have general deficits of attention and working memory rather than a primary working memory deficit that is further exacerbated with increasing working memory demands. Furthermore, they found significant differences between the patients and comparison groups on two of the three measures of executive-functioning working memory. When they examined whether working memory performance was related to intelligence, attention, and pathology, they found a moderate correlation between verbal intelligence scores and the executive-functioning working memory measures for both groups. A trend toward a relationship between working memory performance and negative symptoms in the patients with schizophrenia became stronger when the influence of verbal intelligence was removed. Thus, verbal intelligence did not appear responsible for the relationship between working memory and symptoms. Similarly, attention did not influence the relationship between the executive-functioning working memory tests and symptoms. Based on these results, the authors concluded that patients with schizophrenia indeed have working memory deficits, but that these various working memory tasks measure different, albeit related, aspects of working memory.

## Perseveration

Frontal lobe circuitry dysfunction in schizophrenia may manifest as perseverative behavior. "Perseverations" are defined as unintentional, repetitive activities influenced by recent experiences (Crider, 1997). Perseverations have been considered by some researchers to be the most sensitive and specific phenotypic marker of frontal lobe impairment in schizophrenia (Bilder & Goldberg, 1987; Braff et al., 1991; Koren et al., 1998; Milner, 1963). Furthermore, the degree of perseverative behavior of patients with schizophrenia is similar to that of patients with known frontal lobe pathology (Levin, 1984).

The perseverative behavior that commonly characterizes patients with schizophrenia has been consistently observed on the WCST, which requires individuals to be able to utilize a number of response repertoires. Beyond the WCST, the perseverative behavior of patients with schizophrenia may be observed with a variety of instruments. Perry and Braff (1998) assessed perseverations in patients with schizophrenia and normal comparison subjects using the WCST and a perseveration scale that yields three perseveration scores derived from verbal responses. They applied the perseveration scale to the verbal responses given to Rorschach test protocols, because the Rorschach inkblots are highly abstract and place demands on executive control. They proposed that the demands involved in integrating visually abstract images and a verbal explanation of their relationship to each other taxes frontal–executive abilities. The authors found that, compared to normal comparison subjects, patients with schizophrenia demonstrated a high number of perseverations on both the WCST and the perseveration scale applied to the Rorschach test. Their WCST perseverative responses were significantly correlated with Wechsler Adult Intelligence Scale—Revised (WAIS-R) Vocabulary scores, negative symptom ratings, and a subtype of Rorschach-derived perseverations that are hypothesized to represent DLPFC dysfunction. Finally, the WCST and Rorschach perseveration measures were entered into a logistic regression. The WCST total errors and the three perseveration measures from the Rorschach responses resulted in the correct classification of 89.4% of the total cases, with a sensitivity of 91%, specificity of 91%, and positive predictive power of 87.8%. These authors concluded that perseverative behavior is widely observed in patients with schizophrenia and can be elicited and measured using a variety of instruments.

## Inhibition

Difficulties with inhibition, the process of filtering irrelevant information and preventing it from intruding on conscious awareness or behavior, is hypothesized to be a frontally mediated cognitive process that contributes to the emergence of hallucinations, delusions, and thought disorder in schizophrenia (Frith, 1979). One paradigm used to demonstrate such inhibitory difficulties of patients with schizophrenia is negative priming (Tipper, 1985; for review, see May, Kane, & Hasher, 1995). Normal negative priming occurs in response to a distracter that has been previously ignored. Because the subject has previously inhibited a response to the stimulus, there is an increased (slowed) reaction time to the target that was previously presented as a distracter. The Stroop (1935) task is an illustrative negative priming paradigm. In the Stroop task, responses may include naming the ink color of a rectangle, naming the ink color of letters that together spell a color word (e.g., the word "red" printed in blue ink, an incongruent condition), and naming a color that is the same as the distracting word of the preceding word in a list (e.g., naming the color blue when the word "blue" is ignored in the previous trial). In the latter condition, the subject must utilize inhibitory mechanisms and overcome the previous requirement of responding to the color rather than the word.

Donohoe and Robertson (2003) reviewed 25 studies that administered the Stroop task to patients with schizophrenia. All 25 studies found that patients with schizophrenia had significant impairments on the Stroop task. Furthermore, of the six studies that looked at the relationship of inhibition to symptomatology, all six associated impaired Stroop performance with negative or disorganized symptoms, just as early researchers, such as Frith, had proposed.

An alternative approach to demonstrating inhibition deficits in schizophrenia was carried out in a study by Beech, Powell, McWilliam, and Claridge (1989) who predicted that a deficit in inhibition would lead to a reversed negative priming effect, such that distracters would facilitate rather than impair the reaction to a probe target. Beech et al.'s prediction was tested using a computerized Stroop task in which stimuli were presented for 100 ms and followed by a pattern mask lasting until a response was made. Results revealed that the reaction time required to respond to a previously presented distracter was reduced in patients with schizophrenia compared to normal control subjects. The authors thus concluded that the reduced reaction time in tasks such as the Stroop reflected these patients' inability to inhibit distracter information from the previous trials. These findings were subsequently challenged, however, on the basis that reduced negative priming (i.e., impaired inhibition) was actually due to the use of brief prime presentation time and pattern masking. Moritz and colleagues (2001) administered a negative priming task to patients with schizophrenia but increased presentation times and presented a blank screen rather than a mask followed by a prime presentation. When presentation time was increased and the mask was removed, reduced negative priming did not occur. The authors suggested that the reduced negative priming in schizophrenia may not be due to deficient cognitive inhibition, but rather to difficulties in quickly perceiving visual material and impaired visual processing.

## Fluency

Letter and category fluency tasks involve generation of words beginning with a specific letter or semantic category. According to Lezak (1995), verbal fluency tasks require retrieval of lexically associated words from long-term memory, which puts high demands on frontally mediated strategic processes. Indeed, neuroimaging studies have shown that verbal fluency is associated with left frontal lobe activation (Gourovitch et al., 2000; Mummery, Patterson, Hodges, & Wise, 1996; Paulesu et al., 1997; Pujol et al., 1996) and some studies have found evidence that in addition to the left frontal cortex, there is involvement of the DLPFC, premotor cortex, and right cerebellum (for reviews, see Cabeza & Nyberg, 2000; Indefrey & Levelt, 2000; McGraw, Mathews, Wang, & Phillips, 2001). Other studies have found reduced frontal activity during verbal fluency tasks (Artiges et al., 2000; Curtis et al., 1998; Yurgelun-Todd et al., 1996) and increased activity in the right prefrontal cortex (Crow, 2000; Sommer, Ramsey, & Kahn, 2001; Sommer, Ramsey, Mandl, & Kahn, 2003).

Regardless of the specificity of verbal fluency control within the frontal lobes, patients with schizophrenia consistently demonstrate deficits on verbal fluency tasks. Two hypotheses have been proposed to explain these deficits. One is that disruption in frontal lobe–mediated initiation and search strategies reduces access to semantic memory (Allen, Liddle, & Frith, 1993; Joyce, Collinson, & Crichton, 1996). The other suggests that verbal fluency deficits are due to disorganization of the semantic store,

implicating the temporal lobe structures upon which semantic processing is partially dependent (Goldberg et al., 1998). As a direct test of these competing hypotheses, Giovannetti, Goldstein, Schullery, Barr, and Bilder (2003) compared the animal word-list generation abilities of patients with first-episode schizophrenia to those of controls and a comparison group of individuals with left temporal lobe epilepsy (the latter of whom had known temporal lobe damage and predictable semantic deficits). Both the patients with schizophrenia and those with epilepsy generated fewer words than controls. However, only the patients with epilepsy obtained lower scores on an index of semantic knowledge; patients with schizophrenia did not differ from controls. Based on their findings, the authors posited that verbal fluency deficits in schizophrenia are related to deficient semantic search/access and response monitoring of the frontal lobes rather than temporal lobe dysfunction.

Maron, Carlson, Minassian, and Perry (2004) used an alternative strategy to better understand the contribution of the frontal lobes to verbal fluency impairment in schizophrenia. They posited that since measuring overall performance reveals little about the underlying deficit, types of fluency errors should be delineated. To this end, they assessed the number, length, and type of word clusters produced (e.g., word strings, perseverative responses) and their relationship to the patients' symptoms during both letter and category verbal fluency tasks. They found that patients with schizophrenia demonstrated deficient verbal fluency performance across letter and category tasks, consistent with the literature. Furthermore, they observed a significant reduction in the number of related word clusters on the letter fluency task and a trend for producing fewer clusters on the category fluency task. Despite reduced clustering, however, string length did not differ between groups. The authors reported that their findings provide support for research indicating that problems in frontally mediated organized search and retrieval processes may negatively impact efficient access to the semantic store, and thus do not reflect degradation in the semantic store itself. Furthermore, greater negative symptomatology was correlated with poorer performance, as well as a reduction in the number of strings and clustered words produced on letter, but not category, fluency.

## COGNITIVE NEUROSCIENCE

Cognitive neuroscience serves to link methodologies from neuropsychology and psychophysiology as a means of understanding further the neuroanatomical basis of schizophrenia. Research in the cognitive neurosciences serves to address whether neurocognitive deficits in schizophrenia reflect factors associated with the disease itself or a certain neurobiological vulnerability. It has long been known, at least since the work of Diefendorf and Dodge (1908), that eye movement abnormalities exist in patients with schizophrenia. Ocular movements, such as smooth muscle pursuit and saccadic eye movements, are controlled by the frontal cortex and associated cortical–subcortical circuitry. Thus, by studying oculomotor abnormalities in patients with schizophrenia, new insights have been gained into the role of the frontal lobes in the neurobiology of schizophrenia.

Smooth muscle pursuit involves maintaining a relatively stable image of a target on the retina. Several researchers have since demonstrated that 50% of the first-degree relatives of patients with schizophrenia have dysfunction of the smooth pursuit system, and that these abnormalities correlate with other markers of schizophrenia and symptoms of the disease (Iacono & Clementz, 1993; Levy, Holzman, Matthysse, & Mendell, 1993). Smooth muscle pursuit has, however, been shown to be nonspecific to schizophrenia and has been shown to be highly variable given that it is influenced by a number of factors, such as the individual's level of alertness, age, and drug use (Leigh & Zee, 1991). Saccadic measures that may be more sensitive and specific to schizophrenia have thus received more attention in recent literature. "Saccades" are movements that rapidly redirect gaze to a visual target. At a more cognitively complex level are "antisaccades," which are movements that redirect gaze to the mirror image location of a visual cue. During antisaccade tasks, subjects are first asked to fixate on a central target. The central fixation light is offset simultaneously with the onset of a peripheral cue. Subjects are instructed to look at the mirror image of the cue. Errors occur when subjects are distracted by the target and glance toward it rather than the mirror image. The involvement of the DLPFC in antisaccade tasks was illustrated beautifully in a study comparing antisaccade errors in patients with le-

sions of the DLPFC to patients with lesions in other cortical areas, such as frontal eye fields, supplementary motor areas, and the posterior parietal cortex (Pierrot-Deseilligny, Gaymard, Muri, & Rivaud, 1997). Patients with DLPFC lesions made significantly more antisaccade errors than did the comparison subjects.

Failure to suppress a response tendency toward stimuli that appear suddenly is also commonly observed in schizophrenia (Crawford, Haeger, Kennard, Reveley, & Henderson, 1995; McDowell & Clementz, 1997), supporting the existence of DLPFC pathology in this disease. Patients with schizophrenia, like patients with frontal lobe lesions, commit more antisaccade errors toward a cue (Crawford et al., 1995, Katsanis, Kortenkamp, Iacono, & Grove, 1997; McDowell & Clementz, 1997; Sereno & Holzman, 1995). The first-degree, nonpsychotic relatives of patients with schizophrenia also produce an increased proportion of antisaccade errors (Crawford et al., 1998; Katsanis et al., 1997; McDowell & Clementz, 1997; McDowell, Myles-Worsley, Coon, Byerley, & Clementz, 1999). The latter finding illustrates that, unlike smooth muscle pursuit, saccades and antisaccades are less susceptible to the particular circumstances of a serious mental illness, such as medication, and may therefore be more trait-related. The influence of other factors has been suggested and tested, however. These factors pertain mostly to those considered inherent to the disease itself, such as poor attention or deficient working memory.

Based on computational models of performance on tasks sensitive to prefrontal dysfunction, Roberts, Hager, and Heron (1994) proposed that antisaccade errors are a failure to inhibit a reflexive saccade due to insufficient working memory resources for planning and executing a correct antisaccade. Hutton, Joyce, Barnes, and Kennard (2002) tested this directly by giving patients with schizophrenia saccade tasks under conditions that varied in the amount of working memory required to perform the task. Three paradigms were employed: fixation with distracters, delayed prosaccades, and antisaccades. The fixation task required nothing but inhibition of a prepotent reflex saccade; the delayed prosaccade task required the saccade program to be held in mind until the cue to initiate the saccade was presented; the antisaccade task required that the location of the target be registered and transformed spatially to provide coordinates for the immediate execution of an internally generated saccade to the mirror image location. A simple reflexive saccade paradigm was used as a control task. The performances of 30 patients with schizophrenia who had recently developed the disease were compared to that of 30 normal controls. Results revealed no differences between patients and controls on the fixation distractor task. Patients did, however, make significantly more errors than controls on both the antisaccade and delayed prosaccade task. Furthermore, as competing task demands increased across the paradigms, there was a commensurate increase in the number of saccadic errors in both groups. The authors concluded that "the increased saccadic distractibility in schizophrenia results from an intrinsic deficiency in working memory resources secondary to prefrontal cortex dysfunction" (p. 1733).

Several investigators have revealed normal neuropsychological functioning among a subgroup of patients with schizophrenia (Broerse, Holthausen, van den Bosch, & den Boer, 2001; Palmer et al., 1997). Saccade tasks, according to Reuter and Kathmann (2004), may be particularly useful in detecting subtle deficits in this subgroup of patients with schizophrenia who appear normal on neuropsychological tests. Broerse and colleagues (2001), for example, found that among 24 patients with schizophrenia, schizophreniform disorder, or schizoaffective disorder, 58% could be rated as free of executive deficits on standard neuropsychological tests. When they used saccade tests, however, only 21% were considered to have normal executive functioning. Antisaccade tasks thus show promise as a means of identifying patients with schizophrenia who may predominantly have DLPFC pathology that may or may not otherwise be detected by neuropsychological testing.

## PSYCHOPHYSIOLOGY

Psychophysiological research has led to great advances in our understanding of the anatomical substrates of schizophrenia. As early as the days of Blueler, patients with schizophrenia were observed to have deficits in attention and information processing. Blueler posited that these deficits were due to a reduced ability to filter out irrelevant stimuli. Others (e.g., McGhie & Chapman, 1961) also reported that

patients with schizophrenia were unable to screen out irrelevant sensory stimuli and thus suffered from sensory overload. Disruption of circuits that subserve frontal lobe functions, including the corticostriatal–pallidothalamic (CSPT) circuit (Swerdlow & Koob, 1987) and other cortical–subcortical circuits (Cummings, 1993; Evarts, Kimura, Wurtz, & Hikosaka, 1984), may be at the root of deficient attention and information processing. Swerdlow and Koob (1987) further proposed that because of the interconnectedness of specific neuronal pathways, attention and information-processing deficits may result from dysfunction at any one of the several levels of the CSPT circuit. As Cummings and Benson (1992) explained, disruptions at different points in the circuit can produce similar functional deficits. In the same vein, Brown and Pluck (2000) suggested that reduced function of dopamine-modulated circuits between the frontal cortex and the basal ganglia–thalamus may contribute to the lack of input that contributes to cognitive deficits (such as reduced verbal fluency) in schizophrenia.

Circuitry dysfunction has thus become one of the driving theories behind psychophysiological research in schizophrenia. By studying a psychophysiological function with a known anatomical substrate in the context of clinical symptoms in patients with schizophrenia, the nature of circuitry disruption in schizophrenia may be illuminated. Several investigators have suggested that it is the failure to "gate" or screen out sensory information that leads to the sensory overload, cognitive fragmentation, and thought disorder characteristic of schizophrenia (Perry & Braff, 1994; Venables, 1964). This hypothesis has stimulated a series of studies examining sensorimotor gating in schizophrenia.

One approach commonly utilized to study gating processes is prepulse inhibition (PPI) of the human startle response. Deficits in PPI and habituation are thought to be biological markers of information-processing abnormalities in schizophrenia (Cadenhead, Carasso, Swerdlow, Geyer, & Braff, 1999; Nuechterlein, Dawson, & Green, 1994). The typical paradigm involves administration of a sudden loud tone, bright light, or puff of air. The stimulus normally elicits a series of flexion and extension responses referred to as a startle response. When the startling stimulus is preceded 30 to 500 ms by a weak prestimulus in the same or different modality, the startle response is inhibited, resulting in "prepulse inhibition." At the moment that a prepulse is detected and processed, sensory gating is initiated and buffers responsivity to other sensory stimulation until the prepulse has been completely processed (see Braff, Geyer, & Swerdlow, 2001; McDowd, Filion, Harris, & Braff, 1993). Inhibition of the prepulse startle response is therefore thought to be involved in the earliest stages of information processing. Braff and colleagues (1978) conducted some of the first studies demonstrating PPI deficits in patients with schizophrenia, providing support for the deficit in information processing observed by early clinicians. This finding has since been replicated in patients with schizophrenia (Braff, Grillon, & Geyer, 1992; Filion, Dawson, & Schell, 1998; Grillon, Ameli, Charney, Krystal, & Braff, 1992; Mackeprang, Kristiansen, & Glenthoj, 2002) and other neuropsychiatric disorders such as obsessive–compulsive disorder (Swerdlow, Benbow, Zisook, Geyer, & Braff, 1993), Huntington's disease (Braff et al., 2001; Swerdlow et al., 1995), schizotypal personality disorder (Cadenhead, Geyer, & Braff, 1993), and psychotic disorder (Simons & Giardina, 1992), all of which are characterized by an inability to inhibit redundant or relatively irrelevant sensory, cognitive, or motor information.

PPI has been a useful paradigm for demonstrating correlations between gating deficits and frontally mediated clinical symptoms in schizophrenia. Karper and colleagues (1996) reported that reduced sensorimotor gating in schizophrenia was correlated with distractibility and impaired vigilance. PPI deficits have also been related to positive symptoms (Meincke et al., 2004; Weike, Bauer, & Hamm, 2000). Perry and Braff (1994; Perry, Geyer, & Braff, 1999) demonstrated that patients with schizophrenia who had the poorest PPI showed the highest rates of thought disturbance when presented with complex, cognitive challenge paradigms. Ludewig, Geyer, and Vollenweider (2003) studied PPI and symptomatology in 24 first-episode males with schizophrenia or schizophreniform disorder and 21 age-matched healthy controls. All of the patients were tested during their first psychotic episode, and none had ever been medicated with antipsychotics. No correlations were found between PPI or habituation and clinical characteristics of the patients. Patients did, however, show significant deficits in PPI and habituation of the startle response compared to controls. Their deficits in PPI could therefore not be attributed to the effects of antipsychotic medication, clinical status, or progression of their disease. This and other studies support the notion that reduced PPI is a vulnerability marker of schizophrenia related to genetic and/or neurodevelopmental factors of the disorder. A growing body of literature questions whether deficits in PPI are indeed trait-dependent or whether they are, in contrast, state-dependent. Recent research suggests that the relationship between sensorimotor gating and clinical characteristics such as thought disturbance may be mediated by the acuity of the psychopathology or medication administration. Meincke and associates (2004) examined 36 medicated inpatients with schizophrenia during an acute psychotic episode and then again 2–3 weeks later when psychopathological improvement had been achieved. In keeping with earlier (Perry & Braff, 1994; Perry et al., 1999) findings, more severe thought disorder was correlated with larger PPI deficits. The exception, however, was that this relationship only held during the acute psychotic episode, not when clinical state was improved. The exact nature of the relationship between sensorimotor gating and hallmark characteristics of schizophrenia remains an area inviting exploration. As psychophysiological studies such as these are conducted, we hope that more light may be shed on the relationship between anatomical substrates and the symptoms of schizophrenia.

## CONCLUSION

Our aim in this chapter was to provide a brief rather than exhaustive review of the role of the frontal lobes and frontal lobe circuitry in schizophrenia. Findings from neuropsychology, cognitive neuroscience, and psychophysiology have advanced our understanding of the role of the frontal lobes in schizophrenia. Research in these areas has provided support for theory-based observations of deficits in cognitive functions mediated by the frontal lobes, disruption in neural circuits subserving the frontal lobes, as well as impairments in sensory gating. As research continues to challenge the conclusions of these studies and pose new questions for inquiry, we inch closer toward understanding the nature and extent of frontal lobe impairment in schizophrenia.

## REFERENCES

Addington, J., Addington, D., & Maticka-Tyndale, E. (1991). Cognitive functioning and positive and negative symptoms in schizophrenia. *Schizophrenia Research, 5,* 123–134.

Allen, H. A., Liddle, P. F., & Frith, C. D. (1993). Negative features, retrieval processes and verbal fluency in schizophrenia. *British Journal of Psychiatry, 163,* 769–775.

Andreasen, N. C. Arndt, S., Swayze, V., Cizadlo, T., Flaum, M., O'Leary, D., et al. (1994). Thalamic abnormalities in schizophrenia visualized through magnetic resonance imaging averaging. *Science, 266,* 294–298.

Artiges, E., Martinot, J. L., Verdys, M., Attar-Levy, D., Mazoyer, B., Tzourio, N., et al. (2000). Altered hemispheric functional dominance during word generation in negative schizophrenia. *Schizophrenia Bulletin, 26,* 709–721.

Baddeley, A. (1986). *Working memory.* Oxford, UK: Clarendon Press.

Baddeley. A. (1992). Working memory. *Science, 225,* 556–559.

Baddeley, A., & Hitch, G. (1974). Working memory. In G. A. Bower (Ed.), *Psychology of learning and motivation* (Vol. 8, pp. 47–89). New York: Academic Press.

Basso, M. R., Nasrallah, H. A., Olson, S. C., & Bornstein, R. A. (1998). Neuropsychological correlates of negative, disorganized and psychotic symptoms in schizophrenia. *Schizophrenia Research, 31,* 99–111.

Beech, A., Powell, T., McWilliam, J., & Claridge, G. S. (1989). Evidence of reduced "cognitive inhibition" in schizophrenia. *British Journal of Clinical Psychology, 28,* 109–116.

Bellack, A. S., Mueser, K. T., Morrison, R. L., Tierney, A., & Podell, K. (1990). Remediation of cognitive deficits in schizophrenia. *American Journal of Psychiatry, 147,* 1650–1655.

Berg, E. A. (1948). A simple objective test for measuring flexibility in thinking. *Journal of General Psychology, 39,* 15–22.

Berman, K. F., Zec, R. F., & Weinberger, D. R. (1986). Physiologic dysfunction of dorsolateral prefrontal cortex in schizophrenia: Role of neuroleptic treatment, attention and mental effort. *Archives of General Psychiatry, 45,* 814–821.

Bilder, R. M., & Goldberg, E. (1987). Motor perseverations in schizophrenia. *Archives of Clinical Neuropsychology, 2,* 195–214.

Bogerts, B., Mertiz, E., Schonfeldt, M., & Bausch, R. (1985). Basal ganglia and limbic system pathology in schizophrenia: A morphemetric study of brain volume and shrinkage. *Archives of General Psychiatry, 42,* 784–791.

Braff, D. L., Geyer, M. A., & Swerdlow, N. R. (2001). Human studies of prepulse inhibition of startle: Normal subjects, patient groups, and pharmacological studies. *Psychopharmacology, 156,* 234–258.

Braff, D. L., Grillon, C., & Geyer, M. A. (1992). Gating and habituation of the startle reflex in schizophrenia patients. *Archives of General Psychiatry, 49,* 206–215.

Braff, D. L., Heaton, R., Kuck, J., Cullum M., Moranville, J., Grant, I., et al. (1991). The generalized pattern of neuropsychological deficits in outpatients with chronic schizophrenia with heterogeneous Wisconsin Card Sorting Test results. *Archives of General Psychiatry, 48,* 891–898.

Braff, D. L., Stone, C., Callaway, E., Geyer, M. A., Glick, I. D., & Bali, L. (1978). Prestimulus effects on human startle reflex in normals and schizophrenics. *Psychophyisiology, 14,* 339–343.

Bressi, S., Miele, L., Bressi, C., & Astori, S. (1996). Deficits in central executive component of working memory in schizophrenia. *New Trends in Experimental Clinical Psychiatry, 12,* 243–252.

Broerse, A., Hothausen, E. A. E., van den Bosch, R. J., & den Boer, J. A. (2001). Does frontal normality exist in schizophrenia?: A saccadic eye movement study. *Psychiatry Research, 103,* 167–178.

Brown, R. G., & Pluck, G. (2000). Negative symptoms: The "pathology" of motivation and goal-directed behavior. *Trends in Neurosciences, 23,* 412–417.

Buchanan, R. W., Strauss, M. E., Kirkpatrick, B., Holstein, C., Breier, A., & Carpenter, W. T., Jr. (1994). Neuropsychological impairments in deficit vs. nondeficit forms of schizophrenia. *Archives of General Psychiatry, 51,* 804–811.

Cabeza, R., & Nyberg, L. (2000). Imaging cognition: II. An empirical review of 275 PET and fMRI studies. *Journal of Cognitive Neurosciences, 12,* 1–47.

Cadenhead, K. S., Carasso, B. S., Swerdlow, N. R., Geyer, M. A., & Braff, D. L. (1999). Prepulse inhibition and habituation of the startle response are stable neurobiological measures in a normal male population. *Biological Psychiatry, 45,* 360–364.

Cadenhead, K. S., Geyer, M. A., & Braff, D. L. (1993). Impaired startle prepulse inhibition and habituation in schizoptypal personality disordered patients. *American Journal of Psychiatry, 150,* 1862–1867.

Chen, E. Y., Lam, L. C., Chen, R. Y., Nguyen, D. G., & Chan, C. K. (1996). Prefrontal neuropsychological impairment and illness duration in schizophrenia: A study of 204 patients in Hong Kong. *Acta Psychiatrica Scandinavica, 93,* 144–150.

Chen, Y. L., Chen, E. Y., Chan, C. K., Lam, L. C., & Lieh-Mak, F. (2000). Verbal fluency in schizophrenia: Reduction in semantic store. *Australian and New Zealand Journal of Psychiatry, 34,* 43–48.

Collins, A. A., Remington, G. J., Coulter, K., & Birkett, K. (1997). Insight, neurocognitive function and symptom clusters in chronic schizophrenia. *Schizophrenia Research, 27,* 37–44.

Conklin, H. M., Clayton, E. C., Katsanis, J., & Iacono, W. G. (2000). Verbal working memory impairment in schizophrenia patients and their first-degree relatives: Evidence from the Digit Span task. *American Journal of Psychiatry, 157,* 275–277.

Crawford, T. J., Haeger, B., Kennard, C., Reveley, M. A., & Henderson, L. (1995). Saccadic abnormalities in psychotic patients: I. Neuroleptic-free psychotic patients. *Psychological Medicine, 25,* 461–471.

Crawford, T. J., Sharma, T., Puri, B. K., Murray, R. M., Berridge, D. M., & Lewis, S. W. (1998). Saccadic eye movements in families multiply affected with schizophrenia: the Maudsley Family Study. *American Journal of Psychiatry, 155,* 1703–1710.

Crider, A. (1997). Perseverations in schizophrenia. *Schizophrenia Bulletin, 23,* 63–74.

Crow, T. J. (2000). Invited commentary on functional anatomy of verbal fluency in people with schizophrenia and those at genetic risk: The genetics of asymmetry and psychosis. *British Journal of Psychiatry, 176,* 61–63.

Cummings, J. L. (1993). Frontal–subcortical circuits and human behavior. *Archives of Neurology, 50,* 873–880.

Cummings, J. L., & Benson, F. D. (1992). *Dementia: A clinical approach* (2nd ed.). Boston: Butterworth-Heinemann.

Curtis, V. A., Bullmore, E. T., Brammer, M. J., Wright, I. C., Williams, S. C., Morris, R. G., et al. (1998). Attenuated frontal activation during a verbal fluency task in patients with schizophrenia. *American Journal of Psychiatry, 155,* 1056–1063.

Delahunty, A., & Morice, R. (1996). Rehabilitation of frontal/executive impairments in schizophrenia. *Australian and New Zealand Journal of Psychiatry, 30,* 760–767.

D'Esposito, M., Aguirre, G. K., Zarahn, E., Ballard, D., Shin, R. K., & Lease, J. (1998). Functional MRI studies of spatial and nonspatial working memory. *Cognition and Brain Research, 7,* 1–13.

Diefendorf, A. R., & Dodge, R. (1908). An experimental study of the ocular reactions of the insane from photographic records. *Brain, 31,* 343–489.

Donohoe, G., & Robertson, I. H. (2003). Can specific deficits in executive functioning explain the negative symptoms in schizophrenia?: A review. *Neurocase, 9,* 97–108.

Elliott, R., McKenna, P. J., Robbins, T. W., & Sahakian, B. (1995). Neuropsychological evidence for frontostriatal dysfunction in schizophrenia. *Psychological Medicine, 25,* 619–630.

Evans, J. J., Chua, S. E., McKenna, P. J., & Wilson, B. A. (1997). Assessment of the dysexecutive syndrome in schizophrenia. *Psychological Medicine, 27,* 635–646.

Evarts, E. V., Kimura, M., Wurtz, R. H., & Hikosaka, O. (1984). Behavioral correlates of activity in basal ganglia neurons. *Trends in Neurosciences, 7,* 447–453.

Everett, J., Lavoie, K., Gagnon, J., & Gosselin, N. (2001). Performance of patients with schizophrenia on the Wisconsin Card Sorting Test (WCST). *Journal of Psychiatry and Neuroscience, 26,* 123–130.

Filion, D. L., Dawson, M. E., & Schell, A. M. (1998). The psychological significance of human startle eyeblink modification: A review. *Biological Psychology, 47,* 1–43.

Frith, C. D. (1979). Consciousness, information processing and schizophrenia. *British Journal of Psychiatry, 134,* 225–235.

Frith, C., & Dolan, R. (1996). The role of the prefrontal cortex in higher cognitive functions. *Cognitive Brain Research, 5,* 175–181.

Funuhashi, S., Bruce, C. J., & Goldman-Rakic, P. S. (1989). Mnemonic coding of visual cortex in monkey's dorsolateral prefrontal cortex. *Journal of Neurophysiology, 61,* 331–348.

Funuhashi, S., Bruce, C. J., & Goldman-Rakic, P. S. (1993). Dorsolateral prefrontal lesions and oculomotor delayed response performance: Evidence for mnemonic "scotomas." *Journal of Neuroscience, 13,* 1479–1497.

Fuster, J. M. (1989). *The prefrontal cortex.* New York: Raven.

Giovannetti, T. Goldstein, R. Z., Schullery, M., Barr, W. B., & Bilder, R. M. (2003). Category fluency in first-episode schizophrenia. *Journal of the International Neuropsychological Society, 9,* 384–393.

Gold, J. M., Carpenter, C., Randolph, C., Goldberg, T. E., & Weinberger, D. R. (1997). Auditory working memory and Wisconsin Card Sorting Test performance in schizophrenia. *Archives of General Psychiatry, 54,* 159–164.

Goldberg, T. E., Aloia, M. S., Gourovitch, M. L., Missar, D., Pickar, D., & Weinberger, D. R. (1998). Cognitive substrates of thought disorder: I. The semantic system. *American Journal of Psychiatry, 155,* 1671–1676.

Goldberg, T. E., Torrey, E. F., Gold, J. M., Ragland, J. D., Bigelow, L. B., & Weinberger, D. R. (1993). Learning and memory in monozygotic twins discordant for schizophrenia. *Psychological Medicine, 23,* 71–85.

Goldberg, T. E., & Weinberger, D. R. (1994). Schizophrenia training paradigms, and the Wisconsin Card Sorting Test redux. *Schizophrenia Research, 11,* 291–296.

Goldberg, T. E., Weinberger, D. R., Berman, K. F., Pliskin, N. H., & Podd, M. H. (1987). Further evidence for dementia of the prefrontal type in schizophrenia. *Archives of General Psychiatry, 44,* 1008–1014.

Goldman, R. S. (1994). Approaches to cognitive training in schizophrenia. *Advances in Medical Psychotherapy, 7,* 95–108.

Goldman, R. S., Axelrod, B. N., & Tompkins, L. M. (1992). Effect of structural cues on schizophrenic patients' performance on the Wisconsin Card Sorting Test. *American Journal of Psychiatry, 149,* 1718–1722.

Goldman-Rakic, P. S. (1987). Circuitry of primate prefrontal cortex and regulation of behavior by representational knowledge. In F. Plum & V. Mountcastle (Eds.), *Handbook of physiology: The nervous system* (Vol. 5, pp. 373–417). Bethesda, MD: American Physiological Society.

Goldman-Rakic, P. S. (1991). Prefrontal cortical dysfunction in schizophrenia: The relevance of working memory. In B. Carroll & J. E. Barrett (Eds.), *Psychopathology and the brain* (pp. 1–23). New York: Raven.

Goldman-Rakic, P. S. (1994). Working memory dysfunction in schizophrenia. *Journal of Neuropsychiatry and Clinical Neurosciences, 6*, 348–357.

Gourovitch, M. L., Kirkby, B. S., Goldberg, T. E., Daniel, R., Gold, J. M., Esposito, G., et al. (2000). A comparison of rCBF patterns during letter and semantic fluency. *Neuropsychology, 14*, 353–360.

Green, M. F. (1998). *Schizophrenia from a neurocognitive perspective: Probing the impenetrable darkness*. Boston: Allyn & Bacon.

Green, M. F., & Braff, D. L. (2001). Translating the basic and clinical cognitive neuroscience of schizophrenia to drug development and clinical trials of antipsychotic medications. *Biological Psychiatry, 49*, 374–384.

Green, M. F., Ganzell, S., Satz, P., & Vaclav, J. (1990). Teaching the Wisconsin Card Sorting Test to schizophrenia patients [Letter to the editor]. *Archives of General Psychiatry, 47*, 91–92.

Green, M. F., Satz, P., Ganzell, S., & Vaclav, J. F. (1992). Wisconsin Card Sorting Test performance in schizophrenia: Remediation of a stubborn deficit. *American Journal of Psychiatry, 149*, 62–67.

Grillon, C., Ameli, R., Charney, D. S., Krystal, J., & Braff, D. L. (1992). Startle gating deficits occur across prepulse intensities in schizophrenic patients. *Biological Psychiatry, 32*, 939–943.

Haut, M. W., Cahill, J., Cutlip, W. D., Stevenson, J. M., Makela, E. H., & Bloomfield, S. M. (1996). On the nature of Wisconsin Card Sorting Test performance in schizophrenia. *Psychiatry Research, 65*, 15–22.

Heaton, R. K. (1981). *A manual for the Wisconsin Card Sort Test*. Odessa, FL: Psychological Assessment Resources.

Heaton, R. K., Chelune, G. J., Talley, J. L., Kay, G. G., & Curtiss, G. (1993). *Wisconsin Card Sorting Test manual: Revised and expanded*. Odessa, FL: Psychological Assessment Resources.

Heydebrand, G., Weiser, M., Rabinowitz, J., Hoff, A. L., DeLisi, L. E., & Csernansky, J. G. (2004). Correlates of cognitive deficits in first episode schizophrenia. *Schizophrenia Research, 68*, 1–9.

Huguelet, P., Zanello, A., & Nicastro, R. (2000). A study of visual and auditory verbal working memory in schizophrenic patients compared to healthy subjects. *European Archives of Psychiatry and Clinical Neuroscience, 250*, 79–85.

Hutton, S. B., Joyce, E. M., Barnes, T. R. E., & Kennard, C. (2002). Saccadic distractibility in first-episode schizophrenia. *Neuropsychologia, 40*, 1729–1736.

Iacono, W. G., & Clementz, B. A. (1993). A strategy for elucidating genetic influences on complex psychopathological syndromes. In L. J. Chapman, J. P. Chapman, & D. C. Fowles (Eds.), *Progress in experimental personality and psychopathology research* (pp. 9–24). New York: Springer.

Indefry, P., & Levelt, W. J. M. (2000). The neutral correlates of language production. In M. S. Gazzaniga (Ed.), *The new cognitive neuroscience* (2nd ed., pp. 845–865). Cambridge, MA: MIT Press.

Jernigan, T. L., Zisook, S., Heaton, R. K., Moranville, J. T., Hesselink, J. R., & Braff, D. L. (1991). Magnetic resonance imaging abnormalities in lenticular nuclei and cerebral cortex in schizophrenia. *Archives of General Psychiatry, 48*, 881–890.

Johnstone, E. C., Crow, T. J., Frith, C. D., Husband, J., & Kreel, L. (1976). Cerebral ventricular size and cognitive impairment in chronic schizophrenia. *Lancet, 11*, 924–926.

Joyce, E. M., Collinson, S. L., & Crichton P. (1996). Verbal fluency in schizophrenia: Relationship with executive function, semantic memory and clinical alogia. *Psychological Medicine, 26*, 39–49.

Karper, L. P., Freeman, G. K., Grillon, C., Morgan, C. A., III, Charney, D. S., & Krystal, J. H. (1996). Preliminary evidence of an association between sensorimotor gating and distractibility in psychosis. *Journal of Neuropsychiatry and Clinical Neurosciences, 8*, 60–66.

Katsanis, J., Kortenkamp, S., Iacono, W. G., & Grove, W. M. (1997). Antisaccade performance in patients with schizophrenia and affective disorder. *Journal of Abnormal Psychology, 106*, 468–472.

Keefe, R. S., Lees Roitman, S. E., Harvey, P. D., Blum, C. S., DuPre, R. L., Prieto, D. M., et al. (1995). A pen-and-paper human analogue of a monkey prefrontal cortex activation task: Spatial working memory in patients with schizophrenia. *Schizophrenia Research, 17*, 25–33.

Koren, D., Seidmen, L. J., Harrison, R. H., Lyons, M. J., Kremen, W. S., Caplan, B., et al. (1998). Factor structure of the Wisconsin Card Sorting Test: Dimensions of deficit in schizophrenia. *Neuropsychology, 12*, 289–302.

Kraepelin, E. (1919). *Dementia praecox and paraphrenia* (R. M. Barclay, Trans. & G. M. Robertson, Ed.). Huntington, NY: Robert E. Kreiger.

Lawrie, S. M., Abukmeil, S. S., Chiswick, A., Egan, V., Santosh, C. G., & Berst, J. J. K. (1997). Qualitative cerebral morphology in schizophrenia: A magnetic resonance imaging study and systematic literature review. *Schizophrenia Research, 25*, 155–166.

Leigh, R. J., & Zee, D. S. (1991). *The neurology of eye movements* (2nd ed.). Philadelphia: Davis.

Levin, S. (1984). Frontal lobe dysfunction in schizophrenia: II. Impairments of psychological and brain functions. *Journal of Psychiatric Research, 18*, 57–72.

Levy, D. L., Holzman, P. S., Matthysse, S., & Mendell, N. R. (1993). Eye tracking dysfunction in schizophrenia: A critical perspective. *Schizophrenia Bulletin, 19,* 461–536.

Lezak, M. (1995). *Neuropsychological assessment* (3rd ed.). New York: Oxford University Press.

Liu, Z., Tam, W. C., Xie, Y., & Zhao, J. (2002). The relationship between regional cerebral blood flow and the Wisconsin Card Sorting Test in negative schizophrenia. *Psychiatry and Clinical Neurosciences, 56,* 3–7.

Ludewig, K., Geyer, M. A., & Vollenweider, F. X. (2003). Deficits in prepulse inhibition and habituation in never-medicated, first-episode schizophrenia. *Biological Psychiatry, 54,* 121–128.

Luria, A. R. (1966). *Higher cortical function in man* (B. Haigh, Trans.). New York: Basic Books.

Mackeprang, T., Kristiansen, K. T., & Glenthoj, B. Y. (2002). Effects of antipsychotics on prepulse inhibition of the startle response in drug naive schizophrenic patients. *Biological Psychiatry, 52,* 863–873.

Mahurin, R. K., Velligan, D. I., & Miller, A. L. (1998). Executive–frontal lobe cognitive dysfunction in schizophrenia: A symptom subtype analysis. *Psychiatry Research, 79,* 139–149.

Maron, L. M., Carlson, M. D., Minassian, A., & Perry, W. (2004). A process approach to verbal fluency in patients with schizophrenia [Letter]. Schizophrenia Research, 68, 105–106.

May, C. P., Kane, M. J., & Hasher, L. (1995). Determinants of negative priming. *Psychological Bulletin, 118,* 35–54.

McDowd, J. M., Filion, D. L., Harris, J., & Braff, D. L. (1993). Sensory gating and inhibitory function in late life schizophrenia. *Schizophrenia Bulletin, 19,* 733–746.

McDowell, J. E., & Clementz, B. A. (1997). The effect of fixation condition manipulation on antisaccade performance in schizophrenia: Studies of diagnostic specificity. *Experimental Brain Research, 115,* 333–344.

McDowell, J. E., Myles-Worsley, M., Coon, H., Byerley, W., & Clementz, B. A. (1999). Measuring liability for schizophrenia using optimized antisaccade stimulus parameters. *Psychophysiology, 36,* 138–141.

McGhie, A., & Chapman, J. (1961). Disorders of attention and perception in early schizophrenia. *British Journal of Medical Psychology, 34,* 103–116.

McGraw, P., Mathews, V. P., Wang, Y., & Phillips, M. D. (2001). Approach to functional magnetic resonance imaging of language based on models of language organization. *Neuroimaging Clinics of North America, 11,* 343–353.

Meincke, U., Morth, D., Voss, T., Thelen, B., Geyer, M. A., & Gouzoulis-Mayfrank, E. (2004). Prepulse inhibition of the acoustically evoked startle reflex in patients with an acute schizophrenic psychosis—a longitudinal study. *European Archives of Psychiatry and Clinical Neurosciences, 254,* 415–421.

Metz, J. T., Johnson, M. D., Pliskin, N. H., & Luchins, D. J. (1994). Maintenance of training effects on the Wisconsin Card Sorting Test by patients with schizophrenia or affective disorders. *American Journal of Psychiatry, 151,* 120–122.

Milner, B. (1963). Effect of different brain lesions in card sorting: The role of the frontal lobes. *Archives of Neurology, 9,* 100–110.

Milner, B. (1964). Some effects of frontal lobectomy in man. In: J. M. Warren & K. Akert (Eds.), *The frontal granular cortex and behavior* (pp. 311–334). New York: McGraw-Hill.

Moritz, S., Ruff, C., Wilke, U., Andressen, B., Krausz, M., & Naber, D. (2001). Negative priming in schizophrenia: Effects of masking and prime presentation time. *Schizophrenia Research, 48,* 291–299.

Mummery, C. J., Patterson, K., Hodges, J. R., & Wise, R. J. (1996). Generating "tiger" as an animal name or a word beginning with T: Difference in brain activation. *Proceedings of the Royal Society of London, Series B: Biological Sciences, 263,* 989–995.

Nieuwenstein, M. R., Aleman, A., & de Haan, E. H. F. (2001). Relationship between symptom dimensions and neurocognitive functioning in schizophrenia: A meta-analysis of WCST and CPT studies. *Journal of Psychiatric Research, 35,* 119–125.

Nisbet, H., Siegert, R., Hunt, M., & Fairley, N. (1996). Improving schizophrenic in-patients' Wisconsin card-sorting performance. *British Journal of Clinical Psychology, 35,* 631–633.

Nuechterlein, K. H., Dawson, M. E., & Green, M. F. (1994). Information-processing abnormalities as neuropsychological vulnerability indicators for schizophrenia. *Acta Psychiatrica Scandinavica, 384,* 71–79.

Owen, A. M. (1997). The functional organization of working memory processes within human lateral frontal cortex: The contribution of functional neuroimaging. *European Journal of Neuroscience, 9,* 1329–1339.

Owen, A. M. (2000). The role of the lateral frontal cortex in mnemonic processing: The contribution of functional neuroimaging. *Experimental Brain Research, 133,* 33–43.

Palmer, B. W., & Heaton, R. K. (2000). Executive dysfunction in schizophrenia. In T. Sharma & P. D. Harvey (Eds.), *Cognition in schizophrenia: Impairments, importance and treatment strategies* (pp. 52–72). New York: Oxford University Press.

Palmer, B. W., Heaton, R. K., Paulsen, J. S., Kuck, J., Braff, D., Harris, M. J., et al. (1997). Is it possible to be schizophrenic yet neuropsychologically normal? *Neuropsychology, 11,* 437–446.

Pantelis, C., Barber, F. Z., Barnes, T. Z., Nelson, H. E., Owen, A. M., & Robbins, T. W. (1999). Comparison of set-shifting ability in patients with chronic schizophrenia and frontal lobe damage. *Schizophrenia Research, 37,* 252–270.

Pantelis, C., Harvey, C. A., Plant, G., Fossey, E., Maruff, P., Stuart, G. W., et al. (2004). Relationship of behavioural and symptomatic syndromes in schizophrenia to spatial working memory and attentional set-shifting ability. *Psychological Medicine, 34,* 693–703.

Pantelis, C., & Nelson, H. E. (1994). Cognitive functioning and symptomatology in schizophrenia: The role of frontal–subcortical systems. In A. David & J. C. Cutting (Eds.), *The neuropsychology of schizophrenia* (pp. 215–229). Hove, UK: Erlbaum.

Park, S., & Holzman, P. S. (1992). Schizophrenics show spatial working memory deficits. *Archives of General Psychiatry, 12,* 975–982.

Park, S., Holzman, P. S., & Goldman-Rakic, P. S. (1995). Spatial working memory deficits in the relatives of schizophrenia patients. *Archives of General Psychiatry, 52,* 821–828.

Paulesu, E., Goldacre, B., Scifo, P., Cappa, S. F., Gilardi, M. C., Castiglioni, I., et al. (1997). Functional heterogeneity of left inferior frontal cortex as revealed by fMRI. *NeuroReport, 8,* 2011–2016.

Perlstein, W. M., Carter, C. S., Noll, D. C., & Cohen, J. D. (2001). Relation of prefrontal cortex dysfunction to working memory and symptoms in schizophrenia. *American Journal of Psychiatry, 158,* 1105–1113.

Perry, W., & Braff, D. L. (1994). Information-processing deficits and thought disorder in schizophrenia. *American Journal of Psychiatry, 151,* 363–367.

Perry, W., & Braff, D. L. (1998). A multimethod approach to assessing perseverations in schizophrenia patients. *Schizophrenia Research, 33,* 69–77.

Perry, W., Geyer, M. A., & Braff, D. L. (1999). Sensorimotor gating and thought disturbance measured in close proximity in schizophrenic patients. *Archives of General Psychiatry, 56,* 277–281.

Perry, W., Heaton, R. K., Potterat, E., Roebuck, T., Minassian, A., & Braff, D. L. (2001). Working memory in schizophrenia: Transient "online" storage versus executive functioning. *Schizophrenia Bulletin, 27,* 157–176.

Perry, W., Potterat, E. G., & Braff, D. L (2001). Self-monitoring enhances Wisconsin Card Sorting Test performance in patients with schizophrenia: Performance is improved by simply asking patients to verbalize their sorting strategy. *Journal of the International Neuropsychological Society, 7,* 344–352.

Pierrot-Deseilligny, C., Gaymard, B., Muri, R., & Rivaud, S. (1997). Cerebral ocular motor signs. *Journal of Neurology, 244,* 65–70.

Pujol, J., Vendrell, P., Deus, J., Kulisevsky, J., Marti-Vilalta, J. L., Garcia, C., et al. (1996). Frontal lobe activation during word generation studied by functional MRI. *Acta Neurologica Scandinavica, 93,* 402–410.

Pukrop, R., Matuschek, E., Ruhrmann, S., Brockhaus-Dumke, A., Tendolkar, I., Bertsch, A., et al. (2003). Dimensions of working memory dysfunction in schizophrenia. *Schizophrenia Research, 62,* 259–268.

Reed, R. A., Harrow, M., Herbener, E. S., & Martin, E. M. (2002). Executive function in schizophrenia: Is it linked to psychosis and poor life functioning? *Journal of Nervous and Mental Disease, 190,* 725–732.

Reuter, B., & Kathmann, N. (2004). Using saccade tasks as a tool to analyze executive dysfunction in schizophrenia. *Acta Psychologica, 115,* 255–269.

Roberts, R. J., Hager, L. D., & Heron, C. (1994). Prefrontal cognitive processes: Working memory and inhibition in the antisaccade task. *Journal of Experimental Psychology: General, 123,* 374–393.

Sereno, A. B., & Holzman, P. S. (1995). Antisaccades and smooth pursuit eye movements in schizophrenia. *Biological Psychiatry, 37,* 394–401.

Simons, R. F., & Giardina, B. D. (1992). Reflex modification in psychosis-prone young adults. *Psychophysiology, 29,* 8–16.

Sommer, I. E., Ramsey, N. F., & Kahn, R. S. (2001). Language lateralization in schizophrenia, an fMRI study. *Schizophrenia Research, 52,* 57–67.

Sommer, I. E., Ramsey, N. F., Mandl, R. C., & Kahn, R. S. (2003). Language lateralization in female patients with schizophrenia: An fMRI study. *Schizophrenia Research, 60,* 183–190.

Stroop, J. R. (1935). Studies of interference in serial and verbal reactions. *Journal of Experimental Psychology, 18,* 643–662.

Suddath, R. L., Casanova, M. F., Goldberg, T. E., Daniel, G., Kelsoe, J. R., & Weiinberger, D. R. (1989). Temporal lobe pathology in schizophrenia: A quantitative magnetic resonance imaging study. *American Journal of Psychiatry, 146,* 464–472.

Suddath, R. L., Christison, G. W., Torrey, E. F., Casanova, M. F., & Weinberger, D. R. (1990). Anatomical abnormalities in the brains of monozygotic twins discordant for schizophrenia. *New England Journal of Medicine, 322,* 789–794.

Summerfelt, A. T., Alphs, L. D., Wagman, A. M., Funderburk, F. R., Hierholzer, R. M., & Strauss, M. E. (1991). Reduction of perseverative erros in patients with schizophrenia using monetary feedback. *Journal of Abnormal Psychology, 100,* 613–616.

Swerdlow, N. R., Benbow, C. H., Zisook, S., Geyer, M. A., & Braff, D. L. (1993). A preliminary assessment of sensorimotor gating in patients with obsessive compulsive disorder (OCD). *Biological Psychiatry, 33,* 298–301.

Swerdlow, N. R., & Koob, G. F. (1987). Dopamine, schizophrenia, mania, and depression: Toward a unified hypothesis of cortico-stratio-pallido-thalamic function. *Behavioral and Brain Sciences, 10,* 197–245.

Swerdlow, N. R., Paulsen, J., Braff, D. L., Butters, N., Geyer, M. A., & Swenson, M. R. (1995). Impaired prepulse inhibition of acoustic and tactile startle in patients with Huntington's disease. *Journal of Neurology, Neurosurgery, and Psychiatry, 58,* 192–200.

Tipper, S. P. (1985). The negative priming effect: Inhibitory priming by ignored objects. *Quarterly Journal of Experimental Psychology, A37,* 571–590.

Venables, P. H. (1964). Input dysfunction in schizophrenia. In B. A. Maher (Ed.), *Progress in experimental personality research* (Vol. 1, pp. 1–47). New York: Academic Press.

Vollema, M. G., Geurtsen, G. J., & van Voorst, A. J. P. (1995). Durable improvements in Wisconsin Card Sorting Tests performance in schizophrenic patients. *Schizophrenia Research*, *16*, 209–215.

Weike, A. I., Bauer, U., & Hamm, A. O. (2000). Effective neuroleptic medication removes prepulse inhibition deficits in schizophrenia patients. *Biological Psychiatry*, *47*, 61–70.

Weinberger, D. R., Aloia, M. S., Goldberg, T. E., & Berman, K. F. (1994). The frontal lobes in schizophrenia. *Journal of Neuropsychiatry and Clinical Neurosciences*, *6*, 419–427.

Weinberger, D. R., Berman, K. F., & Zec, R. F. (1986). Physiologic dysfunction of dorsolateral prefrontal cortex in schizophrenia: I. Regional cerebral blood flow evidence. *Archives of General Psychiatry*, *4*, 114–124.

Wilson, F. A., Scalaidhe, S. P., & Goldman-Rakic, P. S. (1993). Dissociation of object and spatial processing domains in primate prefrontal cortex. *Science*, *260*, 1955–1958.

Yurgelun-Todd, D. A., Waternaux, C. M., Cohen, B. M., Gruber, S. A., English, C. D., & Renshaw, P. F. (1996). Functional magnetic resonance imaging of schizophrenic patients and comparison subjects during word production. *American Journal of Psychiatry*, *153*, 200–205.

# CHAPTER 37

# Bipolar Disorder and the Frontal Lobes

*Mary G. DeMay*
*Danijela Pavlic*
*Bruce L. Miller*

## PHENOMENOLOGY

Although Kraepelin in 1913 recognized an association between vascular disease and a manic state, over the early decades of the 20th century, science moved away from exploration of the biological underpinnings of psychiatric illness in favor of psychodynamic and psychological theories of etiology. Recently, there has been a resurgence of interest in psychiatric illness as reflecting a perturbation in brain biology or structure. In this endeavor, the fields of psychiatry and neurology are showing more collaboration, with efforts to correlate anatomically behavioral changes and aberrations with brain abnormality.

Mood disorders secondary to brain injury have long been recognized. Because depression in frontal lobe disease is covered by Lesser and Chung, Chapter 39, this volume, we focus on bipolar illness and specifically, the phenotype of mania.

The core phenomenon of bipolar disorder is the occurrence of mania. The criteria used by the fourth edition of the *Diagnostic and Statistical Manual of Mental Disorders* (DSM-IV; American Psychiatric Association, 1994) are as follows: There must be evidence for a distinct period of abnormally and persistently elevated, expansive, or irritable mood lasting at least 1 week. During the period of mood disturbance, three (or more) of the following symptoms

have persisted (four if the mood is only irritable) and have been present to a significant degree: (1) inflated self-esteem or grandiosity; (2) decreased need for sleep; (3) more talkative than usual or under pressure to keep talking; (4) flighty ideas or subjective experience that thoughts are racing; (5) distractibility (i.e., attention too easily drawn to unimportant or irrelevant external stimuli); (6) increase in goal-directed activity (at work, at school, or sexually) or psychomotor agitation; and (7) excessive involvement in pleasurable activities that have a high potential for painful consequences. DSM-IV criteria also include a requirement for significant psychosocial impairment and the absence of an obvious etiological condition such as amphetamine use or hyperthyroidism (American Psychiatric Association, 1994).

Bipolar disorder is also associated with occurrences of "major depressive episodes," which are defined by DSM-IV as the persistence of either depressed mood or a marked loss of interest in most activities for a period of at least 2 weeks. The episode is associated with at least five symptoms that, in addition to depressed mood and loss of pleasure, consist of (1) significant weight loss when not dieting, or weight gain (e.g., a change of more than 5% of body weight in a month), or decrease or increase in appetite nearly every day; (2) insomnia or hypersomnia nearly every day; (3) psychomotor agitation or retardation nearly every day; (4) fatigue or loss of energy nearly every day; (5) feelings of worthlessness or excessive, or inappropriate, guilt nearly every day; (6) persistent diminished ability to think or concentrate, or indecisiveness; and (7) recurrent thoughts of death (not just fear of dying) or suicidal ideation. Similar to the criteria for mania, there must be significant psychosocial impairment and the absence of an obvious etiological condition, such as treatment with interferon.

Classically, bipolar disorder has recurrences of both mania and depression. However, in unusual cases there are only manic episodes present. In either case, the presence of mania is termed bipolar I disorder. Bipolar II disorder consists of episodes of major depression and subsyndromal mania (e.g., hypomania). Diagnostic criteria for bipolar disorder also include a number of specifiers that include a severity rating, presence of psychotic features, presence of catatonia, postpartum onset, seasonal pattern, or rapid cycling. Currently, this disorder is diagnosed strictly with clinical phenomenology, but someday a biological model will define bipolar disease based on anatomical, neurochemical, and genetic features.

## EPIDEMIOLOGY

Estimates for the lifetime prevalence of bipolar I disorder range from 0.4 to 1.9% of the general population (Jacobi et al., 2004; Judd & Akiskal, 2003; Kessler, Rubinow, Holmes, Abelson, & Zhao, 1997; Regier et al., 1984, 1988; ten Have, Vollebergh, Bijl, & Nolan, 2002). The lifetime prevalence for bipolar II disorder is lower, with current estimates at around 0.5% (Angst, 1998). The largest surveys conducted to date that examine the combined prevalence of bipolar I and II disorder have reported combined rates ranging from 3.9% (Kessler et al., 2005) to 6.4% (Judd & Akiskal, 2003). Unlike other mood disorders, bipolar disorder is equally prevalent in men and women. In women, the postpartum period is a period of enhanced risk for developing manic symptoms (Freeman & Gelenberg, 2005; Jones & Craddock, 2005). There are no known effects of race or ethnicity on lifetime risk for bipolar disorder, although there are geographic pockets with higher rates, probably related to single founders with higher rates of bipolar disease (Mathews et al., 2004).

## LONGITUDINAL COURSE

Most patients diagnosed with bipolar I disorder suffer recurrences of mania and depression when followed prospectively. Although most patients have periods of normal mood (euthymia) interepisodically, a minority have continuous mood instability, and impaired occupational and interpersonal functioning (Zarate, Tohen, Land, & Cavanagh, 2000). Patients with psychotic symptoms are at higher risk for recurrent psychotic symptoms in subsequent episodes and have worse prognoses.

## HERITABILITY

Bipolar I disorder appears to have heritable risk, as demonstrated in a number of monozygotic and dizygotic twin studies (Bertelsen, Harvald, & Hauge, 1977; Kieseppa, Partonen, Haukka, Kaprio, & Lonnqvist, 2004; McGuffin et al., 2003). First-degree relatives of probands with bipolar I disorder have elevated rates of bipolar I disorder (4–24%), bipolar II disorder (1–5%), and major depressive disorder (4–24%) (Mortensen, Pedersen, Melbye, Mors, & Ewald, 2003; Smoller & Finn, 2003).

## EVIDENCE FOR FRONTAL LOBE PATHOLOGY IN BIPOLAR I DISORDER

Many structural neuroimaging studies have demonstrated abnormalities in the frontal lobes in patients diagnosed psychiatrically with bipolar disorder (Blumberg, Charney, & Krystal, 2002; Haldane & Frangou, 2004). Similarly, in patients with classical bipolar illness, magnetic resonance imaging (MRI) studies have shown changes primarily in frontotemporal regions. In particular, reduced gray matter volume in ventral frontal areas appears to be a common abnormality (Drevets et al., 1997). Evidence for both gray and white matter abnormalities in the prefrontal cortex of patients with bipolar disorder (Brambilla et al., 2002; Lopez-Larson, DelBello, Zimmerman, Schwiers, & Strakowski, 2002; Sharma et al., 2003) also exists. Patients with bipolar disorder have more white matter changes suggestive of vascular disease, with these findings replicated to a greater degree in elderly patients with bipolar disorder. This may suggest that white matter disease interrupts neural connections between frontal and temporal regions, resulting in mania. Histologically, changes include vascular malformations, dilated perivascular spaces, infarcts, and necrosis. Basal ganglia, hippocampal, thalamus, and amygdala volumes have been of interest, although findings have been inconsistent. Studies have also found enlargement of the left lateral ventricle in the temporal region. There has been interest in cerebellar volume in bipolar disorder (DelBello, Strakowski, Zimmerman, Hawkins, & Sax, 1999), although no clear-cut associations have been demonstrated. Strakowski and colleagues (2002) studied MRI ventricular and periventricular volumes in patients with first- and multiple-episode bipolar disorder. Patients with multiple episodes had significantly larger lateral ventricles than patients with first episodes or controls. Also, striatal volumes tend to be greater than those seen in normal controls in patients with first-episode bipolar illness. Both unipolar depression and bipolar depression are associated with smaller prefrontal lobe volumes (Strakowski et al., 2002). Interpretation of MRI volumetric analyses is unclear (state vs. trait, reflective of neuronal loss, premorbid risk factor, etc.).

Functional neuroimaging studies, which detect changes in blood flow and glucose metabolism on the scale of seconds, have been performed in patients with bipolar disorder. In general, these studies have shown that several different brain regions (likely networks of neuronal activity) are involved in cognitive processing. Patients with bipolar disorder and depression have shown state-dependent, reduced cortical metabolism relative to controls or patients with unipolar depression (Baxter et al., 1985). Magnetic resonance spectroscopy (MRS) has shown an increase in choline-containing compounds in the basal ganglia of patients with bipolar disorder (Stoll, Renshaw, Yurgelun-Todd, & Cohen, 2000; Strakowski et al., 1993).

## SECONDARY MANIA

Similarly, there is ample evidence to suggest that bipolar syndromes can be induced in association with focal brain injury in previously healthy individuals. When mania is induced by a focal brain injury, the term that has been used is "secondary mania." In 1978, Krauthammer and Klerman defined secondary mania as a manic syndrome without prior history or family history of mania, occurring in the context of an underlying systemic illness or neurological disorder. Secondary mania or bipolar disorder can result from endocrine abnormalities, metabolic disturbances, neoplasm, infection, genetic diseases, toxic–pharmacological effects, vascular changes, infarct or hemorrhage, and traumatic brain injury (Blumberg, Charney, & Krystal, 2002; Gafoor & O'Keane, 2003; Miller, Cummings, McIntyre, Ebers, & Grode, 1986). Bakchine and colleagues (1989) described a manic-like state following bilateral orbitofrontal and right temporoparietal injury that was responsive to treatment with clonidine. Miller and colleagues (1986) reported changes in patients' sexual preference and hypersexuality after brain injury. Starkstein, Boston, and Robinson (1988) reviewed 12 case reports of post–brain injury mania. White matter diseases, including those that undercut frontal lobes, such as CADASIL (cerebral autosomal dominant arteriopathy with subcortical infarcts and leukoencephalopathy) (Ahearn et al., 1998, 2002) have a higher than expected rate of manic-like syndromes. The same is true for neurodegenerative disorders, including Huntington's disease, Creutzfeldt–Jakob disease, and frontotemporal dementia (Mendez, 2000).

More important than the type of injury is the location. Secondary mania is much more common with right-hemisphere lesions than with left and many involve the orbitofrontal, perithalamic, or anterior temporal lobes (Gafoor & O'Keane, 2003). Whether structural or neurodegenerative, the common anatomical theme is either involvement of the orbitofrontal region or brain regions that connect to this area (Starkstein, Boston, & Robinson, 1988). In addition, lesions in the caudate, thalamus, and midbrain are more likely to result in bipolar features than in unipolar manic states.

## NEUROCHEMICAL MECHANISMS

A wide variety of neurochemical abnormalities have been seen in patients with bipolar disorder. Changes in catecholamines seem to represent a core feature of bipolar disease (Schildkraut & Mooney, 2004). Manic states can be reliably precipitated with amphetamines and other compounds that increase noradrenergic brain activity. Dopaminergic excess in

Parkinson's disease triggers similar behaviors (Evans et al., 2004). Similarly, subcortical stimulation with deep brain stimulation in patients with Parkinson's disease has triggered bipolar behavior (Kulisevsky et al., 2002). In contrast, depression is triggered, in part, by catecholamine depletion. The mechanisms for a switch from depressed to manic symptoms still remain largely speculative. Bringing the clinical phenomenology of bipolar disease from biochemistry to anatomy represents a key goal of future research.

## OVERLAP OF BIPOLAR CORE CRITERIA WITH FRONTAL LOBE DISORDERS

It is worthwhile to note that many of the core features of bipolar disorder overlap with known frontal lobe syndromes. Inflated-self-esteem with grandiosity, pressured speech, racing thoughts, distractibility, and excessive involvement in pleasurable activities with a high potential for painful consequences are regular features of patients with injury to the right orbitofrontal or anterior temporal brain regions. It is tempting to speculate about a link between frontal lobe dysfunction and these behavioral features of bipolar illness. Given that features of mania can be seen not only in primary bipolar affective disorder but also in states related to brain injury, vascular disease, toxic–metabolic states, and so forth, the question arises as to whether mania might, at times, represent a phenotype or final common pathway rather than a distinct diagnostic entity. How secondary mania differs etiologically (e.g., structurally, neurochemically) from primary bipolar illness is of great interest. A strong and consistent literature links loss of executive function with bipolar disease. In particular, deficits in set shifting, verbal fluency, planning, attention, and verbal memory are routinely seen during manic, hypomanic, and interepisodic euthymic states (Malhi, Ivanovski, Szekeres, & Olley, 2004; Quraishi & Frangou, 2002). Interestingly, impairment in executive function has been noted in first-degree relatives of both patients with bipolar illness and in patients with unipolar depression (Clark, Sarna, & Goodwin, 2005). Teasing out the components of bipolar disease that represent frontal dysfunction from those that do not represents a future challenge of scientific research into this important and common disease.

## TREATMENT

Lithium remains the initial treatment of choice for manic symptoms such as euphoric mood and irritability (Bauer & Mitchner, 2004). It is the only Food and Drug Administration (FDA)–approved treatment for the maintenance of bipolar disorder. Lithium is the standard by which all other mood stabilizers are evaluated for the treatment of all presentations of mania. It is particularly effective when treatment is initiated early in the course of lifetime illness (Ernst & Goldberg, 2004) and when depression is not a prominent part of the clinical presentation (Goldberg, Harrow, & Leon, 1996). There is some evidence that lithium may be less effective for the treatment of depression versus mania (Geddes, Burgess, Hawton, Jamison, & Goodwin, 2004). Lithium is limited by a small therapeutic index and myriad side effects, including tremor, ataxia, polyuria, polydipsia, and hypothyroidism. Lithium's mechanisms of action, modulation of several second messenger systems, and attenuation of a cell's responsivity to other neurotransmitters (serotonin, $\gamma$-aminobutyric acid [GABA], dopamine) may provide a window into the mechanism of manic states. Lithium appears to reset ionic homeostasis and may be both neuroprotective and stimulate neurogenesis in the hippocampus (Bachmann, Schloesser, Gould, & Manji, 2005; Lagace & Eisch, 2005).

In the past three decades, there has been widespread use of antiepileptic agents for the treatment of mania. These drugs are purported to decrease brain excitation via the blockade of low-voltage sodium-ion channels, which in turn reduces activity of excitatory amino acids such as glutamate and increases activity of the inhibitory neurotransmitter GABA. Divalproex and carbamazepine have been effective in controlled trials for the treatment of mania (Salloum et al., 2005; Swann, Bowden, Calabrese, Dilsaver, & Morris, 1999; Swann et al., 1997). Divalproex may be better tolerated than lithium but still has side effects, including sedation, nausea, weight gain, and alopecia. Divalproex is also associated with an increased risk of hepatic toxicity and thrombocytopenia. Carbamazepine may also be better tolerated than lithium, but its use is complicated by side effects such as sedation, agranulocytosis, and hepatic induction of P450 cytochrome metabolism, which may reduce levels of many other medications. A number of other anticonvulsant mood stabilizers have been found to be useful. Lamotrigine, gabapentin, and topiramate have been used but have not been examined in large-scale, controlled studies. The use of lamotrigine is also limited by concerns about skin rash. There is limited support for the use of omega-3 fatty acids (Stoll et al., 1999).

Typical antipsychotic medications such as chlorpromazine and haloperidol have been used for the treatment of psychosis accompanying mania. Their use is limited by the high risk for extrapyramidal side effects and tardive dyskinesia. The increased tolerability and decreased incidence of dyskinesia in atypical antipsychotics has led to wider use of these antipsychotic medications even in the absence of psychotic symptoms (Citrome & Volavka, 2004). The atypical antipsychotic agents have now been incorporated in recent American Psychiatric Association guidelines (2002) for the treatment of severe mania, and a number of them has been approved by the FDA due to their mood stabilizing effects. The atypical antipsychotic drugs have serotonergic effects (such as agonism of $5\text{-HT}_{1A}$ receptors and antagonism of postsynaptic $5\text{-HT}_{2A}$ receptors) that are thought to underlie their mood-stabilizing and antidepressant effects (Ernst & Goldberg, 2003). The atypical antipsychotics may also increase dopamine neurotransmission in the dorsolateral prefrontal cortex (Youngren, Inglis, Pivirotto, et al., 1999). The atypical antipsychotic agents are limited by a risk for stroke in the elderly and an increased risk of weight gain and diabetes.

Often, single agents are not sufficient to treat mania effectively or prevent recurrence. The FDA has approved combined use of atypical antipsychotic medications with either lithium or divalproex. Large-scale, controlled trials comparing combination treatments have generally not been conducted. Clinicians need to be mindful of possible drug–drug effects with combination therapies.

The treatment of secondary mania always involves treatment of the underlying condition, whenever possible. Thus, it is essential to restore homeostasis by treating infection; correcting electrolyte, metabolic, and endocrinological abnormalities; eliminating offending medications and other toxic agents; and so forth. In the setting of secondary mania due to vascular disease or frontal degenerative disease, however, it may not be possible to correct the underlying abnormality. In the case of vascular disease, it is essential to manage risk factors aggressively to decrease likelihood of progression of disease. In frontotemporal dementia, there is probable benefit to addressing the significant serotonergic deficit (e.g., with selective serotonin reuptake inhibitors). However, in any case, patients may continue to manifest manic or hypomanic symptomatology despite addressing underlying conditions. In such cases, one has little recourse but to treat as if dealing with primary mania or hypomania (i.e., using lithium or other mood stabilizer and atypical antipsychotic agents as needed).

## REFERENCES

Ahearn, E. P., Speer, M. C., Chen, Y. T., Steffens, D. C., Cassidy, F., Van Meter, S., et al. (2002). Investigation of Notch3 as a candidate gene for bipolar disorder using brain hyperintensities as an endophenotype. *American Journal of Medical Genetics, 114,* 652–658.

Ahearn, E. P., Steffens, D. C., Cassidy, F., Van Meter, S. A., Provenzcale, J. M., Seldin, M. F., et al. (1998). Familial leukoencephalopathy in bipolar disorder. *American Journal of Psychiatry, 155,* 1605–1607.

American Psychiatric Association. (2002). *Practice guideline for the treatment of patients with bipolar disorder* (2nd ed.). Washington, DC: Author.

American Psychiatric Association. (1994). *Diagnostic and statistical manual of mental disorders* (4th ed.). Washington, DC: Author.

Angst, J. (1998). The emerging epidemiology of hypomania and bipolar II disorder. *Journal of Affective Disorders, 50,* 143–151.

Bachmann, R. F., Schloesser, R. J., Gould, T. D., & Manji, H. K. (2005). Mood stabilizers target cellular plasticity and resilience cascades: Implications for the development of novel therapeutics. *Molecular Neurobiology, 32,* 173–202.

Bakchine, S., Lacomblez, L., Benoit, N., Parisot, D., Chain, F., Lhermitte, F., et al. (1989). Manic-like state after bilateral orbitofrontal and right temporoparietal injury: Efficacy of clonidine. *Neurology, 39,* 777–781.

Bauer, M. S., & Mitchner, L. (2004). What is a "mood stabilizer"?: An evidence-based response. *American Journal of Psychiatry, 161,* 3–18.

Baxter, L. R., Jr., Phelps, M. E., Mazziotta, J. C., Schwartz, J. M., Gerner, R. H., Selin, C. E., et al. (1985). Cerebral metabolic rates for glucose in mood disorders: Studies with positron emission tomography and fluorodeoxyglucose F 18. *Archives of General Psychiatry, 42*(5), 441–447.

Bertelsen, A., Harvald, B., & Hauge, M. (1977). A Danish twin study of manic–depressive disorders. *British Journal of Psychiatry, 130,* 330–351.

Blumberg, H. P., Charney, D. S., & Krystal, J. H.

(2002). Frontotemporal neural systems in bipolar disorder. *Seminars in Clinical Neuropsychiatry, 7,* 243–254.

Brambilla, P., Nicoletti, M. A., Harenski, K., Sassi, R. B., Mallinger, A. G., Frank, E., et al. (2002). Anatomical MRI study of subgenual prefrontal cortex in bipolar and unipolar subjects. *Neuropsychopharmacology, 27,* 792–799.

Citrome, L., & Volavka, J. (2004). The promise of atypical antipsychotics: Fewer side effects mean enhanced compliance and improved functioning. *Postgraduate Medicine, 116,* 49–51, 55–59, 63.

Clark, L., Sarna, A., & Goodwin, G. M. (2005). Impairment of executive function but not memory in first-degree relatives of patients with bipolar I disorder and in euthymic patients with unipolar depression. *American Journal of Psychiatry, 162,* 1980–1982.

DelBello, M. P., Strakowski, S. M., Zimmerman, M. E., Hawkins, J. M., & Sax, K. W. (1999). MRI analysis of the cerebellum in bipolar disorder: A pilot study. *Neuropsychopharmacology, 21*(1), 63–68.

Drevets, W. C., Price, J. L., Simpson, J. R., Jr., Todd, R. D., Reich, T., Vannier, M., et al. (1997). Subgenual prefrontal cortex abnormalities in mood disorders. *Nature, 386,* 824–827.

Ernst, C. L., & Goldberg, J. F. (2003). Antidepressant properties of anticonvulsant drugs for bipolar disorder. *Journal of Clinical Psychopharmacology, 23,* 182–192.

Ernst, C. L., & Goldberg, J. F. (2004). Antisuicide properties of psychotropic drugs: A critical review. *Harvard Review of Psychiatry, 12,* 14–41.

Evans, A. H., Katzenschlager, R., Paviour, D., O'Sullivan, J. D., Appel, S., Lawrence, A. D., et al. (2004). Punding in Parkinson's disease: Its relation to the dopamine dysregulation syndrome. *Movement Disorders, 19,* 397–405.

Freeman, M. P., & Gelenberg, A. J. (2005). Bipolar disorder in women: Reproductive events and treatment considerations. *Acta Psychiatrica Scandinavica, 112,* 88–96.

Gafoor, R., & O'Keane, V. (2003). Three case reports of secondary mania: Evidence supporting a right frontotemporal locus. *European Psychiatry, 18,* 32–33.

Geddes, J. R., Burgess, S., Hawton, K., Jamison, K., & Goodwin, G. M. (2004). Long-term lithium therapy for bipolar disorder: Systematic review and meta-analysis of randomized controlled trials. *American Journal of Psychiatry, 161,* 217–222.

Goldberg, J. F., Harrow, M., & Leon, A. C. (1996). Lithium treatment of bipolar affective disorders under naturalistic followup conditions. *Psychopharmacology Bulletin, 32,* 47–54.

Haldane, M., & Frangou, S. (2004). New insights help define the pathophysiology of bipolar affective disorder: Neuroimaging and neuropathology findings. *Progress in Neuro-Psychopharmacology and Biological Psychiatry, 28,* 943–960.

Jacobi, F., Wittchen, H. U., Holting, C., Hofler, M., Pfister, H., Muller, N., et al. (2004). Prevalence, comorbidity and correlates of mental disorders in the general population: Results from the German Health Interview and Examination Survey (GHS). *Psychological Medicine, 34,* 597–611.

Jones, I., & Craddock, N. (2005). Bipolar disorder and childbirth: The importance of recognising risk. *British Journal of Psychiatry, 186,* 453–454.

Judd, L. L., & Akiskal, H. S. (2003). The prevalence and disability of bipolar spectrum disorders in the US population: Re-analysis of the ECA database taking into account subthreshold cases. *Journal of Affective Disorders, 73,* 123–131.

Kessler, R. C., Chiu, W. T., Demler, O., Merikangas, K. R., & Walters, E. E. (2005). Prevalence, severity, and comorbidity of 12-month DSM-IV disorders in the National Comorbidity Survey Replication. *Archives of General Psychiatry, 62,* 617–627.

Kessler, R. C., Rubinow, D. R., Holmes, C., Abelson, J. M., & Zhao, S. (1997). The epidemiology of DSM-III-R bipolar I disorder in a general population survey. *Psychological Medicine, 27,* 1079–1089.

Kieseppa, T., Partonen, T., Haukka, J., Kaprio, J., & Lonnqvist, J. (2004). High concordance of bipolar I disorder in a nationwide sample of twins. *American Journal of Psychiatry, 161,* 1814–1821.

Krauthammer, C., & Klerman, G. L. (1978). Secondary mania: Manic syndromes associated with antecedent physical illness or drugs. *Archives of General Psychiatry, 35,* 1333–1339.

Kulisevsky, J., Berthier, M. L., Gironell, A., Pascual Sedano, B., Molet, J., & Pares, P. (2002). Mania following deep brain stimulation for Parkinson's disease. *Neurology, 59,* 1421–1424.

Lagace, D. C., & Eisch, A. J. (2005). Mood-stabilizing drugs: Are their neuroprotective aspects clinically relevant? *Psychiatric Clinics of North America, 28,* 399–414.

Lopez-Larson, M. P., DelBello, M. P., Zimmerman, M. E., Schwiers, M. L., & Strakowski, S. M. (2002). Regional prefrontal gray and white matter abnormalities in bipolar disorder. *Biological Psychiatry, 52,* 93–100.

Malhi, G. S., Ivanovski, B., Szekeres, V., & Olley, A. (2004). Bipolar disorder: It's all in your mind?: The neuropsychological profile of a biological disorder. *Canadian Journal of Psychiatry, 49,* 813–819.

Mathews, C. A., Reus, V. I., Bejarano, J., Escamilla, M. A., Fournier, E., Herrera, L. D., et al. (2004). Genetic studies of neuropsychiatric disorders in Costa Rica: A model for the use of isolated populations. *Psychiatric Genetics, 14,* 13–23.

McGuffin, P., Rijsdijk, F., Andrew, M., Sham, P., Katz, R., & Cardno, A. (2003). The heritability of bipolar affective disorder and the genetic relationship to unipolar depression. *Archives of General Psychiatry, 60,* 497–502.

Mendez, M. F. (2000). Mania in neurologic disorders. *Current Psychiatry Reports, 2,* 440–445.

Miller, B. L., Cummings, J. L., McIntyre, H., Ebers, G., & Grode, M. (1986). Hypersexuality or altered sexual preference following brain injury. *Journal of Neurology, Neurosurgery, and Psychiatry, 49,* 867–873.

Mortensen, P. B., Pedersen, C. B., Melbye, M., Mors, O., & Ewald, H. (2003). Individual and familial risk factors for bipolar affective disorders in Denmark. *Archives of General Psychiatry, 60,* 1209–1215.

Quraishi, S., & Frangou, S. (2002). Neuropsychology of bipolar disorder: A review. *Journal of Affective Disorders, 72,* 209–226.

Regier, D. A., Boyd, J. H., Burke, J. D., Jr., Rae, D. S., Myers, J. K., Kramer, M., et al. (1988). One-month prevalence of mental disorders in the United States: Based on five Epidemiologic Catchment Area sites. *Archives of General Psychiatry, 45,* 977–986.

Regier, D. A., Myers, J. K., Kramer, M., Robins, L. N., Blazer, D. G., Hough, R. L., et al. (1984). The NIMH Epidemiologic Catchment Area program: Historical context, major objectives, and study population characteristics. *Archives of General Psychiatry, 41,* 934–941.

Salloum, I. M., Cornelius, J. R., Daley, D. C., Kirisci, L., Himmelhoch, J. M., & Thase, M. E. (2005). Efficacy of valproate maintenance in patients with bipolar disorder and alcoholism: A double-blind placebo-controlled study. *Archives of General Psychiatry, 62,* 37–45.

Schildkraut, J. J., & Mooney, J. J. (2004). Toward a rapidly acting antidepressant: The normetanephrine and extraneuronal monoamine transporter (uptake 2) hypothesis. *American Journal of Psychiatry, 161,* 909–911.

Sharma, V., Menon, R., Carr, T. J., Densmore, M., Mazmanian, D., & Williamson, P. C. (2003). An MRI study of subgenual prefrontal cortex in patients with familial and non-familial bipolar I disorder. *Journal of Affective Disorders, 77,* 167–171.

Smoller, J. W., & Finn, C. T. (2003). Family, twin, and adoption studies of bipolar disorder. *American Journal of Medical Genetics, 123,* 48–58.

Starkstein, S. E., Boston, J. D., & Robinson, R. G. (1988). Mechanisms of mania after brain injury: 12 case reports and review of the literature. *Journal of Nervous and Mental Disease, 176,* 87–100.

Stoll, A. L., Renshaw, P. F., Yurgelun-Todd, D. A., & Cohen, B. M. (2000). Neuroimaging in bipolar disorder: What have we learned? *Biological Psychiatry 48*(6), 505–517.

Stoll, A. L., Severus, W. E., Freeman, M. P., Reuter, S., Zboyan, H. A., Diamond, E., et al. (2000). Omega 3 fatty acids in bipolar disorder: A preliminary double-blind, placebo-controlled trial. *Archives of General Psychiatry, 56,* 407–412.

Strakowski, S. M., DelBello, M. P., Zimmerman, M. E., Getz, G. E., Mills, N. P., Ret, J., et al. (2002). Ventricular and periventricular structural volumes in first-versus multiple-episode bipolar disorder. *American Journal of Psychiatry, 159,* 1841–1847.

Strakowski, S. M., Wilson, D. R., Tohen, M., Woods, B. T., Douglass, A. W., & Stoll, A. L. (1993). Structural brain abnormalities in first-episode mania. *Biological Psychiatry, 33,* 602–609.

Swann, A. C., Bowden, C. L., Calabrese, J. R., Dilsaver, S. C., & Morris, D. D. (1999). Differential effect of number of previous episodes of affective disorder on response to lithium or divalproex in acute mania. *American Journal of Psychiatry, 156,* 1264–1266.

Swann, A. C., Bowden, C. L., Morris, D., Calabrese, J. R., Petty, F., Small, J., et al. (1997). Depression during mania: Treatment response to lithium or divalproex. *Archives of General Psychiatry, 54,* 37–42.

ten Have, M., Vollebergh, W., Bijl, R., & Nolen, W. A. (2002). Bipolar disorder in the general population in The Netherlands (prevalence, consequences and care utilisation): Results from The Netherlands Mental Health Survey and Incidence Study (NEMESIS). *Journal of Affective Disorders, 68,* 203–213.

Youngren, K. D., Inglis, F. M., Pivirotto, P. J., Jedema, H. P., Bradberry, C. W., Goldman-Rakic, P. S., et al. (1999). Clozapine preferentially increases dopamine release in the rhesus monkey prefrontal cortex compared with the caudate nucleus. *Neuropsychopharmacology, 20,* 403–412.

Zarate, C. A., Jr., Tohen, M., Land, M., & Cavanagh, S. (2000). Functional impairment and cognition in bipolar disorder. *Psychiatric Quarterly, 71,* 309–329.

# CHAPTER 38

# Obsessive–Compulsive Disorder and the Frontal Lobes

*Denys Fontaine*
*Vianney Mattei*
*Philippe H. Robert*

Obsessive–compulsive disorder (OCD) is a mental illness that has been described since the 19th century by several famous clinicians. "Reasoning monomania" (Esquirol in 1838), "madness of doubt" (Falret in 1866), "emotional delirium" (Morel in 1886), and "obsessional neurosis" (Freud in 1894) are some of the designations and concepts by which this nosographic entity was known. Today, OCD is defined by accurate clinical and diagnostic criteria (fourth, text revised edition of the *Diagnostic and Statistical Manual of Mental Disorders* [DSM-IV-TR; American Psychiatric Association, 2000] and *International Classification of Diseases* [ICD-10; World Health Association, 1993]), but the diversity of the explanatory theoretical models makes this disorder difficult to understand. In this context, recent results from functional neuroimaging studies and other areas represent a significant advance in understanding this mental disease, by showing the associations and interactions of frontal and subcortical structures.

After describing the OCD clinical syndrome, our aim in this chapter is to describe the relation between OCD and the frontal lobes through evidence from pharmacological, animal, neuroimaging, and neurosurgical studies.

## CLINICAL DESCRIPTION AND PSYCHOLOGICAL MODELS

OCDs are characterized by the existence of recurrent obsessions and compulsions. Obsessions (from the Latin *obsidere*, to besiege) are thoughts, images, and impulses that are persistent, intrusive, and inappropriate, and that generally result in significant anxiety. The most common obsessions are repeated thoughts of contamination (to be contaminated by touching something or by shaking hands), repeated doubts (e.g., wondering if one has truly carried out an action, such as turning off the gas, locking the door), aggressive impulses (fear of hurting someone), or sexual perceptions. Compulsions (from the Latin *compellere*, to compel) are repetitive behavior (washing one's hands) or mental acts (counting, repeating a phrase) whose goal is to avert or reduce the suffering and anxiety due to the obsessions. The majority of patients are conscious of the abnormal, unreasonable, and excessive nature of these thoughts and behavior. DSM-IV, however, recognizes two types of subjects according to their *insight*: Those who possess bad *insight* do not call into question their beliefs and behavior, in contrast to those who possess good *insight*. On a clinical level, the symptomatology of obsessions and compulsions is rich and varied.

In practice, several categories of patients are described:

- "Washers" present washing rituals with phobic obsessiveness regarding contamination or impurity.
- "Checkers," scared of making a mistake or prejudicing someone against them, thus enact numerous checking rituals.
- "Ruminators" are invaded by obsessions of doubt and indecision, and consequently present with only a few motor rituals.
- "Hoarders" or "accumulators" collect valueless objects in order to restrict their living space to one room or a few square meters.
- In "obsessional slowness" syndrome, subjects are searching for order, symmetry, or perfection.

Mixed forms of OCD are common, and a patient can shift from one form to another during the course of the illness. OCD provokes a loss of time (by definition, more than 1 hour a day). Frequently, the intensity of the symptoms is such that OCD represents a real handicap and is incompatible with a socioprofessional life. Indeed, some patients spend up to 8–10 hours a day mulling over their obsessions and performing compulsive rituals. Thus, some individuals are incapable of leaving their homes or of living autonomously. The recent estimation is that 1.5–2.5% of the general population is affected by OCD (Bebbington, 1998; Hollander, 1997; Karno, Golding, Sorenson, & Burnam, 1988; Nestadt, Samuels, & Romanoski, 1994). OCD typically begins in young adults between ages 20 and 30 (Hantouche, Bourgeois, Bouhassira, & Lancrenon, 1996), rarely during childhood, and even more rarely after 50 years of age (0.01%) (Weiss & Jenike, 2000). Therefore, a late-developing OCD should provoke suspicions of a neurological illness (e.g., Parkinson's disease [Alegret et al., 2001], Huntington's disease [Anderson, Louis, Stern, & Marder, 2001], Sydenham's chorea [Swedo, Rapoport, & Cheslow, 1989], Creutzfeldt–Jakob disease [Lopez, Berthier, Beacker, & Boller, 1997], or cerebral lesions [Etcharry-Bouyx & Dubas, 2000]).

Spontaneous remissions occur in only 12% of cases (Skoog & Skoog, 1999). The average duration of the disorder is estimated at 7.2 years, with 20% of patients having a duration greater than 10 years, and only 30% with less than 1 year (Karno et al., 1988). Overall, the sex ratio is around 1:1, with a predominance of males among children and adolescents. There is frequent comorbidity of OCD with other mental disorders (Welkowitz, Struening, Pittman, & Guardino, 2000), as well as with various neurological pathologies. Table 38.1 indicates OCD's frequent association with major depression and dysthymic disorder (Rasmussen & Eisen, 1998; Welkowitz et al., 2000), and the relatively weak association with the compulsive obsessive personality (Summerfeldt, Huta, & Swinson, 1998). Furthermore, in addition to the similarities between complex tics and compulsions, there is a strong prevalence of OCD (25%) in Tourette's syndrome (Frankel, Cummings, & Robertson, 1986).

Today, therapeutic approaches include clomipramine, selective serotonin reuptake inhibitors (SSRIs), and psychotherapies, among which cognitive-behavioral therapy (CBT) has a privileged position. Using these approaches, approximately 40–60% of patients show a partial improvement, but a few patients remain completely resistant to these treatments (McDougle, Goodman, & Leckman, 1993).

Within the framework of psychological models explaining OCD (Figure 38.1), there are two conflicting perspectives.

**TABLE 38.1. Comorbidity of OCD with Other Psychiatric disorders According to DSM-IV-TR**

| DSM-IV-TR Axis I | | DSM-IV-TR Axis II | |
|---|---|---|---|
| Depression, dysthymia | 30–50% | Avoidant personality | 30% |
| Phobias | 47% | Dependent personality | 10–20% |
| Social phobia | 18% | Histrionic personality | 5–25% |
| Eating disorders | 17% | Schizotypal personality | 15% |
| Panic disorder | 12–14% | Obsessive–compulsive personality | 6% |
| Alcoholism | 14% | Schizophrenia | 12% |

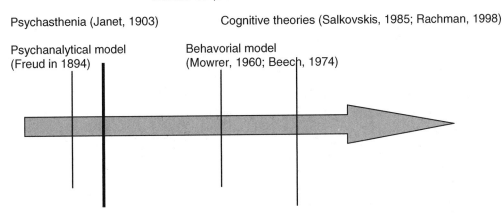

FIGURE 38.1. Chronology of the different psychological models for OCD.

1. The intellectual perspective postulates that the fixed idea is primary, the emotional state simply being a consequence of the ideational disorder. This notion underlies the visionary model of Janet's (1903) psychasthenia, which falls within the more contemporary scope of cognitive theories (Rachman & Shafran, 1998; Salkovskis, 1985). For the theories, the obsessional or intrusive thought, the content of which in general is fairly banal, constitutes an internal stimulus. The negative interpretation of this cognitive stimulus leads to an emotional response of anxiety, secondarily relieved by the realization of the compulsions. The disorder, therefore, resides more in the system of interpretation, directly dependent on the beliefs and cognitive images situated in the long-term memory and established relatively precociously.

2. In opposition, the behavioral model (Beech, 1974; Mowrer, 1960) takes the emotional perspective and considers the anguish to be primary. The rituals are established to reduce the emotional state of anxiety and are maintained by a mechanism of operant conditioning. For the psychoanalytical model, which also defends this perspective, the obsessional symptoms represent the means of neutralizing the effect of the anxiety by specific defense mechanisms.

Among these different models, we have a special interest in psychasthenia, put forward by Janet in 1903. Strongly inspired by Jackson, a contemporary neurologist, Janet defined the psychasthenic state as a deficit of mental energy, innate and/or acquired:

- Leading to a loss of control of voluntary conscious thoughts.
- Favoring the release of thought content (aggressive, sexual, or violent impulses) and stereotypical motor patterns from inferior and subconscious mental structures.
  - Decreasing the expression of appropriate, innovative, or exploratory behavior.
  - Disrupting logical, rational thought and decision-making processes.

It is interesting to compare the psychasthenic model to neuroimaging results. On one hand, they show a hyperfrontality that is believed to reflect the patient's voluntary fight against obsessions. On the other hand, they show a disturbance of the subcortical structures of the caudate nucleus, which is believed to account for the release of stereotyped motor behavior (Cottraux & Gerard, 1998). Obsessions, as well as compulsions, constitute the symptoms of a deficit of cognitive, behavioral, and emotional control usually carried out by the frontal cerebral structures with their subcortical connections.

## NEUROTRANSMITTERS AND OCD

The involvement of the serotoninergic system is suggested by the effectiveness of clomipramine and SSRIs in OCD. There is a positive correlation between the improvement of patients with OCD who are given clomipramine and the decrease of 5-hydroxyindoleacetic acid (5-HIAA) in the cerebrospinal fluid (CSF) and of serotonin (5-HT) in the platelets (Hollander & Cohen, 1996; Thoren, Asberg, & Cronhol, 1980). In addition, administering meta-chlorophenyl-piperazine (m-CPP, a 5-HT antagonist) causes an aggravation of OCD symptoms (Barr, Goodman, Price, McDougle, & Charney, 1992) (for review, see Robert, Benoit, & Caci, Chapter 9, this volume).

However, approximately 40% of patients with OCD do not respond to SSRIs, which leads to the supposition that other neurotransmitters, aside from serotonin, are involved. Several arguments also suggest the implication of dopamine, which is considered to facilitate the activation of behavior and is involved in goal-directed behavior and reward. First, dopaminergic substances (amphetamines, bromocriptine, apomorphine, L-dopa) induce stereotypical movements very similar to those in patients with compulsions (Crum & Anthony, 1993; see review in Riquier, 2003; Stahl, 2002). Second, cocaine increases compulsive symptoms in patients with motor tics in Tourette's syndrome (Daniels, Baker, & Norman, 1996), in which dopaminergic hyperactivity in the putamen and in the caudate nucleus has been demonstrated. OCD is also related to other neurological diseases with dopaminergic dysfunction in the basal ganglia (lethargic encephalitis, Sydenham's chorea, autoimmune attack of the basal ganglia; Swedo, Leonard, & Mittelman, 1997). Finally, in resistant OCD, the relative effectiveness of the association between SSRIs and conventional neuroleptics (McDougle, Barr, Goodman, & Price, 1990), which block the dopaminergic transmission, is an additional argument in favor of the implication of dopamine in the pathophysiology of OCD.

## ANIMAL STUDIES

Repeated, constant, or stereotypical behaviors have been described in several animal species: canine acral lick (large dogs), flank sucking (Dobermans), tail chasing (bull terriers), psychogenic licking alopecia (cats), snout rubbing (pigs), feather picking (parrots), weaving (horses) (Nurnberg, Keith, & Paxton, 1997; Rapoport, Ryland, & Kriete, 1992; Stein, Shoulberg, Helton, & Hollander, 1992). These behaviors, especially the canine behaviors, could correspond to animal equivalents of human stereotypical motor or compulsive disor-ders, and be of interest in evaluating the effect of certain treatments (Nurnberg et al., 1997; Overall, 2000; Rapoport et al., 1992). However, these natural models do not inform us about the pathogenic mechanisms, contrary to the models specifically induced in animals. Compulsive checking behavior has been induced in rats by chronic, subcutaneous injections of quinpirole, a $D_2/D_3$ dopaminergic receptor agonist (Szechtman et al., 2001). Checking behavior of quinpirole-treated rats was partially attenuated by clomipramine and was subject to interruption, which is an attribute characteristic of OCD compulsions. These results suggest that dopaminergic pathways are involved in the pathogenesis of OCD. Recently, stereotypical movements have been induced in monkeys by stereotactic injections of biculline, a γ-aminobutyric acid (GABA) antagonist, in the external globus pallidus (Gpe; Grabli et al., 2004). Anatomical studies have shown that injections were performed in the limbic part of the GPe, a structure receiving inputs from the ventral striatum and projecting to subregions of the subthalamic nucleus, and further toward internal globus pallidus (Gpi) and substantia nigra pars reticulata (SNr) (François et al., 2004). Overall, these data suggest an involvement of the indirect pathway of the corticostriatal–pallidothalamocortical circuits, in the genesis of some behavioral symptoms sharing similar features with symptoms observed in OCD.

## NEUROIMAGING STUDIES

The most interesting data that help us to understand the pathophysiology of OCD come from functional neuroimaging studies (for reviews, see Saxena, Brody, Schwartz, & Baxter, 1998; Saxena & Rauch, 2000) using single-photon emission computed tomography (SPECT), positron emission tomography (PET), or functional magnetic resonance imaging (fMRI). Cerebral function in patients with OCD has been studied in different ways (Table 38.2): (1) in resting conditions, in comparison with normal patients; (2) during symptom provocation, in comparison with resting state; and (3) in resting or symptom provocation studies, comparing the cerebral function before and after treatment.

Most of the resting studies found elevated absolute cerebral blood flow or metabolism in

**TABLE 38.2. Brain Imaging Studies and OCD**

| | | ACC | OFC | DLPFC | Caudate | Put | Thal |
|---|---|---|---|---|---|---|---|
| Resting studies | | | | | | | |
| Baxter et al. (1988) | PET | | ↑ | | ↑ | | |
| Swedo, Schapiro, et al. (1989) | PET | ↑ | ↑ | ↑ | | | |
| Machlin et al. (1991) | SPECT | ↑ | ↑ | | | | |
| Sawle et al. (1991) | PET | | ↑ | ↑ | | | |
| Rubin et al. (1992) | SPECT | | ↑ | ↑ | ↓ | | |
| Lucey et al. (1997) | SPECT | | | ↓ | ↓ | | |
| Lacerda et al. (2003) | SPECT | ↑ | | ↑ | | ↑ | |
| After treatment by SSRI | | | | | | | |
| Benkelfat et al. (1990) | PET | | ↓ | | ↓ | ↓ | |
| Baxter et al. (1992) | PET | ↓ | | | ↓ | ↓ | |
| Swedo et al. (1992) | PET | | ↓ | | | | |
| Saxena et al. (1999) | PET | | ↓ | | ↓ | | |
| Saxena et al. (2002) | PET | | ↓ | | | | ↓ |
| Symptom provocation | | | | | | | |
| Rauch et al. (1994) | PET | ↑ | ↑ | ↑ | ↑ | | |
| McGuire et al. (1994) | PET | | ↑ | | ↑ | | |
| Breiter et al. (1996) | fMRI | ↑ | ↑ | ↑ | ↑ | | |
| Adler et al. (2000) | fMRI | ↑ | ↑ | ↑ | | | |
| Mataix-Cols (2004) | fMRI | ↑ | ↑ | ↑ | | ↑ | ↑ |

*Note.* ACC, anterior cingulate cortex; DLPFC, dorsolateral prefrontal cortex; OFC, orbitofrontal cortex; Put, putamen; Thal, thalamus.

patients with OCD, in comparison with normal controls. In most of the studies, orbitofrontal cortex (OFC) was bilaterally activated (Baxter et al., 1988; Machlin et al., 1991; Nordahl, Benkelfat, Semple, Gross, & King, 1989; Rubin, Villanueva-Meyer, Anath, Trajmar, & Mena, 1992; Sawle, Hymas, Lees, & Frackowiak, 1991; Swedo, Schapiro, et al., 1989). Results are less constant for other brain areas. More often, regional cerebral blood flow (rCBF) or glucose metabolism was increased in the anterior cingulate cortex (ACC; Lacerda et al., 2003; Swedo, Schapiro, et al., 1989) and/or in the dorsolateral prefrontal cortex (DLPFC; Lacerda et al., 2003; Rubin et al., 1992; Sawle et al., 1991; Swedo, Schapiro, et al., 1989). The caudate nucleus was either hyperactivated (Baxter et al., 1988; Molina et al., 1995) or hypoactivated (Lucey et al., 1997; Rubin et al., 1992). Results were more controversial for other areas, including parietal regions, amygdala, hippocampus, thalamus, and basal ganglia, which were inconstantly activated

(Lacerda et al., 2003; Nordahl et al., 1989; Rubin et al., 1992; Swedo, Schapiro, et al., 1989). Finally, concomitant major depression seemed to reduce functional activity in the caudate and thalamus (Saxena et al., 2002). In these resting studies, the cerebral activation might reflect initial abnormalities in brain function, genesis of obsessions and compulsions, mechanisms of resistance to obsessions and compulsions, and/or a chronic cerebral metabolic state resulting from the chronic disease; for example, increased activity in prefrontal cortex has been found in patients resisting obsessions and the urge to ritualize during the PET scanning (Swedo, Schapiro, et al., 1989).

Several PET studies have compared cerebral metabolism in patients with OCD before and after treatment, with slight differences in the findings resulting from various modalities and duration of treatment, scanning conditions, and methods to localize brain regions. In most studies, after successful treatment by SSRIs, regional cerebral metabolism was decreased in the right caudate nucleus (Baxter et al., 1992; Saxena et al., 2002, 2003) or in the left caudate nucleus (Benkelfat et al., 1990), in the bilateral OFC (Benkelfat et al., 1990; Saxena et al., 2002; Swedo et al., 1992), and in the ACC (Baxter et al., 1992). It has been hypothesized that disease response effects are predominant in the caudate nucleus early in treatment (10 weeks) and decrease with time, whereas more conscious cortical mechanisms are involved later (16 weeks to 1 year) through consolidated learning (Baxter et al., 1992). Metabolic changes observed after successful treatment with SSRIs differed in patients with OCD compared to patients with major depression (Saxena et al., 2002, 2003). In patients with concomitant OCD and major depression, glucose metabolic rates were slightly increased in the right caudate nucleus and decreased in ventrolateral prefrontal cortex, after successful treatment. In patients with OCD treated successfully with behavior therapy, glucose metabolism decreased in the right caudate (Baxter et al., 1992) but not significantly in other areas. It is not clear whether the decreased metabolic rate in the caudate nucleus is the cause or the consequence of symptom improvement. Furthermore, glucose metabolism reflects the work of neuronal firing at synaptic nerve terminals, and not the metabolic demands of cell bodies and processes efferent from a structure. Therefore, changes in glucose metabolism in the caudate nucleus might reflect changes in caudate interneurons or changes in structures projecting to caudate nucleus, such as OFC or serotoninergic neurons of the dorsal raphe.

Pretreatment glucose metabolism in PET has been correlated with therapeutic responses. Responders had low pretreatment metabolic rates in the OFC (Rauch et al., 2002; Saxena et al., 1999, 2003; Swedo et al., 1992) and ACC (Swedo et al., 1992), and high pretreatment metabolic rates in the right caudate nucleus (Saxena et al., 2003) and posterior cingulate cortex (Rauch et al., 2002). Preoperative elevated glucose metabolism in the right posterior cingulate cortex was also correlated with significant improvement of OCD symptoms after bilateral, anterior cingulotomy (Rauch et al., 2001). Compared to SSRI treatment, a better response to CBT was correlated with higher pretreatment activation in OFC (Brody et al., 1998).

In symptom provocation studies, patients were exposed successively to individually tailored provocative and innocuous stimuli during fMRI or PET. Symptom provocation induced an increased activation in several regions: bilateral OFC (Adler et al., 2000; Breiter et al., 1996; McGuire et al., 1994; Rauch et al., 1994), right caudate nucleus (Breiter et al., 1996; McGuire et al., 1994; Rauch et al., 1994), ACC (Adler et al., 2000; Breiter et al., 1996; Rauch et al., 1994), DLPFC (Adler et al., 2000; Breiter et al., 1996; Rauch et al., 1994), and inconstantly in the amygdala, hippocampus (Adler et al., 2000; McGuire et al., 1994), anterior temporal cortex (Adler et al., 2000; Breiter et al., 1996), and left posterior cingulate cortex (McGuire et al., 1994). In these studies, functional activation was likely to reflect different processes: genesis of obsessive thoughts, anxiety related to provocative stimuli or modulatory mechanisms, experimental conditions in which compulsions could not be realized. It has been hypothesized that activation in OFC, striatum, and ACC might be related to the urges to ritualize, whereas activation of the hippocampus and posterior cingulate cortex might correspond to the anxiety that accompanied them (McGuire et al., 1994). Higher changes in OCD scores during symptom provocation were correlated with a lower activation in the left OFC, suggesting that the OFC might have an inhibitory role in symptom provocation (Adler et al., 2000; Rauch et al., 1994).

More recently, Mataix-Cols and colleagues (2004) used a symptom provocation paradigm to show that distinct patterns of activation are associated with each symptom dimension of OCD (washing, checking, and hoarding). In response to all types of anxiety, activated regions were the same in patients with OCD as in the controls (Mataix-Cols et al., 2003): visual areas, striatum, thalamus, motor, premotor areas, limbic and paralimbic areas (including ventrolateral prefrontal, OFC, anterior temporal, ACC, insula, hippocampus, amygdala, and DLPFC). During the washing experiment, patients had greater activation than controls in regions involved in the processing of emotions (bilateral OFC, right subgenuate ACC, left medial frontal gyrus, and amygdala) and, specifically, disgust perception (Mataix-Cols et al., 2003; Phillips et al., 1997). During the checking experiment, patients had greater activation than controls predominantly in regions involved in motor and attentional functions: bilateral subthalamic region, right putamen/globus pallidus, right thalamus, DLPFC, and dorsal ACC. During the hoarding experiment, patients had greater activation than controls in left precentral and superior frontal gyrus, and right OFC. Controls showed greater activation than patients in left inferior prefrontal regions during the washing and checking experiments. These regions have also been associated with suppression of negative emotions (Levesque et al., 2003), suggesting that mechanisms regulating anxiety might be more efficient in controls than in patients with OCD.

These findings might explain the discrepancies observed in previous functional imaging studies, in which patients with various symptom dimensions were mixed. They strongly suggest that different symptom dimensions are mediated by relatively distinct components of the associative, limbic, and paralimbic cortico-basal circuits. In regard to these considerations, OCD might be considered as a spectrum of multiple, potentially overlapping syndromes rather than a unitary, nosological entity.

## NEUROSURGICAL PROCEDURES AND DEEP BRAIN STIMULATION

To treat patients with severe, medically intractable OCD, four surgical techniques have been proposed, namely, anterior capsulotomy, cingulotomy, subcaudate tractotomy, and limbic leucotomy, all of which interrupt connections between frontal cortex and subcortical structures (see reviews in Cosgrove & Rauch, 1995; Jenike, 1998).

*Anterior capsulotomy* interrupts fibers in the anterior limb of the internal capsule, connecting the mediodorsal nucleus of the thalamus with the frontal cortex (rostral to areas 6 and 32), and the anterior nuclear group of the thalamus with the cingulate gyrus (areas 23, 24 and 32). The bilateral lesion is produced by either radiofrequency (thermolesion), or stereotactic focal irradiation (radiosurgery). The target is located 5 mm behind the tips of the frontal horn, 20 mm lateral to the midline, at the level of the bicommissural plane. The success of the procedure has been correlated with lesion located on the right side, in the middle of the anterior limb of the internal capsule, at the level of the foramen of Monroe (Lippitz, Mindus, Meyerson, Kihlstrom, & Lindquist, 1999). A prospective study showed that 45% of patients with OCD had an improvement greater than 35% on the Obsessive–

Compulsive subscale of the Comprehensive Psychopathological Rating Scale (CPRS-OC) after capsulotomy (Mindus, Rasmussen, & Lindquist, 1994). The most frequent side effects are transient confusion (86%), nocturnal incontinence lasting several days (27%), and persistent fatigue (32%). The incidence of adverse personality changes after capsulotomy is low and does not increase with time (Mindus, Edman, & Andréevich, 1999).

*Anterior cingulotomy* consists of large thermolesions in the ACC (areas 24 and 32). Bilateral lesions are performed 7 mm lateral to the midline, 20 mm posterior to the tip of the frontal horn, and 1 mm above the roof of the ventricle, sometimes extended superiorly or laterally (Spangler et al., 1996). Initial series reported significant improvement in 57% of patients (Ballantine, Bouckoms, Thomas, & Giriunas, 1987; Jenike et al., 1991). More recently, long-term prospective studies using strict criteria to define treatment response (reduction superior than 35% on the Yale–Brown Obsessive Compulsive Scale [Y-BOCS] and a score of 1 or 2 on Clinical Global Impression—Improvement Scale) showed that 45% of patients were at least partial responders after an average of 32 months (Baer et al., 1995; Dougherty et al., 2002).

*Subcaudate tractotomy* interrupts the connections between the OFC and the ventral striatum by creating a lesion in the substantia innominata under the head of the ventral caudate nucleus. Lesions are placed 7 and 15 mm lateral to the midline in the posteromedial OFC, just inferior to the head of the caudate nucleus. In long-term series, 33–50% of patients were markedly improved (Goktepe, Young, & Bridges, 1975; Hodgkiss, Malizia, Bartlett, & Bridges, 1995). Few side effects have been described: postoperative seizures (2.2%), undesirable personality traits (6.7%), or transient disinhibition.

*Limbic leukotomy* combines bilateral cingulotomy and subcaudate tractotomy, most often in a step-by-step procedure. Patients proposed for a limbic leucotomy were often those for whom bilateral cingulotomy had a poor effect. The aim of this procedure is to disconnect the OFC and the ACC from their reciprocal subcortical striatal and thalamic connections. In a recent study, 42% of patients were considered as responders, but few experienced a marked reduction on Y-BOCS scores (Montoya et al., 2002). Side effects were incontinence (persistent in 14.2% of cases), partial seizures (4.7%), and short-term memory disorder (9.5%).

More recently, *deep brain stimulation* (DBS) has shown efficacy in the treatment of patients with severe and intractable OCD (Aouizerate et al., 2004; Fontaine et al., 2004; Mallet et al., 2002; Nuttin et al., 2003; Sturm et al., 2003). DBS is now widely used to treat Parkinson's disease, the target being either the subthalamic nucleus (STN) or globus pallidus (Deep Brain Stimulation for Parkinson's Disease Study Group, 2001). In these structures, the effect of high-frequency (130 Hz) DBS mimics the effect of a lesion. Considering this action, Nuttin and colleagues (2003) proposed to replace irreversible lesions of anterior cingulotomy by reversible, high-frequency stimulation of the anterior limb of the internal capsule in patients with severe OCD. After the operation, a blinded crossover study of four patients showed that the Y-BOCS score was lower in the stimulator-on condition (mean 19.8) than in the stimulator-off condition (mean 32.3). This stimulation-induced effect was maintained at the mean follow-up of 21 months. Subtraction analysis performed with postoperative and preoperative PET scan showed a marked decrease in frontal glucose metabolism after 3 months of stimulation.

The hypothesis that the effect observed in these patients was due to the stimulation of ventral striatum rather than the stimulation of internal capsule is discussed. First, the best results were obtained in patients in whom the site of stimulation was located more rostrally and medially in the internal capsule, near the ventral striatum. Second, the amplitudes used were very high, leading to an enlargement of the stimulated area. Finally, because high-frequency DBS is supposed to have an inhibitory effect on the cellular bodies of neurons and excitatory effect on fibers (Dostrovsky & Lozano, 2002).

Considering that the ventral caudate nucleus and nucleus accumbens are supposed to be hyperactive in OCD, high-frequency DBS of these structures has been performed in a few patients (Aouizerate et al., 2004; Sturm et al., 2003), leading to improvement of both anxiety and OCD symptoms. In a patient with OCD and major depression, DBS of the ventral caudate nucleus markedly improved symptoms of depression and anxiety until their remission, which was achieved 6 months after surgery (Aouizerate et al., 2004). However, the improvement of OCD symptoms was delayed and partial (Y-BOCS score was 30 before surgery and < 16 after 12 months of DBS). The STN is another potential target to be considered for DBS in OCD. Improvement of obsessive–compulsive personality traits has been observed after STN stimulation in patients with Parkinson's disease who did not have OCD (Alegret et al., 2001). More recently dramatic and early reduction of OCD symptoms has been shown in patients who had both Parkinson's disease and OCD (Fontaine et al., 2004; Mallet et al., 2002). The STN and other striatal structures are divided into distinct but partially overlapping sensorimotor, associative, and limbic territories (Karachi et al., 2002). In several cases, the effect on OCD symptoms was obtained by stimulation of the same STN part that provoked the best improvement of parkinsonian motor signs. Considering the pathophysiology of OCD and the hypothesis of an imbalance between direct and indirect (which include the STN) pathways of the corticostriatal–pallidothalamic cortical loops, improvement of OCD symptoms could be due to the inhibition of the limbic portion of STN or the excitation of excitatory efferent fibers emerging from the STN to the GPi.

## FRONTAL–SUBCORTICAL CIRCUITS AND PATHOPHYSIOLOGICAL MODELS

Alexander described a series of parallel and functionally segregated circuits connecting the frontal cortex, basal ganglia, and thalamus (Alexander, DeLong, & Strick, 1986). Neuroimaging, lesion, and stimulation studies showed that neuroanatomical structures involved in the pathophysiology of OCD belong to three of these circuits, originating, respectively, in the OFC, the ACC, and the DLPFC (Figure 38.2). OCD could result from the dysfunction of one or more of these circuits (Cummings, 1993). Each of these circuits originates in the frontal cortex, projects to the striatum (ventromedial caudate, ventral striatum–nucleus accumbens, dorsolateral caudate, respectively), from striatum to globus pallidus/substantia nigra, from GPi/SNr to thalamus (ventral anterior and mediodorsal nuclei), and finally back to frontal cortex (Alexander et al., 1986). The orbitofrontal circuit mediates empathic, civil, and socially appropriate behavior; the anterior cingulate circuit mediates motivated behavior;

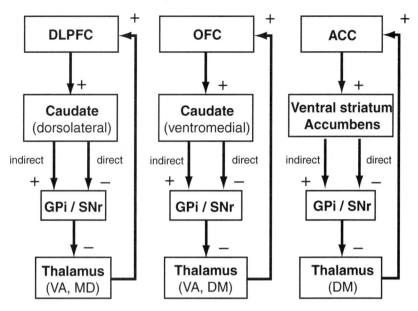

FIGURE 38.2. Parallel frontal–striatal pallidothalamic cortical circuits supposed to be involved in the pathophysiology of OCD, originating respectively in the dorsolateral prefrontal cortex (DLPFC), orbitofrontal cortex (OFC), and anterior cingulate cortex (ACC). Gpi, globus pallidus pars internalis; SNr, substantia nigra pars reticulata; VA, ventral anterior nuclei of the thalamus; MD, dorsomedial nucleus of the thalamus.

the dorsolateral circuit subserves executive functions, including ability to organize a behavioral response to solve a complex problem, independence from environmental contingencies, and shifting to another task (Chow & Cummings, 1999; Cummings, 1993).

Each of these circuits includes two pathways: a direct pathway linking directly the striatum to the GPi/SNr complex, and an indirect pathway projecting to the GPi/SNr complex through GPe and STN (Figure 38.3). These two pathways have opposing effects: Activation of the direct pathway tends to disinhibit the thalamic output target; activation of the indirect pathway tends to inhibit it (Alexander & Crutcher, 1990).

Moreover, the striatum is organized into two different specialized patchy zones: striosomes and matrisomes. The striosomes receive inputs from the limbic system, send projections to the dopaminergic neurons of the SN pars compacta (SNc), and probably play a role in the emotional modulation of information processed in the corticostriatal loops and reward processes (Graybiel & Rauch, 2000). The matrisomes receive inputs from sensorimotor and associative areas and project to output nuclei of the basal ganglia (Graybiel, Aosaki, Flaherty, & Kimura, 1994).

These circuits are modulated by dopaminergic inputs from the SNc and ventral tegmental area, which project to the striatum and frontal–cortical areas. Dopaminergic neurons are involved in the processes of motivation and learning (Bar-Gad & Bergman, 2001). They respond to differences between the prediction of reward and the real, experienced reward by changing their firing rate. The tonically active neurons (TANs) of the striatum, which probably are cholinergic interneurons, show similar responses for predicted and unpredicted rewards. The serotoninergic pathways, originating from the brainstem raphe nuclei, and projecting widely to the limbic structure, including OFC and cingulate cortex, are considered to inhibit these structures.

Several pathophysiological models of OCD, involving a dysfunction of these frontostriatal-pallidothalamic cortical circuits have been proposed (for review, see Aouizerate et al., 2004).

For Modell, Mountz, Curtis, and Greden (1989), OCD symptoms are the consequence of the development of aberrant positive feedback loop in reciprocally excitatory OFC–basal

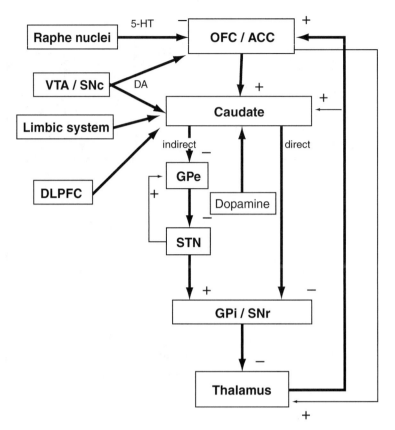

FIGURE 38.3. Schematic synthetic diagram of the ciruits involved in the pathogenesis of OCD and their modulating influences. DLPFC, dorsolateral prefrontal cortex; OFC, orbitofrontal cortex; ACC, anterior cingulate cortex; Gpi, globus pallidus pars internalis; Gpe, globus pallidus pars externalis; SNr, substantia nigra pars reticulata; SNc: substantia nigra pars compacta; VTA, ventral tegmental area; STN, subthalamic nucleus; 5-HT, serotonin; DA, dopamine.

ganglia–thalamic connections associated with dysfunction of modulating influence of the limbic striatopallidal input. However, although many arguments exist in favor of an OFC-circuit hyperactivity, there is no strong argument in favor of either the inhibiting role of the limbic loop or its hypoactivity. Mink (1996) proposed a model for Tourette's syndrome that may be extrapolated to OCD, assuming that when actions, movements, or behaviors are generated by cortical mechanisms, the indirect pathways act broadly to inhibit competing motor–behavioral programs. Simultaneously, the direct pathway focally removes the inhibition from the desired action–movement–behavior. In Tourette's syndrome, tics could result from abnormal and uncontrolled overfunctioning of a group of striatal neurons (matrisomes) belonging to the direct pathway and involved in

the generation of a peculiar motor program (Mink, 2001) that could not be inhibited by the indirect pathway during the realization of the desired motor program. Similarly, OCD could result from the uncontrolled overfunctioning of one of these matrisomes involved in the generation of a peculiar behavioral program or cognitive event.

The Schwartz model is based on the hypothesis of an overfunctioning error detection system, in which OFC, ACC, and striatum are involved (Schwartz, 1998, 1999). This system could be activated repeatedly and inappropriately in response to specific situations, leading to the feeling that "something is wrong," and resulting in the emergence of intrusive and pathological thoughts leading to recurrent compulsive behaviors. Considering this model, Aouizerate and colleagues (2004) proposed that recurrent compulsive behaviors might be considered as excessive expression of reward delivery processes aiming but failing to reduce the internal tension generated by these intrusive thoughts. However, it is not clear whether the overactivity of the dopaminergic–mesocorticolimbic system would be a reinforcing mechanism of such processes or the cause of the obsessions, reflecting excessive computation about predictability of an event.

In the Baxter model, OCD results from an imbalance between direct and indirect striatopallidal pathways (Baxter, 1999; Saxena et al., 1998; Saxena & Rauch, 2000) in OFC and ACC circuits. This model is based on the fact that one of the frontal–subcortical circuit functions is the execution of "prepackaged," complex, sequence-critical response behaviors (i.e., "macros") that, to be adaptive, must be executed quickly in response to specific stimuli. On the one hand, normal activity along the direct pathway would tend to focus behavior toward the execution of the appropriate "macros" during an appropriate amount of time. On the other hand, activation of the indirect pathway could allow suppression of the direct pathway-driven behaviors when switching to another behavior is needed (Saxena & Rauch, 2000). In this model, OCD symptoms could correspond to repetition of stereotyped behaviors executed in loop, without the possibility to switch to others.

For Graybiel and Rauch (2000), OCD results from the dysfunction of the parallel functioning of the corticobasal ganglia loops and the corticothalamic cortical loops. Under normal conditions, both systems acts in parallel during planning, selection, and realization of motor and behavioral programs, with the corticothalamic circuit supporting conscious information processing, and the cortical–basal ganglia circuit supporting automatic processing functions. If corticobasal pathways become abnormal, as supposed in OCD, information normally processed automatically could intrude in the conscious domain as obsessions, and behavioral selection could become narrowed to stereotyped behavior as compulsions.

Progress in the knowledge of frontal cortex and basal ganglia functioning provided cues to understanding the pathophysiology of OCD. However, none of these models is able to explain all the different aspects of OCD pathophysiology. Numerous questions remain unsolved concerning, in particular, the mechanisms and the location of the initial dysfunction within the cortical–subcortical loops, and the unique or multiple character of this mechanism according to the symptoms dimensions.

## REFERENCES

Adler, C., McDonough-Ryan, P., Sax, K., Holland, S., Arndt, S., & Strakowski, S. (2000). fMRI of neuronal activation with symptom provocation in unmedicated patients with obsessive compulsive disorder. *Journal of Psychiatric Research, 34,* 317–324.

Alegret, M., Junqué, C., Valldeoriola, F., Vendrell, P., Marti, M., & Tolosa, E. (2001). Obsessive-compulsive symptoms in Parkinson's disease. *Journal of Neurology, Neurosurgery, and Psychiatry, 70,* 394–396.

Alexander, G., DeLong, M., & Strick, P. (1986). Parallel organization of functionally segregated circuits linking basal ganglia and cortex. *Annals Review of Neuroscience, 9,* 357–381.

Alexander, G., & Crutcher, M. (1990). Functional architecture of basal ganglia circuits: neural substrates of parallel processing. *Trends in Neurosciences, 13,* 266–271.

American Psychiatric Association. (2000). *Diagnostic and statistical manual of mental disorders* (4th ed., text rev.). Washington, DC: Author.

Anderson, K., Louis, E., Stern, Y., & Marder, K. (2001). Cognitive correlates of obsessive and compulsive symptoms in Huntington's disease. *American Journal of Psychiatry, 158,* 799–801.

Aouizerate, B., Cuny, E., Martin-Guehl, C., Guehl, D., Amieva, H., Benazzouz, A., et al. (2004). Deep brain stimulation of the ventral caudate nucleus in the treatment of obsessive–compulsive disorder and major depression. *Journal of Neurosurgery, 101,* 682–686.

Aouizerate, B., Guehl, D., Cuny, E., Rougier, A., Bioulac, B., Tignol, J., et al. (2004). Pathophysiology of obsessive–compulsive disorder: A necessary link between phenomenology, neuropsychology, imagery and physiology. *Progress in Neurobiology, 72,* 195–221.

Baer, L., Rauch, S., Ballantine, H. J., Martuza, R., Cosgrove, G., Cassem, E., et al. (1995). Cingulotomy for intractable obsessive–compulsive disorder. *Archives of General Psychiatry, 52,* 384–392.

Ballantine, H. J., Bouckoms, A., Thomas, E., & Giriunas, I. (1987). Treatment of psychiatric illness by stereotactic cingulotomy. *Biological Psychiatry, 22,* 807–819.

Bar-Gad, I., & Bergman, H. (2001). Stepping out of the box: Information processing in the neural network of the basal ganglia. *Current Opinion in Neurobiology, 11,* 689–695.

Barr, L. C., Goodman, W. K., Price, L. H., McDougle, C. J., & Charney, D. S. (1992). The serotonin hypothesis of obsessive–compulsive disorder: Implications of pharmacological challenge studies. *Journal of Clinical Psychiatry, 53,* 17–28.

Baxter, L., Schwartz, J., Mazziotta, J., Phelps, M., Pahl, J., Guze, B., & Fairbanks, L. (1988). Cerebral glucose metabolic rates in nondepressed patients with obsessive–compulsive disorder. *American Journal of Psychiatry, 145,* 1560–1563.

Baxter, L. (1999). Functional imaging of brain systems mediating obsessive–compulsive disorder: Clinical studies. In D. Charney, E. Nestler, & B. Bunney (Eds.), *Neurobiology of mental illness* (pp. 534–547). New York: Oxford University Press.

Baxter, L. J., Schwartz, J., Bergman, K., Szuba, M., Guze, B., Mazziotta, J., et al. (1992). Caudate glucose metabolic rate changes with both drug and behavior therapy for obsessive–compulsive disorder. *Archives of General Psychiatry, 49,* 681–689.

Bebbington, P. (1998). Epidemiology of obsessive compulsive disorder. *British Journal of Psychiatry, 173,* 2–6.

Beech, H. (1974). *Obsessional states.* London: Methuen.

Benkelfat, C., Nordahl, T., Semple, W., King, A., Murphy, D., & Cohen, R. (1990). Local cerebral glucose metabolic rates in obsessive–compulsive disorder: Patient treated with clomipramine. *Archives of General Psychiatry, 47,* 840–848.

Breiter, H., Rauch, S., Kwong, K., Baker, J., Weisskoff, R., Kennedy, D., et al. (1996). Functional magnetic resonance imaging of symptom provocation in obsessive–compulsive disorder. *Archives of General Psychiatry, 53,* 595–606.

Brody, A., Saxena, S., Schwartz, J., Stoessel, P., Maidment, K., Phelps, M., et al. (1998). FDG-PET predictors of response to behavioral therapy and pharmacotherapy in obsessive compulsive disorder. *Psychiatry Research, 84,* 1–6.

Chow, T. W., & Cummings, J. (1993). Frontal–subcortical circuits. In B. L. Miller & J. L. Cummings (Eds.), *The human frontal lobes* (pp. 3–26). New York: Guilford Press.

Cosgrove, G., & Rauch, S. (1995). Psychosurgery. *Neurosurgery Clinics of North America, 6,* 167–176.

Cottraux, J., & Gerard, D. (1997). Neuroimaging and neuroanatomical issues in obsessive–compulsive disorder: Toward an integrative model—perceived impulsivity. In R. P. Swinson, M. M. Antony, S. Rachman, & M. S. (Eds.), *Obsessive–compulsive disorder: Theory, research, and treatment* (pp. 154–180). New York: Guilford Press.

Crum, R. M., & Anthony, J. C. (1993). Cocaine use and other risk factors for obsessive–compulsive disorder: A prospective study with data from ECA surveys. *Drug and Alcohol Dependence, 31,* 281–295.

Cummings, J. (1993). Frontal–subcortical circuits and human behavior. *Archives of Neurology, 50,* 873–880.

Daniels, J., Baker, D., & Norman, A. (1996). Cocaine-induced tics in untreated Tourette's syndrome. *American Journal of Psychiatry, 153*(7), 965.

Deep Brain Stimulation for Parkinson's Disease Study Group. (2001). Deep-brain stimulation of the subthalamic nucleus or the pars interna of the globus pallidus in Parkinson's disease. *New England Journal of Medicine, 345,* 956–964.

Dostrovsky, J., & Lozano, A. (2002). Mechanisms of deep brain stimulation. *Movement Disorders, 17,* S63–S68.

Dougherty, D., Baer, L., Cosgrove, G., Cassem, E., Price, B., Nierenberg, A., et al. (2002). Prospective long-term follow-up of 44 patients who received cingulotomy for treatment refractory obsessive–compulsive disorder. *American Journal of Psychiatry, 159,* 269–275.

Etcharry-Bouyx, F., & Dubas, F. (2000). Obsessive–compulsive disorders in association with focal brain lesions. In J. Bogouslavsky & J. L. Cummings (Eds.), *Behavior and mood disorder in focal brain lesions* (pp. 304–326). Cambridge, UK: Cambridge University Press.

Fontaine, D., Mattei, V., Borg, M., vonLangsdorff, D., Magnie, M., Chanalet, C., et al. (2004). Effect of subthalamic nucleus stimulation on obsessive–compulsive disorder in a patient with Parkinsons disease. *Journal of Neurosurgery, 100,* 1084–1086.

François, C., Grabli, D., McCairn, K., Jan, C., Karachi, C., Hirsch, E. C., et al. (2004). Behavioural disorders induced by external globus pallidus dysfunction in primates: II. Anatomical study. *Brain, 127,* 2055–2070.

Frankel, M., Cummings, J., & Robertson, M. (1986). Obsessions and compulsions in Gilles de la Tourette's syndrome. *Neurology, 36,* 378–382.

Goktepe, E., Young, L., & Bridges, P. (1975). A further review of the results of stereotactic subcaudate tractotomy. *British Journal of Psychiatry, 126,* 270–280.

Grabli, D., McCairn, K., Hirsch, E., Agid, Y., Féger, J., François, C., et al. (2004). Behavioural disorders induced by external globus pallidus dysfunction in primates: I. Behavioral study. *Brain, 127,* 2037–2054.

Graybiel, A., Aosaki, T., Flaherty, A., & Kimura, M. (1994). The basal ganglia and adaptive motor control. *Science, 265,* 1826–1831.

Graybiel, A., & Rauch, S. (2000). Toward a neurobiology of obsessive–compulsive disorder. *Neuron, 28,* 343–347.

Hantouche, E., Bourgeois, M., Bouhassira, M., & Lancrenon, S. (1996). Aspects cliniques des troubles obsessionnels compulsifs : Résultats de la phase 2 d'une large enquête française [Clinical aspects of OCD: Results of a large phase 2 French survey]. *L'Encéphale, 22,* 225–263.

Hodgkiss, A., Malizia, A., Bartlett, J., & Bridges, P. (1995). Outcome after the psychosurgical operation of stereotactic subcaudate tractotomy, 1979–1991. *Journal of Neuropsychiatry and Clinical Neurosciences, 7,* 230–234.

Hollander, E. (1997). Obsessive compulsive disorder: The hidden epidemic. *Journal of Clinical Psychiatry, 58,* 3–6.

Hollander, M., & Cohen, L. (1996). Psychobiology and psychopharmacology of compulsive spectrum disorders. In J. M. Oldham, E. Hollander, & A. E. Skodol (Eds.), *Impulsivity and compulsivity* (pp. 143–161). Washington, DC: American Psychiatric Publishing.

Janet, P. (1903). *Les obsessions et la psychasthénie*. Paris: Alcan.

Jenike, M., Baer, L., Ballantine, H. J., Martuza, R., Tynes, S., Giriunas, I., et al. (1991). Cingulotomy for refractory obsessive–compulsive disorder. *Archives of General Psychiatry, 48*, 548–555.

Jenike, M. (1998). Neurosurgical treatment of obsessive–compulsive disorder. *British Journal of Psychiatry, 173*, 79–90.

Karachi, C., François, C., Parrain, K., Bardinet, E., Tandé, D., Hirsch, E., et al. (2002). Three-dimensional cartography of functional territories of the human striatopallidal complex by using calbindin immunoreactivity. *Journal of Comparative Neurology, 450*, 122–134.

Karno, M., Golding, J., Sorenson, S., & Burnam, M. (1988). The epidemiology of obsessive compulsive disorder in five US communities. *Archives of General Psychiatry, 45*, 1094–1099.

Lacerda, A., Dalgalarrondo, P., Caetano, D., Camargo, E., Etchebehere, E., & Soares, J. (2003). Elevated thalamic and prefrontal regional cerebral blood flow in obsessive–compulsive disorder: A SPECT study. *Psychiatry Research, 123*, 125–134.

Levesque, J., Eugene, F., Joanette, Y., Paquette, V., Mensour, B., Beaudoin, G., et al. (2003). Neural circuitry underlying voluntary suppression of sadness. *Biological Psychiatry, 53*, 502–510.

Lippitz, B., Mindus, P., Meyerson, B., Kihlstrom, L., & Lindquist, C. (1999). Lesion topography and outcome after thermocapsulotomy or gamma knife capsulotomy for obsessive–compulsive disorder: Relevance of the right hemisphere. *Neurosurgery, 44*, 452–460.

Lopez, O., Berthier, M., Beacker, J., & Boller, F. (1997). Creutzfeldt–Jakob disease with features of obsessive–compulsive disorder and anorexia nervosa: The role of the cortical–subcortical systems. *Neuropsychiatry, Neuropsychology, and Behavioral Neurology, 10*, 120–124.

Lucey, J., Costa, C., Adshead, G., Deahl, M., Busatto, G., Gacinovic, S., et al. (1997). Brain blood flow in anxiety disorders: OCD, panic disorder with agoraphobia, and post-traumatic stress disorder on 99mTcHMPAO single photon emission tomography (SPECT). *British Journal of Psychiatry, 171*, 346–350.

Machlin, S., Harris, G., Pearlson, G., Hoehn-Saric, R., Jeffery, P., & Camargo, E. (1991). Elevated medial frontal cerebral blood flow in obsessive–compulsive disorder: A SPECT study. *American Journal of Psychiatry, 148*, 1240–1242.

Mallet, L., Mesnage, V., Houeto, J., Pelissolo, A., Yelnik, J., Behar, C., et al. (2002). Compulsions, Par-

kinson's disease, and stimulation. *Lancet, 360*, 1302–1304.

Mataix-Cols, D., Cullen, S., Lange, K., Zelaya, F., Andrew, C., Amaro, E., et al. (2003). Neural correlates of anxiety associated with obsessive–compulsive symptom dimensions in normal volunteers. *Biological Psychiatry, 53*, 482–493.

Mataix-Cols, D., Wooderson, W., Lawrence, N., Brammer, M., Speckens, A., & Phillips, M. (2004). Distinct neural correlates of washing, checking, and hoarding symptom dimensions in obsessive–compulsive disorder. *Archives of General Psychiatry, 61*, 564–576.

McDougle, C., Barr, L., Goodman, W., & Price, L. (1990). Neuroleptics addition in fluvoxamine-refractory obsessive–compulsive disorder. *American Journal of Psychiatry, 147*, 652–654.

McDougle, C., Goodman, W., & Leckman, J. (1993). Limited therapeutic effect of addition of buspirone in fluvoxamine-refractory obsessive–compulsive disorder. *American Journal of Psychiatry, 150*, 647–649.

McGuire, P., Bench, C., Frith, C., Marks, I., Frackowiak, R., & Dolan, R. (1994). Functional anatomy of obsessive–compulsive phenomena. *British Journal of Psychiatry, 164*, 459–468.

Mindus, P., Rasmussen, S., & Lindquist, C. (1994). Neurosurgical treatment for refractory obsessive–compulsive disorder: Implications for understanding frontal lobe function. *Journal of Neuropsychiatry and Clinical Neurosciences, 6*, 467–477.

Mindus, P., Edman, G., & Andréevich, S. (1999). A prospective, long term study of personality traits in patients with intractable obsessional illness treated by capsulotomy. *Acta Psychiatrica Scandinavica, 99*, 40–50.

Mink, J. (1996). The basal ganglia: Focused selection and inhibition of competing motor programs. *Progress in Neurobiology, 50*, 381–425.

Mink, J. (2001). Basal ganglia dysfunction in Tourette's syndrome: A new hypothesis. *Pediatric Neurology, 25*, 190–198.

Modell, J., Mountz, J., Curtis, G., & Greden, J. (1989). Neurophysiologic dysfunction in basal ganglia/limbic striatal and thalamo-cortical circuits as a pathogenetic mechanism of obsessive–compulsive disorder. *Journal of Neuropsychiatry and Clinical Neurosciences, 1*, 27–36.

Molina, V., Montz, R., Martin-Loeches, M., Jimenez-Vicioso, A., Carreras, J., & Rubia, F. (1995). Drug therapy and cerebral perfusion in obsessive–compulsive disorder. *Journal of Nuclear Medicine, 36*, 2234–2238.

Montoya, A., Weiss, A., Price, B., Cassem, E., Dougherty, D., Nierenberg, A., et al. (2002). MRI-guided stereotactic limbic leucotomy for treatment of intractable psychiatric disease. *Neurosurgery, 50*, 1043–1052.

Mowrer, O. (1960). *Learning theory and behavior*. New York: Wiley.

Nestadt, G., Samuels, J., & Romanoski, A. (1994). Obsessions and compulsions in the community. *Acta Psychiatrica Scandinavica, 89,* 219–224.

Nordahl, T., Benkelfat, C., Semple, W., Gross, M., King, A., & Cohen, R. M. (1989). Cerebral glucose metabolic rates in obsessive compulsive disorder. *Neuropsychopharmacology, 2,* 23–28.

Nurnberg, H., Keith, S., & Paxton, D. (1997). Considerations of the relevance of ethological animal models for human repetitive behavioral spectrum disorders. *Biological Psychiatry, 41,* 226—229.

Nuttin, B., Gabriels, L., Cosyns, P., Meyerson, B., Andréevich, S., Sunaert, S., et al. (2003). Long-term electrical capsular stimulation in patients with obsessive–compulsive disorder. *Neurosurgery, 52,* 1263–1274.

Overall, K. (2000). Natural models of human psychiatric conditions: Assessment of mechanisms and validity. *Progress in Neuro-Psychopharmacology and Biological Psychiatry, 24,* 727–776.

Phillips, M., Young, A., Senior, C., Brammer, M., Andrew, C., Calder, A., et al. (1997). A specific neural substrate for perception of facial expressions of disgust. *Nature, 389,* 495–498.

Rachman, S., & Shafran, R. (1998). Cognitive and behavioral features of obsessive–compulsive disorder. In R. P. Swinson, M. M. Antony, S. J. Rachman, & M. A. Richter (Eds.), *Obsessive–compulsive disorder: Theory, research and treatment* (pp. 51–78). New York: Guilford Press.

Rapoport, J., Ryland, D., & Kriete, M. (1992). Drug treatment of canine acral lick: An animal model of obsessive compulsive disorder. *Archives of General Psychiatry, 49,* 517–521.

Rasmussen, S., & Eisen, J. (1998). The epidemiology and clinical features of obsessive compulsive disorder. In M. A. Jenike, L. Baer, & W. E. Minichiello (Eds.), *Obsessive compulsive disorders: Practical management* (pp. 11–43). St. Louis, MO: Mosby.

Rauch, S., Jenike, M., Alpert, N., Baer, L., Breiter, H., Savage, C., et al. (1994). Regional cerebral blood flow measured during symptom provocation in obsessive–compulsive disorder using $^{15}$O-labeled $CO_2$ and positron emission tomography. *Archives of General Psychiatry, 51,* 62–70.

Rauch, S., Dougherty, D., Cosgrove, G., Cassem, E., Alpert, N., Price, B., et al. (2001). Cerebral metabolic correlates as potential predictors of response to anterior cingulotomy for obsessive compulsive disorder. *Biological Psychiatry, 50,* 659–667.

Rauch, S., Shin, L., Dougherty, D., Alpert, N., Fischman, A., & Jenike, M. (2002). Predictors of fluvoxamine response in contamination-related obsessive compulsive disorder: A PET symptom provocation study. *Neuropsychopharmacology, 27,* 782–791.

Riquier, F. (2003). Traitements pharmacologiques [Pharmacological treatments]. In Masson (Ed.), *Les troubles obsessionnels compulsifs* [Obsessive-compulsive disorder] (pp. 103–137). Paris: Bouvard.

Rubin, R., Villanueva-Meyer, J., Ananth, J., Trajmar, P.,

& Mena, I. (1992). Regional xenon 133 cerebral blood flow and cerebral Tc99m HMPAO uptake in unmedicated patients with obsessive–compulsive disorder and matched normal control subjects. *Archives of General Psychiatry, 49,* 695–702.

Salkovskis, P. (1985). Obsessional–compulsive problem: A cognitive behavioral analysis. *Behaviour Research and Therapy, 23,* 571–583.

Sawle, G., Hymas, N., Lees, A., & Frackowiak, R. (1991). Obsessional slowness: Functional studies with positron emission tomography. *Brain, 114,* 2191–2202.

Saxena, S., Brody, A., Schwartz, J., & Baxter, L. (1998). Neuroimaging and frontal–subcortical circuitry in obsessive–compulsive disorder. *British Journal of Psychiatry, 173,* 26–37.

Saxena, S., Brody, A., Colgan, M., Maidment, K., Dunkin, J., Alborzian, S., et al. (1999). Localized orbitofrontal and subcortical metabolic changes and predictors of response to paroxetine treatment of obsessive–compulsive disorder. *Neuropsychopharmacology, 21,* 683–693.

Saxena, S., & Rauch, S. (2000). Functional neuroimaging and the neuroanatomy of obsessive–compulsive disorder. *psychiatric Clinics of North America, 23,* 563–586.

Saxena, S., Brody, A., Ho, M., Alborzian, S., Maidment, K., Zohrabi, N., et al. (2002). Differential cerebral metabolic changes with paroxetine treatment of obsessive–compulsive disorder vs. major depression. *Archives of General Psychiatry, 59,* 250–261.

Saxena, S., Brody, A., Ho, M., Zohrabi, N., Maidment, K., & Baxter, L. J. (2003). Differential brain metabolic predictors of response to paroxetine in obsessive–compulsive disorder versus major depression. *American Journal of Psychiatry, 160,* 522–532.

Schwartz, J. (1998). Neuroanatomical aspects of cognitive-behavioural therapy response in obsessive–compulsive disorder: An evolving perspective on brain and behavior. *British Journal of Psychiatry, 35*(Suppl. 35), 38–44.

Skoog, G., & Skoog, I. (1999). A 40-year follow-up of patients with obsessive compulsive disorder. *Archives of General Psychiatry, 56,* 121–127.

Spangler, W., Cosgrove, G., Ballantine, H. J., Cassem, S., Rauch, S., Nierenberg, A., et al. (1996). MRI-guided stereotactic cingulotomy for intractable psychiatric disease. *Neurosurgery, 38,* 1071–1078.

Stahl, S. (2002). Traitements médicamenteux du trouble obsesionnel-compulsif, du trouble panique et des troubles phobiques. In Flammarion-Medecine-Sciences (Ed.), *Psychopharmacologie essentielle* (p. 601). Paris.

Stein, D., Shoulberg, N., Helton, K., & Hollander, E. (1992). The neuroethological approach to obsessive–compulsive disorder. *Comprehensive Psychiatry, 33,* 274–281.

Sturm, V., Lenartz, D., Koulousakis, A., Treuer, H., Herholz, K., Klein, J., et al. (2003). The nucleus accumbens: A target for deep brain stimulation in obsessive–compulsive and anxiety-disorders. *Journal of Chemical Neuroanatomy, 26,* 293–299.

Summerfeldt, L., Huta, V., & Swinson, R. (1998). Personality and obsessive compulsive disorder. In R. P. Swinson, M. M. Antony, S. Rachman, & M. A. Ritcher (Eds.), *Obsessive–compulsive disorder: Theory, research and treatment* (pp. 79–119). New York: Guilford Press.

Swedo, S., Rapoport, J., & Cheslow, D. (1989). High prevalence of obsessive–compulsive symptoms in patients with Syndenham's chorea. *American Journal of Psychiatry, 146,* 246–249.

Swedo, S., Schapiro, M., Grady, C., Cheslow, D., Leonard, H., Kumar, A., et al. (1989). Cerebral glucose metabolism in childhood onset obsessive–compulsive disorder. *Archives of General Psychiatry, 46,* 518–523.

Swedo, S., Pietrini, P., Leonard, H., Schapiro, M., Rettew, D., Goldberger, E., et al. (1992). Cerebral glucose metabolism in childhood-onset obsessive–compulsive disorder: Revisualization during pharmacotherapy. *Archives of General Psychiatry, 49,* 690–694.

Swedo, S., Leonard, H., & Mittelman, B. (1997). Identification of children with pediatric autoimmune neuropsychiatric disorders associated with streptococcal infections by a marker associated with rheumatic fever. *American Journal of Psychiatry, 154*(1), 110–112.

Szechtman, H., Eckert, M., Boersma, J., Bonura, C., McClelland, J., Culver, K., et al. (2001). Compulsive checking behavior of quipirole-sensitized rats as an animal model of obsessive–compulsive disorder. *BMC Neuroscience, 2,* 4.

Thoren, P., Asberg, M., & Cronhol, B. (1980). Clomipramine treatment of obsessive compulsive disorder: II. Biochemical aspects. *Archives of General Psychiatry, 37,* 1289–1294.

Weiss, A., & Jenike, M. (2000). Late-onset obsessive compulsive disorder: A case series. *Journal of Neuropsychiatry and Clinical Neurosciences, 12,* 265–268.

Welkowitz, L., Struening, E., Pittman, J., & Guardino, M. (2000). Obsessive compulsive disorder and comorbid anxiety problems in a national anxiety screening sample. *Journal of Anxiety Disorders, 14,* 471–482.

World Heath Organization. (1993). *CIM-10/ICD-10: Troubles mentaux et troubles du comportement: Descriptions cliniques et directives pour le diagnostic (V)* [ICD-10. Classification of mental behavioral disorders. Clinical description and diagnostic guidelines]. Paris: Masson.

# CHAPTER 39

# Depression and the Frontal Lobes

*Ira M. Lesser*
*Julia A. Chung*

Sadness and depression are perhaps the most common emotions experienced by people. As a brief emotional state, sadness that may occur in response to some external event is typically time-limited. However, a full depressive mood syndrome (i.e., major depressive episode) can be long-lasting, accompanied by significant functional disability, and associated with medical morbidity and mortality. Major depression is a common disorder, with a lifetime prevalence of about 16% (Kessler, Berglund, Demier, Jin, & Walters, 2005). According to a World Health Organization (1996) study, depression causes more disability worldwide than any other illness except cardiovascular disease. In addition to the obvious psychological consequences, the economic impact of depression to individuals and society is enormous. In the year 2000, the economic burden in the United States was estimated to be $83.1 billion (Greenberg et al., 2003). Despite a vast amount of research into depressive illness, there is as yet no clear-cut etiology from a biological or neuropsychiatric perspective to explain the onset or recurrent nature of the disorder.

To diagnose an episode of major depressive disorder (MDD), one must meet the following criteria (DSM-IV-TR; American Psychiatric Association, 2000): depressed mood most of the time and most days and/or diminished interest or pleasure in most activities, plus at least four of the following symptoms occurring most of the time for a 2-week period: significant weight change; sleep disturbance; psychomotor agita-

tion or retardation; fatigue or loss of energy; feelings of worthlessness or inappropriate guilt; trouble thinking or concentrating, or having indecisiveness; and recurrent thoughts of death or suicidal ideation. This symptom picture must cause clinically significant distress or impairment in occupational, social, or other important functions, and must not be solely the direct effect of a known medical illness or substance abuse.

It is well known that applying DSM-IV criteria for depression to medically ill patients may not accurately identify all cases. Some of the symptoms just noted may be part and parcel of the underlying medical illness and/or key symptoms of depression. Whether to "count" them as part of the depressive syndrome, or to think of them as etiologically related to the illness and not part of the depression, has been a matter of debate. Furthermore, reports have differed on factors such as the type of clinical interviews and the scales used to measure depression, on the cutoffs used for these scales to indicate depression in medically ill patients, and on the timing of the assessment in relation to the medical event(s). Questions also have been raised about the validity of using standard interviews and rating scales in medically ill patients, without clear evidence of validity in this population. To complicate matters further, some investigators have reported on major depression, minor depression, or depressive symptoms, without necessarily defining clearly the distinctions between them.

Depression is undoubtedly a heterogeneous condition, with symptoms encompassing abnormalities of mood (feelings of hopelessness, worthlessness, guilt, thoughts of death, suicidal ideation, and dysphoria), motor function (agitation, restlessness, and slowing), cognitive function (ruminations, impairments in attention and short-term memory, and decreased psychomotor speed), and somatic functions (disturbances in sleep, appetite, libido, and energy). The diversity of symptoms present in depression argues against a single etiology, and we know that complex human behavioral disorders such as depression have genetic, constitutional, biological, social, cultural, and interpersonal components that interact in myriad ways leading to the disorder. When we look at one aspect of this, depression and the brain, there is increasing evidence that distributed brain networks, including frontal–subcortical circuits, are involved in at least some patients with depression.

As Cummings (1995) has suggested, there are five parallel frontal–subcortical circuits, each of which links a specific region of the frontal lobes to particular regions of the striatum, the globus pallidus–substantia nigra, and the thalamus. Three of these five circuits appear to play an important role in emotion, including depression: the dorsolateral prefrontal circuit, the orbitofrontal circuit, and the medial frontal circuit. The remaining two circuits are involved in motor and oculomotor functions.

In this chapter, we bring together clinical and experimental data from studies of neuroimaging, neuroanatomy, neuropsychological testing, mood provocation studies, and treatment paradigms in depression. This accumulating body of converging evidence clearly implicates the role of the frontal lobes and their connections in depression.

## NEUROIMAGING

Neuroimaging studies in depression include structural imaging (computerized tomography [CT] and magnetic resonance imaging [MRI]) and functional imaging studies. These investigations have looked at subjects with depression versus control subjects; at the significance of focal brain lesions, such as strokes; at depression in patients with degenerative disorders; and at depression in the older adult.

## Structural Imaging

Structural imaging studies have investigated the differences in regional brain volumes between subjects who are depressed and nondepressed. MRI studies of depression have, in general, revealed reduced volumes in various areas of the brain. For example, Coffey and colleagues (1993) found that inpatients with depression have significantly smaller (7%) frontal lobe volumes compared to healthy controls; Bremner and colleagues (2002) found that patients with MDD had significantly smaller (32%) volumes of the medial orbitofrontal cortex (gyrus rectus) than did healthy control subjects; and the findings of Lacerda and colleagues (2004) suggest that patients with depression have reduced volumes of the lateral and medial orbitofrontal cortices. In an MRI study of women with depression and early-onset depression (onset before age 18 years), Botteron, Raichle, Drevets, Heath, and Todd (2002) found that both patient groups had reduced (average of 19%) left subgenual prefrontal cortex volumes compared to normal controls, whereas Nolan and colleagues (2002) found that children with childhood-onset MDD and nonfamilial depression had significantly larger left-sided prefrontal cortical volumes on MRI than did patients with familial depression or normal controls.

## Functional Imaging

Functional imaging studies using single-photon emission computerized tomography (SPECT) and positron emission tomography (PET) have, in general, shown changes in blood flow or metabolic activity in frontal areas (as well as components of the limbic system) of the brain in individuals with depression (Bench et al., 1992; Drevets, 2000; Lesser et al., 1994; Mayberg, 1994; Milak et al., 2005; Oda et al., 2003; Soares & Mann, 1997). This has been particularly evident in the orbital–inferior prefrontal cortex, and has been found in a variety of studies both of primary and secondary depressions. Findings of generalized reduced regional cerebral blood flow (rCBF) or glucose metabolism (regional cerebral metabolic rate [rCMR]) have been more consistently reported in studies of older individuals with depression compared to younger ones. This may be related to a more global underlying vascular disease in these older patients. There is great consistency, however, in reports of reduced rCBF or rCMR in frontal areas of the brain in both younger and older subjects with depression. It is less clear whether these findings can be consistently localized to particular areas within these frontal systems, or whether they are a state or trait phenomena. As detailed below, there also have been reports of change in these blood flow and metabolic abnormalities with successful treatment of the depression by both pharmacological and psychotherapeutic modalities (Bench, Frackowiak, & Dolan, 1995; Goldapple et al., 2004; Kennedy et al., 2001), implying that they are, in some cases, state-dependent changes.

A different technological approach to understanding brain function is the use of quantitative electroencephalography (QEEG). Studies using QEEG have shown that there are changes in the activity in the prefrontal cortex in patients with depression, and some investigators have correlated this finding with results from studies of brain perfusion (Cook & Leuchter, 2001; Leuchter, Uijtdehaage, Cook, O'Hara, & Mandelkern, 1999). Furthermore, preliminary evidence shows that treatment response to antidepressant medication is associated with changes in the measure of concordance in the prefrontal regions that are distinct from the response to placebo (Leuchter, Cook, Witte, Morgan, & Abrams, 2002).

## NEUROPSYCHOLOGICAL ABNORMALITIES

The performance of patients with depression on standardized neuropsychological tests is impaired in multiple domains that suggest dysfunction of frontal and frontal–subcortical systems. A wide range of disturbances, including deficits in attentional processing, working memory, perceptual functions, and executive functions, has been reported, although results have been inconsistent among studies. Some of these deficits are consistent with dysfunction of the prefrontal cortex, including the areas implicated by structural and functional imaging. Boone and colleagues (1992, 1995) found that in patients with late-onset depression, there were significant deficits in attention and executive functions, particularly in those patients with a large amount of white matter hyperintensities (WMHs). Merriam, Thase, Haas, Keshavan, and Sweeney (1999) found that unmedicated patients with depression had significant performance deficits on the Wisconsin

Card Sorting Test compared to healthy controls, and the deficits correlated with the severity of the depression. These deficits, however, were not as severe as those exhibited by a comparison group of patients with schizophrenia. Herrmann, Ehlis, and Fallgatter (2004), who used near-infrared spectroscopy to study patients with depression performing a verbal fluency task, found significantly reduced increases in patients' frontal oxygenated hemoglobin compared to normal control subjects.

Neuropsychological studies also have demonstrated mood-congruent processing biases in patients with depression. Elliott, Rubinsztein, Sahakian, and Dolan (2002), using functional MRI, found that these patients had differential responses to emotional stimuli in the prefrontal cortices compared to normal controls, including elevated responses to sad target stimuli in the anterior cingulate. We describe more fully the literature on neuropsychological deficits in patients with late-life depression later in this chapter.

## MOOD PROVOCATION STUDIES

Another approach to investigating the brain regions associated with mood changes is the induction of sad mood in experimental subjects. Study designs have included provocation of transient sadness in healthy volunteers and in subjects with major depression, and relapse induction in patients with depression. Despite differences in designs, there is a degree of consensus that the frontal regions play a role in sadness. However, these studies acknowledge that experimentally induced sad mood is not equivalent to the complex syndrome of clinical depression.

Healthy, euthymic volunteers have been studied to examine the cerebral correlates of sad mood. For example, early studies found that experimentally induced sadness was associated with increased activity in paralimbic and inferior–medial prefrontal regions (George et al., 1995; Pardo, Pardo, & Raichle, 1993). More recently, increased rCBF in the left orbitofrontal cortex, right anterior cingulate cortex, and the right midinsular region were found in a SPECT study of sadness induction in healthy women (Ottowitz et al., 2004).

In patients with acute or remitted major depression, similar studies have been done that utilize transient sad mood challenges. For example, Beauregard and colleagues (1998) used an emotional activation paradigm (passive viewing of emotionally laden and emotionally neutral film clips) to study both normal controls and unipolar subjects with acute depression. They found that activation in the medial and inferior prefrontal cortices was present in both subject groups during sadness, but that the subjects with depression had significantly greater activation in the right cingulate gyrus and the left medial prefrontal cortex than the normal controls. Liotti, Mayberg, McGinnis, Brannan, and Jerabek (2002) used autobiographical memory scripts to induce sad mood in groups of subjects with remitted depression, acute depression, and euthymic volunteers with no history of depression. They found that decreased rCBF in the medial orbitofrontal cortex and increased activation in the dorsal anterior cingulate and lateral inferior frontal cortex in subjects with past or current depression distinguished both depressed groups from normal volunteers. The authors proposed that pregenual and orbitofrontal cortex are sites of vulnerability in patients with depression.

A tryptophan-depleting drink was used by Bremner and colleagues (1997, 2003) to induce depression in patients with MDD who were in remission. PET imaging demonstrated decreased brain metabolism in the dorsolateral prefrontal cortex, thalamus, and orbitofrontal cortex in the subjects who relapsed. Additionally, increased baseline metabolism in limbic and prefrontal areas was a predictor of vulnerability to relapse.

## NEUROANATOMY AND NEUROPATHOLOGY

It is one thing to hypothesize about a relationship between depression and frontal lobe dysfunction based on the association of depressive symptoms or disorders with anatomical and functional neuroimaging and/or neuropsychological test results. However, this is quite different from proving it with certainty, because far fewer neuropathological studies have provided conclusive evidence of such a relationship.

With regard to microscopic neuroanatomy, postmortem studies conducted on patients with depression have found morphological changes in the prefrontal cortex. Ongur, Drevets, and Price (1998) reported a reduction in glial density in the subgenual anterior cingulate cortex.

Rajkowska and colleagues (1999) found that, relative to controls, subjects with depression had decreased cortical thickness, reductions in both glial and neuronal cell densities, and decreases in neuronal size in prefrontal regions; these changes differed among specific cortical layers and prefrontal regions. Cotter, Mackay, Landau, Kerwin, and Everall (2001) found evidence of reduced neuronal size and glial density in the anterior cingulate cortex in patients with MDD. In addition to these putative frontal systems abnormalities, various authors have implicated decreased dendritic changes in the hippocampal formation, as well as in the subcortical white matter, as being associated with depression (reviewed by Harrison, 2002). Although the etiology of these neuropathological changes is uncertain, the reductions in cell densities and size may relate to the reduced volumes in these regions on structural imaging, and reduced blood flow and metabolism found on functional imaging.

Preliminary work using advanced neuroimaging techniques (diffusion tensor imaging) has suggested that there are microstructural changes in the white matter of the right superior frontal gyrus in late-life depression (Taylor et al., 2004). This is postulated to lead to functional disconnection of cortical and subcortical circuits, with accompanying changes in mood regulation.

## STROKE AND DEPRESSION

There is a large literature documenting the presence of a depressive syndrome following stroke (Bhogal, Teasell, Foley, & Speechley, 2004; Gainotti, Axxoni, & Marra, 1999; Lyketsos, Treisman, Lipsey, Morris, & Robinson, 1998; Robinson, 1998; Spalletta, Ripa, & Caltagirone, 2005; Starkstein, Robinson, & Price, 1988). A recent meta-analysis of studies conducted between 1977 and 2002 reported a pooled estimate that 33% of all stroke survivors experience depression. The authors reported that, in general, the depression is time-limited, even in the absence of specific treatment (Hackett, Yapa, Parag, & Anderson, 2005), although other studies indicate that treatment of poststroke depression with antidepressants can improve quality of life and perhaps improve survival as well (Jorge, Robinson, Arndt, & Starkstein, 2003). There is a wide range of prevalence figures reported because investigators have studied varied populations, have defined depression in different ways (e.g., major depression vs. subsyndromal depression), have studied patients at various times poststroke, and have utilized various imaging techniques. However, there is little doubt that depression is a common sequela of a cerebrovascular event.

As noted earlier, defining the criteria for or characteristics of patients with poststroke depression has not been an easy task. Whether the depression is related to the stroke itself in some pathophysiological or etiological manner, or whether it is a reaction to the disability and functional limitations (similar to other medical disorders) has been debated (House, 1996; Lyketsos et al., 1998). Robinson, Starkstein, and colleagues have put forth the hypothesis that poststroke depression occurs most frequently with lesions in the frontal lobes, particularly the left frontal pole (Robinson & Starkstein, 1990; Starkstein et al., 1988, 1991). In a large number of patients, these investigators have found a higher prevalence of depression in those with left frontal lesions and, in some cases, a significant correlation between severity of depression scores and distance between the anterior border of the lesion and the frontal pole (higher scores are reflective of more anterior lesions) (Robinson & Starkstein, 1990). Furthermore, they found a high prevalence of poststroke depression after subcortical lesions involving frontal–subcortical circuits (Starkstein, Robinson, & Price, 1987). Others, however, did not find any significant relationship between lesion location, presence of poststroke depression, and time elapsed since stroke (Gainotti et al., 1999). They concluded that their data were more consistent with a psychological, rather than a neurological, model of poststroke depression.

A study that examined the executive dysfunction syndrome in poststroke patients confirmed many of the findings seen with executive dysfunction in older patients with depression who did not have strokes. Vataja and colleagues (2005), using a battery of well-standardized tests of executive function, studied patients with depression 3 months poststroke. All subjects also had an MRI, with assessment of white matter burden. The authors found that about 40% of subjects studied were depressed, and that within this group, about one-half showed depression and executive dysfunction. Those with executive dys-

function had lower scores on measures of cognition and lower complex activities of daily living (ADL) scores. They also had a higher number of brain infarcts in the vascular territory of the left-sided frontal–subcortical structures. These findings support the hypothesis that stroke patients with depression and executive dysfunction are more likely to have structural lesions affecting frontal–subcortical circuitry than those with depression and no executive dysfunction, a finding similar to that of Alexopoulos (2002) in nonstroke older adults with depression.

Several reports on depression and traumatic brain injury also have indicated that patients with depression are more likely to be those with reduced left prefrontal gray matter volumes (Fedoroff et al., 1992; Jorge et al., 2004), adding to the link between frontal systems dysfunction and depression.

## APATHY

In recent years, the syndrome of apathy has received considerable attention from investigators of neuropsychiatric conditions. The symptoms of apathy can overlap with those of depression, yet with careful questioning of patients and collaterals, they often can be distinguished on clinical grounds. Because frontal circuitry has been suggested to play a role in apathy, a brief review of it is appropriate in this chapter on depression.

Apathy is best characterized as a disorder of motivation rather than a disorder of mood per se. This disordered motivation can be seen in decreases in goal-directed activity (e.g., lack of productivity and effort, decreased time spent in activities and socialization); goal-directed thought content (lack of interests or desire to learn new things, decreased curiosity and initiative, lack of concern about personal health); and goal-related emotional responses (unchanging affect, lack of emotional responsivity, flat affect). Investigators have stressed the necessity of meeting all parts of this definition as necessary for the full syndrome of apathy (Marin, 1996, 1997). The Apathy Evaluation Scale, a well-validated measure of apathy, has been used in a variety of studies (Marin, Biedrzycki, & Firinciogullari, 1991).

Apathy has been noted to occur in the context of a variety of neurological disorders: Alzheimer's disease (AD), frontotemporal dementia, delirium, stroke, Parkinson's disease (PD), Huntington's disease (HD), and supranuclear palsy. It has been noted after focal lesions to the mesiofrontal cortex, its connections to the anterior cingulate, or both. It has also been studied in relation to poststroke depression, but the findings have been variable (Duffy & Kant, 1997). Although comparisons among studies are difficult because of differing instruments used to measure apathy and different populations studied, reviews suggest that patients with lesions or dysfunction in frontal areas of the brain have a particularly high prevalence of apathy (van Reekum, Stuss, & Ostrander, 2005).

From a neuroanatomical perspective, the amygdala and its connections with structures subserving memory (the hippocampal complex), somatosensory inputs, and the internal milieu (hypothalamus and posterior orbitofrontal region) have been viewed as having a central role in motivational processes. A neuroanatomical circuit including the nucleus accumbens, the ventral pallidum, and the ventral mesencephalon is postulated to underlie the maintenance of sustaining information of motivational importance. This circuit then receives further input from classical limbic structures and the prefrontal cortex (Duffy, 1997). Disorders interrupting this frontal circuitry (e.g., those noted earlier) can lead to symptoms of apathy, furthering the connection between this brain region and disorders of motivation and mood.

## DEPRESSION AND NEURODEGENERATIVE BRAIN DISORDERS

Another point suggesting an association between frontal–subcortical dysfunction and depression is the fact that depression is more often associated with disorders having known frontostriatal pathology. For example, dementias with subcortical pathology such as PD and HD are more likely to be associated with depression than are cortical dementias such as AD.

PD is a neurodegenerative disorder characterized by degeneration of dopaminergic neurons in the substantia nigra and variable disruptions of other neurotransmitter systems. In addition to the movement disorder, symptoms include executive dysfunction, dementia, and depression. In PD, estimates of comorbid de-

pressive illness are as high as 75%, though many studies indicate a lower prevalence (Edwards et al., 2002). Potential reasons for this association include a reaction to the disability of the disease, a complication of medication usage, and the possibility that the neurodegenerative process of PD also leads to the depression. Data suggest that, on PET imaging, depressed subjects with PD have significantly greater decreases in metabolism in the striatum and orbitofrontal cortex compared to nondepressed patients with PD. In addition, there was a significant inverse correlation between the severity of depression and degree of metabolism in the orbital–inferior frontal lobe. This finding is similar to PET findings in patients with depression without PD (Mayberg et al., 1990).

HD is an inherited neurodegenerative disorder involving the caudate; depression occurs in 9–44% of patients (Mendez, 1994). Mayberg and colleagues (1992) studied patients with early HD with PET and found that selective hypometabolism of the orbitofrontal–inferior prefrontal cortex distinguished depressed patients with HD from nondepressed patients with HD and normal control subjects. Significant caudate, putamen, and cingulate hypometabolism was present in patients with HD, regardless of current mood state, suggesting that depression in HD was due to disruption of the circuits linking the striatum and the frontal lobe regions.

The frontotemporal dementias (e.g., Pick's disease), in which the degenerative disease begins in frontal areas of the brain, typically present with initial behavioral symptoms such as apathy, loss of interest, depressed mood, obsessions, and disinhibition (Kumar & Gottlieb, 1993; Miller, Chang, Mena, Boone, & Lesser, 1993). These personality changes, which are thought to be reflective of frontal systems pathology, often lead to a delay in making the correct diagnosis.

AD is the most common cause of dementia in the elderly, and approximately 10–30% of patients with AD suffer from concurrent depression (Devanand et al., 1997). Hirono and colleagues (1998), who used PET to study patients with probable AD, found that depression was associated with decreased metabolism in the frontal lobe (bilateral superior gyri and the left anterior cingulate gyrus). Lopez and colleagues (2001) similarly studied patients with AD and reported that a patient with major depression had decreased relative rCBF in both the bilateral anterior cingulate and the bilateral superior temporal, left dorsolateral prefrontal, right middle temporal, and right parietal cortices. Other studies of depression in AD, however, have instead demonstrated decreased left temporoparietal blood flow (Starkstein et al., 1995) and decreased metabolism in the parietal lobes (Sultzer et al., 1995).

## DEPRESSION IN THE OLDER ADULT

Depression most commonly presents in young adults, with a second peak incidence in early middle age. Major depression is likely to be a recurrent illness: Among those experiencing their first episode, 50% will have a second episode; among those who have two episodes, about 80% will have a third episode. On the other hand, some people remain depression free until later in life, having their first episode in the seventh decade or later. Much research has been dedicated to examining why these people, who have managed to go through most of their lives without an episode of depression, present with depression at this particular time of their life. Increasing evidence points to a subgroup of older adults who develop depressive illness and who have accompanying cerebrovascular disease. Alexopoulos has termed this "vascular depression," and he and his colleagues have written extensively about it (Alexopoulous, 2002, 2005; Alexopoulos et al., 1997, 2000; Alexopoulos, Kiosses, Klimstra, Kalayam, & Bruce, 2002). A review of this literature indicates that frontal lobe functioning may be disturbed in these patients, and this can serve as a model for understanding the relationship between depression and the frontal lobes.

Our group has been interested in the differential diagnosis of older adults who present with depression for the first time. We were involved in a series of studies using neuroimaging and neuropsychological evaluations to characterize groups of people with late-onset depression (Boone et al., 1995; Lesser et al., 1994, 1996). It had been noted by us and by others (Alexopoulos, Meyers, Young, Mattis, & Kakuma, 1993; Miller et al., 1993) that depression could be the precursor of an illness causing dementia even when the cognitive deficits that occurred during the depression ameliorated as the depression was treated. This led investiga-

tors to look for anatomical or functional deficits that might underlie the clinical symptoms and to attempt to differentiate between depression and early dementia.

Lesser and colleagues (1996) studied a large group of patients with late-onset depression and compared them to both age-matched patients who had experienced a depression earlier in life and control subjects who were never depressed. A subgroup of patients with late-onset depression had larger areas of WMHs compared to both the other groups. Those with the largest amount of white matter involvement also were more severely depressed. Furthermore, they had the most severe of the neuropsychological impairments, which included problems in executive functions (a reflection of frontal lobe dysfunction) (Boone et al., 1992, 1995). Subsequent studies have suggested that the pathophysiology of these WMHs is ischemic in nature, and that they are more frequently located at the level of dorsolateral prefrontal cortex in patients with depression (Thomas et al., 2002).

Other groups, particularly Alexopoulos and colleagues (1997), continued this line of investigation, suggesting that the term "vascular depression" be used to describe patients who had the later onset of depression along with evidence from clinical or radiological/neuroimaging evaluations of cerebrovascular disease. This could include such things as history of stroke or transient ischemic attacks, focal neurological signs, angina, history of myocardial infarction, hypertension, and significant WMHs or areas of infarction on CT or MRI. Furthermore, Alexopoulos and colleagues postulated that there would be a particular clinical picture, with patients demonstrating cognitive impairment, including but not limited to executive function, psychomotor retardation, poor insight, limited guilt or other depressive thinking, and more disability.

Since the publication of this seminal paper, many investigations have been conducted that for the most part have corroborated the initial findings. Much of the work has focused upon defining the anatomical, functional brain impairment, and neuropsychological deficits seen in patients with late-onset depression. There is a reasonable consensus among investigators that older patients' depression is associated with MRI evidence of greater WHMs in frontal areas compared to nondepressed controls (Coffey, Figiel, Djang, & Weiner, 1990;

Firbank, Lloyd, Ferrier, & O'Brien, 2004; Lesser et al., 1996; Steffens, Helms, Krishnan, & Burke, 1999). Similarly, and as discussed earlier, there is consistency in noting reductions in rCBF and rCMR in frontal and prefrontal areas in older subjects with depression.

It appears that a considerable number of these patients who have cerebrovascular disease also have significant cognitive deficits in executive functions, such as difficulties in abstract thinking, sequencing, response inhibition, and sustained effort. In many studies, the degree of cognitive impairment has been related to the severity of the findings in anatomical or functional imaging, as well as the severity of the depression. The fact that these deficits are associated with dysfunction in frontal lobe structures and their subcortical connections adds further evidence linking depression and frontal lobe dysfunction.

## TREATMENT STUDIES

Numerous studies related to antidepressant treatments exist in the literature; some of these focus on changes pre- and posttreatment, whereas others focus on the prediction of treatment response. Treatments studied include pharmacological agents, electroconvulsive therapy (ECT), psychotherapy, sleep deprivation, and cingulotomy. Results of these studies are mixed and at times appear inconsistent; possible reasons for these discrepancies include heterogeneity of the patient population studied (age, gender, duration and severity of illness, depression subtype, treatment history, medication status, family history, comorbid psychiatric disorders, etc.) and differences in study methodology. Despite the lack of clear consistency, the most consistent finding across studies is the association between the frontal lobes and their connections and treatment effects.

Functional imaging paradigms have been used to examine changes in cerebral blood flow and metabolic rates after successful pharmacotherapy for major depression. The sites and directions of change (increases vs. decreases in blood flow or metabolism) reported are inconsistent across studies, although virtually all studies point toward a role for the frontal regions.

Mayberg and colleagues (2000) studied unipolar depression in subjects before, during, and after 6 weeks of treatment with the antidepressant fluoxetine. After 6 weeks of active therapy, responders, compared to nonresponders, demonstrated a pattern of limbic–paralimbic decreases, and brainstem and dorsal cortical increases in regional glucose metabolism. These changes resulted in the correction of prefrontal and parietal hypometabolism seen at baseline, consonant with reports of earlier studies (Baxter et al., 1989; Buchsbaum et al., 1997; Goodwin et al., 1993). In a later study, Kennedy and colleagues (2001) found that successful treatment with paroxetine was associated with a normalization of pretreatment reductions in prefrontal metabolic activity and pretreatment increases in pregenual anterior cingulate activity. Conversely, Brody and colleagues (1999) found that treatment responders to paroxetine had significant posttreatment decreases in orbitofrontal and ventrolateral metabolism compared to nonresponders. Differences among studies include such confounding factors as length of treatment, type of antidepressant medication used, and concomitant use of other psychotropic agents.

Functional neuroimaging also has been used to study the effects of psychotherapy on the brain (Bench et al., 1995; Goldapple et al., 2004; Kennedy et al., 2001). Goldapple and colleagues (2004) used PET imaging pre- and posttreatment to study patients with depression undergoing cognitive-behavioral therapy (CBT) and a comparison group treated with the antidepressant paroxetine. The results suggested that CBT and paroxetine therapy were associated with differential changes in brain metabolism. Responders to CBT had significant increases in hippocampal and dorsal cingulate metabolism, and decreases in the dorsal, ventral, and medial frontal cortex. Medication responders had increased metabolism in the prefrontal cortex and decreased metabolism in the subgenual cingulate and the hippocampus. The authors suggested that these treatment-specific changes support their theory that pharmacological agents work in a so-called "bottom-up" manner (targeting limbic and subcortical regions) and CBT works in a "top-down" manner (targeting medial frontal and cingulate cortices), with both approaches ultimately resulting in an overall modulation of critical circuits involved in depression.

Using another form of psychotherapy for depression, interpersonal psychotherapy (ITP), Martin and colleagues (2001) studied a series of patients treated with either ITP or the antidepressant venlafaxine. Although patients in both treatment arms responded, SPECT scanning revealed differential changes between the two groups, with the venlafaxine group demonstrating activation in the right posterior temporal lobe and right basal ganglia, and the ITP group demonstrating activation in the right posterior cingulate and the right basal ganglia. Brody and colleagues (2001), utilizing PET, studied patients before and after treatment of depression with either ITP or paroxetine, and found that improvement in multiple dimensions of the depression were associated with changes in frontal lobe metabolism.

The effects of ECT on rCBF and rCMR also have been studied. The literature includes inconsistent findings; interpretation of these studies is complicated by a number of factors, such as small sample sizes, differences in patient populations, the timing of studies in relation to the ECT, variations in ECT technique, and other methodological differences. Nevertheless, comparisons between pre- and posttreatment functional imaging studies consistently suggest a relationship between treatment response to ECT and the frontal brain regions.

Many researchers have reported reductions in frontal rCBF or rCMR after successful treatment with ECT (Henry, Schmidt, Matochik, Stoddard, & Potter, 2001; Nobler et al., 1994, 2001). Scott and colleagues (1994) studied patients with unipolar depression before and 45 minutes after a single ECT treatment and on posttreatment SPECT found that a statistically significant reduction in rCBF in the inferior anterior cingulate cortex, and that these changes correlated with the severity of depression. Similarly, Henry and colleagues (2001) examined patients before and after a course of ECT, and found that decreases in metabolic rate in the right parietal, right anterior, and left posterior frontal regions correlated significantly with decreases in depression severity scores.

Not all ECT studies, however, found posttreatment reductions in frontal rCBF or rCMR. Bonne and colleagues (1996) found that responders to ECT had significant increases in rCBF, with the most marked changes in the cingulate gyrus. Awata and colleagues (2002) found that mean rCBF was significantly decreased in subjects with MDD compared to normal controls prior to a course of ECT, and normalized (significantly increased) 2 and 12 weeks after ECT. In another study, Navarro and colleagues (2004) used SPECT to examine subjects with depression pre- and posttreatment with either ECT or antidepressant therapy. During acute depression, both patient subgroups had significant anterior frontal hypoperfusion. After successful treatment with either ECT or medication, both patient subgroups had normalization of these anterior frontal perfusion defects (i.e., significant increases in perfusion).

Studies also have looked at the effects of sleep deprivation used for treatment of depression. Smith and colleagues (1999) used PET to study elderly patients before and after sleep deprivation, and found that improvement in symptoms was associated with reduced metabolism in the right anterior cingulate cortex. Wu and colleagues (1992, 1999) found that patients who responded to sleep deprivation had significant decreases in medial prefrontal cortex and frontal pole metabolic rates, and that lower ratings on the Hamilton Depression Rating Scale correlated significantly with lower metabolic rates in the left medial prefrontal cortex. Responders were found to have higher relative metabolic rates at baseline in the medial prefrontal cortex, ventral anterior cingulate, and posterior subcallosal gyrus than nonreponders and normal controls.

Finally, anterior cingulotomy is a surgical option for patients with particularly severe and treatment-refractory MDD. Dougherty and colleagues (2003) used PET scans to investigate a series of 13 patients and found that postoperative improvement was significantly correlated with high preoperative metabolic rates in the left subgenual prefrontal cortex and the left posterior thalamus. Because surgical interventions for affective disorders are reserved for only the most severe cases, the number of patients studied has been relatively small.

## CONCLUSIONS

Multiple lines of evidence reviewed here lead to the postulate that major depression is associated with frontal lobe/frontal circuit dysfunction. These finding are based upon the clinical association of stroke, traumatic brain injury, and neurodegenerative disorders with depression; anatomical and functional neuroimaging techniques; neuropsychological test findings; experimental mood-inducing paradigms; treatment studies; and emerging neuropathological data. Because the prefrontal cortex is believed to have a major role in volition, working memory, motivation, and mood regulation (all of which are disordered in patients with depression), dysfunction in regional blood flow or metabolism and/or ischemic changes in these area are at least consistent with a role in the pathophysiology of depression (Soares & Mann, 1997). The extent to which this disordered brain function interacts which genetics, environmental insults, aging, and interpersonal issues needs to be more clearly elucidated if we are to truly understand the etiologies of depression.

## REFERENCES

Alexopoulos, G. S. (2002). Frontostriatal and limbic dysfunction in late-life depression. *American Journal of Geriatric Psychiatry, 10*, 687–695.

Alexopoulos, G. S. (2005). Depression in the elderly. *Lancet, 365*, 1961–1970.

Alexopoulos, G. S., Kiosses, D. N., Klimstra, S., Kalayam, B., & Bruce, M. L. (2002). Clinical presentation of the "depression-executive dysfunction syndrome" of late life. *American Journal of Geriatric Psychiatry, 10*, 98–102.

Alexopoulos, G. S., Meyers, B. S., Young, R. C., Campbell, S., Silbersweig, D., & Charlson, M. (1997). The "vascular depression" hypothesis. *Archives of General Psychiatry, 54*, 15–22.

Alexopoulos, G. S., Meyers, B. S., Young, R. C., Kalayam, B., Kakuma T., Gabrielle, M., et al. (2000). Executive dysfunction and long-term outcomes of geriatric depression. *Archives of General Psychiatry, 57*, 285–290.

Alexopoulos, G. S., Meyers, B. S., Young, R. C., Mattis, S., & Kakuma, T. (1993). The course of geriatric depression with "reversible dementia": A controlled study. *American Journal of Psychiatry, 150*, 1693–1699.

American Psychiatric Association. (2000). *Diagnostic and statistical manual of mental disorders* (4th ed., text rev.). Washington, DC: Author.

Awata, S., Konno, M., Kawashima, R., Suzuki, K., Sato, T., Matsuoka, H., et al. (2002). Changes in regional cerebral blood flow abnormalities in late-life depression following response to electroconvulsive therapy. *Psychiatry and Clinical Neurosciences, 56*, 31–40.

Baxter, L. R., Schwartz, J. M., Phelps, M. E., Mazziotta, J. C., Guze, B. H., Selin, C. E., et al. (1989). Reduction of prefrontal cortex glucose metabolism common to three types of depression. *Archives of General Psychiatry, 46*, 243–250.

Beauregard, M., Leroux, J.-M., Bergman, S., Arxoumanian, Y., Beaudoin, G., Bourgouin, P., et al. (1998). The functional neuroanatomy of major depression: An fMRI study using an emotional activation paradigm. *NeuroReport, 9*, 3253–3258.

Bench, C. J., Frackowiak, S. J., & Dolan, R. J. (1995). Changes in regional cerebral blood flow on recovery from depression. *Psychological Medicine, 25*, 247–251.

Bench, C. J., Friston, K. J., Brown, R. G., Scott, L. C., Frackowiak, R. S., & Dolan, R. J. (1992). The anatomy of melancholia—focal abnormalities of cerebral blood flow in major depression. *Psychological Medicine, 22*, 607–615.

Bhogal, S. K., Teasell, R., Foley, N., & Speechley, M. (2004). Lesion location and poststroke depression: Systematic review of the methodological limitations in the literature. *Stroke, 35*, 794–802.

Boone K. B., Lesser, I. M., Miller, B. L., Wohl, M., Berman, N., Lee, A., et al. (1995). Cognitive functioning in older depressed outpatients: Relationship of presence and severity of depression to neuropsychological test scores. *Neuropsychology, 9*, 390–398.

Boone, K. B., Miller, B. L., Lesser, I. M., Hill-Gutierrez, E., Mehringer, C. M., Goldberg, M. A., et al. (1992). Neuropsychological correlates of white matter lesions in normal elderly: A threshold effect. *Archives of Neurology, 49*, 549–554.

Bonne, O., Krausz, Y., Shapira, B., Bocher, M., Karger, H., Gorfine, M., et al. (1996). Increased cerebral blood flow in depressed patients responding to electroconvulsive therapy. *Journal of Nuclear Medicine, 37*, 1075–1080.

Botteron, K. N., Raichle, M. E., Drevets, W. C., Heath, A. C., & Todd, R. D. (2002). Volumetric reduction in left subgenual prefrontal cortex in early onset depression. *Biological Psychiatry, 51*, 342–344.

Bremner, J. D., Innis, R. B., Salomon, R. M., Staib, L. H., Ng, C. K., Miller, H. L., et al. (1997). PET measurement of cerebral metabolic correlates of depressive relapse. *Archives of General Psychiatry, 54*, 364–374.

Bremner, J. D., Vythilingam, M., Ng, C. K., Vermetten, E., Nazeer, A., Oren, D. A., et al. (2003). Regional brain metabolic correlates of alpha-methylparatyrosine-induced depressive symptoms: Implications for the neural circuitry of depression. *Journal of the American Medical Association, 289*, 3125–3134.

Bremner, J. D., Vythilingam, M., Vermetten, F., Nazeer, A., Adil, J., Kahn, S., et al. (2002). Reduced volume of orbitofrontal cortex in major depression. *Biological Psychiatry, 51*, 273–279.

Brody, A. L., Saxena, S., Mandelkern, M. A., Fairbanks, L. A., Ho, M. L., & Baxter, L. R. (2001). Brain metabolic changes associated with symptom factor improvement in major depressive disorder. *Biological Psychiatry, 50*, 171–178.

Brody, A. L., Saxena, S., Silverman, D. H., Alborzian, S., Fairbanks, L. A., Phelps, M. E., et al. (1999). Brain metabolic changes in major depressive disorder from pre- to post-treatment with paroxetine. *Psychiatry Research, 91*, 127–139.

Buchsbaum, M. S., Wu, J., Siegel, B. V., Hackett, E., Trenary, M., et al. (1997). Effect of sertraline on regional metabolic rate in patients with affective disorder. *Biological Psychiatry, 41*, 15–22.

Coffey, C. E., Figiel, G. S., Djang, W. T., & Weiner, R. D. (1990). Subcortical hyperintensity in MRI: A comparison of normal and depressed elderly subjects. *American Journal of Psychiatry, 147,* 187–189.

Coffey, C. E., Wilkinson, W. E., Weiner, R. D., Parashos, I. A., Djang, W. T., Webb, M. C., et al. (1993). Quantitative cerebral anatomy in depression: A controlled magnetic resonance imaging study. *Archives of General Psychiatry, 50,* 7–16.

Cook, I. A., & Leuchter, A. F. (2001). Prefrontal changes and treatment response prediction in depression. *Seminars in Clinical Neuropsychiatry, 6,* 113–120.

Cotter, D., Mackay, D., Landau, S., Kerwin, R., & Everall, I. (2001). Reduced glial cell density and neuronal size in the anterior cingulate cortex in major depressive disorder. *Archives of General Psychiatry, 58,* 545–553.

Cummings, J. L. (1995). Anatomic and behavioral aspects of frontal–subcortical circuits. *Annals of the New York Academy of Sciences, 769,* 1–13.

Devanand, D. P., Jacobs, D. M., Tang, M., Del Castillo-Castaneda, C., Sano, M., Marder, K., et al. (1997). The course of psychopathologic features in mild to moderate Alzheimer disease. *Archives of General Psychiatry, 54,* 257–263.

Dougherty, D. D., Weiss, A. P., Cosgrove, G. R., Alpert, N. M., Cassem, E. H., Nierenberg, A. A., et al. (2003). Cerebral metabolic correlates as potential predictors of response to anterior cingulotomy for treatment of major depression. *Journal of Neurosurgery, 99,* 1010–1017.

Drevets, W. C. (2000). Neuroimaging studies of mood disorders. *Biological Psychiatry, 48,* 813–829.

Duffy, J. D. (1997). The neural substrates of motivation. *Psychiatric Annals, 27,* 24–29.

Duffy, J. D., & Kant, R. (1997). Apathy secondary to neurologic disease. *Psychiatric Annals, 27,* 39–43.

Edwards, E., Kitt, C., Oliver, E., Finkelstein, J., Wagster, M., & McDonald, W. M. (2002). Depression and Parkinson's disease: A new look at an old problem. *Depression and Anxiety, 16,* 39–48.

Elliott, R., Rubinsztein, J. S., Sahakian, B. J., & Dolan, R. J. (2002). The neural basis of mood-congruent processing biases in depression. *Archives of General Psychiatry, 59,* 597–604.

Federoff, J. P., Starkstein, S. E., Forrester, A. W., Geisler, F. H., Jorge, R. E., Arndt, S. V., et al. (1992). Depression in patients with acute traumatic brain injury. *American Journal of Psychiatry, 149,* 918–923.

Firbank, M. J., Lloyd, A. J., Ferrier, N., & O'Brien, J. T. (2004). A volumetric study of MRI signal hyperintensities in late-life depression. *American Journal of Geriatric Psychiatry, 12,* 606–612.

Gainotti, G., Axxoni, A., & Marra C. (1999). Frequency, phenomenology and anatomical–clinical correlates of major post-stroke depression. *British Journal of Psychiatry, 175,* 163–167.

George, M. S., Ketter, T. A., Parekh, P. I., Horwitz, B., Herscovitch, P., & Post, R. M. (1995). Brain activity during transient sadness and happiness in healthy women. *American Journal of Psychiatry, 152,* 341–351.

Goldapple, K., Segal, Z., Garson, C., Lau, M., Bieling, P., Kennedy S., et al. (2004). Modulation of cortical–limbic pathways in major depression: Treatment-specific effects of cognitive behavior therapy. *Archives of General Psychiatry, 61,* 34–41.

Goodwin, G. M., Austin, M. P., Dougall, N., Ross, M., Murray, C., O'Carroll, R. E., et al. (1993). State changes in brain activity shown by the uptake of 99mTc-exametazime with single photon emission tomography in major depression before and after treatment. *Journal of Affective Disorders, 29,* 243–253.

Greenberg, P. E., Kessler, R. C., Birnbaum, H. G., Leong, S. A., Lowe, S. W., Berglund, P. A., et al. (2003). The economic burden of depression in the United States: How did it change between 1990 and 2000? *Journal of Clinical Psychiatry, 64,* 1465–1475.

Hackett, M. L., Yapa, C., Parag, V., & Anderson, C. S. (2005). Frequency of depression after stroke. *Stroke, 36,* 1330–1340.

Harrison, P. J. (2002). The neuropathology of primary mood disorder. *Brain, 125,* 1428–1449.

Henry, M. E., Schmidt, M. E., Matochik, J. A., Stoddard, E. P., & Potter, W. Z. (2001). The effects of ECT on brain glucose: A pilot FDG PET study. *Journal of ECT, 17,* 33–40.

Herrmann, M. J., Ehlis, A.-C., & Fallgatter, A. J. (2004). Bilaterally reduced frontal activation during a verbal fluency task in depressed patients as measured by near-infrared spectroscopy. *Journal of Neuropsychiatry and Clinical Neurosciences, 16,* 170–175.

Hirono, N., Mori, E., Ishii, K., Ikejiri, Y., Imamura, T., Shinomura, T., et al. (1998). Frontal lobe hypometabolism and depression in Alzheimer's disease. *Neurology, 50,* 380–383.

House, A. (1996). Depression associated with stroke. *Journal of Neuropsychiatry, 8,* 453–457.

Jorge, R. E., Robinson, R. G., Arndt, S., & Starkstein, S. (2003). Mortality and poststroke depression: A placebo-controlled trial of antidepressants. *American Journal of Psychiatry, 160,* 1823–1829.

Jorge, R. E., Robinson, R. G., Moser D., Tateno, A., Crespo-Facorro, B., & Arndt S. (2004). Major depression following traumatic brain injury. *Archives of General Psychiatry, 61,* 42–50.

Kennedy, S. H., Evans, K. R., Krüger, S., Mayberg, H. S., Meyer, J. H., McCann S., et al. (2001). Changes in regional brain glucose metabolism measured with positron emission tomography after paroxetine treatment of major depression. *American Journal of Psychiatry, 158,* 899–905.

Kessler, R. C., Berglund, P., Demier, O., Jin, R., & Walters, E. E. (2005). Lifetime prevalence and age-of-onset distributions of DSM-IV disorders in the national comorbidity survey replication. *Archives of General Psychiatry, 62,* 593–602.

Kumar, A., & Gottlieb, G. (1993). Frontotemporal dementias: A new clinical syndrome? *American Journal of Geriatric Psychiatry, 1,* 95–107.

Lacerda, A. L. T., Keshavan, M. S., Hardan, A. Y., Yorbik, O., Brambilla, P., Sassi, R. B., et al. (2004). Anatomic evaluation of the orbitofrontal cortex in major depressive disorder. *Biological Psychiatry, 55,* 353–358.

Lesser, I. M., Boone, K. B., Mehringer, C. M., Wohl, M., Miller, B. L., & Berman, N. (1996). Cognition and white matter hyperintensities in older depressed patients. *American Journal of Psychiatry, 153,* 1280–1287.

Lesser, I. M., Mena, I., Boone, K. B., Miller, B. L., Mehringer, C. M., & Wohl, M. (1994). Reduction in cerebral blood flow in older depressed patients. *Archives of General Psychiatry, 51,* 677–686.

Leuchter, A. F., Cook, I. A., Witte, E. A., Morgan, M., & Abrams, M. (2002). Changes in brain function of depressed subjects during treatment with placebo. *American Journal of Psychiatry, 159,* 122–129.

Leuchter, A. F., Uijtdehaage, S. H., Cook, I. A., O'Hara, R., & Mandelkern, M. (1999). Relationship between brain electrical activity and cortical perfusion in normal subjects. *Psychiatry Research, 90,* 125–140.

Liotti, M., Mayberg, H. S., McGinnis, S., Brannan, S. L., & Jerabek, P. (2002). Unmasking disease-specific cerebral blood flow abnormalities: Mood challenge in patients with remitted unipolar depression. *American Journal of Psychiatry, 159,* 1830–1840.

Lopez, O. L., Zivkovic, S., Smith, G., Becker, J. T., Meltzer, C. C., & DeKostky, S. T. (2001). Psychiatric symptoms associated with cortical–subcortical dysfunction in Alzheimer's disease. *Journal of Neuropsychiatry and Clinical Neurosciences, 13,* 56–60.

Lyketsos, C. G., Treisman, G. J., Lipsey, J. R., Morris, P. L. P., & Robinson R. G. (1998). Does stroke cause depression? *Journal of Neuropsychiatry, 10,* 103–107.

Marin, R. S. (1996). Apathy and related disorders of diminished motivation. In *American Psychiatric Association review of psychiatry* (pp. 205–242). Washington, DC: APA Press.

Marin, R. S. (1997). Apathy—who cares?: An introduction to apathy and related disorders of diminished motivation. *Psychiatric Annals, 27,* 18–23.

Marin, R. S., Biedrzycki, R. C., & Firinciogullari, S. (1991). Reliability and validity of the Apathy Evaluation Scale. *Psychiatry Research, 38,* 143–162.

Martin, S. D., Martin, E., Rai, S. S., Richardson, M. A., & Royall, R. (2001). Brain blood flow changes in depressed patients treated with interpersonal psychotherapy or venlafaxine hydrochloride: Preliminary findings. *Archives of General Psychiatry, 58,* 641–648.

Mayberg, H. S. (1994). Frontal lobe dysfunction in secondary depression. *Journal of Neuropsychiatry and Clinical Neurosciences, 6,* 428–442.

Mayberg, H. S., Brannan, S. K., Tekell, J. L., Silva, J. A., Mahurin, R. K., McGinnis, S., et al. (2000). Regional metabolic effects of fluoxetine in major depression: Serial changes and relationship to clinical response. *Biological Psychiatry, 48,* 830–843.

Mayberg, H. S., Starkstein, S. E., Peyser, C. E., Brandt, J., Dannals, R. F., & Folstein, S. E. (1992). Paralimbic frontal lobe hypometabolism in depression associated with Huntington's disease. *Neurology, 42,* 1791–1797.

Mayberg, H. S., Starkstein, S. E., Sadzot, B., Preziosi, T., Andrezejewski, P. L., Dannals, R. F., et al. (1990). Selective hypometabolism in the inferior frontal lobes of depressed patients with Parkinson's disease. *Annals of Neurology, 28,* 57–64.

Mendez, M. F. (1994). Huntington's disease: Update and review of neuropsychiatric aspects. *International Journal of Psychiatry in Medicine, 24,* 189–208.

Merriam, E. P., Thase, M. D., Haas, G. L., Keshavan, M. S., & Sweeney, J. A. (1999). Prefrontal cortical dysfunction in depression determined by Wisconsin Card Sorting Test performance. *American Journal of Psychiatry, 156,* 780–782.

Milak, M. S., Parsey, R. V., Keilp, J., Oquendo, M. A., Malone, K. M., & Mann, J. J. (2005). Neuroanatomic correlates of psychophathologic components of major depressive disorder. *Archives of General Psychiatry, 62,* 397–408.

Miller, B. L., Chang, L., Mena, I., Boone, K., & Lesser, I. M. (1993). Progressive right fronto-temporal degeneration: Clinical, neuropsychological, and SPECT characteristics. *Dementia, 4,* 204–213.

Navarro, V., Gasto, C., Lomena, F., Mateos, J. J., Portella, M. J., Massana, G., et al. (2004). Frontal cerebral perfusion after antidepressant drug treatment versus ECT in elderly patients with major depression: A 12-month follow-up study. *Journal of Clinical Psychiatry, 65,* 656–661.

Nobler, M. S., Oquendo, M. A., Kegeles, L. S., Malone, K. M., Campbell, C., Sackeim, H. A., et al. (2001). Decreased regional brain metabolism after ECT. *American Journal of Psychiatry, 158,* 305–308.

Nobler, M. S., Sackeim, H. A., Prohovnik, I., Moeller, J. R., Mukherjee, S., Schnur, D. B., et al. (1994). Regional cerebral blood flow in mood disorders: III. Treatment and clinical response. *Archives of General Psychiatry, 51,* 884–897.

Nolan, C. L., Moore, G. J., Madden, R., Farchione, T., Bartoi, M., Lorch, E., et al. (2002). Prefrontal cortical volumes in childhood-onset major depression. *Archives of General Psychiatry, 59,* 173–179.

Oda, K., Okubo, Y., Ishida, R., Murate, Y., Ohta, K., Matsuda, T., et al. (2003). Regional cerebral blood flow in depressed patients with white matter magnetic resonance hyperintensity. *Biological Psychiatry, 53,* 150–156.

Ongur, D., Drevets, W. C., & Price, J. L. (1998). Glial reduction in the subgenual prefrontal cortex in mood disorders. *Proceedings of the National Academy of Sciences of the United States of America, 95,* 13290–13295.

Ottowitz, W. E., Dougherty, D. D., Sirota, A., Niaura,

R., Rauch, S. L., & Brown, W. A. (2004). Neural and endocrine correlates of sadness in women: Implications for neural network regulation of HPI activity. *Journal of Neuropsychiatry and Clinical Neurosciences, 16*, 446–455.

Pardo, J. V., Pardo, P. J., & Raichle, M. E. (1993). Neural correlates of self-induced dysphoria. *American Journal of Psychiatry, 150*, 713–719.

Robinson, R. G. (1998). Treatment issues in poststroke depression. *Depression and Anxiety, 8*, 85–90.

Rajkowska, G., Miguel-Hildago, J. J., Wei, J., Dilley, G., Pittman, S. D., Meltzer, H. Y., et al. (1999). Morphometric evidence for neuronal and glial prefrontal cell pathology in major depression. *Biological Psychiatry, 45*, 1085–1098.

Robinson, R. G., & Starkstein, S. E. (1990). Current research in affective disorders following stroke. *Journal of Neuropsychiatry and Clinical Neurosciences, 2*, 1–14.

Scott, A. I. F., Dougall, N., Ross, M., O'Carroll, R. E., Riddle, W., Ebmeier, K. P., et al. (1994). Short-term effects of electroconvulsive treatment on the uptake of 99mTc-exametazime into brain in major depression shown with single photon emission tomography. *Journal of Affective Disorders, 30*, 27–34.

Smith, G. S., Reynolds, C. F., Pollock, B., Derbyshire, S., Nofzinger, E., Dew, M. A., et al. (1999). Cerebral glucose metabolic response to combined total sleep deprivation and antidepressant treatment in geriatric depression. *American Journal of Psychiatry, 156*, 683–689.

Soares, J. C., & Mann, J. J. (1997). The functional neuroanatomy of mood disorders. *Journal of Psychiatric Research, 31*, 393–432.

Spalletta, G., Ripa, A., & Caltagirone, C. (2005). Symptom profile of DSM-IV major and minor depressive disorders in first-ever stroke patients. *American Journal of Geriatric Psychiatry, 13*, 108–115.

Starkstein, S. E., Bryer, J. B., Berthier, M. L., Cohen, B., Price T. R., & Robinson, R. G. (1991). Depression after stroke: The importance of cerebral hemisphere asymmetries. *Journal of Neuropsychiatry, 3*, 276–285.

Starkstein, S. E., Robinson, R. G., & Price, T. R. (1987). Comparison of cortical and subcortical lesions in the production of post-stroke mood disorders. *Brain, 110*, 1045–1049.

Starkstein, S. E., Robinson, R. G., & Price, T. R. (1988). Comparison of patients with and without poststroke major depression matched for size and location of lesion. *Archives of General Psychiatry, 45*, 247–252.

Starkstein, S. E., Vazquez, S., Migliorelli, R., Teson, A., Petracca, G., & Leiguarda, R. (1995). A SPECT study of depression in Alzheimer's disease. *Neuropsychiatry Neuropsychology and Behavioral Neurology, 8*, 38–43.

Steffens, D. C., Helms, M. J., Krishnan, K. R., & Burke, G. L. (1999). Cerebrovascular disease and depression symptoms in the cardiovascular health study. *Stroke, 30*, 2159–2166.

Sultzer, D. L., Mahler, M. E., Mandelkern, M. A., Cummings, J. L., Van Gorp, W. G., Hinkin, C. H., et al. (1995). The relationship between psychiatric symptoms and regional cortical metabolism in Alzheimer's disease. *Journal of Neuropsychiatry and Clinical Neurosciences, 7*, 476–484.

Taylor, W. D., MacFall, J. R., Payne, M. E., McQuoid, D. R., Provenzale, J. M., Steffens, D. C., et al. (2004). Late-life depression and microstructural abnormalities in dorsolateral prefrontal cortex white matter. *American Journal of Psychiatry, 161*, 1293–1296.

Thomas, A. J., O'Brien, J. T., Davis, S., Ballard, C., Barber, R., Kalaria, R. N., et al. (2002). Ischemic basis for deep white matter hyperintensities in major depression: A neuropathological study. *Archives of General Psychiatry, 59*, 785–792.

Van Reekum, R., Stuss, D. T., & Ostrander L. (2005). Apathy: Why care? *Journal of Neuropsychiatry and Clinical Neuroscience, 17*, 7–19.

Vataja, R., Pohjasvaara, T., Mäntylä, R. Ylikoski, R., Leskelä, M., Kalska, H., et al. (2005). Depression–executive dysfunction syndrome in stroke patients. *American Journal of Geriatric Psychiatry, 13*, 99–107.

World Health Organization. (1996). *Global health statistics: A compendium of incidence, prevalence and mortality estimates for over 200 conditions: The global burden of disease.* Cambridge, MA: Harvard University Press.

Wu, J., Buchsbaum, M. S., Gillin, J. C., Tang, C., Cadwell, S., Wiegand, M., et al. (1999). Prediction of antidepressant effects of sleep deprivation by metabolic rates in the ventral anterior cingulate and medial prefrontal cortex. *American Journal of Psychiatry, 156*, 1149–1158.

Wu, J. C., Gillin, J. C., Buchsbaum, M. S., Hershey, T., Johnson, J. C., & Bunney, W. E., Jr. (1992). Effect of sleep deprivation on brain metabolism of depressed patients. *American Journal of Psychiatry, 149*, 538–543.

# Index

Page numbers followed by *f* indicate figure; *t* indicate table